National Kidney Foundation's PRIMER ON KIDNEY DISEASES

National Kidney Foundation's
PRIMER ON
KIDNEY DISEASES

EIGHTH EDITION

SCOTT J. GILBERT, MD

Professor of Medicine
Tufts University School of Medicine
Nephrologist, Division of Nephrology
Tufts Medical Center
Boston, Massachusetts

DANIEL E. WEINER, MD, MS

Associate Professor of Medicine
Tufts University School of Medicine
Nephrologist, Division of Nephrology
Tufts Medical Center
Boston, Massachusetts

Associate Editors
Andrew S. Bomback, MD, MPH

Associate Professor of Medicine
Department of Medicine, Division of Nephrology
Columbia University College of Physicians and Surgeons
New York, New York

Mark A. Perazella, MD, MS

Professor of Medicine, Section of Nephrology
Yale University School of Medicine
Director, Acute Dialysis Services
Yale–New Haven Hospital
Medical Director, Yale Physician Associate Program
Department of Medicine
Yale University School of Medicine
New Haven, Connecticut

Dena E. Rifkin, MD, MS

Professor of Clinical Medicine
Associate Chief, Medicine Service
VA San Diego
Co-Director, Clinical Foundations Course
Department of Medicine (Nephrology), School of Medicine
Herbert Wertheim School of Public Health and Longevity Science
University of California, San Diego
San Diego, California

ELSEVIER

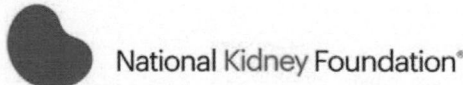

Elsevier
1600 John F. Kennedy Blvd.
Ste 1800
Philadelphia, PA 19103-2899

NATIONAL KIDNEY FOUNDATION'S PRIMER ON
KIDNEY DISEASES, EIGHTH EDITION

ISBN: 978-0-323-79122-9

Notice

Knowledge and best practice in this field are constantly changing. As new research and experience broaden our knowledge, changes in practice, treatment and drug therapy may become necessary or appropriate. Readers are advised to check the most current information provided (i) on procedures featured or (ii) by the manufacturer of each product to be administered, to verify the recommended dose or formula, the method and duration of administration, and contraindications. It is the responsibility of the practitioner, relying on their own experience and knowledge of the patient, to make diagnoses, to determine dosages and the best treatment for each individual patient, and to take all appropriate safety precautions. To the fullest extent of the law, neither the Publisher nor the Authors assume any liability for any injury and/or damage to persons or property arising out of or related to any use of the material contained in this book.

Library of Congress Control Number: 2021947986

Senior Content Strategist: Nancy Anastasi Duffy
Senior Content Development Specialist: Mary Hegeler
Publishing Services Manager: Catherine Jackson
Senior Project Manager: John Casey
Design Direction: Amy Buxton

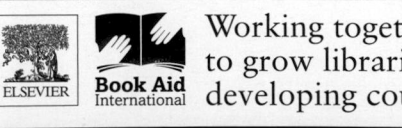

Contributors

Ala Abudayyeh, MD
Associate Professor
Division of Internal Medicine
Section of Nephrology
University of Texas MD Anderson Cancer Center
Houston, Texas

Horacio J. Adrogué, MD
Distinguished Emeritus Professor
Baylor College of Medicine
Department of Medicine
Division of Nephrology
Houston Methodist Hospital
Houston, Texas

Sophia L. Ambruso, DO
Director, Renal Clinic
Rocky Mountain VA Medical Association
Assistant Professor
Division of Hypertension and Renal Diseases
University of Colorado Anschutz Campus
Aurora, Colorado

Shuchi Anand, MD, MS
Assistant Professor of Medicine
Director, Center for Tubulointerstitial Kidney Disease
Stanford University School of Medicine
Palo Alto, California

Amar D. Bansal, MD
Assistant Professor of Medicine
Section of Palliative Care and Medical Ethics
Renal Electrolyte Division
Department of Medicine
University of Pittsburgh School of Medicine
Pittsburgh, Pennsylvania

Jonathan Barratt, PhD, FRCP
The Mayer Professor of Renal Medicine
Department of Cardiovascular Sciences
Honorary Consultant Nephrologist
John Walls Renal Unit
Leicester General Hospital
Head of the Postgraduate Specialty School
    of Clinical Academic Training
Health Education East Midlands
Leicester, United Kingdom

Jonathan W. Bazeley, MD
Assistant Professor of Clinical Medicine
Indiana University School of Medicine
Indianapolis, Indiana

Jeffrey S. Berns, MD
Professor of Medicine and Pediatrics
Renal, Electrolyte and Hypertension
    Division
University of Pennsylvania Perelman School
    of Medicine
Philadelphia, Pennsylvania

Petter Bjornstad, MD
Boettcher Investigator
Assistant Professor of Pediatrics and Medicine
Department of Pediatrics, Section of Endocrinology
Department of Medicine, Division of Renal Diseases
    and Hypertension
University of Colorado School of Medicine
Aurora, Colorado

Shane A. Bobart, MD, FASN
Associate Staff, Associate Program Director
Department of Nephrology and Hypertension
Cleveland Clinic Florida
Weston, Florida

Andrew S. Bomback, MD, MPH
Associate Professor of Medicine
Department of Medicine, Division
    of Nephrology
Columbia University College of Physicians
    and Surgeons
New York, New York

Daniela A. Braun, MD
Department of Internal Medicine D
University Hospital Muenster
Muenster, Germany

Ursula C. Brewster, MD
Associate Professor of Medicine
Section of Nephrology
Department of Internal Medicine
Yale University School of Medicine
New Haven, Connecticut

Daniel C. Cattran, MD, FRCP(C), FACP
Professor of Medicine
Department of Medicine
Senior Scientist
University Health Network
Toronto General Research Institute
Toronto, Ontario, Canada

Anil Chandraker, MD
Medical Director
Kidney and Pancreas Transplantation
Brigham and Women's Hospital
Harvard Medical School
Boston, Massachusetts

Sindhu Chandran, MBBS
Clinical Associate Professor
Division of Nephrology
Department of Medicine
University of California, San Francisco
San Francisco, California

Arlene B. Chapman, MD
Professor of Medicine
Chief, Section of Nephrology
Department of Medicine
Director, Clinical Research Center
Institute for Translational Medicine
Biological Sciences Division
University of Chicago
Chicago, Illinois

David Z. Cherney, MD, PhD
Professor of Medicine
Toronto General Hospital
Department of Medicine, Division of Nephrology
University Health Network
University of Toronto
Toronto, Ontario, Canada

Debbie L. Cohen, MD
Professor of Medicine
Director of Clinical Hypertension Programs
Co-Director of Penn Neuroendocrine Tumor Program
Department of Medicine, Renal Division
University of Pennsylvania
Philadelphia, Pennsylvania

Jared Cook, MD
Assistant Professor
Division of Nephrology
Department of Medicine
University of Alabama at Birmingham
Birmingham, Alabama

Frank B. Cortazar, MD
Chief, Division of Nephrology
Department of Medicine
St. Peter's Hospital
Director, New York Vasculitis and Glomerular Center
New York Nephrology
Albany, New York

Taimur Dad, MD, MS
Assistant Professor of Medicine
Division of Nephrology
Tufts Medical Center
Boston, Massachusetts

Vivette D. D'Agati, MD
Delafield Professor of Pathology and Cell Biology
Columbia University College of Physicians
    and Surgeons
Director, Renal Pathology Laboratory
Columbia University Medical Center
New York, New York

An S. De Vriese, MD, PhD
Professor of Medicine
Department of Nephrology
AZ Sint-Jan
Brugge, Belgium

Vimal K. Derebail, MD, MPH
Associate Professor of Medicine
UNC Kidney Center, Division of Nephrology and Hypertension
University of North Carolina
Chapel Hill, North Carolina

Thomas D. DuBose Jr., MD
Professor Emeritus of Medicine
Wake Forest School of Medicine
Winston-Salem, North Carolina;
Visiting Professor
Department of Medicine
University of Virginia School of Medicine
Charlottesville, Virginia

Lisa Dubrofsky, MDCM, FRCPC
Lecturer
Division of Nephrology
University Health Network
University of Toronto
Toronto, Ontario, Canada

Michael Emmett, MD
Chief of Internal Medicine
Department of Internal Medicine
Baylor University Medical Center
Professor of Internal Medicine
Texas A&M School of Medicine
Clinical Professor of Internal Medicine
University of Texas Southwestern
Dallas, Texas

Pieter Evenepoel, MD, PhD
Microbiology, Immunology, and Transplantation
KU Leuven
Leuven, Belgium

Todd Fairhead, MD, MSc
Assistant Professor
Department of Medicine
University of Ottawa
Ottawa, Ontario, Canada

Antoney J. Ferrey, MD
Assistant Professor
Division of Nephrology, Hypertension, and Kidney
    Transplantation
Department of Medicine
University of California, Irvine
Orange, California

Fernando C. Fervenza, MD, PhD
Professor of Medicine
Department of Nephrology and Hypertension
Mayo Clinic
Rochester, Minnesota

Kevin W. Finkel, MD
Professor of Medicine and Director
Division of Renal Diseases and Hypertension
McGovern Medical School
UT Health Science Center at Houston
Houston, Texas

Ryan P. Flood, DO
Assistant Professor
Division of Renal Diseases and Hypertension
University of Colorado School
    of Medicine
Aurora, Colorado

Manuela Födinger, MD
Professor of Laboratory Medicine
Faculty of Medicine
Sigmund Freud Private University
Institute of Laboratory Diagnostics
Clinic Favoriten
Vienna Health Care Group
Vienna, Austria

Barry I. Freedman, MD, FACP
Professor and Chief
Section on Nephrology
Department of Internal Medicine
Wake Forest School of Medicine
Winston-Salem, North Carolina

Pablo Garcia, MD, MS
Division of Nephrology
Department of Medicine
Stanford University School of Medicine
Palo Alto, California

Joanie M. Garratt, MD
Assistant Professor of Clinical Radiology
Department of Radiology
University of Pennsylvania
Philadelphia, Pennsylvania

Samantha L. Gelfand, MD
Instructor in Medicine
Department of Psychosocial Oncology
    and Palliative Care
Dana-Farber Cancer Institute
Renal Division
Brigham and Women's Hospital
Harvard Medical School
Boston, Massachusetts

Scott J. Gilbert, MD
Professor of Medicine
Tufts University School of Medicine
Nephrologist
Division of Nephrology
Tufts Medical Center
Boston, Massachusetts

Arthur Greenberg, MD
Professor Emeritus of Medicine
Division of Nephrology
Department of Medicine
Duke University Medical Center
Durham, North Carolina

Martin C. Gregory, BM, BCh, DPhil
Professor
Department of Medicine
University of Utah Health
Salt Lake City, Utah

Samantha Gunning, MD
Assistant Professor of Medicine
Section of Nephrology
Department of Medicine
University of Chicago
Chicago, Illinois

Leal Herlitz, MD
Director of Renal Pathology
Department of Anatomic Pathology
Cleveland Clinic
Cleveland, Ohio

Friedhelm Hildebrandt, MD
Chief, Division of Nephrology
Boston Children's Hospital
Boston, Massachusetts

Gerald A. Hladik, MD
Chief, Division of Nephrology and Hypertension
Doc J. Thurston Distinguished Professor of Medicine
UNC School of Medicine
Chapel Hill, North Carolina

Michelle A. Hladunewich, MD, MSc
Professor of Medicine
University of Toronto
Division of Nephrology, Department of Medicine
Toronto, Ontario, Canada

Melanie P. Hoenig, MD
Associate Professor
Harvard Medical School
Division of Nephrology
Beth Israel Deaconess Medical Center
Boston, Massachusetts

Jonathan Hogan, MD
Assistant Professor
Division of Nephrology
Department of Medicine
University of Pennsylvania Perelman School of Medicine
Philadelphia, Pennsylvania

T. Alp Ikizler, MD
Catherine McLaughlin-Hakim Professor of Medicine
Department of Medicine
Vanderbilt University Medical Center
Nashville, Tennessee

Lesley A. Inker, MD, MS
Associate Professor of Medicine
Department of Medicine
Tufts University School of Medicine
Division of Nephrology
Tufts Medical Center
Boston, Massachusetts

Michael G. Ison, MD, MS, FIDSA, FAST
Professor, Divisions of Infectious Diseases and Organ
    Transplantation
Northwestern University Feinberg School of Medicine
Medical Director, Transplant and Immunocompromised Host
    Infectious Diseases Service
Northwestern University Comprehensive Transplant Center
Director, Center for Clinical Research
Northwestern University Clinical and Translational Sciences
    Institute
Chicago, Illinois

Luis A. Juncos, MD
Professor of Medicine
Division of Nephrology/Medicine
University of Arkansas for Medical Sciences
Section Chief
Division of Nephrology/Medicine
Central Arkansas Veterans Healthcare System
Little Rock, Arkansas

Renate Kain, MD, PhD
Professor of Pathology
Department of Pathology
Medical University of Vienna
Vienna, Austria

Jaya Kala, MD
Assistant Professor of Medicine
Division of Renal Diseases and Hypertension
McGovern Medical School
UT Health Science Center at Houston
Houston, Texas

Kamyar Kalantar-Zadeh, MD, MPH, PhD
Professor and Chief
Division of Nephrology, Hypertension, and Kidney
    Transplantation
Department of Medicine
University of California, Irvine
Orange, California;
Staff Physician
Division of Nephrology
Tibor Rubin Veterans Affairs Medical Center
Long Beach, California

Jessica Kendrick, MD, MPH
Professor
Division of Renal Diseases and Hypertension
University of Colorado School of Medicine
Aurora, Colorado

Felix Knauf, MD
Professor
Section of Nephrology
Department of Internal Medicine
Yale University School of Medicine
New Haven, Connecticut

Greg Knoll, MD, MSc, FRCPC
Professor
Head, Division of Nephrology
University of Ottawa and the Ottawa Hospital
Ottawa, Ontario, Canada

Jeffrey B. Kopp, MD
Section Chief
Kidney Disease Section
Kidney Diseases Branch
National Institute of Diabetes and Digestive and Kidney
    Diseases
National Institutes of Health
Bethesda, Maryland

Csaba P. Kovesdy, MD
Fred Hatch Professor of Medicine
Department of Medicine
University of Tennessee Health Science Center
Nephrology Section Chief
Memphis VA Medical Center
Memphis, Tennessee

Jay L. Koyner, MD
Professor of Medicine
Section of Nephrology
Department of Medicine
University of Chicago
Chicago, Illinois

Etty Kruzel-Davila, MD
Department of Nephrology
Galilee Medical Center
Rappaport Faculty of Medicine and Research Institute
Technion-Israel Institute of Technology
Haifa, Israel

Andrew S. Levey, MD
Chief Emeritus
Division of Nephrology
Tufts Medical Center
Professor of Medicine
Tufts University School of Medicine
Boston, Massachusetts

Jian Li, MD
Division of Nephrology and Hypertension
Henry Ford Hospital
Clinical Assistant Professor
Wayne State University
Detroit, Michigan

Stuart L. Linas, MD
Professor of Medicine
University of Colorado School of Medicine
Chief of Nephrology
Department of Medicine
Denver Health and Hospital Authority
Denver, Colorado

Arnaldo Lopez-Ruiz, MD
Assistant Professor
Division of Critical Care Medicine
AdventHealth
Orlando, Florida

Randy L. Luciano, MD, PhD
Associate Professor of Medicine
Section of Nephrology
Department of Internal Medicine
Yale University School of Medicine
New Haven, Connecticut

Valerie A. Luyckx, MD, MSc, PhD
Affiliate Lecturer
Division of Nephrology
Brigham and Women's Hospital
Boston, Massachusetts;
Honorary Associate Professor
Department of Paediatrics and Child Health
University of Cape Town
Cape Town, South Africa;
Nephrologist
University Childrens Hospital
Zurich, Switzerland

Lijun Ma, MD
Section on Nephrology
Department of Internal Medicine
Wake Forest School of Medicine
Winston-Salem, North Carolina

Etienne Macedo, MD, PhD
Assistant Professor
Department of Medicine
University of California, San Diego
San Diego, California

Nicolaos E. Madias, MD
Maurice S. Segal, MD, Professor
    of Medicine
Department of Medicine
Tufts University School of Medicine
Physician, Division of Nephrology
Department of Medicine
St. Elizabeth's Medical Center
Boston, Massachusetts

Ankit N. Mehta, MD, FASN
Program Director
Department of Internal Medicine
Baylor University Medical Center
Clinical Associate Professor of Internal
    Medicine
Texas A&M College of Medicine
Dallas, Texas

Ravindra L. Mehta, MBBS, MD, DM
Professor of Clinical Medicine
Department of Medicine
University of California, San Diego
San Diego, California

Madhukar Misra, MD, FRCP(UK), FACP, FASN
Professor of Medicine
Department of Medicine
University of Missouri
Columbia, Missouri

Matthew A. Morgan, MD
Assistant Professor of Clinical Radiology
Department of Radiology
University of Pennsylvania
Philadelphia, Pennsylvania

Cynthia C. Nast, MD
Professor of Pathology
Director of Renal Pathology
Department of Pathology
Cedars-Sinai Medical Center
Los Angeles, California

Tanun Ngamvichchukorn, MD
Assistant Professor, Renal Division
Department of Internal Medicine
Faculty of Medicine Vajira Hospital
Navamindradhiraj University
Bangkok, Thailand

Thomas D. Nolin, PharmD, PhD
Associate Professor
Department of Pharmacy
    and Therapeutics
University of Pittsburgh School of Pharmacy
Associate Professor
Department of Medicine
University of Pittsburgh School of Medicine
Pittsburgh, Pennsylvania

Ann O'Hare, MD, MA
Staff Physician
Department of Medicine
Department of Veterans Affairs
Professor
Division of Nephrology
Department of Medicine
University of Washington
Seattle, Washington

Kabir O. Olaniran, MD, MPH
Assistant Professor
Division of Nephrology
University of Texas Southwestern Medical Center
Dallas, Texas

Austin R. Pantel, MD, MSTR
Assistant Professor of Radiology
Department of Radiology
University of Pennsylvania
Philadelphia, Pennsylvania

Aldo J. Peixoto, MD
Professor of Medicine
Vice Chair for Quality and Safety
Department of Internal Medicine
Clinical Chief, Section of Nephrology
Yale School of Medicine
New Haven, Connecticut

Mark A. Perazella, MD, MS
Professor of Medicine
Section of Nephrology
Yale University School of Medicine
Director, Acute Dialysis Services
Yale-New Haven Hospital
Medical Director, Yale Physician Associate Program
Department of Medicine
Yale University School of Medicine
New Haven, Connecticut

Dinushi S. Perera, MD
Instructor
Department of Radiology
Beth Israel Deaconess Medical Center
Boston, Massachusetts

Jeffrey Perl, MD, SM, FRCP(C)
Associate Professor of Medicine
Division of Nephrology
Department of Medicine
St. Michael's Hospital
University of Toronto
Toronto, Ontario, Canada

Anja Pfau, MD
Department of Nephrology and Medical Intensive Care
Charité-Universitätsmedizin Berlin
Berlin, Germany

Laura Ferreira Provenzano, MD
Clinical Assistant Professor
Cleveland Clinic Lerner College of Medicine
Department of Nephrology and Hypertension
Cleveland Clinic
Cleveland, Ohio

L. Darryl Quarles, MD
UTMG Professor of Medicine
Department of Medicine
University of Tennessee Health Science Center
Memphis, Tennessee

Jai Radhakrishnan, MD, MS
Professor
Division of Nephrology
Department of Medicine
Columbia University Medical Center
Clinical Director
Division of Nephrology
New York Presbyterian Hospital
New York, New York

Frederic F. Rahbari-Oskoui, MD, MS
Professor of Medicine
Emory University School of Medicine
Atlanta, Georgia

Connie Rhee, MD
Associate Professor
Division of Nephrology, Hypertension, and Kidney
    Transplantation
Department of Medicine
University of California, Irvine
Orange, California

Dana V. Rizk, MD
Professor
Division of Nephrology
Department of Internal Medicine
University of Alabama at Birmingham
Birmingham, Alabama

Avi Z. Rosenberg, MD, PhD
Assistant Professor
Department of Pathology
Johns Hopkins University
Baltimore, Maryland

Mitchell H. Rosner, MD
Professor
Department of Medicine
University of Virginia Health System
Charlottesville, Virginia

Melis Sahinoz, MD
Department of Medicine
Vanderbilt University Medical Center
Nashville, Tennessee

Rosemary V. Sampogna, MD, PhD
Associate Professor of Medicine
Department of Medicine
Columbia University
New York, New York

Paul W. Sanders, MD
Thomas E. Andreoli MD Endowed Chair in Nephrology
Professor, Department of Medicine
University of Alabama at Birmingham
Birmingham Veterans Affairs Health Care System
Birmingham, Alabama

Mark J. Sarnak, MD, MS
Dr. Gerald J. and Dorothy R. Friedman Professor of Medicine
Tufts University School of Medicine
Chief, Division of Nephrology
Tufts Medical Center
Boston, Massachusetts

Steven J. Scheinman, MD
President and Dean
Office of the President
The Commonwealth Medical College
Professor of Medicine
Department of Medical Education
Geisinger Commonwealth School of Medicine
Scranton, Pennsylvania

Jane O. Schell, MD, MHS
Associate Professor of Medicine
Section of Palliative Care and Medical Ethics
Renal Electrolyte Division
Department of Medicine
University of Pittsburgh School of Medicine
Pittsburgh, Pennsylvania

H. William Schnaper, MD
Professor and Vice Chair
Department of Pediatrics
Northwestern University Feinberg School of Medicine
Attending Physician
Division of Kidney Diseases
Ann & Robert H Lurie Children's Hospital of Chicago
Chicago, Illinois

Sarah Schrauben, MD, MSCE
Post-Doctoral Researcher
Renal, Electrolyte and Hypertension Division
University of Pennsylvania Perelman School of Medicine
Philadelphia, Pennsylvania

Brittany L. Schreiber, MD
Fellow, Renal Division
Brigham and Women's Hospital
Boston, Massachusetts

Sanjeev Sethi, MD, PhD
Professor
Department of Laboratory Medicine and Pathology
Mayo Clinic
Rochester, Minnesota

Nikhil Shah, MBBS, DNB
Assistant Clinical Professor
Division of Nephrology and Immunology
Department of Medicine
University of Alberta
Edmonton, Alberta, Canada

Wen Shen, PhD
Assistant Professor
Mechanical and Aerospace Engineering
University of Texas at Arlington
Arlington, Texas

Anushree C. Shirali, MD
Associate Professor
Department of Internal Medicine
Yale University School of Medicine
New Haven, Connecticut

Meghan E. Sise, MD, MS
Assistant Professor
Division of Nephrology
Department of Medicine
Massachusetts General Hospital
Boston, Massachusetts

Vivek Soi, MD
Division of Nephrology and Hypertension
Henry Ford Hospital
Clinical Associate Professor
Wayne State University
Detroit, Michigan

Ian A. Strohbehn, BA
Data Analyst II
Division of Nephrology
Department of Medicine
Massachusetts General Hospital
Boston, Massachusetts

Gere Sunder-Plassmann, MD
Associate Professor of Medicine
Division of Nephrology and Dialysis
Department of Medicine III
Medical University Vienna
Vienna, Austria

Richard W. Sutherland, MD
Professor of Urology
Department of Urology
School of Medicine
University of North Carolina
Chapel Hill, North Carolina

John E. Sy, MD, MAS
Assistant Professor
Division of Nephrology, Department of Medicine
University of California, Irvine
Orange, California;
Staff Physician
Division of Nephrology
Tibor Rubin Veterans Affairs Medical Center
Long Beach, California

Harold M. Szerlip, MD
Clinical Professor of Medicine
Nephrology Division
Medical University of South Carolina
Charleston, South Carolina

Jessica Tangren, MD
Assistant Professor of Medicine
Division of Nephrology, Department of Medicine
Massachusetts General Hospital
Boston, Massachusetts

Navdeep Tangri, MD, FRCPC, PhD
Associate Professor
Department of Medicine
University of Manitoba
Chronic Disease Innovation Centre
Seven Oaks General Hospital
Winnipeg, Manitoba, Canada

Jeffrey M. Testani, MD
Associate Professor of Medicine
Department of Internal Medicine
Section of Cardiovascular Medicine
Yale University
New Haven, Connecticut

Joshua M. Thurman, MD
Professor of Medicine
Department of Internal Medicine
University of Colorado
Aurora, Colorado

Raymond R. Townsend, MD
Professor of Medicine
Department of Medicine
University of Pennsylvania
Philadelphia, Pennsylvania

Howard Trachtman, MD
Director, Division of Nephrology
Department of Pediatrics
NYU Langone Health
New York, New York

Jeffrey M. Turner, MD
Associate Professor of Medicine
Department of Internal Medicine
Section of Nephrology
Yale University
New Haven, Connecticut

Juan Carlos Q. Velez, MD
Chair, Department of Nephrology
Ochsner Medical Center
New Orleans, Louisiana;
Associate Professor of Medicine
Ochsner Clinical School
The University of Queensland
Brisbane, Queensland, Australia

Joseph G. Verbalis, MD
Professor
Department of Medicine
Georgetown University
Chief, Department of Endocrinology
    and Metabolism
Georgetown University Hospital
Washington, DC

Flavio G. Vincenti, MD
Clinical Professor of Medicine and Surgery
Endowed Chair in Kidney Transplantation
Departments of Medicine and Surgery
University of California, San Francisco
San Francisco, California

Marina Vivarelli, MD
Nephrology and Dialysis Unit
Bambino Gesu' Pediatric Hospital IRCCS
Rome, Italy

Bradley A. Warady, MD
Professor
Department of Pediatrics, Division of Nephrology
University of Missouri School of Medicine
Director, Division of Pediatric Nephrology
Director, Dialysis and Transplantation
Department of Pediatrics
Children's Mercy Kansas City
Kansas City, Missouri

Darcy K. Weidemann, MD, MHS
Associate Professor
Department of Pediatrics, Division
    of Nephrology
University of Missouri–Kansas City
Children's Mercy Kansas City
Kansas City, Missouri

Daniel E. Weiner, MD, MS
Associate Professor of Medicine
Tufts University School of Medicine
Nephrologist, Division of Nephrology
Tufts Medical Center
Boston, Massachusetts

Christopher S. Wilcox, MD, PhD
Walters Family Chair in Cardiovascular Medicine
Department of Nephrology and Hypertension
Georgetown University Medical Center
Washington, DC

Jay B. Wish, MD
Professor of Clinical Medicine
Department of Medicine
Indiana University School of Medicine
Chief Medical Officer for Outpatient Dialysis
Department of Nephrology
IU Health
Indianapolis, Indiana

Jerry Yee, MD
Division Head
Nephrology and Hypertension
Henry Ford Hospital
Clinical Professor of Medicine
Department of Internal Medicine
Wayne State University School of Medicine
Detroit, Michigan;
Chief Medical Officer
Greenfield Health Systems
Bingham Farms, Michigan

See Cheng Yeo, MBBS, MRCP (UK), MMED (Int Med), FRCP (London), MD, FAMS
Senior Consultant and Head
Department of Renal Medicine
Tan Tock Seng Hospital
Singapore

Preface

We are excited to present the eighth edition of the *National Kidney Foundation's Primer on Kidney Diseases*. The *Primer* has been a key resource for students, residents, fellows, and clinicians ever since publication of the first edition by Arthur Greenberg and his editorial team in 1993. This eighth edition has been extensively revised and updated to address the quickly changing landscape of clinical nephrology while preserving the accessibility and utility that define the *Primer* as an essential resource for clinical challenges in kidney disease, electrolyte and acid-base disorders, and hypertensive conditions.

This edition brings change to the *Primer*. Dena Rifkin has joined Andrew Bomback and Mark Perazella on our editorial team, providing a breadth of expertise and a wealth of clinical experience to this effort. Our group remains committed to the careful selection of content and a diligent editorial process, stressing usability and clinical applicability.

The past 2 years have been tumultuous, with the COVID pandemic upturning an already changing world. We witnessed the miracles of medicine, with vaccines developed, produced, and administered in record time using new technologies, while also witnessing the limitations of medicine as we all struggled with uncertainty and helplessness in the setting of this new disease. We have realized the need to continue learning, both to improve knowledge and to better apply that knowledge. Despite the pandemic, more than 100 clinicians and researchers devoted considerable time and effort to bring you the eighth edition of the *Primer on Kidney Diseases*, and we are incredibly grateful for their dedication to sharing kidney knowledge.

We would like to dedicate this edition of the *Primer* to front-line healthcare workers, in particular the nephrology team of physicians, researchers, nurses, dialysis technicians, pharmacists, social workers, dieticians, and support colleagues, including transportation and EMS workers, who faced unprecedented challenges in delivering critical care to the sickest and highest risk patients: from dialysis nurses who spent hours in full personal protective gear at the bedside of COVID-19 positive patients with kidney failure; to social workers who reorganized dialysis units to cohort infected patients and protect the vulnerable; to researchers and pharmacists who ensured the safety and efficacy of treatments and vaccines in our unique patients; to coordinators who implemented telehealth systems to maintain care when in-person visits were not possible; to transportation workers and emergency medical technicians who enabled patients to get to the care they needed; and to educators who creatively adapted to ensure the medical workforce would be prepared and available for this and future challenges. Your contributions have not gone unnoticed, and we are all deeply grateful.

Never before in medicine has it been so apparent that we are all in this together. In this spirit, we hope you find the *Primer* to be the same go-to resource clinicians have relied on for the past 30 years to help enable quality medical care.

Scott J. Gilbert, MD
Daniel E. Weiner, MD, MS

Contents

PART 1

Structure and Function of the Kidney

1

Overview of Kidney Structure and Function

MELANIE P. HOENIG, GERALD A. HLADIK

The kidneys play an essential role in normal homeostasis. The key functions of the kidneys include:

1. *Maintenance of normal body fluid composition.* The kidney plays a primary role in the regulation of both the intracellular and extracellular compartments by retention or excretion of water and electrolytes. The concentration of water, sodium, potassium, calcium, phosphate, and hydrogen are tightly regulated within these body compartments to maintain normal cell size and cellular function.

2. *Excretion of waste products of metabolism and excretion of foreign substances.* The kidney is responsible for excretion of nitrogenous waste that is generated primarily in the liver from normal metabolism. In addition, a wide range of pharmacologic and exogenous toxic compounds are excreted in the urine.

3. *Regulation of blood pressure.* Reduced kidney perfusion or activation of the sympathetic nervous system stimulates the release of renin from the juxtaglomerular cells of the kidneys. This enzyme converts angiotensinogen to angiotensin I, which, in turn, is cleaved to form angiotensin II by angiotensin converting enzyme. Angiotensin II is a potent vasoconstrictive agent. In addition, this peptide hormone can stimulate sodium retention throughout the nephron, but especially in the proximal tubule. Angiotensin II also stimulates the release of aldosterone from the zona glomerulosa of the adrenal gland.

4. *Production of hormones*
   a. *Erythropoietin.* Interstitial fibroblasts produce erythropoietin in response to the hypoxia inducible factor (HIF). Erythropoietin is a glycoprotein hormone that promotes maturation of progenitor erythroid cells into mature red blood cells in the bone marrow.
   b. *Activation of vitamin D.* The final hydroxylation of vitamin D to its active form, 1,25-dihydroxy vitamin D, is achieved by the proximal tubule cells in response to parathyroid hormone. This steroid hormone plays an essential role in calcium and phosphate homeostasis, as well as bone metabolism.

The Kidney and Homeostasis

The kidney is the master regulator of homeostasis. Despite substantial variations in intake, environmental conditions, or physical stresses from one individual to another or within the same individual over the course of a few hours, the kidney maintains normal body fluid composition and plasma volume. Important examples include:

- Normal water concentration dictates cell size since water is distributed equally in all body compartments according to the distribution of solute.
- Normal sodium content affects extracellular volume, a key component of which is intravascular volume, organ perfusion, and blood pressure.
- Restriction of potassium primarily to the intracellular space maintains the electrochemical gradient necessary to maintain the negative cell membrane potential required for cells to function normally.
- Normal homeostasis of hydrogen concentration affects protein folding and enzymatic function.
- Since the kidney maintains plasma volume and plays a role in red blood cell production, the kidney also controls the intravascular volume.

Maintenance of Balance

To maintain normal volume and body fluid composition, the kidneys must maintain balance, or "the steady state." Thus, intake and production via metabolism must always equal excretion and consumption. Under normal circumstances, excretion can readily match intake. For example, an increase in water intake normally prompts excretion of water as dilute urine. Intake of a diet rich in potassium can stimulate excretion of a large amount of potassium. Similarly, intake of a high-protein diet can prompt excretion of additional nitrogen and acid, but in the setting of volume depletion or reduced kidney function, these prompt responses may be blunted.

Body Fluid Composition

The human body is composed primarily of water; in adult men, approximately 60% of the lean body weight is water, with a slightly lower percentage in women and children who tend to have slightly more adipose tissue that contains less water than muscle. Water is distributed among the body compartments such that approximately two-thirds is in the intracellular space and one-third in the extracellular space (Fig. 1.1). The extracellular fluid is composed of the interstitium and the vascular fluid. These latter compartments are essentially in continuum; fluid in the vasculature

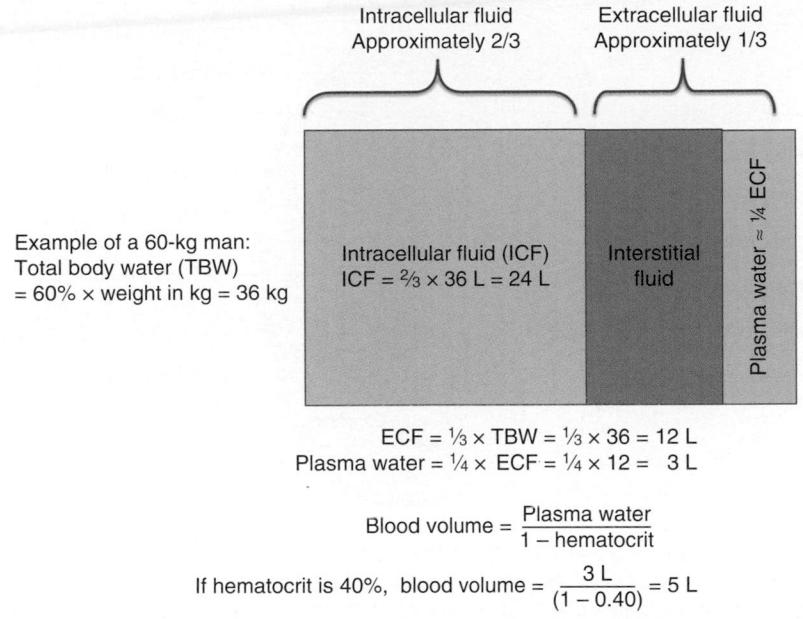

Intracellular fluid
Approximately 2/3

Extracellular fluid
Approximately 1/3

Example of a 60-kg man:
Total body water (TBW)
= 60% × weight in kg = 36 kg

Intracellular fluid (ICF)
ICF = $\frac{2}{3}$ × 36 L = 24 L

Interstitial
fluid

Plasma water ≈ ¼ ECF

ECF = ⅓ × TBW = ⅓ × 36 = 12 L
Plasma water = ¼ × ECF = ¼ × 12 = 3 L

$$\text{Blood volume} = \frac{\text{Plasma water}}{1 - \text{hematocrit}}$$

$$\text{If hematocrit is 40\%, blood volume} = \frac{3 \text{ L}}{(1 - 0.40)} = 5 \text{ L}$$

• **Fig. 1.1** Body fluid compartments, distribution of water, and estimates of compartment volumes. Total body water (TBW) is distributed in the intracellular fluid (ICF) and extracellular fluid (ECF). Plasma water in the vascular space represents approximately one-fourth of the fluid in the ECF. Using this rubric, body fluid compartment volumes can be estimated.

is separated from the interstitium only by small differences in oncotic forces generated by plasma proteins and cells. Typical values for the normal electrolytes in plasma and intracellular fluid are shown in Table 1.1.

TABLE 1.1	Approximate Typical Ion Concentrations, Osmolality, and pH Within the Plasma and Intracellular Fluid	
	Plasma (mEq/L)	Intracellular Fluid (mEq/L)
Cations		
Na^+	138	8
K^+	4	135
Ca^{2+} (ionized)	2	<0.0001
Mg^{2+}	1	2
Total cations	145	145
Anions		
Cl^-	104	4
HCO_3^-	24	10
HPO_4^{2-}, $H_2PO_4^-$	2	40
Protein	10	50
Other (organic anions and SO_4^{2-})	5	41
Total anions	145	145
Osmolality	290 mOsm/L	290 mOsm/L
pH	7.4	7.1

Kidney Structure

The kidneys are positioned along the posterior abdominal wall of the retroperitoneum, each weighing approximately 150 g. Anatomically, the kidneys are divided into two regions: an outer cortex and an inner medulla (Fig. 1.2). The cortex and medulla contain the basic functional units of the kidney, the nephrons, as well as the associated vasculature, nerves, and lymphatic vessels. The nephron consists of the glomerulus, Bowman's capsule, and the renal tubule (Fig. 1.3). On average, each kidney comprises 1 million nephrons, but this number may vary in individuals, from approximately 600,000 to 2 million nephrons per kidney. Distinct functional units form the renal tubule—the proximal tubule, the loop of Henle, the distal convoluted tubule, and the collecting duct. The function and morphology of the tubular epithelium vary in each segment of the nephron (see below). The glomeruli, most of the proximal tubule, and portions of the distal tubule are primarily located in the cortex. The medulla is composed of parallel arrays of the loops of Henle and collecting ducts. On gross inspection, these parallel arrays form the renal pyramids. The rounded apices of the pyramids form the papilla. The urine is maximally concentrated in the renal medulla, and the concentration of solute in the medullary interstitium may exceed that of plasma fourfold.

The process of urine formation begins at the glomerulus. The glomerular filtrate flows into Bowman's capsule and enters into the proximal tubule, where about two-thirds of the filtrate is reabsorbed. Tubular fluid then flows through the thin descending limb of the loop of Henle, and, after a hairpin turn, ascends through the thin ascending limb into the thick ascending limb (TAL) of the loop of Henle. The distal portion of the loop of Henle touches the glomerulus at the juxtaglomerular apparatus (JGA), after which the filtrate flows into the distal convoluted tubule. Fluid in the tubular lumen is maximally dilute at this site. The processed filtrate then flows via the connecting tubule into the cortical and medullary collecting ducts where water is

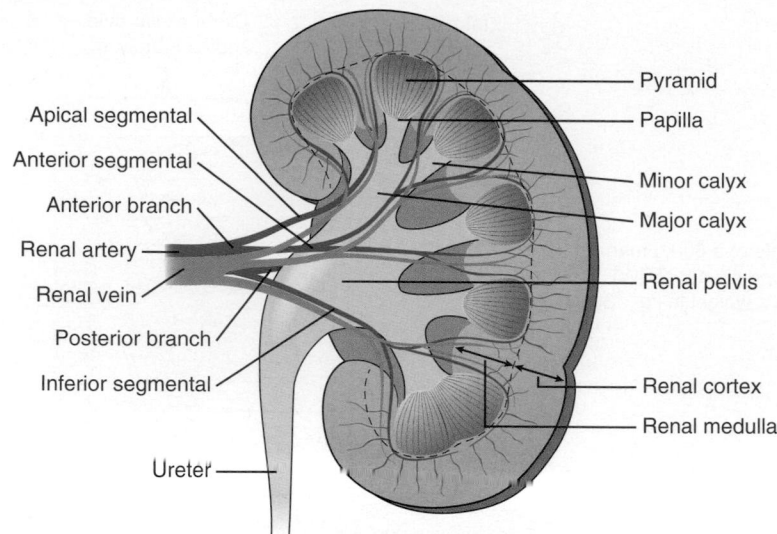

• **Fig. 1.2** The anatomy of the kidney. The cortex is primarily composed of glomeruli, proximal tubules, and portions of the distal tubule. The medulla contains parallel arrays of the loops of Henle tubules and collecting ducts. The renal arteries of the kidney promptly branch into segmental arteries and then interlobar arteries once within the renal parenchyma (see text for additional details). In contrast to the arterial system, the venous system has extensive collaterals for drainage of the kidney; the venous system maps to the arterial system but there is also a subcapsular venous plexus that drains the kidney (not shown). Nevertheless, if there is obstruction or thrombosis of the renal vein, the kidney will swell.

either conserved or excreted. The collecting duct is also the regulatory site of potassium and hydrogen ion secretion. As the filtrate passes through each successive portion of the nephron, a highly orchestrated process of solute reabsorption and secretion occurs that results in the excretion of the precise amount water, acid-base equivalents, and electrolytes necessary to maintain homeostasis. Urine subsequently passes from the papillae (the tips of the pyramids) into the minor calyces, which then converge to form two to three major calyces that configure the renal pelvis. The lining of the renal pelvis, the ureter, bladder, and urethra is comprised of transitional epithelial cells that are impermeable to water. In the urethra, squamous epithelial cells, which are also impermeable to water, line the lumen.

Renal Circulation

Anatomy

The renal circulation is one of the richest vascular beds in the body. The renal arteries originate from the lateral aspect of the aorta and enter the kidneys in the hilum, posterior to the renal veins and anterior to the origin of the ureter. Anatomic variants of the renal arteries and veins are common and can be found in 25% to 40% of patients. During development, blood from transient aortic "sprouts" supplies the kidneys; these degenerate as the kidneys ascend and renal arteries from the lumbar region ultimately perfuse the kidneys. When arteries from earlier in development do not degenerate, there may be residual additional vessels.

The renal arteries enter the kidney in the hilum and then bifurcate first into *segmental arteries* (see Fig. 1.2). The segmental arteries are functional "end arteries" since they serve as the only supply of oxygenated blood to their particular regions of the kidney. The segmental arteries then divide into *interlobar arteries*, and

then *arcuate arteries*, which arch around the kidney as they run between the cortex and the outer medulla; the arcuate arteries give rise to the *interlobular arteries* that extend toward the cortex and, en route, give rise to an array of arterioles. The *afferent arterioles* divide into the glomerular capillaries and then culminate in another arteriole, the *efferent arteriole*. Thus, the glomerular capillary is the only capillary bed in the body flanked by two resistance vessels. Changes in the resistance of the arterioles can affect glomerular pressure and ultimately filtration.

Two Capillary Beds in Series

The efferent arterioles then descend toward the medulla and form a second capillary bed; these capillaries are associated with the proximal tubules and are known as the *peritubular capillaries*. The intimate association between this second capillary bed and the tubules creates a relationship such that filtration and reabsorption can be balanced. For example, if filtration is increased, tubular reabsorption is also increased. This is called *glomerulotubular balance*.

Medullary Blood Supply

The peritubular capillaries continue straight to the medulla and are called the *vasa recta*. The vasa recta then take a hairpin turn and return to the cortex (see Fig. 1.3). This orientation allows the kidney to return electrolytes and water to the circulation while maintaining the concentration gradient that is created by the loops of Henle. Red blood cells that travel in the vasa recta are subjected to very low oxygen tension and a hyperosmotic environment in the medulla. To withstand the osmotic stress, red blood cells have transporters for urea on the cell surface that allow urea to rapidly enter the cells and help maintain cell size and structure (see below).

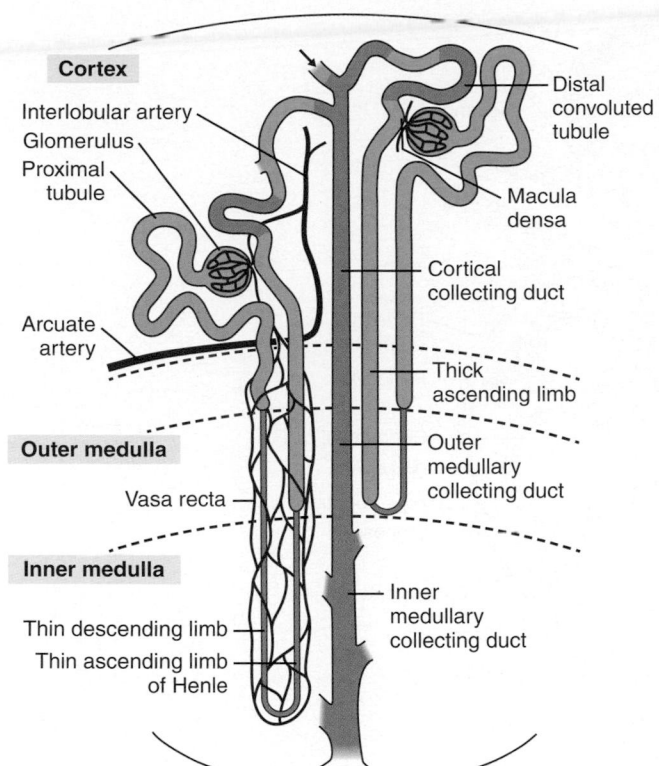

• **Fig. 1.3** **Organization of the nephron.** Each human kidney has approximately 1 million nephrons. Two nephrons are shown here. Each nephron consists of a glomerulus, a proximal convoluted tubule, a thin descending limb and a thin ascending limb of Henle, a thick ascending limb, the macula densa, a distal convoluted tubule, and a connecting tubule. Several nephrons converge and empty into a collecting duct. The collecting duct can be divided into segments based on location: the cortical collecting ducts, the outer medullary collecting duct, and the inner medullary collecting duct. As shown, some glomeruli are deeper and give rise to nephrons with loops of Henle that descend all the way to the papillary tips, whereas more superficial glomeruli have loops of Henle that only reach to the junction of the inner and outer medulla. The interlobular arteries give rise to an array of afferent arterioles, which form the glomerular capillary bundles. Blood exits the glomeruli through the efferent arterioles. These arterioles form a second capillary bed, the peritubular capillaries, which reclaim the fluid and electrolytes reabsorbed in the nephron. In the deeper aspects of the kidney, the peritubular capillaries play a critical role in the maintenance of the osmotic gradient.

Glomerulus

The glomerulus is a complex network of capillaries responsible for the selective ultrafiltration of plasma and the clearance of small solutes. The glomerular capillaries are uniquely interposed between two arterioles: the afferent and efferent arterioles. This anatomic configuration allows for the intricate control of glomerular capillary pressure and the glomerular filtration rate (GFR). The glomerular capillaries form the glomerular filtration barrier (Fig. 1.4), which allows for the selective filtration of small solutes such as water, sodium, and urea, while excluding the passage of cells and large proteins such as albumin. The basement membrane, endothelium, and podocytes confer a net negative charge to the filtration barrier. As a result, negatively charged proteins such as albumin are less likely to pass through the filtration barrier. Under normal conditions, only low-molecular-weight proteins and a small amount of albumin are filtered; these are almost completely

reabsorbed and catabolized by the proximal tubular epithelial cells. This leads to excretion of 40 to 80 mg of protein per day, primarily composed of uromodulin (previously known as *Tamm-Horsfall protein*), a mucoprotein secreted by tubular epithelial cells in the thick ascending loop of Henle.

The glomerulus has four major components: the endothelium, the mesangium, the basement membrane, and the podocytes (Fig. 1.5). In addition to important functional roles, the mesangium and podocytes provide a structural scaffold that supports the glomerular capillaries. The glomerular capillaries have an unusually high proportion of *fenestrae*, or clefts, on the endothelial surface (20% to 50%) that facilitate the efficient trafficking of small solutes and water through the filtration barrier. The glycocalyx is a lattice of negatively charged glycoproteins that overlies the fenestrae that preferentially exclude the passage of negatively charged proteins such as albumin. Aligned between the endothelial cells and the podocytes is the basement membrane. This structure is composed of a network of extracellular matrix proteins that include type IV collagen, laminin, and heparan sulfate-bound proteoglycans. The basement membrane constrains the filtration of proteins in concert with the endothelium and podocytes and has an important role in limiting the flux of solutes and fluids. The visceral epithelium is composed of podocytes, specialized cells named for the foot processes that envelop the glomerular capillaries. The foot processes of one podocyte interdigitate with foot processes from neighboring podocytes to form the filtration slit diaphragm. These specialized intercellular junctions function as a critical barrier to the passage of high-molecular-weight proteins. Podocin and nephrin are two constituent proteins of the filtration slit diaphragm essential for the proper structure and function of the filtration barrier. Inactivating mutations of the genes that encode podocin and nephrin lead to severe proteinuric kidney disease.

Factors That Influence Glomerular Filtration Rate

The GFR is the product of the net filtration pressure along the glomerular capillary (P_{net}) and the surface area of the glomerular capillaries. This relationship can be represented by the following equation:

$$GFR = P_{net} \times Area$$

Transcapillary Starling forces are key determinants of the net filtration pressure. These include the glomerular capillary hydraulic (P_{cap}) and oncotic pressure (π_{cap}) and the interstitial hydraulic (P_{int}) and oncotic pressures (π_{int}). The net filtration pressure can be altered by the permeability of the glomerular capillary (represented by the filtration coefficient, K_f), and the net oncotic pressure may be influenced by the permeability of proteins across the capillary wall, denoted by the refection coefficient (σ). Quantitatively, these forces are related by the following equation:

$$P_{net} = K_f \left[\left(P_{cap} - P_{int} \right) - \sigma \left(\pi_{cap} - \pi_{int} \right) \right]$$

The hydraulic pressure at the origin of the glomerular capillary bed is relatively high, at approximately 60 mm Hg, and exceeds the capillary oncotic pressure throughout the length of the glomerular capillaries. Together with a very high filtration coefficient, the relatively high glomerular capillary pressure favors the net filtration of fluid from the glomerular capillaries into Bowman's space. The capillary oncotic pressure increases along the length of the capillary as filtration of relatively protein-free fluid progresses,

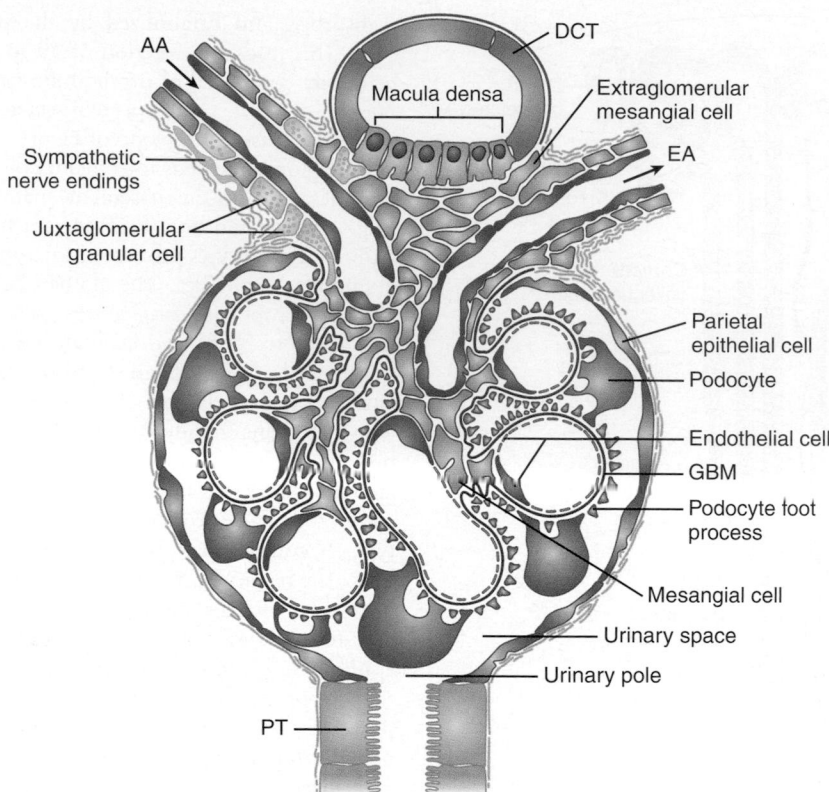

- **Fig. 1.4** Schematic diagram of a section of a glomerulus and its juxtaglomerular apparatus. *AA*, afferent arteriole; *DCT*, distal convoluted tubule; *EA*, efferent arteriole; *GBM*, glomerular basement membrane; *PT*, proximal tubule.

resulting in a gradual fall in net filtration pressure as filtration proceeds toward the efferent arteriole. The GFR typically equals about 20% of the plasma flow rate. Changes in GFR can result from altered glomerular capillary pressure or permeability or from a change in the surface area of the glomerular capillaries. The relative resistance of the afferent and efferent arterioles affects changes in renal plasma flow, net ultrafiltration pressure, and GFR. A number of physiologic mediators can alter the degree of constriction or dilation of these arterioles. Angiotensin II, increased activity of the sympathetic nervous system, and circulating catecholamines cause arteriolar vasoconstriction, whereas prostaglandins, nitric oxide, and bradykinin mediate arteriolar vasodilation. During decreases in renal perfusion, prostaglandins tend to maintain or increase glomerular capillary pressure and GFR by causing afferent arteriolar vasodilatation. Correspondingly, in the normal range of autoregulation of GFR (a perfusion pressure of 80 to 180 mm Hg), angiotensin II maintains glomerular capillary pressure and GFR when there is a relative decline in perfusion by inducing vasoconstriction of the efferent arteriole.

Measurement of Glomerular Filtration Rate

Measurement and estimation of the GFR are extensively reviewed in Chapter 3. The GFR is equal to the total plasma ultrafiltration rate. Normal values are about 120 mL/min/1.73 m² body surface area (BSA) for adult women and 130 mL/min/1.73 m² BSA for adult men, or about 180 L/day. GFR progressively increases with growth during childhood and declines about 1 mL/min/year starting at age 40. GFR can be measured indirectly by determining the clearance of a solute, such as inulin,

that is freely filtered by the glomerulus and is neither secreted nor reabsorbed by the renal tubules. In addition, the solute should not be produced or metabolized by the kidney. When these conditions are met, the filtered load is equivalent to the excreted load, allowing for the calculation of GFR.

Creatinine is an endogenous solute commonly used to estimate GFR. Creatinine clearance is less precise than inulin clearance in determining GFR because approximately 10% to 40% of urinary creatinine is derived from the tubular secretion of creatinine in the proximal convoluted tubule. As a result, creatinine clearance tends to overestimate GFR by about 10% to 15%. The degree of overestimation increases at lower levels of GFR in which the tubular secretion of creatinine is proportionately higher. The serum creatinine level can also be used to assess GFR either alone or through use of estimating equations. As discussed in Chapter 3, the serum creatinine level has limitations for GFR estimation, varying with muscle mass, dietary intake, comorbid illness, age, sex, and volume status. Other filtration markers, like cystatin C, can also be used to estimate GFR. Cystatin C is less influenced by age, sex, and muscle mass compared with serum creatinine and better estimates kidney function at higher levels of GFR.

The Juxtaglomerular Apparatus

The JGA is a conglomeration of structures central to the regulation of GFR, sodium chloride balance, and extracellular fluid volume. The JGA is comprised of:
1. a segment of the distal convoluted tubule called the *macula densa* (see below),
2. the afferent arteriole of its own glomerulus,

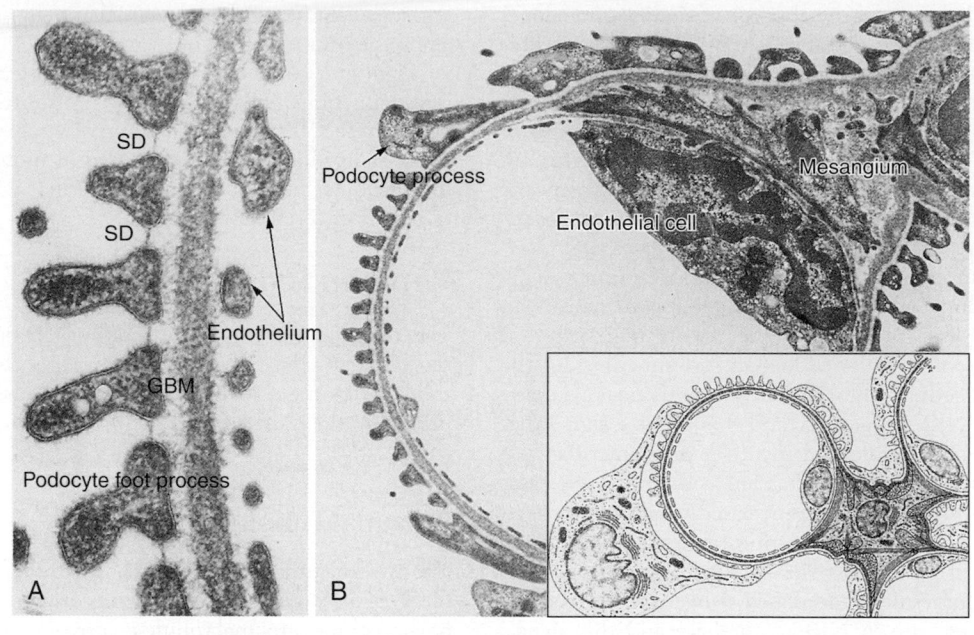

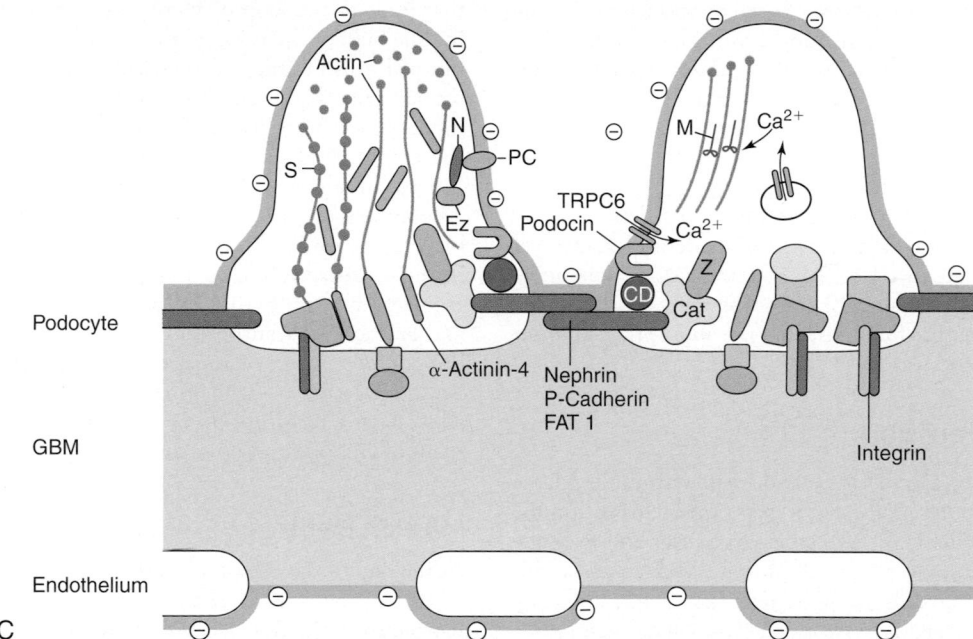

• Fig. 1.5 Structure of the glomerular capillary loop and the filtration barrier. (A) The glomerular filtration barrier consists of endothelial cells, the glomerular basement membrane (GBM), and the filtration slit diaphragms (SD) between podocyte foot processes (×34,000). (B) A single capillary loop demonstrates the fenestrated endothelium, the basement membrane, and the foot processes. The mesangium is contiguous with the subendothelial space and provides structural support that permits the cells to withstand the high pressures characteristic of the glomerular capillaries which favor filtration (×13,000). (C) Schematic diagram of the filtration barrier. The porous endothelium is negatively charged. The GBM is composed of type IV collagen and laminin 521 and other components. The filtration SD are created by podocyte foot processes from distinct cells and various molecule. *Cat*, Catenin; *CD*, CD2-associated protein; *Ez*, Ezrin; *FAT 1*, FAT tumor suppressor homolog 1; *M*, myosin; *N*, NERF2; *PC*, podocalyxin; *S*, synaptopodin; *TRPC6*, transient receptor potential-channel 6; *Z*, ZO1.

3. the smooth muscle cells of these arterioles, and
4. specialized *granular cells* in the wall of the afferent arteriole.

The granular cells release renin in response to decreased perfusion or increased sympathetic tone. In addition, decreased delivery of sodium and chloride to the kidney-specific $Na^+/K^+/2Cl^-$ cotransporter (NKCC2) in the macula densa signals the granular cells to release renin.

Autoregulation of Renal Blood Flow and GFR

The JGA plays an important role in the intrarenal regulation of renal blood flow and GFR. Autoregulatory mechanisms stabilize renal blood flow and GFR during changes in renal perfusion pressure in the range of 80 to 180 mm Hg. Small changes in renal perfusion can influence GFR and potentially cause life-threatening changes in sodium balance. In the absence of significant changes in the effective arterial blood volume (EABV) or underlying kidney disease, two servomechanisms prevent alterations in sodium balance during spontaneous or induced fluctuations in renal perfusion. The first, a rapid myogenic response modulates changes in renal blood flow and GFR after small changes in renal perfusion. Increased hydraulic pressure at the afferent arteriole triggers the intracellular release of calcium that leads to compensatory vasoconstriction. A more delayed mechanism, *tubuloglomerular feedback*, adjusts sodium excretion in response to variations in renal perfusion in the range of renal autoregulation. An increase in renal perfusion pressure will lead to an increase in single-nephron GFR and an increase in the filtered load of sodium chloride. The resultant increase in sodium chloride delivery to the macula densa results in increased NKCC2 activity and this elicits a signal that constricts the afferent arteriole and increases preglomerular vascular resistance. This feedback mechanism counteracts increases in single-nephron GFR arising from increased renal perfusion. In contrast, a decrease in renal perfusion pressure leads to a decrease in the single-nephron GFR and a decrease in the filtered load of sodium chloride. The resultant decreased delivery to the macula densa results in a decrease in NKCC2 activity and this signals the granular cells to release renin. Tubuloglomerular feedback is likely altered in chronic kidney disease based on models of chronic nephron loss. Increased tubular sodium chloride levels at the macula densa, for example, result in increased, not decreased, single-nephron GFR in rats after subtotal nephrectomy.

Tubular Function

The volume of the initial glomerular filtrate is approximately 180 L/day in the setting of a normal GFR as derived above, yet most individuals excrete just 1 to 2 L of urine a day. A circuit of tubules, lined with epithelial cells, reabsorbs the majority of the filtrate and assures that the final urine has the appropriate amount of electrolytes, acid, and water.

Epithelial Cell Transport

Since cells are bound by a lipid bilayer and are impermeable to large molecules, ions, and polar molecules, transport proteins within the epithelial cell membrane help overcome this barrier and facilitate the movement of substances from the filtrate back to the capillaries. The renal tubular cells are polarized cells, characterized by the presence of the Na^+/K^+-ATPase on the basolateral membrane. The Na^+/K^+-ATPase generates an approximately 10-fold higher level of sodium in the extracellular fluid than the intracellular fluid by extruding three intracellular sodium ions in exchange for two extracellular potassium ions with energy derived from the hydrolysis of ATP. This is an example of *primary active transport*. In contrast, transporters on the luminal membrane benefit from the low intracellular concentration of sodium function based on *secondary active transport*. This arrangement allows the kidney to use the concentration gradient created by the low intracellular sodium concentration to reabsorb the majority of sodium in the filtrate.

Movement of sodium into the cell can be achieved with coupled transport of sodium either in the form of cotransport, as with the sodium/glucose cotransporters, or in the form of countertransport, as with the Na^+/H^+-exchanger (see below). Facilitated transport using carriers in the membrane can facilitate the movement of molecules such as glucose and urea. Specialized channels favor movement of specific ions along with their electrochemical

gradient. The aquaporin water channels permit water to move along the osmotic gradient.

Tight junctions are present between the tubular epithelial cells. These junctions limit paracellular transport so that gradients can be established between the urinary filtrate and the interstitium. These tight junctions are composed of multiple proteins, including claudins, occludins, and cadherins, which permit selective transport of certain ions.

Nephron Segments

The tubular segments vary substantially in both function and morphology. The proximal tubule reabsorbs the bulk of the filtrate, the loop of Henle creates the concentration gradient that is present in the medulla, and the distal nephron sets the final urine composition.

Proximal Tubule

The proximal tubule is the workhorse of the kidney, and more than 60% of the filtrate is normally reabsorbed in this region. The first portion of the proximal tubule is convoluted and forms a labyrinth within the renal cortex before transitioning to a straight segment that leads to the loop of Henle. To achieve the task of reabsorbing the bulk of the urinary filtrate, the proximal tubule has a lush luminal brush border of microvilli that increases the surface area dramatically (Fig. 1.6). The primary transporter for sodium on the luminal membrane is the Na^+/H^+-exchanger 3 (NHE3). This antiporter also plays a key role in the reclamation of bicarbonate (see below). In addition, NH_4^+ formed in the proximal tubules from glutamine is excreted via the same transporter, as the molar radius of NH_4^+ is similar to that of H^+. Other important transporters in the proximal tubule include the Na^+/phosphate cotransporters regulated by parathyroid hormone, sodium/glucose transporters, and amino acid transporters. These cells are permeable to water due to the presence of aquaporin 1, and water is reabsorbed in an isosmotic fashion. Tight junctions between proximal tubule cells allow passive reabsorption of water along with paracellular movement of chloride and potassium.

Loop of Henle

At the end of the proximal tubule, the cell type abruptly changes to that of the thin descending limb of Henle (Fig. 1.7). After a hairpin turn, the thin ascending limb of Henle becomes the taller TAL, equipped with the renal-specific NKCC2. NKCC2 requires all four ions for transport. Since the concentration of potassium in the lumen is considerably lower than that of sodium and chloride, additional potassium is supplied by a channel that allows movement of potassium into the lumen, the renal outer medullary potassium channel (ROMK) (Fig. 1.8). NKCC2 plays a critical role in the creation of the medullary concentration gradient. Also of note, the versatile ammonium ion, NH_4^+, can be absorbed by NKCC2 in the K^+ position. The thin limbs are permeable to water, but the TAL cells are not. This differential permeability, along with active transport by the TAL, plays an important role in the development of the medullary gradient within the kidney. For this reason, the loop of Henle is considered the *concentrating segment* of the nephron. The net result is that the concentration of the medulla of the kidney is much higher than the rest of the body. This is the only compartment in the body that has a higher osmolality than serum.

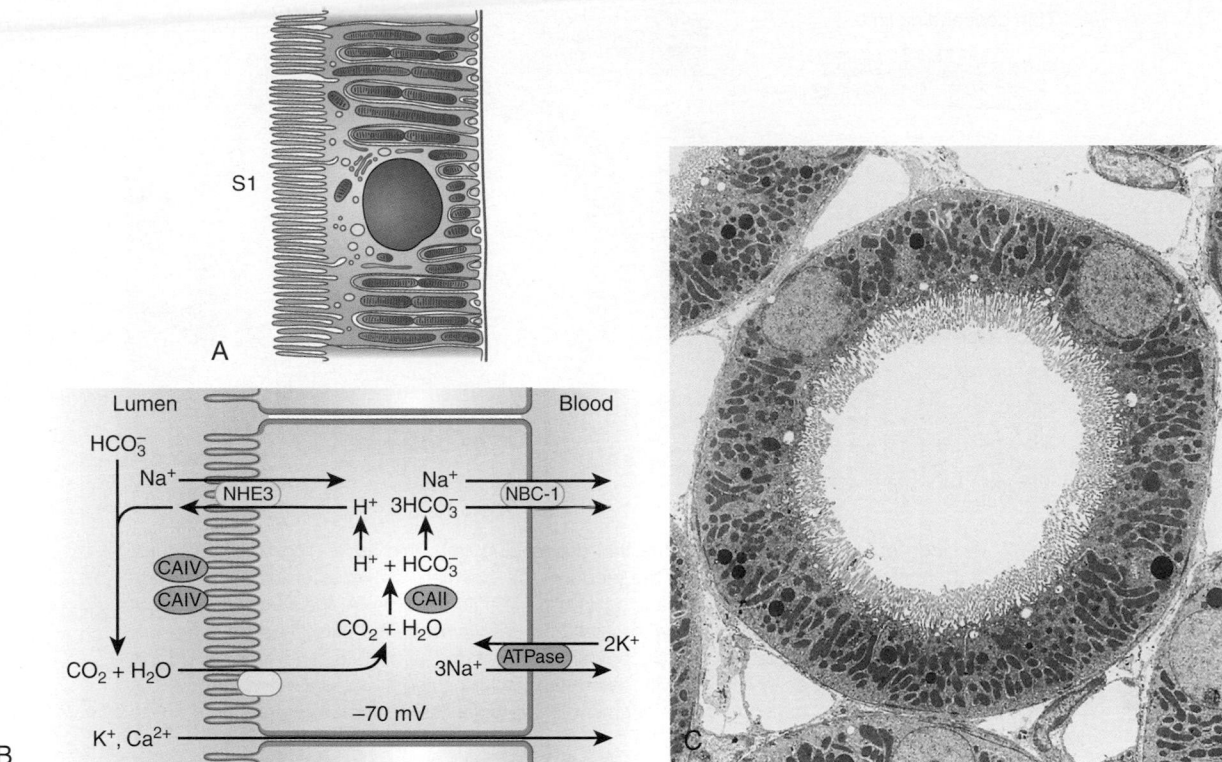

• **Fig. 1.6** Proximal tubule. (A) Schematic diagram of a typical cell of the proximal convoluted tubule, which is characterized by a prominent luminal brush border that increases the membrane surface area about 40-fold. The basolateral infoldings are lined with mitochondria and interdigitate with the basolateral infoldings of adjacent cells (in the image, infoldings from the neighboring cells are depicted in blue). These adaptations are most prominent in convoluted portion of the proximal tubule, S1. (B) The proximal tubule cell has a variety of transport mechanisms to reabsorb the bulk of the initial urinary filtrate. Primary active transport at the basolateral membrane maintains the low intracellular sodium concentration and returns sodium to the peritubular capillaries. The low intracellular concentration facilitates movement of sodium across the luminal membrane from the filtrate. Sodium is reabsorbed from the Na$^+$/H$^+$-exchanger and other transporters on the luminal membrane. (C) Cross section of the S1 segment (×3000). *CAII*, carbonic anhydrase II; *CAIV*, carbonic anhydrase IV; *CO$_2$*, carbon dioxide; *H$^+$*, hydrogen ion; *HCO$_3^-$*, bicarbonate; *H$_2$CO$_3$*, carbonic acid; *H$_2$O*, water; *K$^+$*, potassium; *Na$^+$*, sodium; *NBC-1*, electrogenic sodium bicarbonate cotransporter-1; *OH$^-$*, hydroxyl anion.

When the loop of Henle reaches the cortex, it greets its own glomerulus and transitions into a unique structure called the *macula densa*. Specialized cells in this structure are equipped with the same NKCC that is used here to provide feedback regarding tubular flow to the parent glomerulus as described above.

Distal Nephron

Distal Convoluted Tubule

The distal convoluted tubule is the smallest segment of the nephron, at only 10 to 12 mm long. Cells in this region are also impermeable to water and include a sodium chloride cotransporter, NCC (Fig. 1.9). Removal of solute without water in this region allows the tubular fluid to become dilute; thus, this segment has also been called the *diluting segment*. This segment also has a calcium channel on the luminal membrane, the transient receptor potential channel subfamily V member 5 (TRPV5). In the late portion of the DCT, cells also have transporters that are found in the principal cells (see below).

Collecting Duct

The collecting duct has two populations of cells: the intercalated cells and the principal cells (Fig. 1.10). These cells are interspersed in the collecting duct and act in concert to create the final urine (Fig. 1.11).

The principal cells have two important roles. First, vasopressin stimulation leads to translocation of aquaporin 2 from intracellular vesicles to the luminal membrane. Then, water is reabsorbed along its concentration gradient so that more concentrated urine can be created. Second, under the influence of aldosterone, the epithelial sodium channel (ENaC) facilitates movement of sodium into the cell. This leads to a lumen negative potential, favoring the loss of potassium from the principal cells via ROMK. The neighboring α-intercalated cells are also affected by the luminal negative potential difference as this favors H$^+$ ion secretion via a luminal H$^+$-ATPase. There are also β-intercalated cells that are structurally similar to the α-intercalated cells but with reverse polarity such that the H$^+$-ATPase is on the basolateral membrane and a chloride-bicarbonate exchanger, known as *pendrin*, is on the luminal membrane. These cells play a role in the secretion of bicarbonate in the setting of alkalosis.

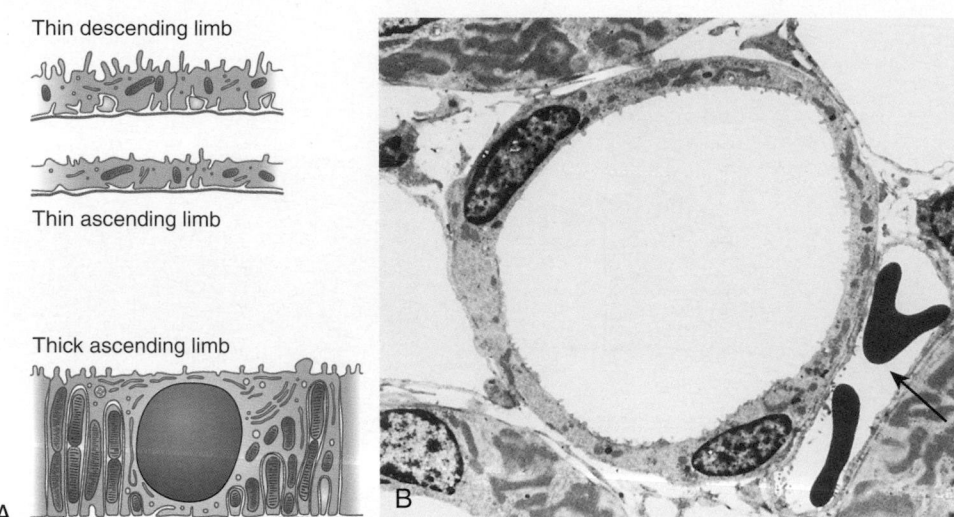

Fig. 1.7 The loop of Henle, composed of the thin descending limb, thin ascending limb, and thick ascending limb, makes a hairpin loop within the medulla. (A) Schematic drawings of the cell morphology. (B) A cross section through the thin descending limb in the outer medulla. At the lower right aspect of the image, a peritubular capillary is seen with red blood cells *(arrow)*. The thin limbs have shallow epithelia without prominent mitochondria and are permeable to water. The thick ascending limb (TAL), in contrast, is composed of taller epithelial cells with basolateral infoldings and prominent mitochondria. The TAL is impermeable to water; transport in this segment is critical for the generation of interstitial solute gradients (×3000).

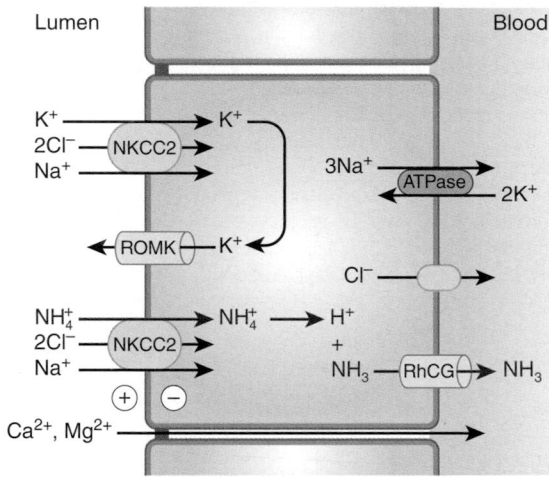

Fig. 1.8 Transport of solutes in the thick ascending limb of Henle. The primary transporter is the sodium-potassium-2 chloride cotransporter (NKCC2) on the luminal membrane, which reabsorbs a significant amount of the filtered load of sodium. In addition, ammonium (NH_4^+) can substitute for potassium (K^+) on the NKCC2. Once in the cell, NH_4^+ dissociates to ammonia (NH_3) because of the higher intracellular pH. NH_3 diffuses into the interstitium through the Rhesus glycoprotein channel (RhCG), where it is then available for secretion into the tubular lumen of a neighboring collecting duct, to act as a buffer for hydrogen ion (H^+). Transport of K^+ into the tubular lumen through ROMK provides K^+ for NKCC2 and generates a lumen-positive charge (+8 mV) that drives the paracellular transport of Ca^{2+} and Mg^{2+}. Molecules and ions that are transported out of the tubular epithelial cells on the basolateral membrane enter the surrounding interstitium and the peritubular capillaries that are in close approximation. *Ca²⁺,* Calcium; *Cl⁻,* chloride; *Mg²⁺,* magnesium; *Na⁺,* sodium; *ROMK,* renal outer medullary potassium channel.

Collecting ducts from neighboring nephrons converge in the papilla and empty into the calyces of the renal pelvis.

Salt and Volume Regulation

The Cellular Basis for Tubular Sodium Reabsorption

As noted earlier, localization of Na^+/K^+-ATPase on the basolateral membrane provides energy for reabsorption of solute from the tubular lumen with the help of a series of sodium transporters on the luminal surface of each nephron segment. The key sodium-dependent transporters, many of which are the target of diuretic agents, are listed below.

1. Proximal tubule:
   a. Na^+/H^+-exchanger 3 (NHE3). This transporter is also essential for the return of filtered bicarbonate back into the systemic circulation.
   b. Carbonic anhydrase. Inhibition of carbonic anhydrase on the luminal brush border of proximal tubular cells by carbonic anhydrase inhibitors limits reabsorption of sodium and bicarbonate in this segment.
2. Thick ascending limb: $Na^+/K^+/2Cl^-$ (NKCC2). This transporter is responsible for the reabsorption of about 25% of filtered sodium. Its activity is inhibited by loop diuretics, such as furosemide, and its actions are disrupted in the genetic condition Bartter syndrome.
3. Distal convoluted tubule: Na^+/Cl^- cotransporter (NCC). This transporter is responsible for about 5% of tubular sodium reabsorption. Thiazide diuretics, like chlorthalidone, inhibit NCC activity and lead to a modest diuresis. Gitelman syndrome is a genetic condition affecting the function of this channel.
4. Collecting duct: epithelial sodium channel (ENaC). The expression and trafficking of this protein channel to the luminal surface of principal cells is primarily activated by aldosterone, whereas its activity is inhibited by the action of atrial natriuretic peptide. Potassium-sparing diuretics, such as amiloride, inhibit ENaC directly, and mineralocorticoid receptor blockers, such spironolactone,

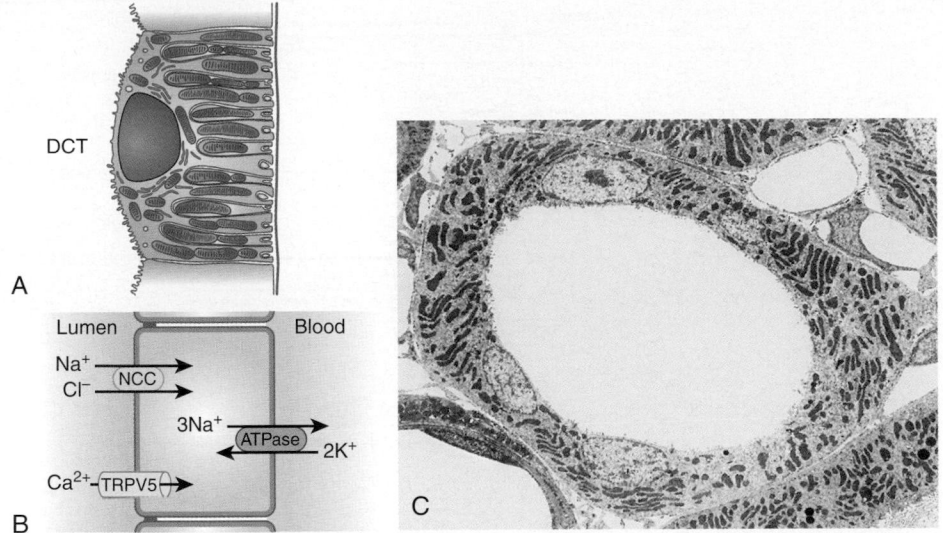

• **Fig. 1.9** Distal convoluted tubule. The distal convoluted tubule (DCT) is the shortest segment in the nephron. The early portion of the DCT features the cells depicted here. The late DCT and the connecting tubule feature cells that are aldosterone responsive and have machinery similar to the principal cells in the collecting duct. (A) Schematic of the cell morphology of the DCT. (B) Schematic of the major transporters on the DCT, which include the sodium/chloride cotransporter (NCC) and the calcium transporter, transient receptor potential channel subfamily V member 5 (TRPV5). Early in the DCT the luminal charge is close to 0 but rises to −30 mV by the end of the DCT as the architecture transitions to the cortical collecting duct (not shown). (C) Cross section of the DCT (×3000).

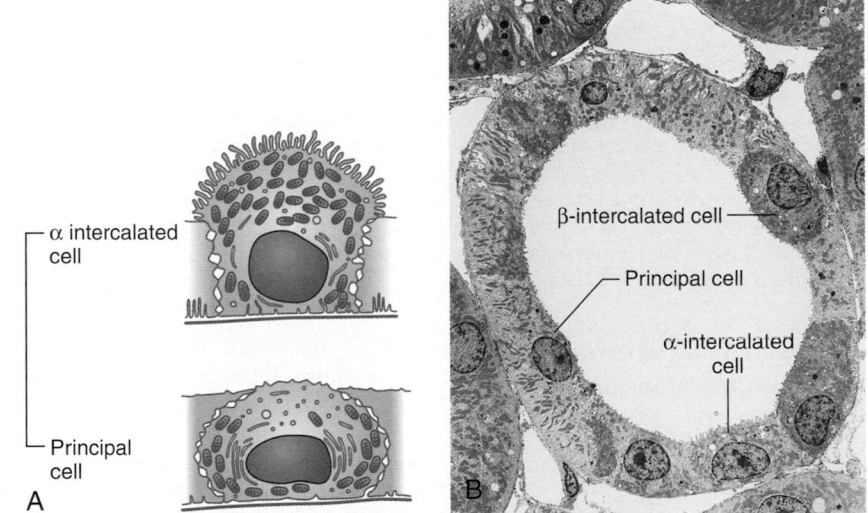

• **Fig. 1.10** The collecting duct features two different cell types interspersed: the principal cells (PC) and the intercalated cells (IC). Since these cells are situated next to each other, the electrochemical gradient created by the PCs affects the ICs. (A) Schematic of the cell morphology. (B) Cross section of the collecting duct (×3000).

indirectly decrease ENaC expression on the luminal membrane of principal cells. Liddle syndrome is an autosomal dominant condition that leads to constitutive activation of ENaC.

The Effective Arterial Blood Volume and Its Relationship to the Extracellular Fluid Volume

About 85% of plasma circulates in the low-pressure venous side of the circulation, with 15% circulating on the high-pressure arterial side. The EABV is the portion of the circulation, predominantly on the arterial side, that is sensed by baroreceptors that control renal sodium handling and extracellular fluid (ECF) volume. Effective arterial blood volume cannot be measured directly but is estimated by integrating clinical features (Table 1.2) with laboratory findings, including the urinary sodium level. A low urinary sodium level (e.g., <20 mEq/L), suggests low EABV and normal tubular function (in the absence of low solute intake or primary polydipsia). The volume of the ECF is largely determined by its content of sodium salts, which, in turn, is controlled by the excretion or retention of sodium by the kidney. Hence, the kidney plays

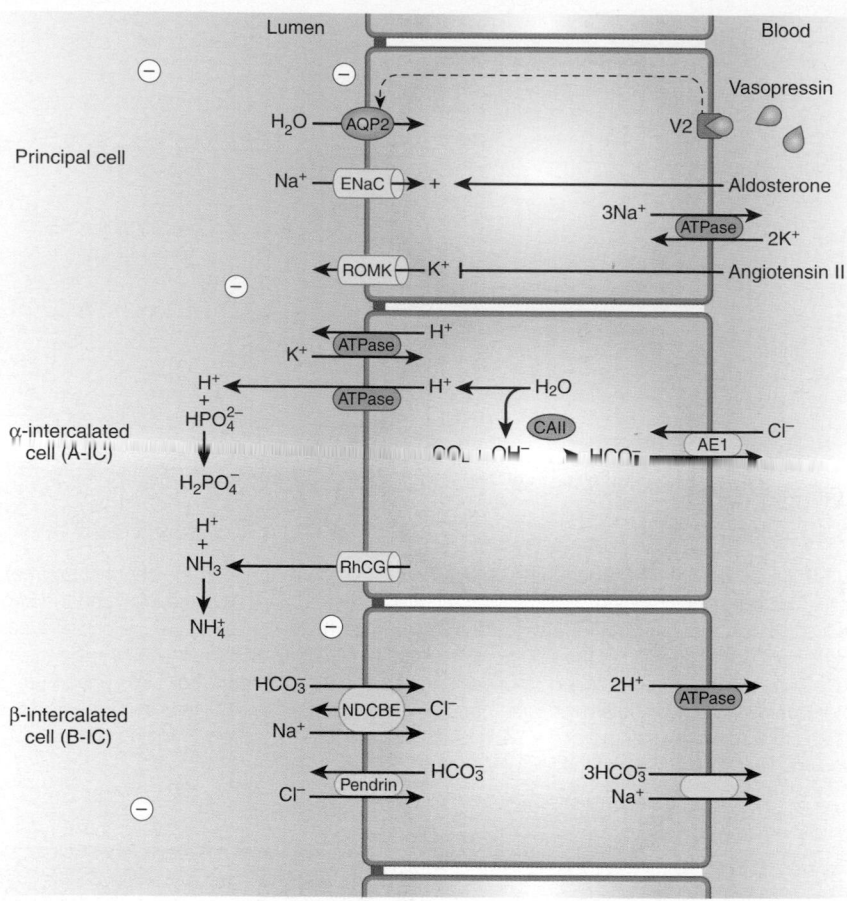

• **Fig. 1.11** The collecting duct cell types: the principal cell, α-intercalated cell (α-IC), and β-intercalated cell (β-IC). The principal cell (PC) is responsive to vasopressin. When vasopressin binds the V2 receptor, an intracellular cascade leads to phosphorylation of intravesicular aquaporins, which are then targeted to the luminal membrane. PC also expresses epithelial sodium channel (ENaC). ENaC is stimulated by aldosterone. When ENaC is active, a lumen-negative potential favors secretion of potassium from the renal outer medullary potassium channel, unless angiotensin II is also present. The electronegative lumen also promotes H+ secretion from the α-IC. This results in the generation of "new bicarbonate," which is extruded from the basolateral membrane by anion exchanger 1 (AE1). The secreted hydrogen can be excreted with titratable acids or ammonia. The β-IC secrete bicarbonate while reabsorbing NaCl.

TABLE 1.2 Effective Arterial Blood Volume and Extracellular Fluid Volume in Common Clinical Scenarios		
Clinical Examples	**Effective Arterial Blood Volume**	**Extracellular Fluid Volume (ECF)**
Gastrointestinal losses (vomiting, nasogastric suction, diarrhea)	Decreased	Decreased
Heart failure, cirrhosis, nephrotic syndrome	Decreased	Increased
Sepsis (ECF volume depends on etiology and resuscitation volume)	Decreased	Normal, decreased, or increased

a pivotal role in regulating ECF volume and maintaining sodium balance.

Normally, the fullness of the EABV parallels that of the ECF volume. However, directional changes in EABV and ECF volume are not always congruent in certain pathologic conditions. For example, the EABV may be decreased in congestive heart failure and cirrhosis, diseases often complicated by increased ECF volume and total body sodium. Decreased EABV in these conditions triggers a cascade of events that cause increased tubular reabsorption of sodium to limit further sodium and water losses. These responses are initially corrective and tend to maintain tissue perfusion. With progression of disease, however, they become maladaptive and result in the formation of edema and excessive activation of the sympathetic nervous system that contributes to increased morbidity and mortality.

The Clinical Assessment of ECF Volume and Total Body Sodium

A thorough history and physical examination are required for the assessment of ECF volume and total body sodium. The presence of edema or ascites indicates increased ECF volume, whereas postural hypotension suggests decreased ECF volume. In general, the status of ECF volume parallels that of total body sodium content. Two exceptions are pure water loss (dehydration) and the syndrome of inappropriate antidiuretic hormone (SIADH) release. In SIADH, total body sodium is slightly decreased despite increased ECF volume, although the ECF volume expansion is too small to discern by physical examination.

Renal Tubular Handling of Sodium

Under normal physiologic conditions, about 67% of the filtered load, or 16,800 mEq of sodium, is reabsorbed in the proximal convoluted tubules; 25% is reabsorbed in the TALs of the loops of Henle; 5% is reabsorbed in distal convoluted tubules; and 3% is reabsorbed in the collecting ducts. Normally, <1% of the filtered load is excreted (50 to 200 mEq/day, depending on dietary sodium intake). The fractional excretion of sodium (FE_{Na}) is the percent of the filtered load of sodium that is excreted in the urine. A simplified equation that is used for calculating the FE_{Na} can be derived as follows:

$$FE_{Na} = Sodium\ excreted\ /\ Filtered\ load\ of\ sodium \times 100$$

$$Sodium\ excreted = U_{Na} \times V$$

$$Filtered\ load\ of\ sodium = GFR \times P_{Na}$$

Using creatinine clearance as a proxy for GFR,

$$Filtered\ load\ of\ sodium = \left(U_{Cr} \times V / P_{Cr}\right) \times P_{Na}$$

Substituting the equation for the filtered load of sodium into the equation for FE_{Na}:

$$FE_{Na} = \left(\frac{\left[U_{Na} \times V\right]}{\left[GFR \times P_{Na}\right]}\right) \times 100$$

$$FE_{Na} = U_{Na} \times \frac{V}{\left[\left(U_{Cr} \times V / P_{Cr}\right) \times P_{Na}\right]} \times 100$$

The volume components cancel out, and the equation can be simplified to:

$$FE_{Na} = \frac{U_{Na} / P_{Na}}{U_{Cr} / P_{Cr}} \times 100\%$$

This equation is useful to decipher the tubular handling of sodium and can be applied to the differential diagnosis of oliguric acute kidney injury. A value of <1% suggests that the kidney is sodium avid and capable of limiting urinary sodium excretion.

Control of Sodium Excretion

The Primacy of the Effective Arterial Blood Volume in Sodium Homeostasis

Under steady-state conditions, urinary sodium excretion matches dietary sodium intake. The slight discrepancy of intake versus urinary excretion stems from extrarenal losses of sodium in the gastrointestinal tract and sweat. The filtered load of sodium is equal to $GFR \times P_{Na}$, where P_{Na} is equal to the plasma sodium concentration and is approximately 25,200 mEq/day (180 L/day × 140 mEq/L). The EABV is the critical component of the circulation that is sensed by baroreceptors and influences renal sodium excretion. An increase in EABV causes increased renal sodium excretion, while decreased EABV causes decreased renal sodium excretion.

The Integrated Compensatory Response

Changes in EABV are sensed by low-pressure baroreceptors in the walls of the right atrium and ventricle of the heart, the central veins, and pulmonary vessels, as well as by high-pressure baroreceptors in the afferent arteriole, the carotid sinus, the left ventricle, and the aortic arch. Baroreceptors are mechanoreceptor sensory neurons that constitute the afferent limb of the compensatory response to changes in EABV. Decreased fullness of the EABV induces changes in glomerular and peritubular hemodynamics and activates neurohumoral signals that act in concert to conserve sodium and maintain the EABV. Key regulatory factors that respond to changes in the EABV are the renin-angiotensin-aldosterone system, the sympathetic nervous system, atrial natriuretic peptide, and vasopressin.

The Sympathetic Nervous System

A decrease in EABV leads to decreased firing of afferent nerves from baroreceptors, thereby activating the sympathetic nervous system. Increased sympathetic outflow through the renal nerves directly increases sodium reabsorption in the proximal tubule and in other nephron segments. Circulating catecholamines and increased sympathetic renal nerve activity stimulate renin release and formation of angiotensin II. Severe decrements in EABV eventually cause intense renal arterial vasoconstriction that, in turn, reduces renal plasma flow and GFR when the renal perfusion pressure is <80 mm Hg. Conversely, decreased sympathetic nerve activation, as a consequence of volume expansion, is permissive with regard to the excretion of excess sodium.

The Renin-Angiotensin System

The renin-angiotensin-aldosterone system regulates both sodium/volume and potassium homeostasis. Angiotensin II and aldosterone have direct effects on the tubular reabsorption of sodium, and angiotensin II has effects on the renal and systemic circulation that tend to maintain or restore the EABV toward normal. Renin is a proteolytic enzyme released from the juxtaglomerular cells of the afferent arterioles in response to three stimuli.

1. Decreased pressure sensed by baroreceptors located within the wall of the afferent arteriole
2. Signals from the macula densa that sense decreased sodium chloride delivery and transport by NKCC2
3. Increased sympathetic outflow

Renin cleaves angiotensinogen, a high-molecular-weight protein that is synthesized predominantly in the liver, to form angiotensin I. Angiotensin I is converted by angiotensin-converting enzyme (produced in the lungs and kidneys) to the biologically active octapeptide angiotensin II. Both angiotensin I and II are degraded by a transmembrane protein ACE 2. Renin catalyzes the rate-limiting step in angiotensin II formation; therefore, plasma levels of renin determine plasma levels of angiotensin II. Angiotensin II directly increases sodium reabsorption in the proximal tubule. In addition, angiotensin II indirectly increases renal sodium reabsorption by altering glomerular hemodynamics and by stimulating the release of aldosterone from the adrenal cortex. Increased systemic levels of angiotensin II also cause systemic vasoconstriction.

Aldosterone

Aldosterone augments sodium reabsorption in the cortical collecting ducts by increasing the activity and expression of ENaCs on the luminal membrane. Aldosterone also plays an important role in stimulating the excretion of potassium (K^+) independent of angiotensin II. The sodium-retaining effects of aldosterone and the effects on K⁺ homeostasis are distinct, modulated by the activity of with no lysine (WNK) kinases. This system allows for the independent activation of maximal sodium reabsorption in hypovolemic states or maximal K⁺ excretion in hyperkalemic states. The importance of WNK kinases was recognized from genetic studies on patients with a Mendelian form of hypertension called *type II pseudohypoaldosteronism*. WNK4 acts as a switch that enables aldosterone to exert paradoxically different effects during hypovolemia compared to hyperkalemia. With hypovolemia, aldosterone induces changes in WNK4 that enhance NCC activity and inhibit ROMK, analogous to observations seen with type II pseudohypoaldosteronism mutant protein. As a result, both sodium and potassium are conserved. With hyperkalemia, aldosterone triggers increased phosphorylation of WNK4 by decreasing intracellular chloride. Phosphorylation of WNK4 releases its inhibition of ENaC and ROMK, leading to increased distal tubular secretion of K⁺.

Atrial Natriuretic Peptide

Pro-atrial natriuretic peptide (pro-ANP) is released from the atria in response to stretching caused by increased ECF volume. Corin, a trypsin-like serine protease, cleaves pro-ANP to form active atrial natriuretic peptide (ANP). ANP dilates the afferent arteriole and constricts the efferent arteriole, increasing glomerular capillary pressure and GFR. ANP also inhibits sodium uptake in all segments of the nephron but most prominently in the collecting ducts where it inhibits the activity of the ENaC. The sum of these effects is a physiologically appropriate natriuresis during volume expansion that restores the ECF volume toward normal.

Vasopressin (Antidiuretic Hormone)

Vasopressin is a neurohypophysial hormone released from the posterior pituitary gland in response to increases in extracellular tonicity and decreased fullness of the EABV. Vasopressin stimulates V_1 receptors on the vasculature, thereby promoting vasoconstriction, and has a pivotal role in maintaining water homeostasis (see below). In addition, vasopressin enhances the reabsorption of sodium in the TAL of the loop of Henle and in the collecting duct.

Water and Osmoregulation

Regulation of Blood Fluid Osmolality

The serum osmolality is regulated within a narrow window based upon the actions of vasopressin on the kidney. The kidney has the ability to excrete water when there is water excess and limit water loss when there is a deficiency of water (dehydration). Importantly, the kidney does not retain sodium or other solutes when there is excess water to restore osmolality; instead, water excretion is the normal response, provided there are no other stimuli for water retention such as volume depletion.

Role of Vasopressin

Vasopressin, also known as *antidiuretic hormone* (ADH), plays a critical role in the regulation of osmolality. An increase in serum osmolality is sensed by specialized cells in the hypothalamus that are equipped with mechanical stretch receptors that depolarize in response to a decrease in cell size in the setting of hyperosmolality. Nonosmotic stimuli for vasopressin release include a decrease in EABV, as noted above, activity of the sympathetic nervous system, pain, nausea, and hypoxia. When vasopressin binds to the V_2

receptors on the basolateral membrane of the principal cells in the kidneys, an intracellular cascade is initiated by cyclic AMP that culminates with the translocation of aquaporin 2 from intracytosolic vesicles to the luminal membrane. The aquaporins on the luminal membrane then permit reclamation of water along the concentration gradient created by the presence of the hypertonic medulla. Vasopressin has a short half-life of just 20 minutes. If the stimulus for vasopressin is removed, the vesicles are targeted for degradation through a complex pathway and the collecting ducts again become impermeable to water.

Medullary Hypertonicity

A hypertonic medulla is necessary to create concentrated urine in the collecting duct. Several mechanisms appear to contribute to the creation of this hypertonic medulla. The NKCC in the TAL promotes the movement of sodium and chloride from the lumen to the interstitial space. In addition, NH_4^+ is also absorbed in this region (see below), where it serves as a pool for subsequent excretion of NH_4^+. A key component of the hypertonic medulla is urea. Although urea has been described as an "ineffective osmole," it is highly polar and, similar to water, crosses cell membranes extremely slowly unless specific transporters are present.

Countercurrent Mechanism

The complex architecture of the renal medulla helps create the concentrated medullary interstitium. The parallel arrangement of the tubules equipped with the hairpin turn results in flow of the urinary filtrate in the descending limb opposite to the flow in the ascending limb. This countercurrent flow multiplies the effect of the active transport of NaCl from the TAL into the interstitium to create the concentrated medulla. Important factors that contribute to the concentrated medulla include:

1. There is active transport of NaCl without water in the thick ascending limb of Henle, which leads to an increase in the osmolality of the surrounding interstitium.
2. The descending limb of Henle has high water permeability, such that water moves down its concentration gradient and out of the lumen. This makes the fluid in the lumen more concentrated.
3. The neighboring vascular bundles, the vasa recta, also make a hairpin turn and return to the cortex in the countercurrent configuration. This arrangement assures that blood flow to the medulla does not wash out the gradient; instead, the descending vasa recta lose water and gain urea, whereas the ascending vessels gain water and lose urea.
4. Urea channels in the collecting duct are activated by vasopressin and increase urea absorption from the collecting duct into the interstitium. This serves two purposes. First, an increase in urea in the interstitium increases its osmolality. Second, the reabsorption of urea from the filtrate limits the loss of water with urea, which can act as an osmotic diuretic.

Tubular Osmolality Throughout the Nephron

Since the initial filtrate from the glomerulus is generated from plasma, it shares the same osmolality, of approximately 290 mOsm/L. As the filtrate moves through the proximal tubule, water is reabsorbed along with solute in an isosmotic fashion so that at the end of the proximal tubule, the luminal fluid still has an osmolality similar to plasma. With the descent into the medulla in the permeable thin descending limb, water leaves the lumen for the hypertonic medulla. By the time the filtrate reaches the hairpin turn of the loop of Henle, the osmolality of the tubular fluid is as high as the surrounding medulla (800 to 1200 mOsm/L). As the fluid ascends in the TAL, which is impermeable to water, solute but not water is removed, so the osmolality decreases. By the time the filtrate reaches the macula densa, it is again similar to plasma. In the distal convoluted tubule, which is also impermeable to water, additional sodium and chloride are removed and the filtrate osmolality can decline to 50 to 100 mOsm/L. In the collecting ducts, if no vasopressin is present, the dilute filtrate created in the distal convoluted tubule is excreted. Depending on the amount of vasopressin present and the osmolality of the medullary interstitium, water leaves the tubular lumen and the final urine becomes more concentrated.

Comparison of Volume Versus Water Regulation

Although osmoregulation and volume regulation have different stimuli, there is considerable overlap. In the setting of volume depletion, the robust and coordinated response by hormones and the sympathetic nervous system prompts reabsorption of both sodium and water regardless of the serum osmolality. In contrast, in the setting of a hyperosmolar state without volume depletion, the sympathetic nervous system and renin-angiotensin-aldosterone axis are not activated, and vasopressin acts alone to facilitate the reabsorption of water without sodium.

Regulation of Body Fluid Acidity and Potassium

The regulation of body-fluid acidity and potassium draws several parallels.

1. The concentrations of potassium (K^+) and hydrogen ion (H^+) are tightly regulated because relatively small perturbations in H^+ and K^+ levels can impair normal cellular function and can result in life-threatening complications.
2. The kidney regulates the excretion of K^+ and H^+ over the course of several hours to days, but immediate extrarenal buffering mechanisms exist to prevent acute life-threatening rises in plasma K^+ and H^+ when there is a surfeit K^+ or H^+.
3. The precise regulation of K^+ and H^+ is coordinated at the same site, the collecting duct. Within the collecting duct, the principal cell is the target of physiologic signals that regulate K^+ secretion and the α-intercalated cell is the site that mediates H^+ secretion.
4. Both K^+ and H^+ secretion is stimulated by the action of aldosterone.
5. Disturbances of K^+ homeostasis may cause or be associated with acid-base disorders, and acid-base disorders may cause abnormalities in K^+ homeostasis.

Sources of Hydrogen Ion

Oxidation of the cationic amino acids, lysine and arginine, as well as the sulfur-containing amino acids, cysteine and methionine, generates fixed acid. A typical diet leads to the liberation of approximately 1 mEq/kg body weight, or 50 to 100 mEq, of fixed acid per day. This H^+ is buffered, in part, by consuming extracellular HCO_3^-. In the absence of a mechanism to excrete the daily fixed acid load, the buffer pool would be depleted, leading to

metabolic acidosis. Hence, the kidney must excrete fixed acid and generate new bicarbonate to replace the bicarbonate consumed to maintain acid-base homeostasis. Metabolism of carbohydrates and fats also generates H^+, but complete oxidation of these compounds leads to the equimolar removal of H^+. Finally, about 15,000 mmol of volatile acid are produced each day from normal metabolism in the form of carbon dioxide (CO_2), the excretion of which is dependent on adequate ventilation.

Regulation of Body Fluid Acidity

The physiologically appropriate concentration of hydrogen ion (H^+) is 1000-fold less than that of most serum electrolytes, on the order of 37 to 43 nanoequivalents per liter (nEq/L). An increase in the hydrogen ion concentration to >100 nEq/L, or a pH of <7.0, if sustained, is not compatible with life because of altered cellular function. Hence, the concentration of H^+ must be precisely maintained and regulated. The maintenance of the arterial pH at 7.40 relies on buffering by the HCO_3^-/CO_2 system and intracellular molecules, the excretion of fixed acid by the kidney, and effective alveolar ventilation.

The HCO_3^-/CO_2 System

The Henderson-Hasselbalch model of acid-base balance emphasizes the importance of the ratio of HCO_3^- to CO_2 as the major determinant of blood pH. The relationship of arterial pH to HCO_3^-/CO_2 is:

$$pH = 6.1 + \log\left(\frac{\left[HCO_3^-\right]}{\left[0.03 \times P_aCO_2\right]}\right)$$

Hence, a decrease in $[HCO_3^-]$ or an increase in P_aCO_2 results in a decrease in arterial pH (acidemia), whereas an increase in $[HCO_3^-]$ or a decrease in P_aCO_2 causes an increase in arterial pH (alkalemia). The kidney regulates the concentration of bicarbonate, while the lungs control the level of arterial PCO_2.

Acid-Base Homeostasis and the Kidney

Proximal Tubular Bicarbonate Reabsorption

Proximal tubular reclamation of bicarbonate does not contribute to fixed acid excretion but is essential for the conservation of filtered bicarbonate. The kidneys filter approximately 4300 mEq of bicarbonate each day. Bicarbonate reabsorption occurs mainly in the proximal tubule, where its transport is governed by the activity of the NHE3 (see Fig. 1.6). H^+ secreted by NHE3 combines with filtered HCO_3^- to form carbonic acid (H_2CO_3), which is then converted to CO_2 and H_2O by carbonic anhydrase IV. CO_2 and H_2O diffuse into the cell through specific channels. Within the cell, water dissociates into OH^- and H^+ while OH^- combines with CO_2 in a reaction catalyzed by carbonic anhydrase II to form HCO_3^-. Intracellular bicarbonate is secreted into the peritubular interstitium by a basolateral sodium/bicarbonate cotransporter 1 (NBC-1, also known as *solute carrier family 4 member 4* [SLC4A4]). Intracellular H^+ is then secreted back into the lumen by NHE3, where it again combines with filtered bicarbonate. Proximal secretion of H^+ in exchange for Na^+ results in a minimal fall in the luminal pH of the proximal convoluted tubule because H_2CO_3 rapidly dissociates to CO_2 and H_2O under the influence of abundant carbonic anhydrase present on the luminal surface of the brush border. In total, this mechanism reclaims filtered bicarbonate back into the systemic circulation. Normal bicarbonate reclamation is sufficient to reclaim all the filtered bicarbonate when the serum bicarbonate is within the normal range. When serum bicarbonate levels exceed normal, the excess bicarbonate overwhelms proximal convoluted tubule reabsorption and is excreted. An exception is in the setting of low EABV when angiotensin II activation of NHE3 increases the proximal reabsorption of sodium and, with it, bicarbonate, regardless of the serum bicarbonate level.

Urinary Acidification

The pH of the tubular lumen progressively decreases and reaches its lowest level in the medullary collecting duct. H^+ excretion is predominantly mediated by an H^+-ATPase located on the luminal surface of α-intercalated cells. For every H^+ excreted, an equimolar quantity of HCO_3^- is released into the systemic circulation. The amount of fixed acid that can be excreted as free H^+ is limited by the minimal urine pH of 4.4. The concentration of H^+ at this pH is 0.04 mEq/L. Therefore, excretion of an average fixed acid load of about 70 mEq/day as free H^+ cannot be attained at an average daily urine volume of 1.5 L (i.e., it would require a urine volume of about 1750 L). How, then, is the fixed acid load excreted? The answer lies in the activity of two urinary buffers: titratable acid, primarily derived from the buffering capacity of dibasic phosphate (HPO_4^{2-}), and ammonia.

H^+ Secretion

Water dissociates into H^+ and OH^- in α-intercalated cells (see Fig. 1.11). The H^+ formed is secreted into the tubular lumen by H^+-ATPase, where it is buffered by dibasic phosphate or ammonia and then excreted in the urine. The OH^- combines with intracellular CO_2 to form HCO_3^- in a reaction catalyzed by carbonic anhydrase II. The newly generated HCO_3^- is then transported into the peritubular capillary interstitium by a chloride/bicarbonate exchanger (AE1; band 3 anion transport protein, also known as *solute carrier family 4 member 1* [SLC4A1]), where it replenishes the HCO_3^- that was consumed by buffering of fixed acid.

Formation and Excretion of Titratable Acid

Dibasic phosphate (HPO_4^{2-}) is freely filtered at the glomerulus and acts as a buffer for H^+ in both the proximal and distal convoluted tubules. The efficacy of HPO_4^{2-} as an effective buffer is explained by the relationship between urine pH and its pK_a. The pK_a of HPO_4^{2-} is 6.8; therefore, about 90% of HPO_4^{2-} buffer capacity occurs above a pH of 5.8. The 30 to 40 mEq of HPO_4^{2-} that are filtered each day account for the excretion of approximately one-half of the daily fixed acid load. The buffering activity of HPO_4^{2-} is called *titratable acid* because it can be measured by titration of the urine with NaOH to a pH of 7.40. The relatively fixed filtered load of HPO_4^{2-} limits the capacity for H^+ excretion as titratable acid. For every H^+ buffered by HPO_4^{2-} and excreted in the urine as (HPO_4^{2-}), a HCO_3^- is generated and released into the plasma.

Formation and Excretion of Ammonium (NH_4^+)

About 30 to 40 mEq of fixed acid per day are excreted in the form of ammonium. During metabolic acidosis, the kidney can increase the generation of ammonium to about 200 mEq/day. Ammonium (NH_4^+) is primarily synthesized in the proximal tubular cells by the deamination of glutamine to glutamate, and further to α-ketoglutarate, yielding two NH_4^+ and two HCO_3^-. Decreased ammoniagenesis

occurs when the GFR falls to <45 mL/min/1.73 m^2 and causes the non-gap component of metabolic acidosis in CKD. NH_4^+ is transported into the interstitium in the TAL, substituting for K^+ on the NKCC2 (see Fig. 1.8). Ammonium then dissociates to ammonia (NH_3) in the medullary interstitium because of the relatively higher pH of this compartment. Ammonia is subsequently transported down its concentration gradient into the lumen of the inner medullary collecting duct via the Rhesus (Rh) glycoprotein (RhCG), present on α-intercalated cells. A low concentration of NH_3 is maintained in the tubular lumen because the low luminal pH and the high pK_a of NH_4^+ (pK_a 9) favors generation of NH_4^+. Indeed, the ratio of NH_3 to NH_4^+ is about 1:1000 at a urine pH of 6 and 1:10,000 at a urine pH of 5.0. New HCO_3^- ions are added to the blood pool for every ammonium cation that is trapped in the lumen and then excreted.

Alkali Excretion

Alkalemia is associated with an increase in the number of the bicarbonate-secreting β-intercalated cells relative to α-intercalated cells in the collecting duct. β-intercalated cells function to excrete excess HCO_3^- during metabolic alkalosis.

Increased alkali associated with a diet enriched in fruits and vegetables leads to the liberation of increased citrate and the generation of organic compounds that are bicarbonate equivalents. Increased urinary excretion of citrate occurs after ingestion of a high alkali diet, thereby limiting the degree of alkalosis through the excretion of base equivalents.

Regulation of Body-Fluid Potassium

Distribution of Potassium Ion in the Body

Potassium (K^+) plays a critical role in determining the resting cell membrane potential. The transcellular distribution of K^+ is largely determined by the Na^+/K^+-ATPase, which transports Na^+ out of cells in exchange for K^+. As a result, the intracellular concentration of K^+ is maintained at a level of approximately 140 mEq/L, where the normal extracellular concentration of K^+ ranges between 3.5 and 5 mEq/L. Both hypokalemia and hyperkalemia can result in potentially life-threatening cardiac dysrhythmias and paralysis by altering the resting potential of skeletal and cardiac muscle. Therefore, tight regulation of the extracellular potassium concentration is of critical importance for the maintenance of normal cellular function. Total body potassium stores average 50 to 60 mEq/kg, or about 3800 mEq for a 70-kg adult, of which 98% is distributed in the intracellular compartment.

K^+ Homeostasis after K^+ Intake

The rise in the serum K^+ level after ingestion of a K^+ load is attenuated by the intracellular uptake of K^+. A potassium-rich meal stimulates the release of insulin and epinephrine, both of which increase the activity of Na^+/K^+-ATPase to promote the intracellular uptake of K^+, predominantly in skeletal muscle. Increased serum K^+ levels also stimulate the release of aldosterone, which upregulates the excretion of K^+ in the collecting duct.

Influence of Acid-Base Status on K^+ Homeostasis

Acid-base status must be considered when interpreting the plasma K^+ level because of the influence of the extracellular H^+ concentration on transcellular potassium flux. Cells buffer increased levels of H^+ in acidemia that results in the shift of K^+ from the intracellular fluid compartment to the extracellular compartment. This occurs to the greatest extent when there is net retention of hydrochloric acid (so-called *mineral acidosis*). Hence, there is a relative increase in the plasma K+ level in acidemia. Despite this relative increase in the serum K+ level, acidosis does not always cause overt hyperkalemia. Individuals with severe diarrhea, for example, are often K+ depleted and have hypokalemia despite the presence of acidemia. K+/H+ exchange occurs to a lesser extent in organic acidoses, such as lactic acidosis. In organic acidoses, H+ enters cells along with an accompanying organic acid via an H+/organic acid transporter, thereby minimizing H+-K+ exchange.

Hyperkalemia can cause metabolic acidosis through two mechanisms. First, K+ entry into cells results in the shift of H+ into the extracellular compartment. Second, hyperkalemia impairs renal ammonium excretion because the intracellular alkalosis generated from potassium/hydrogen ion exchange inhibits ammoniagenesis. In addition, there is decreased availability of ammonia in the medullary interstitium because increased luminal levels of K+ result in the preferential transport of K+ over ammonium by NKCC2 in the TAL of the loop of Henle.

Renal Handling of K+

On average, about 50 to 150 mEq of K+ are excreted in the urine each day, the amount depending on dietary potassium intake. About 90% of filtered K+ is reabsorbed in the proximal nephron and loop of Henle. Most of the K+ excreted in the urine is derived from the secretion of K+ in the cortical collecting duct, the segment of the tubule subject to physiologic regulation. High serum levels of K+ drive increased K+ secretion in the collecting duct, whereas K+ depletion leads to increased reabsorption of K+ at this site.

K+ secretion in the cortical collecting duct is influenced by several major factors.

1. Generation of lumen negative charge. Increased electronegativity in the tubular lumen of the collecting duct promotes K+ excretion by generating a favorable electrochemical gradient for K+ secretion. Increased delivery of sodium, which is rapidly transported into principal cells through ENaC, leaves behind anions, predominantly chloride, that enhance the generation of lumen electronegativity. Increased delivery of nonabsorbable anions such as keto acids or penicillin metabolites also enhances the lumen negative charge and promotes the secretion of K+.
2. Aldosterone. Aldosterone enhances lumen electronegativity by increasing the activity and expression of ENaC on the luminal surface of principal cells. The rapid uptake of Na+ through ENaC exceeds the rate of chloride absorption, thereby generating increased lumen electronegativity. Aldosterone also increases the expression of ROMK on the luminal membrane of principal cells, increasing the permeability to K+ and amplifying the secretion of K+. Finally, aldosterone increases the activity of Na+/K+-ATPase, thus increasing the intracellular potassium content that drives potassium secretion. In addition to facilitating the excretion of K+, the resultant lumen negative charge enhances the secretion of H+ from α-intercalated cells and the addition of new HCO_3^- into the ECF bicarbonate pool. Hence, increased aldosterone also contributes to the development of metabolic alkalosis.
3. Flow-induced potassium secretion. Increased flow through the aldosterone-sensitive portion of the distal convoluted tubule and the cortical collecting duct increases the secretion of K+ from principal cells. Increased flow lowers the concentration of K+ in the tubular lumen, creating a favorable concentration gradient for the secretion of K+ from principal cells via ROMK. In addition, flow-mediated changes in luminal cilia located on principal cells and

α-intercalated cells activate large-conductance calcium, stretch-activated Big Potassium (BK) channels that are expressed on the luminal surface of these cells. Flow-induced K+ secretion accounts for a significant component of increased urinary K+ excretion related to volume expansion, diuretic use, and osmotic diuresis.
4. Increased plasma K+ concentration: Increases in plasma K+ concentrations raise intracellular K+ levels, generating a favorable concentration gradient for the excretion of K+.
5. Metabolic alkalosis: Just as increased concentrations of H+ in acidemia cause the shift of K+ out of cells, decreased extracellular H+ levels in metabolic alkalosis result in increased intracellular levels of K+ that facilitate the secretion of K+.

Renal Handling of Glucose, Amino Acids, Organic Anions, and Cations

Glucose and amino acids are freely filtered by the glomerulus and then reabsorbed nearly completely by the end of the proximal tubule. Glucose reabsorption is achieved by the action of sodium/glucose cotransporters (SGLT1 and SGLT2) on the luminal membrane of the proximal tubules. In the early proximal tubule, high-capacity, low-specificity transporters line the luminal membrane and reabsorb the bulk of the filtered glucose (SGLT2). In the late proximal tubule, low-capacity, high-specificity transporters complete this task (SGLT1). Since the glucose concentration in the filtrate is low in comparison to sodium (glucose concentration of 90 mg/dL is equivalent to 5 mmol/L), there is ample sodium available to reabsorb the majority of the filtered load of glucose. Glucose is transported from the cell back to the circulation via the basolateral transporters GLUT1 and GLUT2. The normal glucose absorptive threshold, or tubular transport maximum (Tm), is about 180 mg/dL, but, in the setting of hyperfiltration, glycosuria may develop at lower serum glucose values (Fig. 1.12).

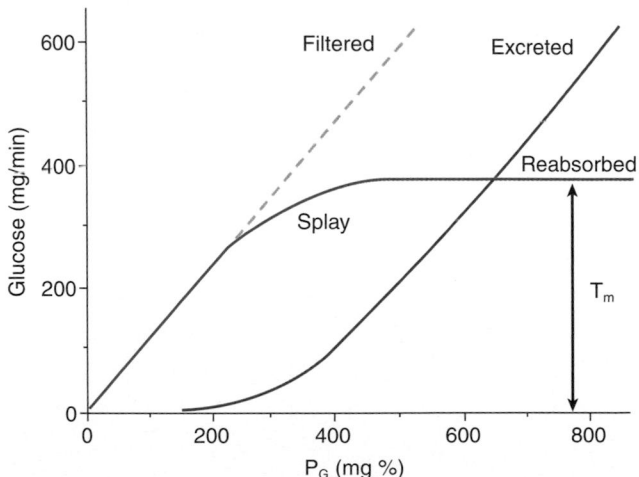

• **Fig. 1.12** Renal glucose reabsorption is related to the filtered load of glucose. When the filtered load of glucose is low, all the glucose is reabsorbed and none is excreted. When the plasma glucose concentration (P_G) and the filtered glucose load rise above the maximum tubular (Tm) resorptive capacity for the glucose transporters, glucose begins to appear in the urine and is excreted. The "splay" reflects the difference between the theoretical curve and actual observations since there is not a sharp cutoff. As individual nephrons may have different thresholds for glucose reabsorption depending on morphologic features, the Tm reflects the average. A similar curve could be drawn for the reabsorption of bicarbonate.

Amino acids are reabsorbed throughout the nephron but primarily in the proximal tubule, with less than 1% of the filtered load of amino acids excreted in the urine. There is a wide array of transporters for amino acids on the luminal and basolateral membranes that have different specificities and different affinities for the neutral, dibasic, and anionic amino acids. Reabsorption of glutamine in the proximal tubule is important for the production of ammonium. A dibasic amino acid transporter is responsible for the reabsorption of the amino acid cystine.

The proximal tubule is also the site of secretion of a wide range of organic cations and anions. These include molecules that are too large for filtration and those that are protein bound. This process is facilitated by an array of organic ion transporters on the basolateral and luminal membranes that function in tandem; molecules are first transported from the basolateral surface into the cell and then secreted into the tubular lumen. These transporters from the solute carrier and ATP binding cassette families can facilitate excretion of a host of different molecules. The organic cation transporters secrete medications such as metformin and trimethoprim as well as endogenous substances like creatinine. The organic anion transporters play a role in the secretion of furosemide, tenofovir, and methotrexate, as well as endogenous substances such as urate and exogenous toxins like mercury.

Bibliography

Carlström M, Wilcox CS, Arendshorst WJ. Renal autoregulation in health and disease. *Physiol Rev.* 2015;95:405–511.

Carrisoza-Gaytan R, Carattino MD, Kleyman TR, Satlin LM. An unexpected journey: conceptual evolution of mechanoregulated potassium transport in the distal nephron. *Am J Physiol Cell Physiol.* 2016;310:C243–C259.

Danziger J, Hoenig MP. The Role of the Kidney in Disorders of Volume Core Curriculum. *Am J Kidney Dis.* 2016;68(5):808–816.

Danziger J, Zeidel ML. Osmotic homeostasis. *Clin J Am Soc Nephrol.* 2015;10:852–862.

Feraille E, Dizin E. Coordinated control of ENaC and Na⁺,K⁺-ATPase in renal collecting duct. *J Am Soc Nephrol.* 2016;27:2554–2563.

Ferenbach DA, Bonventre JV. Kidney tubules: intertubular, vascular, and glomerular cross-talk. *Curr Opin Nephrol Hypertens.* 2016;25:194–202.

McCormick JA, Ellison DH. The Distal Convoluted Tubule. *Compr Physiol.* 2015,5(1):45–98.

Palmer BF, Clegg DJ. Physiology and Pathophysiology of potassium homeostasis: Core Curriculum 2019. Am. *J Kidney Dis.* 2019;74:682–693.

Scott RP, Quaggin SE. Review series: The cell biology of renal filtration. *J Cell Biol.* 2015;209:199–210.

Theilig F, Wu Q. ANP-induced signaling cascade and its implications in renal pathophysiology. *Am J Physiol Renal Physiol.* 2015;308:F1047–F1055.

Weiner ID, Mitch WE, Sands JM. Urea and ammonia metabolism and the control of renal nitrogen excretion. *Clin J Am Soc Nephrol.* 2015;10:1444–1458.

Weiner ID, Verlander JW. Recent advances in understanding renal ammonia metabolism and transport. *Curr Opin Nephrol Hypertens.* 2016;25:436–443.

2

Kidney Development

ROSEMARY V. SAMPOGNA

Development of the Mammalian Kidney

Congenital anomalies of the kidney and urinary tract (CAKUT) are common birth defects that account for 40%-50% of pediatric end-stage kidney disease (ESKD) worldwide. These comprise a wide range of malformations that may be sporadic or inherited. Nephron number can vary up to 10-fold in humans and, although ~40% of variation in creatinine clearance (a proxy for functioning nephrons) is due to inherited alleles, the remaining variation is unaccounted, suggesting that environmental factors, particularly gestational malnutrition, can also "program" long-term metabolic consequences. This chapter addresses the key events that specify normal human kidney development and describes structural and functional consequences of developmental errors. The diagnosis and clinical management of CAKUT is also reviewed.

Overview of Kidney Development

The mammalian kidney is derived from intermediate mesoderm (IM), a primitive tissue that forms on either side of the aorta (Fig. 2.1). Three pairs of excretory organs of increasingly advanced design develop in a craniocaudal and overlapping temporal sequence. (1) The pronephros originates on day 22 of gestation, as the mesonephric duct emerges via epithelialization of the mesoderm. Primitive tubules join this duct and disappear by day 25. (2) The mesonephros is comprised of excretory units that resemble primitive nephrons and produce small amounts of urine that contribute to the amniotic fluid. By week 16, these regress in females and give rise to elements of the genital duct system in males. (3) The metanephros (definitive kidney) initiates around day 28–32, when a single epithelial outgrowth from the mesonephric duct known as the ureteric bud (UB) invades neighboring metanephric mesenchyme (MM) (see Fig. 2.1A). The MM is a condensation of IM-derived undifferentiated cells that release inductive molecular signals required for initial UB outgrowth and subsequent branching propagation, as well as inhibitory signals that restrict the site of UB outgrowth to a single location. In turn, signals that emanate from the UB instruct the conversion of undifferentiated MM to epithelial structures. Repetitive bi-directional inductive signals help prevent ectopic branching events and drive the UB to arborize into the collecting system. Concomitantly, the MM proliferates and differentiates to form epithelial tubules (mesenchymal-to-epithelial transition) that span from glomerulus to distal convoluted tubule. Thus, these two synchronized processes, nephrogenesis (MM-derived) and branching morphogenesis (UB-derived), shape human kidney development, a process thought to be complete by week 36.

Repeating Branching Morphogenesis Establishes the Kidney Collecting System

Active UB branching within the kidney's periphery (the nephrogenic zone) ultimately gives rise to the collecting duct system. (Note that the kidney calyces, sinus, and ureter are also derived from UB epithelia). The number of repeating branching events is a key determinant of final nephron number as UB tips induce discrete subsets of MM cells to undergo nephrogenesis (see Fig. 2.1C). In humans, branching morphogenesis is thought to be complete by week 20–22 of gestation. Thereafter, collecting duct development occurs by extension of peripheral branch segments and new nephrons form predominantly around the tips of terminal collecting duct branches.

Distinct peripheral (cortical) and central (medullary) domains of the developing kidney are established between gestational weeks 22 and 34. The kidney cortex, comprising 70% of total kidney volume at birth, becomes organized as a relatively compact, circumferential layer at the periphery, while the medulla (30% of total volume) has a modified pyramidal shape with a broad base adjacent to the cortex. These well-differentiated zones can be discerned on fetal ultrasound by week 20 to 25. The apex of the cone is formed by convergence of collecting ducts in the inner medulla known as the *papilla*. Distinct morphologic differences also emerge between medullary and cortical collecting ducts. The former organize into elongated, relatively unbranched linear arrays, which converge centrally in a region devoid of glomeruli. In contrast, developing cortical collecting ducts continue to induce MM at the nephrogenic zone. The most central segments of the collecting duct system, formed from the first several generations of UB branching, undergo remodeling by combination of growth, apoptosis, and tubule dilatation to form the pelvis and calyces.

As above, the UB arises from the mesonephric duct in response to MM-derived inductive signals. Failure of UB induction results in kidney agenesis, while erroneous outgrowth of multiple UBs can result in kidney malformations including collecting system and/or ureter duplication. The precise position at which the UB is induced is critical to the nature of UB-MM reciprocal interactions, and ectopic positioning can be associated with malformations (kidney dysplasia) or compromise the integrity of the ureterovesical junction.

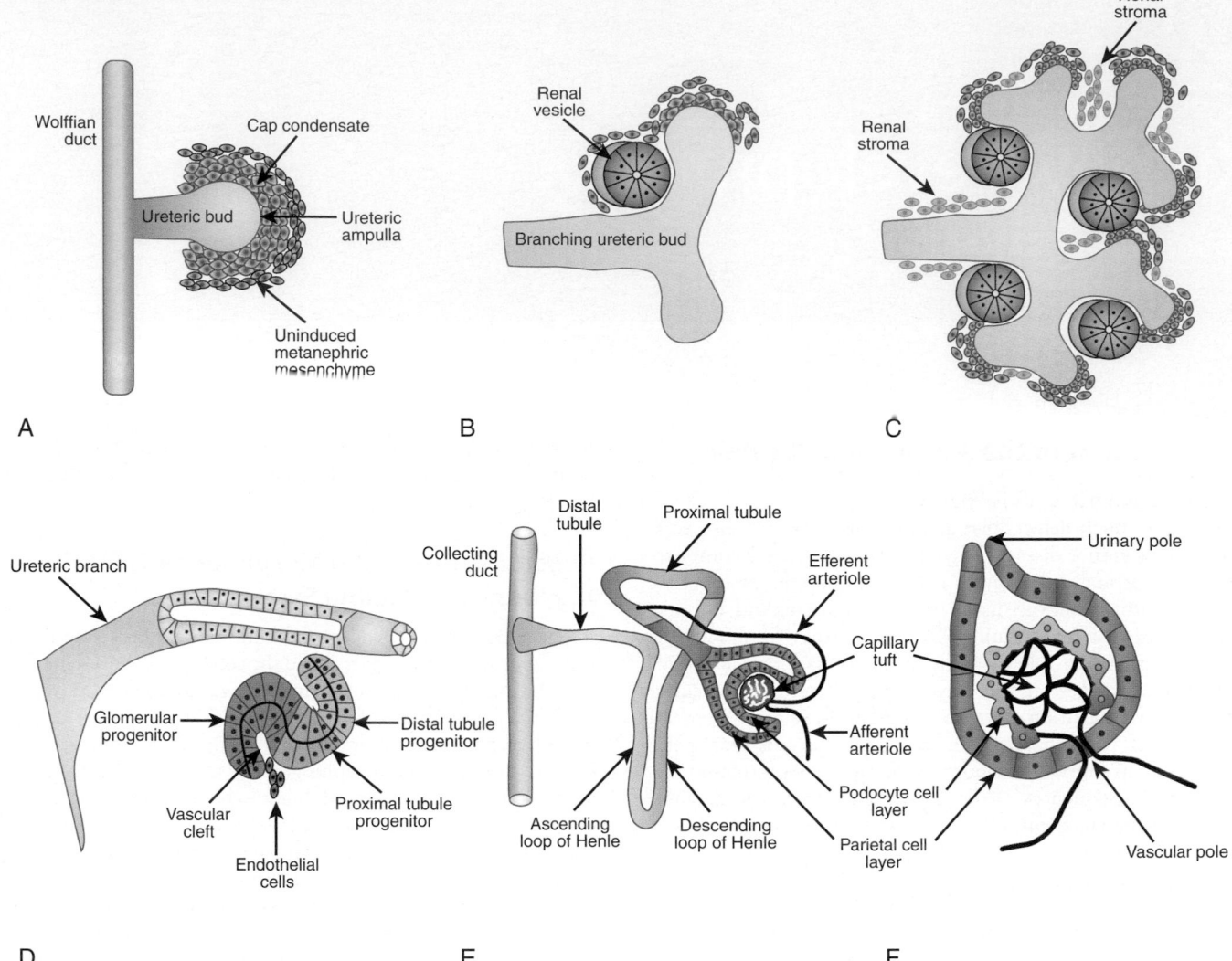

• **Fig. 2.1** Stages of kidney formation. (A) Induction of the metanephric mesenchyme by the ureteric bud promotes aggregation of mesenchyme cells around the tip of the ureteric bud. (B) Polarized renal vesicles are formed. (C) Stromal cells secrete factors that influence nephrogenesis and branching morphogenesis. (D) Formation of the S-shaped body involves the formation of a proximal cleft that is invaded by angioblasts. (E) The complete nephron is joined to the collecting duct. (F) Glomerulus demonstrating organization of the capillary tuft, podocytes, and parietal epithelial cells.

Formation of the Nephron (Nephrogenesis)

Signals transmitted from the UB induce adjacent MM to undergo a mesenchymal-to-epithelial transformation (MET). Initially, mesenchyme cells condense around the ampulla of the advancing UB (see Fig. 2.1A), then form an oval mass called a *pretubular aggregate* (see Fig. 2.1B). An internal cavity forms within this developing renal vesicle, which is comprised of multipotent precursors that give rise to all of the nephron epithelial cell types. Nephron segmentation into glomerular and tubular domains is initiated by the sequential formation of two clefts in the renal vesicle. The lower (*vascular*) cleft gives way to the comma-shaped body and subsequent generation of an upper cleft leads to formation of an S-shaped body, which is characterized by three segments or limbs (see Fig. 2.1D). The middle limb gives rise to the proximal convoluted tubule and the upper limb to the descending and ascending limbs of the loops of Henle and the distal convoluted tubule.

Formation of the glomerulus begins as the vascular cleft broadens while the lower limb of the S-shaped body forms a cup-shaped structure (see Fig. 2.1D and F). Epithelial cells lining the inner wall of this cup will comprise the visceral glomerular epithelium, or podocyte layer. Cells lining the outer wall of the cup will form the parietal glomerular epithelium that lines the Bowman capsule (see Fig. 2.1F). The glomerular capillary tuft is formed via recruitment and proliferation of endothelial and mesangial cell precursors. Recruitment of angioblasts and mesangial precursors into the vascular cleft form a primitive vascular plexus (see Fig. 2.1E). Podocytes of these capillary loop stage glomeruli lose mitotic capacity and begin to form actin-based cytoplasmic extensions, or foot processes, and specialized intercellular junctions, termed *slit diaphragms*. Subsequent development of the glomerular capillary tuft involves a poorly defined sequence of capillary branching and formation of endothelial fenestrae. Mesangial cells, in turn, populate the core of the tuft and provide structural support to capillary

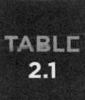

TABLE 2.1 Systemic Syndromes, Chromosomal Abnormalities, and Metabolic Disorders with Kidney or Urinary Tract Malformation

Syndromes

Beckwith-Wiedemann

Cerebro-oculo-renal

CHARGE

DiGeorge

Ectrodactyly, ectodermal dysplasia, and cleft/lip palates

Ehlers-Danlos

Fanconi pancytopenia syndrome

Fraser

Fryns

Meckel

Marfan

MURCS association

Oculo-auriculo-vertebral (Goldenhar)

Oculo-facial-digital (OFD)

Pallister-Hall

Kidney cyst and diabetes

Simpson-Golabi-Behmel (SGBS)

Tuberous sclerosis

Townes-Brock

VATER

WAGR

Williams-Beuren

Zellweger (cerebrohepatorenal)

Chromosomal Abnormalities

Trisomy 21

Klinefelter

DiGeorge, 22q11

45, X0 (Turner)

(XXY) Klinefelter

Tri 9 mosaic, Tri 13, Tri 18, del 4q, del 18q, dup 3q, dup 10q

Triploidy

Metabolic Disorders

Peroxisomal

Glycosylation defect

Mitochondriopathy

Glutaric aciduria type II

Carnitine palmitoyltransferase II deficiency

loops via deposition of extracellular matrix. The full complement of glomeruli in the fetal human kidney is attained by 32–36 weeks. It should be kept in mind that the process of nephrogenesis at each UB tip occurs approximately 1 million times in each kidney. Moreover, the requirement for reciprocal induction implies that signaling defects in either compartment can have pleiotropic effects across the entire urinary tract.

Kidney Malformations

Definition and Overview

Urinary tract malformations are classified under the overall term *Congenital Anomalies of the Kidney and Urinary Tract* (CAKUT). These malformations are the most frequently detected abnormalities during intrauterine life (0.1 to 0.7 pregnancies) and are the major cause of childhood kidney failure. In 30% of affected patients, CAKUT occur in combination with nonkidney malformations as part of a genetic syndrome. Over 200 distinct syndromes feature some type of kidney and urinary tract malformation (Table 2.1).

CAKUT represent a spectrum of developmental malformations including:
- Aplasia (agenesis): congenital absence of kidney tissue
- Simple hypoplasia: kidney length > 2 standard deviations below the mean for age with reduced nephron number but normal kidney architecture
- Dysplasia ± cysts: malformation of tissue elements
- Isolated dilatation of the kidney pelvis ± ureters (collecting system)
- Anomalies of position including ectopic and fused (horseshoe) kidney

These malformations may be unilateral or bilateral and are associated with structural abnormalities of the lower urinary tract in 50% of affected patients. These ureteral abnormalities include vesicoureteral reflux (VUR) (25% of cases), ureteropelvic junction obstruction (11%), and ureterovesical junction obstruction (11%). Kidney dysplasia is a polymorphic disorder characterized at the microscopic level by abnormal differentiation of mesenchymal and epithelial elements, decreased nephron number, loss of the demarcating zone between the cortex and the medulla, and metaplastic transformation of mesenchyme to cartilage and bone. Dysplastic kidneys range in size from large, distended kidneys with multiple large cysts to small kidneys, with or without cysts. A small dysplastic kidney without macroscopic cysts, imaged by ultrasound, is classified as hypoplastic/dysplastic in the absence of a pathologic examination, which distinguishes between simple hypoplasia and dysplasia. The multicystic dysplastic kidney (MCDK) is an extreme form of kidney dysplasia.

Etiology of Human Urinary Tract Malformation

Advances in chromosomal microarrays and next-generation sequencing have implicated over 50 genes in syndromic and nonsyndromic forms of CAKUT. Familial forms comprise up to 20% of cases (Table 2.2), but most are sporadic with no obvious syndrome or Mendelian pattern of inheritance. Moreover, malformations can affect one or more urologic structures and show variable penetrance between individuals carrying the same mutation. In probands with bilateral kidney agenesis or dysgenesis, and without evidence of a genetic syndrome or a family history, 9% of

TABLE 2.2   Human Gene Mutations Exhibiting Defects in Kidney Morphogenesis

Primary Disease	Gene(s)	Kidney Phenotype
Alagille syndrome	JAGGED1, NOTCH2	Cystic dysplasia
Apert syndrome	FGFR2	Hydronephrosis
Bardet-Biedl syndrome	BBS1	Cystic dysplasia
Beckwith-Wiedemann syndrome	$p57^{KIP2}$	Medullary dysplasia
Branchio-oto-renal (BOR) syndrome	EYA1, SIX1, SIX5	Unilateral or bilateral agenesis/dysplasia, hypoplasia, collecting system anomalies
Cenani-Lenz syndrome	LRP4	Agenesis, ureteropelvic junction obstruction
Campomelic dysplasia	SOX9	Dysplasia, hydronephrosis
Duane radial ray (Okihiro) syndrome	SALL4	Unilateral agenesis, VUR, malrotation, cross-fused ectopia, pelviectasis
Fraser syndrome	FRAS1, FREM2, GRIP1	Agenesis, dysplasia
Hirschsprung disease	GDNF, RET	Agenesis, hypodysplasia
Hypoparathyroidism, sensorineural deafness and renal anomalies (HDR) syndrome	GATA3	Dysplasia
Kallmann syndrome	KAL1, FGFR1, PROK2, PROK2R, SEMA3A	Agenesis
Meckel-Gruber syndrome	MKS1, MKS3, NPHP6, NPHP8	Cystic dysplasia
Nephronophthisis	CEP290, GLIS2, RPGRIP1L, NEK8, SDCCAG8, TMEM67, TTC21B	Cystic dysplasia
Okihiro syndrome	SALL4	Unilateral agenesis, VUR, malrotation, ectopia
Pallister-Hall syndrome	GLI3	Dysplasia
Prune belly syndrome	CHRM3 (reported in 1 family)	Megaureters, agenesis, hypodysplasia
Renal-coloboma syndrome	PAX2	Hypoplasia, VUR
Kidney dysplasia, isolated	DACH1, CDC5L	Dysplasia, VUR
Kidney hypoplasia, isolated	BMP4, RET, DSTYK	Hypoplasia
Renal tubular dysgenesis	RAS components	Tubular dysplasia
Kidney cysts and diabetes syndrome	HNF1B	Dysplasia, hypoplasia
Rubinstein-Taybi syndrome	CREBBP	Agenesis, hypoplasia
Simpson-Golabi-Behmel syndrome	GPC3	Medullary dysplasia
Smith-Lemli-Opitz syndrome	DHCR7	Agenesis, dysplasia
Townes-Brock syndrome	SALL1	Hypoplasia, dysplasia, VUR
VACTERL	TRAP1	VUR, duplex kidney, cystic dysplasia, agenesis
Zellweger syndrome	PEX1	VUR, cystic dysplasia

VUR, Vesicoureteral reflux.

first-degree relatives have kidney and/or lower urinary tract malformations apparent on ultrasound.

The leading genetic syndromes associated with CAKUT are trisomies 21, 18, and 13. Gene-disrupting copy number variants (CNVs) also have been found to contribute to CAKUT, particularly Chr.17q12 (renal cyst and diabetes syndrome; RCAD), Chr.22q11.2 deletion (DiGeorge/velocardiofacial syndrome), and Chr.1q21.1. The important role of rare point mutations in the pathogenesis of CAKUT is derived from analysis of large-scale cohort studies of children with recognizable nonsyndromic CAKUT, as well as syndromic disorders that are attributable to dominant mutations and that co-present with specific extrarenal manifestations (e.g., *PAX2, HNF1B, SALL1, WT1, SIX1, EYA1*). Finally, although rare, many recessive forms of CAKUT have been reported. These usually involve loss of function; for example, recessive loss-of-function mutations in *FRAS1, FREM1, FREM2,* and *GRIP1* may cause Fraser syndrome, characterized by genital anomalies, cryptophthalmos, and CAKUT.

TABLE 2.3	Clinical Indications to Evaluate for a Kidney Anomaly

History of Teratogen Exposure

ACE inhibitors and angiotensin receptor blockers

Alcohol

Alkylating agents

Illicit drugs

Radiation exposure

Trimethadione

Vitamin A congeners

Physical Examination Findings

High imperforate anus

Abnormal external genitalia

Supernumerary nipples

Preauricular pits and ear tags, cervical cysts or fistula

Hearing loss

Aniridia

Coloboma or optic disk dysplasia

Hemihypertrophy

ACE, Angiotensin-converting enzyme.

CAKUT also can be induced by environmental factors such as prenatal exposure to a variety of prescription and nonprescription drugs (Table 2.3). Angiotensin-converting enzyme inhibitors and angiotensin II receptor blockers cause a particular form of CAKUT termed *renal tubular dysgenesis* (RTD), which is a severe perinatal disorder characterized by an absence or paucity of differentiated proximal tubules, early severe oligohydramnios, and perinatal death. RTD may also be caused by mutations in the genes that encode renin, angiotensinogen, angiotensin-converting enzyme, and angiotensin II receptor type 1. Additional potential risk factors for kidney birth defects include pregestational diabetes, smoking, and binge drinking during the first trimester.

Clinical Management of Congenital Anomalies of the Kidney and Urinary Tract

Major Considerations During the Antenatal Period

CAKUT are identified in >1% of overall live births, and the sensitivity of prenatal ultrasound screening at 23 weeks' gestation is ~80%. Assessment of amniotic fluid volume is a key element of the antenatal evaluation. Fetal urine production begins at 9 weeks of gestation, and by 20 weeks, 90% of the amniotic fluid volume is generated by fetal urine production. Thus, decreased amniotic fluid volume (*oligohydramnios*) at or beyond the 20th week of gestation is a nonspecific marker of fetal kidney dysfunction;

oligohydramnios also can be associated with severe intrauterine growth restriction, urinary outflow obstruction, and premature rupture of membranes. Bilateral kidney agenesis (absence of both kidneys) is incompatible with extrauterine life because absence of amniotic fluid results in pulmonary hypoplasia, leading to severe respiratory insufficiency at birth. In the presence of a solitary kidney, oligohydramnios is typically caused by kidney dysgenesis or obstruction of urinary outflow. Poor postnatal outcome is associated with the presence of severe oligohydramnios and small, hyperechogenic kidneys. When chronic kidney failure is present at birth, mortality rates reach a striking 93% within the first year of life, and children who survive infancy have a 30-fold higher mortality as compared to age-matched children without chronic kidney failure.

Management after Birth

The postnatal clinical presentation of kidney malformations depends upon the amount of functioning kidney mass, the degree of bilateral urinary tract obstruction, and the complication of urinary tract infection. Unilateral kidney agenesis is usually accompanied by compensatory hypertrophy in the existing kidney and remains asymptomatic. Severe hypoplasia or dysplasia usually presents soon after birth with decreased kidney function that may be accompanied by oliguria or polyuria. Alternatively, patients may present with a flank mass or an asymptomatic abnormality detected by kidney imaging.

A detailed history and careful physical examination should be performed for all infants with antenatally detected CAKUT (see Table 2.3). Because sufficient volume and fluid dynamics of amniotic fluid is required for proper lung maturation, the physical examination should focus on the pulmonary system, with careful evaluation for pneumothorax associated with pulmonary hypoplasia. Examination of the abdomen may reveal an MCDK-associated mass, an obstructed kidney, or an obstructed bladder (e.g., posterior urethral valves). A single umbilical artery is associated with CAKUT, particularly VUR. An infant with prune belly syndrome, a multisystem disease of unclear genetic etiology that usually affects males, will have deficient abdominal wall musculature and undescended testes. Various frequently observed abnormalities include abnormal positioning of the anal orifice, abnormal external genitalia, periauricular pits, and coloboma.

Urine output should be carefully documented; this can be done by weighing wet diapers. Ultrasound examination of the upper and lower urinary tract should be performed within the first 24 hours of life in newborns with a history of oligohydramnios, progressive hydronephrosis, distended bladder, or bilateral severe hydroureteronephrosis on antenatal sonograms. In male infants, a distended bladder and bilateral hydroureteronephrosis may be secondary to posterior urethral valves, a condition that requires immediate intervention. Kidney ultrasound for unilateral hydronephrosis is not recommended within the first 72 hours of life because urine output gradually increases over the first 24 to 48 hours of life as renal plasma flow and glomerular filtration rate (GFR) increase. Thus, the degree of urinary tract dilatation can be underestimated during this period of transition.

Measurement of serum creatinine should be considered in the postnatal period in the setting of bilateral kidney disease or an affected solitary kidney. Because newborn serum creatinine reflects maternal levels in the first day after birth, measurement should be delayed for 24 hours. Neonatal serum creatinine declines to 0.3 to 0.5 mg/dL (27 to 44 μmol/L) within approximately 1 week in term infants and 2 to 3 weeks in preterm infants.

Clinical Approach to Specific Malformations

Fetal Echogenic Kidney

Increased echogenicity of one or both kidneys is a frequent presentation of kidney disease in the fetus. Deletions in *TCF2* are the most frequent mutations identified in the fetal echogenic kidney. Other genetic causes include autosomal-recessive and autosomal-recessive forms of polycystic kidney disease. Mutations in *TCF2* are also associated with other malformations such as kidney hypoplasia and dysplasia, MCDK, kidney agenesis, horseshoe kidney, and ureteropelvic junction obstruction (UJO). Newborns with an antenatal history of hyperechoic kidneys should be studied with a kidney ultrasound to further define the phenotype. At this point, polycystic kidney disease may be obvious. A genetic metabolic disorder may be indicated by non-renal findings. In the absence of such findings, a careful physical examination and pelvic ultrasound should be performed to rule out genital abnormalities.

Unilateral Kidney Agenesis

The estimated general incidence of unilateral kidney agenesis is 1 in ~2000 live births. One-third of these have associated CAKUT, of which vesicoureteral reflux is most frequently identified (24%). Thus, diagnosis requires ultrasound verification that a second ectopic kidney is not present (e.g., pelvis) as well as lower urinary tract evaluation. A voiding cystourethrogram (VCUG) is indicated in cases that are characterized by hydronephrosis and/or hydroureter. Management of affected patients involves determining the functional status of the existing kidney; if serum creatinine is normal, the long-term prognosis is excellent. However, various studies suggest that some patients ultimately will develop proteinuria and hypertension. Accordingly, it is reasonable to propose that individuals with a single functioning kidney should have periodic blood pressure measurement, evaluation for proteinuria, and monitoring of comorbidities including body weight.

Kidney Dysplasia

The most common form of kidney dysplasia is the *hypodysplastic kidney*, which has been observed in over 200 genetic syndromes (see Tables 2.1 and 2.2). Thought to arise from errors in branching and nephrogenesis, kidneys are small for age with reduced nephron number. The kidney parenchyma is abnormal, containing primitive tubules and interstitial fibrosis. However, large dysplastic kidneys with decreased nephron number also have been described. Cystic elements can generate a large kidney, the most extreme example being the MCDK. In addition, large dysplastic kidneys are a feature of somatic overgrowth syndromes including Beckwith-Wiedemann syndrome and Simpson-Golabi-Behmel syndrome. During the antenatal period, dysplastic kidney(s) is/are likely to be discovered as an incidental finding. After birth, bilateral kidney dysplasia is associated with a variable degree of decreased kidney function proportional to severity. Postnatal ultrasonography reveals increased echogenicity, loss of corticomedullary differentiation, and cortical cysts. Clinical follow-up involves serial measurement of kidney function. Because kidney dysplasia is associated

with lower urinary tract abnormalities including posterior urethral valves (PUV), vesicoureteral reflux (VUR), and ureteropelvic junction obstruction (UPJO), imaging of the lower urinary tract should be considered, particularly if hydronephrosis and/or hydroureter are detected.

Multicystic Dysplastic Kidney

MCDK is a severe form of kidney dysplasia that may present as a flank mass and usually occurs unilaterally. Ultrasound demonstrates an enlarged, misshapen kidney with large, randomly distributed, unconnected cysts, and compensatory hypertrophy in the contralateral kidney. A paucity of intervening solid tissue gives the appearance of a "cluster of grapes" and the kidney is nonfunctional. Bilateral MCDK gives rise to Potter syndrome, characterized by widely separated eyes with epicanthal folds, a broad nasal bridge, low-set ears, and a receding chin. Rare complications of MCDK include hypertension and urinary tract infection. Wilms tumor and renal cell carcinoma have also been described, but the incidence of malignant complications is not significantly different from the general population. Contralateral urinary tract abnormalities are detected in approximately 25% of cases and include rotational or positional anomalies, kidney hypoplasia, VUR, and UPJO. The presence of hydronephrosis or hydroureter warrants evaluation for VUR and UPJO, as well as blood pressure monitoring.

The natural history of MCDK is a progressive reduction in kidney size. In general, kidney ultrasound is recommended every 3 months for the first year of life and then every 6 months up to involution of the mass or at least up to 5 years of age. By age 2, 60% of kidneys will contract and 20% to 25% will be undetectable by ultrasound. Increase in the size of the MCDK is unusual but should prompt consideration of nephrectomy to rule out malignant transformation, especially if hypertension is present.

Kidney Ectopia

Kidney ectopia can occur when the kidney does not ascend to its normal position within the retroperitoneal fossa at the level of the second lumbar vertebra. As the kidney ascends, it rotates 90 degrees such that the kidney hilum becomes directed medially. Migration and rotation are complete by 8 weeks of gestation.

The pelvic kidney is the most common ectopic presentation. A kidney also may cross the midline, with or without fusion to the contralateral kidney, known as *crossed kidney ectopia*. The majority of patients with kidney ectopia are asymptomatic, and diagnosis is often made coincidentally during routine antenatal or postnatal ultrasound, or a pelvic mass may be palpated on physical examination. Lower urinary tract anomalies are frequently present; VUR is most common and is present in 20% of crossed kidney ectopia, 30% of simple (ipsilateral) kidney ectopia, and 70% of bilateral simple kidney ectopia. Other associated abnormalities include contralateral kidney dysplasia (4%), cryptorchidism (5%), hypospadias (5%), and uterine and vaginal agenesis, as well as adrenal, cardiac, and skeletal anomalies.

Identification of an ectopic kidney requires careful physical examination for other anomalies and monitoring of kidney function. A normal-appearing contralateral kidney with no evidence of hydronephrosis typically does not require further evaluation. Presence of a dilated collecting system should be evaluated with a VCUG to rule out associated VUR. A 99mTc–dimercaptosuccinic acid (DMSA) scan is also recommended to assess for differential kidney function, and decreased GFR or abnormal appearance indicates a need for continued follow-up. If the ectopic kidney is severely hydronephrotic and the VCUG examination is normal, then a diuretic renogram with a MAG-3 or diethylenetriaminepentaacetic acid (DTPA) scan should be performed to further assess the degree of obstruction; in the setting of mild or moderate hydronephrosis, serial ultrasound is suggested.

Kidney Fusion

Fusion is thought to occur prior to kidney ascent from the pelvis, thus kidneys are typically ectopic and supplied by anomalous vessels such as the iliac arteries. Horseshoe kidney is the most common form, in which fusion occurs at one pole of each kidney, usually the lower pole. The fused kidney may lie in the midline (symmetric), or lateral to the midline (asymmetric), and each kidney most often retains separate collecting systems and ureters. A crossed, fused ectopic kidney may occur if one kidney crosses the midline to fuse with the contralateral kidney.

Associated urogenital anomalies include ureteral duplication, ectopic ureter, retrocaval ureter, bicornuate and/or septate uterus, hypospadias, and undescended testis. Other involved organ systems include the gastrointestinal tract (anorectal malformations such as imperforate anus, malrotation, and Meckel diverticulum), the central nervous system (neural tube defects), and the skeleton (rib defects, clubfoot, or congenital hip dislocation).

Although most patients with a horseshoe kidney are asymptomatic and diagnosed incidentally, some present with pain and/or hematuria due to hydronephrosis with or without obstruction or infection. Causes of hydronephrosis include VUR, obstructive kidney calculi, UPJO, or external ureteric compression by an aberrant vessel. Infection and calculi likely are due to increased urinary stasis. Postnatal ultrasound should be performed to confirm the initial diagnosis and identify any associated urogenital abnormalities. A VCUG is indicated when it is clinically important to rule out VUR and, if obstruction is observed, serum creatinine should be measured.

Complete bibliography is available at Elsevier eBooks for Practicing Clinicians.

Key Bibliography

Abdelhak S, Kalatzis V, Heilig R, et al. A human homologue of the *Drosophila eyes absent* gene underlies Branchio-Oto-Renal (BOR) syndrome and identifies a novel gene family. *Nat Genet.* 1997;15:157–164.

Bamshad M, Lin RC, Law DJ, et al. Mutations in human TBX3 alter limb, apocrine and genital development in ulnar-mammary syndrome. *Nat Genet.* 1997;16(3):311–315.

Barbaux S, Niaudet P, Gubler M-C, et al. Donor splice-site mutations in WT1 are responsible for Frasier syndrome. *Nat Genet.* 1997;17:467–470.

Blake J, Rosenblum ND. Renal branching morphogenesis: morphogenetic and molecular mechanisms. *Semin Cell Dev Biol.* 2014;36C:2–12.

Cain JE, Di Giovanni V, Smeeton J, Rosenblum ND. Genetics of renal hypoplasia: insights into mechanisms controlling nephron endowment. *Pediatr Res.* 2010;68(2):91–98.

Cano-Gauci DF, Song HH, Yang H, et al. Glypican-3-deficient mice exhibit the overgrowth and renal abnormalities typical of the Simpson-Golabi-Behmel syndrome. *J Cell Biol.* 1999;146:255–264.

Cheng HT, Kim M, Valerius MT, et al. Notch2, but not Notch1, is required for proximal fate acquisition in the mammalian nephron. *Development.* 2007;134(4):801–811.

Franco B, Guioli S, Pragliola A, et al. A gene deleted in Kallmann's syndrome shares homology with neural cell adhesion and axonal pathfinding molecules. *Nature.* 1991;353:529–536.

Hatada I, Ohashi H, Fukushima Y, et al. An imprinted gene p57KIP2 is mutated in Beckwith Wiedemann syndrome. *Nat Genet.* 1996;14(2):171–173.

Kang S, Graham JM Jr, Olney AH, Biesecker LG. GLI3 frameshift mutations cause autosomal dominant Pallister-Hall syndrome. *Nat Genet.* 1997;15(3):266–268.

Kohlhase J, Wischermann A, Reichenbach H, Froster U, Engel W. Mutations in the SALL1 putative transcription factor gene cause Townes-Brocks syndrome. *Nat Genet.* 1998;18:81–83.

Kreidberg JA. Podocyte differentiation and glomerulogenesis. *J Am Soc Nephrol.* 2003;14(3):806–814.

Li W, Hartwig S, Rosenblum ND. Developmental origins and functions of stromal cells in the normal and diseased mammalian kidney. *Dev Dyn.* 2014;243(7):853–863.

McDonald SP, Craig JC, et al. Long-term survival of children with end-stage renal disease. *N Engl J Med.* 2004;350(26):2654–2662.

McGregor L, Makela V, Darling SM, et al. Fraser syndrome and mouse blebbed phenotype caused by mutations in FRAS1/Fras1 encoding a putative extracellular matrix protein. *Nat Genet.* 2003;34(2):203–208.

Oda T, Elkahloun AG, Pike BL, et al. Mutations in the human Jagged1 gene are responsible for Alagille syndrome. *Nat Genet.* 1997;16:235–242.

Porteous S, Torban E, Cho N-P, et al. Primary renal hypoplasia in humans and mice with PAX2 mutations: evidence of increased apoptosis in fetal kidneys of Pax2[1Neu] +/− mutant mice. *Hum Mol Genet.* 2000;9:1–11.

Sakaki-Yumoto M, Kobayashi C, Sato A, et al. The murine homolog of SALL4, a causative gene in Okihiro syndrome, is essential for embryonic stem cell proliferation, and cooperates with Sall1 in anorectal, heart, brain and kidney development. *Development.* 2006;133(15):3005–3013.

Sanna-Cherchi S, Westland R, Ghiggeri GM, et al. Genetic basis of human congenital anomalies of the kidney and urinary tract. *J Clin Invest.* 2018;128(1):4–15.

Weber S, Moriniere V, Knuppel T, et al. Prevalence of mutations in renal and developmental genes in children with renal hypodysplasia: results of the ESCAPE study. *J Am Soc Nephrol.* 2006;17(10):2864–2870.

3

Assessment of Kidney Function in Acute and Chronic Settings

LESLEY A. INKER, ANDREW S. LEVEY

Excretory function of the kidney occurs by glomerular filtration of plasma followed by selective tubular reabsorption or secretion of water and solutes to maintain homeostasis. Because glomerular filtration rate (GFR) is generally considered the best overall assessment of kidney function, this chapter focuses on GFR and its assessment, with other functions of the kidney reviewed elsewhere in the *Primer*.

Glomerular Filtration Rate

GFR is the product of the average filtration rate of each single nephron (the filtering unit of the kidneys) multiplied by the number of nephrons in both kidneys. The normal GFR level varies considerably according to age, sex, body size, physical activity, diet, pharmacologic therapy, and physiologic states such as pregnancy. For GFR to be standardized for differences in kidney size (kidney size is proportional to body size), GFR is typically indexed for body surface area, which is computed from height and weight, and then expressed per 1.73 m² surface area, which was the mean body surface area of young men and women at the time indexing was first proposed. Normal average GFR values are approximately 130 and 120 mL/min/1.73 m² for young men and women, respectively.

Reductions in GFR can be due to a decline in the nephron number or a decline in the average single-nephron GFR resulting from physiologic or hemodynamic alterations. However, a rise in single-nephron GFR due to increased filtration pressure (e.g., increased glomerular capillary pressure) or surface area (e.g., glomerular hypertrophy) can compensate for decreases in nephron number; therefore, the level of GFR may not reflect the loss of nephrons. As a result, there may be substantial kidney damage before GFR decreases.

GFR cannot be measured directly in humans; thus, "true" GFR cannot be known with certainty. However, GFR can be assessed from clearance measurements (measured GFR [mGFR]) or serum levels of endogenous filtration markers (estimated GFR [eGFR]).

Measurement of the Glomerular Filtration Rate

Classically, "measured" GFR is determined from the urinary clearance of an "ideal" filtration marker (inulin). Urinary clearance is calculated as the product of the urinary flow rate (V) and the urinary concentration (U$_x$) divided by the average plasma concentration (P$_x$) during the clearance period. Urinary excretion of a substance depends on filtration, tubular secretion, and tubular reabsorption. Substances that are filtered but neither secreted nor reabsorbed by the tubules are ideal filtration markers because their urinary clearance equals GFR. Alternative exogenous filtration markers include iothalamate, iohexol, ethylenediaminetetraacetic acid, and diethylenetriaminepentaacetic acid, which are often chelated to radioisotopes for ease of detection but may differ in their renal handling from inulin. Urinary clearance requires a timed urine collection for measurement of urine volume, and special care must be taken to avoid incomplete urine collections, which will limit the accuracy of the clearance calculation. Plasma clearance is an alternative method to measure GFR and has the advantage of avoiding the need for a timed urine collection but is also affected by extrarenal elimination. All these considerations mean that measured GFR may differ from true GFR.

Estimation of the Glomerular Filtration Rate

Because of the difficulties with measurement, GFR is often estimated with serum level endogenous filtration markers. For markers that are freely filtered, the plasma level is related to the reciprocal of the level of GFR, but the plasma level of many filtration markers is also influenced by generation, tubular secretion and reabsorption, and extrarenal elimination; these are collectively termed *non-GFR determinants* of the plasma concentration (Fig. 3.1). In the steady state, a constant plasma level is maintained because generation is equal to urinary excretion and extrarenal elimination. Estimating equations incorporate demographic and clinical variables as surrogates for the non-GFR determinants and provide a more accurate estimate of GFR than the reciprocal of the plasma concentration alone. Estimated GFR may differ from measured GFR if GFR is in the nonsteady state or if there is a discrepancy between the true and average value for the relationship of the surrogate to the non-GFR determinants of the filtration marker. Other sources of error include measurement error in the endogenous filtration marker (including failure to calibrate the assay for the filtration marker to the assay used in the development of the equation) or measurement error in GFR in developing the equation. In principle, the magnitude of all these errors is likely greater at higher measured GFR, although such errors may be more clinically significant at lower measured GFR.

Creatinine is the most commonly used endogenous filtration marker in clinical practice, and cystatin C is now recommended as

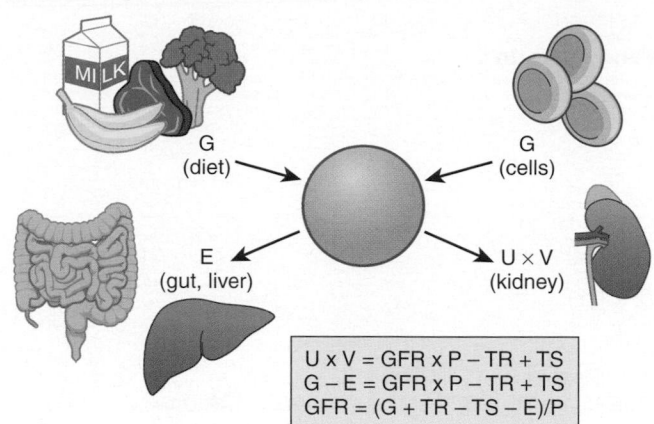

$$U \times V = GFR \times P - TR + TS$$
$$G - E = GFR \times P - TR + TS$$
$$GFR = (G + TR - TS - E)/P$$

• **Fig. 3.1** Determinants of the serum level of endogenous filtration markers. The serum level (P) of an endogenous filtration marker is determined by its generation (G) from cells and diet, extrarenal elimination (E) by gut and liver, and urinary excretion (U × V) by the kidney. Urinary excretion is the sum of filtered load (glomerular filtration rate [GFR] × P), tubular secretion (TS), minus reabsorption (TR). In the steady state, urinary excretion equals generation and extrarenal elimination. By substitution and rearrangement, GFR can be expressed as the ratio of the non-GFR determinants (G, TS, TR, and E) to the serum level. (Adapted from Stevens LA, Levey AS. Use of measured GFR as a confirmatory test. *J Am Soc Nephrol.* 2009;20:2305–2313.)

a confirmatory test and shows promise for wider use. In the past, urea was widely used. The concepts discussed later are relevant for children and adults; however, the specifics of the following discussion focus on estimating GFR in adults. Table 3.1 includes the two most commonly used GFR estimating equations for children, as well as recently developed equations that perform well in young adults (CKiD U25).

Endogenous Filtration Markers

Creatinine

Metabolism and Excretion

Creatinine, an end product of muscle catabolism, has a molecular mass of 113 Da. It is derived by the metabolism of phosphocreatine in muscle and distributed throughout extracellular fluid. Generation can be increased by creatine intake in meat or dietary supplements. Advantages of creatinine are that it is freely filtered and is easily measured at low cost. The main disadvantage of creatinine is the large number of factors other than GFR that may affect its serum level (termed *non-GFR determinants*), meaning that a given serum creatinine level may correspond to a wide range of true GFRs (see Fig. 3.1 and Table 3.2). The effect of tubular secretion and extrarenal elimination on the serum level of creatinine is greater in patients with reduced GFR. Clinically, it can be difficult to distinguish a rise in serum creatinine due to inhibition of creatinine secretion or extrarenal elimination from a decline in GFR, but these causes should be suspected if the serum level of other filtration markers remains unchanged.

Creatinine Clearance

Creatinine clearance is usually computed from the creatinine excretion in a 24-hour urine collection and a single measurement of serum creatinine in the steady state. There are expected values for creatinine excretion, and deviations from these expected values can provide some indication of errors in timing or completeness of urine collection. Creatinine clearance systematically overestimates GFR because of tubular creatinine secretion. In the nonsteady state (e.g., in acute kidney disease or between dialysis treatments), it is necessary to obtain additional blood samples during the urine collection for more accurate estimation of the average serum concentration.

Equations for Estimating Glomerular Filtration Rate from Serum Creatinine

GFR can be estimated from serum creatinine (eGFRcr) with equations that consider age, sex, race, and body size as surrogates for creatinine generation (see Table 3.1). Despite increasing accuracy of creatinine-based estimating equations over the past several years, all equations are limited by variation in non-GFR determinants of serum creatinine (see Fig. 3.1). In particular, none of these equations will perform well in patients with extreme levels of creatinine generation, such as amputees, very large or small individuals, patients with muscle-wasting conditions, or people with high or low levels of dietary meat intake (see Table 3.2). Because of differences in diet and body composition across populations and geographical regions, it is unlikely that equations developed in a single racial or ethnic group or geographic area will be accurate across multiple populations.

The Kidney Disease Improving Global Outcomes Chronic Kidney Disease (KDIGO CKD) 2013 clinical practice guidelines, as well as other guidelines and commentaries on these guidelines, concur in their recommendation for the use of the Chronic Kidney Disease Epidemiology (CKD-EPI) 2009 creatinine equation, or other equations if they have been shown to be more accurate in specific populations. In particular, this recommendation replaces prior recommendations from the KDOQI CKD 2002 clinical practice guidelines for use of the Cockcroft-Gault formula and Modification of Diet in Renal Disease (MDRD) Study equations. However, the MDRD Study equation is still used by many clinical laboratories, and the Cockcroft-Gault formula is still used by some for drug dosing (see later in this chapter).

The CKD-EPI 2009 equation was developed using a large database of participants from research studies and patients from clinical populations with diverse characteristics, including people with and without kidney disease, diabetes, and a history of organ transplantation. The equation includes age, sex, and race (grouped as people who self-identified as black or other) in addition to creatinine. The CKD-EPI equation was developed with serum creatinine assays standardized to international reference standards and GFR measured by urinary clearance of iothalamate, which overcomes limitations of the Cockcroft-Gault formula. The CKD-EPI equation uses a two-slope "spline" to model the relationship between GFR and serum creatinine, providing more accurate GFR estimates than the MDRD Study equation at higher GFRs (>60 mL/min/1.73 m²). The CKD-EPI equation is more accurate than the Cockcroft-Gault formula and MDRD Study equation across a wide range of characteristics, including age, sex, race, body mass index, and presence or absence of diabetes or history of organ transplantation. With the CKD-EPI equation, it is now reasonable to report eGFR across the entire range of values without substantial bias, and many clinical laboratories have begun to do so.

The CKD-EPI 2021 equation was developed from the same dataset used for development of the 2009 equation without inclusion of a term for Black race in response to the call

TABLE 3.1	GFR Estimating Equations Based on Serum Creatinine and Cystatin C

Creatinine-Based Equations

Cockcroft-Gault Formula

C_{cr} (mL/min) = (140 − age) × weight/72 × Scr × 0.85 [if female]

MDRD Study Equation for Use With Standardized Serum Creatinine (Four-Variable Equation)

GFR (mL/min/1.73 m²) = 175 × $S_{Cr}^{-1.154}$ × $age^{-0.203}$ × 0.742 [if female] × 1.210 [if Black]

2009 CKD-EPI Equation for Use With Standardized Serum Creatinine

GFR (mL/min/1.73 m²) = 141 × min (Scr/κ, 1)α × max(Scr/κ, 1)$^{1.209}$ × 0.993^{Age} × 1.018 [if female] × 1.157 [if Black]
where κ is 0.7 for females and 0.9 for males, α is −0.329 for females and −0.411 for males, min indicates the minimum of Scr/κ or 1, and max indicates the maximum of Scr/κ or 1

2021 CKD-EPI Equation for Use With Standardized Serum Creatinine

GFR (mL/min/1.73 m²) = 142 x min (Scr/κ,1)^{α} x max(Scr/κ,1)$^{-1.200}$ x 0.9938^{age} x 1.012 [if female]
where κ is 0.7 for females and 0.9 for males, α is -0.241 for females and -0.302 for males, min indicates the minimum of Scr/κ or 1, max indicates the maximum of Scr/κ or 1

Schwartz Formula (Younger Than 18 Years of Age)

GFR = 0.413 × ht/Scr
GFR = 40.7 × [HT/Scr]$^{0.640}$ × [30/BUN]$^{0.202}$

CKiD U25 Creatinine Equation (Pediatric and Young Adults to Age 25)

GFR = K × height/Scr
where K for males 1–11 y, 39 × $1.008^{(age − 12)}$; 12–17 y, 39 × $1.045^{(age − 12)}$; 18–25 y, 50.8;
and K for females: 1–11 y, 36.1 × $1.008^{(age − 12)}$; 12–17 y, 39 × $1.023^{(age − 12)}$; 18–25 y, 41.4

Cystatin C-Based Equations

CKiD U25 Cystatin C Equation (Pediatric and Young Adults to Age 25)

GFR = K × 1/Scys
where K for males 1–14 y, 87.2 × $1.011^{(age − 15)}$; 15–17 y, 87.2 × $0.960^{(age − 15)}$; 18–25 y, 77.1; and K for females: 1–11 y, 79.9 × $1.004^{(age − 12)}$; 12–17 y, 79.9 × $0.974^{(age − 12)}$; 18–25 y, 68.3

2012 CKD-EPI Cystatin C Equation

133 × min (Scys/0.8, 1)$^{-0.499}$ × max (Scys/0.8, 1)$^{-1.328}$ × 0.996^{Age} × 0.932 [if female]
where Scys is serum cystatin C, min indicates the minimum of Scr/κ or 1, and max indicates the maximum of Scr/κ or 1

Creatinine-Cystatin C-Based Equations

2012 CKD-EPI Creatinine-Cystatin C Equation

135 × min(Scr/κ, 1)α × max (Scr/κ, 1)$^{-0.601}$ × min (Scys/0.8, 1)$^{-0.375}$ × max (Scys/0.8, 1)$^{-0.711}$ × 0.995^{Age} × 0.969 [if female] × 1.08 [if black]
where Scr is serum creatinine, Scys is serum cystatin C, κ is 0.7 for females and 0.9 for males, α is −0.248 for females and −0.207 for males, min indicates the minimum of Scr/κ or 1, and max indicates the maximum of Scr/κ or 1

2021 CKD-EPI Creatinine-Cystatin C Equation

GFR (mL/min/1.73 m²) = 135 x min (Scr/k,1)^{α} x max (Scr/k,1)$^{-0.544}$ × min (Scys/0.8,1)$^{-0.323}$ × max (Scys/0.8,1)$^{-0.778}$ × 0.9961^{age} × 0.963 [if female]
where k is 0.7 for females and 0.9 for males, α is -0.219 for females and -0.144 for males, min indicates the minimum of Scr/κ or 1, max indicates the maximum of Scr/κ or 1

Schwartz Formula (Younger Than 18 Years of Age)

39.1 × (HT/Scr)$^{0.516}$ × (1.8/cysC)$^{0.294}$ × (30/BUN)$^{0.169}$ × (HT/1.4)$^{0.188}$ × 1.099 [if male]

to remove race from clinical algorithms in medicine. It is less accurate than the CKD-EPI 2009 equation but sufficiently accurate for use in clinical practice and more accurate than prior equations. It avoids potential for misclassification by race in a diverse population. The CKD-EPI 2021 equation is now recommended for use by the American Society of Nephrology (ASN) and the National Kidney Foundation (NKF). Other equations have been developed in selected populations. For example, the Berlin Initiative Study (BIS) developed an equation in elderly white Germans, the revised Lund-Malmö (LMR) equation was developed in Swedish adults, and the Full Age Spectrum (FAS) equation was developed in Caucasian European and North American populations. These equations are not more accurate than the CKD-EPI equation. They did not include multiple race and ethnic groups in their development, limiting their generalizability.

Cystatin C

Metabolism and Excretion

Cystatin C is a 122 amino acid protein with a molecular mass of 13 kDa. Cystatin C is generated by all cells and distributed throughout intravascular fluid. After filtration, approximately 99% of the filtered cystatin C is reabsorbed and catabolized by the proximal tubular cells. There is some evidence for the existence of tubular secretion and extrarenal elimination, which has been estimated at 15% to 21% of renal clearance.

Because cystatin C is not excreted in the urine, it is difficult to study its generation and renal handling. Thus, understanding non-GFR determinants of cystatin C other than GFR relies on epidemiologic associations. Table 3.2 describes some of the key factors thought to be related to cystatin generation. Studies indicate that cystatin C is less affected by muscle metabolism than serum creatinine; thus, serum levels of cystatin C are less affected by age, sex, race, and diet than creatinine levels. However, factors other than GFR and muscle mass should be considered when cystatin C levels are interpreted.

Equations for Estimating Glomerular Filtration Rate from Serum Cystatin C

GFR estimates based on cystatin C (eGFRcys) alone are not more accurate than creatinine-based estimating equations (eGFRcr) overall, but it may be more accurate in selected clinical settings (see Table 3.2); rather, it is the combination of the two markers (eGFRcr-cys) that generally results in the most accurate estimate in populations with and without CKD. The CKD-EPI 2012 cystatin C and creatinine-cystatin C equations (see Table 3.1) were developed with cystatin C that was measured with assays traceable to the international reference standard in a large database of subjects with diverse characteristics. KDIGO guidelines recommend use of the CKD-EPI 2012 equations if cystatin C is measured. Other equations, such as the BIS and the Caucasian, Asian, Pediatric, and Adults (CAPA) and FAS equations, were also developed with standardized cystatin C alone or in combination with creatinine, but their performance is not superior to the CKD-EPI equations. The 2021 CKD-EPI creatinine-cystatin C was developed without a term for Black race. Its use is also recommended by the ASN and NKF.

Urea

The serum urea nitrogen concentration has limited value as an index of GFR because of widely variable non-GFR determinants, primarily urea generation and tubular reabsorption. Urea, an end product of protein catabolism by the liver, has a molecular mass of 60 Da. Reduced kidney perfusion and states of antidiuresis (such as volume depletion or heart failure) are associated with increased urea reabsorption. This leads to a greater decrease in urea clearance than the concomitant decrease in GFR. When measured GFR is less than approximately 20 mL/min/1.73 m^2, the overestimation of GFR by creatinine clearance due to creatinine secretion is approximately equal to the underestimation of GFR by urea clearance due to urea reabsorption; accordingly, the average of the urea clearance and the creatinine clearance provides a reasonable approximation of the measured GFR. This average clearance can be a useful clinical tool as patients approach ESKD. Factors

TABLE 3.2   Primary Use of Estimated Glomerular Filtration Rate Using Creatinine or Cystatin C and Sources of Error in Interpretation

Primary Use	eGFRcr	eGFRcys
	Initial Test for Assessment of GFR	**Confirmatory Test for Assessment of GFR**
Nonsteady state (AKI)	Change in eGFR lags behind the change in mGFR (eGFR overestimates mGFR when mGFR is declining and underestimates mGFR when mGFR is rising)	Change in eGFR lags behind the change in mGFR (eGFR overestimates mGFR when mGFR is declining and underestimates mGFR when mGFR is rising)
Non-GFR determinants[a]	Directly measured in clinical studies	Hypothesized from clinical observations and epidemiologic studies
Factors affecting generation	Decreased by large muscle mass, high-protein diet, ingestion of cooked meat and creatine supplements Increased by small muscle mass, limb amputation, muscle-wasting diseases	Decreased in hyperthyroidism, glucocorticoid excess, and possibly obesity, inflammation, and smoking Increased in hypothyroidism
Factors affecting tubular reabsorption or secretion	Decreased by drug-induced inhibition of secretion (trimethoprim, cimetidine, fenofibrate)	NA
Factors affecting extrarenal elimination	Decreased by inhibition of gut creatininase by antibiotics Increased by dialysis, large losses of extracellular fluid (drainage of pleural fluid or ascites)	Increased by large losses of extracellular fluid (drainage of pleural fluid or ascites)
Range	Less precise at higher GFR, due to higher biological variability in non-GFR determinants relative to GFR and larger measurement error in Scr and GFR	Less precise at higher GFR, due to higher biological variability in non-GFR determinants relative to GFR, and larger measurement error in Scys and GFR
Interference with assays	Spectral interferences (bilirubin, some drugs) Chemical interferences (glucose, ketones, bilirubin, some drugs)	NA

[a]Errors in eGFRcrcys related to non-GFR determinants of creatinine or cystatin are hypothesized to be less than for eGFRcr and eGFRcys alone. Effects of factors affecting non-GFR determinants refer to effects on eGFR.

AKI, acute kidney injury; *eGFRcr,* glomerular filtration rate estimates based on serum creatinine; *eGFRcys,* glomerular filtration rate estimates based on cystatin C; *GFR,* glomerular filtration rate; *mGFR,* measured glomerular filtration rate; *Scr,* serum creatinine; *Scys,* serum cystatin C.

associated with increased generation of urea include protein loading from hyperalimentation or absorption of blood after gastrointestinal hemorrhage. Catabolic states due to infection, corticosteroid administration, or chemotherapy also increase urea generation. Decreased urea generation is seen in severe malnutrition and liver disease.

Novel Filtration Markers and Panel eGFR

Other markers are under investigation for use in estimating GFR instead of or in addition to creatinine and cystatin C. Beta-2-microglobulin (B2M) and beta trace protein (BTP) are low-molecular-weight serum proteins that undergo renal handling similar to cystatin C. The CKD-EPI recently published equations with these markers in diverse cohorts. A four-marker panel that includes age and sex but not race was as accurate as eGFRcr-cys. Another area of research investigation is discovery of novel metabolites as filtration markers using global metabolomics. A four-marker panel without creatinine, age, sex, or race was as accurate as eGFRcr-cys.

Clinical Application of Estimated Glomerular Filtration Rate

Routine Evaluation: Initial Testing With eGFRcr with Confirmation by Other Measures

Creatinine is inexpensive and widely available, and many precise assays exist. The KDIGO CKD 2013 guidelines thus recommended using eGFRcr as an initial test. However, eGFRcr, regardless of the equation, will be less accurate in people with factors affecting serum creatinine other than GFR (see Fig. 3.1). In these situations, confirmation of the eGFRcr is advised (Fig. 3.2). Confirmatory tests could include eGFRcr-cys or eGFRcys or a clearance measurement using either an exogenous filtration marker or a timed urine collection for creatinine clearance. The need for confirmatory tests is determined by the accuracy of eGFRcr in the specific clinical setting and whether clinical decision making requires a more accurate estimate than eGFRcr. Examples of how eGFRcr alone or in combination with confirmatory tests are used in clinical practice are discussed in the following sections. Concerns about the accuracy of GFR evaluation and how to best evaluate it are appropriate indications for referral to a nephrologist.

GFR Evaluation in Chronic Kidney Disease

The level of GFR is used to define and stage CKD. Thus, evaluation of GFR is necessary for the detection, evaluation, and management of CKD. In many circumstances, eGFRcr is sufficient for diagnosis, evaluation, and management. However, there are some circumstances where confirmation of eGFRcr may be helpful (see Fig. 3.2). For example, in some patients, moderate-to-severe decrease in eGFRcr (45 to 59 mL/min/1.73 m^2) may be the only indication for the diagnosis of CKD (patients without albuminuria or other markers of kidney disease). In these patients, eGFRcr-cys confirms the presence of low GFR and provides prognostic information. A recent KDIGO controversy conference on early CKD identification and intervention concluded that, for people with diabetes and hypertension or other risk conditions for CKD, yearly measurement of both creatinine and cystatin C should be performed to confirm the presence or absence of low

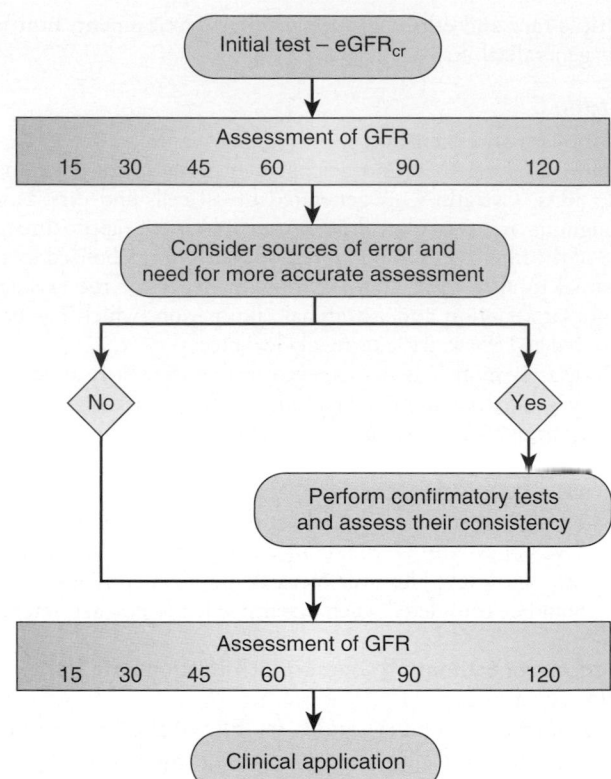

• **Fig. 3.2** An approach to the evaluation of GFR. Our approach is to use initial and confirmatory testing to develop a final assessment of true glomerular filtration rate (GFR) and to apply it in individual decision making. We would initially estimate GFR using serum creatinine level (eGFRcr) — the findings from this assessment must be interpreted in light of its limitations. Estimation of GFR based on serum cystatin C (eGFRcys), both creatinine and cystatin C (eGFRcr-cys), and measured creatinine clearance (mClcr) are useful confirmatory tests in some circumstances, and measured GFR (mGFR) is an appropriate confirmatory test, if available and performed using an accurate procedure. We recommend using the most convenient confirmatory test that will enable clinical decision making, recognizing that more than one confirmatory test might be required. Clinical application of the findings requires additional clinical information, for example, a clinical action plan based on chronic kidney disease GFR categories, drug-dosing recommendations or use in predictive instruments (Adapted from Levey AS, Coresh J, Tighiouart H, Greene T, Inker LA. Measured and estimated glomerular filtration rate: current status and future directions. *Nat Rev Nephrol.* 2020;16(1):51-64)

GFR. Confirmation of the level of GFR may be particularly helpful in deciding whether to avoid agents and medications that are toxic to the kidneys (e.g., iodinated radiocontrast, nonsteroidal antiinflammatory drugs, aminoglycoside antibiotics) or in deciding to initiate dialysis or list for transplant.

GFR Evaluation in Acute Kidney Disease

Acute kidney injury (AKI) is defined and staged according to the rate of rise in serum creatinine rather than the level of GFR. AKI is one of a number of acute kidney diseases in which GFR may be changing and serum creatinine concentrations are not in the steady state. In the nonsteady state, there is a lag before the rise in the serum marker because of the time required for retention of an endogenous filtration marker, during which eGFR is

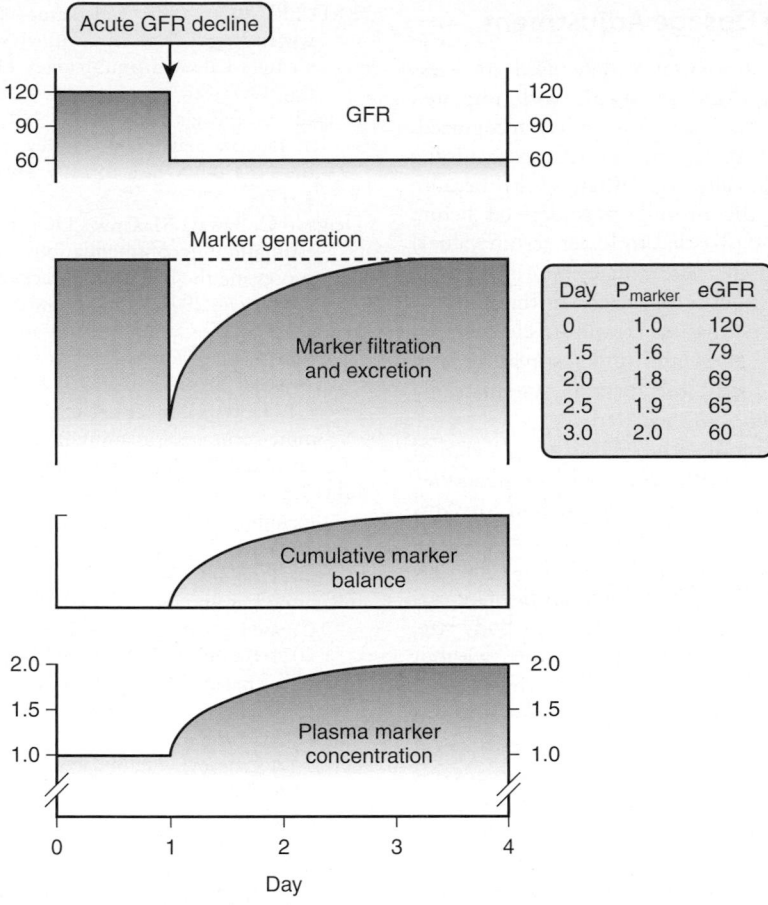

Day	P_{marker}	eGFR
0	1.0	120
1.5	1.6	79
2.0	1.8	69
2.5	1.9	65
3.0	2.0	60

• **Fig. 3.3** Effect of an acute glomerular filtration rate (GFR) decline on generation, filtration, excretion, balance, and serum level of endogenous filtration markers. After an acute GFR decline, generation of the marker is unchanged, but filtration and excretion are reduced, resulting in retention of the marker (a rising positive balance) and a rising plasma level (nonsteady state). During this time, estimated GFR (eGFR) is greater than true GFR (or measured GFR). Although true GFR remains reduced, the rise in plasma level leads to an increase in filtered load (the product of GFR times the plasma level) until filtration equals generation. At that time, cumulative balance and the plasma level plateau at a new steady state. In the new steady state, eGFR approximates true GFR (or measured GFR). GFR is expressed in units of mL/min/1.73 m^2. Tubular secretion, reabsorption, and extrarenal elimination are assumed to be zero. (Adapted from Stevens LA, Levey AS. Use of measured GFR as a confirmatory test. *J Am Soc Nephrol.* 2009;20:2305–2313.)

higher than true GFR (Fig. 3.3). Conversely, following recovery of the GFR, there is a lag before the excretion of the retained marker, during which eGFR is lower than true GFR. During this time, neither the serum level of the marker nor eGFR accurately reflects true GFR. Nonetheless, a change in eGFR in the nonsteady state can be a useful indication of the magnitude and direction of the change in true GFR. If eGFR is falling, the decline in eGFR is less than the decline in true GFR. Conversely, if eGFR is rising, the rise in eGFR is lower than the rise in true GFR. The more rapid the change in estimated GFR, the larger the change in true GFR. A kinetic equation for change in GFR is available and which allows estimation of the true GFR given the rate of change in eGFR and assumed creatinine generation rate.

Serum cystatin C increases more rapidly than serum creatinine when true GFR declines, likely because of its smaller volume of distribution. More data are required to establish whether eGFRcys is a more sensitive indicator of a rapid GFR decline than eGFRcr.

GFR Evaluation in Reduced Muscle Mass

In certain populations, such as in children, the elderly, and patients with chronic diseases (heart failure, liver failure, organ transplant recipients), neuromuscular diseases, limb amputation, or eating disorders, eGFRcys has been hypothesized to be more accurate than eGFRcr. In patients in whom eGFRcr is likely to be inaccurate because of non-GFR determinants affecting serum creatinine or interference with creatinine assays and in whom there are minimal non-GFR determinants likely affecting cystatin C, it may be preferable to rely on eGFRcys rather than eGFRcr-cys. For example, one study describes better performance of eGFRcys versus eGFRcr or eGFRcr-cys in amputees. However, the cause of large discrepancies between eGFRcr and eGFRcys has not been systematically evaluated; if greater certainty in GFR evaluation is needed, a clearance measurement should be considered.

GFR Evaluation in Drug Dosage Adjustment

The Cockcroft-Gault formula has been widely used to assess pharmacokinetic properties of drugs in people with impaired kidney function, but its limitations are now widely recognized. The Cockcroft-Gault formula was derived to estimate creatinine clearance and, hence, it systematically overestimates GFR because of creatinine secretion. Also, the formula was derived before creatinine standardization (which has led to lower serum values) and, therefore, it also systematically overestimates creatinine clearance. In addition, inclusion of a term for weight in the numerator leads to systematically overestimating creatinine clearance in patients who are edematous or obese and underestimating it in those who are thin or frail. Finally, the formula systematically underestimates creatinine clearance in the elderly.

In part because of these limitations, the KDIGO 2011 clinical update on drug dosing in patients with acute and chronic kidney diseases recommended using the most accurate method for GFR evaluation for each patient (rather than limiting the evaluation to the Cockcroft-Gault formula) and specifically mentioned consideration of eGFR as it is reported by clinical laboratories (see earlier in this chapter). Because drug dosing is based on body size, it is important to express GFR as milliliter per minute, without indexing for body surface area (BSA), for dosing adjustment based on GFR. Converting eGFR from mL/min/1.73 m^2 to mL/min requires multiplication by BSA/1.73 m^2, and the accuracy of non-BSA-indexed eGFR compared to non-BSA-indexed mGFR appears to be similar as the accuracy of BSA-indexed eGFR to BSA-indexed mGFR. The few studies that have compared the efficacy or safety outcomes associated with dosing have suggested superiority or equivalence of GFR-estimating equations to the Cockcroft-Gault formula. For drugs with potential for severe toxicity and for which excretion by the kidney is quantitatively important, it would be prudent to confirm eGFRcr by a clearance measurement.

GFR Evaluation in Kidney Donor Evaluation

US policies require mGFR or measured creatinine clearance for kidney donor evaluation, but screening is usually performed using eGFR. Current guidelines recommend decision making about donor candidacy based both on the level of GFR and the risk of kidney failure following kidney donation. We recommend a strategy for GFR evaluation that includes consideration of prior probability of measured GFR, possible errors in estimated and measured GFR, and consistency of all test results to determine the level of GFR.

Complete bibliography is available at Elsevier eBooks for Practicing Clinicians.

Key Bibliography

Bjork J, Nyman U, Larsson A, Delanaye P, Pottel H. Estimation of the glomerular filtration rate in children and young adults by means of the CKD-EPI equation with age-adjusted creatinine values. *Kidney Int.* 2021;99(4):940–947.

CKD-EPI 2020. GFR Calculator—CKD-EPI. N.p., 2020. https://www.tuftsmedicalcenter.org/Research-Clinical-Trials/Institutes-Centers-Labs/Chronic-Kidney-Disease-Epidemiology-Collaboration/Overview.

Delgado C, Baweja M, Burrows NR, et al. Reassessing the inclusion of race in diagnosing kidney diseases: an interim report from the NKF-ASN task force. *J Am Soc Nephrol.* 2021;32(6):1305–1317.

Delgado C, Baweja M, Crews DC, et al. A unifying approach for GFR estimation: recommendations of the NKF-ASN task force on reassessing the inclusion of race in diagnosing kidney disease. *Am J Kidney Dis.* 2021;S0272-6386(21)00828–3.

Fan L, Levey AS, Gudnason V, et al. Comparing GFR estimating equations using cystatin C and creatinine in elderly individuals. *J Am Soc Nephrol.* 2015;26:1982–1989.

Freed TA, Coresh J, Inker LA, et al. Validation of a metabolite panel for a more accurate estimation of glomerular filtration rate using quantitative LC-MS/MS. *Clin Chem.* 2019;65(3):406–418.

Inker LA, Couture SJ, Tighiouart H, et al. A new panel estimated GFR, including B(2)-microglobulin and B-Trace protein and not including race, developed in a diverse population. *Am J Kidney Dis.* 2021;77(5):673–683.

Inker LA, Eneanya ND, Coresh J, et al. New creatinine- and cystatin C-based equations to estimate GFR without race. *N Engl J Med.* 2021;10.1056/NEJMoa2102953.

Inker LA, Titan S. Measurement and estimation of GFR for use in clinical practice: Core Curriculum 2021. *Am J Kidney Dis.* 2021;S0272-6386(21)00707–1.

Levey AS, Coresh J, Tighiouart H, Greene T, Inker LA. Measured and estimated glomerular filtration rate: current status and future directions. *Nat Rev Nephrol.* 2020;16(1):51–64.

Levin A, Stevens PE, Bilous RW, et al. Kidney disease: improving global outcomes (KDIGO) CKD work group. KDIGO 2012 clinical practice guideline for the evaluation and management of chronic kidney disease. *Kidney Int.* 2013;3:1–150.

Liu X, Foster MC, Tighiouart H, et al. Non-GFR determinants of low-molecular-weight serum protein filtration markers in CKD. *Am J Kidney Dis.* 2016;68:892–900.

Pierce CB, Munoz A, Ng DK, Warady BA, Furth SL, Schwartz GJ. Age- and sex-dependent clinical equations to estimate glomerular filtration rates in children and young adults with chronic kidney disease. *Kidney Int.* 2021;99(4):948–956.

Pottel H, Bjork J, Courbebaisse M, et al. Development and validation of a modified full age spectrum creatinine-based equation to estimate glomerular filtration rate: a cross-sectional analysis of pooled data. *Ann Intern Med.* 2021;174:183–191.

Powe NR. Black kidney function matters: use or misuse of race? *JAMA.* 2020;324:737–738.

Schwartz GJ, Schneider MF, Maier PS, et al. Improved equations estimating GFR in children with chronic kidney disease using an immunonephelometric determination of cystatin C. *Kidney Int.* 2012;82(4):445–453. doi:10.1038/ki.2012.169.

Soveri I, Berg UB, Bjork J, et al. Measuring GFR: a systematic review. *Am J Kidney Dis.* 2014;64(3):411–424.

Stevens LA, Coresh J, Greene T, Levey AS. Assessing kidney function—measured and estimated glomerular filtration rate. *N Engl J Med.* 2006;354:2473–2483.

Titan S, Miao S, Tighiouart H, et al. Performance of indexed and nonindexed estimated GFR. *Am J Kidney Dis.* 2020;76:446–449.

4

Urinalysis and Urine Microscopy

ARTHUR GREENBERG

The relatively simple chemical tests performed during routine urinalysis rapidly provide important information about a number of primary kidney and systemic disorders. The microscopic examination of the urine sediment is an indispensable part of the evaluation of patients with reduced glomerular filtration, proteinuria, hematuria, urinary tract infection, or nephrolithiasis, and the urine sediment provides valuable clues about the kidney parenchyma.

Urine dipstick tests can be readily automated, and most high-throughput clinical laboratories rely on computerized optical scanning or flow cytometry with automated instruments to perform microscopic urinalyses. Red blood cells (RBCs) and white blood cells (WBCs) can be counted with precision, and reasonable results are obtainable for squamous epithelial cells. However, these methods cannot reliably identify important elements such as renal tubular epithelial cells, oval fat bodies, crystals, or casts. Their accuracy for detection even of RBCs and WBCs decreases with specimen aging, and sensitivity is reduced within as little as 2 hours after voiding. The interval between collection of a "routine" urine specimen, delivery to the lab, and processing may vary considerably.

When a primary kidney disorder is suspected, the automated urinalysis should be regarded only as a screening test. It does not supplant careful examination under the microscope of a specimen picked up promptly at the bedside, spun down, and examined at once. This task of careful review of the urine under the microscope must not be delegated; it should be performed personally by specialists experienced in examining the urine. Studies show both that a urinalysis performed by a nephrologist is more likely to aid in reaching a correct diagnosis than a urinalysis reported by a clinical chemistry laboratory and that urinalyses performed by physicians without special training are more often inaccurate. The features of a complete urinalysis are listed in Box 4.1.

Specimen Collection and Handling

Urine should be collected with a minimum of contamination. A clean-catch midstream sample is preferred. If this is not feasible, bladder catheterization is appropriate in adults; the risk of inducing a urinary tract infection with a single in-and-out catheterization is negligible. Suprapubic aspiration is used in infants. In the uncooperative male patient, a clean, freshly applied condom catheter and urinary collection bag may be used. Urine in the collection bag of a patient with an indwelling bladder catheter is subject to stasis, but a sample suitable for examination may be collected by withdrawing urine from above a clamp placed on the tube that connects the catheter to the drainage bag.

The chemical composition of the urine changes with standing, and the formed elements within a urine sample degenerate over time. The urine is best examined when fresh. A brief period of refrigeration is acceptable but risks precipitation of crystals. Because bacteria multiply at room temperature, bacterial counts from unrefrigerated urine are unreliable. High urine osmolality and low pH favor cellular preservation, and these two characteristics of the first-voided morning urine give it particular value in cases of suspected glomerulonephritis. Some experts favor use of the second morning urine to avoid effects of overnight bladder stasis. However, the most important goal is examination without delay, irrespective of what specimen is used.

Physical and Chemical Properties of the Urine

Appearance and Odor

Normal urine is clear with a faint yellow tinge due to the presence of urochrome. As the urine becomes more concentrated, its color deepens. Bilirubin, other pathologic metabolites, and a variety of drugs may discolor the urine or change its smell. Suspended erythrocytes, leukocytes, or crystals may render the urine turbid. Conditions associated with a change in the appearance or odor of the urine are listed in Table 4.1.

Specific Gravity

The specific gravity of any fluid is the ratio of that fluid's weight to the weight of an equal volume of distilled water. The urine specific gravity is a conveniently determined but inaccurate surrogate for osmolality. Specific gravities of 1.001 to 1.035 correspond to an osmolality range of 50 to 1000 mOsm/kg. A specific gravity near 1.010 connotes isosthenuria, with a urine osmolality matching that of plasma. Relative to osmolality, the specific gravity is elevated when dense solutes, such as protein, glucose, or radiographic contrast agents, are present.

Three methods are available for specific gravity measurement. The hydrometer is the reference standard but requires both a sufficient volume of urine to allow flotation of the hydrometer and equilibration of the specimen to the calibrated temperature. The second method is based on the well-characterized relationship between urine specific gravity and refractive index. Refractometers calibrated in specific gravity units are commercially available and require only a drop of urine. Finally, the specific gravity may also be estimated by dipstick.

BOX 4.1

Routine Urinalysis

Appearance and Odor
Specific Gravity
Chemical Tests (Dipstick)

pH
Protein
Glucose
Ketones
Blood
Urobilinogen
Bilirubin
Nitrites
Leukocyte esterase

Microscopic Examination (Formed Elements)

Crystals: urate; calcium phosphate, oxalate, or carbonate; triple
    phosphate; cystine; drugs
Cells: leukocytes, erythrocytes, renal tubular cells, oval fat bodies,
    transitional epithelium, squamous cells
Casts: hyaline, granular, red blood cell, white blood cell, tubular cell,
    degenerating cellular, broad, waxy, lipid laden
Infecting organisms: bacteria, yeast, *Trichomonas,* nematodes
Miscellaneous: spermatozoa, mucous threads, fibers, starch, hair, and
    other contaminants

The specific gravity is used to determine whether the urine is concentrated. During a solute diuresis accompanying hyperglycemia, diuretic therapy, or relief of obstruction, the urine is isosthenuric. In contrast, with a water diuresis caused by overhydration or diabetes insipidus, the specific gravity is typically 1.004 or lower. In the absence of proteinuria, glycosuria, or iodinated contrast administration, a specific gravity of more than 1.018 implies preserved concentrating ability. Iodinated radiographic contrast is very dense, and if the specific gravity is supraphysiologic (i.e., >1.035), one should suspect that contrast is responsible. Measurement of specific gravity is useful in differentiating between prerenal azotemia and acute tubular necrosis (ATN) and in assessing the significance of proteinuria observed in a random voided urine sample. Because the protein indicator strip responds to the concentration of protein, the significance of a borderline reading depends on the overall urine concentration.

Routine Dipstick Methodology

The urine dipstick is a plastic strip to which absorbent tabs impregnated with chemical reagents have been affixed. The reagents in each tab are chromogenic. After timed development, the color is compared with a chart or read by a colorimetric instrument. Some reactions are highly specific. Others are affected by the presence of interfering substances or extremes of pH. Discoloration of the urine with bilirubin or blood may obscure the color changes.

pH

Test pads for pH use indicator dyes that change color with pH. The physiologic urine pH ranges from 4.5 to 8. The determination is most accurate if performed promptly because growth of

TABLE 4.1 Selected Substances That May Alter the Physical Appearance or Odor of the Urine

Color Change	Substances
White	Chyle, pus, calcium phosphate crystals, triple phosphate (struvite) crystals, propofol
Pink/red/brown	Erythrocytes, hemoglobin, myoglobin, porphyrins, beets, blackberries, senna, cascara, levodopa, methyldopa, deferoxamine, phenolphthalein and congeners, food colorings, metronidazole, phenacetin, anthraquinones, doxorubicin, phenothiazines, propofol, triple phosphate (struvite) crystals (salmon colored)
Yellow/orange/brown	Bilirubin, urobilin, phenazopyridine urinary analgesics, senna, cascara, mepacrine, iron compounds, nitrofurantoin, riboflavin, rhubarb, sulfasalazine, rifampin, fluorescein, phenytoin, metronidazole
Brown/black	Methemoglobin, homogentisic acid (alcaptonuria), melanin (melanoma), levodopa, methyldopa
Blue or green, green/brown	Biliverdin, *Pseudomonas* infection, dyes (methylene blue and indigo carmine), triamterene, vitamin B complex, methocarbamol, indican, phenol, chlorophyll, propofol, amitriptyline, triamterene
Purple staining of indwelling plastic urine collection devices	Infection with *Escherichia coli, Pseudomonas, Enterococcus,* others

Odor	Substance or Condition
Sweet or fruity	Ketones
Ammoniac	Urea-splitting bacterial infection
Fetid, pungent	Asparagus (sulfurous breakdown products)
Maple syrup	Maple syrup urine disease
Musty or mousy	Phenylketonuria
"Sweaty feet"	Isovaleric or glutaric acidemia, or excess butyric or hexanoic acid
Rancid	Hypermethioninemia, tyrosinemia

urea-splitting bacteria and loss of dissolved carbon dioxide raise the pH. In addition, bacterial metabolism of glucose may produce organic acids that lower pH. These strips are not sufficiently accurate to be used for the diagnosis of renal tubular acidosis. A specimen collected anaerobically under mineral oil should be promptly assayed with a pH electrode when precision is required.

Protein

Protein measurement uses the protein-error-of-indicators principle. The pH at which some indicators change color varies with the protein concentration of the bathing solution. Protein indicator strips are buffered at an acid pH near their color change point. Wetting them with a protein-containing specimen induces a color change. The protein reaction may be scored from trace to 4+ or by protein concentration. Their equivalence is approximately as follows:

Trace	5–20 mg/dL
1+	30 mg/dL
2+	100 mg/dL
3+	300 mg/dL
4+	>2000 mg/dL

Highly alkaline urine, especially after contamination with quaternary ammonium skin cleansers or from patients who abuse sodium bicarbonate, may produce false-positive reactions by overwhelming the pH buffer of the chromogenic tab.

Protein strips are highly sensitive to albumin but less so to globulins, hemoglobin, or light chains. If light chain proteinuria is suspected, assays that are more sensitive should be used. With acid precipitation tests, an acid that denatures protein (i.e., sulfosalicylic acid) is added to the urine specimen, and the density of the precipitate is related to the protein concentration. Urine that is negative by dipstick but positive by sulfosalicylic acid precipitation is highly suspicious for the presence of light chains. Tolbutamide, high-dose penicillin, sulfonamides, and radiographic contrast agents may yield false-positive turbidimetric reactions. More sensitive and specific tests for light chains, such as immunoelectrophoresis or immunonephelometry, are preferred and necessary for confirmation and more definitive diagnosis.

If the urine is very concentrated, the presence of a modest protein reaction is less likely to correspond to significant proteinuria in a 24-hour collection or when assessed by spot urine protein-to-creatinine ratio. Even so, it is unlikely that a 3+ or 4+ reaction would be seen solely because of a high urine concentration or, conversely, that the urine would be dilute enough to yield a negative reaction despite significant proteinuria. The protein indicator used for routine dipstick analysis is neither sufficiently sensitive nor specific for albuminuria in the moderately increased (30 to 299 mg/g) or high normal range (10 to 29 mg/g).

Blood

Reagent strips for blood rely on the peroxidase activity of hemoglobin to catalyze an organic peroxide with subsequent oxidation of an indicator dye. Free hemoglobin produces a homogeneous color. Intact red cells cause punctate staining if present only in a small quantity. False-positive reactions occur if the urine is contaminated with other oxidants, such as povidone-iodine, hypochlorite, or bacterial peroxidase. Ascorbate yields false-negative results. Myoglobin is also detected because it has intrinsic peroxidase activity. A urine sample that is positive for blood by dipstick analysis but shows no red cells on microscopic examination is suspect for myoglobinuria or hemoglobinuria. A specific assay for urine myoglobin can be used to confirm the diagnosis, if required.

Specific Gravity

Specific gravity reagent strips measure ionic strength using indicator dyes with ionic strength-dependent dissociation constants (pKa). They do not detect glucose or nonionic radiographic contrast agents.

Glucose

Dipstick reagent strips are specific for glucose, relying on glucose oxidase to catalyze the formation of hydrogen peroxide, which then reacts with peroxidase and a chromogen to produce a color change. High concentrations of ascorbate or ketoacids reduce test sensitivity; however, the degree of glycosuria occurring in diabetic ketoacidosis is sufficient to prevent false-negative results despite ketonuria.

Ketones

Ketone reagent strips depend on the development of a purple color after acetoacetate reacts with nitroprusside. Some strips can also detect acetone, but none react with β-hydroxybutyrate. False-positive results may occur in patients who are taking levodopa or drugs such as captopril or mesna that contain free sulfhydryl groups.

Urobilinogen

Urobilinogen is a colorless pigment produced in the gut from the metabolism of bilirubin. Some is excreted in feces and the rest is reabsorbed and excreted in the urine. In obstructive jaundice, bilirubin does not reach the bowel and urinary excretion of urobilinogen is diminished. In other forms of jaundice, urobilinogen is increased. The urobilinogen test is based on the Ehrlich reaction in which diethylaminobenzaldehyde reacts with urobilinogen in acid medium to produce a pink color. Sulfonamides may produce false-positive results and degradation of urobilinogen to urobilin may yield false-negative results. Better tests are available to diagnose obstructive jaundice.

Bilirubin

Bilirubin reagent strips rely on the chromogenic reaction of bilirubin with diazonium salts. Conjugated bilirubin is not normally present in the urine. False-positive results may be observed in patients receiving chlorpromazine or phenazopyridine. False-negative results occur in the presence of ascorbate.

Nitrite

The nitrite screening test for bacteriuria relies on the ability of gram-negative bacteria to convert urinary nitrate to nitrite, which activates a chromogen. False-negative results occur with infection with enterococcus or other organisms that do not produce nitrite, when ascorbate is present, or when urine has not been retained in the bladder long enough (approximately 4 hours) to permit sufficient production of nitrite from nitrate.

Leukocyte Esterase

Granulocyte esterases can cleave pyrrole amino acid esters, producing free pyrrole that subsequently reacts with a chromogen. The test threshold is 5 to 15 WBCs per high-power field (WBCs/HPF). False-negative results occur with glycosuria, high specific gravity, ascorbate, phenazopyridine, some antibiotics, or excessive oxalate excretion. Contamination with vaginal material may yield a positive test result without true urinary tract infection.

Albumin Dipsticks

Albumin-selective dipsticks are available for screening for moderately elevated albuminuria in the range of 30 to 299 μ/mg creatinine. The most accurate screening occurs when first morning specimens are examined as exercise can increase albumin excretion. One type of dipstick uses colorimetric detection of albumin bound to gold-conjugated antibody. Normally, the urine albumin concentration is less than the 20 μg/L detection threshold for these strips. Unless the urine is very dilute, a patient with no detectable albumin by this method is unlikely to have elevated albumin excretion. However, because urine concentration varies widely, this assay has the same limitations as any test that only measures concentration. It is useful only as a screening test, and more formal testing is required if albuminuria is detected.

A second type of dipstick has tabs for measurement of both albumin and creatinine concentration, permitting estimation of the albumin-to-creatinine ratio. In contrast to the other dipstick tests described in this chapter, these strips cannot be read by simple visual comparison with a color chart. An instrument is required, but this system is suitable for point-of-care testing. When present on more than one determination, an albumin-to-creatinine ratio of 30 to 300 mg/g signifies moderately increased albuminuria. Details on the interpretation of urine albumin concentration are provided in Chapters 5 and 26.

Microscopic Examination of the Spun Urinary Sediment

Specimen Preparation and Viewing

The contents of the urine are reported as the number of cells or casts per HPF ($\times$ 400) after resuspension of the centrifuged pellet in a small volume of urine. The accuracy and reproducibility of this semiquantitative method depend on using the correct volume of urine. Twelve milliliters of urine should be spun in a conical centrifuge tube for 5 minutes at 1500 to 2000 rpm (450 g). After centrifugation, the tube is inverted and drained. The pellet is resuspended in the few drops of urine that remain in the tube after inversion by flicking the base of the tube gently with a finger or with the use of a pipette. Care should be taken to suspend the pellet fully without excessive agitation.

A drop of urine is poured or transferred by pipette onto a microscope slide. The drop should be of sufficient size that a standard 22 $\times$ 22-mm coverslip just floats on the urine with a thin rim of urine at the edges. If too little is used, the specimen rapidly dries. If an excess of urine is applied, it will spill onto the microscope objective or stream distractingly under the coverslip. Commercial urine stains or the Papanicolaou stain may be used to enhance detail. Most nephrologists prefer the convenience of viewing unstained urine. Subdued light is necessary. When conventional microscopy is used, the condenser and diaphragm are adjusted to maximize contrast and definition. When the urine is dilute and few formed elements are present, detection of motion of objects suspended in the urine ensures that the focal plane is correct. One should scan the urine at low power ($\times$ 100) to obtain a general impression of its contents before moving to high power ($\times$ 400) to look at individual fields and identify specific elements. It is useful to scan large areas at low power and then move to high power when an item of interest is located. Cellular elements should be quantitated by counting or estimating the number in at least 10 representative HPFs. Casts may be quantitated by counting the number per low-power field, although most observers use less-specific terms, such as *rare, occasional, few, frequent,* and *numerous.*

Cellular Elements

The principal formed elements of the urine are listed (see Box 4.1). The figures in this chapter constitute an atlas of selected formed elements.

Erythrocytes

RBCs (Fig. 4.1A and B) may find their way into the urine from any source between the glomerulus and urethral meatus. The presence of more than two to three erythrocytes per HPF is considered pathologic. Erythrocytes are biconcave disks 7 μm in diameter. They become crenated in hypertonic urine. In hypotonic urine, they swell or burst, leaving ghosts. Erythrocytes originating in the renal parenchyma are dysmorphic, with spicules or blebs (acanthocytes), submembrane cytoplasmic precipitation, membrane folding, and vesicles. Those originating in the collecting system retain their uniform shape. Studies suggest good separation between urologic and intrarenal pathology when phase contrast microscopy is used by experienced observers. In one study, up to 85% of patients with nondysmorphic microscopic hematuria had a urologic disorder, whereas 87.5% of those with dysmorphic hematuria had glomerular disease. Cutoff points for deciding that hematuria is dysmorphic depend on the method used. The number of dysmorphic RBCs as a fraction of total RBCs required to reach the threshold for deciding if hematuria is dysmorphic is lower for conventional than phase contrast microscopy. The presence of proteinuria by dipstick may corroborate the presence of glomerular kidney disease, and the combination of hematuria with proteinuria predicts glomerular disease with high specificity. Of course, many glomerular and tubular disorders do not cause proteinuria and many glomerular diseases do not cause hematuria. Studies comparing urinalysis results to kidney biopsy findings disclose that sensitivity of dysmorphic hematuria as a predictor of glomerular disease is low when non-proliferative forms of glomerular disease are included.

Leukocytes

Polymorphonuclear leukocytes (PMNs) (see Fig. 4.1C) are approximately 12 μm in diameter and are most readily recognized in a fresh urine sample before their multilobed nuclei or granules have degenerated. Swollen PMNs with prominent granules displaying Brownian motion are termed *glitter* cells. PMNs may indicate urinary tract inflammation, intraparenchymal diseases such as glomerulonephritis or interstitial nephritis, or upper or lower urinary tract infection. Periureteral inflammation, as in regional ileitis or acute appendicitis, may also cause pyuria.

Renal Tubular Epithelial Cells

Tubular cells (see Fig. 4.1D) are larger than PMNs, ranging from 12 to 20 μm in diameter. Proximal tubular cells are oval or egg shaped and tend to be larger than the cuboidal distal tubular cells. However, because size varies with urine osmolality, these cells cannot be reliably differentiated. In hypotonic urine, it may be difficult to distinguish tubular cells from swollen PMNs. A few tubular cells may be seen in a normal urine sample. More commonly, these cells indicate tubular injury or inflammation from ATN or interstitial nephritis.

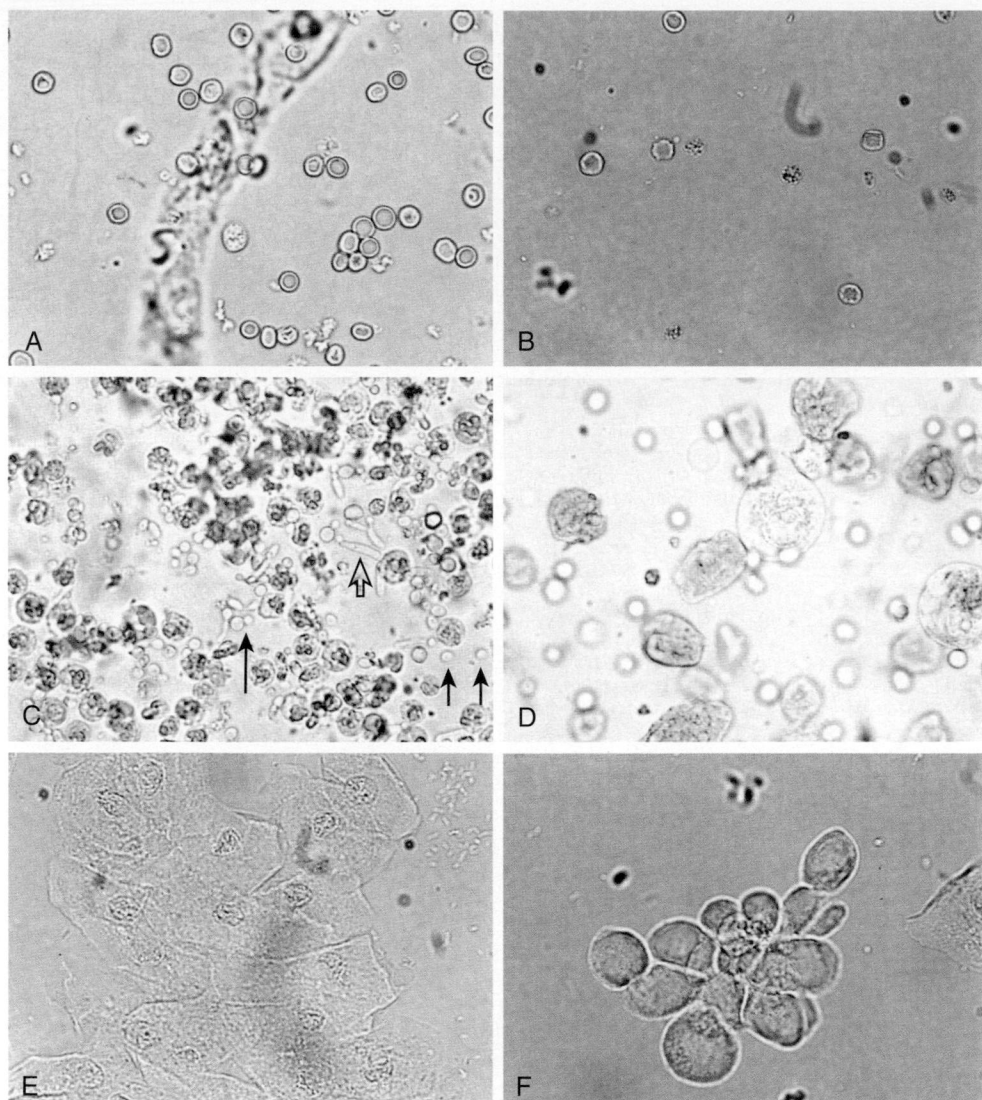

• **Fig. 4.1** Cellular elements in the urine. In this and subsequent figures, all photographs were made from unstained sediments and photographed at ×400 original magnification. (A) Nondysmorphic red blood cells (RBCs). They appear as uniform, biconcave disks. (B) Dysmorphic RBCs from a patient with immunoglobulin A nephropathy. Their shape is irregular, with membrane blebs and spicules. (C) Urine obtained from a patient with an indwelling bladder catheter. Innumerable white blood cells as well as individual *(small arrows)*, budding *(single thick arrow)*, and hyphal *(open arrow)* fungal forms are present. (D) Renal tubular epithelial cells. Note the variability of shape. The erythrocytes in the background are much smaller. (E) Squamous epithelial cells. (F) Transitional epithelial cells in a characteristic clump.

Other Cells

Squamous cells (see Fig. 4.1E) of urethral, vaginal, or cutaneous origin are large, flat cells with small nuclei. Transitional epithelial cells (see Fig. 4.1F) line the renal pelvis, ureter, bladder, and proximal urethra. They are rounded cells, several times the size of leukocytes, and often occur in clumps. In hypotonic urine, they may be confused with swollen tubular epithelial cells.

Casts and Other Formed Elements

Based on their shape and origin, casts are appropriately named. Immunofluorescence studies demonstrate that they consist of a matrix of Tamm-Horsfall urinary glycoprotein (uromodulin)

in the shape of the distal tubular or collecting duct segment where they were formed. The matrix has a straight margin that is helpful in differentiating casts from clumps of cells or debris. Use of phase contrast microscopy facilitates identification of casts.

Hyaline Casts

Hyaline casts (Fig. 4.2A) consist of protein alone. Because their refractive index is close to that of urine, they may be difficult to see with conventional microscopy, requiring subdued light and careful manipulation of the iris diaphragm to increase diffraction and visual contrast. Hyaline casts are nonspecific. They occur in concentrated urine from healthy individuals, as well as in numerous pathologic conditions.

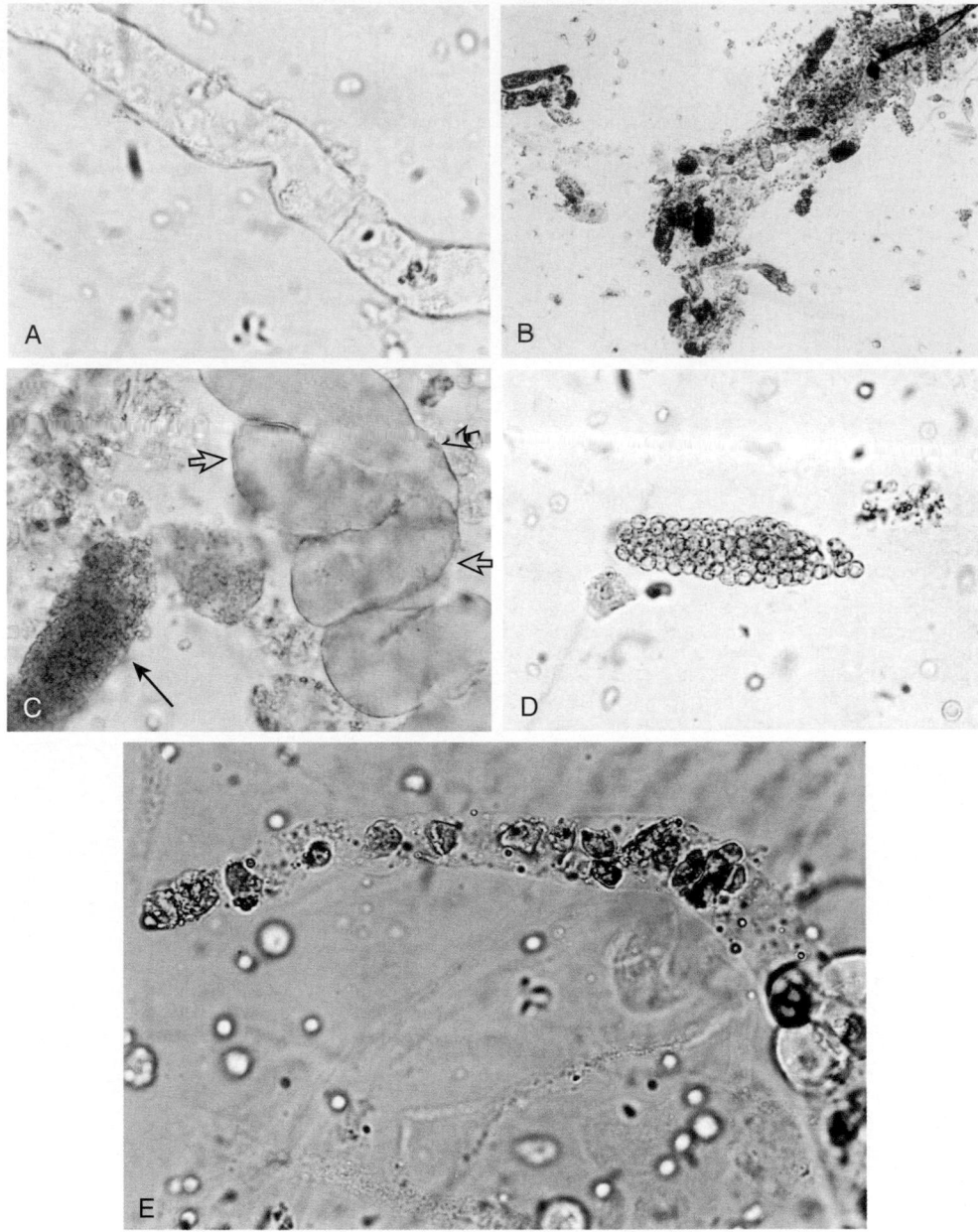

• **Fig. 4.2** Casts. All images photographed at an original magnification ×100. (A) Hyaline cast. (B) Muddy brown granular casts and amorphous debris from a patient with acute tubular necrosis. (C) Waxy cast *(open arrows)* and granular cast *(solid arrow)* from a patient with lupus nephritis and a telescoped sediment. Note background hematuria. (D) Red blood cell cast. Background hematuria is also present. (E) Tubular cell cast. Note the hyaline cast matrix.

Granular Casts

Granular casts (see Fig. 4.2B) consist of finely or coarsely granular material. Immunofluorescence studies show that the fine granules are derived from altered proteins. Coarse granules may result from degeneration of embedded cells. Granular casts are nonspecific but usually pathologic. They may be seen after exercise or with simple volume depletion and as a finding in ATN, glomerulonephritis, or tubulointerstitial disease.

Waxy Casts

Waxy casts, or broad casts (see Fig. 4.2C), are made of hyaline material with a much greater refractive index than hyaline casts—hence, their description as waxy. They behave as though they are more brittle than hyaline casts and they frequently have fissures along their edges. In a systematic review, waxy casts were more common in postinfectious glomerulonephritis, amyloidosis, and individuals with reduced kidney function of either short or long duration. They are rare in membranous nephropathy and focal segmental glomerulopathy. Broad casts form in tubules that have become dilated and atrophic and, from their presence, one can infer that the patient has chronic parenchymal disease.

Red Blood Cell Casts

RBC casts indicate intraparenchymal bleeding. The hallmark of glomerulonephritis, they are seen less frequently with tubulointerstitial disease, including allergic interstitial nephritis and with anticoagulant (warfarin)-induced acute kidney injury (AKI). RBC casts have been described along with hematuria in healthy

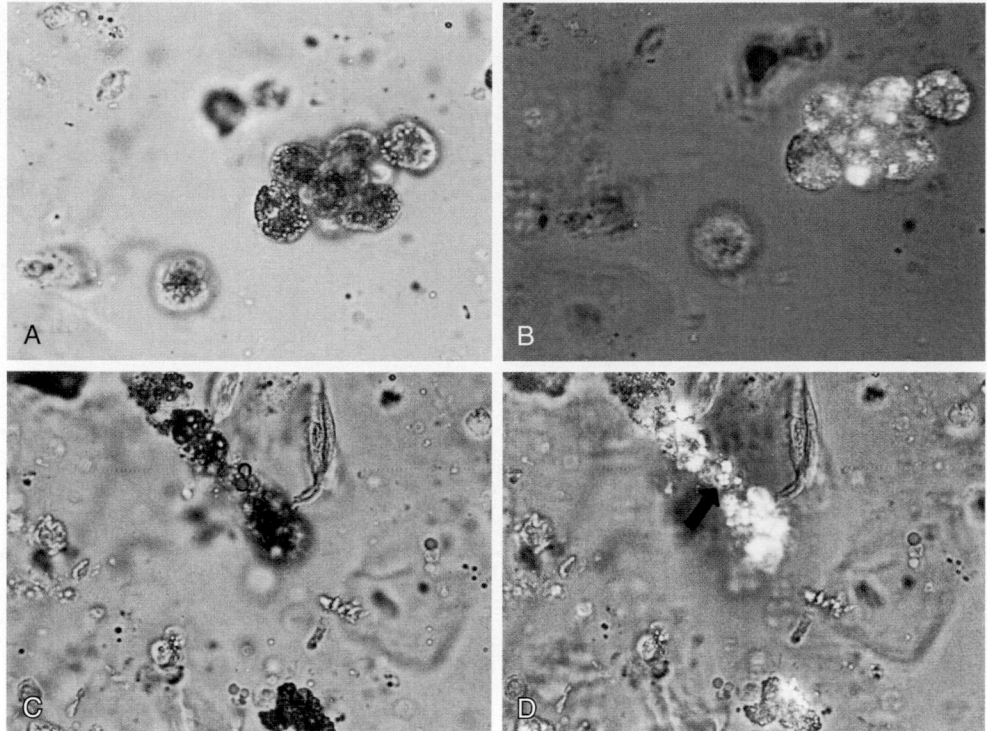

• **Fig. 4.3** Lipid. (A) Oval fat bodies, as seen by bright-field illumination. (B) Same field as in (A) viewed under polarized light. (C) Lipid-laden cast, bright-field illumination. (D) Same field as in (C) viewed under polarized light. Arrow points to characteristic Maltese cross.

individuals after exercise. Fresh RBC casts (see Fig. 4.2D) retain their brown pigment and consist of readily discernible erythrocytes in a tubular cast matrix. Over time, the heme color is lost, along with the distinct cellular outline. With further degeneration, RBC casts are difficult to distinguish from coarsely granular casts. RBC casts may be diagnosed by the company they keep; they appear in a background of hematuria with dysmorphic red cells, granular casts, and proteinuria. Occasionally, the evidence for intraparenchymal bleeding is a hyaline cast with embedded red cells. These have the same pathophysiologic implication as RBC casts. When only a few RBCs are noted as part of a cast, it is important to focus up and down on the cast to ensure that the RBCs are actually within the cast rather than merely adherent to its surface.

White Blood Cell Casts

WBC casts consist of WBCs in a protein matrix. They are characteristic of interstitial inflammation and are useful in distinguishing pyelonephritis from lower urinary tract infection. They may also be seen with interstitial nephritis and other tubulointerstitial disorders.

Tubular Cell Casts

Tubular cell casts (see Fig. 4.2E) can consist either of a few tubular cells in a hyaline matrix or a dense agglomeration of sloughed tubular cells. They occur in concentrated urine but are more characteristically seen with the sloughing of tubular cells that occurs early in the course of ATN.

Bacteria, Yeast, and Other Infectious Agents

Bacillary or coccal forms of bacteria may be discerned even on an unstained urine sample. Examination of a Gram stain preparation of unspun urine allows estimation of the bacterial count.

One organism per HPF of unspun urine corresponds to 20,000 organisms per cubic millimeter. Budding yeasts and hyphal forms occur with *Candida* infection or colonization. *Candida* organisms are similar in size to erythrocytes, but have a greenish hue and are not biconcave disks. When budding forms or hyphae are present, yeast is obvious (see Fig. 4.1C). *Trichomonas* organisms are identified by their teardrop shape and motile flagellum.

Lipiduria

In the nephrotic syndrome with lipiduria, tubular cells reabsorb luminal fat. Sloughed tubular cells containing fat droplets are called *oval fat bodies*. Fatty casts contain lipid-laden tubular cells or free lipid droplets. By light microscopy, lipid droplets appear round and clear with a green tinge. Cholesterol esters are anisotropic, and cholesterol-containing droplets rotate polarized light to produce a "Maltese cross" appearance. Triglycerides appear similar by light microscopy but are isotropic. Crystals, starch granules, mineral oil, and other urinary contaminants are also anisotropic. Before concluding that anisotropic structures are lipid, the observer must compare polarized and bright-field views of the same object (Fig. 4.3).

Crystals

Crystals may be present spontaneously or may precipitate with refrigeration of a specimen. They can be difficult to type because they have similar shapes; the common urinary crystals are described in Table 4.2. The pH is an important clue to identity because the solubility of many urinary constituents is pH dependent. The three most distinctive crystal forms are cystine, calcium oxalate, and magnesium ammonium (triple) phosphate. Cystine

TABLE 4.2 Common Naturally Occurring Urinary Crystals

Description	Composition	Comment
Crystals Found in Acid Urine		
Amorphous	Uric acid Sodium urate	Cannot be distinguished from amorphous phosphates except by urine pH; may be orange tinted by urochrome
Rhomboid prisms	Uric acid	—
Rosettes	Uric acid	—
Bipyramidal	Calcium oxalate	Also termed *envelope shaped*
Dumbbell shaped	Calcium oxalate	—
Needles	Uric acid	—
Hexagonal plates	Cystine	Presence may be confirmed with nitroprusside test
Crystals Found in Alkaline Urine		
Amorphous	Phosphates	Indistinguishable from urates except by pH
"Coffin lid" (beveled rectangular prisms)	Magnesium ammonium (triple) phosphate	Seen with urea-splitting infection and bacteriuria
Granular masses or dumbbells	Calcium carbonate	Larger than amorphous phosphates
Yellow-brown masses with or without spicules	Ammonium biurate	—

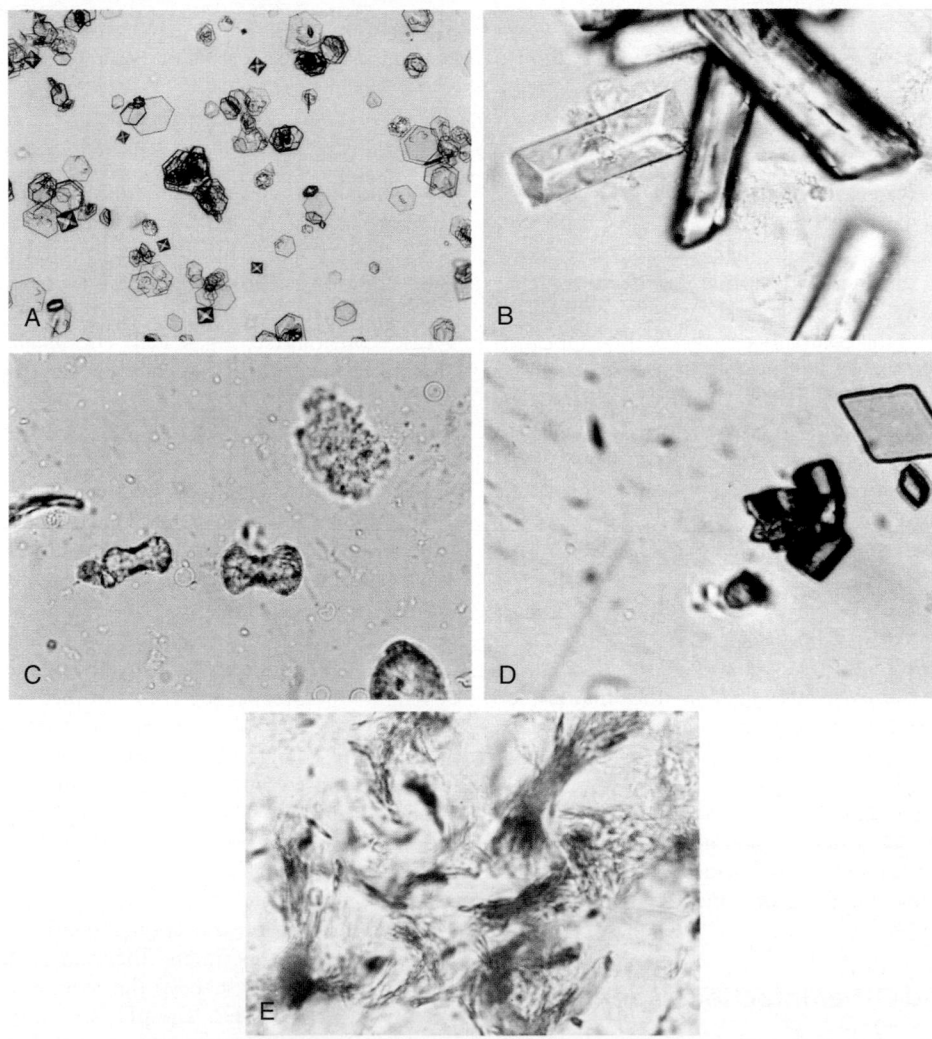

• **Fig. 4.4** Crystals. (A) Hexagonal cystine and bipyramidal or envelope-shaped oxalate. (B) Coffin lid-shaped triple phosphate. (C) Dumbbell-shaped oxalate. (D) Rhomboid urate. (E) Needle-shaped urate. (A, Courtesy Dr. Thomas O. Pitts.)

TABLE 4.3	Drug-Induced Crystalluria	
Drug	**Description**	**Comment**
Amoxicillin	Straw floor broom	—
Ciprofloxacin	Needle or starburst	—
Indinavir	Platelike rectangles, fan shaped, starburst	Causes nephrolithiasis or renal colic. In vitro solubility increased at very low pH. The lowest urine pH achievable in vivo may not actually be acidic enough to lessen crystalluria.
Sulfa drugs	Needles or sheaves of wheat, dumbbell	Reduced solubility at low pH
Radiographic contrast	Needles	Reduced solubility at low pH
Acyclovir, valacyclovir	Needles (birefringent)	—
Methotrexate	Clumped plates (yellow brown)	Reduced solubility at low pH
Triamterene	Spherical (birefringent)	Reduced solubility at low pH
Atazanavir	Needles	More likely at high urine pH
Darunavir	—	—
Orlistat	—	See oxalate, Table 4.2
Ethylene glycol	—	See oxalate, Table 4.2

crystals (Fig. 4.4A) are hexagonal plates that resemble benzene rings. Calcium oxalate dihydrate crystals (see Fig. 4.4A) are classically described as "envelope shaped" but when viewed as they rotate in the urine under the microscope appear bipyramidal. Coffin lid-shaped triple phosphates (see Fig. 4.4B) are rectangular with beveled ends. Oxalate monohydrate (see Fig. 4.4C) may also occur as a dumbbell-shaped crystal. Urate may have several forms, including rhomboids (see Fig. 4.4D) or needles (see Fig. 4.4E).

Drugs excreted in the urine may form crystals, as listed in Table 4.3. Determination of their appearance under polarized light can be informative. Confirmation of the identity of drug crystals requires spectroscopic analysis, which is seldom available clinically. However, review of the patient's drug list combined with a literature search for descriptions of crystals associated with those drugs may be very helpful in determining which drug is responsible for crystalluria, crystal-related AKI, or nephrolithiasis.

Characteristic Urine Sediments

The urine sediment is a rich source of diagnostic information. Occasionally a single finding (e.g., cystine crystals) is pathognomonic. More often, the sediment must be considered as a whole and interpreted in conjunction with other clinical and laboratory findings. Several patterns bear emphasis.

In acute glomerulonephritis, the urine may be pink or pale brown and turbid. Blood and moderate proteinuria are detected by dipstick analysis. The microscopic examination shows dysmorphic

RBCs and RBC casts, as well as granular and hyaline casts; WBC casts are rare.

In the nephrotic syndrome, the urine is clear or yellow. Foaminess may be noted because the elevated protein content alters the urine surface tension. In comparison with the sediment of patients with glomerulonephritis, the nephrotic sediment is bland. Hyaline casts and lipiduria with oval fat bodies or lipid-laden casts predominate. Granular casts and a few tubular cells may also be present, along with a few RBCs.

With some forms of chronic glomerulonephritis, a "telescoped" sediment is observed (see Fig. 4.2C). This term refers to the presence of the elements of a glomerulonephritis sediment together with waxy or broad casts, the latter indicative of tubular atrophy. Dipstick findings of heavy proteinuria may be present.

In pyelonephritis, WBC casts and innumerable WBCs are present, along with bacteria. In lower tract infections, WBC casts are absent.

The sediment in ATN (see Fig. 4.2B) characteristically shows tubular cells, tubular cell casts, and muddy brown granular casts. Few diagnoses in medicine have more immediacy than confirmation of the presence of ATN in a patient with suggestive clinical findings when these elements are noted in the first low-power field to come into focus as the microscope is adjusted. A urine sediment score, derived by totaling points given for the number of renal tubular epithelial cells observed per HPF and the number of granular casts observed per low-power field, has been found in a single-center study to be useful in differentiating ATN from other etiologies of AKI. At least one other similar index has been proposed, but no scoring system has been widely validated or gained general acceptance. The use of novel urinary biomarkers to predict onset or severity of AKI has received much ongoing attention. Combining measurement of these markers with suggestive findings on conventional urine microscopy may have additive predictive value, but this also remains a work in progress. The typical urinary findings in individual kidney disorders are discussed in their respective chapters.

Bibliography

Becker GJ, Garigali G, Fogazzi GB. Advances in urine microscopy. *Am J Kidney Dis*. 2016;67:954–964.

Birch DF, Fairley KF, Becker GJ, et al. *A Color Atlas of Urine Microscopy*. New York: Chapman & Hall; 1994.

Cameron JS. A history of urine microscopy. *Clin Chem Lab Med*. 2015;53(Suppl):S1453–S1464.

Canaris CJ, Flach SD, Tape TG, et al. Can internal medicine residents master microscopic urinalysis? Results of an evaluation and teaching intervention. *Acad Med*. 2003;78:525–529.

Cavanaugh C, Perazella MA. Urine sediment examination in the diagnosis and management of kidney disease: core curriculum 2019. *Am J Kidney Dis*. 2019;73:258–272.

Claure-Del Granado R, Macedo E, Mehta RL. Urine microscopy in acute kidney injury: time for a change. *Am J Kidney Dis*. 2011;57:657–660.

Dolscheid-Pommerich RC, Klarmann-Schulz U, Conrad R, Stoffel-Wagner B, Zur B. Evaluation of the appropriate time period between sampling and analyzing for automated urinalysis. *Biochem Med*. 2016;26:82–89.

Fogazzi GB, Verdesca S, Carigali G. Urinalysis: core curriculum 2008. *Am J Kidney Dis*. 2008;51:1052–1067.

Foot CL, Fraser JF. Uroscopic rainbow: modern matula medicine. *Postgrad Med J*. 2006;82:126–129.

Hamadah M, Gharaibeh K, Mara KC, Thompson KA, Lieske JC, Said S, Nasr SH, Leung N. Urinalysis for the diagnosis of glomerulonephritis: role of dysmorphic red blood cells. *Nephrol Dial Transplant*. 2018;33:1397–1403.

Kincaid-Smith P. Haematuria and exercise-related haematuria. *Br Med J*. 1982;285:1595–1597.

Lamchiagdhase P, Preechaborisutkul K, Lomsomboon P, Srisuchart P, Tantiniti P, Ra N, Preechaborisutkul B. Urine sediment examination: a comparison between the manual method and the iQ200 automated urine microscopy analyzer. *Clin Chim Acta*. 2005;358:167–174.

Martinez MG, dos Silva S, do Valle AP, Amaro CR, Corrente JE, Martin LC. Comparison of different methods of erythrocyte dysmorphism analysis to determine the origin of hematuria. *Nephron Clin Pract*. 2014;128:88–94.

Perazella MA. Crystal-induced acute renal failure. *Am J Med*. 1999;106:459–465.

Perazella MA. The urine sediment as a biomarker of kidney disease. *Am J Kidney Dis*. 2015;66:748–755.

Raymond JR, Yarger WE. Abnormal urine color: differential diagnosis. *South Med J*. 1988;81:837–841.

Rutecki GJ, Goldsmith C, Schreiner GE. Characterization of proteins in urinary casts: fluorescent-antibody identification of Tamm-Horsfall mucoprotein in matrix and serum proteins in granules. *N Engl J Med*. 1971;284:1049–1052.

Spinelli D, Consonni D, Garigali G, Fogazzi GB. Waxy casts in the urinary sediment of patients with different types of glomerular diseases: results of a prospective study. *Clin Chim Acta*. 2013;424:47–52.

Tsai JJ, Yeun JY, Kumar VA. Comparison and interpretation of urinalysis performed by a nephrologist versus a hospital-based clinical laboratory. *Am J Kidney Dis*. 2005;46:820–829.

Unic A, Gabaj NN, Miller M, Culej J, Lisac A, Horvat A, Vrkic N. Ascorbic acid-a black hole of urine chemistry screening. *J Clin Lab Anal*. 2018;32:e22390.

Voswinckel P. A marvel of colors and ingredients: the story of urine test strips. *Kidney Int*. 1994;46(suppl):3–7.

5

Hematuria and Proteinuria

TAIMUR DAD, SCOTT J. GILBERT

Kidney disease is defined by a reduction in the glomerular filtration rate (GFR), impairment of tubular function, or damage to kidney structure. This damage manifests as loss of the integrity of the filtration barrier, impairment of tubular function, or changes in other processes that interfere with normal kidney function. Urinalysis and urine sediment examination are useful tools to detect this damage, and both hematuria and proteinuria are important biomarkers of kidney disease. The appearance of red blood cells (RBCs) in the urine and the presence and type of proteinuria may point to the site of nephron damage and inform the subsequent diagnostic evaluation. For example, blebs on the surface of RBCs in the urine sediment can indicate glomerular bleeding as these cells undergo morphologic changes when forced across the glomerular basement membrane (GBM); albuminuria often reflects damage to the filtration barrier with a loss of the charge and size selectivity of the membrane; and low-molecular-weight proteinuria, such as β-2 microglobulin (β2M), retinol-binding protein (RBP), and α–1 microglobulin (α1M), identifies a failure of proximal tubular protein reabsorption or excessive filtration of pathologic molecules. The persistence of hematuria and the level of proteinuria provide prognostic information as well as an assessment of continued disease activity and response to treatment.

As early kidney damage may occur without clinical correlations, screening for hematuria and proteinuria is encouraged in high-risk populations, such as those with diabetes, hypertension, autoimmune conditions, or a family history of kidney disease. The detection of abnormal levels of these biomarkers warrants a full and complete evaluation. This chapter explores the significance of hematuria and proteinuria, the mechanisms of their development, the evaluation of these findings, and treatment options.

Hematuria

Hematuria is defined by the presence of RBCs in the urine. This can be divided into macroscopic (also known as *gross* or *visible*) and microscopic hematuria. Macroscopic hematuria is visible to the naked eye while microscopic hematuria requires urine sediment evaluation. As little as 1 mL of blood in a liter of urine can result in discoloration of the urine. Urine can appear on a spectrum from light pink to dark red/cola colored depending on the concentration of RBCs.

Definition

On microscopic evaluation, the presence of three or more RBCs per high-power (400×) field in a centrifuged urine sample is generally considered abnormal. However, there is no absolute cutoff, and lowering this cutoff results in more false-positive results, while increasing this cutoff will result in more false-negative results for any given etiology.

Etiology

Hematuria can be due to RBC loss anywhere along the genitourinary tract, ranging from the glomerulus to the urethra (Table 5.1). Glomerular hematuria may be distinguished from other causes of hematuria using RBC morphology in the urine sediment and the presence and amount of albuminuria. The most common glomerular causes of asymptomatic hematuria include IgA nephropathy and thin basement membrane disease (TBMD). In about half of affected individuals, immunoglobulin A (IgA) nephropathy can present with macroscopic hematuria following upper respiratory tract infections, although this should be differentiated from post-infectious glomerulonephritis (PIGN). PIGN typically has a longer lag than IgA nephropathy between the infection and the onset of hematuria. TBMD results from genetic defects in type IV collagen that make up the GBM. The inheritance pattern is autosomal dominant, resulting in multiple family members with microscopic hematuria, often without progressive kidney disease. Conversely, a family history of hematuria and progressive kidney disease, hearing loss, and ocular abnormalities suggest Alport syndrome, a genetic condition similar to TBMD in which affected individuals can progress to kidney failure.

Inflammatory diseases of the glomerulus also cause glomerular hematuria. These include lupus nephritis, membranoproliferative glomerulonephritis (MPGN), antineutrophil cytoplasmic antibody-associated (ANCA) vasculitis, and antiglomerular basement membrane disease, among others. Glomerular diseases that lack significant inflammation but result in increased GBM permeability, such as focal segmental glomerulosclerosis (FSGS), minimal change disease (MCD), and membranous nephropathy, primarily cause proteinuria, but can also have hematuria. Hematuria has been reported as an uncommon finding in diabetic kidney disease. In addition, direct barotrauma in the setting of hypertensive emergency can result in hematuria. Lastly, glomerular hematuria

TABLE 5.1	**Causes of Hematuria**

Glomerular

- Pauci-immune (ANCA related) vasculitis/anti-GBM disease
- Alport syndrome
- Thin basement membrane disease
- IgA nephropathy
- Associated with other glomerular diseases (FSGS, MCD, membranous nephropathy)
- Diabetic kidney disease
- Hypertensive emergency
- Exercise induced

Tubular/Interstitial

- Interstitial nephritis
- Papillary necrosis

Urothelial

- Malignancy (involving the kidney, ureters, bladder, or prostate)
- Nephrolithiasis
- Nephrocalcinosis
- Hypercalciuria
- Hyperoxaluria
- Strictures
- Bladder or ureteral polyps

Medications

- Cyclophosphamide/ifosfamide
- Anticoagulation associated[a]

Structural Kidney Diseases

- Acquired or hereditary cystic disease
- Medullary sponge kidney

Other Causes

- Infection (pyelonephritis, cystitis, urethritis, prostatitis, schistosomiasis, TB, polyoma virus)
- Rejection or trauma in a kidney transplant
- Pelvic radiation
- Sickle cell disease/trait
- Thrombotic microangiopathy
- Post instrumentation of the urinary tract or trauma
- Contamination from menstrual bleeding

Rare Causes

- Analgesic nephropathy
- Renal vein thrombosis
- Renal infarct/necrosis
- Endometriosis of the urinary tract
- Loin pain hematuria syndrome
- Nutcracker syndrome
- Arteriovenous malformations

[a]Also shown to cause glomerular bleeding.

ANCA, Antineutrophil cytoplasmic antibodies; *FSGS*, focal segmental glomerulosclerosis; *GBM*, glomerular basement membrane; *MCD*, minimal change disease; *TB*, tuberculosis.

or chronic tubulointerstitial disease should be considered, with the latter including analgesic nephropathy. Although rare in the United States, infections such as tuberculosis or schistosomiasis can cause pyuria and hematuria with sterile bacterial cultures in endemic countries.

Macroscopic hematuria with passage of blood clots in the urine is most often of urothelial (non-glomerular) origin, with the risk of malignancy generally increasing in older individuals. Other risk factors for urothelial carcinoma include exposure to cigarette smoking, occupational carcinogens, radiation, or medications such as cyclophosphamide. In older men, prostatic hypertrophy can be a cause of hematuria, but caution should be used to exclude malignancy. Hematuria associated with renal colic can be from nephrolithiasis; however, blood clots causing urinary obstruction can cause similar pain. Risk factors for crystalluria and nephrolithiasis, such as hypercalciuria and hyperoxaluria, have also been identified as causes of microscopic hematuria. Anticoagulation can result in hematuria originating in the urothelial tract and has also been implicated, albeit rarely, in glomerular bleeding.

Medications that directly cause hematuria are uncommon, with the exception of several chemotherapeutic agents. Conversely, many medications cause discoloration of urine without actual RBCs or free heme pigment in the urine (Table 5.2). Causes include certain foods such as beets and metabolites such as porphyrins, bile pigments, and methemoglobin.

Mechanical trauma to the genitourinary tract, including with instrumentation such as the placement of a bladder catheter, is commonly associated with hematuria. Similarly, papillary infarction or necrosis (more frequently seen in individuals with sickle cell disease and in a subset of individuals with analgesic nephropathy), kidney infarcts, damage from radiation, or structural kidney disease can all result in hematuria. In addition to causes already mentioned, hematuria in kidney transplant patients can be due to BK polyoma virus infection, rejection, recurrence of original kidney disease (if associated with hematuria), trauma, or structural/anastomotic problems.

TABLE 5.2	**Common Medications Causing Urine Discoloration Mimicking Hematuria**

Red

- Phenytoin
- Phenazopyridine
- Deferoxamine

Red-Brown

- Metronidazole
- Levodopa

Brown

- Nitrofurantoin
- Chloroquine

Dark Appearing

- Metronidazole
- Methyldopa
- Imipenem-cilastatin

Red-Orange

- Rifampin

can be found in healthy individuals after intense exercise; this is a diagnosis of exclusion and typically benign in nature.

The presence of pyuria in the setting of hematuria, along with specific symptoms, can point to infection or inflammation being the cause. Numerous bacterial pathogens can cause infectious cystitis. Without infectious symptoms and with sterile cultures, acute

Detection

Evaluation typically starts with a urine dipstick test when there is discoloration of the urine or when there is concern for hematuria. The dipstick relies on the peroxidase activity of the heme molecule, which results in a detectable change in color on an impregnated indicator pad. This sensitive reaction can detect very small amounts of heme in the urine in the form of intact RBCs or heme pigment from either free hemoglobin (e.g., intravascular hemolysis) or myoglobin (e.g., rhabdomyolysis) in the urine. False-positive results can be due to the presence of semen, bacterial peroxidase, or highly alkaline urine, or after cleaning the perineum with oxidizing agents. False-negative results can occur in cases of high vitamin C intake.

Evaluation

The evaluation of hematuria (Fig. 5.1) begins with a careful personal and family history that can provide clues to the possible etiology. Personal history should include prior episodes of hematuria, antecedent travel, upper respiratory tract infection before the onset of hematuria, recent strenuous exercise, history of renal colic or previous nephrolithiasis, passage of blood clots in the urine, pelvic radiation, recent trauma or instrumentation, and initiation of new medications or use of anticoagulants. Hematuria in the setting of menstruation should always be interpreted with caution because of the risk of contamination of the urine sample. Family history should include the presence of hematuria, hearing or ocular disorders, progressive kidney disease, and hematologic abnormalities such as sickle cell disease/trait or coagulation disorders. Physical examination should explore signs of infection (for pyelonephritis, cystitis, or prostatitis), severe hypertension, edema pointing to possible accompanying hypoalbuminemia from nephrotic syndrome, masses in the setting of kidney or prostatic malignancy, or enlarged kidneys from autosomal dominant polycystic kidney disease (ADPKD).

The next step involves examination of a freshly voided urine sample. Once there is confirmation of heme positivity with a urinary dipstick, the urine should be centrifuged. A dark pellet at the bottom of the tube with clear appearing supernatant indicates the presence of RBCs in the urine. A dark supernatant raises suspicion of free heme pigment, as seen in hemoglobinuria or myoglobinuria, and should prompt evaluation for either intravascular hemolysis or rhabdomyolysis, respectively. This can also be seen if the

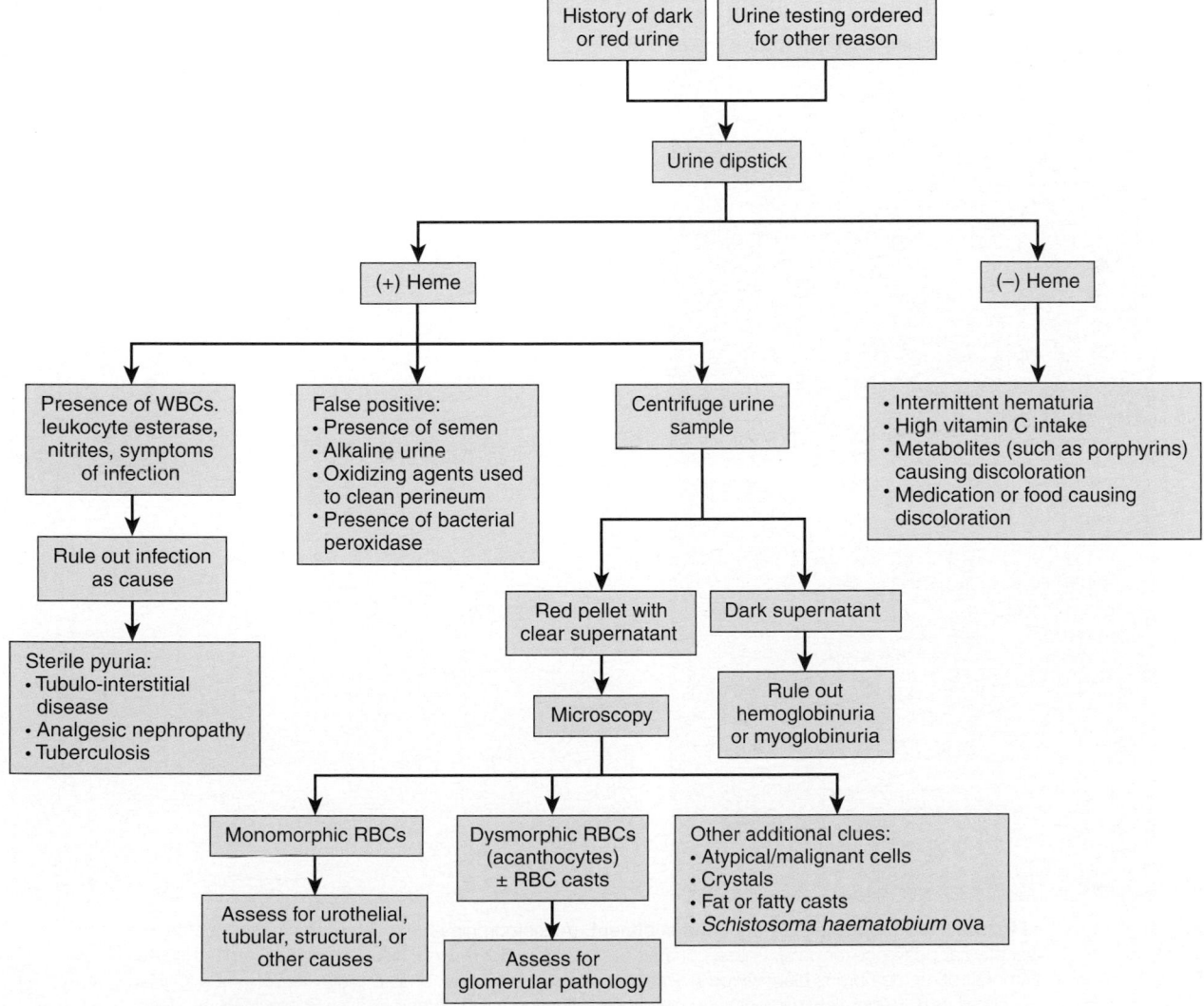

• **Fig. 5.1** Clinical approach to hematuria. *RBCs*, Red blood cells; *WBCs*, white blood cells.

urine is dilute and has been sitting for a period of time, resulting in osmotic lysis of RBCs. The pellet formed after centrifugation should be re-suspended and evaluated under the microscope. This is generally done with bright-field microscopy, although superior evaluation of RBC morphology can be performed with phase-contrast microscopy. Normal RBC shape results in a biconcave disk appearance. RBCs can appear distorted in the urine for a variety of reasons, resulting in "dysmorphic" RBCs. A specific kind of dysmorphic RBC, called an *acanthocyte*, has characteristic vesicle-like protrusions and is particularly indicative of glomerular hematuria. Acanthocytes should be distinguished from crenated RBCs, which are frequently seen and have spicules thought to be from RBC shrinkage in concentrated urine (Fig. 5.2). An acanthocyte threshold of greater than 5% is typically used for diagnosing glomerular hematuria with high specificity but low sensitivity. The presence of RBC casts and albuminuria further strengthens the diagnosis of glomerular hematuria. Other than RBC morphology, urine microscopy can provide additional clues, such as fat or fatty casts in the setting of accompanying heavy proteinuria, crystals in the setting of nephrolithiasis, tubular epithelial cells with intranuclear inclusions (decoy cells) in the presence of BK nephropathy, or atypical appearing cells in the setting of

malignancy. The more common test to assess for atypical cells, a stained urine cytology exam by a pathologist, lacks sensitivity and is, therefore, not recommended.

Laboratory testing should be tailored to the suspected etiology of hematuria. For example, in the setting of a suspected glomerular cause, serum creatinine, electrolytes, and albumin should be measured. Serologic testing can also be performed in the setting of glomerular pathology. Blood counts and coagulation panel can be assessed to identify the presence of anemia, hemolysis, and coagulation abnormalities.

Imaging plays a vital role in the workup for hematuria. Ultrasound of the kidneys can be used to evaluate kidney structure without exposure to radiation. More sensitive imaging can be performed with computed tomography (CT) scans either with or without intravenous contrast depending on the suspected etiology. Cystoscopy with direct visualization of the urothelial mucosa remains the gold standard for evaluation of the lower urinary tract. Magnetic resonance imaging (MRI) is less frequently used in the evaluation of hematuria. Finally, kidney biopsy can be performed in the setting of hematuria to achieve a definitive kidney disease diagnosis. Even with the availability of these studies, the etiology of microscopic hematuria may not be identified in a significant

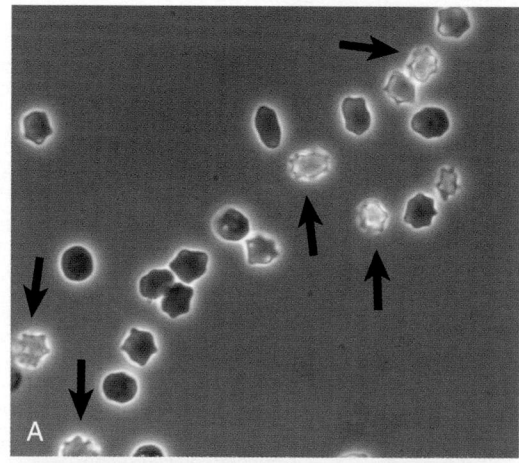
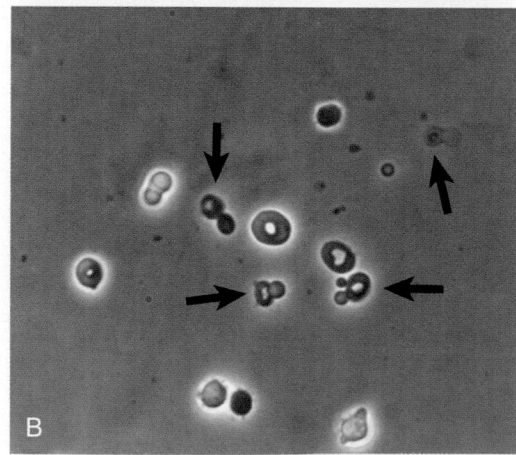
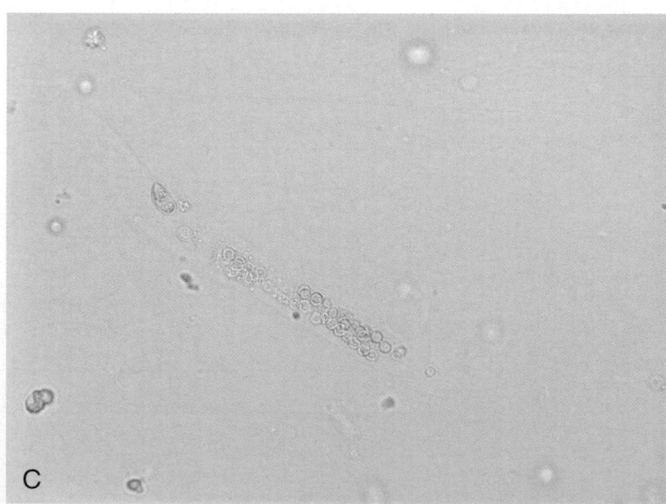

• **Fig. 5.2** **Red blood cells in the urine sediment.** (A) Isomorphic erythrocytes, some of which have a crenated appearance *(arrows)*. Phase-contrast microscopy, original magnification ×400. (B) Acanthocytes demonstrating membrane blebs *(arrows)*. Phase-contrast microscopy, original magnification ×400 (C) Red blood cell cast. Bright-field microscopy, original magnification ×100. (A and B, from Fogazzi GB, Verdesca S, Garigali G. Urinalysis: core curriculum 2008. *Am J Kid Dis*. 2008;51:1052–1067.)

proportion of patients. Follow-up evaluation of such patients remains an area of uncertainty.

Management

The management of hematuria depends on the underlying causes, which are discussed elsewhere in the *Primer*. Many of the causes described above may require co-management with urology.

PROTEINURIA

With an intact glomerular filtration barrier and functioning tubules, the amount of protein normally present in the urine is less than 150 mg/day. Increased levels of proteinuria can indicate kidney damage, and the quantity and type of protein in the urine are tools to identify the site and cause of kidney damage. Albuminuria is a marker of damage to the filtration barrier, whereas low-molecular-weight proteins in the urine often indicate tubular injury or overflow proteinuria. Levels of proteinuria in excess of 3.5 g/day (nephrotic range) suggest a number of disease processes including FSGS, MCD, membranous nephropathy, and amyloidosis that are distinct from diseases with less than 2 g/day of proteinuria.

The quantification of proteinuria has additional value in assessing prognosis and response to therapy. Higher levels of proteinuria are associated with higher risk of death, more rapid GFR decline, and increased risk of kidney failure in both diabetic and nondiabetic kidney disease, and lowering of proteinuria through renin-angiotensin blockade, SGLT2 inhibitor use, or disease-specific directed therapies is associated with lower rates of progressive GFR loss and kidney failure. Furthermore, the presence of albuminuria, even at low levels of 30 mg/day, is associated with increased all-cause and cardiovascular mortality, left ventricular hypertrophy (LVH), stroke, and vascular calcification, independent of the underlying disease process or the level of kidney function. This was clearly shown in the work of the Chronic Kidney Disease Epidemiology Collaboration (CKD-EPI) consortium (Fig. 5.3). As a result, proteinuria and albuminuria are often monitored as evidence of response to therapy in many primary and secondary kidney diseases, including diabetic kidney disease.

Definition

Normal levels of protein in the urine are less than 150 mg/day. This protein is primarily composed of uromodulin (also known as *Tamm-Horsfall protein*), with less than 30 mg/day of albumin

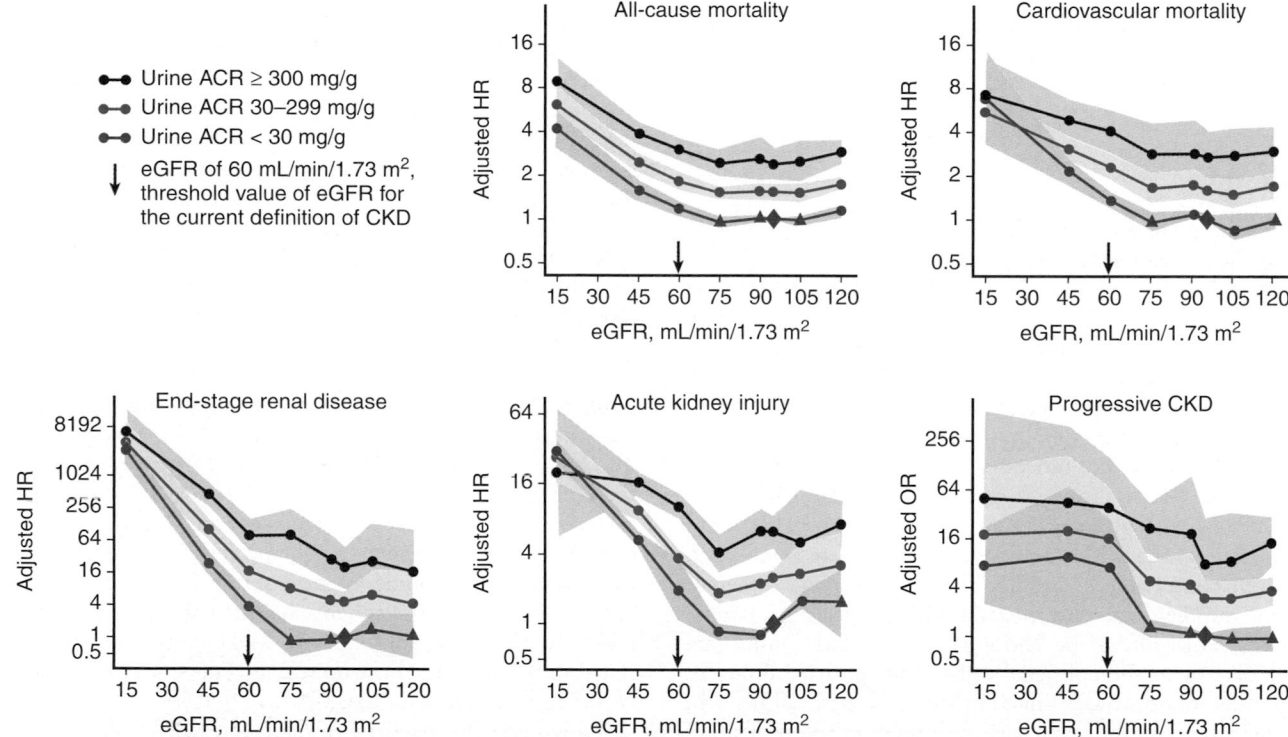

• **Fig. 5.3** Summary of continuous meta-analysis for general population cohorts with albumin-to-creatinine ratio (ACR). Mortality is reported for general population cohorts assessing albuminuria as urine ACR. Kidney outcomes are reported for general population cohorts assessing albuminuria as either urine ACR or reagent strip. Estimated glomerular filtration rate (eGFR) is expressed as a continuous variable. The three lines represent urine ACR of < 30, 30–299, and ≥300 mg/g (<3, 3–29, and ≥30 mg/mmol, respectively) or reagent strip negative and trace, 1+ positive, ≥2+ positive. All results are adjusted for covariates and compared to reference point of eGFR of 95 mL/min per 1.73 m² and ACR of less than > 30 mg/g (<3 mg/mmol) or reagent strip negative (diamond). Each point represents the pooled relative risk (RR) from a meta-analysis. Solid circles indicate statistical significance compared to the reference point (*P* < .05); triangles indicate non-significance. Red arrows indicate eGFR of 60 mL/min per 1.73 m², threshold value of eGFR for the current definition of CKD. *CKD*, chronic kidney disease; *HR*, hazard ratio; *OR*, odds ratio. (From Levey AS, Coresh J. Chronic kidney disease. *Lancet*. 2012;379:165–180.)

excreted in the urine. Clinical practice guidelines identify levels of albuminuria greater than 30 mg/day that persist for more than 3 months as defining chronic kidney disease (CKD). Urine albumin levels between 30 and 300 mg/day are referred to as *moderately increased albuminuria* (previously *microalbuminuria*), whereas levels greater than 300 mg/day are referred to as *severely increased albuminuria* (previously *macroalbuminuria*).

Isolated proteinuria is defined by greater than 300 mg of protein excretion per day in the absence of abnormalities in the urine sediment, GFR loss, or comorbid conditions (diabetes, hypertension, rheumatologic or infectious diseases). This is often detected incidentally without evidence of edema or nephrotic syndrome.

Proteinuria can also be typed according to its mechanism: *glomerular*, *tubular*, *overflow*, and *postrenal*. These are discussed below under Physiology.

Albuminuria greater than 30 mg/day is present in 6.7% of the US general population, with a higher prevalence in the elderly and in individuals with comorbidities. The prevalence of albuminuria in individuals with diabetes is 28.8%, and 16% of individuals with hypertension have albuminuria. The prevalence of albuminuria increases after the age of 40, with 3.3% of the adult population with a normal GFR having persistent albuminuria. Albuminuria is 50% more common in women than men (9.7% vs. 6.1%). It is also more common in individuals of African and Mexican ancestry as compared to non-Hispanic Whites. This likely reflects an increased prevalence of diseases associated with proteinuria in individuals of African ancestry, including diabetes, hypertension, primary glomerular diseases, and the risk allele of *APOL1*.

Physiology

Because of the structure of the GBM, small amounts of protein are filtered at the glomerulus by processes of diffusion and convection with the vast majority then reabsorbed through receptor-mediated endocytosis, primary in the proximal convoluted tubule (PCT). A more modest amount of protein, primarily uromodulin, is secreted by the tubule.

The glomerular filtration barrier is comprised of a fenestrated endothelium, a basement membrane, and an epithelial covering derived from podocyte foot processes and linking slit diaphragms. The endothelial fenestrations are pores of less than 100 nm in diameter coated with glycocalyx that represent the first barrier to protein filtration. The GBM includes a matrix of type IV collagen and laminin comprising a middle lamina densa, with adherent polyanionic proteoglycans like heparan sulfates creating a lamina rara interna (adjacent to the endothelial cells) and lamina rara externa (adjacent to the epithelial cells). The epithelial lining of interdigitating foot processes linked by slit diaphragms of nephrin and podocin provide the final barrier through creation of pores 7 nm in diameter. Together, the intact glomerular filtration barrier provides a size- and charge-specific barrier than allows passage of small (0 to 35 nm) and uncharged or cationic molecules but reflects molecules of larger size and increasingly anionic charge (Table 5.3).

The primary plasma protein is albumin, a 70-kD molecule with a diameter of 6 nm and an anionic charge (isoelectric point [pI] –4.5). This results in a sieving coefficient of 0.00062 and filtration of between 4 and 8 g of albumin by the glomerulus each day under normal circumstances. Nearly all of this is reabsorbed by the PCT through receptor-mediated endocytosis such that less than 20 mg of albumin is excreted in the urine. Megalin

TABLE 5.3	Filtration Across the Glomerular Basement Membrane by Size	
Substance	Molecular Weight (g/mol)	Sieving Coefficient
Sodium	23	1.0
Glucose	180	1.0
Inulin	5,500	1.0
Myoglobulin	17,000	0.75
Albumin	69,000	0.0006

and cubilin are key factors in this process. An increase in urinary protein excretion occurs with defects in the glomerular filtration barrier, impairment of tubular reabsorption of filtered protein, or an excessive load of filtered proteins that overwhelm the reabsorptive capacity of the tubule.

Glomerular proteinuria is largely albumin and other macromolecules, and related to defects in the size- and charge-selective barrier that normally reflect these larger, anionic molecules. This can occur with structural changes seen with inflammation, scarring, deposition, or genetic conditions that affect the integral proteins of the filtration barrier (such as nephrin and podocin). Albuminuria typically exceeds 400 mg/day.

Tubular proteinuria is composed of low-molecular-weight proteins (<25 kD), such as β-2-microglobulin, retinol-binding protein, immunoglobulin light chains, and polypeptide fragments, and it is thus unlikely to be identified by the traditional urine dipstick that detects intact albumin. These smaller molecules are normally filtered by the glomerulus and then reabsorbed by the tubule. With tubular pathology seen in tubulointerstitial nephritis, tubular toxicity from heavy-metal poisoning, Dent disease, and Lowe syndrome, the low-molecular-weight proteins are not reabsorbed and appear in the urine. Tubular proteinuria typically occurs at a level of 200 to 2000 mg/day with albuminuria below 400 mg/day, but larger amounts of albuminuria can be seen with coexisting glomerular disease. Urine protein electrophoresis is often used to identify these proteins.

Overflow proteinuria occurs when overproduction and excessive filtration of low-molecular-weight proteins exceed the reabsorptive capacity of the tubule. This can result in the appearance in the urine of immunoglobulin light chains (with multiple myeloma), lysozyme (with myelomonocytic leukemia), myoglobin (with rhabdomyolysis or intrinsic muscle disorders), or free hemoglobin (with intravascular hemolysis).

Proteinuria can occur with damage to the collecting system, often referred to as *postrenal proteinuria*. This is seen in conditions including inflammation, irritation, infection, or cancer of the renal pelvis, ureters, bladder, and prostate. The protein in these cases is typically nonalbumin (i.e., immunoglobulins), levels are often low, and the duration may be transient.

Detection

Proteinuria is most commonly detected with a semi-quantitative urine dipstick and then confirmed with quantitative measures. Confirmation on repeat testing will exclude false positives and transient proteinuria.

Semi-Quantitative Methods

Two semi-quantitative methods of detecting proteinuria are available. The urine dipstick uses pads impregnated with indicator dyes that undergo a colorimetric reaction with albumin in the urine. The common dyes, tetrabromophenol blue and bromocresol green, are very specific but lack sensitivity in the setting of dilute urine or nonalbumin proteins such as immunoglobulin light chains. The reaction on the pad is scored:

Trace	15–30 mg/dL
1+	30–100 mg/dL
2+	100–300 mg/dL
3+	300–1000 mg/dL
4+	>1000 mg/dL

Interpretation must account for urinary concentration (often estimated by the specific gravity). Scores of 2+ and greater are highly suggestive of significant proteinuria, but scores of trace or 1+ are only predictive when the specific gravity is less than 1.025. In addition to urine concentration, the sensitivity and specificity of the urine dipstick is affected by the presence of other chemicals. False positives are seen with alkaline urine (pH >8) that overwhelms the buffer, drugs (tolbutamide, cephalosporins, chlorhexidine, benzalkonium) that interfere with the reaction, and iodinated radiocontrast agents. As mentioned, false negatives are seen in dilute urine or in the presence of nonalbumin proteins.

A second semi-quantitative method relies on the biuret reaction of urinary proteins with sulfosalicylic acid (SSA). This reaction occurs with all proteins at a sensitivity of 5 to 10 mg/dL. Thus, a strongly positive reaction with SSA in the setting of a negative urine dipstick indicates the presence of a nonalbumin protein in the urine, such as immunoglobulin light chains in multiple myeloma. The SSA test is scored:

0	No turbidity (0 mg/dL)
Trace	Slight turbidity (1–10 mg/dL)
1+	Turbidity through which print can be read (15–30 mg/dL)
2+	White cloud without precipitate through which heavy black lines on a white background can be seen (40–100 mg/dL)
3+	White cloud with fine precipitate through which heavy black lines cannot be seen (150–350 mg/dL)
4+	Flocculent precipitate (>500 mg/dL)

False positives with SSA test are seen after iodinated radiocontrast administration.

Quantitative Methods

Quantification of urinary protein excretion is important in individuals with persistent proteinuria to help narrow the spectrum of kidney injury (benign proteinuria vs. non-nephrotic proteinuria vs. nephrotic syndrome) and to monitor progression of disease and response to treatment over time. Two quantitative assessments of proteinuria are available.

The standard for measuring proteinuria is a timed, usually 24-hour, urine collection. These collections are cumbersome to collect, difficult to transport, and often inaccurate because of improper or incomplete collection. Timed collections are particularly challenging for individuals with persistent proteinuria who require frequent measurements. Collections of shorter duration (6 or 12 hours) suffer from wider variability. The completeness of a collection can be assessed by assuming women below the age of 50 excrete 15 to 20 mg creatinine per kilogram lean body mass per day, while men excrete 20 to 25 mg creatinine per kilogram lean body mass. Creatinine production and, therefore, excretion decline with advancing age.

An alternative is the measurement in a spot urine collection of the ratio of protein or albumin to creatinine. The urine protein-to-creatinine ratio (UPCR) and urine albumin-to-creatinine ratio (UACR) correct the protein and albumin measurements (in mg/dL) for urinary concentration or dilution by standardizing for 1g of daily creatinine excretion. This is expressed in units of mg/g and correlates with the daily protein and albumin excretion (Fig. 5.4). Care must be used in interpreting the results in groups that do not meet population norms, such as younger, muscular, and athletic individuals who excrete more than 1 g of creatinine per day (thus underestimating protein excretion), or older, slight, and more frail individuals who excrete less creatinine (thus overestimating protein excretion). In children, the normal value for the protein-to-creatinine ratio is <200 mg/g over the age of 2 years and <500 mg/g in infants and toddlers between 6 and 24 months of age, reflecting lower creatinine generation. Given diurnal variations in protein excretion, repeat measurements should ideally be performed at the same time each day. Furthermore, changes in creatinine filtration, as seen in acute kidney injury (AKI) and variability in tubular creatinine secretion impact the accuracy of the ratio. Nevertheless, the use of UPCR and UACR are supported by Kidney Disease: Improving Global Outcomes (KDIGO) guidelines.

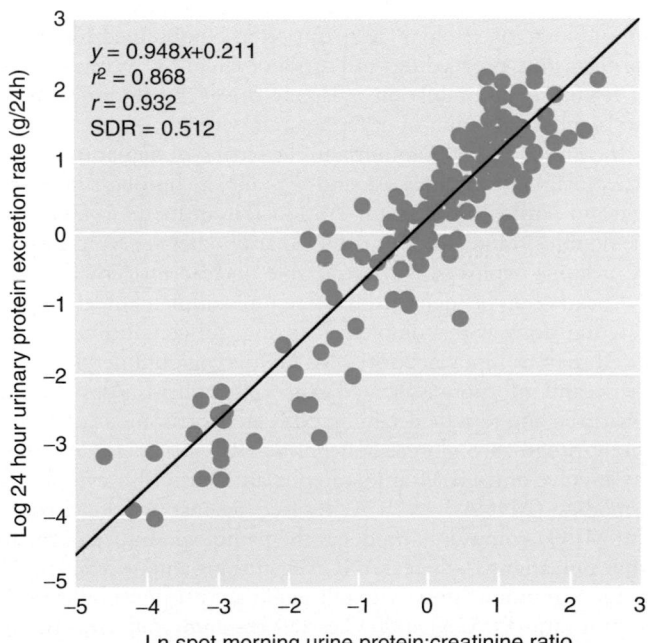

• **Fig. 5.4** Correlation between log spot morning urine protein:creatinine ratio and log 24-hour urinary protein in 177 nondiabetic patients with chronic nephropathies and persistent clinical proteinuria, showing regression equation and line. *r,* Correlation coefficient; *r²,* determination coefficient; *SDR,* ln SD of regression line. (From Ruggenenti P, Gaspari F, Perna A, Remuzzi G. Cross-sectional longitudinal study of spot morning urine protein:creatinine ratio, 24-hour urine protein excretion rate, glomerular filtration rate, and end-stage renal failure in chronic renal disease in patients without diabetes. *BMJ.* 1998;316:504–509.)

Evaluation

Once proteinuria has been detected and quantitated, the evaluation requires a careful history, complete physical exam, and directed laboratory testing. The history must include factors associated with kidney disease such as age, prior kidney injury, comorbid conditions such as diabetes, hypertension, cancer, and autoimmune diseases, and family history of kidney disease. The physical exam should measure blood pressure, assess for LVH, and evaluate for lymphadenopathy, splenomegaly, edema, arthritis, rash, and sinus disease. A fundoscopic examination is useful for detecting small vessel disease. On laboratory testing, quantification of and typing of proteinuria, examination of the urine sediment for cells and casts, estimation of kidney function, measurement of electrolytes and assessment of serologic markers and infection are performed. Electrocardiogram and echocardiogram are useful in identifying LVH.

Younger individuals are more likely to have benign proteinuria or transient proteinuria. *Transient proteinuria* is a common phenomenon affecting 4% of men and 7% of women. Fever and vigorous exercise are often responsible, and reassessment should occur when the patient is well (free of fever) and after avoidance of vigorous exercise.

Orthostatic proteinuria is seen in children and adolescents (2% to 5%) but is rare in adults over 30 years of age. It can be assessed by doing a split urine collection that includes a supine and an upright collection. The protein content of the upright collection is greater than the supine collection with poor understanding of the mechanism. This is a benign condition with an excellent prognosis and requires no follow-up once identified.

Persistent proteinuria less than 2000 mg/day without features of hematuria, GFR loss, rheumatologic conditions, or abnormal immunologic or serologic tests can often be observed for several months before proceeding with further evaluation. With concerning features, the evaluation is largely driven by findings on the history, physical exam, or other laboratory tests.

The presence of albuminuria in the setting of hematuria is suggestive of glomerular disease and warrants a thorough immunologic and serologic evaluation. Antinuclear antibodies (ANA) and anti-double-stranded DNA (dsDNA) antibodies are typically present in lupus nephritis, and extractable nuclear antigens (Ro, Sm, RNP) can often be identified. Low serum complement levels identify conditions with complement-fixing antigen-antibody complexes, such as lupus nephritis, MPGN, cryoglobulinemic kidney disease, and infection-associated glomerulonephritis. Albuminuria, hematuria, and rapidly declining GFR are worrisome features of a rapidly progressive glomerulonephritis (RPGN), many of which may involve anti-GBM antibodies or antineutrophil cytoplasmic antibodies (ANCAs). ANCA directed against myeloperoxidase (anti-MPO) commonly produces the pathologic injury of microscopic polyangiitis, whereas ANCA against proteinase 3 (anti-PR3) produces granulomatosis with polyangiitis. Anti-phospholipase A2 receptor (anti-PLA2R) antibodies and less commonly anti-thrombospondin type-1 domain-containing 7A (THSD7A) antibodies are found in idiopathic membranous nephropathy.

Glomerular proteinuria can also be seen with a number of systemic infections. Hepatitis C (HCV) infection can induce rheumatoid factor (RF) and cryoglobulinemic kidney disease. Hepatitis B (HBV) infection has been associated with membranous glomerulopathy, MPGN, and polyarteritis nodosa (PAN). Human immunodeficiency virus (HIV) infection is associated with the collapsing variant of FSGS.

Older subjects with an active cancer, a history of cancer, or biomarkers of cancer activity are at risk for membranous nephropathy, MPGN (breast, colon, stomach, lung cancer), or MCD (Hodgkin and non-Hodgkin lymphomas).

Tubular proteinuria is suggested by the presence of nonalbumin protein in the urine. For example, an elevated ratio of β-2-microglobulin to albumin in the urine would warrant evaluation for Sjögren syndrome, malignancy, medication toxicity, and heavy metal exposure.

Finally, overflow proteinuria occurs from myoglobinuria after muscle damage from drugs, traumatic injury, or inherited muscle enzyme disorders; hemoglobinuria with intravascular hemolysis or paroxysmal nocturnal hemoglobinuria (PNH); immunoglobulin light chains with multiple myeloma; or lysozyme with myelomonocytic leukemia. These proteins can be measured directly or detected by electrophoresis.

A kidney biopsy is usually reserved for:
- Proteinuria associated with a declining GFR
- Proteinuria in the nephrotic range (greater than 3500 mg/day)
- Proteinuria with features of a glomerular (albuminuria, acanthocytes, RBC casts) or tubular (low-molecular-weight proteins) source
- Persistent proteinuria in a patient with systemic lupus erythematosus (SLE) or other rheumatologic condition

Patients with diabetes and nephrotic-range proteinuria are not usually biopsied given the frequency of diabetic kidney disease in this population, but dramatic increases in proteinuria that was previously stable may suggest a superimposed condition. Biopsy surveys of diabetic patients identify an alternative etiology in 30% of cases.

Management

Treatment of proteinuria includes disease-specific and general interventions. Disease-specific treatments are discussed elsewhere in the *Primer*, with the objective of targeting the underlying condition to reduce the damage to the kidney and the loss of protein in the urine. General interventions include use of renin-angiotensin blockade that alters glomerular hemodynamics and mediators of fibrosis. The consequences of significant protein loss in the urine, including hyperlipidemia, hypercoagulability, impaired immunologic response, and malnutrition, must not be overlooked.

Complete bibliography is available at Elsevier eBooks for Practicing Clinicians.

Key Bibliography

Becker GJ, Garigali G, Fogazzi GB. Advances in urine microscopy. *Am J Kidney Dis.* 2015;67:954–964.

Boulware LE, Jaar BG, Tarver-Carr ME, Brancati FL, Powe NR. Screening for proteinuria in US adults: a cost-effectiveness analysis. *JAMA.* 2003;290:3101–3114.

Cohen RA, Brown RS. Microscopic hematuria. *N Engl J Med.* 2003;348:2330–2338.

Fotheringham J, Campbell MJ, Fogarty DG, El Nahas M, Ellam T. Estimated albumin excretion rate versus urine albumin-creatinine ratio for the estimation of measured albumin excretion rate: derivation and validation of an estimated albumin excretion rate equation. *Am J Kidney Dis.* 2014;63:405–414.

Ginsberg JM, Chang BS, Matarese RA, Garella S. Use of single voided urine samples to estimate quantitative proteinuria. *N Engl J Med.* 1983;309:1543–1546.

Halpern JA, Chugtai B, Ghomrawi H. Cost-effectiveness of common diagnostic approaches for evaluation of asymptomatic microscopic hematuria. *JAMA Intern Med*. 2017;177(6):800–807.

Hausmann R, Kuppe C, Egger H, et al. Electrical forces determine glomerular permeability. *J Am Soc Nephrol*. 2010;21:2053–2058.

Hogan MC, Reich HN, Nelson PJ, et al. The relatively poor correlation between random and 24-hour urine protein excretion in patients with biopsy-proven glomerular diseases. *Kidney Int*. 2016;90:1080.

Kohler H, Wandel E, Brunck B. Acanthocyturia—a characteristic marker for glomerular bleeding. *Kidney Int*. 1991;40:115–120.

Levey AS, Coresh J. Chronic kidney disease. *Lancet*. 2012;379:165–180.

Microhematuria Guidelines from the American Urologic Association 2020. Microhematuria Guidelines from the American Urologic Association (2020). https://www.auanet.org/guidelines/microhematuria.

Merrill AE, Khan J, Dickerson JA, et al. Method-to-method variability in urine albumin measurements. *Clin Chim Acta*. 2016;460:114.

Ohisa N, Yoshida K, Matsuki R, et al. A comparison of urinary albumin–total protein ratio to phase-contrast microscopic examination of urine sediment for differentiating glomerular and nonglomerular bleeding. *Am J Kidney Dis*. 2008;52:235–241.

Praga M, Alegre R, Hernández E, et al. Familial microscopic hematuria caused by hypercalciuria and hyperuricosuria. *Am J Kidney Dis*. 2000;35:141.

Raymond JR, Yarger WE. Abnormal urine color: differential diagnosis. *South Med J*. 1988;81:837–841.

Sharp VJ, Barnes KT, Erickson BA. Assessment of asymptomatic microscopic hematuria in adults. *Am Fam Physician*. 2013;88:747–754.

Tangri N, Grams ME, Levey AS, et al. multinational assessment of accuracy of equations for predicting risk of kidney failure: a meta-analysis. *JAMA*. 2016;315:164.

Tryggvason K, Patrakka J. Thin basement membrane nephropathy. *J Am Soc Nephrol*. 2006;17:813–822.

Waldman M, Crew RJ, Valeri A, et al. Adult minimal-change disease: clinical characteristics, treatment, and outcomes. *Clin J Am Soc Nephrol*. 2007;2:445–453.

Ying T, Clayton P, Naresh C, Chadban S. Predictive value of spot versus 24-hour measures of proteinuria for death, end-stage kidney disease or chronic kidney disease progression. *BMC Nephrol*. 2018;19:55.

6

Imaging of the Kidneys

DINUSHI S. PERERA, JOANIE M. GARRATT, AUSTIN R. PANTEL, MATTHEW A. MORGAN

Introduction

Visualizing the genitourinary system was one of the first goals of the nascent radiological sciences at the turn of the 20th century. It was a fortuitous discovery that the sodium iodide patients were taking for syphilis made their bladder denser ("opacified") on x-ray imaging. The development of organic iodine agents that could be administered intravenously and would be excreted in the urine advanced the field of kidney imaging. This created an image of the kidneys, ureter, and bladder that could be captured on x-ray film. Although intravenous contrast opacifies every organ receiving blood flow, the development of contrast agents for genitourinary radiology and the fact that these agents were excreted through the kidneys have linked the two ever since.

Kidney imaging has evolved at a tremendous rate, and evaluating kidney disease in the modern era often relies on gathering information from multiple different imaging techniques.

Imaging Modalities

Conventional Radiography and Intravenous Urography/Pyelography (IVU/IVP)

Conventional radiography (x-rays) of the kidneys has limited value for most kidney disease processes. Radiography has excellent contrast resolution for calcium and gas, so kidney stones or gas-containing infections can be seen. However, it has poor resolution for soft tissues, and at best the outline of the kidney appears like a "ghost" on a radiograph.

Intravenous urography (or intravenous pyelography) addresses the visibility problem when an injected iodine "contrast" collects in the kidney parenchyma and is then excreted (Fig. 6.1). The technique is close to a hundred years old and has been almost completely supplanted by CT urography, which is faster and more versatile, with much better ability to visualize the kidney parenchyma (in addition to other abdominal organs).

Computed Tomography (CT)

Computed tomography administers x-rays at different angles around an arc (tomography) to build a sinogram of different attenuation values. This sinogram is then deconvoluted by a computer to provide two-dimensional images of a patient (Fig. 6.2B); these can be reconstructed into three-dimensional images, if desired (Fig. 6.2C).

CT scans can be performed without contrast, particularly if evaluating for stones (Fig. 6.3), but they may also employ the same iodinated contrast used in intravenous urography. CT scans with contrast can also be protocoled to scan at multiple different time points to gather more information about the kidney parenchyma or the enhancement pattern of kidney masses (Fig. 6.4).

Although far more powerful than traditional radiographic techniques, CT administers a higher radiation dose. Whether the absolute value of the radiation dose is significant in a patient's lifetime is debated and depends on the patient's age and the number of studies performed.

Ultrasound (US)

Ultrasound is conceptually similar to sonar and uses non-ionizing sound waves to construct an image (Fig. 6.5A). It has a number of qualities that stand out as an imaging technique. It is portable, creates images quickly, and can display them in real time. Its ability to image continuously also allows it to detect Doppler shift in soundwaves and provides valuable information about movement, such as the flow of blood through vessels (Fig. 6.5B).

Ultrasound also has its limitations. Unlike traditional radiographic techniques, calcium and gas are poorly imaged and anything behind them is blocked from view. Large patient habitus also limits ultrasound visualization.

Development of contrast microbubbles for ultrasound (contrast-enhanced ultrasound, CEUS) now permits evaluation of perfusion of the kidney parenchyma and kidney masses. The enhancement is analogous to iodinated contrast media for CT (Fig. 6.6), but the limitations of body habitus, gas, and calcifications remain.

Magnetic Resonance Imaging (MRI)

Magnetic resonance imaging (MRI) takes advantage of the spin of protons (usually hydrogen ions) in different microenvironments in order to generate image contrast. MRI employs time-varying magnetic fields and radio frequency electromagnetic radiation, but, unlike CT, ionizing radiation is not needed. A set of magnetic field gradients and radio wave pulses is called a *sequence*, and these sequences can be modified to take advantage of different types of tissue contrast (Fig. 6.7). Sequences can range from less than a minute in length to several minutes long. These sequences are arranged in protocols and the type of protocol is tailored to answer a specific clinical question.

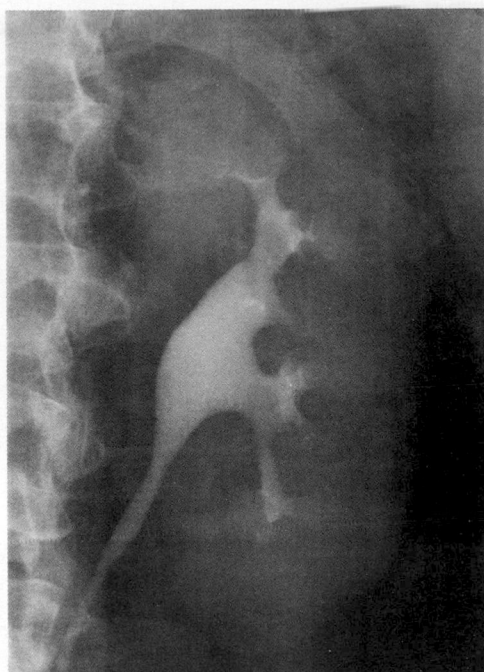

• **Fig. 6.1** A normal kidney as visualized by an intravenous urogram. The intravenous contrast opacifies the kidney parenchyma, allowing visualization on an x-ray. Contrast is beginning to be excreted into the collecting system.

MRI is a very powerful imaging tool for illustrating different kinds of tissue contrast within the kidneys. Spatial resolution is usually quite good if the patient can participate in a breath hold, but it is usually not as good as CT. This is why CT is preferred for evaluation of the collecting system, which often requires fine detail for detecting small urothelial lesions.

Besides the excellent tissue contrast, another advantage of MRI is that it does not require iodinated contrast, so hypersensitivity

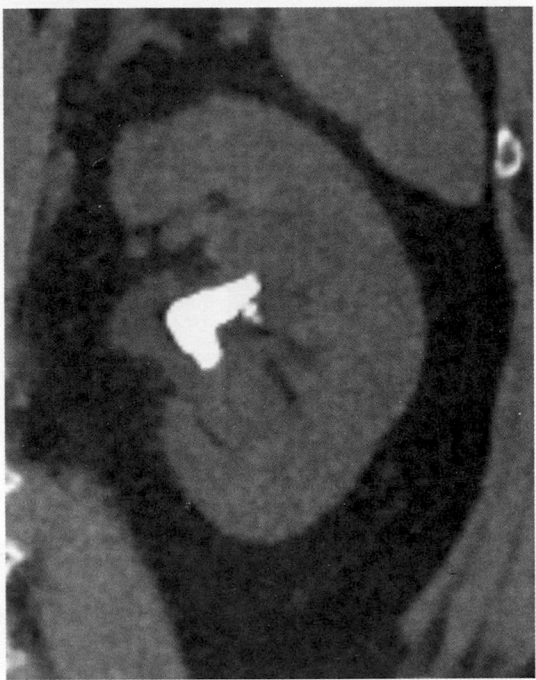

• **Fig. 6.3** Staghorn calculus in the kidney pelvis on a noncontrast CT.

to iodine-containing compounds is not an issue. MRI can often answer clinical questions without contrast, but, if contrast is needed, a gadolinium-containing contrast can be used (discussed later in chapter).

The drawbacks to MRI include the longer duration of the exam, which can be difficult for patients to tolerate, especially since the bore of the MRI is narrow to improve the magnetic field strength and the machine can be loud as the magnetic gradients are shifting. Open design MRI machines are available, but these often yield suboptimal images, limiting their utility. Patients must also be capable of holding their breath, since motion artifact from breathing will degrade MRI

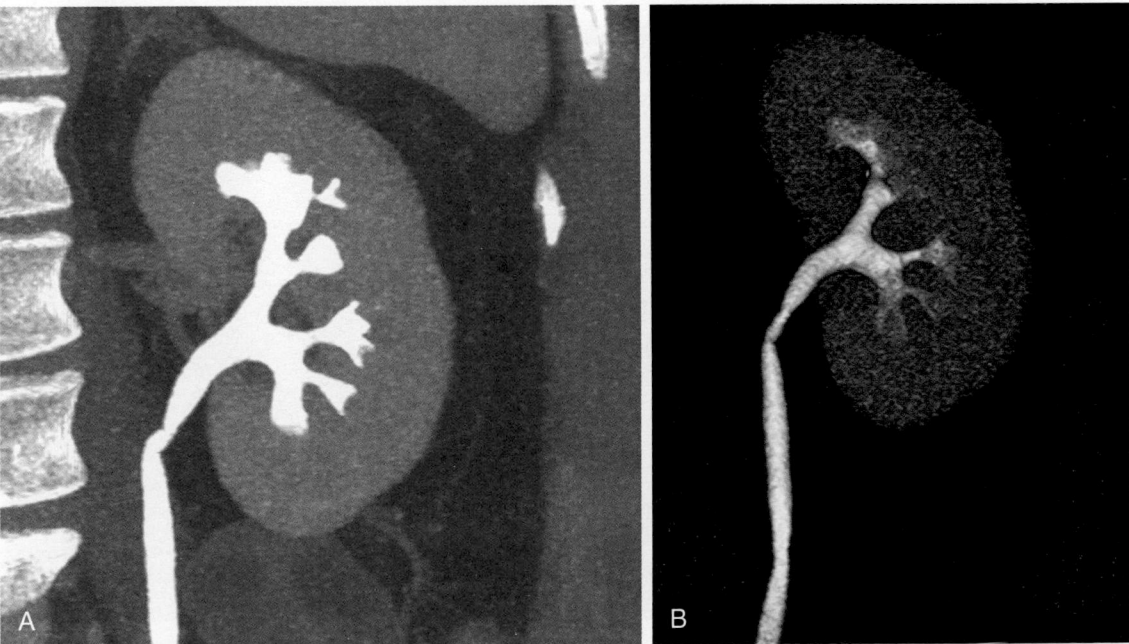

• **Fig. 6.2** (A) Normal kidney is shown in the coronal plane during the excretion phase of a CT urogram. This same kidney has been modeled in 3D using the source CT images (B).

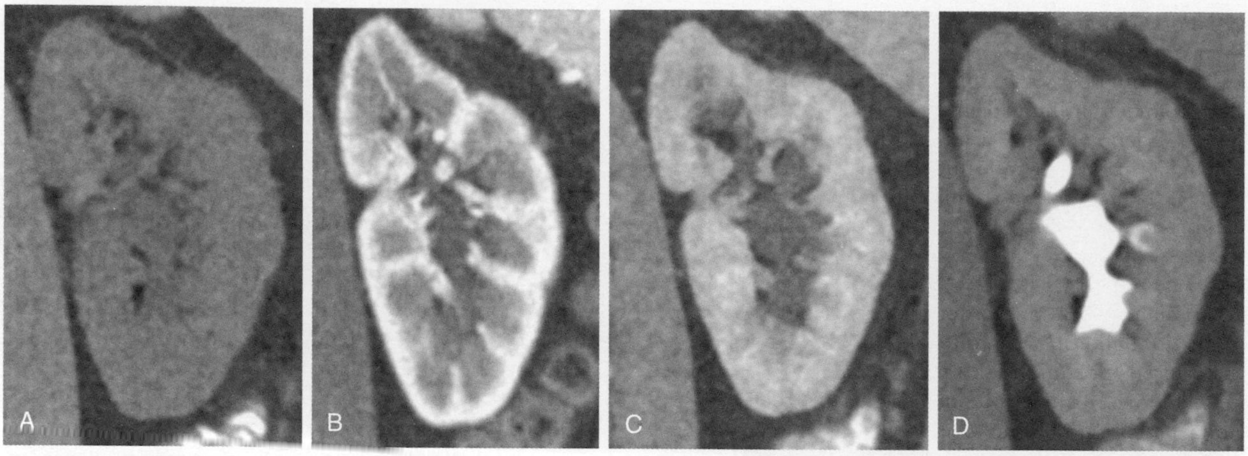

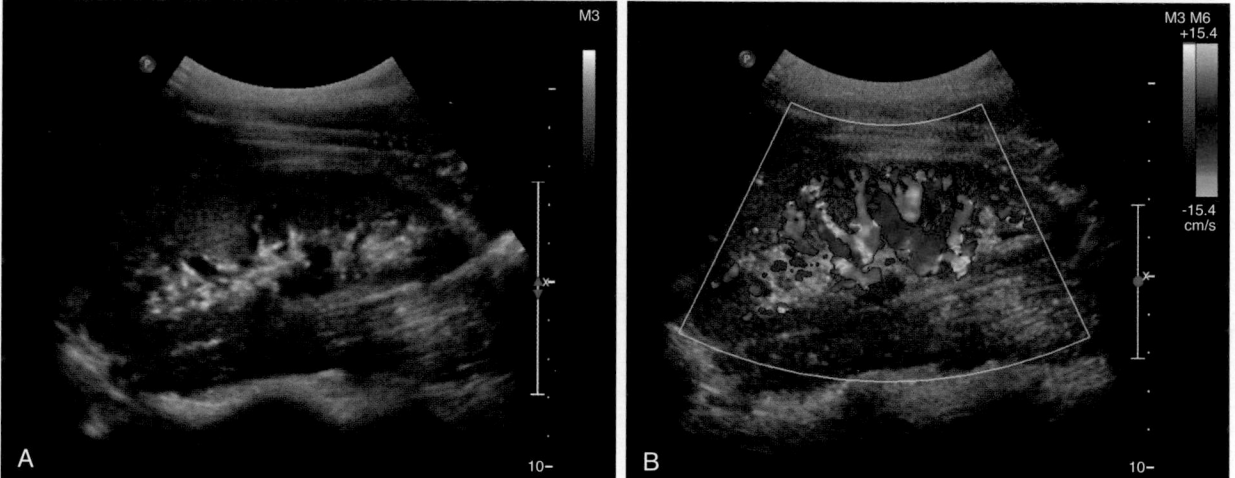

• **Fig. 6.4** A normal kidney imaged with CT in four different phases of contrast (A–D, left to right): noncontrast, corticomedullary phase, nephrographic phase, and excretory phase.

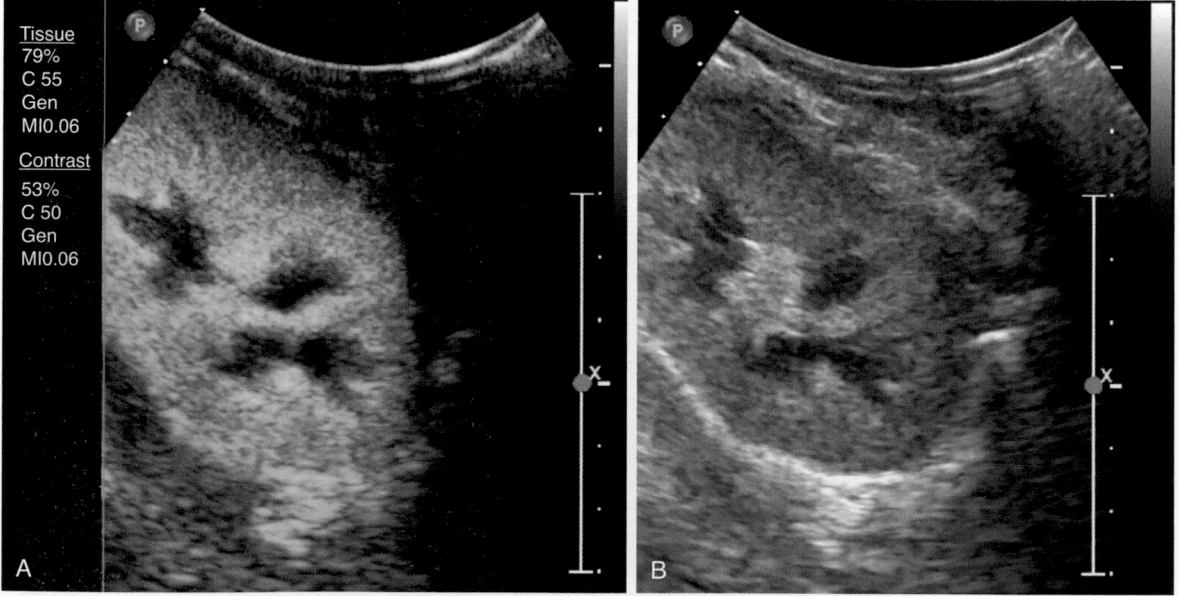

• **Fig. 6.5** A normal kidney imaged with ultrasound. (A) The kidney is imaged in long axis with grayscale imaging only. (B) A color Doppler map overlays the grayscale image, showing vascular flow through the kidney.

• **Fig. 6.6** A contrast-enhanced image of a normal kidney transplant. The grayscale appearance of the kidney is on the right. The matching, enhanced image on the left shows homogeneous enhancement of the transplant, indicating normal perfusion.

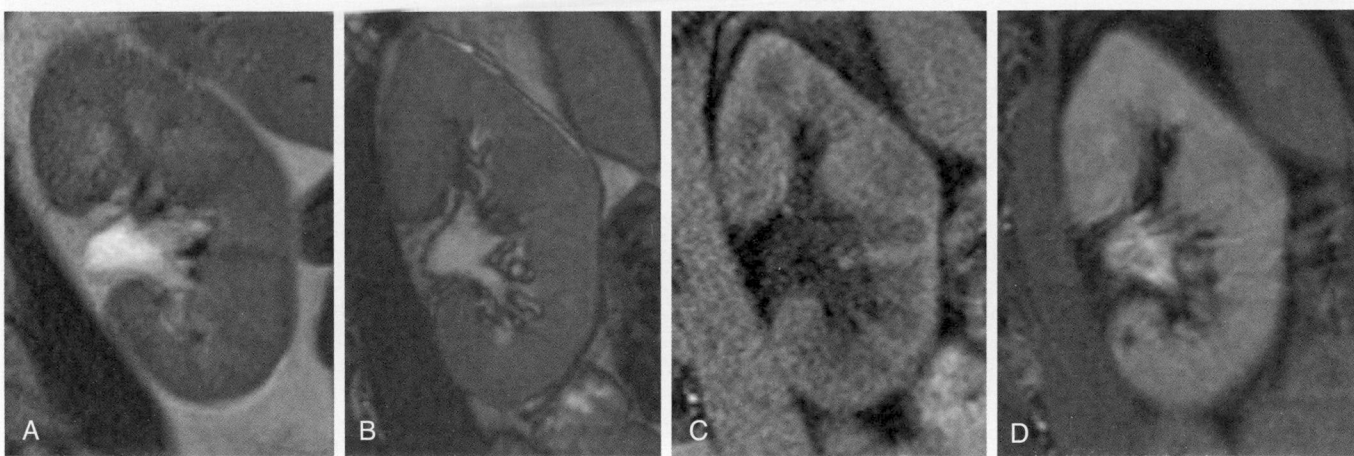

• **Fig. 6.7** Four coronal images of the same normal kidney with different MRI sequences (A-D, left to right): T2-weighted sequence, balanced steady state free procession sequence, T1-weighted sequence, postcontrast T1-weighted sequence.

images. Finally, cost and availability can be issues: MRI machines are expensive and require a great deal of maintenance, so the cost of these exams is greater than with other imaging modalities.

Kidney Scintigraphy

Kidney scintigraphy was developed early in the history of kidney imaging and remains a powerful technique for quantifying excretory function of the kidneys, particularly differential function between kidneys and assessing how much obstruction is occurring in a dilated collecting system.

The method of imaging is different than the techniques previously described. Whereas other techniques pass radiation *through* a

patient to generate an image, in kidney scintigraphy a radiotracer – a compound labeled with a radionuclide – *emits* radiation from within the patient and images are generated by a special camera that detects the radiation (Fig. 6.8A). These emissions can be tracked over time to indicate a tracer's passage within and through the kidney (Fig. 6.8B).

The biology of the radiotracer should inform the selection of the agent for specific clinical applications. For instance, a commonly used radiotracer, Technetium 99m-mercaptoacetyltriglycine (Tc-99m MAG3), is secreted by the proximal tubules, improving imaging in patients with reduced kidney function compared to other agents.

Although the quantitative abilities of kidney scintigraphy give it a special place within kidney imaging, scintigraphy also has some drawbacks. The radiotracers emit ionizing radiation, similar

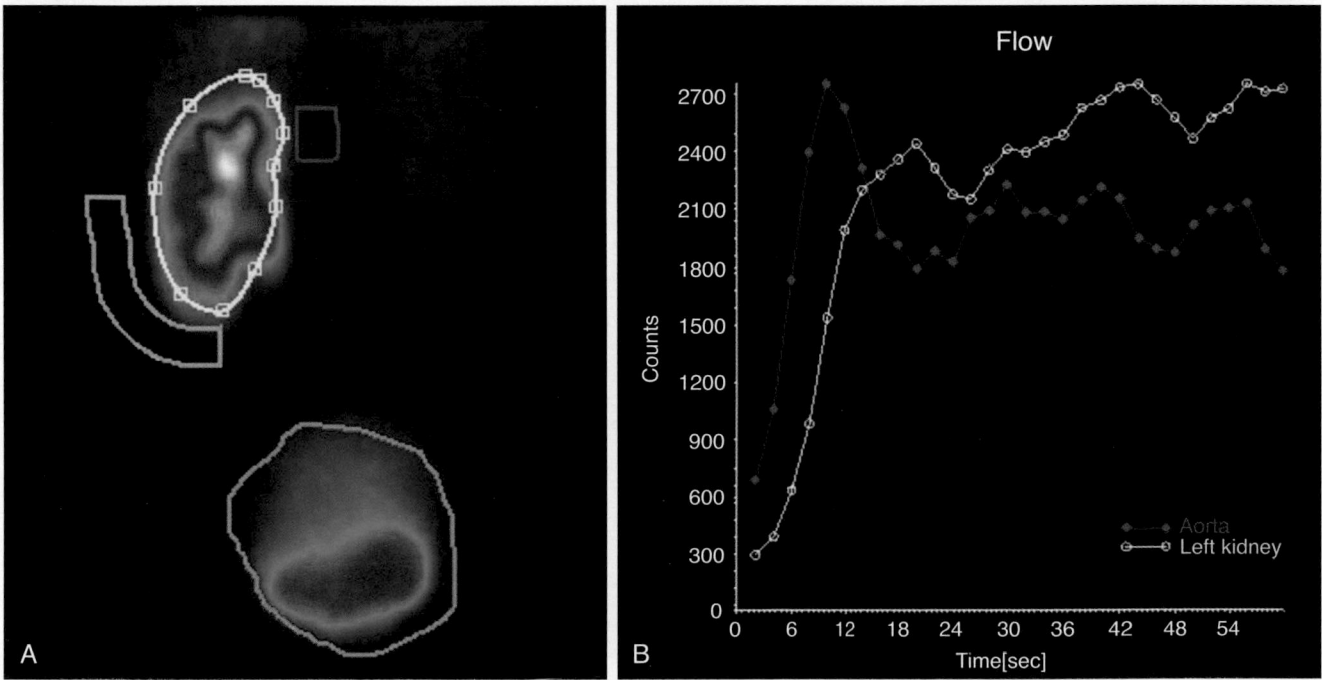

• **Fig. 6.8** Kidney scintigraphic evaluation of a solitary left kidney using Tc99m-MAG3 radiotracer. (A) Radiotracer is being excreted out of the normal kidney (yellow region of interest around the kidney). (B) Blood flow to the kidney is compared to the flow in the aorta, graphing the number of scintillations in the respective region of interest ("counts") on the y axis against time in seconds on the x axis.

to CT, but usually at a lower dose. The spatial resolution of the imaging is also poor relative to other imaging techniques, so kidney scintigraphy is often combined with ultrasound, CT, or MRI to appreciate both structure and function of the kidneys.

Kidney Cysts and Masses

Kidney cysts are commonly encountered lesions in general radiology practice. The term "cyst" encompasses epithelial cysts, peri/parapelvic cysts, and caliceal diverticula, which are benign and of no clinical consequence. On ultrasound, simple cysts are well-marginated, anechoic lesions with a thin wall. Simple cysts measure near water attenuation (range of 0-20 Hounsfield units) on CT, are hyperintense on T2-weighted images (similar to CSF or other fluid intensity structures) on MRI, and do not enhance with contrast.

The Bosniak classification, first described in 1986 and refined over time, has been widely used by radiologists and urologists to stratify the risk of cystic kidney lesions for malignancy based on contrast-enhanced CT characteristics (Fig. 6.9). Silverman et al. (2019) proposed an update to the Bosniak classification to better define imaging terms, formally incorporate MRI into the classification system, and improve sensitivity and specificity for malignancy. A simple cyst is categorized as Bosniak I. A Bosniak II lesion is a minimally complicated but benign cyst with few thin septa. A Bosniak IIF lesion is a complicated cyst with multiple thin septa or minimally thickened septa or wall. The "F" refers to "follow-up," as these lesions

are usually benign, but the risk of malignancy is non-zero; therefore imaging surveillance with ultrasound, CT, or MRI is recommended, reasonably at 6 months. A Bosniak III lesion has thick or irregular septa or wall. A Bosniak IV lesion has one or more enhancing nodules. Bosniak III and IV lesions are typically resected. In the 2019 update to the Bosniak classification, "few" has been defined as one to three and "multiple" as four or more, with regard to number of septa. The terms "thin," "minimally thickened," and "thick" have been assigned measurements of ≤2 mm, 3 mm, and ≥4 mm, respectively. The terms "irregular" and "nodule" also have defined imaging features and measurements. Calcifications of any morphology along septa or wall are now placed in the Bosniak II category, as these are not, as an isolated feature, predictive of malignancy.

Autosomal Dominant Polycystic Kidney Disease

Autosomal dominant polycystic kidney disease (ADPKD) is the most common hereditary cystic kidney disorder and typically leads to chronic kidney disease (CKD) in adulthood. Kidney cysts are both cortical and medullary in location and increase in size and number over time. The kidneys eventually become massively enlarged and replaced by innumerable cysts of varying sizes, with little identifiable normal kidney parenchyma (Fig. 6.10). Since kidney cysts are ubiquitous in practice, thresholds for considering a diagnosis of ADPKD have been devised that depend on age and whether or not the patient has a family history of the disease. If

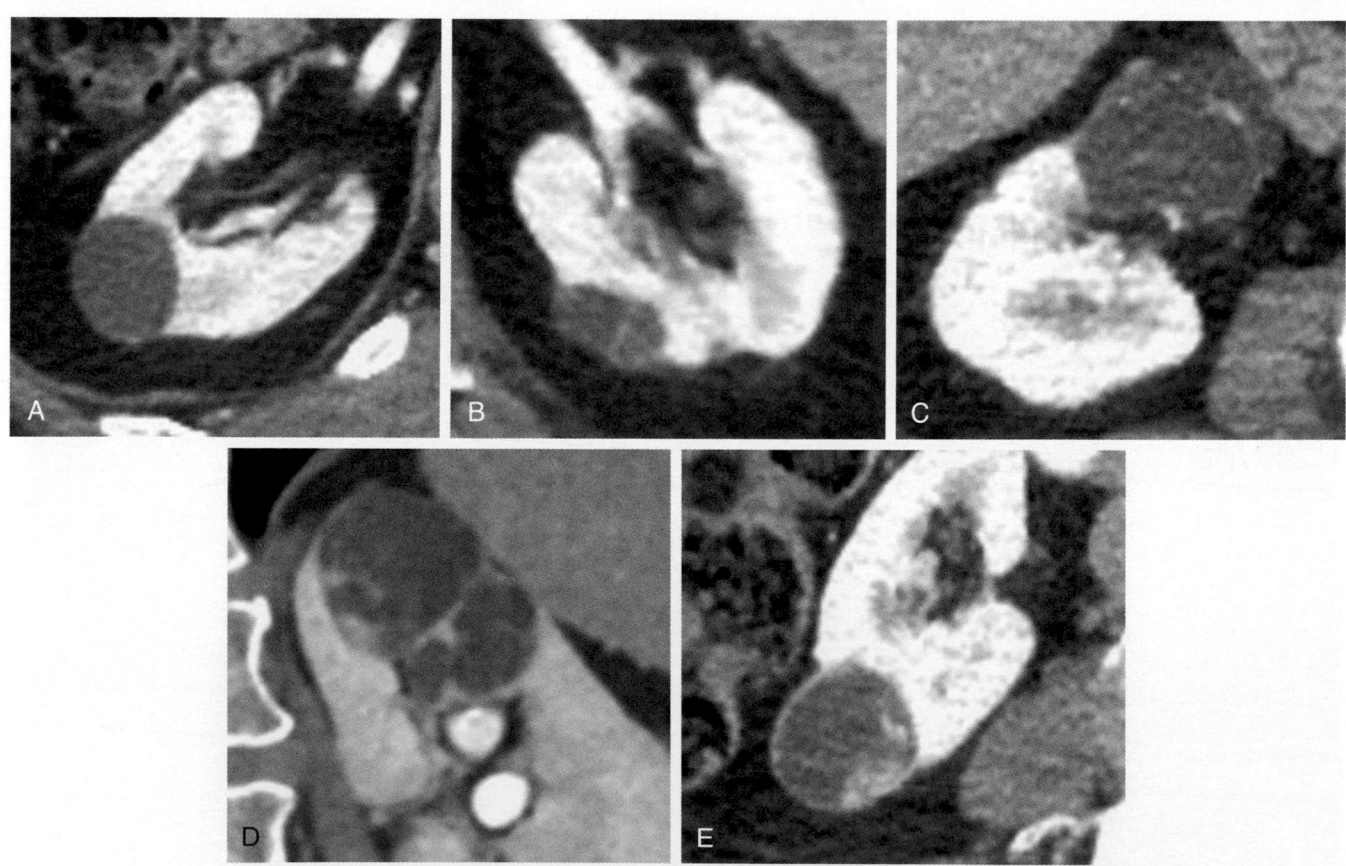

• **Fig. 6.9** Images of kidney cysts with varying degrees of complexity. The likelihood of cystic renal cell carcinoma based on the imaging appearance is captured in the Bosniak criteria. (A) Simple kidney cyst, Bosniak I. (B) Kidney cyst with a thin septation, Bosniak II. (C) Kidney cyst with multiple thin and minimally thickened septations, Bosniak IIF. (D) Kidney cyst with irregular enhancing septations, Bosniak III. (E) Kidney cyst with an enhancing mural nodule, Bosniak IV.

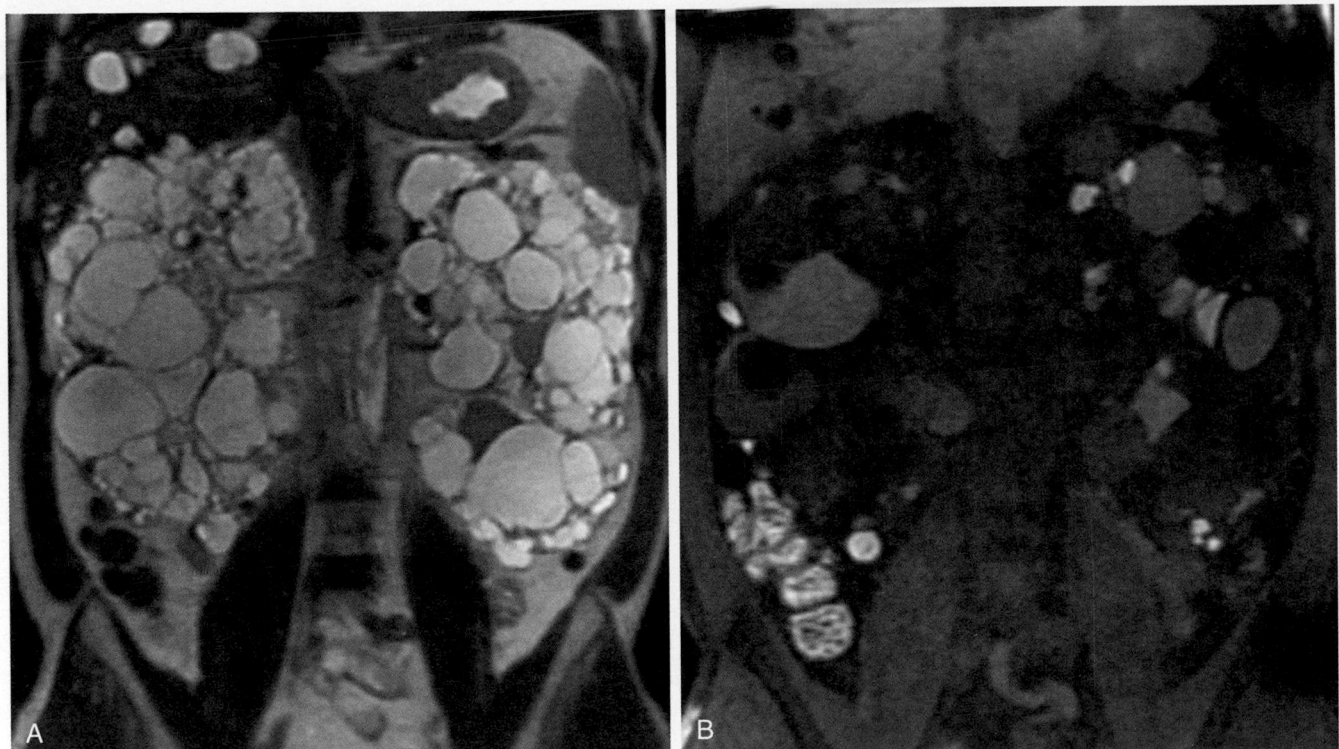

• **Fig. 6.10** Autosomal dominant polycystic kidney disease. (A) Coronal T2-weighted MR image demonstrates markedly enlarged kidneys with innumerable cysts. Most cysts are T2 hyperintense, indicating simple fluid, but others have variable intensity. (B) Coronal MR T1-weighted precontrast image demonstrates T1 hyperintensity of some cysts, indicating proteinaceous or hemorrhagic content.

the patient has a family history of ADPKD, and if the patient is less than 40 years of age, then three cysts bilaterally suggest the diagnosis; if 40-60 years old, then four cysts bilaterally; and if greater than 60 years old, then eight cysts bilaterally. If the patient has no family history of ADPKD, then ≥20 cysts distributed bilaterally is suggestive of the diagnosis.

While cysts are well seen by ultrasound, evaluation is challenging due to the large size of the kidneys, and evaluation is also limited by patient body habitus and operator experience. The Consortium for Radiologic Imaging Studies of Polycystic Kidney Disease (CRISP) has shown that total kidney volume (TKV), measured by MRI or CT, is a prognostic biomarker in assessing disease progression and treatment response. The gold standard for measuring TKV is manual segmentation, which is labor-intensive and requires radiological expertise and specialized computer software. The Mayo Clinic imaging classification (MCIC) risk assessment uses an ellipsoid formula, requiring only measurement of the three orthogonal axes of each kidney, which is more practical and still accurate. CT is a good modality to assess for complications such as hemorrhage, infection, or malignancy. The risk of renal cell carcinoma is not increased in ADPKD. However, MRI remains the preferred modality for identifying a solid mass among numerous cysts, due to superior soft tissue contrast, even without intravenous gadolinium.

Acquired Cystic Disease of Dialysis

Acquired cystic disease refers to the development of kidney cysts in patients with end-stage kidney disease, in the absence of a hereditary cystic kidney disorder. Cysts can be cortical or medullary in location, and the incidence increases with length of time on dialysis. Kidneys are small and echogenic on ultrasound. CT and MRI

better demonstrate cysts of varying size and complexity, typically less than <3 cm in diameter. There is an increased risk of developing renal cell carcinoma, which occurs in approximately 7% of patients. Kidney cysts regress after kidney transplant, but the increased risk of malignancy in the native kidneys persists. Screening of asymptomatic patients for malignancy is controversial.

Lithium-Induced Nephropathy

Lithium-induced nephropathy is a well-known entity seen in patients on long-term lithium therapy, with a characteristic imaging appearance. On ultrasound, kidneys are normal in size with numerous punctate echogenic foci. Abundant 1-2 mm T2 hyperintense cysts are seen in the kidney cortex and medulla on MRI (Fig. 6.11). Findings correspond to distal tubular dilatation with microcyst formation on pathology.

Glomerulocystic Disease

Glomerulocystic disease is a rare cystic kidney disorder characterized histologically by cystic dilatation of Bowman capsule. Kidneys are enlarged with multiple, mostly subcentimeter cortical cysts in a predominantly subcapsular distribution. Tiny cortical cysts are not discretely visible by ultrasound; rather, increased cortical echogenicity and loss of normal corticomedullary differentiation is typically seen.

Angiomyolipoma

Angiomyolipoma (AML) is a benign tumor composed of variable amounts of smooth muscle, blood vessels, and fat. Imaging diagnosis is based on the detection of fat. On ultrasound, AMLs are

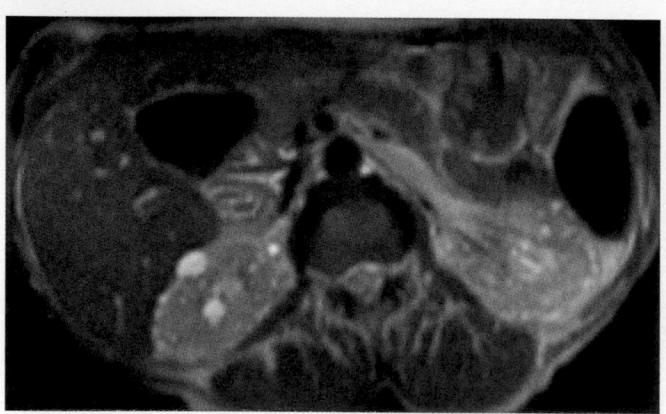

• **Fig. 6.11** Axial T2-weighted MR image of the kidneys, showing numerous tiny bright cysts in this patient with lithium-induced nephropathy.

including artifact, calcification, or complex cyst. Fat components are hypodense on CT, similar to intraabdominal fat. On MRI, angiomyolipomas follow the signal of intraabdominal fat on all sequences and lose signal on fat-saturated sequences (Fig. 6.12B-D). Non-fat components enhance avidly. Approximately 4% of angiomyolipomas are "fat poor" and cannot be differentiated from renal cell carcinoma. Angiomyolipomas are at risk for hemorrhage when large; therefore, referral to interventional radiology for embolization is suggested when these lesions reach 4 cm.

Renal Cell Carcinoma

Renal cell carcinoma (RCC) is the most common malignant neoplasm of the kidneys and is often incidentally identified on imaging studies performed for other reasons. Renal cell carcinoma has a varied appearance on ultrasound and can be solid, cystic with complex features, and hyper-, iso-, or hypoechoic relative to kidney parenchyma. The sensitivity of ultrasound is low for detecting small lesions. Characterization of kidney masses is usually done with multiphasic contrast-enhanced CT or MRI (Fig. 6.13). Clear cell RCC, the most common subtype, demonstrates avid

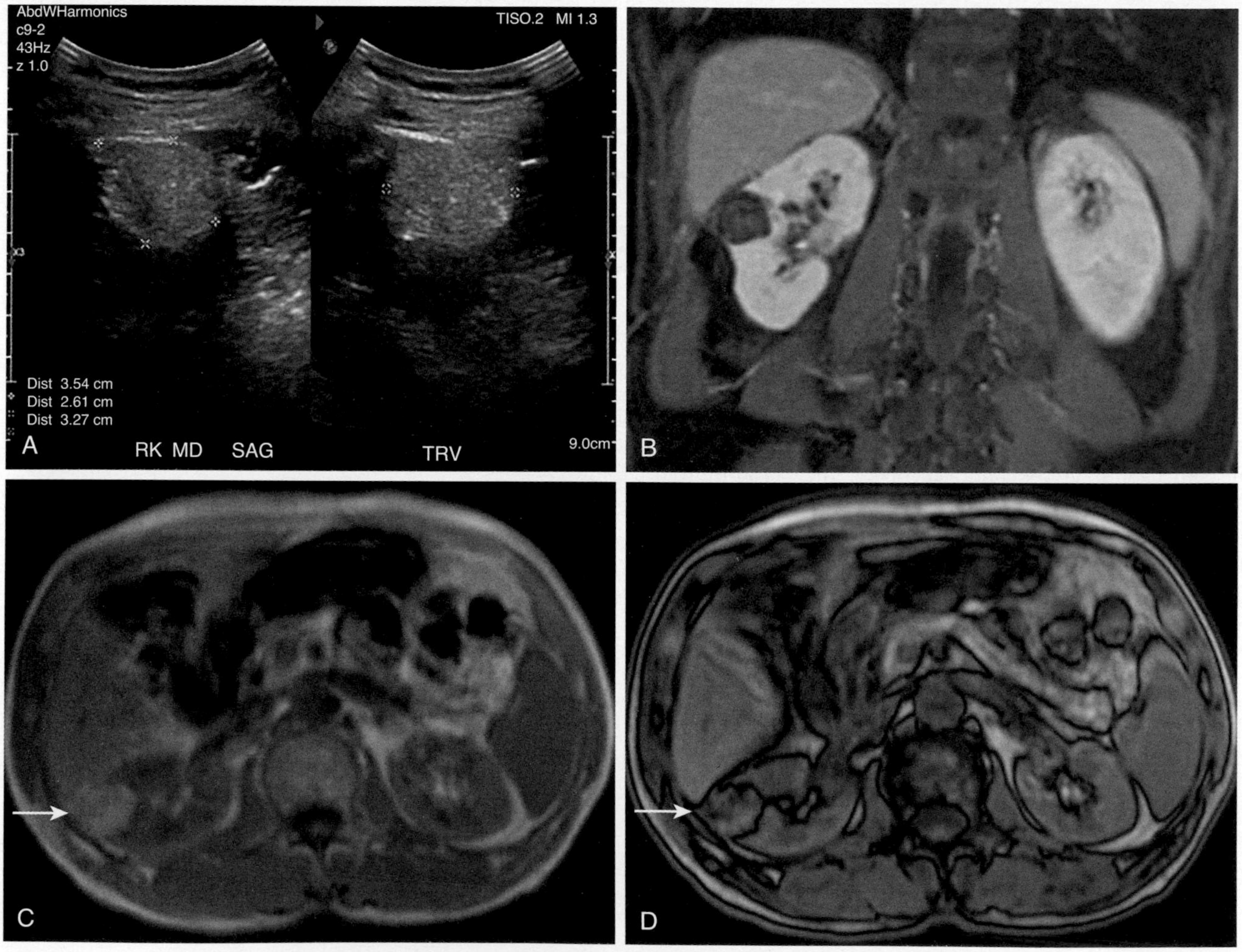

solid, echogenic lesions, with density similar to kidney sinus fat (Fig. 6.12A). Renal cell carcinomas can also appear echogenic on ultrasound. A vast majority of subcentimeter echogenic lesions are clinically insignificant, with differential considerations also

• **Fig. 6.12** Angiomyolipoma. (A) An echogenic mass is seen in the right kidney. (B) The mass demonstrates heterogeneous enhancement on the postcontrast T1-weighted sequence. (C, D) The mass follows signal intensity of intraabdominal fat on T1-weighted in- and out-of-phase GRE sequences. India ink artifact on the out-of-phase sequence (*arrow*) indicates a fat-water interface between the mass and the kidney parenchyma. The presence of bulk fat is diagnostic of an angiomyolipoma.

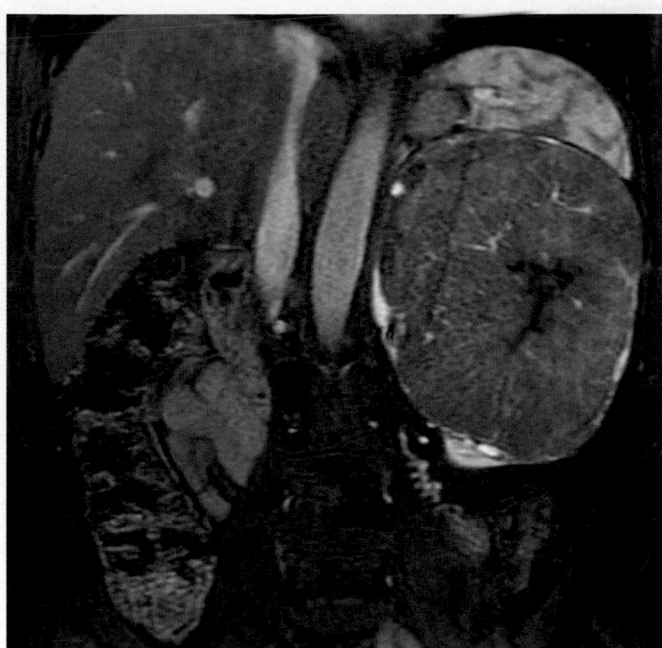

• **Fig. 6.13** Coronal postcontrast T1-weighted MR image shows a large hypoenhancing mass with a central scar arising from the left kidney, consistent with chromophobe subtype renal cell carcinoma.

enhancement in the corticomedullary phase and becomes hypoenhancing in the nephrographic phase. Chromophobe RCC also demonstrates avid enhancement in the corticomedullary phase, but to a lesser degree than the clear cell subtype. Papillary RCC is typically hypointense on T2-weighted imaging and hypoenhancing on all postcontrast phases. Contrast-enhanced CT and MRI yield similar information; however, MRI is more sensitive for identifying complex features within cysts, such as wall thickening or septations, as well as detecting enhancement through the use of subtraction imaging.

Contrast-enhanced ultrasound is a relatively new and inexpensive tool for characterizing kidney masses, with advantages over the traditional imaging modalities. The contrast agent is comprised of microbubbles that are non-toxic to the kidneys, making CEUS an attractive option for patients with a reduced glomerular filtration rate (GFR). Clear cell RCC demonstrates avid early enhancement, a pseudocapsule, and early washout. Papillary RCC is, again, hypoenhancing on all phases. Larger lesions typically enhance more heterogeneously than small lesions.

Kidney Lymphoma

Kidney lymphoma typically occurs in the setting of widespread non-Hodgkin lymphoma. Primary kidney lymphoma (isolated to kidneys with no systemic manifestations) accounts for <1% of extranodal lymphoma and is thought to originate from the lymphatic-rich kidney capsule or perinephric fat or arise from lymphocytes present in areas of chronic inflammation. Imaging patterns of lymphoma are variable and include multiple masses (most common), solitary masses, direct extension from retroperitoneal lymphadenopathy, diffuse infiltration and nephromegaly, and perirenal soft tissue.

Other Kidney Imaging Findings

Nephrolithiasis

Urolithiasis affects up to 6% to 12% of Americans during their lifetimes and costs billions of dollars each year. Acute abdominal pain accounts for up to 10% of all emergency department visits, with about a third of those attributed to kidney "colic."

Because of its high sensitivity and specificity, availability, and ease of performance, unenhanced CT is frequently the primary imaging modality for evaluation of kidney stone disease (Fig. 6.14). Technological advances, including tube current modulation and iterative reconstruction, have reduced the ionizing radiation dose while maintaining diagnostic imaging quality, often referred to as "low-dose kidney protocol" studies. The anatomic definition of CT allows direct visualization of a calculus within the urinary tract; if a calculus is not directly visualized, findings of dilation of the urinary collecting system or infection are secondary signs of urolithiasis.

Radiography, specifically IVU (intravenous urography) and KUB abdominal radiographs (kidney ureter bladder), was previously the mainstay for kidney stone evaluation (Fig. 6.15); however, radiography is not as sensitive or specific as CT because overlapping structures can obscure kidney stones. While also less sensitive than CT, ultrasound does not utilize ionizing radiation and remains useful in the evaluation of kidney stone disease (Fig. 6.16), particularly in patients who are young, pregnant, or have recurrent stone disease. The use of MR in the setting of kidney colic is still evolving, as many calculi do not produce MR signal.

Obstructive Uropathy

Urinary tract obstruction is common and can lead to GFR loss, termed *obstructive nephropathy*; approximately 10% of all kidney failure cases result from obstructive uropathy. Numerous pathologic processes can impede urine flow.

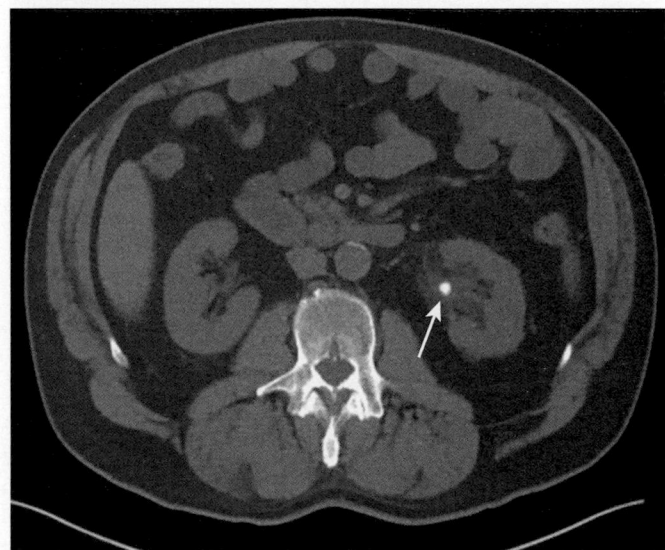

• **Fig. 6.14** Unenhanced axial CT image shows an 8-mm obstructing calculus at the left ureteropelvic junction (*arrow*) with associated inflammatory changes.

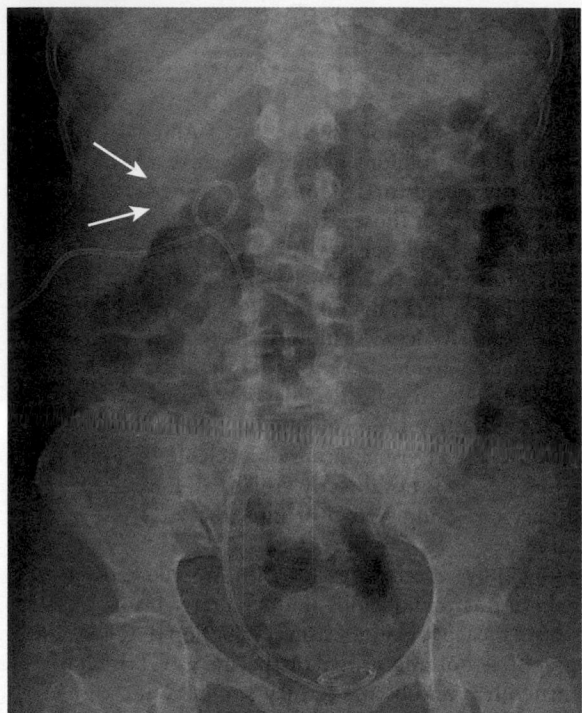

• **Fig. 6.15** Abdominal radiograph shows two adjacent calcifications overlying the upper aspect of the right kidney shadow, consistent with kidney calculi (*arrows*). A right percutaneous nephroureterostomy catheter, seen looped in the kidney pelvis, follows the course of the ureter, and terminates in the bladder.

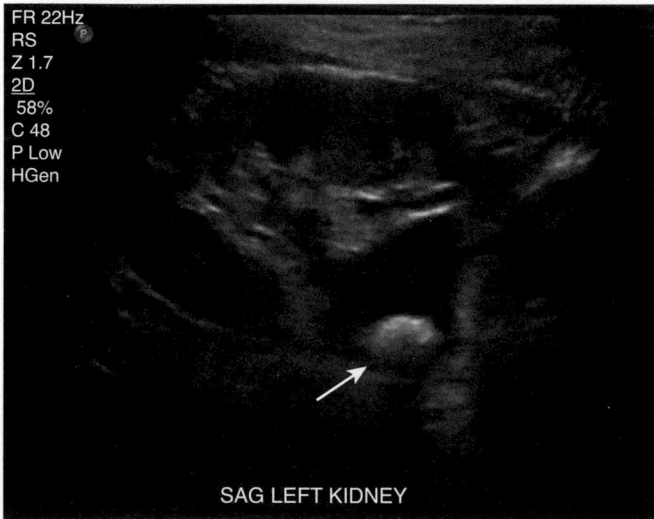

• **Fig. 6.16** Long axis ultrasound image of the left kidney shows a shadowing calculus (*white arrow*) at the left ureteropelvic junction (UPJ). Associated mild hydronephrosis suggests obstruction.

While often the primary imaging study because of low cost and lack of ionizing radiation, kidney ultrasound will be normal in about 50% of cases of acute urinary obstruction. Also, anatomical hydronephrosis on ultrasound suggests but does not indicate underlying urinary tract obstruction. Many patients will have a CT or CT urography during the work-up for obstructive uropathy.

Benign prostatic hypertrophy, urolithiasis, cancer, ureteral/urethral stricture, and ureteropelvic junction stenosis are common

etiologies of urinary tract obstruction. Ureteral obstruction may result from less common entities, such as from a blood clot, sloughed papilla, fungus ball, or bezoar. Ureteral clot, for instance, is the consequence of intraureteral hemorrhage, such as from calculi, underlying tumor, or trauma; hyperattenuating blood within a collecting system or ureter is best appreciated on unenhanced CT images and will not enhance on a contrast-enhanced study (Fig. 6.17).

Kidney Infection

Urinary tract infections (UTIs) are the most common bacterial infection. UTIs accounted for approximately 10.5 million office visits and 2 to 3 million ED visits in the United States in 2007. Both pyelonephritis and kidney abscess usually result from retrograde bladder infection.

Imaging Features of Pyelonephritis

Ultrasound is insensitive in detecting pyelonephritis, with abnormalities identified in about 25% of patients. Sonographic findings include abnormal echogenicity of the kidney parenchyma, specifically hypoechoic areas of edema or hyperechoic areas of hemorrhage; associated hypoperfusion of these regions may be detected with color Doppler imaging. The anatomic detail of CT and MRI enable increased sensitivity and specificity for detection of pyelonephritis. Kidney enlargement, wedge-shaped areas of hypoenhancement extending through the cortex (striated nephrogram), and perinephric inflammatory changes are findings that suggest pyelonephritis (Fig. 6.18).

Imaging Features of Kidney Abscess

On ultrasound, a kidney abscess is a circumscribed hypoechoic mass that demonstrates posterior acoustic enhancement but is without internal vascularity on color Doppler ultrasound; solid masses, by comparison, will typically have internal vascularity. A peripherally enhancing kidney mass that is centrally hypoattenuating on contrast-enhanced CT indicates a kidney abscess. Additional findings on MRI are central diffusion restriction and heterogeneity on T1- and T2-weighted images from internal debris (Fig. 6.19).

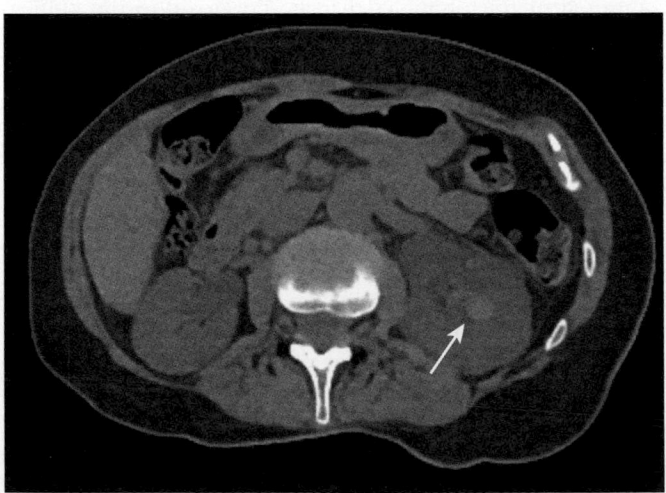

• **Fig. 6.17** Unenhanced axial CT image shows a hyperattenuating focus in the left kidney pelvis (*arrow*), which was confirmed as a blood clot. Mild left kidney enlargement and hydronephrosis from additional left ureteral clot (not shown).

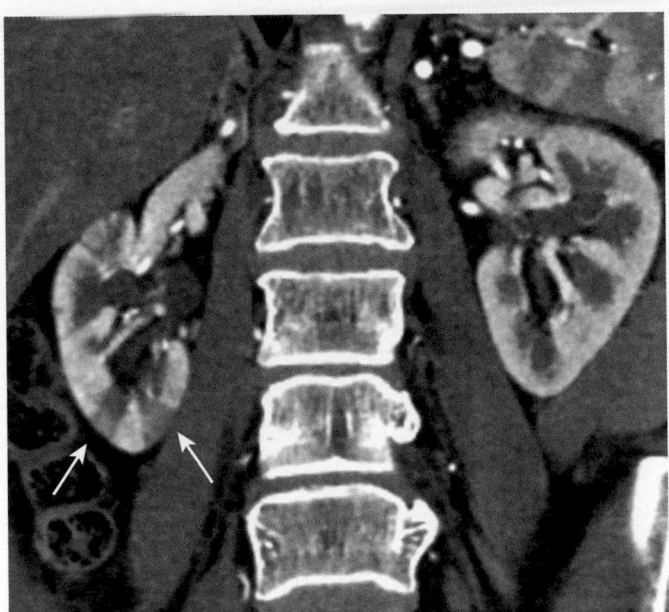

• **Fig. 6.18** Contrast-enhanced coronal CT image showing the wedge-shaped hypoenhancing areas (*white arrows*) of the right kidney, known as a *striated nephrogram*, in this patient with pyelonephritis. Normal corticomedullary enhancement of the left kidney.

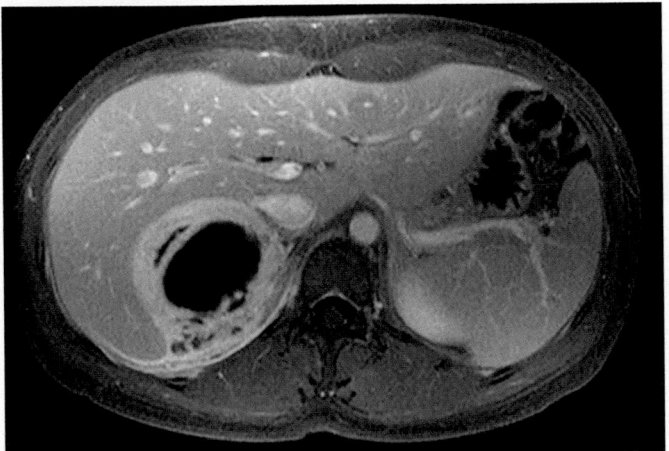

• **Fig. 6.19** Axial postgadolinium axial MR images of a patient with a right upper pole kidney abscess that extends into the perirenal space.

Radionuclide Kidney Evaluation and Obstruction

Nuclear imaging of the kidneys enables real-time visualization of kidney physiology through the detection of emissions from injected radiotracers. By analyzing the uptake and excretion of the radiotracer, several diagnoses can be made. With advances in other radiologic modalities (such as ultrasound, CT, and MRI), kidney scintigraphy is now most often utilized in the evaluation of obstruction in non-pediatric medicine. In this section, we will discuss specific kidney radiotracers, imaging protocols, and imaging interpretation, with a focus on assessment of kidney obstruction.

Several radiotracers are currently utilized to image the kidneys, with the specific clinical indication matched to radiotracer biology:

1. ^{99m}Tc-Dimercaptosuccinic Acid (DMSA): This agent binds to the proximal tubule to enable static imaging of the kidney cortex. ^{99m}Tc-DMSA is primarily used in pediatric patients to detect areas of decreased radiotracer uptake in the kidney cortex representing scarring from pyelonephritis.
2. ^{99m}Tc-Diethylenetriaminepentaacetic Acid (DTPA): This agent is filtered by the glomeruli and not secreted. ^{99m}Tc-DTPA can be used to measure GFR and image for obstruction.
3. ^{99m}Tc-Mercaptoacetyltriglycine (MAG3): This agent is predominately bound to plasma proteins and excreted through tubular secretion. Compared to ^{99m}Tc-DTPA, ^{99m}Tc-MAG3 has a greater extraction fraction and is the preferred agent for patients with reduced GFR and in the evaluation of obstruction.

The imaging protocol to evaluate for obstruction includes several basic elements, with numerous variations. After the intravenous injection of the radiotracer, images are taken posteriorly, owing to the retroperitoneal location of the kidneys. Immediate imaging with short frame captures kidney perfusion. Frame duration is then increased, and imaging continues for approximately 20 minutes. Kidney split function is calculated between 1-3 minutes by dividing the counts in each kidney by the sum of the counts in both kidneys. This early time period is chosen so that the radiotracer has been taken up by the kidney cortex but not yet excreted into the collecting system. A diuretic may then be given, and imaging continued for another 20 minutes. The patient is then asked to void and additional images are then obtained.

The diagnosis of kidney obstruction is made through visual inspection of the radiotracer uptake and excretion by the kidneys over time. Time-activity curves depicting the number of counts in the kidney as a function of time and various quantitative metrics can aid in making a diagnosis. A normal non-obstructed kidney demonstrates prompt blood flow, corticomedullary transit, and clearance of radiotracer from the collecting system prior to diuretic administration, with augmentation thereafter (Fig. 6.20). Obstruction is characterized by radiotracer delivery to a kidney without excretion over the imaging interval, even after diuretic administration (Fig. 6.20D-F); a post-void image demonstrates radiotracer retention. Without appropriate medical intervention, obstruction may result in GFR loss. Of note, the evaluation of obstruction is precluded in a poorly functioning kidney. A non-obstructed but patulous collecting system would demonstrate poor excretion prior to diuretic excretion, but brisk excretion after a diuretic challenge (Fig. 6.20G-I).

By imaging kidney physiology through detection of radiotracer emissions, nuclear imaging retains a specific niche in the evaluation of certain kidney pathology, including obstruction.

Diffuse Kidney Parenchymal Disease

Ultrasound is often ordered in the setting of decreased estimated GFR, either acute or chronic, with the intention of identifying urinary obstruction manifesting as hydronephrosis. Although valuable for this indication, imaging can also show changes from diffuse kidney parenchymal disease in patients.

One common manifestation of chronic kidney damage on imaging is parenchymal thinning. Normal kidney parenchyma is at least 1.5 cm in thickness. If one can resolve the cortex from the medulla, then the normal cortical thickness is at least 1 cm. The kidney usually measures >10 cm in length in a patient <60 years of age, so decreased kidney size, particularly in the craniocaudal dimension, is often a marker of CKD. Reduced visual differentiation between the cortex and medulla is also thought to be a sign of diffuse kidney disease.

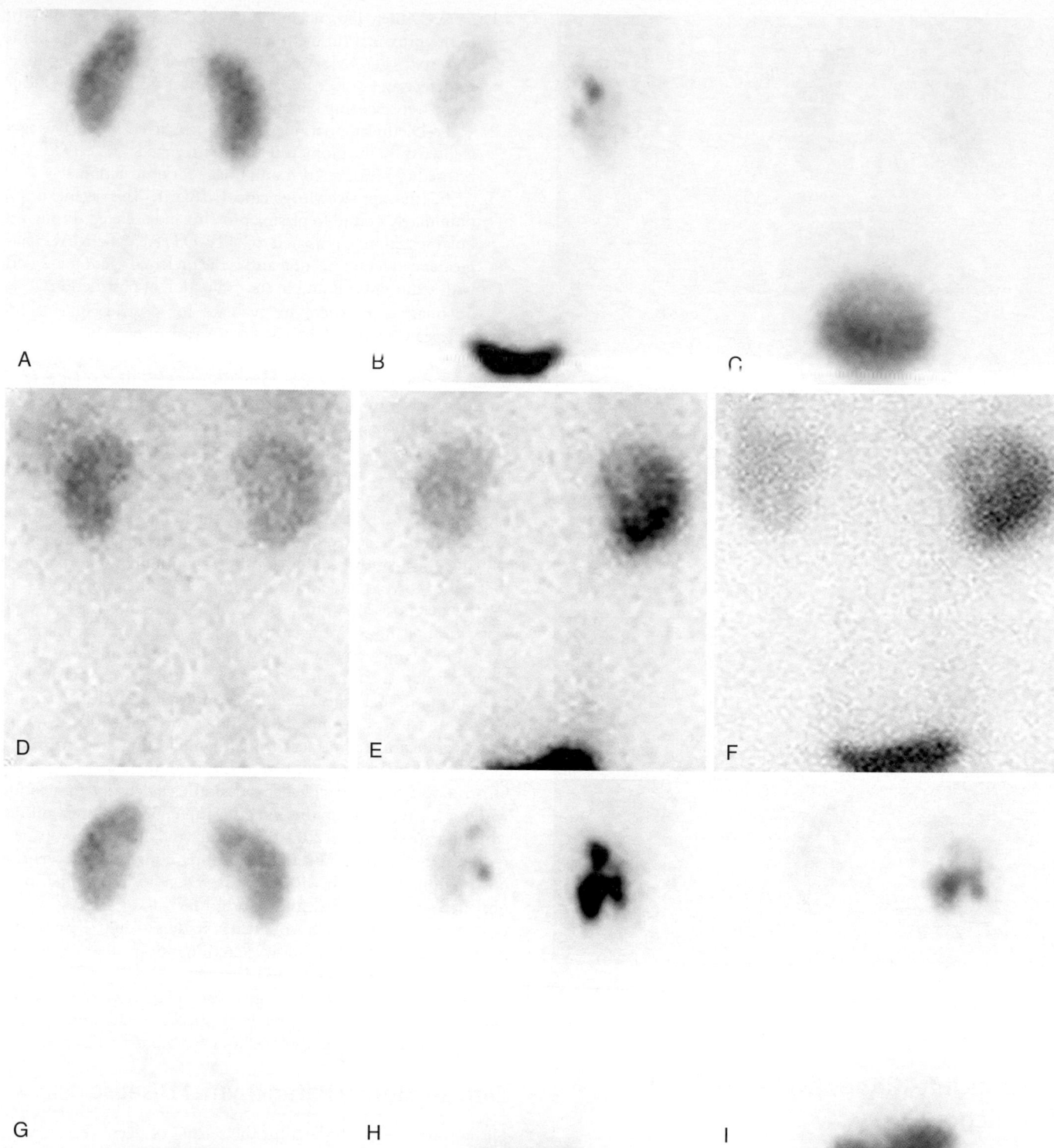

• **Fig. 6.20** (A–C) Normal diuretic renogram demonstrates relatively equal differential function (A at 2 min) and excretion prior to (B at 20 min) and after furosemide administration at 20 min (C at 39 min). (D-F) Obstructive diuretic renogram demonstrates relatively equal differential function (D at 2 min) without significant excretion from the right kidney before or after furosemide was given at 20 min (E at 40.5 min and F after voiding). (G-I) Diuretic renogram of a non-obstructed, dilated collecting system demonstrates relatively equal differential function (G at 2 min) with progressive radiotracer accumulation in the collecting system prior to furosemide administration (H at 20 min). After furosemide administration at 20 min, there is prompt clearance from the collecting system (I at 39 min).

It is not uncommon to see some areas of thinning within the kidney parenchyma, whereas other areas are of normal thickness. This is often a result of focal scarring from old infectious or inflammatory events. More severe and extensive thinning suggests a history of untreated vesico-ureteral reflux.

Parenchymal or cortical thickness can be assessed in CT, MRI, or ultrasound, but a finding specific to the ultrasound evaluation of CKD is increased echogenicity of the kidney cortex (Fig. 6.21). The increased brightness of the cortex is thought to result from a combination of sclerosis, focal tubular atrophy, and hyaline casts, and is not specific to any particular kidney disease.

There are some problems with using cortical echogenicity to evaluate for kidney disease, however. One is that the "brightness" of the parenchyma is a qualitative finding. This can be addressed by comparing the right kidney echogenicity against the adjacent liver, presupposing that the liver is normal; the liver, too, can become bright, for instance, if there is liver steatosis. Another problem is that making a reliable judgment about kidney echogenicity requires careful attention to the ultrasound technique. Accidentally using the wrong settings on the machine can spuriously increase the echogenicity in the cortex and result in a false imaging diagnosis. Finally, increased echogenicity is usually associated with more advanced disease. Early kidney parenchymal disease is often difficult, if not impossible, to detect.

Although not in routine use, color Doppler has been investigated as a way to evaluate for damaged microcirculation in the kidneys and to use this as a marker for diffuse parenchymal disease. Similarly, ultrasound elastography has been suggested as a tool to evaluate for diffuse parenchymal disease but is still investigational.

Renal Artery Stenosis

Imaging for renal artery stenosis usually occurs in a setting in which there is presumed renovascular disease, but in which blood pressure is not well controlled with medications. In this situation, imaging can help determine if there is renal artery narrowing, if it is bilateral, and whether it is high grade.

Renal artery stenosis, particularly from atherosclerosis, can be suggested on CT angiography, but this is through morphologic findings of the renal artery, the downstream kidney, and secondary signs of decreased blood flow. MRI angiography can also be useful for morphologic evaluation of the renal arteries (Fig. 6.22). One of the more useful functions of cross-sectional imaging may be in identifying features of the affected kidney that indicate longstanding disease (such as decreased kidney size) and a low likelihood of benefit of intervention. Indirect evaluation of a blood pressure gradient across a renal artery lesion is tricky on cross-sectional imaging, however. Special MRI sequences to evaluate cortical hypoxia (BOLD-MRI) are possible, but not common in clinical use.

Because of this limitation, a more common screening study for renal artery stenosis is Doppler ultrasound, even though it is thought to be less accurate overall relative to CT angiography. The idea is that even if a pressure/flow-limiting stenosis in the main renal artery may not be seen on ultrasound, it should cause sufficient change to a spectral Doppler waveform to allow detection (Fig. 6.23). Assessment of the main renal artery waveform is thought to be more reliable than evaluation of the parenchymal waveforms, and a peak systolic velocity of 100-200 cm/s in the main renal artery is a common threshold for a diagnosis of flow-limiting renal artery stenosis. The sensitivity and specificity of this cutoff will vary depending on the threshold one chooses, and the higher the velocity, the more assured one can be that there is a flow-limiting stenosis. Other Doppler parameters have been investigated, but none has currently supplanted peak systolic velocity. Contrast-enhanced ultrasound has also been evaluated, but its diagnostic role is currently undefined and it is not routinely used in clinical practice.

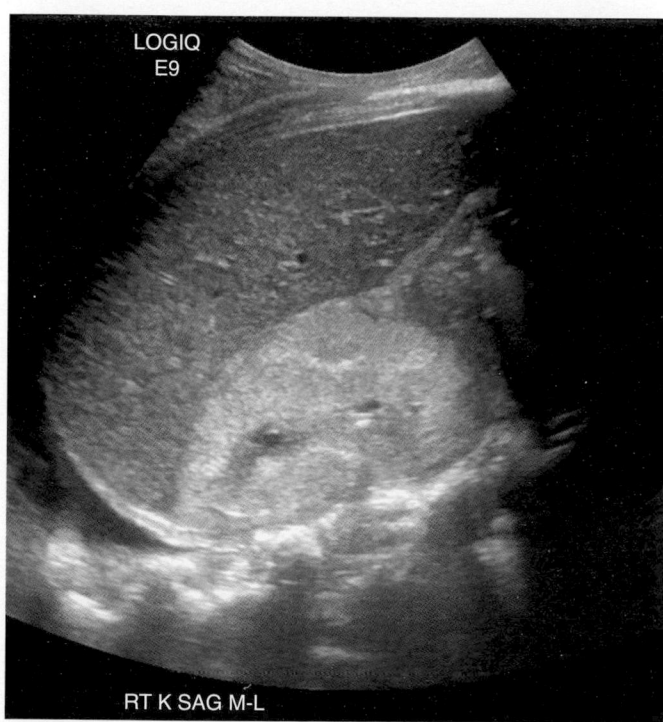

• **Fig. 6.21** A long axis image of the right kidney shows that the parenchyma is brightly echogenic relative to the overlying liver, indicating chronic parenchymal injury in a patient with longstanding HIV nephropathy.

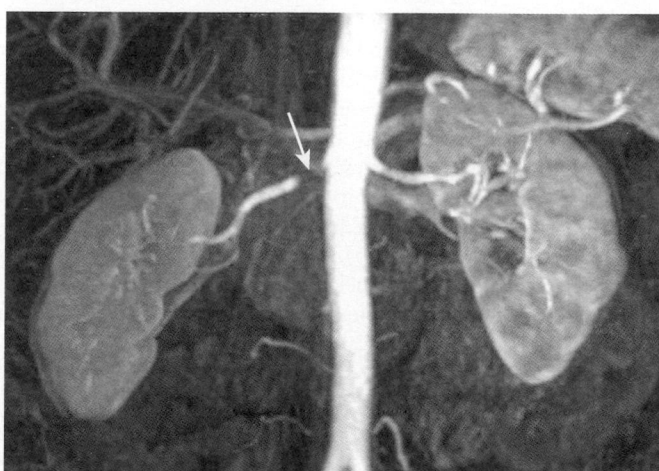

• **Fig. 6.22** Coronal maximum intensity projection (MIP) MRI image. Gadolinium contrast was administered. There is a tight stenosis at the origin of the right renal artery (*arrow*). There is contrast distal to the stenosis, suggesting that the stenosis is not completely occlusive, although this tiny amount of flow is obscured. The right kidney is hypoenhancing relative to the left, suggesting that this stenosis is flow limiting.

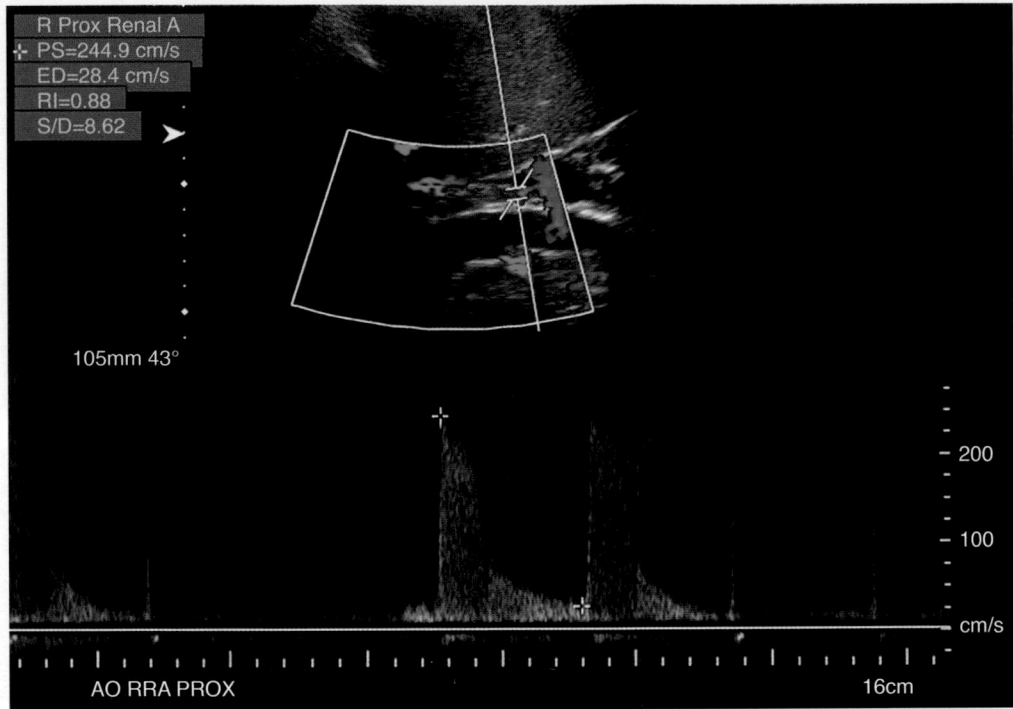

• **Fig. 6.23** An example of renal artery stenosis on spectral Doppler evaluation. The spectrum at the bottom of the image shows a peak systolic velocity of 245 cm/s, compatible with severe renal artery stenosis. The color Doppler image at the top shows the vessel from which the spectrum is being acquired.

There are other drawbacks to ultrasound evaluation, however, in addition to the decreased accuracy relative to cross-sectional angiography. Although there is no ionizing radiation involved, which is ideal for a screening procedure, it is one of the most technically demanding studies for a sonographer to perform, contributing to the heterogeneity in accuracy in practice. It is also limited by bowel gas and patient body habitus, particularly when evaluating the origins of the renal arteries. Finally, ultrasound is limited in detection of fibromuscular dysplasia and accessory/polar arteries relative to CT and MRI angiography.

Conventional angiography with measurement of the pressure gradient over a stenosis is the gold standard for imaging evaluation (Fig. 6.24). A decrease in kidney pressure sufficient to activate the RAAS pathway usually requires >60% luminal narrowing, and because of the small artery size, the degree of spatial resolution on cross-sectional imaging is not as great as that with catheter-based angiography. Nevertheless, agreement between angiograph and CT angiography is high. Because of the invasive nature of catheter-based angiography, it usually is reserved for a preinterventional evaluation (Fig. 6.25).

Captopril renography, a nuclear medicine technique, has been performed in the past for evaluation of renal artery stenosis, but it is no longer in common clinical use.

Imaging in Kidney Transplant

Ultrasound is the primary imaging technique for evaluating a kidney allograft. It can image the transplant morphology with grayscale imaging and assess perfusion with color Doppler without requiring intravenous contrast. Spectral Doppler evaluation, interpreting velocity of blood flow through Doppler shifts, is particularly valuable for assessing acute complications of transplantation, which are frequently due to problems with the vascular anastomosis. Spectral Doppler can also signal more diffuse parenchymal abnormalities after the initial postsurgical period, such as that of chronic transplant rejection.

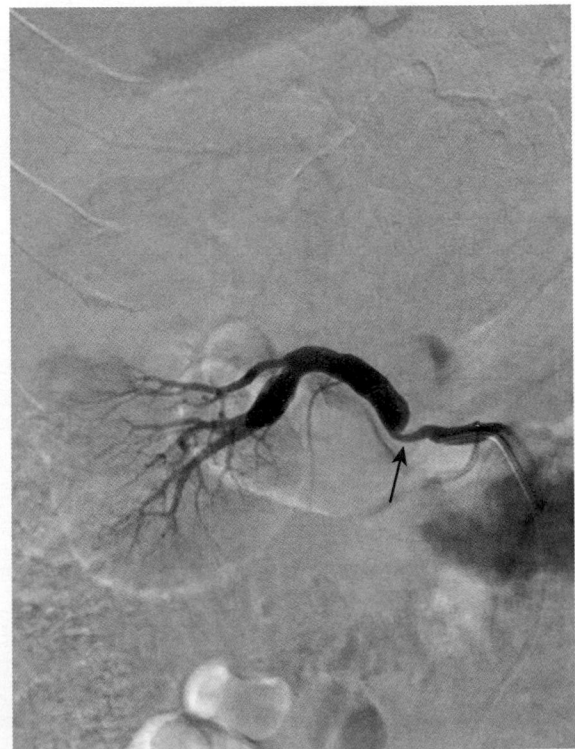

• **Fig. 6.24** Catheter angiogram of renal artery stenosis. The region of narrowing in the renal artery is indicated by the arrow. The catheter is positioned in front of the narrowing.

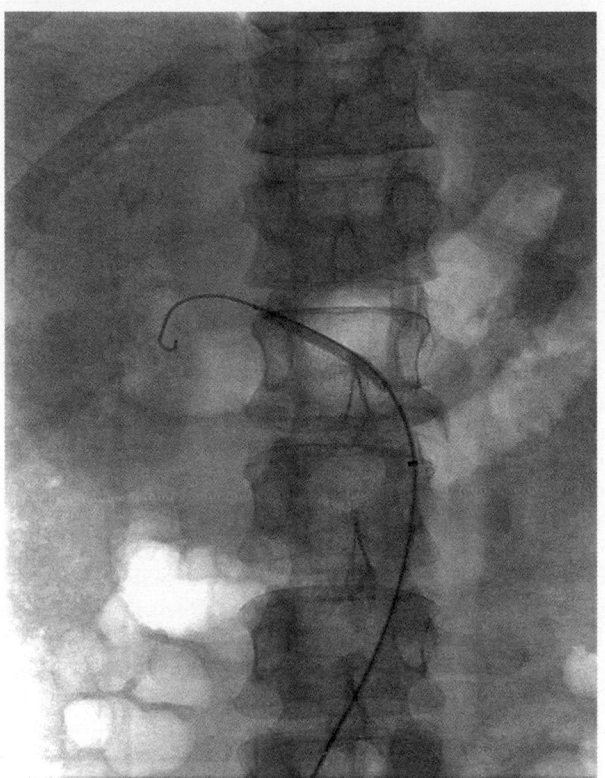

• **Fig. 6.25** A wire has been passed across the right renal artery stenosis and a balloon has been inflated as part of an angioplasty procedure.

Early postoperative complications include renal artery and renal vein thrombosis, acute compartment syndrome, and peritransplant fluid collections, such as a hematomas or urine leaks. Later, transplant rejection (particularly T-cell-mediated rejection) as well as interstitial fibrosis and tubular atrophy are more of a concern. Problems at the vascular anastomoses, including thrombosis and stenosis, are usually evaluated directly, and an elevated velocity across an anastomosis signals flow-limiting stenosis similar in concept to evaluation for renal artery stenosis in a native kidney (above). The transplant parenchymal resistive indices have been relied upon as a screening marker for rejection. Increasing resistive indices to greater than 0.80 is consistent with transplant rejection that may warrant confirmation with a transplant biopsy.

Ultrasound has limitations over CT and MRI. For instance, bowel gas (or postsurgical gas in an acute setting) blocks sound waves and may obscure the kidney. Deeper structures may be harder to resolve, such as deep pelvic collections or complex vascular anastomoses. Similarly, transplants in patients with an expanded abdominal mass may be harder to resolve clearly.

Doppler also has some limitations. Although a powerful tool for evaluating flow in the major kidney vessels and at the periphery, it may struggle to detect small (or sometimes large) areas of decreased perfusion. Contrast-enhanced ultrasound will likely improve evaluation of perfusion. The accuracy of kidney resistive indices for detecting rejection has also been debated.

Another limitation of ultrasound is that it can only imply the function of the transplant through a combination of grayscale and Doppler findings. Nuclear medicine studies, however, are capable of evaluating transplant function by examining the clearance of a radiotracer.

Other imaging techniques such as fluoroscopy, CT, and MRI can be used for evaluating other issues in kidney transplants. MRI can obtain excellent tissue contrast without IV contrast agents, whereas CT often needs iodinated contrast agents to adequately distinguish the allograft. This distinction has become less of an issue with the rise of group II gadolinium-based contrast agents (see the following section).

Despite these focused applications, however, ultrasound is the primary tool in kidney transplant imaging and likely will be for the foreseeable future, especially as ultrasound contrast agents are likely to become more common.

Contrast Agents for Imaging

Intravascular contrast agents are a critical component of imaging to help delineate the structure of organs and to develop a differential diagnosis. Because most contrast agents are excreted by the kidneys, they also draw special attention from the nephrologist.

Currently, there are three types of contrast agents in common clinical use. Iodinated contrast agents are designed to interact with an x-ray beam and are employed in CT imaging. Gadolinium-based contrast agents are designed to affect the spin of nearby surrounding protons and are used in MR imaging. Ultrasound contrast agents are a species of "microbubble" comprised of gas trapped within a protein, lipid, or polymer shell.

Iodinated Contrast Agents

Iodinated contrast agents have received special attention from clinicians because of their potential for nephrotoxicity and hypersensitivity reactions after intravascular administration.

Administration of any contrast agent should be evaluated as a risk versus benefit tradeoff, similar to the administration of any medication. For iodinated contrast agents, the benefits are significant. Iodinated agents allow accurate visualization of vessels and allow the radiologist to assess how tissues are being perfused, markedly expanding and improving a differential diagnosis. For kidney imaging in particular, iodinated contrast helps differentiate kidney inflammation from other processes, and relative excretion can be assessed in a qualitative way. CT angiograms evaluate vessel patency. For urologic imaging, excreted iodinated contrast is invaluable for CT urograms that evaluate kidney masses, ureters, and the bladder.

Iodinated contrast agents are excreted by the kidney and have been associated with reduced GFR. Historically, this has been described as "contrast-induced nephropathy" (CIN), although the pathophysiology of CIN is unclear and a direct causal link between administration of intravenous contrast and nephropathy is not always clear. More recently, the American College of Radiology adopted the term "postcontrast acute kidney injury" (PC-AKI) as a more general means to describe a decrease in kidney function (usually indicated by elevation in serum creatinine) after administration of contrast. CIN would be included as a subset of PC-AKI in which the causal relationship between the iodinated contrast and the depressed kidney function is clear and direct. Intraarterial administration of iodinated contrast, such as with fluoroscopic angiography, is also thought to have more nephrotoxic effect than intravenous administration, which is typical for CT imaging. Decreased kidney function can occasionally be seen on CT when contrast is "trapped" in the kidney (Fig. 6.26) and not being effectively excreted. This appearance is not truly specific for CIN.

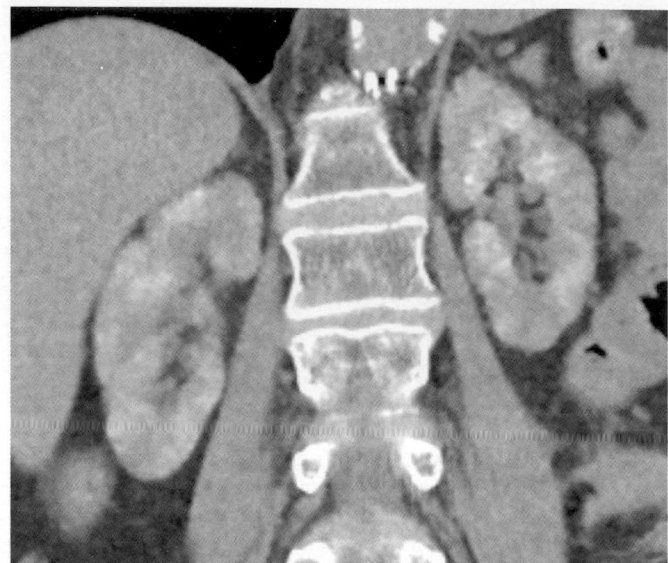

• **Fig. 6.26** Retained contrast in the kidneys, indicating a marked decrease in urinary excretory function and kidney injury. In this coronal CT image, patchy areas of contrast can be seen in both kidney parenchyma; however, no contrast has been given for this abdominal study. Instead, the patient received iodinated contrast for a CT angiogram of the head and neck 16 hours earlier.

Advanced CKD is considered a risk factor for the development of CIN, but there is no agreed-upon serum creatinine or eGFR threshold that defines a patient at risk. Administration of iodinated contrast in patients with reduced GFR should be thought of as a spectrum along a risk/benefit decision. Serum creatinine above 1.5 to 2.0 mg/dL or an eGFR below 30 mL/min are commonly used thresholds to reconsider risk and benefit. Other risk factors have been suggested, including age >60 years, heart failure, diabetes mellitus, anemia, and volume and route of administered contrast, but these have not been clearly shown to be independent risk factors for development of CIN.

Kidney protective maneuvers from iodinated contrast have been extensively studied, including sodium bicarbonate, N-acetylcysteine, and diuretics, but the effectiveness of these appears minimal, if they are effective at all. Intravenous fluids before administration of iodinated contrast are thought to be the most protective maneuver, but the ideal rate and volume, as well as the actual benefit, is unclear.

Another concern is hypersensitivity and allergic reactions to iodinated contrast. This is a real cause for concern in at-risk patients, although true allergic reactions are uncommon. An important consideration is any prior reaction to iodinated contrast since a mild allergic reaction does not exclude that the next reaction may be severe. Radiology departments have premedication protocols for these patients that usually include steroids and/or diphenhydramine, but, as with PC-AKI, the best prevention is to avoid contrast exposure with alternative studies or protocols.

Gadolinium-Based Contrast Agents

Gadolinium-based agents are usually used for MRI contrast, and, like iodinated contrast, most are predominantly excreted by the kidney. Although potentially nephrotoxic, the doses needed for MR imaging are an order of magnitude less than iodinated contrast. At these smaller doses, gadolinium is not thought to be nephrotoxic.

One of the key concerns with gadolinium contrast is triggering nephrogenic systemic fibrosis (NSF) when the contrast is administered to patients with reduced kidney function. This is thought to be due to gadolinium ions dissociating from their ligand when clearance is reduced. Although rare, the concern about NSF had limited use of gadolinium contrast in patients with eGFR less than 30 mL/min.

Importantly, the relatively recent division of gadolinium contrast agents into three groups has changed thinking about the risk of NSF (Table 6.1). The concern for NSF has markedly diminished with the development of "Group II" gadolinium contrast agents that are now in common clinical use.

Ultrasound Contrast Agents

The last type of intravascular contrast is ultrasound contrast agents, a species of "microbubble." These consist of a gas (such as sulfur hexafluoride, perflutren, or air) surrounded by a shell of protein, lipid, or polymer. These are injected intravenously, and the ultrasound beam strongly reflects off the bubbles, resulting in a bright signal. The contrast kinetics and enhancement patterns are similar to iodinated or gadolinium-based contrast. The regions that can be evaluated are still limited by factors that otherwise limit ultrasound (bowel gas, bone, metal, large patient body habitus).

Importantly, these bubbles are not excreted by the kidney and are not nephrotoxic. Instead, the bubbles eventually rupture and are exhaled. The risk of hypersensitivity and adverse reactions are also minimal. The role for these agents was muted with the development of group II contrast agents, but they will likely play an increasingly important role in kidney imaging.

Complete bibliography is available at Elsevier eBooks for Practicing Clinicians.

TABLE 6.1	**Grouping of Gadolinium-Based MRI Contrast Agents Based on Nephrogenic Systemic Fibrosis (NSF) Risk**	
Group I	Agents that have been associated with the greatest number of NSF cases. Older restrictions on kidney function still apply, and these agents are no longer advertised in the United States.	Gadodiamide, Gadoversetamide, Gadopentetate dimeglumine
Group II	Agents associated with few, if any, unconfounded cases of NSF.	Gadobenate dimeglumine, Gadoteridol, Gadobutrol, Gadoterate meglumine, Gadoterate meglumine
Group III	Agents for which insufficient information has been gathered to classify as group I or II but for which few, if any, unconfounded cases of NSF have been reported. These are treated as Group I agents out of caution.	Gadoxetate disodium

With group I and III agents, if the patient is receiving dialysis or has acute kidney injury, he/she is considered at risk for developing NSF after administration, and these agents are not typically administered. An eGFR of <30 mg/dL is thought to confer risk. For all inpatients, for outpatients and emergency department patients with most recent prior eGFR below 45 mL/min, or for patients with risk factors (such as diabetes mellitus, hypertension, or a history of kidney disease), a repeat eGFR within 2 days of the planned administration of contrast is usually recommended.

Key Bibliography

Craig WD, Wagner BJ, Travis MD. Pyelonephritis: radiologic-pathologic review. *Radiographics*. 2008;28(1):255–277, quiz 327-8.

Davenport MS, Perazella MA, Yee J, et al. Use of intravenous iodinated contrast media in patients with kidney disease: consensus statements from the American College of Radiology and the National Kidney Foundation. *Kidney Med*. 2020 Jan 22;2(1): 85–93.

Davenport MS, Asch D, Cavallo J, et al. Nephrogenic systemic fibrosis (NSF). In: ACR manual on contrast media: version 10.3. American College of Radiology; 2020. https://www.acr.org/-/media/ACR/Files/Clinical-Resources/Contrast_Media.pdf. Accessed December 2021.

Dillman JR, Trout AT, Smith EA, Towbin AJ. Hereditary renal cystic disorders: imaging of the kidneys and beyond. *Radiographics*. 2017;37(3):924–946.

Durand E, Prigent A. The basics of renal imaging and function studies. *Q J Nucl Med*. 2002;46(4):249–267.

Fried JG, Morgan MA. Renal imaging: core curriculum 2019. *Am J Kidney Dis*. 2019;73(4):552–565.

Kazmierski B, Deurdulian C, Tchelepi H, Grant EG. Applications of contrast-enhanced ultrasound in the kidney. *Abdom Radiol (NY)*. 2018;43(4):880–898.

Quaia E, Correas JM, Mehta M, Murchison JT, Gennari AG, van Beek EJR. Gray scale ultrasound, color Doppler ultrasound, and contrast-enhanced ultrasound in renal parenchymal diseases. *Ultrasound Q*. 2018;34(4):250–267.

Schieda N, Krishna S, Davenport MS. Update on gadolinium-based contrast agent-enhanced imaging in the genitourinary system. *AJR Am J Roentgenol*. 2019;212:1223–1233.

Silverman SG, Pedrosa I, Ellis JH, et al. Bosniak classification of cystic renal masses, version 2019: an update proposal and needs assessment. *Radiology*. 2019;292(2):475–488.

Taylor AT. Radionuclides in nephrourology, part 1: Radiopharmaceuticals, quality control, and quantitative indices. *J Nucl Med*. 2014;55(4):608–615.

Weinreb JC, Rodby RA, Yee J, et al. Use of intravenous gadolinium-based contrast media in patients with kidney disease: consensus statements from the American College of Radiology and the National Kidney Foundation. *Kidney Med*. 2021;3:142–150.

PART 2

Acid-Base and Electrolytes

7

Hyponatremia and Hypoosmolar Disorders

JOSEPH G. VERBALIS

The incidence of hyponatremia depends on the population screened and the criteria used to define the disorder. Hospital incidences of 15% to 22% are common if hyponatremia is defined as any serum sodium concentration ([Na$^+$]) of less than 135 mmol/L, but in most studies only 1% to 4% of patients have a serum [Na$^+$] lower than 130 mmol/L, and fewer than 1% have a value lower than 120 mmol/L. Multiple studies have confirmed prevalence ranging from 7% in ambulatory populations up to 38% in acutely hospitalized patients. Older individuals are particularly susceptible to hyponatremia, with reported incidence as high as 53% among institutionalized geriatric patients. Although most cases are mild, hyponatremia is important clinically because (1) acute severe hyponatremia can cause substantial morbidity and mortality; (2) mild hyponatremia can progress to more dangerous levels during management of other disorders; (3) general mortality is higher in hyponatremic patients across a wide range of underlying comorbidities; and (4) overly rapid correction of chronic hyponatremia can produce severe neurologic complications and death.

Definitions

Hyponatremia is of clinical significance only when it reflects corresponding plasma hypoosmolality. Plasma osmolality (P$_{osm}$) can be measured directly by osmometry and is expressed as milliosmoles per kilogram of water (mOsm/kg H$_2$O). P$_{osm}$ can also be calculated from the serum [Na$^+$], measured in millimoles per liter (mmol/L), and the glucose and blood urea nitrogen (BUN) levels, both expressed as milligrams per deciliter (mg/dL), as follows:

$$P_{osm} = 2 \times \text{Serum } [Na^+] + \text{Glucose} / 18 + \text{BUN} / 2.8$$

Because the glucose and BUN concentrations are normally dwarfed by the sodium concentration, osmolality often is estimated simply by doubling the serum [Na$^+$]. All three methods produce comparable results under most conditions. However, total osmolality is not always equivalent to *effective osmolality*, which is sometimes referred to as the *tonicity* of the plasma. Solutes that are predominantly compartmentalized in the extracellular fluid (ECF) are effective solutes because they create osmotic gradients across cell membranes and lead to osmotic movement of water from the intracellular fluid (ICF) compartment to the ECF compartment. In contrast, solutes that permeate cell membranes (e.g., urea, ethanol, methanol) are not

effective solutes, because they do not create osmotic gradients across cell membranes, and therefore they are not associated with secondary water shifts. Only the concentration of effective solutes in plasma should be used to determine whether clinically significant hypoosmolality is present. In most cases, these effective solutes include sodium, its associated anions, and glucose (but only in the presence of insulin deficiency, which allows the development of an ECF/ICF glucose gradient); importantly, urea, a solute that penetrates cells, is not an effective solute.

Hyponatremia and hypoosmolality are usually synonymous, with two important exceptions. First, *pseudohyponatremia* can be produced by marked elevation of serum lipids or proteins. In such cases, the concentration of Na$^+$ per liter of serum water is unchanged, but the concentration of Na$^+$ per liter of serum is artifactually decreased because of the increased relative proportion occupied by lipid or protein. Although measurement of serum or plasma [Na$^+$] by ion-specific electrodes, currently used by most clinical laboratories, is less influenced by high concentrations of lipids or proteins than is measurement of serum [Na$^+$] by flame photometry, such errors nonetheless can still occur when serum samples are diluted before measurement in autoanalyzers. However, because direct measurement of P$_{osm}$ is based on the colligative properties of only the solute particles in solution, increased lipids or proteins will not affect the measured P$_{osm}$. Second, high concentrations of effective solutes other than Na$^+$ can cause relative decreases in serum [Na$^+$] despite an unchanged P$_{osm}$; this commonly occurs with marked hyperglycemia. Misdiagnosis can be avoided again by direct measurement of P$_{osm}$ or by correcting the serum [Na$^+$] by 1.6 mmol/L for each 100 mg/dL increase in blood glucose concentration greater than 100 mg/dL (although some studies have suggested that 2.4 mmol/L may be a more accurate correction factor, especially when the glucose is very high).

Pathogenesis

The presence of significant hypoosmolality always indicates an excess of water relative to solute in the ECF. Because water moves freely between the ICF and ECF, this also indicates an excess of total body water relative to total body solute. Imbalances between water and solute can be generated initially either by *depletion* of body solute more than body water or by *dilution* of body solute because of increases in body water out of proportion to body solute (Box 7.1). However, this distinction represents

BOX 7.1

Pathogenesis of Hypoosmolar Disorders

Solute Depletion (Primary Decreases in Total Body Solute + Secondary Water Retention)[a]

Kidney Solute Loss
Diuretic use
Solute diuresis (glucose, mannitol)
Salt-wasting nephropathy
Mineralocorticoid deficiency

Non-Kidney Solute Loss
Gastrointestinal (diarrhea, vomiting, pancreatitis, bowel obstruction)
Cutaneous (sweating, burns)
Blood loss

Dilution (Primary Increases in Total Body Water ± Secondary Solute Depletion)[b]

Impaired Kidney Free Water Excretion
Increased proximal reabsorption
    Hypothyroidism
Impaired distal dilution
    SIADH
    Glucocorticoid deficiency
Combined increased proximal reabsorption and impaired distal dilution
    Congestive heart failure
    Cirrhosis
    Nephrotic syndrome
Decreased urinary solute excretion
    Beer potomania
    Low protein/solute diet

Excess Water Intake
Primary polydipsia
Dilute infant formula
Fresh water drowning

[a]Virtually all disorders of solute depletion are accompanied by some degree of secondary retention of water by the kidneys in response to the resulting intravascular hypovolemia; this mechanism can lead to hypoosmolality, even when the solute depletion occurs via hypotonic or isotonic body fluid losses.

[b]Disorders of water retention primarily cause hypoosmolality in the absence of any solute losses, but, in some cases of SIADH, secondary solute losses occur in response to the resulting intravascular hypervolemia and can further aggravate the hypoosmolality. (However, this pathophysiology probably does not contribute to the hyponatremia of edema-forming states such as congestive heart failure and cirrhosis, because, in these cases, multiple factors favoring sodium retention result in an increased total body sodium load.)

SIADH, Syndrome of inappropriate antidiuretic hormone secretion.

Modified from Verbalis JG. The syndrome of inappropriate antidiuretic hormone secretion and other hypoosmolar disorders. In: Coffman TM, Falk RJ, Molitoris BA, Neilson EG, Schrier RW, eds. *Diseases of the Kidney and Urinary Tract.* 9th ed. Philadelphia: Lippincott Williams and Wilkins; 2013:2012–2054.

Differential Diagnosis

The diagnostic approach to hypoosmolar disorders should include a careful history (especially concerning medications and diet); physical examination with emphasis on clinical assessment of ECF volume status, including measurement of orthostatic vital signs, and a thorough neurologic evaluation; measurement of serum or plasma electrolytes, glucose, BUN, creatinine, and uric acid; calculated and/or directly measured P_{osm}; and determination of simultaneous urine sodium and osmolality. Although the prevalence varies according to the population being studied, multiple studies indicate that euvolemic hyponatremia generally constitutes the largest single group of hyponatremic patients found in this setting. A definitive diagnosis is not always possible at the time of presentation, but an initial categorization based on the patient's clinical ECF volume status allows selection of appropriate initial therapy in most cases (Fig. 7.1).

Decreased Extracellular Fluid Volume (Hypovolemia)

Clinically detectable hypovolemia, determined most sensitively by careful measurement of orthostatic changes in blood pressure and pulse rate, usually indicates some degree of solute depletion. Elevations of the BUN and uric acid concentrations are useful laboratory correlates of decreased ECF volume. Even isotonic or hypotonic volume losses can lead to hypoosmolality if water or hypotonic fluids are ingested or infused as replacement. A low urine sodium concentration (U_{Na}) in such cases suggests a non-kidney cause of solute depletion, whereas a high U_{Na} suggests kidney causes of solute depletion (see Box 7.1). Diuretic use is the most common cause of hypovolemic hypoosmolality, and thiazides are much more commonly associated with severe hyponatremia than loop diuretics.

Although diuretics represent a prime example of solute depletion, the pathophysiologic mechanisms underlying diuretic-associated hypoosmolality are complex and have multiple components, including sodium depletion with secondary stimulation of arginine vasopressin (AVP) secretion and impaired diluting ability of the inner medullary collecting duct, both leading to significant degrees of free water retention. Many patients do not manifest clinical evidence of marked hypovolemia, in part because ingested water has been translocated to the ICF in response to nonosmotically stimulated secretion of AVP, as is generally true for all disorders of solute depletion. To complicate diagnosis further, the U_{Na} may be high or low depending on when the last diuretic dose was taken. Consequently, any suspicion of diuretic use mandates careful consideration of this diagnosis. A low serum [K⁺] is an important clue to diuretic use because few other disorders that cause hyponatremia and hypoosmolality also produce appreciable hypokalemia. Whenever the possibility of diuretic use is suspected in the absence of a positive history, a urine screen for diuretics should be performed.

Most other causes of kidney or non-kidney solute losses resulting in hypovolemic hypoosmolality will be clinically apparent, although some cases of salt-wasting nephropathies (e.g., chronic interstitial nephropathy, polycystic kidney disease, obstructive uropathy, Bartter syndrome) or mineralocorticoid deficiency (e.g., Addison disease) can be challenging to diagnose during the early phases of the disease.

A controversial cause of hypovolemic hyponatremia is cerebral salt wasting (CSW), in which some patients with intracranial

an oversimplification, because most hypoosmolar states include variable contributions of both solute depletion and water retention. For example, isotonic solute losses occurring during an acute hemorrhage do not produce hypoosmolality until the subsequent retention of water from ingested or infused hypotonic fluids causes a secondary dilution of the remaining ECF solute. Nonetheless, this concept has proved useful because it provides a logical framework for understanding the diagnosis and treatment of hypoosmolar disorders.

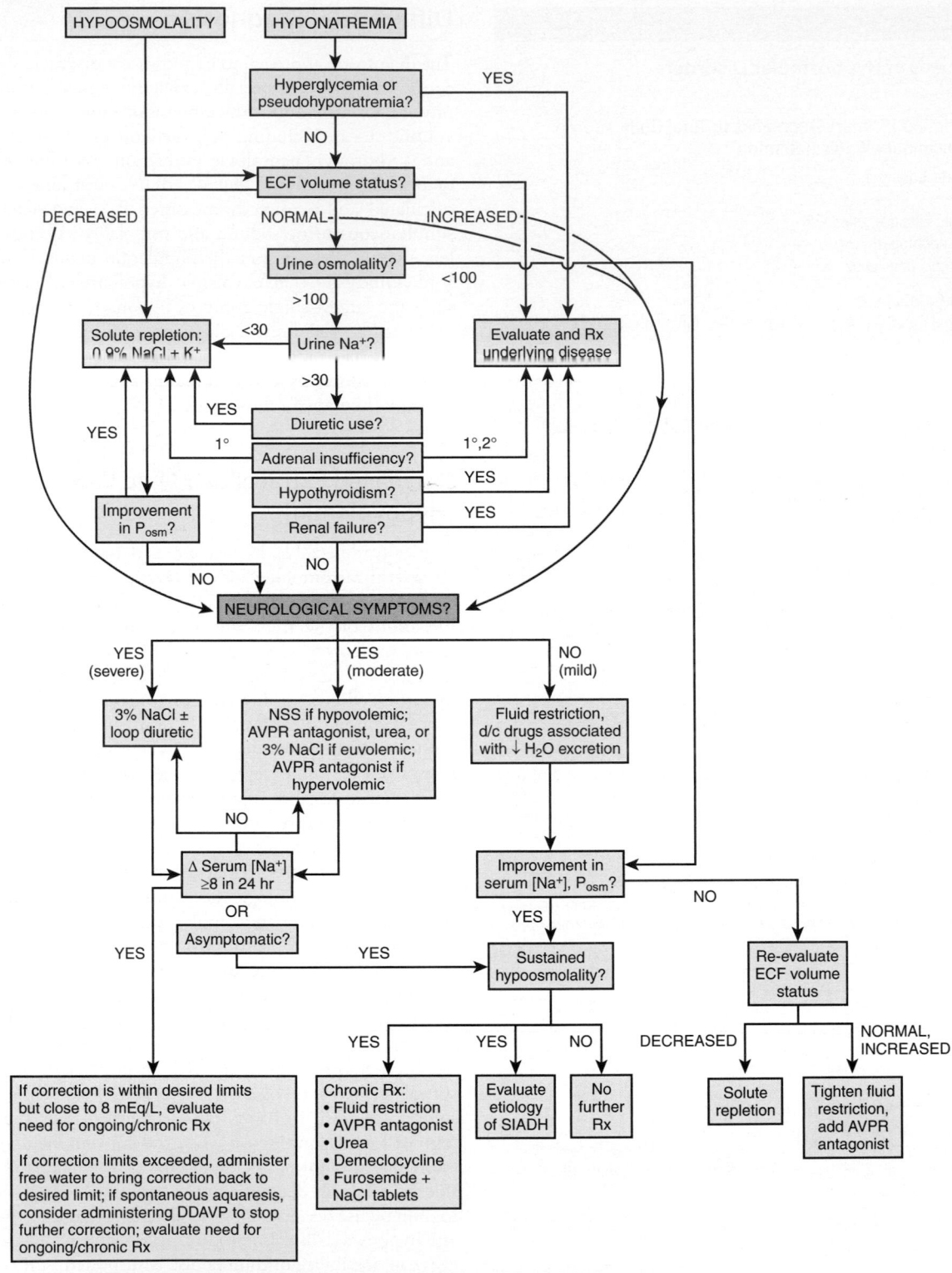

• **Fig. 7.1 Algorithm for evaluation and treatment of hypoosmolar patients.** The brown arrows and brown box in the center emphasizes that the presence of central nervous system dysfunction resulting from hyponatremia should always be assessed immediately, so that appropriate therapy can be started as soon as possible in significantly symptomatic patients, even while the outlined diagnostic evaluation is proceeding. Values for osmolality are in mOsm/kg H_2O, and those referring to serum [Na$^+$] are in mmol/L. Δ, Change (in concentration); *1°*, primary; *2°*, secondary; *AVPR*, arginine vasopressin receptor; *d/c*, discontinue; *DDAVP*, desmopressin; *ECF*, extracellular fluid volume; P_{osm}, plasma osmolality; *Rx*, treatment; *SIADH*, syndrome of inappropriate antidiuretic hormone secretion. (Modified from Verbalis JG. The syndrome of inappropriate antidiuretic hormone secretion and other hypoosmolar disorders. In: Coffman TM, Falk RJ, Molitoris BA, Neilson EG, Schrier RW, eds. *Diseases of the Kidney and Urinary Tract*. 9th ed. Philadelphia: Lippincott Williams and Wilkins; 2013:2012–2054.)

diseases may have a primary natriuresis leading to ECF and/or intravascular volume contraction, with elevated plasma AVP levels that are physiologically appropriate for hypovolemia. Some have suggested that this syndrome also encompasses patients without cerebral disorders and propose adding "renal salt wasting" (RSW) to the descriptor: that is, CSW/RSW. Reports on the prevalence of this disorder have varied greatly (from 94% to 0% of patients with subarachnoid hemorrhage), mainly based on the criteria used to assess ECF volume status.

Normal Extracellular Fluid Volume (Euvolemia)

Virtually any disorder associated with hypoosmolality can manifest with an ECF volume status that appears normal by standard methods of clinical evaluation. Because clinical assessment of ECF volume status is not very sensitive, normal or low levels of serum BUN and uric acid are helpful laboratory correlates of relatively normal ECF volume.

Conversely, a low U_{Na} suggests a depletional hypoosmolality secondary to ECF losses with subsequent volume replacement by water or other hypotonic fluids; as discussed earlier, such patients may appear euvolemic by all the usual clinical parameters used to assess ECF volume status. Primary dilutional disorders are less likely in the presence of a low U_{Na} (<30 mmol/L), although this pattern can occur in hypothyroidism as well.

A high U_{Na} (≥30 mmol/L) generally suggests a dilutional hypoosmolality such as the *syndrome of inappropriate antidiuretic hormone secretion* (SIADH; see Box 7.1). SIADH is the most common cause of euvolemic hypoosmolality in clinical practice. The criteria necessary for a diagnosis of SIADH remain essentially unchanged since defined by Bartter and Schwartz in 1967 (Box 7.2), but several points deserve emphasis. First, true hypoosmolality must be present, and hyponatremia secondary to pseudohyponatremia or hyperglycemia must be excluded.

Second, the urinary osmolality (U_{osm}) must be inappropriate for the low P_{osm}. This does not require that the U_{osm} be greater than P_{osm} but merely that the urine not be maximally dilute (i.e., U_{osm} should not exceed 100 mOsm/kg H_2O in adults, although this may be somewhat higher in older adults and patients with advanced CKD). U_{osm} need not be inappropriately elevated at all levels of P_{osm} but simply at some level of P_{osm} less than 275 mOsm/kg H_2O. This is evident in patients with a reset osmostat who suppress AVP secretion at some level of P_{osm}, resulting in maximal urine dilution and free water excretion at plasma osmolalities falling below this level. Although some consider a reset osmostat to be a separate disorder rather than a variant of SIADH, such cases nonetheless illustrate that some hypoosmolar patients can exhibit an appropriately dilute urine at some, although not all, plasma osmolalities.

Third, clinical euvolemia must be present to diagnose SIADH, and this diagnosis cannot be made in a hypovolemic or significantly edematous patient. Importantly, this does not mean that patients with SIADH cannot become hypovolemic for other reasons, but in such cases it is impossible to diagnose the underlying SIADH until the patient is rendered euvolemic.

The fourth criterion, RSW, has probably caused the most confusion regarding SIADH. The importance of this criterion lies in its usefulness in differentiating hypoosmolality caused by a decreased effective intravascular volume (in which case kidney Na⁺ conservation occurs) from dilutional disorders in which urinary Na⁺ excretion is normal or increased because of ECF volume expansion. However, U_{Na} can also be high in kidney

---

BOX 7.2

Criteria for the Diagnosis of the Syndrome of Inappropriate Antidiuretic Hormone Secretion

Essential Criteria

1. Decreased effective osmolality of the ECF (P_{osm} less than 275 mOsm/kg H_2O)
2. Inappropriate urinary concentration (U_{osm} greater than 100 mOsm/kg H_2O with normal kidney function) at some level of plasma hypoosmolality
3. Clinical euvolemia, as defined by the absence of signs of hypovolemia (orthostasis, tachycardia, decreased skin turgor, dry mucous membranes) or hypervolemia (subcutaneous edema, ascites)
4. Elevated urinary sodium excretion despite a normal salt and water intake
5. Normal thyroid, adrenal, and kidney function

Supplemental Criteria

1. Abnormal water load test (inability to excrete at least 80% of a 20-mL/kg water load in 4 hr and/or failure to dilute U_{osm} to less than 100 mOsm/kg H_2O)
2. Plasma vasopressin (AVP) level inappropriately elevated relative to plasma osmolality
3. No significant correction of serum sodium concentration ([Na⁺]) with volume expansion but improvement after fluid restriction

AVP, Arginine vasopressin; *ECF,* extracellular fluid; P_{osm}, plasma osmolality; U_{osm}, urinary osmolality.

Modified from Verbalis JG. The syndrome of inappropriate antidiuretic hormone secretion and other hypoosmolar disorders. In: Coffman TM, Falk RJ, Molitoris BA, Neilson EG, Schrier RW, eds. *Diseases of the Kidney and Urinary Tract.* 9th ed. Philadelphia: Lippincott Williams and Wilkins; 2013:2012–2054.

---

causes of solute depletion, such as diuretic use or Addison disease, and, conversely, patients with SIADH can have a low urine Na⁺ excretion if they subsequently become hypovolemic or solute depleted, conditions sometimes produced by imposed salt and water restriction. Consequently, although high urine Na⁺ excretion is generally the rule in patients with SIADH, its presence does not necessarily confirm this diagnosis, nor does its absence exclude it.

The final criterion emphasizes that SIADH remains a diagnosis of exclusion, and the absence of other potential causes of hypoosmolality must always be verified. Glucocorticoid deficiency and SIADH can be especially difficult to distinguish, because either primary or secondary hypocortisolism can cause elevated plasma AVP levels and, in addition, can have direct kidney effects to prevent maximal urine dilution. Therefore, no patient with chronic hyponatremia should be diagnosed as having SIADH without a thorough evaluation of adrenal function, either via a cortisol level ≥18 μg/dL or a rapid adrenocorticotropin (ACTH) stimulation test using the same cortisol cutoff; acute hyponatremia of obvious origin, such as that occurring postoperatively or in association with pneumonitis, may be treated without adrenal testing as long as there are no other clinical signs or symptoms suggestive of adrenal dysfunction. Many different disorders have been associated with SIADH, and these can be divided into several major etiologic groups (Box 7.3).

Some cases of euvolemic hyponatremia do not fit particularly well into either a dilutional or a depletional category. Chief among these is the hyponatremia that occurs in patients who ingest large

BOX 7.3

Common Causes of the Syndrome of Inappropriate Antidiuretic Hormone Secretion

Tumors

Pulmonary/mediastinal (bronchogenic carcinoma, mesothelioma, thymoma)
Nonchest (duodenal carcinoma, pancreatic carcinoma, ureteral/prostate carcinoma, uterine carcinoma, nasopharyngeal carcinoma, leukemia)

Central Nervous System Disorders

Mass lesions (tumors, brain abscesses, subdural hematoma)
Inflammatory diseases (encephalitis, meningitis, lupus cerebritis, acute intermittent porphyria, multiple sclerosis)
Degenerative/demyelinative diseases (Guillain-Barré, spinal cord lesions)
Miscellaneous (subarachnoid hemorrhage, head trauma, acute psychosis, delirium tremens, pituitary stalk section, transsphenoidal adenomectomy, hydrocephalus)

Drugs

Stimulated AVP release (nicotine, phenothiazines, tricyclic antidepressants)
Direct kidney effects and/or potentiation of AVP antidiuretic effects (desmopressin, oxytocin, prostaglandin synthesis inhibitors)
Mixed or uncertain actions (ACE inhibitors, carbamazepine and oxcarbazepine, chlorpropamide, clofibrate, clozapine, cyclophosphamide, 3,4-methylenedioxymethamphetamine ["Ecstasy"], omeprazole, serotonin reuptake inhibitors, tacrolimus, vincristine)

Pulmonary Diseases

Infections (tuberculosis, acute bacterial or viral pneumonia, aspergillosis, empyema)
Mechanical/ventilatory (acute respiratory failure, COPD, positive-pressure ventilation)

Other

HIV and AIDS
Prolonged strenuous exercise (marathon, triathlon, ultramarathon, hot-weather hiking)
Postoperative state
Senile atrophy
Idiopathic

ACE, Angiotensin-converting enzyme; *AIDS,* acquired immunodeficiency syndrome; *AVP,* arginine vasopressin; *COPD,* chronic obstructive pulmonary disease.

Modified from Verbalis JG. The syndrome of inappropriate antidiuretic hormone secretion and other hypoosmolar disorders. In: Coffman TM, Falk RJ, Molitoris BA, Neilson EG, Schrier RW, eds. *Diseases of the Kidney and Urinary Tract.* 9th ed. Philadelphia: Lippincott Williams and Wilkins; 2013:2012–2054.

volumes of beer with little food intake for prolonged periods, called *beer potomania.* Even though the volume of fluid ingested may not seem sufficiently excessive to overwhelm kidney diluting mechanisms, in these cases free water excretion is limited by very low urinary solute excretion, resulting in water retention and dilutional hyponatremia. However, because such patients have very low sodium intakes as well, it is likely that relative depletion of body Na^+ stores also contributes to the hypoosmolality in some cases. A similar pathophysiology can occur in patients on vegetarian diets with insufficient protein and sodium intake.

Increased Extracellular Fluid Volume (Hypervolemia)

The presence of hypervolemia, as detected clinically by the presence of significant edema and/or ascites, indicates whole-body sodium excess, and hypoosmolality in these patients suggests a relatively decreased effective intravascular volume or perfusion pressure leading to water retention as a result of both elevated plasma AVP levels and decreased distal delivery of glomerular filtrate. Such patients usually have a low U_{Na} because of secondary hyperaldosteronism, but under certain conditions the U_{Na} may be elevated (e.g., glucosuria in diabetics, diuretic therapy). Hyponatremia generally does not occur until fairly advanced stages of diseases such as congestive heart failure, cirrhosis, and nephrotic syndrome, so the diagnosis is usually not difficult. Kidney failure can also cause retention of both sodium and water, but in this case, the factor limiting excretion of excess body fluid is not decreased effective circulating volume but rather decreased glomerular filtration.

It should be remembered that even though many edema-forming states have secondary increases in plasma AVP levels as a result of decreased effective arterial blood volume, they are nonetheless not classified as SIADH because they fail to meet the criterion of clinical euvolemia (see Box 7.2). Although it can be argued that this distinction is semantic, this criterion remains important because it allows segregation of identifiable etiologies of hyponatremia that are associated with different methods of evaluation and therapy.

Several situations can cause hyponatremia because of acute water loading in excess of kidney excretory capacity. Primary polydipsia can cause hypoosmolality in a small subset of patients with some degree of underlying SIADH, particularly psychiatric patients with long-standing schizophrenia who are taking neuroleptic drugs or, rarely, patients with normal kidney function in whom the volumes ingested exceed the maximum kidney free water excretory rate of approximately 500 to 1000 mL/h.

Endurance exercising, such as marathon or ultramarathon racing, has been associated with sometimes fatal hyponatremia, primarily as a result of ingestion of excessive amounts of hypotonic fluids during the exercise that exceed the water excretory capacity of the kidney. This is called *exercise-associated hyponatremia* (EAH). Many athletes with EAH have met diagnostic criteria for SIADH immediately following prolonged exercise, which serves to decrease further their free water excretory capacity both during and following exercise. Although the stimuli for AVP secretion during endurance exercise have not been fully elucidated, potential candidates include baroreceptor activation, nausea, cytokine release from muscle rhabdomyolysis, and exercise itself. Most cases of EAH are associated with weight gain, reflecting the excess water retention, but patients are usually classified as clinically euvolemic, because water retention alone without sodium excess, as observed in these patients, does not generally produce clinical manifestations of hypervolemia such as edema or ascites. Rarely, cases of EAH may present as hypovolemic with hypotension and tachycardia as a result of under-replaced sodium losses in sweat.

Clinical Manifestations of Hyponatremia

Hypoosmolality is associated with a broad spectrum of neurologic manifestations, ranging from mild, nonspecific symptoms (e.g., headache, nausea) to more significant deficits (e.g., disorientation, confusion, obtundation, focal neurologic deficits, and seizures). In the most severe cases, death can result from respiratory arrest after tentorial herniation with subsequent brainstem compression. This neurologic symptom complex, termed *hyponatremic encephalopathy*, primarily reflects brain edema resulting from osmotic water shifts into the brain caused by the decreased effective P_{osm}. Significant symptoms generally do not occur until the serum [Na⁺] falls to less than 125 mmol/L, and the severity of symptoms can be roughly correlated with the degree of hypoosmolality. However, individual variability is marked, and the level of serum [Na⁺] at which symptoms will appear cannot be accurately predicted for any individual patient.

Several factors other than the severity of hypoosmolality also affect the degree of neurologic dysfunction. Most important is the rate at which hypoosmolality develops. Rapid development of severe hypoosmolality is frequently associated with marked neurologic symptoms, whereas gradual development over several days or weeks is often associated with relatively mild symptomatology despite achievement of an equivalent degree of hypoosmolality. This occurs because the brain can counteract osmotic swelling by secreting intracellular solutes, both electrolytes and organic osmolytes, via a process called *brain volume regulation*. Because this is a time-dependent process, rapid development of hypoosmolality can result in brain edema before adaptation can occur; with slower development of hypoosmolality, brain cells can lose solute at a sufficient rate to prevent the development of brain edema and subsequent neurologic dysfunction.

Underlying neurologic disease also can significantly affect the level of hypoosmolality at which central nervous system symptoms appear. For example, moderate hypoosmolality is usually not of major concern in an otherwise healthy patient, but it can precipitate seizure activity in a patient with underlying epilepsy. Non-neurologic metabolic disorders (e.g., hypoxia, hypercapnia, acidosis, and hypercalcemia) similarly can affect the level of P_{osm} at which central nervous system symptoms occur. Recent studies suggest that some people may be susceptible to a vicious cycle in which hypoosmolality-induced brain edema causes noncardiogenic pulmonary edema, and the resulting hypoxia and hypercapnia then further impair the ability of the brain to volume regulate, leading to more brain edema, neurologic deterioration, and death in some cases. Other clinical studies suggest that menstruating women and young children may be particularly susceptible to the development of neurologic morbidity and mortality during hyponatremia, especially in the acute postoperative setting. The true clinical incidence and underlying pathophysiologic mechanisms responsible for these sometimes-catastrophic outcomes remain to be determined.

Finally, the issue of whether mild to moderate hyponatremia is truly "asymptomatic" has been challenged by recent studies showing subtle defects in cognition and gait stability in hyponatremic patients that appear to be reversed by correction of the disorder. The functional significance of the gait instability was illustrated in a study of Belgian patients with hyponatremia who were judged to be "asymptomatic" at the time of presentation to an emergency department (ED). These patients demonstrated a markedly increased incidence of falls, despite being apparently "asymptomatic." The clinical significance of the gait instability and fall data has been further evaluated by multiple independent studies that have shown increased bone fractures in hyponatremic subjects. More recent studies have shown that hyponatremia is associated with increased bone loss in experimental animals and a significant increase in odds ratio for osteoporosis and fractures in humans. Thus, the major clinical significance of chronic hyponatremia may lie in the increased morbidity and mortality associated with falls and fractures in older populations.

Treatment

Although various authors have published recommendations for the treatment of hyponatremia, no standardized treatment algorithms are universally accepted, with many differences of opinion regarding best practices. There is a dearth of evidence-based data on which to base true guidelines, and most of the literature reflects expert opinions. A synthesis of several expert recommendations for treatment of hyponatremia is illustrated in Fig. 7.1. This algorithm is based primarily on the neurologic symptomatology of hyponatremic patients rather than the serum [Na⁺] or on the chronicity of the hyponatremia, which is often difficult to ascertain.

If any degree of clinical hypovolemia is present, the patient should be considered to have a solute depletion-induced hypoosmolality and should be treated with isotonic (0.9%) NaCl at a rate appropriate for the estimated volume depletion. If diuretic use is known or suspected, fluid therapy should be supplemented with potassium (30 to 40 mmol/L), even if the serum [K⁺] is not low because of the propensity of such patients to have total-body potassium depletion. Patients with diuretic-induced hyponatremia usually respond well to isotonic NaCl and do not require 3% NaCl unless they exhibit severe neurologic symptoms. However, such patients often have an electrolyte-free water diuresis (termed *aquaresis*) after their ECF volume deficit has been corrected, because normalization of the ECF volume removes the hypovolemic stimulus to AVP secretion, resulting in a more rapid correction of the serum [Na⁺] as a result of increased free water excretion than predicted from the rate of saline infusion.

Most often, the hypoosmolar patient is clinically euvolemic, but several situations dictate a reconsideration of potential solute depletion, even in the patient without clinically apparent hypovolemia. These include low U_{Na} (<20 to 30 mmol/L), any history of recent diuretic use, and any suggestion of primary adrenal insufficiency. Whenever a reasonable likelihood of depletion, rather than dilution, hypoosmolality exists, it is appropriate to treat initially with isotonic NaCl. If the patient has SIADH, no significant harm will have been done with a limited (1 to 2 L) saline infusion, because such patients will excrete excess NaCl without markedly changing their P_{osm}. However, this therapy should be abandoned if the serum [Na⁺] does not improve because longer periods of continued isotonic NaCl infusion can worsen hyponatremia by virtue of cumulative water retention.

Treatment of euvolemic hypoosmolality varies depending on the presentation. If all criteria for SIADH are met, except that the U_{osm} is low, the patient should simply be observed, because this presentation may represent spontaneous reversal of a transient form of SIADH. If there is any suspicion of either primary or secondary adrenal insufficiency, glucocorticoid replacement should be started immediately after completion of a rapid ACTH stimulation test. Prompt water diuresis after initiation of glucocorticoid treatment strongly supports glucocorticoid deficiency, but the absence of a quick response does not exclude this diagnosis, because several days of glucocorticoid therapy may be necessary for normalization of P_{osm}.

Hypervolemic hypoosmolality is usually treated initially with diuretics and other measures directed at the underlying disorder. Such patients rarely require any therapy to increase P_{osm} acutely, but often benefit from varying degrees of sodium and water restriction to reduce body fluid retention. However, worsened hyponatremia following administration of aggressive loop diuretic therapy in combination with continued or increased fluid intake and/or ineffectiveness of fluid restriction sometimes necessitates additional treatment of the hyponatremia, particularly via vasopressin receptor antagonists (vaptans), because saline administration can worsen fluid retention.

Goals and Limits of Serum [Na⁺] Correction

In any case of significant hyponatremia, one is challenged by how quickly the serum [Na⁺] should be corrected. Although hyponatremia is associated with a broad spectrum of neurologic symptoms, sometimes leading to death in severe cases, too rapid correction of severe hyponatremia can produce the *osmotic demyelination syndrome (ODS)*, a brain demyelinating disease that also can cause substantial neurologic morbidity and mortality. Clinical and experimental results suggest that optimal treatment of hyponatremia must entail balancing the risks of hyponatremia against the risks of correction for each patient. Multiple factors should be considered: the severity of the hyponatremia, the duration of the hyponatremia, the patient's symptom burden, and the presence of other risk factors for ODS. Neither sequela from hyponatremia itself nor ODS after therapy is very likely in a patient whose serum [Na⁺] is greater than 125 mmol/L, although, in some cases, significant symptoms can develop even with serum [Na⁺] greater than 125 mmol/L if the rate of fall of serum [Na⁺] has been rapid. The importance of the duration and symptom burden of hyponatremia relates to how well the brain has volume regulated in response to the hyponatremia and, consequently, to the degree of risk for demyelination with rapid correction.

Cases of acute hyponatremia (somewhat arbitrarily defined as hyponatremia of less than 48-hour duration) are usually symptomatic if the hyponatremia is severe (i.e., <125 mmol/L). These patients are at greatest risk from neurologic complications caused by the hyponatremia itself, and the risk of ODS is low since brain volume regulation has not been completed. Consequently, the serum [Na⁺] should be corrected to higher levels promptly, most often with the use of 3% NaCl unless the patient is undergoing a spontaneous aquaresis, in which case the correction will occur without intervention (see Fig. 7.1). For most such cases, specific limits to the magnitude of correction are not necessary (Fig. 7.2).

Patients with more chronic hyponatremia (greater than 48-hour duration) and mild or no neurologic symptoms are at little immediate risk from complications of hyponatremia itself but can develop ODS after overly rapid correction. There is no indication to correct the serum [Na⁺] in these patients rapidly, and slower acting therapies that correct serum [Na⁺] over 24 to 72 hours should be employed, such as fluid restriction or discontinuing drugs that limit free water excretion (see Fig. 7.1).

Although these situations have reasonably clear treatment indications, most patients have hyponatremia of indeterminate duration and varying degrees of neurologic impairment. This group presents the most challenging treatment decision because the hyponatremia may have been present sufficiently long to allow some degree of brain volume regulation but not long enough to prevent an element of brain edema and neurologic symptoms. Most authors recommend prompt treatment for such patients because of their symptoms but with methods that allow a controlled and limited correction of their hyponatremia (see Fig. 7.1). Reasonable correction parameters consist of a rate of correction of serum [Na⁺] that results in a total magnitude of correction that does not exceed 10-12 mmol/L during the first 24 hours and 18 mmol/L throughout the first 48 hours of correction. However, the correction goal

should be set lower than the limit (i.e., 6-8 mmol/L) in order to reduce the chance of exceeding the limit (see Fig. 7.2). If the correction limit is exceeded, consideration should be given to administration of hypotonic fluid (e.g., D₅W) to bring the correction magnitude back to the limit (see Fig 7.2).

Maximum correction rates should be even lower (no > 8 mmol/L/24 hr) if risk factors for the development of ODS are present, including alcoholism, liver disease, malnutrition, hypokalemia, and a very low serum [Na⁺] (≤105 mmol/L). In such cases, goals should be commensurately lower (i.e., 4-6 mmol/L) and, if the correction rate is exceeded, water should be administered, with or without desmopressin, to bring the correction magnitude back to the limit (see Fig. 7.2). Recent studies have verified that ODS is uncommon even in patients corrected >8 mmol/L/24 hr (0.5% of patients with a serum [Na⁺] ≤120 mmol/L), but this complication occurred more frequently in patients with hypokalemia and chronic alcoholism.

To follow these recommendations, serum [Na⁺] levels must be carefully monitored at frequent intervals during the active phases of treatment (every 2 to 4 hours for 3% NaCl administration; every 6 to 8 hours for vaptan administration) to adjust therapy so that the correction stays within desired limits. It cannot be emphasized too strongly that it is necessary to correct the serum [Na⁺] acutely only to a safe range rather than to normal levels. As a practical point, after an acute correction has reached 8 mmol/L, the need for continued acute therapy should be carefully assessed, because ongoing correction may result in an overcorrection by the time the next serum [Na⁺] is available (see Fig. 7.1). In some situations, patients may spontaneously correct their hyponatremia via a water diuresis. If the hyponatremia is acute (e.g., psychogenic polydipsia with water intoxication), such patients do not appear at risk for ODS. However, if the hyponatremia has been chronic (e.g., hypocortisolism, diuretic therapy), intervention should be considered to limit the magnitude of correction of serum [Na⁺], such as infusion of hypotonic fluids to match urine output and/or administration of desmopressin 1 to 2 µg IV every 8 hours, using the same therapeutic endpoints as for active corrections.

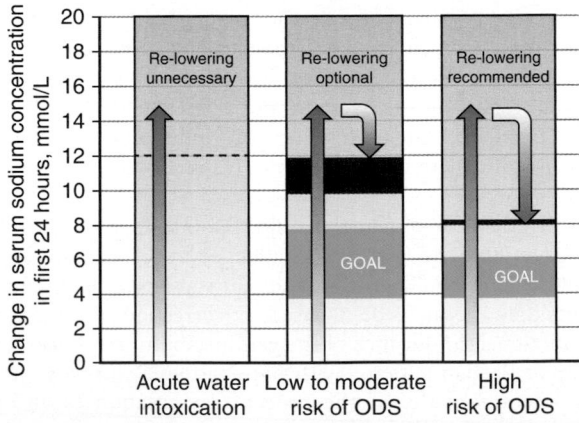

• **Fig. 7.2** Limits and goals of sodium correction in hypoosmolar patients. Limits (*red*) and goals (*green*) of sodium correction in the first 24 hours for patients presenting with a serum [Na⁺] <120 mmol/L. The blue arrows show recommendations for re-lowering of the serum [Na⁺] back to the 24-hour limit when the recommended limit is exceeded. *L*, Liter; *mmol*, millimole; *ODS*; osmotic demyelination syndrome (Modified from Verbalis JG, Goldsmith SR, Greenberg A, et al. Diagnosis, evaluation, and treatment of hyponatremia: expert panel recommendations. Am J Med. 2013;126(10 suppl 1):S1–S42.)

Specific Current Therapies

Controlled correction of hyponatremia is best accomplished with hypertonic (3%) NaCl solution, because patients with euvolemic hypoosmolality (e.g., SIADH) usually will not respond to isotonic NaCl. An initial infusion rate can be estimated by multiplying the patient's body weight (in kilograms) by the desired rate of increase in serum $[Na^+]$ in mmol per liter per hour (e.g., in a 70-kg patient, increasing serum $[Na^+]$ by approximately 1 mmol/L/h will require an infusion of 3% NaCl at 70 mL/h). An alternative option for more emergent situations is administration of a 100-mL bolus of 3% NaCl, repeated two or three times if there is no clinical improvement within 30 minutes. Intravenous administration of this volume of hypertonic saline raises the serum $[Na^+]$ by an average of 2-4 mmol/L, well below the recommended maximal 24-hour increase of 10-12 mmol/24 hr or 18 mmol/48 h. Because the brain can only accommodate an average increase of approximately 8%-10% in brain volume before herniation occurs, quickly increasing the serum $[Na^+]$ by as little as 2-4 mmol/L in acute hyponatremia can effectively reduce brain swelling and intracranial pressure. The efficacy of this method was shown in a recent clinical trial from Ireland, which demonstrated that boluses of 3% NaCl corrected the serum $[Na^+]$ more quickly than continuous infusion in historical controls and resulted in a more rapid improvement of the Glasgow Coma Scale score.

Vasopressin receptor antagonists ("*vaptans*") can be used to increase the serum $[Na^+]$ by stimulating kidney free water excretion, or *aquaresis*, thereby leading to increased serum $[Na^+]$ in the majority of patients with hyponatremia resulting from SIADH, congestive heart failure, or cirrhosis. Although the optimal use of AVP receptor antagonists in any setting has not yet been fully determined, the US Food and Drug Administration (FDA) has approved conivaptan and tolvaptan for the treatment of euvolemic and hypervolemic hyponatremia; tolvaptan has been approved by the European Medicines Agency (EMA) and elsewhere for treatment of SIADH. Specific administration instructions for both vaptans can be found in prescribing information. Although general principles of vaptan use are similar, there are also some important differences:

1. Conivaptan is a parenteral drug whereas tolvaptan is administered orally.
2. Conivaptan therapy is limited to a maximum duration of 4 days because of drug-interaction effects with other agents metabolized by the CYP3A4 hepatic isoenzyme, whereas tolvaptan therapy is not limited (in the U.S., the FDA recommends use for only 30 days based on the duration of the phase 3 trials of tolvaptan, but in many other countries there is no such recommendation).
3. For all vaptans, it is critical that the serum $[Na^+]$ concentration is measured frequently during the active phase of correction of the hyponatremia (a minimum of every 6 to 8 hours but more frequently in patients with risk factors for development of ODS) with appropriate measures as discussed above to limit overly rapid correction.
4. Up-titration of vaptan dose can be done if the increase in serum $[Na^+]$ has been <5 mmol/L in the previous 24 hours.
5. Fluid restriction should not be used during the active phase of a vaptan correction, thereby allowing the patient's thirst to compensate for an overly vigorous aquaresis.
6. Although vaptans are not contraindicated with decreased kidney function, these agents generally will not be effective if the serum creatinine is greater than 2.5 mg/dL.
7. Tolvaptan is contraindicated in patients with cirrhosis or liver failure because of some cases of reversible hepatotoxicity using this drug at high doses in clinical trials of polycystic kidney disease, but whether this is true of conivaptan as well has not been studied.

Urea may be an alternative oral treatment for SIADH and other hyponatremic disorders. The mechanism of action is to correct hypoosmolality not only by increasing solute-free water excretion but also by decreasing urinary sodium excretion. Doses of 15 to 60 g/day are generally effective; the dose can be titrated in increments of 15 g/day at weekly intervals as necessary to achieve normalization of the serum $[Na^+]$. Uncontrolled trials have suggested adequate efficacy and safety of urea, but there is no FDA-approved form of the agent. The disadvantages associated with the use of urea include poor palatability (though flavored preparations are now available), the development of azotemia at higher doses, and lack of long-term studies in patients with chronic hyponatremia.

Isotonic saline ($[Na^+]$ = 154 mmol/L) is the treatment of choice for solute depletion hyponatremia (i.e., hypovolemic hyponatremia). This initial therapy is appropriate for patients who either have clinical signs of hypovolemia or in whom a spot urine $[Na^+]$ is <20-30 mmol/L. However, this therapy is ineffective for most cases of dilution hyponatremia such as SIADH, and continued inappropriate administration of isotonic saline to euvolemic patients may worsen their hyponatremia, and/or cause fluid overload in patients with hypervolemic hyponatremia.

Fluid restriction has been the most popular and most widely accepted treatment for patients with chronic hyponatremia. When SIADH is present, fluids should generally be limited to 500–1000 mL/24 hr. Because fluid restriction increases the serum $[Na^+]$ largely by under-replacing the excretion of fluid by the kidneys in combination with insensible fluid loses, some have advocated an initial restriction to 500 mL less than the 24-hour urine output. When instituting a fluid restriction, it is important for the nursing staff and the patient to understand that this includes all fluids that are consumed, not just water. Restricting fluid intake can be effective when properly applied and managed in selected patients, but serum $[Na^+]$ is generally increased only slowly (1–2 mmol/L/day) even with severe fluid restriction. In addition, this therapy is often poorly tolerated because of an associated increase in thirst, leading to poor adherence with long-term therapy. Recent observational registries and randomized controlled trials have indicated that significantly less than 50% of hospitalized patients placed on a fluid restriction achieved a ≥5 mmol/L increase in serum $[Na^+]$. Consequently, in patients with characteristics suggestive of fluid restriction failure (low urine volume, high urine osmolality, elevated urine:plasma electrolyte ratio), consideration should be given to use of more effective pharmacologic or saline treatment strategies. In addition, fluid restriction is not practical for some patients, particularly patients in intensive care settings who often require administration of significant volumes of fluids as part of their therapies.

Chronic Hyponatremia Treatment

Some patients will benefit from continued treatment of hyponatremia following discharge from the hospital. One exception is patients with the reset osmostat syndrome; because the hyponatremia of such patients is not progressive but rather fluctuates around their reset level of serum $[Na^+]$, no therapy is generally required. For most other cases of mild to moderate SIADH, fluid restriction represents the least toxic therapy and it should be tried as the initial therapy, with pharmacologic intervention reserved for refractory cases in which the degree of fluid restriction required to avoid hypoosmolality is so severe that the patient is unable, or unwilling, to maintain it.

If pharmacologic treatment is necessary, the choices include urea, furosemide in combination with NaCl tablets, demeclocycline, and the vasopressin receptor antagonists. Although each of these treatments can be effective in individual circumstances, the only drugs currently approved by the regulatory agencies for treatment of hyponatremia are vasopressin receptor antagonists. For patients who have responded to either conivaptan or tolvaptan in the hospital, consideration should be given to continuing tolvaptan as an outpatient. In patients with established chronic hyponatremia, tolvaptan has been shown to be effective at maintaining a normal [Na$^+$] for as long as 4 years on continued daily therapy. However, many patients with hospitalized hyponatremia have a transient form of SIADH without the need for long-term therapy. In the conivaptan open-label study, approximately 70% of patients treated as an inpatient for 4 days had normal serum [Na$^+$] concentrations 7 and 30 days after cessation of the vaptan therapy in the absence of chronic therapy for hyponatremia.

Deciding which patients with hospitalized hyponatremia are candidates for long-term therapy should be based on the etiology of the SIADH, because patients with some causes of SIADH (e.g., non-resectable tumors) are more likely to experience persistent hyponatremia that may benefit from long-term treatment with tolvaptan. Nonetheless, for any individual patient this simply represents an estimate of the likelihood of requiring long-term therapy. In all cases, consideration should be given to a trial of stopping the drug at 2-4 weeks following discharge to see if hyponatremia recurs. Seven days is a reasonable period of tolvaptan cessation to evaluate the presence of continued SIADH, because this period was sufficient to demonstrate recurrence of hyponatremia in the tolvaptan SALT clinical trials. Barriers to effective use of vaptans for chronic hyponatremia include high cost (though generic versions of tolvaptan became available in 2020) and FDA recommendations against use beyond 30 days.

Guidelines for the appropriate treatment of chronic hyponatremia, and particularly the role of vaptans relative to other treatments such as oral urea, are still evolving. Of special interest will be studies to assess whether more effective treatment of hyponatremia can reduce the incidence of falls and fractures in older patients, the use of health care resources for both inpatients and outpatients with hyponatremia, and the increased morbidity and mortality of patients with hyponatremia associated with multiple disease states. Consequently, the indications for treatment of water-retaining disorders in patients without symptomatic hyponatremia must await further studies specifically designed to assess the effects of treatment on clinically relevant outcomes, as well as

clinical experience that better delineates efficacies and potential toxicities of all treatments for hyponatremia.

Complete bibliography is available at Elsevier eBooks for Practicing Clinicians.

Key Bibliography

Adrogué HJ, Madias NE. Diagnosis and treatment of hyponatremia. *Am J Kidney Dis*. 2014;64:681–684.

Berl T. Vasopressin antagonists. *N Engl J Med*. 2015;372:2207–2216.

Berl T, Quittnat-Pelletier F, Verbalis JG, et al. Oral tolvaptan is safe and effective in chronic hyponatremia. *J Am Soc Nephrol*. 2010;21:705–712.

Corona G, Giuliani C, Parenti G, et al. Moderate hyponatremia is associated with increased risk of mortality: evidence from a meta-analysis. *PLoS ONE*. 2013;0.c00451.

Ellison DH, Berl T. Clinical practice. The syndrome of inappropriate antidiuresis. *N Engl J Med*. 2007;356:2064–2072.

Fenske W, Stork S, Koschker AC, et al. Value of fractional uric acid excretion in differential diagnosis of hyponatremic patients on diuretics. *J Clin Endocrinol Metab*. 2008;93:2991–2997.

Greenberg A, Verbalis JG, Amin AN, et al. Current treatment practice and outcomes. Report of the hyponatremia registry. *Kidney Int*. 2015;88:167–177.

Hawkins RC. Age and gender as risk factors for hyponatremia and hypernatremia. *Clin Chim Acta*. 2003;337:169–172.

Hoorn EJ, Rivadeneira F, van Meurs JB, et al. Mild hyponatremia as a risk factor for fractures: the Rotterdam Study. *J Bone Miner Res*. 2011;26:1822–1828.

Renneboog B, Musch W, Vandemergel X, et al. Mild chronic hyponatremia is associated with falls, unsteadiness, and attention deficits. *Am J Med*. 2006;119:71–78.

Rosner MH, Kirven J. Exercise-associated hyponatremia. *Clin J Am Soc Nephrol*. 2007;2:151–161.

Schrier RW, Gross P, Gheorghiade M, et al. Tolvaptan, a selective oral vasopressin V2-receptor antagonist, for hyponatremia. *N Engl J Med*. 2006;355:2099–2112.

Spasovski G, Vanholder R, Allolio B, et al. Clinical practice guideline on diagnosis and treatment of hyponatraemia. *Nephrol Dial Transplant*. 2014;29(suppl 2):1–139.

Sterns RH. Disorders of plasma sodium. *N Engl J Med*. 2015;372:1267–1269.

Sterns RH, Nigwekar SU, Hix JK. The treatment of hyponatremia. *Semin Nephrol*. 2009;29:282–299.

Usala RL, Fernandez SJ, Mete M, et al. Hyponatremia is associated with increased osteoporosis and bone fractures in a large U.S. health system population. *J Clin Endocrinol Metab*. 2015;100:3021–3031.

Verbalis JG. Brain volume regulation in response to changes in osmolality. *Neuroscience*. 2010;168:862–870.

Verbalis JG, Barsony J, Sugimura Y, et al. Hyponatremia-induced osteoporosis. *J Bone Miner Res*. 2010;25:554–563.

Verbalis JG, Goldsmith SR, Greenberg A, et al. Diagnosis, evaluation, and treatment of hyponatremia: expert panel recommendations. *Am J Med*. 2013;126(10 suppl 1):S1–S42.

Wald R, Jaber BL, Price LL, et al. Impact of hospital-associated hyponatremia on selected outcomes. *Arch Intern Med*. 2010;170:294–302.

8

Hypernatremia and Hyperosmolar Disorders

SOPHIA L. AMBRUSO, STUART L. LINAS

The serum sodium concentration ([Na+]) is the ratio of sodium to water in the extracellular fluid (ECF) compartment. It is determined by the relationship among total body sodium, potassium, and water, the last of which typically is the main determinant. Dysnatremias, or derangements in serum [Na+], include both hyponatremia and hypernatremia. This chapter focuses on the etiology and management of hypernatremia, a hyperosmolar state defined by serum [Na+] exceeding 145 mEq/L.

Hypernatremia itself is not a disorder but rather a laboratory abnormality caused by an underlying pathologic process. The diagnostic approach to hypernatremia must consider the determinants of the serum [Na+]. Although excesses in total body sodium and, very rarely, excesses in total body potassium can lead to hypernatremia, the majority of cases result from deficits in total body water (TBW).

To simplify the management of hypernatremia, this chapter considers the balance of TBW and sodium separately. This important concept will be illustrated by dividing the water and sodium components of the ECF compartment into separate theoretical beakers (Fig. 8.1). The goal is to determine appropriate, timely therapies for a disorder that is associated with a high degree of morbidity and mortality.

Definitions

Normal serum [Na+] is 135 to 145 mEq/L. This range is generally maintained despite large individual variations in salt and water intake. Hypernatremia is *always* a water problem and sometimes also a salt problem. There is no predictable relationship between serum [Na+] (a measure of osmolality and tonicity) and total body salt or volume status. More specifically, although hypernatremia confirms the presence of a relative water deficit, the isolated laboratory finding of a serum [Na+] greater than 145 mEq/L does not reveal anything about a person's volume status. As a result, hypernatremia may occur in the setting of hypovolemia, euvolemia, or hypervolemia, as indicated in Fig. 8.1.

Dehydration and Volume Depletion

Comparing the terms "dehydration" and "volume depletion" illustrates the distinction between water and sodium balance. Although *dehydration* is commonly used to describe a person's volume status, this use is inaccurate. Dehydration does not equal volume depletion.

Rather, *dehydration* is a description of water balance, whereas *volume depletion* refers to a person's sodium balance. Although these two clinical scenarios may coexist, they should not be confused. It is important that the two terms are not used interchangeably and that a patient's water and sodium balance be considered independently when addressing dysnatremias clinically.

Hyperosmolality and Hypertonicity

Hypernatremia always reflects a hyperosmolar state, whereas the reverse is not always true. For example, hyperosmolality may also be a consequence of severe hyperglycemia or elevated blood urea nitrogen, as is seen in kidney failure. Furthermore, hyperosmolality does not necessarily mean hypertonicity. For example, uremia is a hyperosmolar but not a hypertonic state. Urea is an ineffective osmole because it can freely cross cell membranes, unlike sodium; therefore, urea contributes to osmolality but not to tonicity. In contrast to urea, sodium, which is unable to cross cell membranes freely, is an effective osmole and is the primary cation that affects plasma osmolality (P_{osm}). Hypernatremia is a hypertonic state in which water will flow from the intracellular to the extracellular space, resulting in cellular dehydration and shrinkage.

Background

Hypernatremia is all about water. A more accurate term for hypernatremia might be "hypoaquaremia" because it literally means a state in which there is too little water in the intravascular space and, therefore, too little water in the intracellular space. To begin any discussion of hypernatremia (or hyponatremia), it is important to understand that dysnatremias are actually disorders of water homeostasis.

Water distributes throughout all body compartments, with two-thirds in the intracellular and one-third in the extracellular compartment. Three-quarters of the water in the extracellular compartment is located in the interstitial space, and one-quarter is in the intravascular space (Fig. 8.2). Water is lost (or gained) in the same proportions as it is distributed throughout all body compartments. Pure water loss does not affect plasma volume status or hemodynamics significantly until very late because of the normal distribution of water throughout all body compartments. For example, for every 1 L of water deficit, only approximately 80 mL is lost from the intravascular (plasma) compartment.

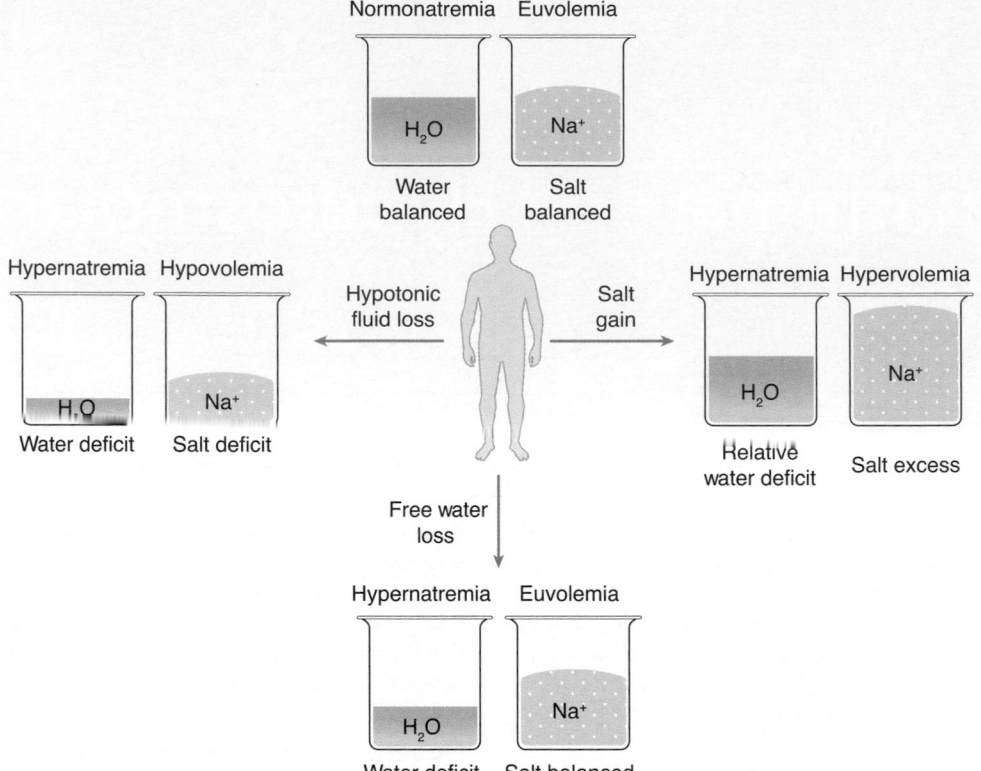

• **Fig. 8.1 Diagnostic approach to hypernatremia.** The pathophysiology of hypernatremia is best understood by separating water and salt balance, done so here by theoretical beakers. Water balance determines the serum sodium concentration, whereas salt balance determines volume status. The beakers at the top of the figure represent normal physiology with water and salt in balance. In the three remaining cases of hypernatremia there is a water deficit with varying degrees of salt balance or volume status. Refer to Table 8.1 for further details regarding the specific causes of hypernatremia for each group of salt balance.

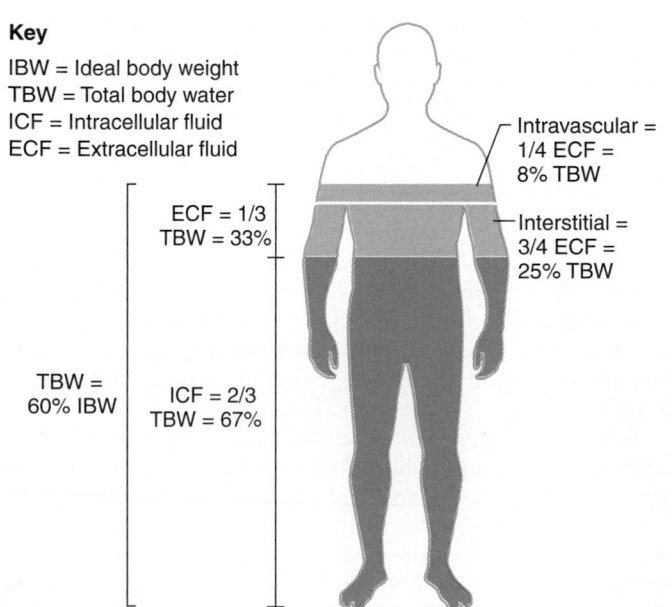

Key

IBW = Ideal body weight
TBW = Total body water
ICF = Intracellular fluid
ECF = Extracellular fluid

• **Fig. 8.2 Normal water distribution.** Total body water (TBW) is 60% of a person's ideal body weight. Of that, two-thirds (66%) is distributed to the intracellular space (ICF) and one-third (33%) to the extracellular space (ECF). Three-quarters of the extracellular space, approximately 25% of TBW, is interstitial, whereas one-quarter, approximately 8% of TBW, is intravascular.

Epidemiology

The incidence of hypernatremia in all hospitalized patients ranges from less than 1% to approximately 3%. However, in critically ill patients, the overall prevalence of hypernatremia ranges between 9% and 26% and is hospital acquired in approximately 80% of these cases. Hypernatremia present at the time of hospital admission is primarily a disease of older adults and of those with mental illness or impaired sensorium. Most patients with hypernatremia on admission to the hospital have concomitant infections. Hypernatremia that is present on hospital admission is generally treated earlier than hypernatremia that develops during the hospital course, most likely because of increased attention paid to individual laboratory values and volume status on hospital admission.

In contrast, hospital-acquired hypernatremia is typically seen in patients who are younger than those with hypernatremia on admission, with an age distribution similar to that of the general hospitalized population. Hospital-acquired hypernatremia is largely iatrogenic from inadequate and/or inappropriate fluid prescription and, therefore, is largely preventable. It results from a combination of decreased access to water, disease processes that may increase insensible losses or interfere with the thirst mechanism, and administration of loop diuretics. Approximately half of patients with hospital-acquired hypernatremia are intubated and, therefore, have no free access to water. Of the remainder, most have altered mental status.

Patients at highest risk for hospital-acquired hypernatremia are those at the extremes of age (infants and older adults), those with altered mental status, and those without access to water (i.e., intubated or debilitated patients). In addition to the impaired thirst and decreased urinary concentrating ability that accompany advanced age, older patients have a lower baseline TBW content, making smaller changes in water balance more clinically relevant.

Clinical Manifestations

Symptoms

Clinical symptoms related to hypernatremia can be attributed to cellular dehydration and shrinkage due to the loss of intracellular water. Loss of intracellular water occurs throughout the body, but the primary symptoms are neurologic. The severity of neurologic symptoms is more dependent on the rate of rise in serum [Na$^+$] than on the absolute value. Polyuria and polydipsia are frequently the presenting symptoms of diabetes insipidus (DI), with or without the presence of hypernatremia.

Neurologic symptoms comprise a continuum that begins with fatigue, lethargy, irritability, and confusion and progresses to seizures and coma. Additional symptoms of hypernatremia include anorexia, nausea, vomiting, and generalized muscle weakness. Altered mental status can be both a cause and an effect of hypernatremia, and consequently can be difficult to distinguish clinically. In addition, cellular dehydration and shrinkage can lead to rupture of cerebral veins because of traction, which results in focal intracerebral and subarachnoid hemorrhages; this occurs more often in infants than in adults.

Signs

Signs of hypernatremia depend, in part, on its cause and severity. Abnormal subclavicular and forearm skin turgor and altered sensorium are commonly found in patients with hypovolemic or euvolemic hypernatremia, whereas patients with hypervolemic hypernatremia typically have classic signs of volume overload, such as elevated neck veins and edema.

Pathophysiology

A sound understanding of the normal physiology of water and salt balance is integral to the understanding and management of dysnatremias. The intracellular and extracellular body compartments exist in osmotic equilibrium. The development of hypernatremia is most commonly the result of increased water losses combined with inadequate intake. Rarely does hypernatremia occur as a consequence of excessive sodium intake.

Regulation of plasma [Na$^+$] is determined by the regulation of P$_{osm}$, of which plasma [Na$^+$] is the primary determinant. Normal P$_{osm}$ is between 285 and 295 mOsm/kg. If the P$_{osm}$ varies by 1% to 2% in either direction, physiologic mechanisms are in place to return the P$_{osm}$ to normal. In the case of hypernatremia or hyperosmolality, receptor cells in the hypothalamus detect increases in P$_{osm}$; in response, they stimulate thirst to increase water intake and simultaneously stimulate antidiuretic hormone (ADH) release to limit urinary water losses (by increasing water reabsorption in the collecting duct). Under normal conditions, the body is able to maintain the serum osmolality under tight control. The goal of "normonatremia" is to avoid changes in cellular volume and thereby prevent potential disruptions in cellular structure and function. The body's normal physiologic defense against hypernatremia is twofold: an endogenous thirst stimulus and renal conservation of water.

As with other electrolyte disturbances, the pathophysiology of hypernatremia can be easily categorized into two phases—an initiation phase and a maintenance phase. Simply stated, the initiation, or generation, phase must be caused by a net water loss or, less commonly, a net sodium gain. For hypernatremia to exist as anything more than a transient state, there must be a maintenance phase, defined necessarily by inadequate water intake.

Water metabolism is primarily controlled by arginine vasopressin (AVP) or *ADH*, as it is commonly termed. ADH is produced in the hypothalamus (supraoptic and paraventricular nuclei) and is stored in and secreted by the posterior pituitary. ADH release can be stimulated by either increases in P$_{osm}$ or decreases in mean arterial pressure or blood volume. In the setting of hypernatremia, the primary stimulus for the release of ADH comes from osmoreceptors located in the hypothalamus. ADH acts on the vasopressin type 2 (V$_2$) receptors in the collecting duct to cause increased water reabsorption from the tubular lumen via insertion of aquaporin-2 channels (Fig. 8.3).

The kidney's primary role in hypernatremia is to concentrate the urine maximally, preventing further loss of electrolyte-free fluid. For the kidney to do so, the following must be present: (1) a concentrated medullary interstitium, (2) ADH to insert aquaporin-2 channels into the apical membranes of the collecting duct, and (3) the ability of collecting duct cells to respond to ADH.

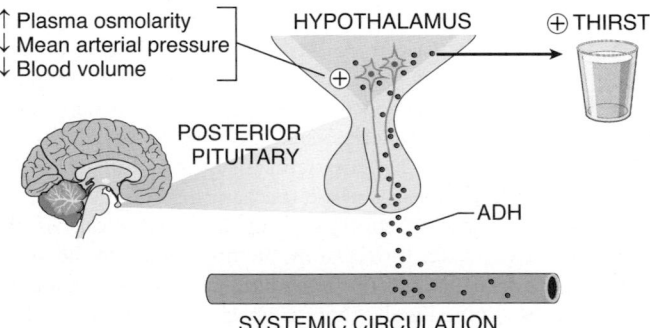

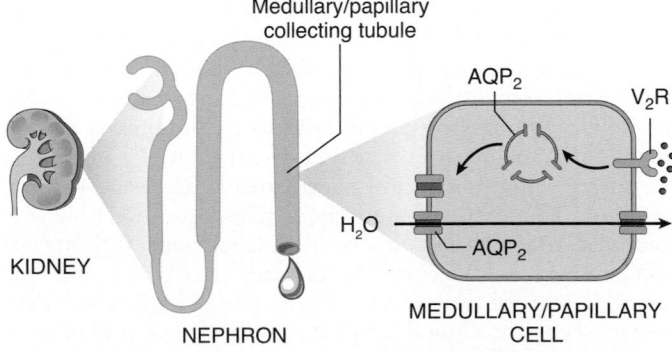

• **Fig. 8.3** ADH stimulus, release, and activity. ADH release is stimulated by an increase in plasma osmolality, decrease in mean arterial pressure, or decrease in blood volume. In hypernatremia, osmoreceptors in the hypothalamus directly stimulate the thirst mechanism while inducing ADH release from the posterior pituitary. ADH acts on the vasopressin type 2 (V$_2$) receptors in the medullary and papillary collecting ducts, upregulating AQP$_2$ channel production and insertion into the apical membrane, leading to increased water reabsorption from the tubular lumen. ADH, antidiuretic hormone; AQP$_2$, aquaporin-2; V$_2$R, vasopressin type 2 receptor.

In a steady state, water intake must equal water output. Obligatory kidney water loss is directly dependent on solute excretion and urinary concentrating ability. Also recall that solute intake must equal solute excretion. Therefore, if a person has to excrete, for example, 700 mOsm of solute per day (primarily Na^+, K^+, and urea), and his or her urine concentration capability is impaired, as reflected by a maximum urinary osmolality (U_{osm}) of 100 mOsm/kg, then the minimum urine output requirement will be 7 L (see calculation below).

Required urine output (L)

= solute excretion (mOsm)/urine osmolality (mOsm/kg)

However, if the kidneys are able to concentrate the urine to a U_{osm} of 700 mOsm/kg, urine output would need to be only 1 L.

Thirst, on the other hand, is an ADH-independent mechanism of defense against hypertonicity. Like ADH release, thirst is triggered by osmoreceptors located in the hypothalamus. The intense thirst stimulated by hypernatremia may be impaired or absent in patients with altered mental status or hypothalamic lesions and in older adults. It is important to note that patients with moderate to severe increases in electrolyte-free water losses may maintain eunatremia because of the powerful thirst mechanism. For example, a patient with nephrogenic DI may maintain a normal serum [Na^+] if given unlimited access to water but may develop marked hypernatremia in situations in which access to water is restricted (e.g., altered mental status, mechanical ventilation, nothing-by-mouth status during hospitalization).

Although ADH activity is a pivotal physiologic defense against hyperosmolality, only an increase in water intake can replace a water deficit. An increase in ADH activity in collecting tubules can only help to decrease ongoing water losses but cannot replace water that has already been lost. Therefore, both ADH-dependent and ADH-independent mechanisms are integral to the body's efforts to protect against hypernatremia or hyperosmolality.

The brain has multiple defense mechanisms designed to protect it from the adverse effects of cellular dehydration. As the serum [Na^+] rises, water moves from the intracellular to the extracellular space to equalize the osmolalities in the body compartments. Almost immediately, there is an increase in the net leak of serum electrolytes (primarily Na^+ and K^+) into the intracellular space, which increases intracellular osmolality. In addition, there is an increased production of cerebrospinal fluid, with movement into the interstitial areas of the brain. Within approximately 24 hours, brain cells generate *osmolytes* or *idiogenic osmoles* (e.g., amino acids, trimethylamines, myoinositol) to increase intracellular osmolality to return water intracellularly. This process restores intracellular volume over a period of days, thereby decreasing the adverse clinical impact of hypernatremia (i.e., cellular dehydration). The increase in transcellular transport of electrolytes is somewhat transient because over time it interferes with normal cellular function. Idiogenic osmoles clearly serve a protective role, but their removal is also slow (days) when isotonicity has been reestablished. The clinical implications of slow removal of idiogenic osmoles from the perspective of hypernatremia correction varies based on patient population. Previously, recommendations for slow serum sodium correction due to assumed risk of cellular swelling and cerebral edema were based on pediatric data. However, a more recent prospective analysis of critically ill adult patients with hypernatremia demonstrated no association between rate of correction and cerebral edema, seizures, and/or alteration of consciousness. Therefore, in adult populations, more rapid hypernatremia correction is recommended.

Pathogenesis and Diagnostic Approach

Hypernatremia most commonly results from the combination of increased water loss and decreased water intake. Any clinical condition associated with increased water loss or decreased water intake predisposes to hypernatremia. In general, for hypernatremia to occur, the rate of water excretion must exceed that of water intake. Hypernatremia secondary to sodium loading, which is less common, is an exception to this basic principle.

Water losses occur via the genitourinary and gastrointestinal tracts, as well as via the skin and respiratory tract as insensible losses. DI and osmotic diuresis result in excess urinary loss of water, and excess water is lost via stool in severe diarrhea. Conditions that increase insensible losses include fever, burns, open wounds, and hyperventilation.

Although hypernatremia is due to an imbalance of water homeostasis, there may be a concomitant salt disturbance. After a thorough clinical history is obtained and a complete physical examination performed, the first decision point in the evaluation of any patient with hypernatremia is to determine the patient's sodium balance or volume status (see Fig. 8.1). Hypernatremia can be seen in patients whose sodium balance is negative (hypovolemic), normal (euvolemic), or positive (hypervolemic), but in all cases a negative water balance is present. Determining the patient's sodium balance is essential to planning the appropriate therapy.

Negative Sodium Balance

Hypernatremia due to the loss of hypotonic fluids is associated with both a negative sodium balance and a negative water balance (Table 8.1). In such cases, hypernatremia develops because the sustained loss of water exceeds that of sodium. These patients usually manifest typical signs of sodium depletion, or hypovolemia, such as tachycardia and orthostatic hypotension. Determination of the urine sodium concentration ([U_{Na}]) can help distinguish between kidney losses, such as from diuretics or osmotic diuresis ([U_{Na}] >20 mEq/dL), and extrarenal losses, such as from diarrhea or vomiting ([U_{Na}] <20 mEq/dL).

Normal Sodium Balance

Hypernatremia in patients with a normal sodium balance results from the loss of electrolyte-free fluid, or pure water (see Table 8.1). These patients have a normal total body sodium (and are therefore euvolemic) but are TBW depleted. The causes of hypernatremia in patients with a normal sodium balance may be kidney or extrarenal. In these cases, urine osmolality (U_{osm}), which reflects ADH levels and function, is often more helpful than U_{Na}. A low U_{osm} is consistent with kidney losses and, therefore, with low ADH levels or function (DI), whereas a high U_{osm} suggests extrarenal losses of free water and intact secretion of and response to ADH.

Etiologies of DI may be central, nephrogenic, or gestational (Box 8.1). The key diagnostic step in determining a central versus a nephrogenic cause is based on the response to exogenous hormone replacement (i.e., vasopressin). A finding of little or no increase in U_{osm} after administration of exogenous vasopressin is diagnostic of nephrogenic DI. However, it is important to remember that central or nephrogenic DI may be partial: Either ADH is present but in insufficient quantity (partial central DI) or there is an incomplete response to ADH in the collecting duct (partial nephrogenic DI). Distinguishing between nephrogenic DI and central DI has historically required the administration of desmopressin

TABLE 8.1   Causes of Hypernatremia

Kidney Causes of Water Deficit

Salt Deficit *(Urine [Na⁺] >20 mEq/dL)*	Salt Balanced *(U_{osm}/P_{osm} <1)*	Salt Excess
Diuresis	***Diabetes Insipidus (See Box 8.1)***	Mineralocorticoid excess
Medication (loop diuretic)	ADH-dependent	
Post-AKI	Central	
Postobstructive	Nephrogenic	
Osmotic (glucose, urea, mannitol)	Acquired	
	ADH-independent	
	Electrolyte disturbance	
	Drug-induced	
	Chronic kidney disease	
	Malnutrition	

Extrarenal Causes of Water Deficit

Salt Deficit *(Urine [Na⁺] <20 mEq/dL)*	Salt Balanced *(U_{osm}/P_{osm} <1)*	Salt Excess
Gastrointestinal	***Increased Insensible Losses***	***Excessive Na⁺ Intake***
Vomiting	Cutaneous (fever, sweating, increased temperature, burns)	Saline
Diarrhea	Respiratory (tachypnea)	Bicarbonate
Nasogastric suction	***Decreased Intake***	Salt ingestion
Enterocutaneous fistula	Primary hypodipsia (older adults, hypothalamic, or osmoreceptor dysfunction)	Hyperalimentation/TPN
Cutaneous	Reset osmostat	Hypertonic dialysate
Sweating	Limited access to water (altered mental status, iatrogenic)	
Burns	***Intracellular Shift***	
	Seizures	
	Severe exercise	

ADH, antidiuretic hormone; *AKI,* acute kidney injury; *[Na⁺],* sodium ion concentration; *P_{osm},* plasma osmolality; *U_{osm},* urine osmolality, *TPN,* total parenteral nutrition.

acetate (dDAVP), a synthetic analogue of ADH, with subsequent surveillance of the kidney response via urine osmolality measurements. Unfortunately, difficulties in interpreting these results remain. Furthermore, direct measurement of ADH remains technically difficult; thus, it has not been widely adopted in clinical practice. More recently, direct measurement of plasma copeptin, the C-terminal segment of ADH with good ex-vivo stability, has demonstrated diagnostic accuracy after hypertonic saline infusion.

One rare form of DI is gestational, or pregnancy-related, DI, which is caused by production of placental vasopressinase that metabolizes ADH. Gestational DI should be evident from the clinical history. The manifestations are similar to those of nephrogenic DI in that there is little or no increase in U_{osm} with exogenous vasopressin; however, gestational DI responds to dDAVP, which is unaffected by vasopressinase.

Nephrogenic DI can be either hereditary (genetic defect of the V_2 receptor gene or aquaporin water channel) or acquired. Acquired nephrogenic DI may be reversible and includes any clinical condition in which the kidney is unable to maximally concentrate the urine. The mechanisms of acquired nephrogenic DI are ADH independent. The most common cause of acquired nephrogenic DI is chronic lithium use. The mechanism of lithium-induced nephrogenic DI includes both a decrease in density of V_2 receptors and decreased expression of aquaporin-2 channels. Hypercalcemia, hypokalemia, and severe malnutrition are other common examples of reversible nephrogenic DI. Hypercalcemia can induce a reversible nephrogenic DI through inhibition of sodium reabsorption in the loop of Henle, which impairs the generation of an adequate medullary gradient and reduces concentrating ability. In addition, dysregulation of the aquaporin-2 channel can be seen with hypercalcemia. Hypokalemia causes

nephrogenic DI by decreasing collecting tubule responsiveness to ADH. Decreased protein intake leads to decreased urea production and, therefore, a decreased medullary gradient with inability to maximally concentrate the urine.

A high U_{osm} suggests extrarenal losses as the cause of euvolemic hypernatremia. To generate a high U_{osm}, the kidney must be able to concentrate the urine, an ability that requires intact ADH-dependent mechanisms. Insensible losses are the primary source of electrolyte-free water loss in this subgroup of patients. Increased insensible losses occur via the skin (burns, sweat), respiratory tract (tachypnea), or both.

Finally, patients with hypodipsia or adipsia may develop euvolemic hyponatremia. Most often, they have normally functioning kidneys but lack adequate water intake. These patients typically have a high U_{osm} and low urine output. Idiopathic hypodipsia occurs, but identification of an impaired thirst mechanism as the primary disorder causing hypernatremia should lead to a more thorough neurologic investigation to rule out the presence of hypothalamic tumors or disorders. An impaired thirst mechanism or limited access to water in the setting of DI can result in severe hypernatremia and can be life threatening.

Positive Sodium Balance

Hypernatremia resulting from total body sodium gain is the least common type of hypernatremia (see Table 8.1). In these cases, total body sodium is uniformly increased, but TBW may be increased or unchanged, depending on the cause. An increase in extracellular volume should be readily identifiable by the presence of hypervolemia on clinical examination. This clinical presentation is usually iatrogenic, resulting from hypertonic fluid administration (saline or bicarbonate), and it reflects a gain of sodium without an appropriate gain of water. Excess mineralocorticoid activity can also result in hypernatremia with a positive sodium balance, and, in the absence of typical iatrogenic risk factors, should alert the clinician to evaluate for potential causes of mineralocorticoid excess.

An example of hypernatremia in the setting of positive sodium balance is the hemodynamically stable hypernatremic patient with acute respiratory distress syndrome (ARDS) and an elevated central venous pressure. This relative hypervolemic hypernatremic state reflects an imbalance of both water and salt. Commonly, the physician might be concerned that administration of the free water necessary to correct the serum [Na$^+$] (e.g., 3 L) would cause the patient to become fluid overloaded. This would be in direct contrast to the goal of a net negative fluid balance for optimal management of ARDS. However, as normal distribution of water dictates that less than 10% of TBW is distributed into the intravascular space, <300 mL of 3 L of administered free water (intravenously or enterally) would remain in the vascular space; therefore, the fluid administration would not materially impact

the patient's volume status. In addition, it is imperative to understand that further diuresis to obtain a net negative sodium balance, in the absence of water administration, will exacerbate the hypernatremia by increasing free water urinary losses.

Treatment

Treatment goals of hypernatremia include both replacement of the free water deficit and prevention or reduction of ongoing water loss. The amount, route, and rate of replacement depend on the severity of symptoms, rate of onset, concurrent clinical conditions, and the patient's sodium balance (volume status). Correction of the latter in a hemodynamically unstable patient is always a priority, no matter how severe the hypernatremia. In this setting, ECF depletion should always be corrected with 0.9% saline before the water deficit is addressed. After the patient is hemodynamically stable, it is important to focus on the treatment of the water deficit because the complications of hypernatremia frequently result from its inappropriate correction or treatment, not the electrolyte disturbance itself. Management of hypernatremia should include identification of the underlying cause in addition to correction of the hypertonic state. Treatment of hypernatremia can, most often, be broken down into the following seven steps (Box 8.2).

Step 1.   Determine Sodium Balance. Evaluation of the patient's sodium balance, or volume status, is a critical first step for both appropriate diagnosis and treatment of hypernatremia. This information should be obtained through a thorough history and physical examination. If the patient is hemodynamically unstable from sodium depletion, this should be addressed first with the administration of isotonic saline.

Step 2.   Calculate Free Water Deficit. Before initiating therapy, it is both prudent and appropriate to quantify the deficit and develop a treatment plan for the individual patient. Calculation of the water deficit represents only a snapshot in time. If it were possible to prevent any further water losses, insensible or otherwise, the calculated water deficit would be the amount that must be administered to normalize the serum [Na$^+$], as shown in Box 8.3, Formula 1:

$$\text{Water deficit} = \text{TBW} \times \left(\text{plasma} \left[\text{Na}^+ \right] / 140 - 1 \right)$$
$$= \left(0.5 \text{ or } 0.6 \right) \times \text{lean body weight} \times$$
$$\left(\text{plasma} \left[\text{Na}^+ \right] / 140 - 1 \right)$$

where the lean body weight is expressed in kilograms. TBW is generally considered to be 50% of lean body weight in women and 60% in men. In this equation, 140 may be replaced by the target serum [Na$^+$]. For example, if the current [Na$^+$] is 160 mEq/L and the goal

---

BOX 8.3

Important Water Balance Formulas

Formula 1   Water deficit = TBW × (plasma [Na⁺] / 140 − 1)

   = (0.5 or 0.6) × lean body weight

   × (plasma [Na⁺] / 140 − 1)

Formula 2 $\Delta[Na^+]_s = [Na^+]_{inf} − [Na^+]_s / TBW + 1$

Formula 3   Urine output = $C_{electrolytes} + C_{electrolyte-free}$
or

   $C_{electrolyte-free} = V \times [1 − \{(U_{Na} + U_K) / P_{Na}\}]$

---

is to reduce the [Na⁺] by 10 mEq/L in 24 hours, then 150 mEq/L is substituted for 140 in the equation. This method may be used to calculate the water deficit for any target serum [Na⁺].

Step 3.   Choose a Replacement Fluid. The choice of fluid for repletion of a free water deficit depends on the clinical assessment of the patient's sodium balance. Specifically, a key determination is whether the deficit is the result of a pure water loss, requiring only water repletion, or a hypotonic fluid loss, which requires both water and salt repletion. In general, patients with a pure water loss should be repleted with the use of enteral free water (oral or nasogastric tube) or by intravenous administration of 5% dextrose in water (D_5W). Patients with a deficit of both salt and water should be repleted with a combination of salt and water. This correction may be accomplished by the administration of 0.2% or 0.45% saline or with the use of separate intravenous solutions, one for water repletion (D_5W) and one for correction of the salt deficit (0.9% saline). The potential advantage of using two separate infusions is the avoidance of continued salt repletion after the volume deficit has been corrected.

The route of repletion must also be determined. As with nutritional repletion, the enteral route for repletion of free water is preferable; however, it is not always an option as patients commonly have altered mental status. Water can be repleted through a nasogastric tube if gut function is not compromised. The enteral route is preferable because it avoids the administration of the dextrose required to provide water intravenously. Dextrose may increase serum osmolality via hyperglycemia, which can lead to an osmotic diuresis and the unwanted kidney clearance of additional electrolyte-free water. Most commonly, correction of the free water deficit will be done, at least initially, via the intravenous route.

Step 4.   Determine Rate of Repletion. The rate of correction of serum [Na⁺] is recommended to be approximately 0.5 mEq/L/h, or a decrease of 10 to 12 mEq/L in a 24-hour period. No human studies have been performed to substantiate the appropriateness of this rate. However, based on animal studies, this reflects the observed rate of cerebral de-adaptation, or the rate at which the brain is able to shed electrolytes and idiogenic osmoles acquired in the adaptive response to cellular dehydration. An important exception to this recommended rate of correction occurs in acutely symptomatic patients who have seizures or acute obtundation, potentially requiring intubation for airway protection. In these circumstances, the rate of correction can be 1 to 2 mEq/L/h initially, with the

overall rate still not to exceed the recommended 10 to 12 mEq/L in 24 hours. Furthermore, acute symptoms suggest that the hypernatremia developed rapidly, and, consequently, the brain has not had time to adapt. If adaption to hypernatremia has not yet occurred, the risk that cerebral edema will complicate rapid correction is minimal. If the duration of hypernatremia is unknown, the clinician should err on the side of caution and avoid rapid correction. However, if the onset is known to be acute (i.e., developing within the past 24 hours), the serum [Na⁺] can be corrected more quickly because brain adaptation does not occur this quickly.

The calculation of water deficit shown in Step 2 (see Box 8.3, Formula 1) is particularly useful for hypernatremia caused by pure water losses. However, in multiple observational studies a concomitant sodium deficit is present in more than 50% of hypernatremia cases. For this reason, it is frequently necessary to replace both water and sodium deficits, which may be accomplished with 0.2% or 0.45%. Table 8.2 lists the sodium concentrations of commonly used intravenous fluids. Formula 2 can be clinically useful for predicting the change in serum [Na⁺] that will occur with infusion of 1 L of a particular fluid and, accordingly, choosing an appropriate rate of infusion.

$$\Delta[Na^+]_s = [Na^+]_{inf} − [Na^+]_s / TBW + 1$$

where $\Delta[Na^+]_s$ is the change in serum [Na⁺] per liter of fluid infused, $[Na^+]_{inf}$ is the concentration of sodium in the infusate, $[Na^+]_s$ is the patient's current concentration of sodium, and TBW is 50% of ideal body weight for women, or 60% for men, expressed in liters (L).

Step 5.   Estimate Ongoing "Sensible" Losses. The formulas presented for calculation of the water deficit (see Step 2) and estimation of the impact of a particular infusate on serum [Na⁺] (see Step 4) both assume a closed system. They do not account for any ongoing kidney or extrarenal losses. In patients with DI or an osmotic diuresis due to hyperglycemia or administration of mannitol, ongoing urinary water losses can be significant. Formula 3 is clinically useful in estimating the amount of ongoing kidney water

TABLE 8.2   Distribution of Commonly Used Fluids[a]

Fluid	Infusate [Na⁺] (mEq/L)	ECF Distribution (%)[a]	Intravascular Distribution (%)[a]
D_5W	0	33	8
0.225% NaCl in D_5W	38.5	50	12.5
0.45% NaCl	77	62.5	15.5
Lactated Ringer solution	130	100	25
0.9% NaCl in water	154	100	25

[a]The distribution of water is assumed to be two-thirds intracellular and one-third extracellular, with the extracellular distribution being one-quarter intravascular and three-quarters interstitial.

D_5W, 5% dextrose in water; ECF, extracellular fluid; [Na⁺], sodium ion concentration; NaCl, sodium chloride.

losses, based on clearance (C) of the electrolyte and electrolyte-free components of the urinary fluid:

$$\text{Urine output} = C_{\text{electrolytes}} + C_{\text{electrolyte-free}}$$

or

$$C_{\text{electrolyte-free}} = V \times \left[1 - \left\{ (U_{Na} + U_K) / P_{Na} \right\} \right]$$

where U_{Na} is the urine sodium concentration, U_K is the urine potassium concentration, and P_{Na} is the plasma sodium concentration, all expressed in milliequivalents per liter (mEq/L). Volume (V) may be expressed in any increment of time, with subsequent extrapolation to a 24-hour period.

The following example illustrates the utility of this free water clearance formula. If the random U_{Na} is 25 mEq/L, U_K is 15 mEq/L, and P_{Na} is 160 mEq/L, then 25% of the urine output can be attributed to the clearance of electrolytes, and 75% is electrolyte-free water. In the setting of a serum [Na$^+$] of 160 mEq/L, urine with 75% electrolyte-free water clearance is inappropriate. The U_{osm} can help to distinguish whether the high free water clearance represents an osmotic diuresis or DI. A high U_{osm} would be consistent with an osmotic diuresis (from glucose, urea, or mannitol), whereas a low U_{osm} would be consistent with DI.

Step 6. Estimate Ongoing "Insensible" Losses. Ongoing losses include urine and stool output as well as losses from the skin and respiratory tract, termed *insensible losses*. It is reasonable to assume insensible losses of 10 to 15 mL/kg/day for women and 15 to 20 mL/kg/day for men, with factors such as fever, ambient temperature, infection, burns, open wounds, and tachypnea causing an increase in insensible losses.

Step 7. Identify and Treat Underlying Causes. Although the mainstay of treatment of hypernatremia is repletion of the water deficit, attempts to prevent additional losses should be undertaken. In central DI, for example, treatment with a V_2 agonist (i.e., desmopressin) is critical. Nephrogenic DI is considerably more difficult to treat, but treatment can include administration of a thiazide diuretic to create a mildly volume-depleted state and, consequently, decreased water delivery to the collecting ducts. Low-protein and low-sodium diets can also help to decrease the amount of obligatory solute clearance and thereby decrease the urine output. See Box 8.4 for further condition-specific treatment recommendations.

The treatment approach described earlier applies primarily to hypernatremia in the setting of normal or negative sodium balance. Treatment of hypernatremia with a positive sodium balance is quite different and relies primarily on correction of the hypervolemic state with diuretics. An important consideration in this clinical scenario is that, although gain of sodium is the primary disturbance, there is still a relative lack of water. Diuresis in the absence of water repletion will exacerbate the hypernatremia. Loop diuretics interfere with the concentrating mechanism of the kidneys and, therefore, cause an inappropriate loss of electrolyte-free water in addition to the desired natriuresis. For this reason, it is imperative to replete the free water deficit in these patients and to calculate their ongoing losses using Formula 3 (see Step 5) to achieve adequate repletion. This is of particular concern in those patients who are without free access to water.

Undercorrection, a common mistake encountered in the treatment of hypernatremia, is most commonly caused by underestimation of ongoing sensible and insensible losses. Formula 3 allows the clinician to obtain a more accurate reflection of ongoing kidney electrolyte-free

---

BOX 8.4

Special Considerations for Treatment of Hypernatremia

Negative Sodium Balance
Correct water and salt deficit
Treat underlying condition (e.g., hyperglycemia, urinary obstruction)

Normal Sodium Balance
Correct water deficit
CDI: administer dDAVP and correct underlying disorder
GDI: administer dDAVP (vasopressinase does not cleave dDAVP)
NDI (reversible): remove offending medication, correct electrolyte abnormality
NDI (irreversible): thiazide diuretic, NSAIDs, decrease salt intake
NDI (lithium-related): amiloride and thiazide diuretic, acetazolamide

Positive Sodium Balance
Correct water deficit and sodium/volume overload
Diuretics
Dialysis if concurrent kidney failure is present

CDI, central diabetes insipidus; *dDAVP*, desmopressin; *GDI*, gestational diabetes insipidus; *NDI*, nephrogenic diabetes insipidus; *NSAIDs*, nonsteroidal antiinflammatory drugs.

---

water loss. In addition, it is important to identify and account for insensible losses applicable to the individual patient. It was previously believed that overcorrection, or overly rapid correction, placed the patient at increased risk of cellular swelling and cerebral edema. While this may be true in the pediatric population, the rapid correction of hypernatremia in adult populations has not been shown to be associated with neurologic complications. Because the formulas described here are only a guide and lack precision for individual patients, it is critical that serum chemistry values be checked frequently to ensure that the expected and actual rates of correction are similar to allow appropriate and timely adjustments to the treatment decisions, therefore avoiding additional neurologic compromise.

All formulas used to facilitate treatment of hypernatremia have limitations. Specifically, the formulas do not factor in ongoing sensible or insensible losses and use TBW, which is an imprecise term. These formulas should be considered as adjunctive tools but should not replace sound clinical judgment. The isolated use of these formulas to guide therapy could prove deleterious to the patient if used in lieu of appropriate clinical assessment and reassessments. For these reasons, it is critical that serum [Na$^+$] be measured frequently (typically, every 2 hours initially) to assess whether the patient is responding as predicted. This is particularly important for patients with significant unmeasurable losses (e.g., diarrhea, burns) and for those patients with particularly high, ongoing, measurable losses (as frequently occurs with DI).

Complications of Hypernatremia

In several large observational studies, hypernatremia is independently associated with both an increased length of hospital stay and increased mortality. It is unclear whether hypernatremia is simply a marker of illness severity or it contributes directly to an increase in mortality. Acute (≤24 hours) hypernatremia with serum [Na$^+$] levels greater than 160 mEq/L is associated with a 75% mortality rate in adults, whereas chronic hypernatremia is associated with a much lower rate of approximately 10%. Even modest hospital-acquired

BOX 8.5

Hypernatremia Key Points

- Hypernatremia always reflects a hyperosmolar state.
- Hypernatremia is always a water problem, and sometimes a salt problem.
- Patients must have a defect in their thirst mechanism or limited access to free water for hypernatremia to persist.
- The sodium concentration itself does not provide any information about total body salt or volume status.
- A calculation of the water deficit represents only a snapshot in time.
- Formulas should be considered an adjunct tool, not a substitute for sound clinical judgment and frequent monitoring of the serum [Na⁺].
- Failure to consider ongoing sensible and insensible losses is the most common cause of undercorrection.

hypernatremia has been associated with increased mortality in patients with serum [Na⁺] greater than 150 mEq/L, demonstrating a severity of illness-adjusted relative risk of 2.6 for death. Increased mortality and increased length of stay in patients with hypernatremia have been seen across a broad spectrum of patient populations, including both medical and surgical intensive care patients. A decreased level of consciousness occurring as a complication of hypernatremia is an important prognostic indicator associated with mortality. Although the mechanism of the high mortality is not known, it is clear that a judicious approach to diagnosis and treatment of hypernatremia is imperative (Box 8.5).

In addition to the adverse central nervous system effects, hypernatremia also inhibits insulin release and increases insulin resistance, thereby predisposing patients to hyperglycemia. Hypernatremia also decreases hepatic gluconeogenesis, lactate clearance, and cardiac function. A patient's level of consciousness, rather than the absolute serum [Na⁺], is a more important prognostic indicator of mortality.

Adverse sequelae associated with hypernatremia are often underappreciated and frequently lead to a delay in treatment. Studies have shown that fewer than 50% of patients with hospital-acquired hypernatremia receive free water replacement within 24 hours of the first identified elevated serum [Na⁺], and the majority take longer than 72 hours to treat. Furthermore, patients whose hypernatremia is corrected within 72 hours have a lower mortality than those whose hypernatremia is not corrected within 72 hours. In light of the significant associations with adverse physiologic sequelae, increased length of stay, and increased mortality seen with hospital-acquired hypernatremia, hypernatremia should not be viewed as an incidental or negligible electrolyte abnormality.

Complete bibliography is available at Elsevier eBooks for Practicing Clinicians.

Key Bibliography

Adler SM, Verbalis JG. Disorders of body water homeostasis in critical illness. *Endocrinol Metab Clin North Am.* 2006;35:873–894.

Adrogue HA, Madias NE. Aiding fluid prescription for the dysnatremias. *Intensive Care Med.* 1997;23:309–316.

Adrogue HJ, Madias NE. Hypernatremia. *N Engl J Med.* 2000;342:1493–1499.

Alshayeb HM, Showkat A, Babar F, et al. Severe hypernatremia correction rate and mortality in hospitalized patients. *Am J Med Sci.* 2011;341:356–360.

Berl T, Robertson G. Pathophysiology of water metabolism. In: Brenner BM, ed. *The Kidney.* 6th ed. Philadelphia: WB Saunders; 2000: 866–893.

Chassagne P, Druesne L, Capet C, et al. Clinical presentation of hypernatremia in elderly patients: a case control study. *J Am Geriatr Soc.* 2006;54:1225–1230.

Chauhan K, Pattharanitima P, Patel N, et al. Rate of correction of hypernatremia and health outcomes in critically ill patients. *Clin J Am Soc Nephrol.* 2019;14(5):656–663.

Darmon M, Timsit J, Francais A, et al. Association between hypernatraemia acquired in the ICU and mortality: a cohort study. *Nephrol Dial Transplant.* 2010;25:2502–2510.

de Groot T, Sinke AP, Kortenoeven MLA, et al. Acetazolamide attenuates lithium-induced nephrogenic diabetes insipidus. *J Am Soc Nephrol.* 2016;27:2082–2091.

Fenske W, Refardt J, Chifu I, et al. A copeptin-based approach in the diagnosis of diabetes insipidus. *N Engl J Med.* 2018;379: 428–439.

Funk G, Lindner G, Druml W, et al. Incidence and prognosis of dysnatremias present on ICU admission. *Intensive Care Med.* 2010;36: 304–311.

Hall JB, Schmidt GA, Wood LDH. Electrolyte disorders in critical care. In: Hall JB, Schmidt GA, Wood LDH, eds. *Principles of Critical Care.* 3rd ed. New York: McGraw-Hill; 2005:1161–1166.

Hoorn EJ, Betjes M, Weigel J, et al. Hypernatraemia in critically ill patients: too little water and too much salt. *Nephrol Dial Transplant.* 2008;23:1562–1568.

Liamis G, Kalogirou M, Saugos V, et al. Therapeutic approach in patients with dysnatraemias. *Nephrol Dial Transplant.* 2006;21:1564–1569.

Lien YH, Shapiro JI, Chan L. Effect of hypernatremia on organic brain osmoles. *J Clin Invest.* 1990;85:1427–1435.

Lindner G, Funk G, Lassnigg A, et al. Intensive care-acquired hypernatremia after major cardiothoracic surgery is associated with increased mortality. *Intensive Care Med.* 2010;36:1718–1723.

Lindner G, Funk G, Schwarz C, et al. Hypernatremia in the critically ill is an independent risk factor for mortality. *Am J Kidney Dis.* 2007;50:952–957.

Nguyen MK, Kurtz I. Analysis of current formulas used for treatment of the dysnatremias. *Clin Exp Nephrol.* 2004;8:12–16.

Palevsky PM. Hypernatremia. *Semin Nephrol.* 1998;18:20–30.

Rose BD, Post TW. *Clinical Physiology of Acid-Base and Electrolyte Disorders.* 5th ed. New York: McGraw-Hill; 2001.

9

Volume, Edema, and the Clinical Use of Diuretics

VIVEK SOI, JIAN LI, JERRY YEE

Edema represents expansion of the interstitial volume and is a common phenotypic presentation of multiple pathologic processes. The word *diuretic* is derived from the Greek roots *dia* "thoroughly" and *ourein* "urine." Consequently, the term *diuretic* is defined by its ability to amplify urine output and treat edema. Historically, "dropsy" was coincidentally alleviated by various plant and mineral compounds, including mercurial agents such as calomel and novasurol. Subsequently, the primacy of salt retention's role in edema formation led to the development of agents that generated urinary sodium loss. Chlorothiazide, which became available in 1958, ushered in the modern era of targeted diuretic therapy, initially as therapy of edematous states and shortly afterward as treatment of essential hypertension. These agents' capacity to reduce blood pressure (BP) and thus decrease the morbidity and mortality associated with uncontrolled hypertension makes diuretics one of several first-line therapies for treatment of hypertension. Diuretics are also requisite treatment tools in volume overload states, including chronic kidney disease (CKD), nephrotic syndrome, cirrhosis, and heart failure (HF) where they facilitate decongestion. This chapter reviews the various diuretic classes, respective mechanisms of action, and physiologic adaptations that ensue from prolonged use.

Diuretic Classes

The predominant nephron sites of action of the various diuretic classes are illustrated in Fig. 9.1. The diuretic classes include inhibitors of sodium reabsorption in the proximal tubule (PT) where approximately 65% occurs, thick ascending loop of Henle (TALH) where up to 25% occurs, distal convoluted tubule (DCT) where approximately 5% to 10% occurs, and epithelial sodium channel (ENaC) that are, along with mineralocorticoid receptor antagonists (MRAs), potassium-sparing agents that act in the collecting tubule. Osmotic diuretics exert their effect at several points in the nephron that are highly water permeable. SGLT2 inhibitors have a diuretic effect, which may be a major contributor to their other benefits, as discussed in Chapter 26.

Carbonic Anhydrase Inhibitors

Carbonic anhydrase inhibitors (CAIs), represented by acetazolamide (ACZ), produce a brisk alkaline diuresis, impairing sodium reabsorption by decreasing generation of intracellular hydrogen ion (see Fig. 9.1). As a result, there is diminution of sodium reabsorption via the apical PT sodium-hydrogen exchanger (NHE-3). Although NHE3 accounts for nearly one-third of PT sodium reabsorption, CAIs do not produce a proportional loss of sodium because downstream sodium reabsorption increases at the TALH and collecting duct (CD), and glomerular filtration is reduced by tubuloglomerular feedback with a reduction in filtered sodium load. ACZ also facilitates diuresis by inducing kidney vasodilation and inhibiting the bicarbonate-chloride exchanger pendrin, localized to type B-interacted cells of the distal nephron.

ACZ is currently the only CAI used as a diuretic; other CAIs are used as topical formulations for glaucoma therapy. ACZ is readily absorbed and eliminated by tubular secretion (≈50%). However, its use is constrained by its transient action and because prolonged use produces hypokalemia and metabolic acidosis, among other side effects. These side effects can be used to therapeutic advantage: ACZ (daily dosage range, 250–500 mg) corrects the metabolic alkalosis that occurs with thiazide or loop diuretic therapy. ACZ can also attenuate lithium-induced nephrogenic diabetes insipidus. By inhibiting carbonic anhydrase (CA), ACZ decreases intracellular lithium content, resulting in greater urine osmolality with reduced urine volumes. ACZ must be employed cautiously in advanced CKD because systemic accumulation may lead to neurologic side effects. The anticonvulsant topiramate inhibits CA and may cause metabolic acidosis, high urine pH, and kidney phosphate stone formation. Administration of topiramate to patients with a history of kidney stone disease or renal tubular acidosis must be done with caution, if at all, and only when other treatment options are exhausted.

SGLT-2 Inhibitors

Glucose filtered through glomeruli is primarily reabsorbed by the PT sodium-glucose cotransporter-2 (SGLT2) (see Fig 9.1). Blockade by SGLT2 inhibitors (SGLT2i) or "flozins," including canagliflozin, dapagliflozin, empagliflozin, and ertugliflozin, reduce glycemia in type 2 diabetes by enhancing glucose excretion, which produces natriuresis via osmotic diuresis. Resultant natriuresis with reduction in extracellular fluid volume (ECFV) is accompanied by modest BP reduction and restoration of tubuloglomerular feedback that is frequently impaired in diabetic kidney disease. The diuretic effect of SGLT2i is heterogeneous. An initial polyuria is transient, with subsequent reduction of urine output

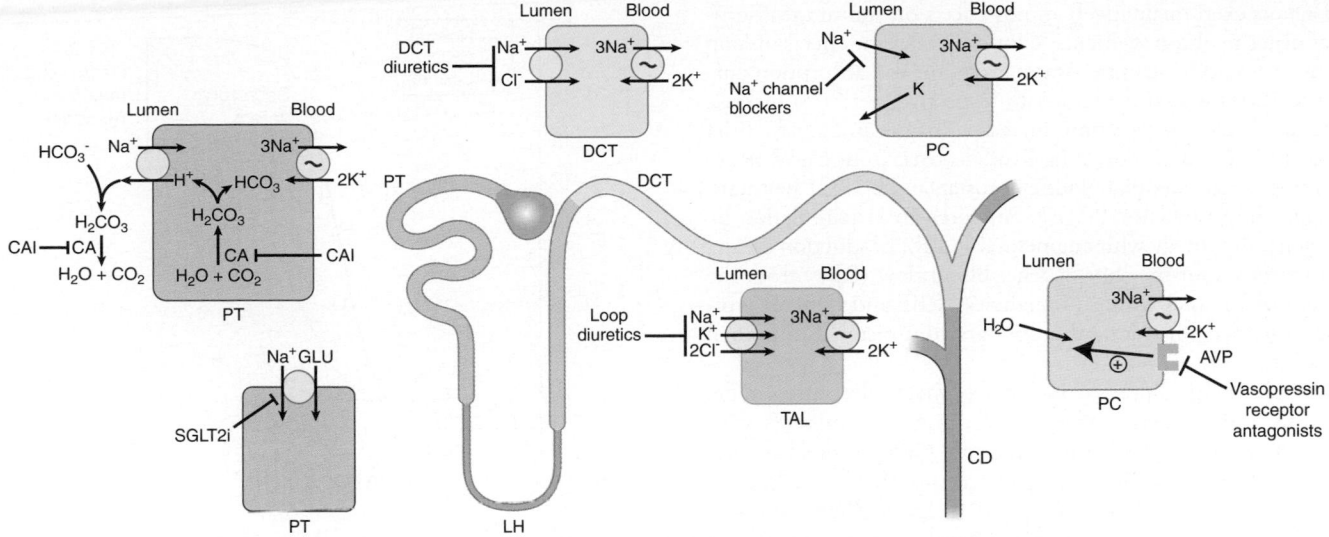

• **Fig. 9.1** Predominant sites and mechanisms of action of clinically important diuretic drugs. Patterns identify sites of action along the nephron and corresponding cell types affected. The proximal tubule (PT, purple segment) is represented by a typical PT cell. The sodium hydrogen exchanger (NHE-3) and sodium glucose cotransporter 2 (SGLT2) are responsible for the majority of sodium reclamation in the PT. The loop of Henle (LH) includes a thick ascending limb (TAL, green segment), and a typical TAL cell is shown in green. The sodium-potassium-2 chloride cotransporter (NKCC2) absorbs sodium via the luminal aspect of the membrane. The distal convoluted tubule (DCT, blue segment) is represented by a typical DCT cell in blue. The sodium chloride cotransporter (NCC) and epithelial sodium transporter (ENaC) regulate sodium reabsorption at this level. The collecting duct (CD, yellow and orange segments) includes principal cells (PC), shown in yellow. Note that, for clarity, two principal cells are shown. Both water and salt pathways exist in the same cells. Both intracellular and luminal actions of carbonic anhydrase (CA) inhibitors in suppressing CA are important in their ability to reduce sodium reabsorption by the kidney proximal tubule. Note that sodium channel blockers probably act along the last half of the DCT and in the connecting tubule as well as in the CD. Spironolactone and eplerenone (not shown) are competitive mineralocorticoid receptor antagonists and act primarily in the cortical collecting tubule. Aquaretics, such as conivaptan or tolvaptan, inhibit water reabsorption by PC by blocking the action of arginine vasopressin on V2 receptors. V2 receptors facilitate insertion of aquaporin 2 water channels in the luminal membrane.

attributable to upregulated sodium, water, and urea reabsorption along the remaining nephron and by renin-angiotensin-aldosterone system (RAAS) activation.

Several trials of SGLT2i demonstrated reductions in cardiovascular (CV) events and rate of progression of CKD, and are discussed in Chapter 26. Sodium accumulation in extravascular tissues such as skin and muscle is associated with volume expanded states, and SGLT2i were shown to reduce cutaneous sodium in patients with type 2 diabetes, supporting the thesis that SGLT2 inhibitors reduce cardiovascular disease (CVD) by decreasing interstitial fluid sodium and volume.

Distal Convoluted Tubule Diuretics

The major site of action of thiazide and thiazide-like diuretics is the early DCT. Here, these agents inhibit coupled, electroneutral sodium and chloride reabsorption by the sodium chloride cotransporter (NCC). Water-soluble thiazides like hydrochlorothiazide (HCTZ) inhibit CA at high doses, which augments sodium excretion. Thiazides also inhibit sodium chloride and water reabsorption in the medullary CD, thereby impairing maximal urinary dilution. Additional drug effects include reductions of uric acid and calcium excretion, elevated urinary magnesium excretion, and impairment of potassium-mediated insulin secretion. The most widely prescribed agent in this class is HCTZ, with an onset of diuresis by

2 hours and peak effect within 3 to 6 hours of administration that dose-dependently continues for up to 12 hours. The half-life of HCTZ is prolonged in decompensated HF and kidney failure, and dosages from 100 to 200 mg daily are required for adequate diuresis of CKD patients. Cumulative natriuresis is arbitrated by the filtered sodium load. Historically, thiazides were eschewed at glomerular filtration rates (GFRs) less than 30 mL/min because of lower efficacy, but more recent data support the use of thiazide diuretics as antihypertensive agents in more advanced stages of CKD.

The concept of "class effect" among thiazide (HCTZ) and thiazide-like diuretics (chlorthalidone [CTD]) has been debated relative to BP reduction and CV outcomes. Although structurally similar, CTD and HCTZ differ pharmacokinetically. CTD has a longer half-life of 40 to 60 hours versus 3.2 to 13.1 hours for HCTZ and larger volume of distribution due to extensive partitioning into red blood cells that serve as a drug depot. The prolonged plasma half-life of CTD likely accounts for its greater potency on a milligram-per-milligram basis compared to HCTZ.

Loop Diuretics

Loop diuretics act predominantly at the luminal TALH membrane where they compete with chloride ion binding to a kidney-specific sodium-potassium-2-chloride cotransporter (NKCC2). Consequently, loop agents inhibit sodium chloride reabsorption.

Loop agents exert qualitatively minor effects on sodium reabsorption at other nephron segments. Clinically relevant effects of loop diuretics are a decrease in free water excretion and absorption during water loading and dehydration, respectively; a 30% increase in fractional calcium excretion; increased magnesuria; and a brief increase followed by a more long-lived decrease in uric acid excretion. Loop agents stimulate kidney prostaglandin (PG) synthesis, especially the vasodilator PG E2. Angiotensin II stimulation by loop agents in synergy with augmented PG E2 production are the probable causes for the shift of renal blood flow (RBF) from the inner to outer kidney cortex. Nonetheless, RBF and GFR are typically maintained when loop diuretics are administered to normal individuals.

Available loop diuretics include bumetanide, furosemide, torsemide, and ethacrynic acid (the last preferred for those with a true sulfa allergy). These compounds are highly protein bound, mainly to albumin. Therefore, to gain access to their site of action, loop agents undergo PT secretion, as do thiazide diuretics, via an organic anion transporter-dependent process. Tubular secretion of loop diuretics is impeded by elevated levels of endogenous organic acids, some of which increase in CKD, and agents that utilize the same transporter, for example, salicylates and nonsteroidal antiinflammatory drugs (NSAIDs). Uremic toxins and fatty acids can decrease loop diuretic protein binding and alter pharmacokinetics.

Diuretic excretion rates and natriuretic response approximate drug delivery to the medullary TALH. This relationship is exemplified by a sigmoidal curve. A normal dose-response relationship (typically observed in untreated hypertension patients) may be shifted (downward and rightward) by a variety of clinical conditions, ranging from ECFV depletion to HF or nephrotic syndrome and drug therapy (Fig. 9.2). One example of the latter is the blunting of diuretic effect via inhibition of prostaglandin synthesis by NSAIDs.

Furosemide is the most widely used loop diuretic. Efficacy is complicated by its variable absorption, with bioavailability ranging from 12% to 112%. The coefficient of variation for absorption varies from 25% to 43% for different furosemide products; exchanging one furosemide formulation for another will not standardize patient absorption and/or response to oral furosemide. Bumetanide and torsemide have superior gut absorption compared to furosemide. The consistency of torsemide absorption and its longer duration of action are features to consider when loop diuretic therapy is required for chronic HF patients and/or CKD patients. Loop diuretics are common therapy in CKD, with the kidney drug clearance reduced in parallel with declining kidney function. Generally, furosemide pharmacokinetics are more significantly changed in CKD than the other loop diuretics because its kidney metabolism and intact clearance is reduced in CKD. Alternatively, bumetanide and torsemide undergo significant hepatic metabolism that is marginally reduced by CKD. In CKD, pharmacokinetic profiles change only as the result of decreased kidney drug clearance.

Potassium-Sparing Diuretics

Potassium-sparing diuretics are divided into two subclasses: MRAs that target the apical mineralocorticoid receptor and ENaC inhibitors that inhibit the luminal namesake channel, resulting in more downstream terminal effects.

The ENaC inhibitors, amiloride and triamterene, diminish sodium reabsorption at the late DCT and CD, thereby reducing basolateral sodium-potassium ATPase activity with consequent reduction in the intracellular potassium concentration. The net

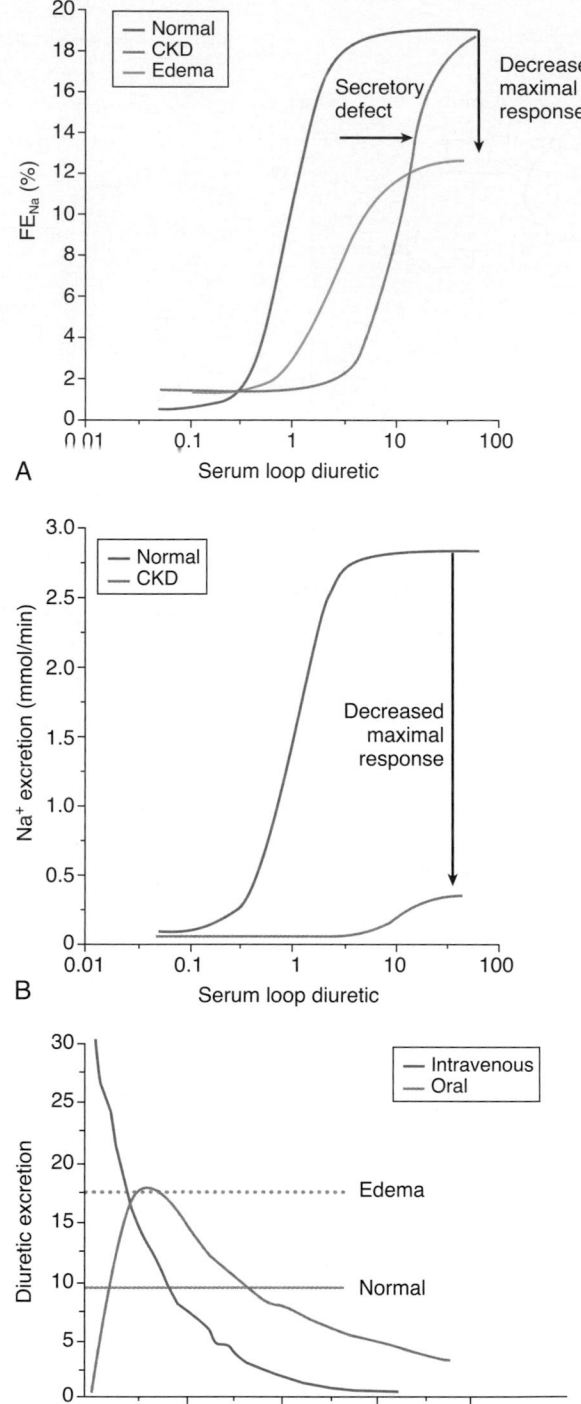

• **Fig. 9.2** (A) Comparison of effects of chronic kidney disease (CKD) and conditions marked by edema on the loop diuretic dose response, expressed as fractional sodium excretion (FE$_{Na}$). Diuretic delivery via secretion into the lumen is impaired in CKD (pharmacokinetic abnormality), whereas the response to delivered drug is diminished with edema (pharmacodynamic defect). (B) Effect of CKD on the absolute response to a loop diuretic; compare (A). (C) Pharmacokinetics of intravenous and oral loop diuretics. The diuretic thresholds for normal and edematous individuals are shown as horizontal lines; whereas a normal individual responds appropriately to either an intravenous or oral diuretic, some edematous individuals can only reach threshold excretion with intravenous diuretic administration. (From Ellison DH. Treatment of disorders of sodium balance in chronic kidney disease. Adv Chronic Kidney Dis. 2017;24(5):332-341.)

effect is reduction of potassium secretion into the tubular lumen. ENaC-directed potassium-sparing diuretics are modestly natriuretic; thus, clinical utility resides primarily in their ability to counterbalance potassium loss, particularly when more proximally acting diuretics increase distal sodium delivery. As a result, ENaC inhibitors are often marketed in combination with thiazide diuretics to avoid the need for potassium supplementation. These drugs are actively secreted by PT cationic transporters and possess modest natriuretic effect. These cationic compounds interfere with the PT secretion of creatinine. Thus, mild serum creatinine elevations may accompany their administration. Amiloride and triamterene undergo extensive kidney clearance and will accumulate with repetitive dosing in settings of reduced GFR.

The MRAs, spironolactone, eplerenone, and finerenone, differ from ENaC inhibitors not only in their site and mechanism of action, but also in clinical use as adjunctive therapy for congestive heart failure. The RAAS is pathologically upregulated in patients with chronic HF with reduced ejection fraction (HFrEF). The addition of MRAs to other approved HF medications has improved clinical outcomes in patients with HFrEF with mild to severe symptoms and also in patients with left ventricular dysfunction after myocardial infarction. Spironolactone is a well-absorbed, highly protein-bound, lipid-soluble MRA with a 20-hour half-life. Its onset of action is slow, with peak response occurring 48 hours or more after initial dosing. 7α-thiomethylspirolactone and canrenone are the two main metabolites of spironolactone and account for most of the drug's effect. Spironolactone, unlike amiloride and triamterene, remains biologically active as a diuretic and antihypertensive agent at low GFRs because active drug enters the basolateral space before engaging the mineralocorticoid receptor to blockade aldosterone. Eplerenone is a highly selective MRA. Thus, its much lower affinity for "off target" androgen and progesterone receptors produces undesirable effects such as gynecomastia less often compared to spironolactone. Typically, eplerenone is at best a very mild diuretic; its antihypertensive effect originates from nondiuretic aspects of its action. Finerenone is also an MRA, but it has enhanced receptor affinity compared to eplerenone in vivo. Consequently, this agent has potent antiproteinuric effects without significant BP lowering or hyperkalemia.

Osmotic Diuretics

Mannitol is a low-molecular-weight, uncharged polysaccharide, administered by the intravenous route. It undergoes unimpeded glomerular filtration and acts as an osmotic diuretic. Essentially non-reabsorbed along the nephron, mannitol exerts a dose-dependent effect, effectively trapping water and solutes in the tubular fluid, with augmented excretion of sodium, potassium, and chloride. Its onset of action is relatively rapid, between 30 and 60 minutes, and its diuretic action is brief. Although mannitol has been tried to prevent AKI by delivery pre-cardiopulmonary bypass, during rhabdomyolysis, or after radiocontrast media exposure, the literature does not support these practices. Because mannitol expands the ECFV en route to its diuretic site of action, it may precipitate pulmonary edema in HF patients and must be used cautiously in this circumstance, if at all. The receipt of excessive mannitol, especially in settings of reduced GFR, can cause dilutional hyponatremia, hyperkalemia, and/or AKI. The last adverse effect is attributable to dose-dependent afferent arteriolar vasoconstriction that is correctable with extracorporeal mannitol elimination of the surfeit, that is, hemodialysis.

Kidney urea transporters (UTs) reside in the descending limb of the loop of Henle (UT-A2), inner medullary CD (UT-A1 and UT-A3), and descending vasa recta (UT-B1). UTs contribute to maintenance of the corticomedullary osmotic gradient, and UT-A1 is regulated by arginine vasopressin. Knockout of mouse urea transporter genes diminishes urinary concentrating capacity and diuresis. Extrapolation of these observations has provoked development of UT inhibitors. Currently, none is available for clinical application.

Adaptation to Diuretic Therapy

Diuretic-induced inhibition of sodium reabsorption in one nephron segment elicits counter-regulatory adaptations by other segments. This adaptation not only limits the antihypertensive effect and ECFV depletion of diuretics but also contributes to development of side effects. Although some degree of diuretic resistance is associated with prolonged use, intractable disease state-related diuretic resistance may occur with HF, cirrhosis, or nephrotic syndrome.

The initial dose of a diuretic typically produces a brisk increase of urine output succeeded by a new equilibrium state with body weight stabilization. Daily fluid and electrolyte excretion either matches or is less than intake. In nonedematous patients treated with thiazide or loop diuretic, this adaptation, known as the "braking phenomenon," occurs within 1 to 2 days and limits net weight loss to 1 to 2 kg. This event is most evident in normal subjects given a loop diuretic. For example, furosemide administered orally to subjects ingesting a high daily sodium diet of 270 mmol produces rapid natriuresis, with negative sodium balance after 6 hours. During the next 18 hours, positive sodium balance occurs with no net weight reduction. This phenomenon has been replicated for 3 consecutive days (Fig. 9.3) and is reproducible even after a 1-month hiatus from drug exposure. Thus, single, daily furosemide dosing will generally not achieve negative sodium balance, unless a most stringent regimen of sodium restriction is followed.

The mechanistic basis of the braking phenomenon is complex. The sigmoidal relationship between natriuresis and furosemide excretion rate is shifted rightward in subjects ingesting a low sodium diet, denoting blunted tubular response. The importance of ECFV depletion in the process of postdiuretic sodium retention has been clearly demonstrated. However, there is an ECFV-independent component to this process unrelated to aldosterone; that is, no effect on sodium balance following spironolactone administration. In rats, cellular hypertrophy of the distal nephron follows prolonged exposure to loop diuretic infusions and is marked by aldosterone-independent processes of amplified sodium chloride reabsorption and enhanced potassium secretion. These biological adaptations manifest as postdiuretic sodium retention and diuretic tolerance in humans, plausibly explaining why sodium retention may persist for up to 2 weeks following cessation of loop diuretic agents.

Neurohumoral Response to Diuretics

Plasma renin activity and aldosterone concentrations rise within minutes of receipt of an intravenous diuretic, a process independent of volume loss and/or sympathetic nervous system (SNS) activation. This elevation of plasma renin activity is generated by inhibition of NaCl reabsorption at the macula densa, in conjunction with loop diuretic stimulation of kidney prostaglandin release. This first wave of neurohumoral effects transiently increases afterload and may lessen the antihypertensive efficacy of a loop diuretic

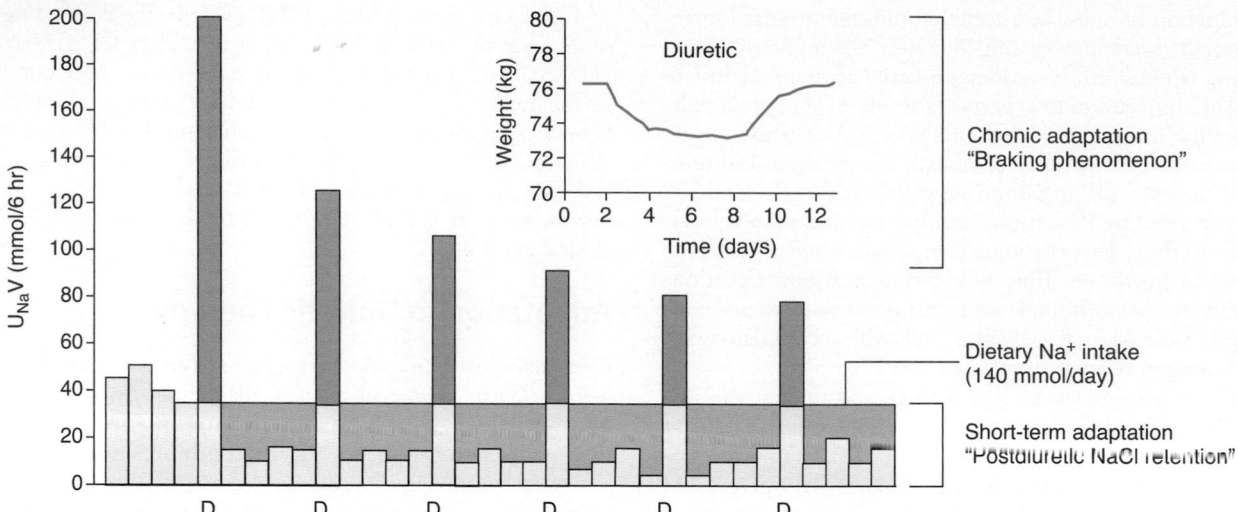

• **Fig. 9.3 Effect of a loop diuretic on urinary sodium excretion.** Each bar represents a 6-hour time interval. Purple bars indicate periods during which urinary sodium excretion ($U_{Na}V$) exceeds that of dietary intake. Blue areas indicate periods of postdiuretic sodium retention, during which dietary sodium intake exceeds urinary sodium excretion. The horizontal black line indicates dietary sodium intake per 24-hour period. Changes in the magnitude of the natriuretic response over several days are reflective of the "braking phenomenon." Inset shows the effect of diuretics on weight (and extracellular fluid volume) during several days of diuretic administration. (Data from Wilcox CS, Mitch WE, Kelly RA, et al. Response of the kidney to furosemide: I. Effects of salt intake and renal compensation. J Lab Clin Med. 1983;102:450–458.)

briefly. Shortly after this initial rise in renin activity, diuretics induce a more sustained increase in renin activity and aldosterone, attributable to an increase in SNS activity (β-agonism) and decline of ECFV. An increase in kidney prostaglandin production and nitric oxide is the likely explanation for the preload reduction and decrease in ventricular filling pressures that occur within 15 minutes of loop diuretic administration.

Diuretic Treatment of Edema

The pathophysiology of sodium and water retention in edematous patients is characterized by a complex interchange of hemodynamic and neurohumoral factors. For example, systemically perceived arterial underfilling sets into motion related sodium and water retention in HF patients. The level of neurohormonal activation, degree of kidney vasoconstriction, and extent to which kidney perfusion pressure is reduced modulate this process. In other instances, such as in the patient with a reduced GFR and/or nephrotic syndrome, sodium and water retention derive from a more primary set of kidney processes. In each circumstance, efforts should be directed toward correction of the underlying disease state as diuretic use is contemplated.

Two important considerations that must always accompany diuretic therapy at both initiation and during continuation are dietary sodium restriction (2 g sodium per day) and dose reduction/elimination of drugs that foster sodium retention, including NSAIDs, nonspecific vasodilators such as hydralazine and minoxidil, and high-dose β-blockers or central α-agonists. After diuretic initiation, choice of drug, dosage, and dosing frequency are subjective processes that focus on etiology and extent of ECFV overload. There is a treatment hierarchy among the thiazide diuretics; longer-acting compounds such as chlorthalidone or metolazone are preferred in edematous patients. CTD can be quite effective in the setting of mild-to-moderate edema given once or twice daily in the 25- to 50-mg/day range. When the underlying disease state worsens and/or dietary sodium

restriction is not adequately maintained, conversion to a loop diuretic-based regimen is the more practiced approach. Combination diuretic therapy can be subsequently considered because severity of edema requires "sequential nephron blockade" or the underlying disease state is exceptionally responsive to diuretics other than loop agents, such as spironolactone (range, 50–400 mg/day) in patients with advanced liver disease.

Determining the minimally effective dose for a diuretic effect is a necessary clinical exercise, specifically for individuals with reduced GFR (see Fig. 9.2). Gradually increasing a diuretic dose until an adequate diuretic response occurs establishes the "threshold" dose; thereafter, dosing frequency is defined by clinical circumstances. The initial dose from which dose titration proceeds is influenced by level of kidney function and severity of edema. If kidney function is reduced, the diuretic dose-response curve shifts rightward and maximal effectiveness, based on absolute sodium excretion rate, is significantly reduced. Therefore, dietary sodium restriction becomes even more important. In a patient with CKD and edema, initial loop agent doses are furosemide 40 mg, torsemide 10 mg, and bumetanide 1 to 2 mg. Each agent should be administered twice daily, and the starting dose is titrated upward until desired efficacy is attained. Often, the dose that elicits an increase in urine output can be continued indefinitely unless the underlying disease state worsens and/or dietary sodium intake supervenes diuretic effect. Conversely, a diuretic dose that establishes "euvolemia" may occasionally be lowered due to strict dietary adherence to sodium intake. Diuretic dose reduction must always be contemplated because this maneuver minimizes loss of potassium, magnesium, and, in the case of loop diuretics, calcium.

Diuretic Resistance: Causes and Treatment

ECFV regulation in most edematous patients is achievable with organized application of diuretic therapy principles. "Diuretic-resistant" patients abound in ambulatory and inpatient settings.

Among hospitalized individuals, diuretic resistance is frequently linked to the complex nature of the sodium-retentive state, with multiple organ systems at play and acuity of illness as the major determinant. In diuretic-resistant ambulatory patients, excessive sodium intake is a key pathogenic factor often overlooked. Several features are important when determining the "dry" or "target" weight in edematous patients, including symptom relief that incorporates patient input into the treatment equation, extent of comorbid illnesses, and realistic appreciation of the limits of treatment. A systematic approach to safe and maximally effective diuretic treatment is outlined (Fig. 9.4).

Poorly regulated sodium intake can scuttle the net negative sodium balance that characterizes a well-planned dietary and diuretic regimen. A 24-hour urine sodium excretion that exceeds 100 mmol is a reasonable marker of adequate diuretic action; however, obtaining a complete 24-hour urine collection may be problematic. An alternative approach that evaluates diuretic adequacy is calculation of the fractional sodium excretion 1–2 hours after administration of a well-absorbed diuretic. True diuretic resistance is unlikely if the fractional excretion of sodium exceeds 2%. However, diuretic resistance may be misconstrued when there is inconsistent drug absorption, especially with respect to furosemide—a problem circumventable by intravenous delivery of 80 to 120 mg, typically.

In CKD, reduced diuretic clearance mitigates efficacy; tubular secretion of loop agents is slowed, so larger doses must be provided to achieve the drug threshold. Conversion from the intravenous to oral route is often arbitrary. The oral agent has a wide coefficient

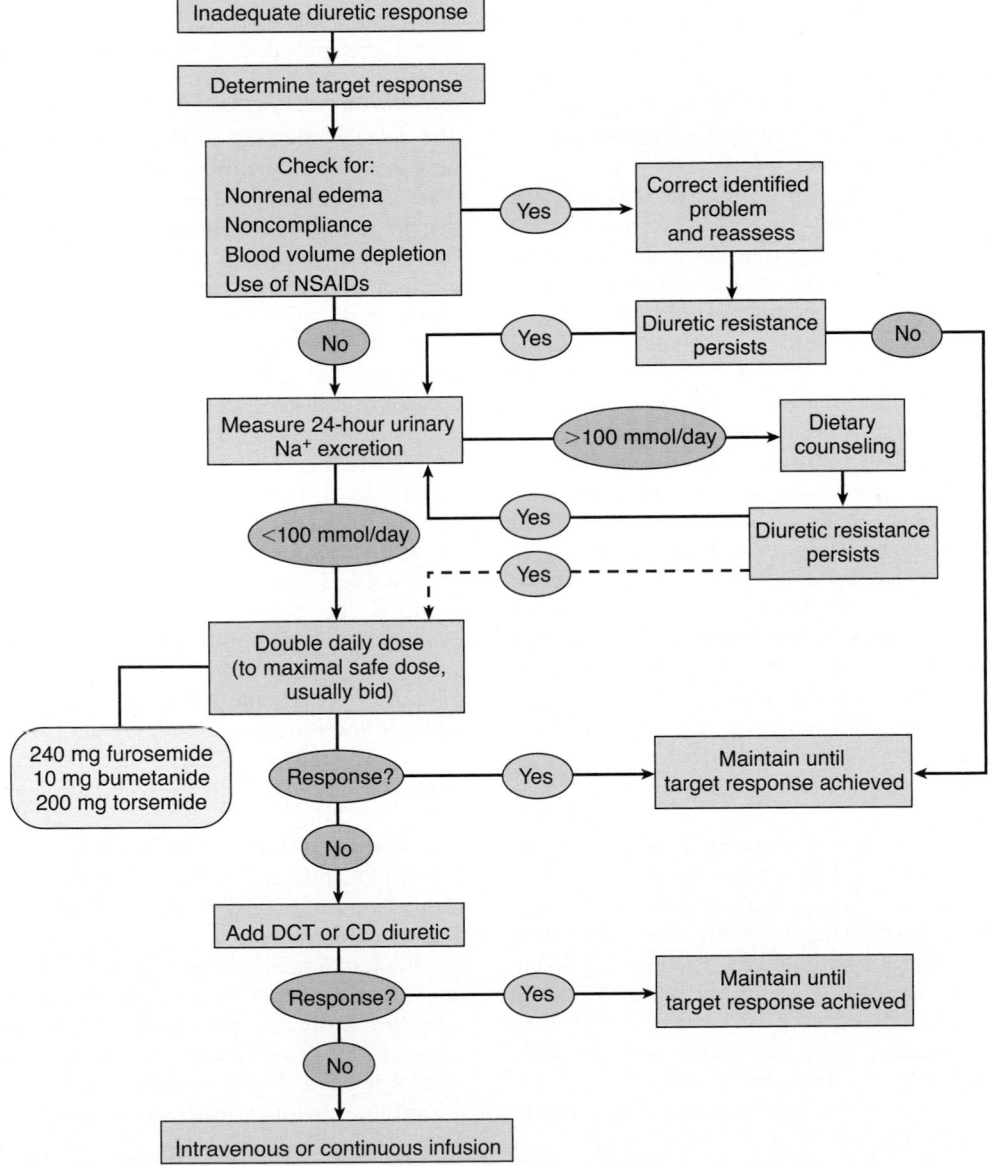

• **Fig. 9.4** **Algorithm for the treatment of the diuretic-resistant patient.** Combination diuretic regimens are addressed in the text. Maximal recommended loop diuretic doses given as monotherapy are provided in the yellow box. Note that higher doses are recommended for patients with acute kidney injury (AKI). Larger doses may improve the natriuretic response because of a lengthier duration of action; however, this can occur at the cost of increased side effects. *CD,* Collecting duct; *DCT,* distal convoluted tubule; *NSAIDs,* nonsteroidal antiinflammatory drugs. (Modified from Wilcox CS. Diuretics. In: Brenner B, ed. Brenner and Rector's The Kidney. 5th ed. Philadelphia: WB Saunders; 1996.)

of variation for gut absorption; however, oral furosemide, with mean gut absorption of 50%, should be prescribed at twice the intravenous dose.

The pathophysiology of edema formation in nephrotic syndrome is complex and incompletely understood. The "underfill" theory posits that low plasma oncotic pressure from hypoalbuminemia promotes egress of fluid from the vascular space to the interstitial space, with consequent kidney retention of salt and water via activation of the sympathetic nervous system, vasopressin, and RAAS. However, the alternative "overfill" theory is now considered the principal mechanism for edema formation. In this schema, the kidneys retain sodium independently of circulating plasma volume. Data from experimental animals with unilateral nephrotic syndrome or glomerulonephritis suggests that primary sodium retention in these disorders is from augmented distal CD sodium reabsorption by the CD. Recently, the serine protease plasminogen has been identified as a pathogenetic factor. Its aberrant appearance in urine in experimental and human nephrotic syndrome and subsequent activation to plasmin by urokinase-type plasminogen activator (uPA) amplifies ENaC-regulated sodium. Thus, amiloride may attenuate a portion of the excessive sodium reabsorption in nephrotic syndrome.

Nephrotic syndrome often presents as a diuretic-resistant state. Alterations in the pharmacokinetics and pharmacodynamics of loop diuretics account for this tempering effect. Loop diuretic delivery is impaired in hypoalbuminemic individuals as diuretic secretion is highly contingent on prevailing plasma albumin concentrations. In decompensated nephrotic syndrome, the diuretic dose-response relationship shifts rightward (higher threshold for effect) and downward (reduced maximal response or decreased sensitivity). Diuretics binding to albumin in tubular fluid reduce the proportion of unbound, active drug. At urine albumin concentrations exceeding 4 g/L, up to 65% of diuretic may be albumin bound. Accordingly, starting doses that are two- to threefold greater than normal oral starting doses are recommended.

Administration of anti-RAAS agents to reduce albuminuria are always a consideration in the edema-reduction strategy of nephrotic syndrome. Nonetheless, the cornerstone of therapy remains restriction of sodium intake, which typically is accompanied by diuretic therapy. However, the "reduced" diuretic responsiveness inherent to nephrotic syndrome typically mandates more frequent loop diuretic dosing. Another therapeutic option for treatment of ECFV overload includes diuretic combination regimens of 2 or 3 agents.

Hemodynamic abnormalities are frequent in diuretic-resistant patients, especially if HF and/or reduced ejection fraction is present. Accordingly, inotropic agents such as dobutamine may augment RBF and diuretic action in systolic HF. Permissive elevation of BP and/or the strategic withholding of RAAS inhibitors may restore diuretic efficacy as these agents may lower BP below a critical threshold for diuretic effect, particularly when small or large vessel disease is present in kidney vascular beds. In addition, diuretics should not be administered in temporal proximity to anti-RAAS agents because of the latter's potential to abruptly lower BP.

Special Diuretic Dosing Strategies

Additional approaches to overcoming diuretic resistance, aside from increasing dosing frequency, include high-dose oral loop diuretic therapy, diuretic combinations, continuous infusion therapy, albumin plus furosemide infusions for those with severe hypoalbuminemia, and high-dose loop diuretic and hypertonic saline coadministration (see Fig. 9.4). These strategies are not mutually exclusive and generally employed empirically with limited scientific foundation. A major limiting factor of "diuresing" the volume-overloaded patient is the consequential reduction of GFR. Obtaining effective control of ECFV surfeit requires careful timing of the ongoing diuresis to avoid subsequent response-limiting reductions of GFR and electrolyte complications.

High-Dose Oral Loop Diuretics

Remarkably high doses of loop diuretics are an alternative tactic for management of diuretic resistance. Although this approach has been used with some trepidation, presumably because of concern for ototoxicity, it has been successful in the ambulatory setting. Oral furosemide at daily dosages of 500 mg is a safe and effective decongestion therapy for advanced HF patients. In such patients, drug absorption may be delayed and/or incomplete from gut wall edema, thereby reducing peak plasma drug concentrations.

Combination Diuretic Therapy

The role of diuretic combinations in diuretic-resistant states such as nephrotic syndrome or HF is predicated on the ability of diuretics of different classes to effect sequential nephron blockade, thereby providing enhanced effectiveness. ACZ has been used in combination with loop agents to inhibit proximal sodium reabsorption, enhancing delivery of water and solute to the loop of Henle for subsequent inhibition of reabsorption by a loop agent.

The addition of a thiazide diuretic may overcome loop diuretic resistance. During chronic administration of a loop agent, development of cell hypertrophy occurs in the DCT, with intensified sodium reabsorption. This adaptation is partially suppressed by addition of thiazide. Although multiple combinations of diuretics have been used, pairing of thiazide and loop agent, with or without a potassium-sparing diuretic, is the most frequently successful combination. Furthermore, a metolazone-furosemide combination is commonly used when significant ECFV reduction is critical. The onset of an augmented diuretic response to this combination is often unpredictable, owing to potentially erratic absorption of metolazone. Achieving adequate systemic concentrations of metolazone to potentiate a loop diuretic may require multiple doses and several hours to days of therapy. If an oral thiazide is precluded for whichever reason, intravenous chlorothiazide (500–1000 mg/day) can be synergistically applied with a loop agent.

In the ambulatory setting, a starting dose of between 2.5 and 5.0 mg of metolazone daily or every other day can be administered with a loop diuretic. With initiation of combination therapy, the dose of a loop diuretic is usually kept constant until an adequate diuretic response is evident. Thereafter, frequency of administration of metolazone is reduced; the dose of loop agent may also be decreased. In all instances, careful monitoring of diuretic response is mandatory to avoid overt ECFV depletion and/or significant electrolyte losses. If either transpires, both medications should be discontinued, with corrective measures taken, as necessary.

Diuretic Infusions

In diuretic resistance, pharmacokinetic and pharmacodynamic considerations have implied theoretical advantage of continuous loop diuretic infusion compared with repeated bolus administration. Notably, studies that have attempted to delineate differences between infusion and bolus therapy have been heterogeneous and confounded by variables of study size, level of kidney function, BP, concomitant vasoactive therapies, and differing primary disease states. Some clarity, however, has been given to this controversy. In the Diuretic Optimization Strategies Evaluation (DOSE) trial of acute decompensated HF that compared intravenous furosemide bolus therapy to continuous infusion, there was no improvement in global symptom assessment with continuous infusion. In general, the use of loop diuretic infusions is a matter of preference.

Albumin and Furosemide Coadministration

In patients with severe nephrotic syndrome, the best method for delivery of loop diuretic has been deliberated, and two options are prevalent: intravenous albumin and furosemide as separate infusions or an ex vivo premixing of both components pre-injection. Severely hypoalbuminemic patients who have failed traditionally aggressive diuretic approaches are candidates for an albumin infusion plus intravenous loop agent. Albumin exerts its maximal intravascular volume expansion within 30 to 60 minutes of administration. The tactic of premixed loop diuretic and albumin was evaluated in cirrhotic patients with ascites (40 mg furosemide with 25 g albumin) but was not superior to furosemide (40 mg) alone. Overall, this tactic is not superior to loop diuretic alone.

Hypertonic Saline and Loop Diuretic Therapy

This combination appears counterintuitive based in the presence of a volume-expanded state. The rationale is an osmotic effect of hypertonic saline promoting rapid fluid mobilization from "third" spaces into the vascular compartment, thereby enhancing the probability of diuretic efficacy via improved hemodynamics. Correspondingly, there is an upward and leftward shift in the loop diuretic dose-response curve. A regimen of furosemide (250–1000 mg twice daily, IV) plus hypertonic saline (150 mL water with NaCl 1.4% to 4.6%) was shown safe and effective compared to repeated paracentesis, in hospitalized patients with cirrhosis and refractory ascites. Limitations and concern regarding net sodium accumulation make this approach difficult to extrapolate to a noncirrhotic patient population and requires greater experience and analysis.

Vasopressin Receptor Antagonists

Vasopressin receptor antagonists, so-called "vaptans," block engagement of the arginine vasopressin receptor 2 (AVPR2) by its natural ligand AVP in the DCT and CD. Vaptans increase free water clearance to a greater extent than sodium excretion and are therapeutically applied in heart failure, cirrhosis, and the syndrome of inappropriate ADH. Vaptans have also been considered for addition to loop diuretic-based regimens to intensify overall diuretic effect without amplifying neurohumoral status or worsening RBF or GFR. The vaptans do not have a well-established role in the outpatient management of diuretic resistance unless hyponatremia precludes the administration of more conventional combination diuretic regimens.

Special Considerations in Edema Management

Isolated Ultrafiltration

The advent of simple, portable ultrafiltration devices sparked renewed interest in this therapeutic possibility. Accordingly, extracorporeal, isolated venovenous ultrafiltration (UF) by peripheral vein has been applied in selected patients with diuretic-resistant, decompensated HF. The Ultrafiltration versus Intravenous Diuretics for Patients Hospitalized for Acute Decompensated CHF (UNLOAD) trial was the first landmark study demonstrating that isolated UF might provide greater fluid removal than diuretic therapy. UF provided improved quality of life, more rapid symptomatic improvement, and reduced hospital readmission. Despite initial enthusiasm, subsequent studies failed to validate the UNLOAD results and highlighted worsening kidney function as a limitation. At least two questions must be answered before widespread advocacy of this therapy: (1) Do beneficial effects such as improvement in ECFV status and decrements of neurohormonal activation persist? and (2) Is diuretic resistance mitigated by this modality?

End-Stage Kidney Disease

Some patients with end-stage kidney disease (ESKD) develop high interdialytic weight gains. Such persons are candidates for loop diuretic therapy when sufficient residual kidney function is present to facilitate a meaningful diuretic response. When loop agents are considered a therapeutic option in long-term hemodialysis patients, high doses of a loop agent or combination diuretic therapy are generally preferred. An loop diuretic can reduce interdialytic weight gains, with improved clinical outcomes. Individuals with urine outputs exceeding 200 mL/day on diuretic therapy are nearly twice as likely to retain residual kidney function after 1 year of dialytic therapy compared to untreated subjects.

Hemodialytic Removal

High plasma protein binding is common with loop diuretics. Less than 10% of total body stores of any loop diuretic is cleared from plasma during a routine hemodialysis session. Therefore, diuretic dosing in ESKD patients with residual kidney function is feasible.

Diuretic-Related Adverse Events

Diuretic-related side effects are divided into those of known etiology, including electrolyte and/or metabolic aberrations, and those of more obscure origin. Electrolyte changes are the most common side effects and occur more commonly with more potent loop diuretics. However, diuretic potency may be outweighed by duration of action. For example, thiazide-type diuretics such as chlorthalidone and metolazone, while less potent than a loop diuretic, may still produce significant hypokalemia and hypomagnesemia, owing to their relatively longer durations of action.

Hyponatremia

Hyponatremia is a potentially serious complication of diuretic therapy and usually occurs within a few weeks after start of treatment. Thiazide diuretics are more apt to cause hyponatremia than loop diuretics due to impairment of urinary dilution at the cortical CD. Furthermore, upregulation of ADH due to relative decreases in effective circulatory volume may independently lower sodium due to increased free water reabsorption. Treatment with CTD imposes a 70% greater risk for hospitalization for hyponatremia than HCTZ. Thiazide-treated elderly women are most susceptible to thiazide-induced hyponatremia, probably due to relatively smaller total body water volumes and low dietary osmolar intake. Withholding thiazide, restricting free water intake, providing nutritional support, and normalizing hypokalemia when present are usually adequate treatment measures. Severely symptomatic hyponatremia with seizures requires emergent correction; however, overly rapid correction or overcorrection of hyponatremia must be avoided to prevent a potentially devastating osmotic demyelination syndrome.

Hypokalemia and Hyperkalemia

Hypokalemia occurs frequently in patients treated by loop and/ or thiazide agents. The pathophysiology of the potassium deficit includes flow-dependent potassium secretion in the distal nephron, increase of distal tubular luminal chloride concentration, metabolic alkalosis, and stimulation of distal potassium secretion via enhanced aldosterone and/or vasopressin levels. Notably, serum potassium levels less than 3.0 mmol/L are uncommon in diuretic-treated outpatients, unless there is excessive dietary sodium intake, administration of a long-acting diuretic such as CTD or metolazone, or hyperaldosteronism. Although diuretic-induced hypokalemia in the range of 3.0 to 3.5 mmol/L may be associated with increased ventricular ectopy and altered glucose homeostasis, the cardiac ramifications of mild diuretic-induced hypokalemia are debatable. Profound hypokalemia with serum potassium concentrations <2.5 mmol/L produces generalized muscle weakness, induces *torsades de pointes*, and predisposes rhabdomyolysis with potential for acute kidney injury (AKI).

Potassium-sparing diuretics, such as triamterene and amiloride, and MRAs, such as spironolactone and eplerenone, reduce urinary potassium and magnesium excretion. Therefore, their use with a thiazide or loop diuretic is complementary. However caution must be exercised because significant potassium retention may occur during potassium-sparing diuretic treatment, but is typically encountered when one or more other risk factors for development of hyperkalemia are present: preexisting low GFR (i.e., <20 mL/ min), AKI superimposed on CKD, concurrent and/or inadvertent potassium supplementation, ingestion of potassium-containing salt substitutes, treatment with an anti-RAAS agent, NSAID treatment, or hyperchloremic metabolic acidosis in association with hyporeninemic hypoaldosteronism. Therapy with trimethoprim-sulfamethoxazole or heparin may also reduce urinary potassium excretion and provoke hyperkalemia.

Acid-Base Changes

Mild metabolic alkalosis is a common complication of thiazide therapy, especially when higher doses are used. Severe alkalosis is encountered more frequently during loop diuretic treatment. Generation of a metabolic alkalosis with diuretic therapy occurs primarily from ECFV contraction. The alkalosis is repaired by administration of lost electrolytes, potassium, sodium, and chloride. However, this approach must be altered in ECFV-expanded patients such as those with HF. Here, a potassium-sparing diuretic or ACZ may be appropriate. Metabolic alkalosis can attenuate the natriuresis of a loop agent, a factor of some relevance to diuretic-resistant individuals. CAIs can lead to a nonanion gap metabolic acidosis mimicking proximal renal tubular acidosis. All potassium-sparing diuretics can induce metabolic acidosis that occurs more commonly in the elderly and patients with CKD. Recovery from metabolic acidosis may require several days following discontinuation of a potassium-sparing diuretic.

Hypomagnesemia

Loop diuretics inhibit magnesium reabsorption at the loop of Henle where nearly 65% of the filtered magnesium load undergoes reclamation. All potassium-sparing diuretics attenuate the heightened magnesium excretion that results from thiazide or loop diuretic therapy. Cellular magnesium depletion occurs in 20% to 50% of patients on thiazide therapy, principally with long-acting, thiazide-type diuretics like CTD. Hypomagnesemia-related symptoms include depression, muscle weakness, and a host of neurological symptoms. Refractory hypokalemia, hypocalcemia, and an array of atrial/ventricular arrhythmias including *torsades de pointes* may occur. Many of these abnormalities, particularly refractory hypokalemia and hypocalcemia, are rapidly corrected by supplementation of magnesium.

Hyperuricemia

There is ongoing debate regarding the pathogenetic potential of hyperuricemia regarding CVD and CKD. Thiazide therapy dose-dependently increases serum urate levels by as much as 35%, attributable to reduced kidney urate clearance. This increase may stem from increased urate reabsorption from ECFV contraction and/or competition for tubular secretion of urate and diuretic via the organic anion transporter pathway. Serum uric acid levels may be measured periodically, but concurrent antihyperuricemic therapy in absence of symptomatic gout is not recommended.

Hyperglycemia

Prolonged thiazide treatment impairs glucose tolerance and can lead to diabetes mellitus. Hyperglycemia/glucose intolerance has been linked to diuretic-induced hypokalemia, with subsequent inhibition of pancreatic β cell–mediated insulin secretion, a likely dose-dependent effect that is potentially reversible upon withdrawal of the offending agent. This is less frequent with loop agents. In the Systolic Hypertension in the Elderly Program (SHEP) trial, the risk of new-onset diabetes with CTD was 45% higher per 0.5 mEq/L decline of serum potassium concentration. Although data regarding reversibility in HCTZ-treated patients appeared conflicting, long-term therapy produced minor, if any, changes in fasting serum glucose concentrations. This effect is plausibly correctable by concurrent potassium-sparing diuretic administration.

Hyperlipidemia

Short-term thiazide diuretic therapy can dose-dependently elevate total serum cholesterol levels, modestly increase low-density lipoprotein (LDL) cholesterol, and elevate triglyceride levels. There is minimal alteration of high-density lipoprotein (HDL) cholesterol concentrations. All diuretics, including loop agents, induce these lipid alterations, with the possible exception of indapamide. The mechanism of diuretic-induced dyslipidemia remains uncertain, but putative mechanisms are ascribed to insulin resistance and/ or reflex activation of the RAAS and SNS consequent to reduced ECFV. Long-term thiazide diuretic treatment is associated with normalization of total cholesterol levels to baseline within one year of treatment.

Ototoxicity

Loop diuretics may cause ototoxicity by inhibition of the NKCC2 in marginal and dark cells of the stria vascularis that produce endolymph and generate the endocochlear potential. Loop agents decrease this potential, raising acoustic thresholds, that is, deafness. This effect, which is infusion rate- and peak plasma concentration-dependent (<50 mg/mL), may occur within 20 minutes of infusion. Ototoxicity is usually reversible, but permanent deafness has been reported, especially after treatment with ethacrynic acid. Slow, continuous furosemide infusions (<4 mg/min) versus bolus injection and divided oral dose regimens may avert this complication. Patients with advanced kidney disease simultaneously treated with an aminoglycoside and furosemide harbor great risks for the complication of ototoxicity.

Drug Hypersensitivity

Photosensitivity dermatitis occurs rarely during treatment with furosemide or thiazide. HCTZ is more frequently associated with photosensitivity than its related compounds. Acute allergic interstitial nephritis (AIN), manifested by fever, rash, and/or eosinophilia, is an uncommon complication of diuretics. However, AIN may produce significant kidney injury/failure if drug exposure is prolonged. This phenomenon may emerge abruptly or insidiously, sometimes occurring months after initiation of therapy with a thiazide or loop agent. Early changes in kidney function in diuretic-treated patients may be ascribed to diuretic-induced ECFV lowering instead of AIN, thus permitting unchecked immunologic damage. Ethacrynic acid differs structurally from loop diuretics and represents a nontoxic replacement for individuals who have experienced thiazide- or loop diuretic-related AIN.

Adverse Drug Interactions

By causing hypokalemia and/or hypomagnesemia, diuretics also increase digitalis toxicity. During diuretic therapy associated with significant ECFV contraction, plasma lithium concentrations may increase. The concentration increase is variable and unpredictable. Therefore, lithium levels should be carefully monitored in patients treated with diuretics and lithium. NSAIDs can dose-dependently attenuate diuretic effects and predispose individuals to an AKI that is often reversible. The combination of indomethacin and triamterene is notably hazardous and associated with prolonged AKI. The relatively insoluble triamterene may cause a crystal nephropathy characterized by brown, spherical crystals that assume a Maltese cross-like appearance when viewed with polarized light. This nephropathy responds to urinary alkalinization. Kidney stone formation is less common with triamterene than crystalluria. Individuals treated with agents that inhibit one or more components of RAAS may develop a typically reversible form of AKI when excessively diuresed.

Bibliography

Brater DC. Diuretic therapy. *N Engl J Med*. 1998;339:387–395.

Chalasani N, Gorski JC, Horlander JC, et al. Effects of albumin/furosemide mixtures on responses to furosemide in hypoalbuminemic patients. *J Am Soc Nephrol*. 2001;12:1010–1016.

Costanzo MR, Ronco C. Isolated ultrafiltration in heart failure patients. *Curr Cardiol Rep*. 2012;14:254–264.

Ellison DH. Treatment of disorders of sodium balance in chronic kidney disease. *Adv Chronic Kidney Dis*. 2017;24(5):332–341.

Felker GM, Lee KL, Bull DA, et al. NHLBI Heart Failure Clinical Research Network. Diuretic strategies in patients with acute decompensated heart failure. *N Engl J Med*. 2011;364:797–805.

Fliser D, Schröter M, Neubeck M, Ritz E. Co-administration of thiazides increases the efficacy of loop diuretics even in patients with advanced renal failure. *Kidney Int*. 1994;46:482–488.

Freda BJ, Slawsky M, Mallidi J, Braden GL. Decongestive treatment of acute decompensated heart failure: cardiorenal implications of ultrafiltration and diuretics. *Am J Kidney Dis*. 2011;58:1005–1017.

Goldsmith SR, Gilbertson DT, Mackedanz SA, Swan SK. Renal effects of conivaptan, furosemide, and the combination in patients with chronic heart failure. *J Card Fail*. 2011;17:982–989.

Hari P, Bagga A. Co-administration of albumin and furosemide in patients with the nephrotic syndrome. *Saudi J Kidney Dis Transpl*. 2012;23:371–372.

Hix JK, Silver S, Sterns RH. Diuretic-associated hyponatremia. *Semin Nephrol*. 2011;31:553–566.

Karadsheh F, Weir MR. Thiazide and thiazide-like diuretics: an opportunity to reduce blood pressure in patients with advanced kidney disease. *Curr Hypertens Rep*. 2012;14:416–420.

Kassamali R, Sica D. Acetazolamide—a forgotten diuretic agent. *Cardiol Rev*. 2011;19:276–278.

Rosner MH, Gupta R, Ellison D, Okusa MD. Management of cirrhotic ascites: physiological basis of diuretic action. *Eur J Intern Med*. 2006;17:8–19.

Shankar SS, Brater DC. Loop diuretics: from the Na-K-2Cl transporter to clinical use. *Am J Physiol Renal Physiol*. 2003;284:F11–F21.

Sica DA. Metolazone and its role in edema management. *Congest Heart Fail*. 2003;9:100–105.

Sica DA. Diuretic use in chronic kidney disease. *Nat Rev Nephrol*. 2011;8:100–109.

Sica DA, Gehr TW. Diuretic combinations in refractory oedema states: pharmacokinetic-pharmacodynamic relationships. *Clin Pharmacokinet*. 1996;30:229–249.

Sica DA, Gehr TW. Diuretic use in stage five chronic kidney disease and end-stage renal disease. *Curr Opin Nephrol Hypertens*. 2003;12:483–490.

Svenningsen P, Bistrup C, Friis UG, et al. Plasmin in nephrotic urine activates the epithelial sodium channel. *J Am Soc Nephrol*. 2009;20:299–310.

Tuttolomondo A, Pinto A, Parrinello G, Licata G. Intravenous high-dose furosemide and hypertonic saline solutions for refractory heart failure and ascites. *Semin Nephrol*. 2011;31:513–522.

Wilcox CS. New insights into diuretic use in the patient with chronic renal disease. *J Am Soc Nephrol*. 2002;13:798–805.

Zillich AJ, Garg J, Basu S, Bakris GL, Carter BL. Thiazide diuretics, potassium, and the development of diabetes: a quantitative review. *Hypertension*. 2006;48:219–224.

10

Disorders of Potassium Metabolism

CSABA P. KOVESDY

Introduction

Dyskalemias (i.e., hypo- and hyperkalemia) are common abnormalities that occur frequently in patients with chronic kidney disease and are associated with increased morbidity and mortality. Due to their acute effects on cardiac arrhythmias, severe hypo- and hyperkalemia are medical emergencies that require immediate intervention. Because of their potential for recurrence, dyskalemias require long-term interventions to minimize their recurrence. The recent development of newer potassium binders has resulted in a re-evaluation of the optimal strategies for the chronic management of hyperkalemia.

Potassium Homeostasis

Total body potassium is about 3500 mmol. Approximately 98% of this total is intracellular, primarily in skeletal muscle and, to a lesser extent, in the liver. The remaining 2% (about 70 mmol) is in the extracellular fluid. Two homeostatic systems help maintain potassium homeostasis. The first system regulates potassium excretion from the kidney and gut. The second regulates potassium distribution between the extracellular and intracellular fluid compartments.

External Potassium Balance

The average American diet contains about 100 mmol (4 g) of potassium per day, with higher average potassium intake in women compared to men, older individuals compared to younger, and Caucasians compared to African-Americans. Dietary potassium intake may vary widely from day to day. To stay in potassium balance, it is necessary to increase potassium excretion when dietary potassium increases and decrease potassium excretion when dietary potassium decreases. Normally the kidneys excrete 90% to 95% of dietary potassium, with the remaining 5% to 10% excreted by the gut. Potassium excretion by the kidney is a relatively slow process, requiring 6 to 12 hours to eliminate an acute load.

Kidney Handling of Potassium

To understand the physiologic factors that determine kidney excretion of potassium, it is critical to review the main features of tubular potassium handling. Plasma potassium is freely filtered across the glomerular capillary into the proximal tubule. The majority of filtered potassium is subsequently reabsorbed by the proximal tubule and loop of Henle. In the distal tubule and the collecting duct, potassium is secreted into the tubular lumen. For practical purposes, urinary excretion of potassium reflects potassium secretion into the lumen of the distal tubule and collecting duct. Thus, any factor that stimulates potassium secretion increases urinary potassium excretion; conversely, any factor that inhibits potassium secretion decreases urinary potassium excretion.

Physiologic Regulation of Kidney Potassium Excretion

Five major physiologic factors stimulate distal potassium secretion (i.e., increase excretion): aldosterone, high distal sodium delivery, high urine flow rate, high [K$^+$] in tubular cells, and metabolic alkalosis (Table 10.1). Aldosterone directly increases the activity of Na$^+$/K$^+$-adenosine triphosphatase (ATPase) in the collecting duct cells, thereby stimulating secretion of potassium into the tubular lumen. Medical conditions that impair aldosterone production or secretion (e.g., diabetic nephropathy, chronic interstitial nephritis) or drugs that inhibit aldosterone production or action (e.g., nonsteroidal antiinflammatory drugs [NSAIDs], angiotensin-converting enzyme [ACE] inhibitors, angiotensin receptor blockers [ARBs], heparin, spironolactone) decrease potassium secretion by the kidney. Conversely, medical conditions associated with increased aldosterone levels and distal sodium delivery (primary hyperaldosteronism, secondary hyperaldosteronism due to diuretics or vomiting) increase potassium loss in the urine. Although there is profound secondary hyperaldosteronism in congestive heart failure and cirrhosis, each of these conditions may be associated with hyperkalemia rather than hypokalemia because of decreased delivery of sodium to the distal nephron. Many diuretics increase kidney potassium excretion by a number of mechanisms, including high distal sodium delivery, high urine flow rate, metabolic alkalosis, and hyperaldosteronism due to volume depletion. Poorly controlled diabetes commonly increases urinary potassium excretion due to osmotic diuresis with high urinary flow rate and enhanced distal delivery of sodium.

Reabsorption of sodium in the collecting duct occurs through selective sodium channels. This creates an electronegative charge within the tubular lumen relative to the tubular epithelial cell. This, in turn, promotes secretion of cations (K$^+$ and H$^+$) into the lumen. Therefore, drugs that block the sodium channel in the collecting duct decrease potassium secretion. Conversely, in Liddle syndrome, a rare genetic disorder in which the sodium channel is constitutively open, avid sodium reabsorption results in excessive potassium secretion.

An increase in dietary potassium causes an inhibition of the thiazide-sensitive NaCl cotransporter in the distal convoluted tubule through an enteric sensing mechanism, prior to a detectable rise in plasma potassium concentration. This leads to increased flow

TABLE 10.1	Physiologic Factors Increasing Kidney Potassium Excretion		
Factor	Mechanism	Medical Conditions Affecting It	Drugs Affecting It
Aldosterone	Increase Na$^+$/K$^+$-ATPase activity in collecting duct	Diabetic nephropathy Interstitial nephritis Primary hyperaldosteronism Secondary hyperaldosteronism	NSAIDs ACE inhibitors ARBs Heparin Spironolactone
Distal Na$^+$ delivery	Create electrochemical gradient	Uncontrolled diabetes	Loop diuretics Thiazide diuretics
Urine flow	Increase concentration gradient	Uncontrolled diabetes	Loop diuretics Thiazide diuretics
Tubular [K$^+$]	Increase concentration gradient	Hyperkalemia	—
Metabolic alkalosis	Decreased proximal Na$^+$ reabsorption	Primary hyperaldosteronism	Loop diuretics Thiazide diuretics

ACE, angiotensin converting enzyme; *ARB*, angiotensin receptor blocker; *NSAIDs*, nonsteroidal antiinflammatory drugs.

and delivery of sodium to the downstream distal nephron and increased potassium secretion.

Adaptation in Chronic Kidney Disease

In patients with chronic kidney disease (CKD), three major mechanisms protect against hyperkalemia: (1) increased kidney potassium excretion mediated by aldosterone, (2) increased intestinal potassium excretion, and (3) increased potassium excretion per nephron. The kidney compensates for reduced nephron number in CKD by increasing the efficiency of potassium excretion. Clearly, there is a limit to kidney compensation, and a significant loss of kidney function impairs the ability to excrete potassium, thereby predisposing to a positive potassium balance and a tendency toward hyperkalemia. A normal plasma potassium concentration is typically maintained under steady state circumstances (i.e., stable dietary potassium intake), but the kidneys' ability to acutely dispose of increased potassium loads diminishes significantly in patients with advanced stages of CKD, who experience increasing frequencies of hyperkalemic episodes. Serum aldosterone levels are elevated in many patients with CKD. Aldosterone stimulates the activity of both Na$^+$/K$^+$-ATPase and H$^+$/K$^+$-ATPase, thereby promoting secretion of potassium in the collecting duct and defending against hyperkalemia. These adaptive mechanisms are less effective in patients with acute kidney injury (AKI) as compared with CKD, and severe hyperkalemia occurs more frequently in patients with AKI as compared with those with CKD. Moreover, patients with AKI are often hypotensive, resulting in hypoperfusion and release of potassium from ischemic tissues.

A subset of patients with CKD fails to increase aldosterone levels appreciably; as a result, they develop hyperkalemia at moderate levels of GFR loss (<50 mL/min), typically in association with nonanion gap metabolic acidosis (type IV renal tubular acidosis). This condition is most commonly encountered with diabetic nephropathy and chronic interstitial nephritis. Moreover, administration of drugs that inhibit aldosterone production or secretion (e.g., ACE inhibitors, ARBs, NSAIDs, heparin) may provoke hyperkalemia in patients with mild to moderate CKD.

Intestinal Potassium Excretion

Like the collecting duct, the small intestine and colon secrete potassium in response to aldosterone. In normal individuals, intestinal potassium excretion plays a minor role in potassium homeostasis, accounting for about 10% of total potassium excretion. However, in patients with significant GFR loss, intestinal potassium secretion is increased three- to fourfold providing a significant contribution to potassium homeostasis. This adaptation is limited and is inadequate to compensate for the loss of urinary excretion in patients with advanced kidney disease but is a significant contributor to the potassium balance in patients with kidney failure on dialysis.

Internal Potassium Balance

Extracellular fluid [K$^+$] is approximately 4 mEq/L, whereas the intracellular [K$^+$] is approximately 150 mEq/L. Because of the uneven distribution of potassium between the fluid compartments, a relatively small net shift of potassium from the intracellular to the extracellular fluid compartment produces marked increases in plasma potassium. Conversely, a relatively small net shift from the extracellular to the intracellular fluid compartment produces a marked decrease in plasma potassium. Unlike kidney excretion of potassium that requires several hours, potassium shift between the extracellular and intracellular fluid compartment (also referred to as extrarenal potassium disposal) is extremely rapid, occurring within minutes.

Extrarenal potassium disposal plays a critical role in the prevention of life-threatening hyperkalemia following potassium-rich meals. The following example will illustrate this important principle. Suppose that a 70-kg anephric patient with a plasma potassium of 4.5 mmol/L eats 1 cup of pinto beans, which contains 35 mmol of potassium. Initially, the dietary potassium is absorbed into the extracellular fluid compartment (20% × 70 kg = 14 L). This amount of dietary potassium will increase the plasma potassium by 2.5 mmol/L (35 mmol/14 L). In the absence of extrarenal potassium disposal, the patient's plasma potassium would rise acutely to 7.0 mmol/L, a level frequently associated with serious ventricular arrhythmias. In practice, the increase in plasma potassium is much smaller because of efficient physiologic mechanisms that promote potassium shifts into the intracellular fluid compartment.

Effects of Insulin and Catecholamines on Extrarenal Potassium Disposal

The two major physiologic factors that stimulate transfer of potassium from the extracellular to the intracellular fluid compartments are insulin and epinephrine. The stimulation of extrarenal potassium disposal by insulin and beta-2 adrenergic agonists is mediated by stimulation of the Na^+/K^+-ATPase activity, primarily in skeletal muscle cells. Interference with these two physiologic mechanisms (insulin deficiency/resistance or beta-2 adrenergic blockade, respectively) predisposes to hyperkalemia. On the other hand, excessive insulin or epinephrine levels predispose to hypokalemia.

The potassium-lowering effect of insulin is dose related within the physiologic range of plasma insulin and is independent of its effect on plasma glucose. Even the low physiologic levels of insulin present during fasting promote extrarenal potassium disposal. In nondiabetic individuals, hyperglycemia stimulates endogenous insulin secretion, thereby decreasing the plasma potassium. In insulin-dependent diabetics, endogenous insulin production is limited and significant hyperglycemia may occur. Hyperglycemia results in plasma hypertonicity, which promotes potassium shifts out of the cells and produces paradoxical hyperkalemia.

The potassium-lowering action of epinephrine is mediated by beta-2 adrenergic stimulation and is blocked by nonselective beta-blockers but not by selective beta-1 adrenergic blockers. Alpha-adrenergic stimulation promotes shifts of potassium *out of cells* into the extracellular fluid compartment, leading to an increase in plasma potassium. Epinephrine is a mixed alpha-adrenergic and beta-adrenergic agonist, such that its net effect on plasma potassium reflects the balance between its beta-adrenergic (potassium-lowering) and alpha-adrenergic (potassium-raising) effects. In normal individuals, the beta-adrenergic effect of epinephrine predominates over the alpha-adrenergic effect, such that the plasma potassium decreases. In contrast, the alpha-adrenergic effect of epinephrine on potassium shifts is much more prominent in patients with severe kidney failure; as a result, patients undergoing dialysis are refractory to the potassium-lowering effect of epinephrine.

Effect of Acid-Base Disorders on Extrarenal Potassium Disposal

Acid-base disorders produce internal potassium shifts in a less predictable manner. As a general rule, metabolic alkalosis shifts potassium into cells, whereas metabolic acidosis shifts potassium out of cells. However, the nature of the metabolic acidosis determines its effect on plasma potassium. Cells are relatively impermeable to chloride. With mineral acidoses, the entry of protons (but not chloride) into cells results in a reciprocal release of potassium from cells to maintain electro-neutrality. In contrast, cells are highly permeable to organic anions. The addition of an organic acid to the extracellular fluid results in parallel shifts of protons and organic anions into the cells, with no net change in the electric balance; as a result, potassium is not released from cells. Thus, mineral acidoses (i.e., hyperchloremic, normal anion gap metabolic acidosis) typically result in hyperkalemia, whereas organic metabolic acidoses (e.g., lactic acidosis) do not affect the plasma potassium.

Laboratory Tests to Evaluate Potassium Disorders

Serum or plasma measurements are both used to measure potassium concentration. While both are acceptable, knowledge of the method that was applied for an individual measurement is important, since serum potassium is, on average, 0.1–0.7 mmol/L higher than plasma potassium.

Differential Diagnosis of Hypokalemia and Hyperkalemia

The clinical history, medication review, family history, and physical examination are sufficient to create a rapid differential diagnosis of most potassium disorders. In selected patients, the etiology of hypokalemia or hyperkalemia is not apparent and additional specialized laboratory tests may be useful. Measurement of the fractional excretion of potassium (FE_K) may help distinguish between kidney and non-kidney etiologies of hyperkalemia and hypokalemia. The general principle underlying this test is that the kidney compensates for hyperkalemia by increasing potassium excretion and compensates for hypokalemia by decreasing potassium excretion. In contrast, when potassium excretion is inappropriate for the plasma potassium, this suggests a kidney etiology. The optimal use of FE_K to inform the differential diagnosis requires that this value be obtained before the potassium abnormality (hyperkalemia or hypokalemia) is corrected.

Fractional Excretion of Potassium

FE_K is the percent of potassium filtered into the proximal tubule that appears in the urine. It represents potassium clearance corrected for GFR, or Cl_K/Cl_{Cr}. Since the clearance of any substance can be calculated from UV/P, this ratio can be algebraically transformed to:

$$\left[\left(U_K V / P_K \right) / \left(U_{Cr} V / P_{Cr} \right) \right] \times 100\%$$

The Vs in the numerator and denominator cancel out, giving a simplified formula:

$$\left[\left(U_K / P_K \right) / \left[U_{Cr} / P_{Cr} \right) \right] \times 100\%$$

where U_K and U_{Cr} are the concentrations of potassium and creatinine in the urine, respectively, and P_K and P_{Cr} are the corresponding plasma concentrations. For an individual with normal kidney function on a typical dietary potassium intake, the FE_K is approximately 10%. When hypokalemia is a result of extrarenal causes (e.g., low potassium diet, gastrointestinal losses, potassium shifts into cells), the kidney conserves potassium and the FE_K is low. In contrast, hypokalemia due to kidney potassium losses is associated with an increased FE_K. Similarly, in the setting of hyperkalemia, a high FE_K suggests an extrarenal etiology, whereas a low FE_K is consistent with a kidney etiology. If a urine creatinine measurement is not available, one can often use U_K alone to differentiate between kidney and extrarenal causes of hyperkalemia. Specifically, in a hypokalemic patient, $U_K > 20$ mEq/L suggests a kidney etiology, whereas $U_K < 20$ mEq/L suggests an extrarenal etiology.

Several factors limit the utility of the FE_K in the differential diagnosis of potassium disorders. The FE_K is increased when dietary potassium is increased, and it is decreased when dietary potassium is decreased. Furthermore, in patients with CKD, there is an adaptive increase in potassium excretion per functioning nephron, such that FE_K increases. This means that the "normal" value for a given individual can vary substantially, making it difficult to determine the significance of a high or low FE_K.

Hypokalemia

Hypokalemia Versus Potassium Deficiency

It is important to distinguish between potassium deficiency and hypokalemia. Potassium deficiency is the state resulting from a persistent negative potassium balance (i.e., potassium excretion exceeding potassium intake). Hypokalemia refers to a low plasma potassium concentration. Hypokalemia can be due to either potassium deficiency (inadequate potassium intake or excessive potassium losses) or net potassium shifts from the extracellular to the intracellular fluid compartment. A patient may have severe potassium deficiency without manifesting hypokalemia. An important example is a patient presenting with diabetic ketoacidosis. Such patients have typically had severe hyperglycemia with osmotic diuresis for several days, leading to high levels of kidney potassium excretion and potassium deficiency. However, as a result of insulin deficiency and hyperglycemia-induced hyperosmolality, there is a concomitant shift of potassium out of the cells into the extracellular fluid compartment. At presentation to the hospital, such patients are frequently normokalemic or even hyperkalemic. Once they are treated with exogenous insulin, there is a rapid shift of potassium back into the cells and, within a few hours, the patients develop significant hypokalemia. Conversely, patients hospitalized with an acute myocardial infarction commonly have hypokalemia due to stress-induced catecholamine release and enhanced extrarenal potassium disposal, even though they have a normal external potassium balance.

Clinical Disorders Associated with Hypokalemia

Table 10.2 provides a list of the most common causes of hypokalemia. The kidney can avidly conserve potassium, such that hypokalemia due to inadequate potassium intake is a rare event requiring prolonged starvation ("tea and toast diet"). Therefore, hypokalemia is usually due to excessive potassium losses from the gut or the kidney, or to potassium shifts from the extracellular to the intracellular fluid compartments. Prolonged vomiting causes potassium losses, in part due to potassium present in gastric secretions (~10 mEq/L) but primarily due to kidney losses because of secondary hyperaldosteronism from volume depletion. Severe diarrhea, either due to disease or laxative abuse, results in significant potassium excretion in the stool. Patients undergoing bowel preparation for colonoscopy are at high risk for hypokalemia, especially those who have other risk factors (e.g., concomitant diuretic use).

Hypokalemia due to excessive kidney potassium losses is seen with a number of clinical syndromes. Conceptually, it is useful to classify hypokalemia as associated with hypertension or with normal blood pressure (Fig. 10.1). When hypokalemia is associated with hypertension, measurements of plasma renin and aldosterone may be helpful in the differential diagnosis. Several physiologic observations are relevant in this regard. First, aldosterone, a mineralocorticoid, stimulates sodium reabsorption and potassium secretion in the collecting duct. Second, the physiologic stimulus for aldosterone secretion is activation of the renin-angiotensin axis. Moreover, aldosterone-induced sodium retention suppresses the renin-angiotensin axis by negative feedback. Third, glucocorticoids at high concentrations

TABLE 10.2	Causes of Hypokalemia

Inadequate potassium intake (severe malnutrition)

Extrarenal potassium losses
- Vomiting
- Diarrhea

Hypokalemia due to urinary potassium losses
- Diuretics (loop diuretics, thiazides, acetazolamide)
- Osmotic diuresis (e.g., hyperglycemia)
- Hypokalemia with hypertension
  - Primary hyperaldosteronism
  - Glucocorticoid-remediable hyperaldosteronism
  - Malignant hypertension
  - Renovascular hypertension
  - Renin-secreting tumor
  - Essential hypertension with excessive diuretics
  - Liddle syndrome
  - 11β hydroxysteroid dehydrogenase deficiency
    - Genetic
    - Drug induced (chewing tobacco, licorice, some French wines)
  - Congenital adrenal hyperplasia
- Hypokalemia with a normal blood pressure
  - Distal renal tubular acidosis (type I)
  - Proximal renal tubular acidosis (type II)
  - Bartter syndrome
  - Gitelman syndrome
  - Hypomagnesemia (cis-platinum, alcoholism, diuretics)

Hypokalemia due to potassium shifts
- Insulin administration
- Catecholamine excess (acute stress)
- Familial periodic hypokalemic paralysis
- Thyrotoxic hypokalemic paralysis

bind to mineralocorticoid receptors and mimic their physiologic actions. And fourth, glucocorticoids are stimulated by adrenocorticotropic hormone (ACTH) and suppress ACTH production by negative feedback.

Primary hyperaldosteronism is due to autonomous (non-renin-mediated) secretion of aldosterone by the adrenal cortex. This results in avid sodium retention and potassium secretion by the distal nephron. Patients present with volume-dependent hypertension, hypokalemia, and metabolic alkalosis. Biochemical evaluation reveals a *high serum aldosterone level and suppressed plasma renin*. An abdominal computed tomography (CT) scan reveals either a unilateral adrenal adenoma or bilateral adrenal hyperplasia. The former is treated surgically and the latter with aldosterone antagonism. *Glucocorticoid-remediable hyperaldosteronism* (GRA) is a rare, autosomal dominant condition in which there is fusion of the 11β-hydroxylase and aldosterone synthase genes. As a result, aldosterone production is stimulated by ACTH; abnormally high levels of aldosterone result from physiologic levels of ACTH but can be suppressed by dexamethasone. Patients with GRA have a very similar clinical presentation to those with primary hyperaldosteronism (volume-dependent hypertension, hypokalemia, high serum aldosterone, and low serum renin), except that they are younger and have a family history of hypertension.

Patients with *renovascular hypertension, renin-secreting tumors*, and severe *malignant hypertension* may also present with severe hypertension and hypokalemia. In contrast to patients with

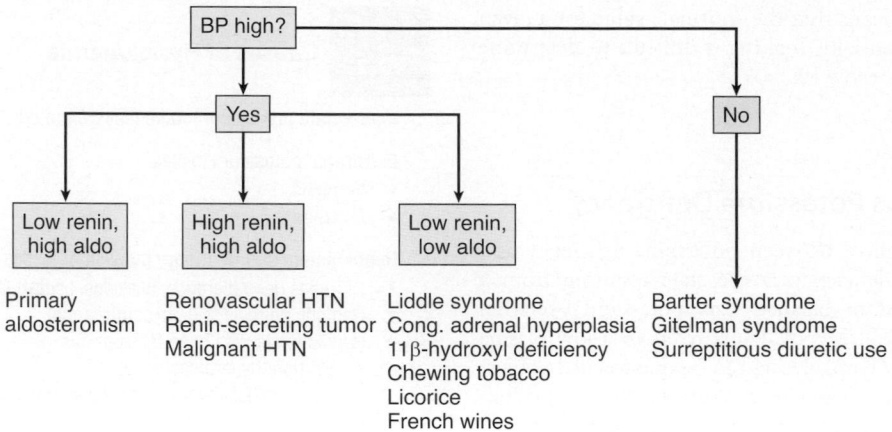

• **Fig. 10.1** Differential diagnosis of hypokalemia, using blood pressure (BP) and plasma renin and aldosterone (aldo). *HTN,* hypertension.

primary hyperaldosteronism, these patients have secondary hyperaldosteronism (i.e., *high serum renin and aldosterone levels*). Of course, patients with essential hypertension may also have hypokalemia and high plasma renin and aldosterone levels if they are treated with loop or thiazide diuretics.

Patients with *11β-hydroxysteroid dehydrogenase deficiency*, a rare genetic disorder, have a defect in the conversion of cortisol to cortisone in the peripheral tissues. This results in high tissue cortisol levels that activate the mineralocorticoid receptors, producing hypokalemia and hypertension. Such patients have *low serum renin and aldosterone levels*. Chewing tobacco, certain brands of licorice, and some French red wines contain *glycyrrhizic acid*, which inhibits 11β-hydroxysteroid dehydrogenase. Ingestion of these foods may produce hypokalemia, volume-dependent hypertension, and low serum renin and aldosterone levels, similar to the clinical presentation of congenital 11β-hydroxysteroid dehydrogenase deficiency.

Patients with *congenital adrenal hyperplasia* have a deficiency of 11β-hydroxylase, an enzyme required in the common pathways for mineralocorticoids and glucocorticoids. These patients have low serum renin and aldosterone levels, high levels of DOCA (deoxycorticosterone acetate, a mineralocorticoid), and high levels of androgen. Boys exhibit early puberty and girls exhibit virilization with hirsutism and clitoromegaly. This condition improves with exogenous corticosteroids to suppress ACTH.

Liddle syndrome is a rare autosomal dominant disorder caused by a defect of the sodium channel, such that there is increased sodium absorption and potassium secretion in the collecting duct. Patients present with hypokalemia, hypertension, and volume overload. Their biochemical profile reveals a *low serum renin and aldosterone*. The patients' blood pressure and plasma potassium improve dramatically after inhibiting the sodium channel with amiloride.

Hypokalemia due to excessive kidney potassium excretion is also seen in a number of clinical conditions in which hypertension is infrequent. Both distal (type I) and proximal (type II) renal tubular acidoses (RTA) are associated with kaliuresis and hypokalemia; both conditions present with a normal anion gap metabolic acidosis. *Distal RTAs* are frequently associated with hypercalciuria and calcium oxalate kidney stones. *Proximal RTAs* are rare in adults and often associated with a generalized defect in proximal tubular function (Fanconi syndrome), manifesting with glycosuria (with a normal blood glucose),

hypophosphatemia with phosphaturia, and a low serum uric acid with uricosuria.

Bartter syndrome is a rare familial disease characterized by hypokalemia, metabolic alkalosis, hypercalciuria, normal blood pressure, and high plasma renin and aldosterone levels. Serum magnesium is usually normal. It has been associated with a number of mutations that inhibit active sodium reabsorption in the thick ascending limb of the loop of Henle, including mutations in the $Na^+/K^+/2Cl^-$-cotransporter, ClC-Kb, and ROMK (see Chapter 37). These patients act as if they are chronically ingesting loop diuretics; for this reason, they are difficult to distinguish clinically from patients with surreptitious diuretic ingestion. Patients with *Gitelman syndrome* differ in that they have hypocalciuria and hypomagnesemia. Gitelman syndrome has been linked to a mutation in the thiazide-sensitive Na^+/K^+-cotransporter. These patients handle potassium as if they are chronically ingesting thiazide diuretics.

Familial hypokalemic periodic paralysis is a rare, autosomal dominant disorder in which affected individuals develop periodic episodes of severe muscle weakness in association with profound hypokalemia, due to rapid shifts of potassium from the extracellular to the intracellular fluid compartment. Interestingly, even when the patient has complete paralysis, the diaphragm and bulbar muscles are spared, such that the patient is able to breathe, swallow, talk, and blink. The paralysis resolves within hours of potassium ingestion. The patients are asymptomatic with normal plasma potassium levels in between the acute episodes. *Thyrotoxic hypokalemic paralysis* is an unusual manifestation of hyperthyroidism, seen primarily in Asian patients. The clinical presentation is similar to that of hypokalemic periodic paralysis, except that the paralytic episodes cease when the hyperthyroidism is corrected.

Drug-Induced Hypokalemia

A number of drugs have the potential to cause hypokalemia, either by stimulating kidney potassium excretion or by blocking extrarenal disposal. Exogenous mineralocorticoids mimic the effects of aldosterone, thereby stimulating distal potassium secretion. High doses of glucocorticoids possess some mineralocorticoid activity and have a similar effect. Most diuretics, including loop diuretics, thiazide diuretics, and acetazolamide, increase kidney potassium excretion. A number of drugs, including alcohol, diuretics, and cis-platinum, cause kidney magnesium wasting and hypomagnesemia. For reasons that are not well understood, hypomagnesemia impairs kidney potassium conservation. Thus, these patients may have associated hypokalemia that is refractory to potassium supplementation until the magnesium deficit is corrected.

Drugs that promote extrarenal potassium disposal may also result in hypokalemia. This phenomenon can be seen after the administration of an acute dose of insulin. Similarly, beta-2 agonists (either intravenous or nebulized), including albuterol and terbutaline, frequently result in acute hypokalemia.

Clinical Manifestations of Hypokalemia

Hypokalemia may produce electrocardiographic abnormalities, including a flattened T wave and a U wave (Fig. 10.2). Hypokalemia also appears to increase the risk of ventricular arrhythmias in patients with ischemic heart disease or patients taking digoxin. Severe hypokalemia is associated with variable degrees of skeletal muscle weakness, even to the point of paralysis. Rarely, diaphragmatic paralysis from hypokalemia can lead to respiratory arrest. There may also be decreased motility of smooth muscle, manifesting as ileus or urinary retention. Severe hypokalemia may occasionally produce rhabdomyolysis.

Profound hypokalemia also interferes with the urinary concentrating mechanism in the distal nephron, resulting in nephrogenic diabetes insipidus. Such patients have a low urine osmolality in the face of high serum osmolality and are refractory to vasopressin.

Over time, tubulointerstitial nephritis due to hypokalemia can progress to interstitial fibrosis.

Treatment of Hypokalemia

The acute treatment of hypokalemia requires potassium supplementation, either intravenously or orally. The correlation between plasma potassium and total potassium deficit in hypokalemic patients is quite poor. A given patient's plasma potassium is a reflection of both external potassium balance and transcellular potassium shifts. The percent of administered exogenous potassium that remains in the extracellular fluid compartment is variable. Thus, it is difficult to predict how much potassium replacement will be required for a particular patient. If the patient is hypokalemic in the setting of potassium deficiency, a relatively large amount of potassium replacement is needed. In contrast, hypokalemia that is primarily due to transcellular potassium shifts requires relatively little potassium repletion. Without adequate monitoring, it is possible to give too much potassium and make the patient hyperkalemic. Therefore, one should give multiple small doses of potassium, with frequent checks of plasma potassium values.

Oral potassium administration is safer than the intravenous route and less likely to produce an overshoot in the plasma potassium. Each oral dose should not exceed 20 to 40 mEq of potassium. Intravenous potassium chloride should be reserved for severe, symptomatic hypokalemia (<3.0 mEq/L) or for patients who cannot ingest oral potassium. Intravenous potassium chloride should not be given any faster than 10 mmol/hour in the absence of continuous EKG monitoring. The plasma potassium should be rechecked every 2 to 3 hours to confirm a clinical response and avoid an overshoot.

Correction of the underlying medical condition may prevent recurrence of hypokalemia after its correction. If the patient has a chronic condition associated with persistent urinary or gastrointestinal potassium losses such that hypokalemia is likely to recur, the patient should be encouraged to increase the intake of foods high in potassium (especially fresh fruits, nuts, and legumes). In some patients, chronic oral potassium supplementation may be necessary.

Hyperkalemia

Pseudohyperkalemia is a factitious elevation of the plasma potassium caused by in vitro release of potassium from blood cells or platelets. It may be seen with in vitro hemolysis, thrombocytosis, or severe leukocytosis. Pseudohyperkalemia due to hemolysis is readily apparent because the serum is pink. Pseudohyperkalemia due to severe thrombocytosis or leukocytosis can be confirmed by drawing simultaneous blood samples in tubes with and without anticoagulant; if potassium in the latter (serum) is higher than in the former (plasma), the diagnosis is confirmed.

True hyperkalemia is caused by a positive potassium balance (increased potassium intake or decreased potassium excretion) or an increase in net potassium shift from the intracellular to the extracellular fluid compartment. Table 10.3 provides a list of the most common causes of hyperkalemia. In practice, most patients who develop severe hyperkalemia have multiple contributory factors. For example, a patient with CKD due to diabetic nephropathy may be treated with an ACE inhibitor and have mild hyperkalemia. However, when he or she is started on indomethacin for acute gouty arthritis, the patient rapidly develops severe hyperkalemia.

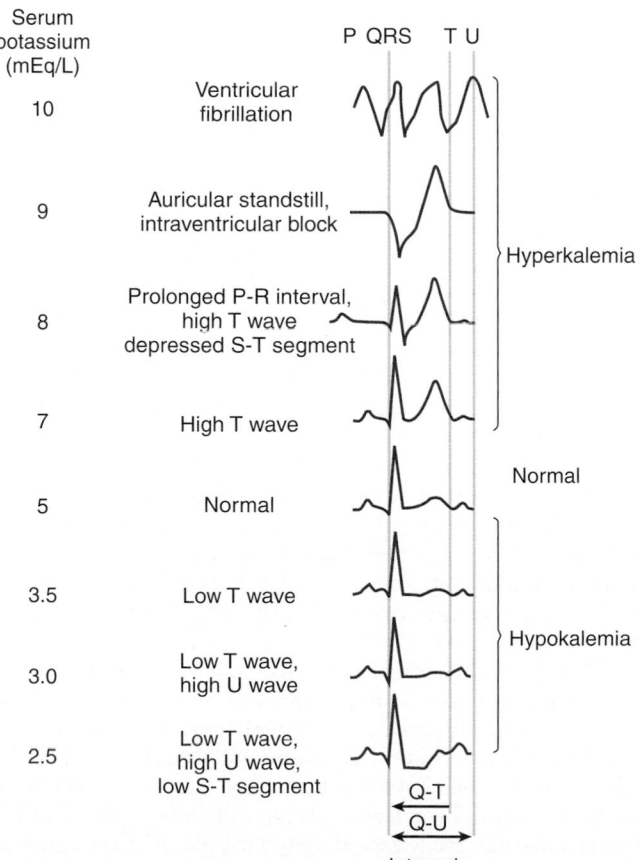

• **Fig. 10.2** Typical electrocardiographic changes associated with hypokalemia and hyperkalemia.

TABLE 10.3 **Causes of Hyperkalemia**

Pseudohyperkalemia

- Hemolysis
- Thrombocytosis
- Severe leukocytosis
- Fist clenching

Decreased kidney excretion

- Acute or chronic kidney disease
- Aldosterone deficiency (e.g., type IV renal tubular acidosis, diabetic nephropathy, chronic interstitial nephritis, or obstructive nephropathy)
- Adrenal insufficiency (Addison disease)
- Drugs that inhibit potassium excretion
- Kidney diseases that impair distal tubule function
  - Sickle cell anemia
  - Systemic lupus erythematosus

Abnormal potassium distribution

- Insulin deficiency
- Beta-blockers
- Metabolic or respiratory acidosis
- Familial hyperkalemic periodic paralysis

Abnormal potassium release from cells

- Rhabdomyolysis
- Tumor lysis syndrome

TABLE 10.4 **Mechanisms for Drug-Induced Hyperkalemia**

Decrease kidney potassium excretion

Block sodium channel in the distal nephron
- Potassium-sparing diuretics: amiloride, triamterene
- Antibiotics: trimethoprim, pentamidine

Block aldosterone production
- ACE inhibitors (e.g., captopril, enalapril, lisinopril, benazepril)
- Angiotensin receptor blockers
- NSAIDs and COX-2 inhibitors
- Heparin
- Tacrolimus

Block aldosterone receptors
- Spironolactone
- Eplerenone

Block Na⁺/K⁺-ATPase activity in the distal nephron
- Cyclosporine

Inhibit extrarenal potassium disposal

- Block beta-2 adrenergic–mediated extrarenal potassium disposal: nonselective beta-blockers (e.g., propranolol, nadolol, timolol)
- Block Na⁺/K⁺-ATPase activity in skeletal muscles: digoxin overdose (not therapeutic doses)
- Inhibit insulin release (e.g., somatostatin)

Potassium release from injured cells

- Drug-induced rhabdomyolysis (e.g., lovastatin, cocaine)
- Drug-induced tumor lysis syndrome (chemotherapy agents in acute leukemias and high-grade lymphomas)
- Depolarizing paralytic agents (e.g., succinylcholine)

Drug-induced acute kidney injury

ACE, Angiotensin converting enzyme; *NSAIDs*, nonsteroidal antiinflammatory drugs.

Drug-Induced Hyperkalemia

A large number of drugs have the potential to cause hyperkalemia, either by inhibiting kidney potassium excretion or by blocking extrarenal disposal (Table 10.4). Most individuals taking these drugs will not develop hyperkalemia. Patients with advanced CKD are at the highest risk, especially if they have a high dietary potassium intake or are taking additional medication that predisposes to hyperkalemia. Most diuretics (loop diuretics, thiazide diuretics, acetazolamide) increase urinary potassium excretion and tend to cause hypokalemia. However, potassium-sparing diuretics inhibit urinary potassium excretion and predispose to hyperkalemia by one of two mechanisms. Spironolactone and eplerenone are competitive inhibitors of aldosterone; they bind to the aldosterone receptors in the collecting duct, thereby inhibiting Na⁺/K⁺-ATPase activity and indirectly limiting potassium secretion. The immunosuppressive drug, cyclosporine, also blocks Na⁺/K⁺-ATPase activity in the distal nephron. Two other potassium-sparing diuretics, amiloride and triamterene, bind to the sodium channel in the collecting duct. This inhibits sodium reabsorption in the distal nephron and thereby limits the establishment of an electrochemical gradient required for potassium secretion. Interestingly, two antibiotics, trimethoprim (one of the components of Bactrim) and pentamidine, have also been shown to block the sodium channel in the collecting duct and, therefore, predispose patients to hyperkalemia. In addition, trimethoprim has been shown to inhibit the collecting tubule H⁺/K⁺-ATPase.

Because aldosterone plays an important role in enhancing enteric potassium excretion in patients with kidney failure, drugs that inhibit aldosterone production (either directly or indirectly) predispose such patients to hyperkalemia. Angiotensin II is a potent stimulator of aldosterone production in the adrenal cortex. ACE inhibitors inhibit the production of angiotensin II, thereby decreasing aldosterone levels. Similarly, angiotensin II receptor blockers

also inhibit aldosterone production. Prostaglandins stimulate renin production, and prostaglandin inhibitors (NSAIDs) inhibit the production of renin, thereby indirectly decreasing aldosterone production. This effect is seen even with "kidney-sparing NSAIDs," such as sulindac (a nonselective COX-1 and COX-2 inhibitor). Hyperkalemia may also be caused by selective COX-2 inhibitors. Heparin has been shown to directly inhibit the production of aldosterone in the kidney cortex, primarily by decreasing the number and affinity of angiotensin II receptors in the zona glomerulosa. This effect occurs even with the low doses of subcutaneous heparin or enoxaparin used for prophylaxis of venous thrombosis in hospitalized patients (e.g., 5000 units twice daily). Tacrolimus, an immunosuppressant drug, may also cause hyperkalemia by inhibiting aldosterone synthesis. Oral contraceptives containing drospirenone (a progestin) inhibit kidney potassium excretion and may provoke hyperkalemia in women with CKD.

Given the stimulation of extrarenal potassium disposal by beta-adrenergic agonists, it is not surprising that beta-2 antagonists can predispose to hyperkalemia. This effect is seen primarily with nonselective beta-blockers (e.g., propranolol, nadolol, carvedilol), rather than beta-selective blockers (e.g., atenolol, metoprolol), and the severity of hyperkalemia is typically mild with increases in plasma potassium rarely exceeding 0.5 mEq/L. There is significant systemic absorption of topical beta-blockers, and hyperkalemia may rarely be provoked by timolol eye drops. Drugs inhibiting endogenous insulin release, such as somatostatin, have been rarely implicated as a cause of hyperkalemia in patients with kidney failure. Presumably, long-acting somatostatin analogs, such as octreotide, would have a similar effect on plasma potassium. *Digoxin overdose* causes inhibition of Na^+/K^+-ATPase activity in skeletal muscle cells and may manifest with hyperkalemia. This effect is rarely seen at therapeutic doses of the drug. Depolarizing paralytic agents used for general anesthesia, such as *succinylcholine*, can occasionally produce hyperkalemia by causing potassium to leak out of the cells.

Finally, drugs can also induce hyperkalemia indirectly by causing release of intracellular potassium from injured cells (e.g., rhabdomyolysis with *statins* and *cocaine*, or tumor lysis syndrome when chemotherapy is administered in patients with acute leukemia or high-grade lymphoma). Moreover, drug-induced AKI may be associated with secondary hyperkalemia.

A common clinical dilemma occurs when patients with CKD develop hyperkalemia after being started on an ACE inhibitor or ARB. One would like to continue this drug due to its renoprotective benefit. Therapeutic options for this scenario include reducing the dose of ACE inhibitor or ARB, starting or increasing the dose of a loop or thiazide diuretic, discontinuing other medications that promote hyperkalemia, reinforcing dietary potassium restriction, and adding a potassium binder. Fludrocortisone (0.1 to 0.2 mg daily) can be tried in refractory cases, although it may promote peripheral edema and hypertension resulting from avid sodium retention, and its use is generally discouraged. Finally, the patient should be questioned about constipation, as the addition of laxatives may promote fecal potassium excretion.

Fasting Hyperkalemia in Patients Undergoing Dialysis

Prolonged fasting decreases plasma insulin concentrations, thereby promoting potassium shifts from the intracellular to the extracellular fluid compartments. In normal individuals, the excess potassium is excreted in the urine such that the plasma potassium remains constant. In kidney failure, the potassium entering the extracellular fluid compartment during fasting cannot be excreted, thereby resulting in progressive hyperkalemia. The phenomenon of fasting hyperkalemia may be clinically significant in patients undergoing dialysis who fast longer than 8 to 12 hours before a surgical or radiologic procedure. Occasionally, such patients develop life-threatening hyperkalemia during a prolonged fast. The hyperkalemia can be prevented by the administration of intravenous dextrose (to stimulate endogenous insulin secretion) for the duration of the fast. If the patient is diabetic, insulin must be added to the dextrose infusion to prevent paradoxical hyperkalemia.

Clinical Manifestations of Hyperkalemia

Hyperkalemia may produce progressive electrocardiographic abnormalities, including peaked T waves, flattening or absence of P waves, widened QRS complexes, and sine waves (see Fig. 10.2). The major risk of severe hyperkalemia is the development of life-threatening ventricular arrhythmias.

Severe hyperkalemia, like severe hypokalemia, can cause skeletal muscle weakness, even to the point of paralysis and respiratory failure. Hyperkalemia impairs urinary acidification by decreasing collecting tubule apical H^+/K^+-ATPase, which may result in a renal tubular acidosis (type IV RTA). Hyperkalemia stimulates endogenous aldosterone secretion but not insulin secretion.

Treatment of Hyperkalemia

Severe hyperkalemia associated with electrocardiographic changes is a life-threatening state requiring emergent intervention (Fig. 10.3). There is no single plasma potassium concentration that defines severe hyperkalemia, although values above 6-6.5 mEq/L would typically elicit emergency interventions. The presence of EKG findings typical of hyperkalemia should render any plasma potassium value "severe" and requires emergent management:

1. *The first step is to stabilize the cardiac electrophysiology.* Acute administration of intravenous calcium gluconate does not change plasma potassium but does transiently improve the EKG. The effect of 10 mL of 10% calcium gluconate solution over 1 minute is almost immediate. If there is no improvement in the EKG appearance within 3 to 5 minutes, the dose should be repeated. Although calcium chloride has more elemental calcium per ampule than calcium gluconate, it is generally avoided in patients with a peripheral venous access as it may cause skin necrosis if it infiltrates.

2. *The second step is to shift potassium* from the extracellular to the intracellular fluid so as to rapidly decrease the plasma potassium concentration. This involves administration of insulin and/or a beta-2 agonist.

   a. *Intravenous insulin* is the fastest way to lower the plasma potassium. The plasma potassium starts to decrease within 15 minutes. Intravenous glucose is given concurrently to prevent hypoglycemia. Regular insulin is administered as 10 units along with a 50-mL bolus of 50% dextrose (1 ampule of D_{50}), followed by a continuous infusion of 5% dextrose at 100 mL/hour to prevent late hypoglycemia. Hypoglycemia is a common complication of intravenous insulin therapy, especially in patients with kidney failure in whom the half-life of insulin is increased; hence, close monitoring of blood glucose concentration is necessary. Hypoglycemia in patients with kidney failure may be less frequent with short-acting synthetic insulins (lispro and aspart), which are not metabolized by the kidney. In patients with diabetes, if the blood glucose concentration is >300 mg/dL, one can administer the intravenous insulin without concomitant 50% dextrose. One should never give dextrose without insulin for the acute treatment of hyperkalemia; in patients with inadequate endogenous insulin production, the resulting hyperglycemia can produce a paradoxical increase in plasma potassium.

   b. *Beta-agonists*. One should give 20 mg of albuterol (a $beta_2$-agonist) by inhalation over 10 minutes. The onset of action is 30 minutes; the concentrated form of albuterol (5 mg/mL) should be used to minimize the inhalation volume. The dose required to lower plasma potassium is considerably higher than that used to treat asthma, because only a small fraction of nebulized albuterol is absorbed systemically. Thus, 0.5 mg of intravenous albuterol (available in Europe but not in the United States) produces a comparable change in plasma potassium to that seen after 20 mg of nebulized albuterol. The potassium-lowering effect of albuterol is additive to that of insulin.

3. Once the previous temporizing measures have been performed, further interventions are done to *remove potassium from the body*.

   a. *Diuretics*. Loop and thiazide diuretics work if the patient has adequate kidney function.

   b. *Sodium bicarbonate* administration can lower plasma potassium by enhancing kidney potassium excretion in

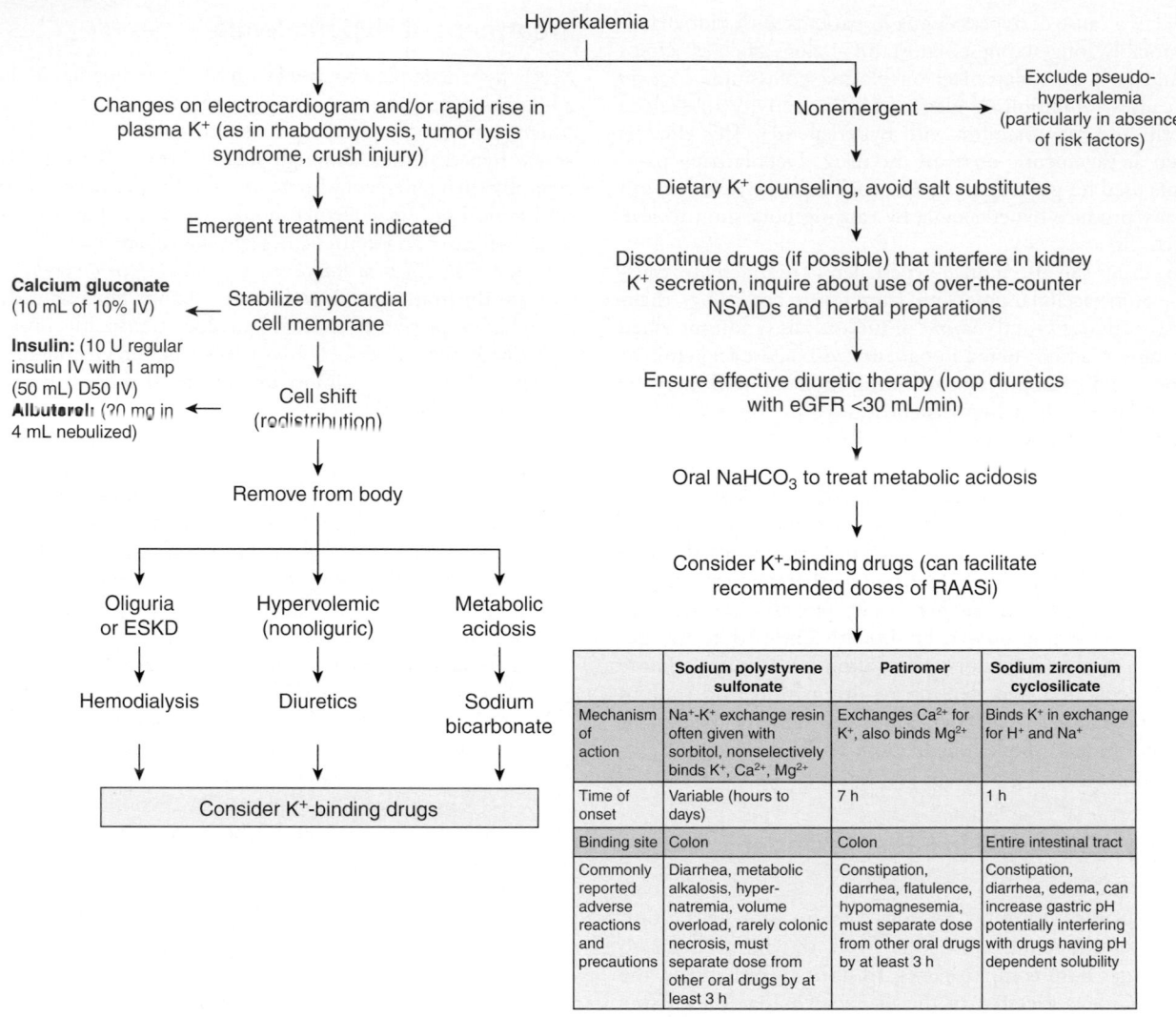

• **Fig. 10.3** Approach to treatment of hyperkalemia. (From Palmer BF, Clegg DJ. Physiology and Pathophysiology of Potassium Homeostasis: Core Curriculum 2019. Am J Kidney Dis. 2019;74(5):682-695.)

patients with normal kidney function and in those with CKD who are not yet on dialysis. However, bicarbonate administration is of dubious value for treatment of hyperkalemia in patients without residual kidney function and should not be routinely used for emergency treatment of hyperkalemia. Moreover, bicarbonate administration does not enhance the potassium-lowering effects of insulin or albuterol. Bicarbonate administration is still indicated if the patient has severe metabolic acidosis (serum bicarbonate <10 mmol/L).

c. Dialysis is indicated in patients who lack kidney function (severe acute kidney injury or end-stage kidney disease). Dialysis is the most effective way to correct hyperkalemia but can seldom be initiated quickly enough to preclude the administration of the other emergency measures listed above.

d. Potassium binders are typically administered following other emergency interventions as an adjunct and/or as a means to transition to chronic (preventative) therapy of hyperkalemia.
  i. Sodium polystyrene sulfate (SPS, *Kayexalate*) is a resin exchanger that moves potassium from the blood into the gut, in exchange for an equal amount of sodium. It is relatively slow acting, requiring several hours before

plasma potassium decreases. Each gram of SPS removes 0.5 to 1.0 mmol of potassium. It is administered as 50 g in 30 mL sorbitol by mouth or 50 g in a retention enema. The rectal route is faster and more reliable. The studies documenting the efficacy of SPS for treatment of hyperkalemia are generally small and of relatively low quality. A recent randomized, double-blinded clinical trial of 31 patients with CKD and mild hyperkalemia allocated patients to receive SPS or placebo for 7 days. Those treated with SPS had a mean decrease in plasma potassium of about 1.0 mmol/L. Controlled studies of the efficacy and safety of SPS therapy over longer durations are not available, and SPS is not approved for chronic management of hyperkalemia. The use of SPS has been associated with colonic necrosis in rare cases, particularly when combined with sorbitol, leading to a "black box" warning by the FDA.
  ii. Two new potassium binders are available. *Patiromer* is a polymer that binds potassium in exchange for calcium in the colon that is approved for chronic management of hyperkalemia. Patiromer should not be used as an emergency treatment of hyperkalemia except as an adjunct to the first-line interventions mentioned above.

Patiromer has been compared to placebo in several randomized, double-blinded clinical trials of patients with CKD and hyperkalemia, many of whom had diabetes or heart failure and were receiving concomitant mineralocorticoid receptor antagonist, ACE inhibitor, or ARB treatment. Studies of both short-term (28 days) and long-term (up to 1 year) duration demonstrated a significant (~1 mmol/L) and sustained reduction in plasma potassium in patients receiving patiromer. The safety profile was excellent, with the exception of gastrointestinal complications and mild hypomagnesemia in a minority of patients. Serum magnesium concentration should be monitored and patiromer should be avoided in patients with severe constipation, bowel obstruction, or impaction. The starting dose of patiromer is 8.4 grams once daily, with dose titrations recommended at weekly intervals until the desired plasma potassium concentration is achieved. Concern exists about the binding of patiromer to other oral medication, and dosing should be spaced by 3 hours from other medications.

iii. *Zirconium cyclosilicate* is a cation (sodium-potassium) exchanger that has a 9-fold higher potassium-binding capacity (per gram) than SPS. Zirconium cyclosilicate has a crystal structure that selectively binds potassium in exchange of sodium across the intestinal tract and is approved for chronic management of hyperkalemia. Similar to patiromer, zirconium cyclosilicate is also not indicated as monotherapy for emergency treatment of hyperkalemia but can be used as an adjunct to first-line interventions. The efficacy and safety of zirconium cyclosilicate in patients with hyperkalemia has been shown in several randomized controlled trials of medium- to long-term duration. Zirconium cyclosilicate lowered plasma potassium concentration by 0.5-1 mEq/L, with greater declines seen in patients with more severe hyperkalemia. Control of plasma potassium concentration was maintained for the duration of the therapy. Zirconium cyclosilicate was well tolerated. The most important adverse effect was mild to moderate edema, as each 5-g dose of zirconium cyclosilicate contains 400 mg of sodium; edema occurred more frequently in patients taking the highest dose (15 g) of the drug. Zirconium cyclosilicate should be avoided in patients with severe constipation, bowel obstruction, or impaction, and edema should be monitored. The starting dose of zirconium cyclosilicate is 10 g thrice daily for up to 48 hours, followed by once-daily dosing and weekly-dose titration for chronic administration. Zirconium cyclosilicate is also approved for treating chronic hyperkalemia in chronic hemodialysis patients, in whom it should be administered once daily on non-dialysis days only. Other oral medications should be spaced by 2 hours.

For patients with moderate hyperkalemia not associated with electrocardiographic changes, it is frequently sufficient to identify and eliminate the predisposing factor(s) responsible for the elevated plasma potassium. The same measures should also be considered after the emergency interventions used in patients with severe hyperkalemia.

1. Counsel the patient on dietary potassium restriction of 40 to 60 mEq (1.5 to 2.5 g) per day (Table 10.5).
2. Avoid medications that interfere with kidney excretion of potassium (see Table 10.3). ACE inhibitors and ARBs play a

TABLE 10.5	Potassium Content of Selected Foods	
Food	Potassium (mg)	Potassium (mEq)
Pinto beans (1 cup)	1370	35
Raisins (1 cup)	1106	28
Honeydew (1/2 melon)	939	24
Nuts (1 cup)	688	18
Black-eyed peas (1 cup)	625	16
Collard greens (1 cup)	498	13
Banana (1 medium)	440	11
Tomato (1 medium)	366	9
Orange (1 large)	333	9
Milk (1 cup)	351	9
Potato chips (10)	226	6

major role in slowing the progression of CKD. For this reason, when patients on these medications develop hyperkalemia, one should first attempt to decrease dietary potassium intake; treat constipation, if present, to maximize gastrointestinal excretion of potassium; stop other drugs contributing to hyperkalemia; add a diuretic; or add a potassium binder such as patiromer or zirconium cyclosilicate. Only if all other measures fail to control the hyperkalemia, should the ACE inhibitor or ARB be discontinued.

3. If clinically indicated, chronic medication with diuretics can be used to stimulate urinary potassium excretion. In patients with advanced CKD, loop diuretics are usually necessary.
4. Administer sodium bicarbonate in patients with chronic metabolic acidosis. Chronic sodium bicarbonate therapy may also be renoprotective in patients with CKD.
5. When other measures have failed, the chronic use of binders such as patiromer or zirconium cyclosilicate can be used to avoid hyperkalemia. The use of these agents can be particularly helpful in patients with frequent episodes of recurrent severe hyperkalemia, such as those with advanced CKD.
6. Specific therapy may be indicated for the underlying etiology, when available. For example, patients with *adrenal insufficiency* require replacement with exogenous glucocorticoids and mineralocorticoids. In patients with *hyperkalemic periodic paralysis* (a rare, autosomal dominant disorder in which affected individuals develop periodic episodes of severe muscle weakness in association with profound hyperkalemia), prophylactic aerosolized albuterol can prevent both exercise-induced hyperkalemia and muscle weakness.

Complete bibliography is available at Elsevier eBooks for Practicing Clinicians.

Key Bibliography

Clase CM, Carrero JJ, Ellison DH, et al. Potassium homeostasis and management of dyskalemia in kidney diseases: conclusions from a Kidney Disease: Improving Global Outcomes (KDIGO) controversies conference. *Kidney Int.* 2020;97(1):42–61 Jan.

Cupisti A, Kovesdy CP, D'Alessandro C, Kalantar-Zadeh K. Dietary approach to recurrent or chronic hyperkalaemia in patients with decreased kidney function. *Nutrients*. 2018 Feb 25;10(3):261.

Epstein M, Lifschitz MD. Potassium homeostasis and dyskalemias: the respective roles of renal, extrarenal and gut sensors in potassium handling. *Kidney Int Suppl*. 2016;6:7–15.

Kovesdy CP. Management of hyperkalaemia in chronic kidney disease. *Nat Rev Nephrol*. 2014;10(11):653–662 Nov.

Kovesdy CP, Appel LJ, Grams ME, et al. Potassium homeostasis in health and disease: a scientific workshop cosponsored by the National Kidney Foundation and the American Society of Hypertension. *Am J Kidney Dis*. 2017;70(6):844–858.

Krishna GG, Steigerwalt SP, Pikus R, et al. Hypokalemic states. In: Narins RG, ed. *Clinical Disorders of Fluid and Electrolyte Metabolism*. New York: McGraw-Hill; 1994:659–696.

Kurtz I. Molecular pathogenesis of Bartter's and Gitelman's syndromes. *Kidney Int*. 1998;54:1396–1410.

Lifton RP, Dluhy RG, Powers M, et al. A chimaeric 11 beta-hydroxylase/aldosterone synthase gene causes glucocorticoid-remediable aldosteronism and human hypertension. *Nature*. 1992;355:262–265.

Palmer BF. Potassium binders for hyperkalemia in chronic kidney disease-diet, renin-angiotensin-aldosterone system inhibitor therapy, and hemodialysis. *Mayo Clin Proc*. 2020;95(2):339–354.

Palmer BF, Clegg DJ. Physiology and pathophysiology of potassium homeostasis: core curriculum 2019. *Am J Kidney Dis*. 2019;74(5):682–695.

Shimkets RA, Warnock DG, Bositis CM, et al. Liddle's syndrome: heritable human hypertension caused by mutations in the beta subunit of the epithelial sodium channel. *Cell*. 1994;79:407–414.

11

Disorders of Calcium, Phosphorus, and Magnesium Homeostasis

RYAN P. FLOOD, JESSICA KENDRICK

Disorders of mineral metabolism (calcium, phosphorus, magnesium) are common, especially in hospitalized patients. The extracellular concentrations of these ions are less than 1% of total body stores, and the principal site of storage is bone. Thus, serum levels may not always reflect underlying pathology. Knowledge of the complex homeostasis of these ions is critical in formulating the differential diagnosis of disorders affecting these ions and in directing appropriate treatment. This regulation occurs in four major target organs (intestine, kidney, parathyroid glands, and bone) via the complex integration of four hormones (parathyroid hormone [PTH], vitamin D and its derivatives, fibroblast growth factor 23 [FGF23], and α-klotho, hereafter called *klotho*). An understanding of normal physiology is necessary to accurately diagnose and treat disorders of calcium, phosphorus, and magnesium.

Normal Physiology

Parathyroid Hormone

PTH is released in response to hypocalcemia (Fig. 11.1) and maintains calcium homeostasis by three mechanisms: (1) increasing bone mineral dissolution, thus releasing calcium and phosphorus; (2) increasing kidney reabsorption of calcium and excretion of phosphorus; and (3) enhancing the gastrointestinal absorption of both calcium and phosphorus indirectly through its effects on the synthesis of $1,25(OH)_2$-vitamin D. In healthy individuals, the increase in serum PTH level in response to hypocalcemia effectively restores serum calcium levels while maintaining normal serum phosphorus levels.

PTH enhances the conversion of 25(OH)-vitamin D [calcidiol] to $1,25(OH)_2$-vitamin D [calcitriol], with the latter decreasing PTH secretion at the level of the parathyroid glands and completing a typical endocrine feedback loop. In primary hyperparathyroidism, PTH is secreted autonomously from adenomatous glands without regard to physiologic stimuli. In contrast, in secondary hyperparathyroidism, the glands initially respond appropriately to low levels of ionized calcium; however, after a prolonged period of chronic kidney disease (CKD) and secondary hyperparathyroidism, the hyperplastic glands become adenomatous and therefore unresponsive to stimuli that would normally suppress PTH secretion (sometimes called *tertiary hyperparathyroidism*). After entering the circulation, PTH binds to PTH receptors located throughout the body. Therefore, disorders of PTH excess or insufficiency not only affect serum levels of calcium and phosphorus but also lead to bone, cardiac, skin, and neurologic manifestations.

PTH is cleaved from a precursor preprohormone to an 84-amino-acid protein in the parathyroid gland, where it is stored with other PTH-protein fragments in secretory granules for release. After release, the circulating 84-amino-acid protein has a half-life of 2 to 4 minutes. It is then further cleaved into N-terminal, C-terminal, and mid-region fragments of PTH, which are finally metabolized in the liver and kidneys. PTH secretion can be triggered by hypocalcemia, hyperphosphatemia, or calcitriol deficiency, whereas profound hypomagnesemia can reduce PTH release. The extracellular concentration of ionized calcium is the most important determinant of temporal PTH levels. Active secretion of PTH from stored granules in response to hypocalcemia is controlled by the calcium-sensing receptor (CaSR), and mutations of the CaSR gene can lead to syndromes of hypercalcemia or hypocalcemia through dysregulated PTH release. The CaSR is expressed in thyroid C-cells and in the kidney, where it controls excretion of calcium in the thick ascending limb of the loop of Henle in response to changes in serum calcium concentration.

Through the years, a succession of increasingly sensitive assays has been developed to measure PTH. A major difficulty in measuring PTH accurately with the first-generation assay is the cross-reactivity with inactive, circulating PTH-protein fragments that may accumulate in CKD. These early assays targeted the C-terminus but were inaccurate in patients with kidney disease because of accumulation of these fragments. Subsequent N-terminus assays resulted in similar problems. Accuracy was improved by the development of a second-generation two-site antibody test (commonly called the "INTACT" assay) to detect full-length (1–84, or active) PTH molecules. In this assay, a capture antibody binds to the N-terminus, and a second antibody binds to the C-terminus. However, because the N-terminal antibody is at amino acid 7 instead of amino acid 1, this intact assay still detects some retained C-terminal fragments, albeit less than the older assays. These fragments accumulate in CKD, leading to falsely elevated values in assays of intact PTH such that values above the normal range are associated with complications of hypoparathyroidism at the level of bone. A third-generation assay was developed, which directed antibody binding to the proximal N-terminus portion 1-4 of the PTH molecule thought to be the most "biologically active" while not binding to PTH fragments. It detects 95% of circulating PTH in patients with normal kidney function and 85% in patients with CKD, as compared

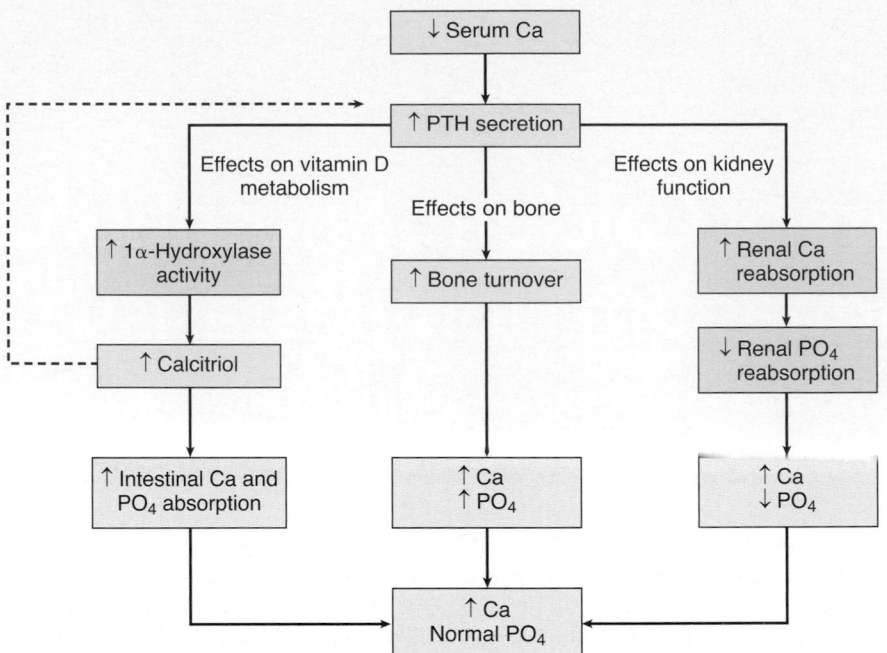

• Fig. 11.1 Normal homeostatic response to hypocalcemia. In the presence of hypocalcemia, secretion of parathyroid hormone (PTH) is increased. PTH acts on three target organs. PTH works at the intestine indirectly by first increasing the 1α-hydroxylase activity in the kidney; this enzyme converts calcidiol to calcitriol, which increases intestinal absorption of both calcium and phosphorus. Calcitriol then negatively feeds back on the parathyroid glands to suppress PTH release (*dotted line*). In bone, PTH increases bone turnover, resulting in a release of calcium and phosphorus. Last, PTH works directly on the kidney to increase kidney calcium reabsorption and to decrease kidney phosphorus reabsorption. The net effect is a rise in serum calcium but no net change in serum phosphorus. The blue boxes indicate homeostatic steps in the kidney that are abnormal in people with chronic kidney disease. Because of diminished kidney mass, conversion of calcidiol to calcitriol and phosphorus excretion are impaired.

to 80% and 50%, respectively, with the second-generation assay. However, given the widely available and more robustly evaluated second-generation assay, the 2017 Kidney Diseases Improving Global Outcomes (KDIGO) guidelines continue to suggest using the second-generation assay for PTH monitoring. Additionally, it is recommended to use the same lab for all PTH assays and evaluating trends in PTH levels rather than isolated values.

Vitamin D

Vitamin D is called a "vitamin" because it is an essential nutrient that must come from an exogenous source if it cannot be endogenously manufactured in sufficient quantity; however, this is a misnomer, because vitamin D is a hormone that can be synthesized in the skin. Vitamin D_2 (ergocalciferol) from plants and vitamin D_3 (cholecalciferol) primarily from oily fish are the main exogenous sources in a Western diet outside of supplementation in food products. In the skin, 7-dehydrocholesterol is converted to vitamin D_3 in response to sunlight, which is inhibited by sunscreen of skin protection factor (SPF) 8 or greater. After entering the blood, vitamins D_2 and D_3 from diet or skin bind to vitamin D–binding protein and are carried to the liver, where they are hydroxylated to yield 25(OH)D, often called *calcidiol*; accordingly, blood calcidiol levels are a direct assessment of the nutritional (dietary) intake and skin conversion of vitamin D. Some clinical assays measure hydroxylated forms of both D_2 and D_3, whereas others measure the total level of 25(OH)D ($D_2 + D_3$). 25(OH)D (calcidiol) is then

converted in the kidney to 1,25(OH)$_2$D (calcitriol) by the action of 1α-hydroxylase (the CYP27B1 isoenzyme of the cytochrome P-450 system). In the kidney, CYP27B1 activity is affected by almost every hormone involved in calcium homeostasis. Its activity is stimulated by PTH, estrogen, calcitonin, prolactin, growth hormone, low serum calcium, and low serum phosphorus, and inhibited by calcitriol and FGF23 providing feedback loops of regulation. FGF23 also stimulates CYP24, leading to accelerated degradation of both calcidiol and calcitriol, and thus contributing to the known vitamin D deficiency of CKD.

Calcitriol circulates in the bloodstream bound to vitamin D–binding protein. The free form of 1,25(OH)$_2$D enters the target cell, where it interacts with its nuclear vitamin D receptor (VDR). This complex then combines with the retinoic acid X receptor to form a heterodimer, which in turn interacts with the vitamin D response element (VDRE) on the target gene. The major functions of 1,25(OH)$_2$D are carried out in three target organs: (1) the small intestine, where it regulates the intestinal absorption of calcium and, to a lesser degree, phosphorus and possibly magnesium; (2) the parathyroid gland, where it inhibits PTH synthesis at the level of messenger RNA transcription; and (3) the osteoblast/osteocytes in bone, where it directly stimulates the secretion of FGF23. Importantly, the kidney CYP27B1 is essential for the feedback loops between calcitriol and both PTH and FGF23.

In addition to the role of vitamin D in mineral metabolism, the VDR is expressed in multiple organs, and 1α-hydroxylase activity can be detected in extrarenal tissues including immune cells, muscle cells, and myocardiocytes. Both 25(OH)D and 1,25(OH)$_2$D can be taken up by extrarenal cells, with the former then converted intracellularly to 1,25(OH)$_2$D. These features may mediate autocrine or paracrine effects of vitamin D outside its classic target tissues, especially effects on cell differentiation and proliferation and immune function. Recent studies in both normal and CKD patients have demonstrated widespread vitamin D (calcidiol) insufficiency and deficiency. Low levels of this precursor to calcitriol are associated with hyperparathyroidism, falls, fractures, cardiovascular disease, mortality, and cancers in the general population. However, repletion has not yet been shown to improve clinical outcomes in CKD.

Fibroblast Growth Factor 23

FGF23 is a phosphatonin, which is a group of proteins that were identified from the study of genetic disorders characterized by hypophosphatemia from urinary phosphate wasting and cases of FGF23-producing tumor-induced osteomalacia associated with urinary phosphate wasting. FGF23 is made by osteocytes, a subgroup of osteoblasts that are interconnected through a series of canaliculi within cancellous (trabecular) bone. FGF23 directly inhibits the conversion of 25(OH)D to 1,25(OH)$_2$D through downregulation of the CP27B1 in the kidney and increases the catabolism of both forms of vitamin D through stimulation of CYP24. FGF23 also inhibits PTH, while 1,25(OH)D and PTH stimulate FGF23, completing a feedback loop (Fig. 11.2). Thus, FGF23 provides the key PTH-bone link and kidney-bone link. Levels of FGF23 are elevated as early as CKD stage 2 and are associated with left ventricular hypertrophy and increased mortality. In the kidney, FGF23 acts through the FGF receptor and its coreceptor klotho; however, in cardiomyocytes, FGF23 acts independently of klotho. In addition to FGF23, there are other phosphatonins, such as matrix extracellular phosphoglycoprotein (MEPE), that may provide an intestine-kidney link.

Klotho

Alpha-klotho null mice have apparent premature aging: early demise, infertility, arteriosclerosis and arterial calcification, osteoporosis, hyperphosphatemia, emphysema, and skin atrophy, paralleling observations of FGF23 null mice. It was thus named klotho after the Greek goddess who spins the thread of life. Alpha-klotho is a 130-kDa transmembrane protein that is predominantly expressed in the distal tubule of the kidney but also in multiple other tissues. The extracellular domain is also cleaved by proteases including a disintegrin and metalloproteinase (ADAM10 and ADAM17) and secreted into the blood, urine, and cerebrospinal fluid where it functions as a hormone. Thus, there is both tissue klotho and secreted (soluble or circulating) klotho. In the kidney, tissue klotho serves as a coreceptor for FGF23, and receptor activation leads to increased urinary excretion of phosphorus. Klotho also stimulates calcium reabsorption in the distal tubule by preventing endocytosis (stabilizing) of the major calcium channels, TRPV5 and TRPV6. Therefore, klotho may work with FGF23 to increase urinary phosphorus content but also ensures that the urine with high phosphorus does not also have high calcium, preventing supersaturation of the urine. Both FGF23 (from bone) and klotho (in the kidney) are stimulated by 1,25(OH)$_2$D, and both FGF23 and klotho stimulate kidney 1-alpha hydroxylase (CYP27B1) to complete the endocrine feedback loop. In addition, cleaved/soluble klotho stimulates FGF23 secretion from bone and can affect kidney phosphate homeostasis even in the absence of membrane klotho. Thus, klotho joins FGF23, PTH, and calcitriol in a series of feedback loops that ensure optimal concentrations of calcium and phosphorus in bone and blood.

Calcium

Serum calcium levels are tightly controlled within a narrow range, usually 8.5 to 10.5 mg/dL (2.1 to 2.6 mmol/L). However, the serum calcium level is a poor reflection of overall total body calcium

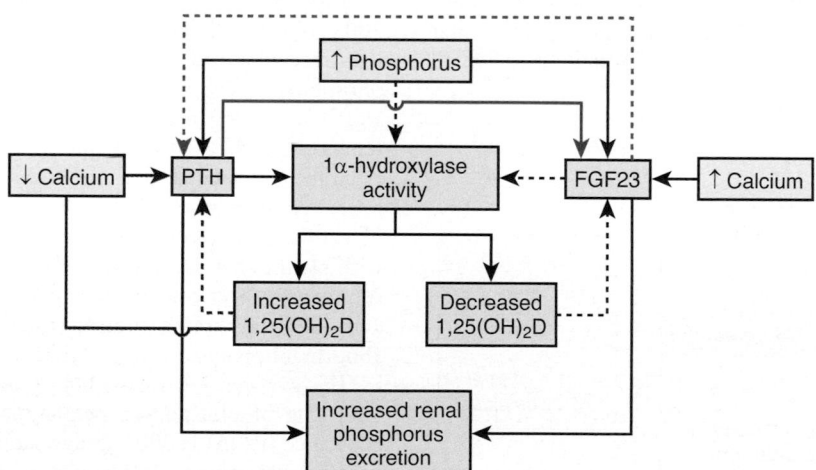

• **Fig. 11.2 Hormonal control of phosphorus.** In the setting of increased phosphorus intake or hyperphosphatemia, both parathyroid hormone (PTH) and fibroblast growth factor 23 (FGF23) are stimulated and induce kidney phosphorus excretion. However, PTH and FGF23 have opposing effects on the CYP27B1 (1α-hydroxylase) to increase and decrease 1,25(OH)$_2$D (calcitriol) production, respectively. The increased calcitriol then feeds back to inhibit PTH, and the decreased calcitriol then feeds back to inhibit FGF23 (as calcitriol normally stimulates FGF23). Hypocalcemia also stimulates PTH, and recent data suggest hypercalcemia stimulates FGF23. The solid lines represent an increase in levels; the dotted lines represent a decrease or inhibition of levels. (Adapted from Moe SM, Sprague SM. Chronic kidney disease–mineral bone disorder. In: Taal MW, Chertow GM, Marsden PA, Skorecki K, Yu ASL, Brenner BM, eds. *Brenner and Rector's the Kidney.* 9th ed. Philadelphia: Elsevier Saunders; 2012:2023.)

because the intravascular space contains only 0.1% to 0.2% of extracellular calcium, which in turn represents only 1% of total body calcium, with nearly all total body calcium stored in bone. Only ionized calcium, approximately 50% of total serum calcium, is physiologically active, with the remaining 50% of total serum calcium bound to albumin or anions such as citrate, bicarbonate, and phosphorus (Fig. 11.3).

Calcium absorption across the intestinal epithelium occurs via a vitamin D–dependent, saturable (transcellular) and vitamin D–independent, nonsaturable (paracellular) pathway. In states of adequate dietary calcium, the paracellular mechanism prevails, but the vitamin D–dependent pathways are critical in calcium-deficient states. Usually, the dietary intake of calcium is about 600 to 1000 mg/day in healthy adults. Out of every 1 g of ingested calcium, 600 mg is excreted in feces and 200 mg via the urine, thus leading to a net absorption of approximately 200 mg/day. The duodenum is the major site of calcium absorption, although the other segments of the small intestine and the colon also contribute to calcium absorption. In addition, there is secretion of calcium into the lumen of the mid- to distal- small and large intestine via paracellular transport contributing to fecal calcium losses. The heterogeneous distribution of calcium absorption and secretion along the small and large intestines creates a mechanism to respond to changes in physiologic stimulation to manage calcium homeostasis.

In the intestine and in the kidney, transcellular absorption occurs via three steps: (1) the entry of calcium from the lumen into the cells via transient receptor potential vanilloid (TRPV) channels, (2) the intracellular calcium then associates with calbindin to be "ferried" to the basolateral membrane, and (3) calcium is removed from the enterocytes predominantly via the calcium-ATPase, with the Na/Ca exchanger (NCX) playing a minor role. All of the key regulatory components of active calcium transport, TRPV, calbindin, Ca-ATPase, and NCX, are upregulated by calcitriol. At the level of the kidney, vitamin D and PTH work together to control calcium reabsorption and excretion.

In the kidney, the majority (60% to 70%) of calcium is reabsorbed passively in the proximal tubule, driven by a gradient that is generated by reabsorption of sodium and water. In the thick ascending limb, another 20% to 30% of calcium is reabsorbed via paracellular transport driven by the lumen positive net charge. The remaining 10% of calcium reabsorption occurs in the distal convoluted tubule, the connecting tubule, and the initial portion of the cortical collecting duct. The final regulation of urinary calcium excretion is carried out in these distal segments. Patients with CKD are at risk for maladaptive mineral bone metabolism and abnormal calcium homeostasis. Studies have demonstrated that patients suffering from CKD managed with oral calcium replacement or increased dietary calcium intake were shown to have a net positive calcium balance with a hypothetically increased risk for tissues' deposition and vascular calcification. Therefore, in 2017 KDIGO changed its recommendation of maintaining a normal serum calcium level in CKD to avoiding hypercalcemia and treatment of symptomatic hypocalcemia on an individualized basis, as patients with CKD are at risk for increased morbidity and mortality related to cardiovascular complications in the setting of vascular calcifications.

Phosphorus

Inorganic phosphorus is critical for numerous normal physiologic functions, including skeletal development, cell membrane phospholipid content and function, cell signaling, platelet aggregation, and energy transfer through mitochondrial metabolism. Normal homeostasis maintains serum concentrations between 2.5 and 4.5 mg/dL (0.81 to 1.45 mmol/L). The terms *phosphorus* and *phosphate* are often used interchangeably, but, strictly speaking, "phosphate" refers to the inorganic form that is in equilibrium (pK 6.8) between HPO_4^{2-} and $H_2PO_4^-$ at physiologic pH in a ratio of about 4:1. For that reason, phosphorus is usually expressed in millimoles (mmol) rather than milliequivalents (mEq) per liter (L); however, as most laboratories report this inorganic component as "phosphorus," we will use this term in the remainder of this chapter. Levels are highest in infants and decrease with growth, reaching adult levels in the late teenage years.

Total adult body stores of phosphorus are approximately 700 g, of which 85% is contained in bone. Of the remainder, 14% is intracellular and only 1% is extracellular. Of this extracellular phosphorus, 70% is organic and contained within phospholipids and 30% is inorganic. Of the latter, 15% is protein bound and the remaining 85% is either complexed with sodium, magnesium, or calcium or is circulating as the free monohydrogen or dihydrogen forms. Accordingly, only 0.15% of total body phosphorus (15% of extracellular phosphorus) is freely circulating and measured with serum chemistries. Therefore, as with calcium, serum measurements reflect only a small fraction of total body phosphorus and do not accurately indicate total body stores in the setting of abnormal homeostasis (e.g., CKD).

The average American diet contains approximately 1000 to 1400 mg of phosphorus per day, and the recommended daily allowance (RDA) is 800 mg/day. Approximately two-thirds of the ingested phosphorus is excreted in the urine and the remaining one-third in stool. In general, high-protein foods and dairy products contain the most phosphorus, whereas fruits and vegetables contain the least. In addition, grain-based (e.g., soy) protein contains phosphorus bound with phytate, making it less bioavailable. Many prepackaged and fast foods contain extra phosphorus as a preservative, which may not be identified on food labels and vary from lot to lot. An often surreptitious and unquantified source of dietary phosphorus is that which exists in prescription medications. A recent evaluation of commonly prescribed anti-hypertensive

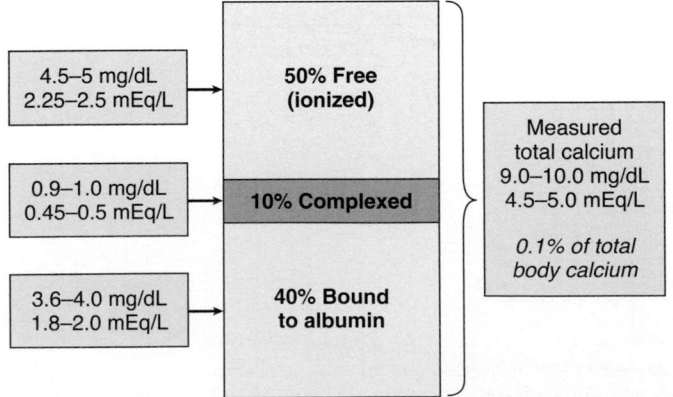

• **Fig. 11.3 Distribution of extracellular calcium.** Only 0.1% of the total body calcium is in the extracellular space; the other 99.9% is localized in bone. The serum calcium concentration reported by the clinical laboratory is total serum calcium. However, only approximately 50% of this total calcium is the physiologically active ionized component. The other 50% of serum calcium is composed of the 10% of the total calcium that is complexed to anions such as bicarbonate, phosphate, and citrate and the 40% that is bound to albumin.

medication, multivitamins, and anti-depressants found they have significant quantities of phosphorus, up to 20 to 40 mg per pill, depending on their manufacturer. Therefore, it is difficult to accurately predict the dietary intake based on food type and medications alone.

Between 60% and 70% of dietary phosphorus is absorbed by the gut, in all intestinal segments. Medications that bind dietary phosphorus can decrease the net amount of phosphorus absorbed by decreasing the amount of free phosphorus available for absorption. In patients with CKD, such phosphate binders are used to compensate for the loss of kidney phosphorus excretion.

Passive enteric absorption (which is dependent on the luminal phosphorus concentration) occurs via the epithelial brush border sodium-phosphate cotransporter (NPT2b), driven by the sodium gradient created by the basolateral Na^+/K^+-ATPase transporter. The NPT2b sits in the terminal web, just below the brush border in "ready-to-use" vesicles that traffic to the brush border in response to acute and chronic changes in phosphorus concentration. Calcitriol can upregulate the NPT2b and thereby actively increase phosphorus absorption.

Most inorganic phosphorus is freely filtered by the glomerulus. Approximately 70% to 80% of the filtered load is reabsorbed in the proximal tubule, the primary site of regulated phosphorus reabsorption in the kidney, with the remaining 20% to 30% reabsorbed in the distal tubule. Hypophosphatemia stimulates CYP27B1, thereby increasing conversion of calcidiol to calcitriol, which in turn increases intestinal phosphorus absorption. Calcitriol also stimulates kidney tubular phosphorus reabsorption, leading to a reduction in urinary phosphorus excretion. In the presence of hyperphosphatemia, there is a rapid increase in urinary excretion of phosphorus, mediated by the levels of serum phosphorus, PTH, and FGF23. Although the effects are more minor, kidney phosphorus excretion is also increased by volume expansion, metabolic acidosis, glucocorticoid exposure, and calcitonin, and is decreased by growth hormone and thyroid hormone. Because of the capacity of the kidney to increase urinary phosphorus excretion, sustained hyperphosphatemia is not seen clinically without impairment of kidney function.

Magnesium

Magnesium plays an important role in neuromuscular function, control of cardiac excitability and vasomotor tone, mitochondrial function and energy metabolism, and DNA and protein synthesis. Magnesium is also a cofactor for many transporters involved in the regulation of sodium, potassium, and calcium. Normal magnesium levels are 0.7 to 1.1 mmol/L (1.4 to 2.2 mEq/L). Magnesium storage is located primarily in the hydroxyapatite mineral component of bone, accounting for 50%-60% of total body stores, while 40%-50% is located in muscle and non-muscular soft tissues. The large bone reserve provides an exchangeable source of magnesium to respond to changes in serum magnesium concentrations.

At this time, there are no known hormones that specifically regulate magnesium homeostasis or balance. Approximately 30% of the dietary magnesium is absorbed, mostly in the small intestine via paracellular pathways with a smaller contribution in the colon. In the colon, absorption from the lumen is predominantly active via transient receptor potential melastatin type 6 channel (TRPM6) and TRPM7, the activity of which is downregulated by increased intracellular magnesium and is independent of vitamin D. Extrusion of magnesium from the basolateral side may be through the Na^+/Mg^{2+} exchanger CNNM4 based on data from rodent models. However, humans with VNNM4 mutations do not have hypomagnesemia.

About 10% to 20% of filtered magnesium is reabsorbed in the proximal convoluted tubule, and reabsorption decreases with extracellular volume expansion in parallel with that of sodium and calcium. Unlike other divalent ions, most (75%) magnesium is reabsorbed passively through paracellular pathways in the thick ascending limb of the loop of Henle, driven by a lumen-positive voltage in a specific cation-permeable channel formed by the tight junction proteins Claudin-16 (formerly called *paracellin*), Claudin-14, and Claudin-19. Mutations of the last proteins have a role in the development of familial hypomagnesemia with hypercalciuria and nephrocalcinosis. About 5% to 10% of magnesium is reabsorbed in the distal convoluted tubule, driven primarily by the luminal membrane potential established by the voltage-gated potassium channel and facilitated by TRMP6, which is located at the luminal membrane of the distal convoluted tubule. Estrogen, insulin, magnesium, and pH may alter expression or function of this transporter.

Bone

The majority of the total body stores of calcium and phosphorus are located in bone in the form of hydroxyapatite [$Ca_{10}(PO_4)_6(OH)_2$]. Trabecular (cancellous) bone comprises 15% to 20% of bone. Trabecular bone is located predominantly in the epiphyses of the long bones and serves a metabolic function. There is a relatively rapid exchange of calcium between trabecular bone and plasma (days to weeks), as evidenced by a short turnover rate of the radioisotope[45] calcium. In contrast, cortical (compact) bone is located in the shafts of long bones and comprises 80% to 90% of bone. This bone serves primarily a protective and mechanical function and it has a calcium turnover rate of months. The nonmineral component of bone consists principally (90%) of highly organized cross-linked fibers of type I collagen; the remainder consists of proteoglycans and "noncollagen" proteins such as osteopontin, osteocalcin, osteonectin, and alkaline phosphatase. The predominant cell types involved in bone turnover are osteoclasts, the bone-resorbing cells derived from circulating hematopoietic cells, and osteoblasts, the bone-forming cells derived from the marrow. These cells are important in bone remodeling, which occurs in response to hormones, cytokines, and changes in mechanical forces and can in turn affect calcium and phosphorus homeostasis.

Disorders of Mineral Metabolism

Hypercalcemia

Hypercalcemia is defined as elevated serum calcium. Ionized calcium represents the biologically active fraction of total serum calcium. In the presence of hypoalbuminemia, there is a proportionate increase in ionized calcium relative to total calcium, so that measurements of total serum calcium in patients with hypoalbuminemia may underestimate the amount of physiologically active (ionized) calcium. A commonly used formula to estimate ionized calcium from total serum calcium is to add 0.8 mg/dL to the total calcium value for every 1 mg/dL decrease in serum albumin below 4 mg/dL. In certain circumstances, such as the presence of increased concentrations of albumin or molecules capable of binding calcium (e.g., phosphate and citrate), paraproteinemias, or abnormally high or low blood pH, direct measurement of serum-ionized calcium is essential, especially if intravenous (IV) calcium infusion is contemplated. In patients with advanced CKD on dialysis, this estimating formula is not very accurate.

Clinical Manifestations of Hypercalcemia

The severity of symptoms caused by hypercalcemia depends on the degree and rate of rise in serum calcium. Gastrointestinal symptoms such as nausea, vomiting, constipation, abdominal pain, and, rarely, peptic ulcer disease may occur. Neuromuscular involvement includes altered mentation, impaired concentration, fatigue, lethargy, and muscle weakness. Hypercalcemia can impair kidney water handling by inducing nephrogenic diabetes insipidus and sodium wasting. The resulting diuresis worsens the hypercalcemia, because volume depletion limits the protective hypercalciuria and exacerbates the volume-dependent proximal tubule reabsorption of calcium. In addition, volume depletion may lead to acute kidney injury, which further limits calcium excretion and favors an additional increase in serum calcium. The hypercalciuria associated with prolonged hypercalcemia can rarely lead to nephrolithiasis and nephrocalcinosis. Cardiovascular effects include hypertension and shortening of the QT interval on the electrocardiogram (ECG). Although cardiac arrhythmias are uncommon, hypercalcemia can trigger digitalis toxicity.

Differential Diagnosis of Hypercalcemia

The most common causes of hypercalcemia are malignancy and hyperparathyroidism; in most series, these two diagnoses account for more than 90% of cases. The remaining causes are listed in Box 11.1, with key causes discussed in more detail in the following paragraphs.

Malignancy

Malignancy is the most common cause of hypercalcemia in hospitalized patients, and the presence of hypercalcemia in cancer patients confers a poor prognosis. Hypercalcemia can result from

---

BOX 11.1

Causes of Hypercalcemia

Malignancy
    Local osteolytic hypercalcemia
    Humoral hypercalcemia of malignancy (PTHrp)
    Hematologic malignancies such as lymphoma where there is ectopic
        calcitriol synthesis
Hyperparathyroidism
Thyrotoxicosis
Granulomatous diseases (sarcoidosis, histoplasmosis, tuberculosis)
Drug-induced
    Vitamin D
    Thiazide diuretics
    Estrogens and antiestrogens
    Androgens (breast cancer therapy)
    Vitamin A
    Lithium
Immobilization
Total parenteral nutrition
Impaired kidney function (AKI or CKD), usually in the setting of
    medications such as calcium-containing phosphate binders or
    calcitriol or its analogues

AKI, Acute kidney injury; *CKD,* chronic kidney disease; *PTHrp,* parathyroid hormone–related peptide.

---

direct invasion of bone by metastatic disease, referred to as *local osteolytic hypercalcemia* (LOH). In LOH, tumor cells within the bone marrow space produce a variety of inflammatory cytokines, collectively termed *osteoclast-activating factors,* which lead to net bone resorption, calcium release, and hypercalcemia. PTH levels are suppressed in response to the hypercalcemia. This mechanism is common with hypercalcemia resulting from breast cancer or multiple myeloma. Hypercalcemia can also result from the production of circulating factors that stimulate osteoclastic resorption of bone. Humoral hypercalcemia of malignancy is caused by secretion of parathyroid hormone–related peptide (PTHrp) by tumor cells. PTHrp bears similarity to PTH only in the initial 8-amino-acid sequence, but this homology permits binding to the PTH receptor, leading to increased bone turnover and hypercalcemia. Specific assays are available to distinguish circulating PTHrp from PTH. Finally, hypercalcemia in malignancy can result from increased production of calcitriol, which stimulates gastrointestinal absorption of calcium. Various lymphoid tumors, most notably Hodgkin lymphoma, have been shown to synthesize large quantities of calcitriol.

Hyperparathyroidism

The incidence of *primary hyperparathyroidism* has declined over the past 30 years, but it is still the second most common cause of hypercalcemia. In most cases, primary hyperparathyroidism is caused by a benign adenoma of a single parathyroid gland that autonomously secretes PTH. The disorder may be sporadic, familial, or inherited as a component of the constellation of multiple endocrine neoplasia (MEN). The elevation in PTH results in increased intestinal absorption of calcium through stimulation of calcitriol production, increased osteoclastic bone resorption, and increased kidney tubular reabsorption of calcium. However, because of the elevation in serum calcium, the filtered load of calcium exceeds the ability of the kidney to reabsorb calcium, leading to hypercalciuria and potentially to nephrolithiasis. *Secondary hyperparathyroidism* is caused by diffuse hyperplasia of all four glands in response to ongoing stimuli such as hypocalcemia or hyperphosphatemia. Iatrogenic hypercalcemia may occur in patients with secondary hyperparathyroidism treated with calcium-based phosphate binders or calcitriol and its derivatives. Secondary hyperparathyroidism can also cause hypercalcemia via increased bone resorption when the glands become adenomatous and no longer respond to the change in calcium—a stage often called *tertiary hyperparathyroidism.*

Lithium may interfere with the CaSR, leading to a "resetting" of the parathyroid gland sensitivity such that higher levels of calcium are needed to decrease PTH. Clinically, these patients may appear to have hyperparathyroidism, but hypercalcemia resolves when lithium is stopped.

Vitamin D Excess

Hypercalcemia from excessive intake of native vitamin D supplements (ergocalciferol and cholecalciferol) is rare, because 1α-hydroxylase (CYP27B1) activity is tightly regulated by calcium levels. In contrast, the excessive administration of calcitriol or of other active vitamin D analogues, such as paricalcitol or doxercalciferol, which bypass this regulatory step at the level of the kidney, can lead to hypercalcemia. These drugs are commonly used in the treatment of secondary hyperparathyroidism in CKD. An endogenous source of excess calcitriol is production by non-kidney tissue like lymphomas and granulomatous diseases, including sarcoidosis, tuberculosis, endemic fungal infections, and berylliosis. Hypercalcemia manifests secondary to pulmonary and lymph node monocyte and macrophage activation and conversion of calcidiol to calcitriol via 1α-hydroxylase activity. Patients with these disorders can often present with asymptomatic or symptomatic hypercalcemia, hypercalciuria, nephrocalcinosis, chronic kidney disease, nephrogenic diabetes insipidus, and nephrolithiasis. Sarcoidosis, being the most common and well evaluated of the granulomatous disorders, hypercalcemia has been reported in up to 63% in a case series of patients. Given the heterogenous nature of granulomatous disorders, special attention must be paid to the patient's history and risk factors, as management is focused on the treatment of the causative condition.

Familial Hypocalciuric Hypercalcemia

Inactivating mutations of the CaSR cause familial hypocalciuric hypercalcemia (FHH), a rare hereditary disease with autosomal-dominant transmission. Calcium is unable to activate the mutant receptor in the kidney, leading to increased kidney reabsorption of calcium into the blood from the tubular fluid and hypocalciuria, usually with urine calcium excretion less than 100 mg/day. Because this mutation may also affect the receptor at the level of the parathyroid gland, PTH may be slightly elevated out of proportion to the degree of hypercalcemia. Other clues pointing to this diagnosis include a family history of asymptomatic hypercalcemia.

Probands are often discovered after parathyroidectomy fails to correct hypercalcemia.

Approach to the Patient With Hypercalcemia

Clinicians may approach patients with hypercalcemia by considering the diagnoses in Box 11.1. An alternative approach is to formulate a differential diagnosis based on the physiology of calcium homeostasis (Fig. 11.4) and tailoring diagnostic studies to the suspected pathophysiology.

Parathyroid Glands

The normal response to hypercalcemia is suppression of PTH secretion. Interpretation of a PTH level (normal: 10 to 65 pg/mL) must always be performed in conjunction with a simultaneously measured calcium level. For example, if the serum calcium level is 11.5 mg/dL and the PTII is 50 pg/mL, the circulating level of PTH is inappropriately high, suggesting hyperparathyroidism. Conversely, if the calcium is 8.5 mg/dL and the PTH is 70 pg/mL, then the elevated PTH is appropriate. Because PTH increases urinary phosphorus excretion, a normal or high-normal PTH level with hypercalcemia and a low or low-normal phosphorus level are essentially diagnostic of primary hyperparathyroidism, but only when kidney function is normal. Radionuclide sestamibi imaging may be helpful in localizing an adenomatous gland; however, there is a high risk of false-negative scans, and an experienced parathyroid surgeon can usually locate the enlarged gland. Rarely,

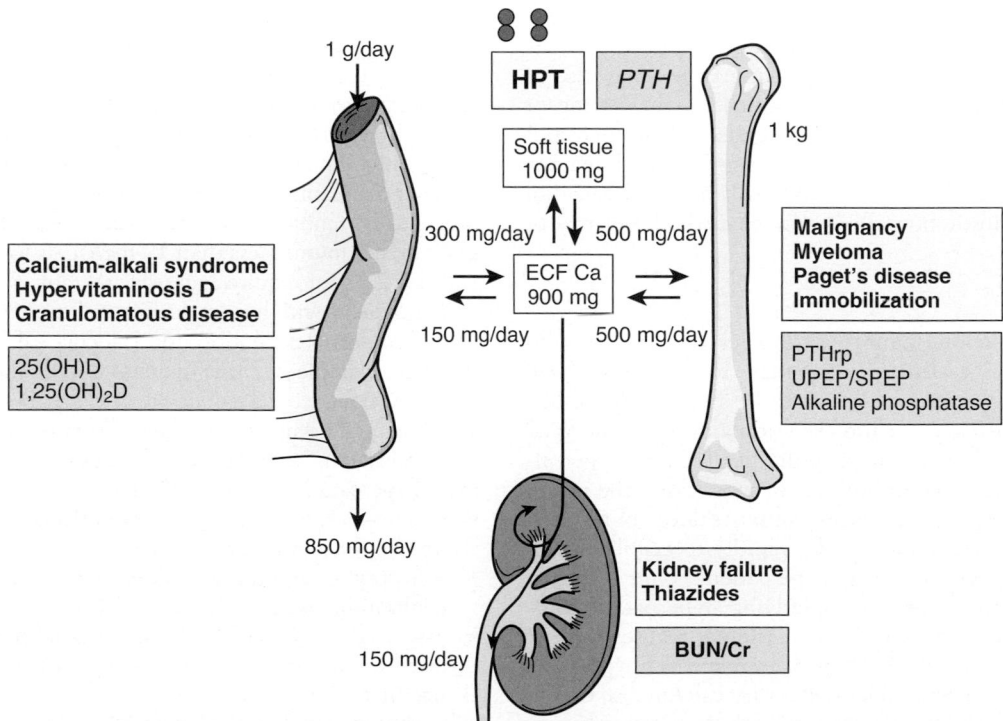

• **Fig. 11.4 Approach to a patient with hypercalcemia.** The normal daily calcium balance is shown, demonstrating the fluxes between the serum compartment and intestine and bone as well as the excretion of calcium. The patient with hypercalcemia must have an abnormality at the parathyroid glands *(top)*, intestine *(left)*, bone *(right)*, or kidney *(bottom)*. The yellow boxes represent causes of hypercalcemia that are associated with abnormalities at each of these target organs. The blue boxes indicate diagnostic tests that may be abnormal in these disorders. *BUN,* Blood urea nitrogen; *Cr,* creatinine; *ECF,* extracellular fluid; *HPT,* hyperparathyroidism; *PTH,* parathyroid hormone; *PTHrp,* parathyroid hormone–related peptide; *SPEP,* serum protein electrophoresis; *UPEP,* urine protein electrophoresis.

glands are found in the mediastinum. Parathyroid cancers secrete excess PTH, leading to severe hyperparathyroidism, and marked hypercalcemia may be present.

Bone

Hypercalcemia of bony origin occurs either because of enhanced bone turnover (osteoclast activity exceeding osteoblast activity, or net bone resorption exceeding bone formation) caused by local tumor invasion or increased secretion of hormonal factors by tumor cells (PTHrp, calcitriol, and PTH). Alternatively, immobilization may lead to the release of calcium from the bone, especially in the setting of excess turnover. Diagnostic studies for bone-induced hypercalcemia include PTH, PTHrp, urine and serum protein electrophoresis and immunofixation (to diagnose myeloma), and alkaline phosphatase, The last is markedly elevated in Paget disease and other high bone turnover states.

Intestine

Enhanced intestinal absorption of calcium can occur in conditions that result in elevated circulating levels of calcidiol or calcitriol. This can occur because of vitamin D toxicity with very high calcidiol levels, calcitriol therapy in patients with secondary hyperparathyroidism, calcitriol-producing granulomatous diseases and lymphomas, and hyperparathyroidism, which in turn increases calcitriol synthesis. In addition, excess calcium ingestion, especially with alkali, can lead to hypercalcemia. This is now referred to as *calcium-alkali syndrome* and was previously called *milk-alkali syndrome,* named for the combination of therapies used to treat peptic ulcer disease (sodium bicarbonate and milk) before the advent of proton pump blockers. To detect vitamin D toxicity, levels of both 25(OH)vitD (calcidiol) and 1,25(OH)$_2$vitD (calcitriol) should be measured. This is particularly important as many patients are taking large quantities of cholecalciferol in supplements and vitamins. In the setting of exogenous vitamin D intake, calcidiol levels will be high and calcitriol levels normal to high. In the setting of granulomatous production of calcitriol, calcitriol levels will be high; calcidiol levels are nondiagnostic but will usually be at the lower end of normal to low.

Kidneys

With volume depletion, serum calcium levels rise and mild hypercalcemia results. Thiazide diuretics, by blocking distal tubular sodium reabsorption, enhance the NCX. This results in a reduction in urinary calcium excretion and hypercalcemia. These effects are used to advantage in the treatment of hypercalciuria in patients with nephrolithiasis. In most cases, the rise in serum calcium in response to thiazide diuretics does not result in clinical hypercalcemia, and any rise is rapidly reversible. When thiazides induce hypercalcemia and the patient is not clinically volume depleted, there may be underlying hyperparathyroidism. PTH acts at the kidney to increase tubular reabsorption of calcium. Even so, patients with hypercalcemia from hyperparathyroidism tend to have an elevated urine calcium excretion, because the filtered load of calcium is so high. In primary hyperparathyroidism, the urinary calcium/creatinine ratio is usually greater than 0.2 (mg/mg), whereas, in patients with FHH, the urinary calcium/creatinine ratio is less than 0.01 mg/mg. Ideally, a 24-hour urine collection should be measured, but a spot collection may differentiate primary hyperparathyroidism from FHH and should be considered before parathyroidectomy in unclear cases.

Treatment of Symptomatic Hypercalcemia

The ultimate goal of therapy is to remedy the underlying cause of hypercalcemia; however, patients who present with acute symptoms of hypercalcemia require immediate treatment to reduce the serum level. The safest and most effective treatment in patients with normal cardiac and kidney function is volume expansion with IV normal saline, which reduces proximal tubular reabsorption of sodium, water, and calcium. Most patients with symptomatic hypercalcemia are volume depleted at presentation because of the polyuria and natriuresis induced by hypercalcemia. In severe cases, very aggressive volume resuscitation may be required, with close attention to the patient's cardiopulmonary status to avoid volume overload. After volume expansion is achieved, calcium reabsorption can be further reduced with IV loop diuretics, such as furosemide, that block the Na$^+$-K$^+$-2Cl$^-$ cotransporter in the thick ascending limb, thus disrupting the favorable electrochemical gradient for passive (paracellular) calcium reabsorption. As patients must be adequately hydrated before the diuretic is administered to avoid worsening hypovolemia and hypercalcemia, accurate assessment of intake and output is critical to optimize this treatment approach.

If these conservative treatments fail to restore normocalcemia, other pharmacologic options should be used (Table 11.1). Because the response to these agents is not immediate, their use in patients with severe symptoms of hypercalcemia may be appropriate early in the course of management. In the United States, the bisphosphonates pamidronate and zoledronic acid are approved for the treatment of malignancy-associated hypercalcemia. These agents block osteoclast-mediated bone resorption by inducing osteoclast apoptosis. Typically, a clinical response is seen within 2 to 4 days, with a nadir in serum calcium within 4 to 7 days. Caution is required, because acute kidney injury has been reported with rapid administration of bisphosphonates or in settings of volume depletion. Calcitonin has the advantage of a rapid reduction of serum calcium, but its use is limited by a short duration of action and tachyphylaxis. Glucocorticoids are effective first-line agents, along with saline diuresis, when the hypercalcemia is mediated by elevated circulating levels of calcitriol due to granulomatous disorders or lymphoma. Mild hypercalcemia, defined as a corrected calcium for albumin less than 12 mg/dL, is usually not symptomatic and may not require aggressive therapy.

For patients with hypercalcemia and confirmed primary hyperparathyroidism, evaluation for evidence of end-organ damage should be completed. This includes a 24-hour urine calcium and creatinine collection, a baseline dual X-ray absorptiometry (DXA), and imaging to evaluate for nephrolithiasis, nephrocalcinosis, and vertebral fractures. The criteria for operative management of primary hyperparathyroidism includes:

- Calcium >1.0 mg/dL (0.25 mmol/L) over the upper limit of normal for standardized lab value
- A history of symptomatic kidney stones or imaging-confirmed nephrolithiasis or nephrocalcinosis
- T-score on DXA at lumbar spine, total hip, femoral neck, or distal one-third radius or imaging with evidence of vertebral fractures
- Creatinine clearance less than 60 mL/min
- 24-hour urine calcium greater than 400 mg/dL (10 mmol/d) and increased stone risk with a kidney stone risk profile
- Age less than 50 years
- Desire not to participate in longitudinal observation

For a patient who meets one or more of the above criteria, a preoperative localization nuclear medicine study followed by surgical parathyroidectomy is recommended. For patients who do not meet

TABLE 11.1	Treatments for Hypercalcemia	
Agent	**Mode of Action**	**Dose**
IV saline	Increases tubular flow and excretion of calcium	Based on patient's cardiovascular status and level of kidney function; 200–500 mL/hr
IV furosemide or loop diuretics	Block NKCC2 channel in loop of Henle, thus reducing positive electrochemical gradient for passive calcium reabsorption	20–40 mg intravenously after volume resuscitation; dose may need to be adjusted based on level of kidney function
IV bisphosphonates	Inhibit osteoclastic activity	Pamidronate, 60–90 mg over 4 hr or Zoledronate, 4–8 mg over 15 min; dose may need to be adjusted based on level of kidney function
Calcitonin	Inhibits bone resorption and enhances calcium excretion	4–12 IU/kg IM/SQ every 12 hr
Glucocorticoids	Inhibit conversion of 25(OH)D to 1,25(OH)$_2$D	Prednisone 20 mg PO daily for 10-14 days with 5 mg weekly taper pending clinical response
Cinacalcet	Allosteric activator of CaSR, mimicking increased calcium to reduce PTH	30 mg daily to twice daily, to a maximum dose of 90 mg twice daily; give with food to reduce nausea
Denosumab	Receptor activator of RANK ligand inhibitor; Inhibits osteoclasts resulting in decreased bone resorption	Hypercalcemia of malignancy: 120 mg subcutaneous every 4 weeks*

CaSR, Calcium-sensing receptor; *IV*, intravenous; *NKCC2*, Na^{2+}/K$^+$/2Cl$^2-$–cotransporter; *PTH*, parathyroid hormone.

*Caution: need to monitor for evidence of hypocalcemia, which can be severe, especially in CKD patient population.

one of the above criteria, surveillance with annual calcium and kidney function measurement, DXA every 1 to 2 years, and surveillance for vertebral fracture or nephrolithiasis are recommended.

An alternative to surgical parathyroidectomy in older patients or those not good candidates for surgery is the use of cinacalcet, a calcimimetic. This agent is an allosteric activator of the CaSR that "mimics" higher levels of calcium, thereby decreasing PTH secretion and serum calcium. For primary hyperparathyroidism, the dose is usually 30 mg twice daily, titrating up to 90 mg twice daily.

Hypocalcemia

With true hypocalcemia, the ionized calcium concentration is low; however, in patients with hypoalbuminemia, there is a decrease in total calcium but not necessarily a decrease in ionized calcium. In patients with excess citrate (from blood transfusions) or acute administration of bicarbonate, the percentage of calcium that is bound to these anions increases; this reduces the free ionized calcium, usually with only a minimal change in total calcium. Acute respiratory alkalosis also lowers the ionized calcium as a decrease in the hydrogen ion concentration leads to protons dissociating from binding sites on other proteins. This increases protein binding of ionized calcium, thereby decreasing ionized calcium. Because the actual magnitude of any change in these circumstances may be hard to predict, the ionized calcium concentration is best measured directly. False hypocalcemia (due to reduced serum albumin level) can be excluded by correcting the calcium for albumin or by directly measuring the ionized calcium concentration. Consider false hypocalcemia in patients with malnutrition, chronic illness, cirrhosis, and/or nephrotic syndrome.

Clinical Manifestations of Hypocalcemia

Symptoms only occur with changes in the free ionized calcium, and most patients with mild hypocalcemia exhibit very few symptoms. Large or abrupt changes in ionized calcium may lead to symptoms including perioral numbness and spasms of the hands and feet. In some patients, progression to tetany or seizures occurs. This increased neuromuscular reactivity can be demonstrated by eliciting the Chvostek sign or Trousseau sign. The Chvostek sign is tested by tapping on the facial nerve near the temporal mandibular joint and watching for grimacing caused by spasm of the facial muscles. The Trousseau sign is tested by inflating a blood pressure cuff to a pressure greater than the systolic blood pressure for 3 minutes and watching for spasm of the outstretched hand. Of these two signs, Trousseau is more specific. If these clinical signs are positive, hypocalcemia should be confirmed by measurement of ionized calcium.

Differential Diagnosis of Hypocalcemia

The causes of hypocalcemia are best organized mechanistically.

Vitamin D Deficiency

Vitamin D, once activated to calcitriol, is the primary determinant of intestinal calcium absorption. Individuals may be deficient in vitamin D because of poor absorption from dietary sources (e.g., malabsorption, short bowel, poor nutrition), lack of sun exposure, abnormal conversion of D2/D3 to calcidiol in the liver (cirrhosis, some drugs), or decreased kidney conversion of calcidiol to calcitriol (CKD). These patients have low levels of vitamin D and an increase in PTH.

Hypoparathyroidism

Deficiency or inactivity of PTH results in hypocalcemia. This may be caused by inadvertent removal of the parathyroid glands during thyroid surgery or by radiation therapy, congenital defects, or autoimmune disease. These patients have an inappropriately low PTH for their low calcium levels. In the absence of PTH, the only mechanism to increase serum calcium is via intestinal absorption stimulated by the administration of vitamin D (usually in the active form, calcitriol) and oral calcium. Hypomagnesemia may also cause resistance to PTH as well as suppression of PTH release.

Pseudohypoparathyroidism

The term *pseudohypoparathyroidism* describes a group of disorders that are characterized by hypocalcemia and hypophosphatemia, elevated PTH levels, and lack of tissue responsiveness to PTH. The magnesium and calcidiol levels are normal. A PTH infusion test can confirm the tissue resistance. IV administration of PTH normally results in increased urinary cyclic adenosine monophosphate (cAMP) and phosphorus excretion, but patients with pseudohypoparathyroidism lack this response. The most common form of pseudohypoparathyroidism is type Ia, Albright hereditary osteodystrophy, which is also associated with short stature, round facies, obesity, brachydactyly, and other defects.

Tissue Consumption of Calcium

Hypocalcemia may result from the precipitation of calcium into extraskeletal tissue, such as occurs in pancreatitis. In addition, excess bone formation in some malignancies with osteoblastic bone metastases may cause the bone to take up excess calcium acutely. After parathyroidectomy, there is an acute drop in serum calcium and phosphorus because of the "hungry bone syndrome," wherein calcium and phosphorus are rapidly taken up because of the sudden reduction in PTH. Preoperative calcitriol use (if serum calcium is low or normal) for several days prior to surgery is often effective in preventing hungry bone syndrome, as is correction of vitamin D deficiency. The use of bisphosphonates before surgery has been shown in small studies to minimize the drop in serum calcium levels. It is more controversial whether calcimimetics need to be stopped prior to surgery. Many protocols stop this medication at least the day before surgery. Hungry bone syndrome is more severe and more protracted in patients with kidney failure who are undergoing parathyroidectomy as a treatment for severe secondary hyperparathyroidism and these patients warrant close postoperative monitoring. In acute hyperphosphatemia caused by rhabdomyolysis or tumor lysis syndrome, phosphorus binds to calcium, leading to a fall in ionized calcium. Similarly, the infusion of citrate, a preservative in blood and plasma transfusions, can reduce ionized calcium, as discussed earlier. Last, sepsis is also associated with hypocalcemia, although the mechanism is not clear.

Treatment of Hypocalcemia

IV calcium infusions are indicated only in the setting of symptomatic hypocalcemia and they should not be administered to patients with severe hyperphosphatemia because of the risk of ectopic precipitation of calcium phosphate. IV calcium comes in two forms: calcium gluconate (10-mL vial = 94 mg elemental calcium) and calcium chloride (10-mL vial = 273 mg elemental calcium). Calcium chloride is typically used only during cardiopulmonary resuscitation because its infusion is painful and can cause vein sclerosis. Importantly, patients who are not symptomatic should be repleted with oral, not IV, calcium. The most common oral supplement is calcium carbonate, starting with 1 to 2 g of elemental calcium three times daily (1250 mg calcium carbonate = 500 mg elemental calcium), given away from meals. The amount of calcium absorbed will be increased if calcitriol (0.25 μg twice daily to start) is coadministered. Any hypomagnesemia should be treated concomitantly, and, if appropriate, patients may be changed from loop to thiazide diuretics to decrease urinary calcium excretion. The use of calcium supplementation in patients with CKD is discussed in Chapter 53.

Hyperphosphatemia

Hyperphosphatemia can result from increased intestinal absorption, from cellular release or rapid shifts of phosphorus from the intracellular to the extracellular compartment, or from decreased kidney excretion. Persistent hyperphosphatemia (>12 hours) occurs almost exclusively in the setting of impaired kidney function.

Increased intestinal absorption is usually caused either by the use of phosphate-containing oral purgatives or enemas or by vitamin D overdoses. Increased tissue release of phosphorus is commonly seen in acute tumor lysis syndrome, rhabdomyolysis, hemolysis, hyperthermia, profound catabolic stress, or acute leukemia. These disorders can also lead to acute kidney injury, limiting kidney phosphate excretion and further exacerbating the hyperphosphatemia. Rarely, thyrotoxicosis or acromegaly leads to hyperphosphatemia. Acute hyperphosphatemia usually does not cause symptoms unless there is a significant reciprocal reduction of serum calcium. The treatment of acute hyperphosphatemia includes volume expansion, dialysis, and administration of phosphate binders. In the setting of normal kidney function, or even mild to moderate kidney disease, hyperphosphatemia is usually self-limited because of the capacity of the kidney to excrete a phosphorus load. Sequelae and treatment of hyperphosphatemia related to CKD, including bone disease and cardiovascular disease, are discussed in detail in Chapter 53.

Hypophosphatemia

Hypophosphatemia can occur with decreased phosphorus intake (decreased intestinal absorption or increased gastrointestinal losses) or with excess kidney wasting because of tubular defects or hyperparathyroidism. In addition, low serum phosphorus levels may also occur in the setting of extracellular-to-intracellular shifts. In the case of cellular shifts, total body phosphorus may not be depleted. By convention, hypophosphatemia is often graded as mild (<3.5 mg/dL), moderate (<2.5 mg/dL), or severe (<1.0 mg/dL). Moderate and severe hypophosphatemia usually occur only if there are multiple causes (Box 11.2). A special population of interest is

---

BOX 11.2

Causes of Hypophosphatemia

Decreased Intestinal Absorption

Antacid abuse or excessive calcium supplement use
Malabsorption and chronic diarrhea
Vitamin D deficiency
Starvation or anorexia
Alcoholism

Increased Urinary Losses

Primary hyperparathyroidism
Following kidney transplantation
Extracellular volume expansion
Glucosuria (after treatment of DKA)
Postobstructive or post ATN solute diuresis
Acetazolamide
Fanconi syndrome
X-linked and vitamin D–dependent rickets
Oncogenic osteomalacia

Redistribution

Respiratory alkalosis
Alcohol withdrawal
Severe burns
Postfeeding syndrome
Leukemic blast crisis
Treatment of hyperglycemia

ATN, Acute tubular necrosis; *DKA,* diabetic ketoacidosis.

kidney transplant patients as they are at increased risk for post-transplant hypophosphatemia as they often suffer from moderate to severe secondary hyperparathyroidism. With a functional allograft, in the presence of persistently elevated parathyroid hormone and fibroblast growth factor 23, they have increased urinary phosphate losses and can suffer from hypophosphatemia. If severe, this can lead to respiratory failure and impaired myocardial performance, so postoperative monitoring is paramount.

Clinical Manifestations of Hypophosphatemia

Hypophosphatemia is fairly common, observed in approximately 3% of all hospitalized patients, 10% of hospitalized alcoholic patients, and 70% of mechanically ventilated patients. Symptoms include muscle weakness (and difficulty weaning from the ventilator), hemolysis, impaired platelet and white blood cell function, rhabdomyolysis, and, in moderate to severe cases, neurologic disorders. Hypophosphatemia is probably overtreated in the intensive care unit, where the "difficult to wean" patient may be given phosphorus when the low phosphorus levels are actually caused by cellular shifts due to respiratory alkalosis. A careful review of the trend in serum phosphorus with arterial blood pH can help discern which patients need to be treated.

Differential Diagnosis of Hypophosphatemia

The differential diagnosis and treatment approach are based on the cause and site of phosphate loss. The cause is usually clinically apparent, but if it is not, the simplest test is measurement of the 24-hour urine phosphorus excretion or the fractional excretion of phosphate ($FEPO_4$) from a random urine sample. The expected kidney response to hypophosphatemia is avid reabsorption. If the urinary excretion is less than 100 mg/24 hours or the $FEPO_4$ is <5%, then the kidney is responding appropriately to hypophosphatemia and the cause must be impaired intake, gastrointestinal losses, or extracellular-to-intracellular shifts. The $FEPO_4$ is calculated as follows:

$$FEPO_4 = \frac{U_{PO4} \times P_{Cr}}{P_{PO4} \times U_{Cr}} \times 100$$

where U and P are urinary and plasma concentrations of phosphorous (PO_4) and creatinine (Cr).

Decreased Oral Intake

The average American diet contains excessive amounts of phosphorus. All proteins and dairy products contain phosphorus, and phosphorus is used as a preservative in most processed foods. Decreased intake of phosphorus is usually seen only with generalized poor oral intake, gastrointestinal losses from diarrhea and malabsorption, or alcoholism. Occasionally, antacid abuse or excessive calcium supplements will lower absorption by binding phosphorus.

Redistribution

Approximately 15% of the extraskeletal phosphorus is intracellular, and hypophosphatemia may result from a shift from extracellular to intracellular stores. In most situations, this shift is not clinically detectable; however, if there is underlying phosphate depletion, more profound hypophosphatemia may be observed. The most common clinical cause of this form of hypophosphatemia is hyperglycemia with or without ketoacidosis. The glucose-induced osmotic diuresis results in a net deficit of phosphorus, whereas cellular glucose uptake stimulated by insulin during treatment further causes a shift of the extracellular phosphorus into cells as glycogen stores are repleted. In this setting, hypophosphatemia is usually transient and, in general, should not be treated. In patients who are malnourished, sudden "refeeding" may shift phosphorus into cells, which can be lethal in severe starvation or anorexia nervosa. Respiratory, but not metabolic, alkalosis also increases the intracellular flux of phosphorus. Even in normal subjects, severe hyperventilation (to a carbon dioxide tension [PCO_2] of <20 mm Hg) may lower serum phosphorus concentrations to less than 1.0 mg/dL. Therefore, in ventilated patients, arterial blood gases may be helpful in differentiating shifts resulting from true phosphorus depletion. Last, in hungry bone syndrome after parathyroidectomy (described earlier), there is increased bone uptake of phosphorus and resultant hypophosphatemia.

Increased Urinary Losses

Phosphorus clearance by the kidney is primarily determined by the phosphorus concentration, urinary flow, PTH, and FGF23 and other phosphatonins. Patients who are significantly volume-expanded exhibit less proximal tubular reabsorption of phosphorus in parallel with reduced proximal sodium and water reabsorption. Similarly, patients with glucosuria and postobstructive diuresis experience increased urinary flow and phosphorus losses. In primary hyperparathyroidism, there is increased urinary phosphorus excretion caused by elevated PTH levels. Both congenital and acquired Fanconi syndrome are characterized by increased urinary phosphorus excretion because of defects in proximal tubule reabsorption, together with glucosuria, hypouricemia, aminoaciduria, and, potentially, proximal (type 2) renal tubular acidosis. Acquired forms of Fanconi syndrome may be seen in multiple myeloma and after administration of some chemotherapy agents (cisplatin, ifosfamide, and 6-mercaptopurine), outdated tetracycline, or the antiretroviral agent tenofovir.

Rickets and Osteomalacia

Hypophosphatemia can lead to impaired bone mineralization. Several genetic disorders are associated with hypophosphatemia and rickets in children. Autosomal dominant hypophosphatemic rickets (ADHR) is rare and associated with a mutation that limits normal degradation of FGF23. Autosomal recessive hypophosphatemic rickets (ARHR), also rare, is caused by a mutation in the gene encoding dentine matrix protein (DMP), a locally produced inhibitor of FGF23. X-linked hypophosphatemic rickets (XLH), the most common form of rickets, is due to a mutation called *PHEX* (phosphate regulating gene with homologies to endopeptidases located on the X chromosome), which normally degrades FGF23. Mutations in PHEX, therefore, lead to inappropriate levels of FGF23. Thus, several discrete disorders are now linked to abnormalities in FGF23. In tumor-induced osteomalacia, tumors of mesenchymal origin secrete phosphatonins such as FGF23, MEPE, or FRP4, which upregulate the sodium phosphate cotransporter with resultant urinary phosphate wasting.

Treatment of Hypophosphatemia

Treatment is usually necessary for patients with moderate to severe hypophosphatemia. Increasing oral phosphorus intake is the preferred treatment because IV administration of phosphate complexes with calcium and can lead to extraskeletal calcifications. Oral supplementation can be given with skim milk (1000 mg/quart), whole milk (850 mg/quart), Neutra-Phos K capsules (250 mg/capsule; maximum dose, three tabs every 6 hours), or Neutra-Phos solution (128 mg/mL). Oral phosphorus may induce or exacerbate diarrhea. Milk is much better tolerated, is a source of protein, and is cheaper. The concomitant administration of vitamin

D may enhance its absorption. If necessary, phosphorus may be repleted intravenously as potassium phosphate (3 mmol/mL of phosphorus, 4.4 mEq/mL of potassium) or sodium phosphate (3 mmol/mL of phosphorus, 4.0 mEq/mL of sodium) in a single administration, usually mixed in 50 mL of normal saline.

For patients suffering from XLH, pharmaceutical advances have been made to address the limitations of traditional therapies of oral phosphate and active vitamin D replacement. In 2019, a phase III clinical trial was conducted using a fully human monoclonal antibody against FGF23, burosumab. When compared with conventional therapy, burosumab demonstrated improved radiographic findings, decreased limb deformity, improved growth and mobility, normalization of serum phosphate, and reduced alkaline phosphatase. These findings are encouraging for reducing long-term consequences associated with XLH.

Hypermagnesemia

Hypermagnesemia is present when the serum magnesium level is greater than 2.9 mg/dL (1.2 mmol/L), although clinical manifestations typically do not occur until serum levels are greater than 4 mg/dL (1.6 mmol/L). Signs and symptoms include hyporeflexia (usually the first sign) and weakness that may progress to paralysis and can involve the diaphragm. Cardiac findings are bradycardia, hypotension, and cardiac arrest. ECG findings include prolonged PR, QRS, and QT intervals, and complete heart block may occur when the levels are as high as 15 mg/dL (6.2 mmol/L). Of note, moderate hypermagnesemia can inhibit the secretion of PTH, which may lead to hypocalcemia and subsequent prolonged QT interval.

Differential Diagnosis of Hypermagnesemia

Because hypermagnesemia appears to stimulate kidney excretion, it is "self-regulating," and prolonged hypermagnesemia generally occurs only when there is reduced kidney function. Hypermagnesemia is usually iatrogenic from laxatives, antacids, or intravenous magnesium administration. Levels will be purposefully elevated in the treatment of preeclampsia and eclampsia, but they resolve quickly with cessation of therapy because of kidney excretion. Other causes of a mild elevation of magnesium include theophylline intoxication, tumor lysis syndrome, acromegaly, FHH, and adrenal insufficiency.

Treatment of Hypermagnesemia

Treatment begins with avoiding magnesium-containing medications, including some laxatives and antacids, in patients with reduced kidney function. In the presence of normal kidney function, asymptomatic hypermagnesemia will resolve spontaneously and no treatment is indicated. If hypermagnesemia is symptomatic, IV administration of calcium gluconate (~90 to 180 mg of elemental calcium) over 10 to 20 minutes will help antagonize the effect of the excessive magnesium. Supportive therapy may include mechanical ventilation and the placement of a temporary pacemaker. With adequate kidney function, volume expansion with IV saline facilitates kidney excretion of magnesium. In the case of kidney failure, dialysis is required.

Hypomagnesemia

Serum magnesium less than 1.3 mg/dL (0.53 mmol/L) defines hypomagnesemia. Similar to calcium and phosphorus, a minority of magnesium is in the extracellular space; however, unlike calcium there is no "ionized" magnesium measurement available. Therefore, when blood magnesium levels are normal, this does not exclude magnesium deficiency. On the other hand, when there is severe magnesium deficiency, there is almost always hypomagnesemia. In patients with normal magnesium levels but clinical suspicion of hypomagnesemia, urine magnesium should be checked. If low, this confirms magnesium depletion.

Kidney wasting of magnesium can be diagnosed in the presence of hypomagnesemia if there is more than 24 mg of magnesium in the 24-hour urine collection or if the fractional excretion of magnesium is greater than 2%. The fractional excretion of magnesium is calculated as follows:

$$FEM_g = \frac{U_{Mg} \times P_{Cr}}{(P_{Mg} \times 0.7) \times U_{Cr}} \times 100$$

where U and P are urinary and plasma concentrations of magnesium (Mg) and creatinine (Cr). The plasma concentration is multiplied by 0.7 since only 70% of circulating magnesium is not bound to albumin and able to be filtered across the glomerulus.

Clinical Manifestations of Hypomagnesemia

Hypomagnesemia is seen in 10% of hospitalized patients and 20% of patients in the ICU. Forty percent of patients with hypomagnesemia will have hypokalemia, and 20% will have hypocalcemia, hypophosphatemia, or hyponatremia. Notably, hypokalemia may appear refractory to potassium replacement until the magnesium is repleted, believed to be secondary to intracellular magnesium changes that alter renal outer medullary potassium channel (ROMK) potassium reabsorption, although this may not be the only mechanism. Thus, magnesium levels should be evaluated in hypokalemia. Patients with severe hypomagnesemia may have clinical neurologic or cardiovascular abnormalities. Symptoms include muscle cramps, generalized fatigue, and ileus. With more severe depletion, confusion, ataxia, nystagmus, tremor, hyperreflexia, fasciculations, tetany, and seizures may occur. Cardiac arrhythmia can be seen, particularly with patients on digoxin, with ECG changes including prolonged PR and QT intervals with a widened QRS complex. Torsades de pointes is the other classic finding. Magnesium levels are not generally included on routine blood chemistry panels and, thus, patients at risk (malnutrition, chronic diarrhea, alcoholism, use of diuretics or digoxin) should be specifically tested for hypomagnesemia.

Differential Diagnosis of Hypomagnesemia

Hypomagnesemia may be caused by (1) decreased intake, as in chronic alcoholism and malabsorption syndromes; (2) increased gastrointestinal losses; (3) increased urinary losses; or (4) intravascular chelation and extravascular deposition, as seen with hypocalcemia (Box 11.3). The last can occur when substances that complex with magnesium become available, such as fatty acids released in acute pancreatitis and citrate loading with blood product transfusions. It also occurs in the hungry bone syndrome following parathyroidectomy. Urinary losses occur in the presence of hypercalcemia (where calcium competes with magnesium to be reabsorbed in the thick ascending limb), osmotic diuresis, volume expansion (because of the decreased magnesium reabsorption associated with the increased tubular flow), and genetic disorders or drugs that lead to defects in tubular magnesium transport. Culprit drugs include diuretics, aminoglycosides, amphotericin B, cisplatin, calcineurin inhibitors such as cyclosporine and tacrolimus, and proton pump inhibitors, making it important to monitor

BOX 11.3

Causes of Hypomagnesemia

Decreased Intake

Prolonged fasting
Chronic alcoholism
Protein-calorie malnutrition
Inadequate parenteral nutrition

Gastrointestinal Losses

Chronic diarrhea
Laxative abuse
Malabsorption syndromes
Massive resection of the small intestine
Neonatal hypomagnesemia

Kidney Losses

Drugs
  Diuretics
  Amphotericin B
  Aminoglycosides
  Cisplatin
  Pentamidine
  Proton pump inhibitors
  Cyclosporine
  Tacrolimus
  Foscarnet
  Cetuximab
High urinary output states
  Postobstructive diuresis
  Post ATN solute diuresis
  Posttransplantation polyuria
Inherited hypomagnesemia
  Gitelman syndrome
  Bartter syndrome
  Other genetic transient receptor potential abnormalities
Primary hyperaldosteronism
Hypercalcemic states
Phosphate depletion
Chronic metabolic acidosis
Idiopathic kidney wasting

Miscellaneous

Acute pancreatitis
Hungry bone syndrome
Diabetic ketoacidosis
Acute intermittent porphyria

TABLE 11.2 Examples of Magnesium Supplementation

Source	Mass of Elemental Magnesium[a]
Mag-Ox 400 PO (Mg oxide)	240 mg per tablet = 20 mEq per tablet
Uro-Mag 140 PO (Mg oxide)	85 Mg = 7 mEq
Magnesium gluconate 500 (tablet or liquid)	27 Mg = 2.3 mEq
Slow-Mag PO (Mg chloride)	64 Mg = 5.3 mEq
MagTab SR (84 Mg elemental mg per tab)	84 Mg tablet = 7 mEq
Magnesium sulfate 1 g IV	96 Mg = 8 mEq

[a]Mg of magnesium per tablet = mEq magnesium per tablet.
IV, Intravenous.

dysfunction. In asymptomatic hypomagnesemia, up to 720 mg of oral elemental magnesium can be given per day, although oral magnesium salts are associated with gastrointestinal symptoms including diarrhea. In some cases, amiloride may be effective in reducing kidney wasting. In severe symptomatic hypomagnesemia, 1 to 2 g (8 to 16 mEq) of IV magnesium sulfate may be administered over 15 to 30 minutes, followed by an infusion of 5 to 6 g (40 to 48 mEq) over 24 hours, with levels checked daily (but as far away from the last infusion as possible) to avoid overrepletion. As only a portion of intravenously administered magnesium is retained, repeat magnesium levels several days later are needed to determine the efficacy of repletion. Dosing for IV and oral administration of magnesium is presented in Table 11.2.

Bibliography

de Baaij JH, Hoenderop JG, Bindels RJ. Magnesium in man: implications for health and disease. *Physiol Rev.* 2015;95:1–46.

Favus MJ. Factors that influence absorption and secretion of calcium in the small intestine and colon. *Am J Physiol.* 1985;248(2 Pt 1): G147–G157.

Glendenning P, Chew GT. Controversies and consensus regarding vitamin D deficiency in 2015: whom to test and whom to treat?. *Med J Aust..* 2015;202:470–471.

Grober U, Schmidt J, Kisters K. Magnesium in prevention and therapy. *nutrients.* 2015;7:8199–8226.

Hansen KE, Johnson MG. An update on vitamin D for clinicians. *Curr Opin Endocrinol Diabetes Obes.* 2016;23:440–444.

Hill Gallant KM, Spiegel DM. Calcium balance in chronic kidney disease. *Curr Osteoporos Rep.* 2017;15(3):214–221.

Hu MC, Kuro-o M, Moe OW. Renal and extrarenal actions of Klotho. *Semin Nephrol.* 2013;33:118–129.

Huang CL, Kuo E. Mechanism of hypokalemia in magnesium deficiency. *J Am Soc Nephrol.* 2007;18:2649–2652.

Jahnen-Dechent W, Ketteler M. Magnesium basics. *Clin Kidney J.* 2012;5(Suppl 1):i3–i14 .

KDIGO 2017. Clinical practice guideline update for the diagnosis, evaluation, prevention, and treatment of chronic kidney disease–mineral and bone disorder (CKD-MBD). *Kidney International Supplements.* 2017;7:1–59.

Kelly A, Levine MA. Hypocalcemia in the critically ill patient. *J Intensive Care Med.* 2013;28:166–177.

magnesium blood levels when these drugs are used. Similar to calcium and phosphorus, shifts from the extracellular to intracellular space can occur, particularly with treatment of diabetic ketoacidosis and alcohol withdrawal. In contrast to the rapid shifts of calcium and phosphorus from bone to maintain serum levels, this potential compensatory mechanism for magnesium may take weeks and, thus, is not a factor in acute homeostasis of blood levels.

Treatment of Hypomagnesemia

Counseling and education should be provided for patients to increase their intake of high-magnesium-containing foods, which include seeds (pumpkin, almond, and cashew), legumes, soy products, whole grains, spinach, Swiss chard, apricots, and avocados. Magnesium should be administered cautiously in the presence of kidney

Marcocci C, Cetani F. Clinical practice. Primary hyperparathyroidism. *N Engl J Med*. 2011;365:2389–2397.

Messa P, Cafforio C, Alfieri C. Calcium and phosphate changes after renal transplantation. *J Nephrol*. 2010 (suppl:16):S175–S181.

Moe SM. Calcium homeostasis in health and in kidney disease. *Compr Physiol*. 2016;6:1781–1800.

Olauson H, Larsson TE. FGF23 and Klotho in chronic kidney disease. *Curr Opin Nephrol Hypertens*. 2013;22:397–404.

Pham P-CT, Pham SV, Miller JM, Pham P-TT. Hypomagnesemia in patients with type 2 diabetes. *Clin J Am Soc Nephrol*. 2007;2(2):366-373.

Sherman RA, Ravella S, Kapoian T. A dearth of data: the problem of phosphorus in prescription medications. *Kidney Int*. 2015;87(6):1097–1099.

Zhu CY, Sturgeon C, Yeh MW. Diagnosis and management of primary hyperparathyroidism. *JAMA*. 2020;323(12):1186–1187.

12

Approach to Acid-Base Disorders

ANKIT N. MEHTA, MICHAEL EMMETT

Acid-base disorders can have major clinical and diagnostic implications. If they generate extreme acidemia or alkalemia, the abnormal pH itself may result in pathophysiologic consequences. For example, the tertiary structure of proteins is altered by extreme pH conditions, potentially affecting the activity of enzymes and ion transport systems. Consequently, every metabolic pathway may be impacted by acidemia or alkalemia. In addition, extreme acidemia can depress cardiac function, impair the vascular response to catecholamines, and cause arteriolar vasodilation and venoconstriction, with resultant systemic hypotension and pulmonary edema. Insulin resistance, reduced hepatic lactate uptake, and accelerated protein catabolism are other effects of acidemia. Alkalemia can generate cardiac arrhythmias, produce neuromuscular irritability, and contribute to tissue hypoxemia. In alkalemic patients, cerebral and myocardial blood flow falls and respiratory depression occurs. Potassium disorders, a common accompaniment of acid-base perturbations, also contribute to the morbidity.

Although mild and moderate acid-base disorders may not directly affect physiologic function, the identification of such disorders may be an important diagnostic clue to the existence of serious medical conditions. Whenever an acid-base disorder is identified, the underlying cause should be sought. This diagnostic imperative often overrides the importance of any therapeutic intervention directed at the pH itself. The situation is analogous to the discovery of fever or hypothermia. Although very high or very low temperatures can themselves be dangerous and require aggressive therapy directed at restoration of a more normal temperature, often more important is the effort to identify and treat the underlying cause of the abnormal temperature. Similarly, the recognition of an acid-base disorder must generate a search for its clinical cause or causes, and recognition of a mixed acid-base disorder should trigger an investigation to determine the etiology of each component.

The acid-base status of the extracellular fluid (ECF) is carefully regulated to maintain the arterial pH in a narrow range between 7.36 and 7.44 (hydrogen ion concentration [H^+] 44 to 36 nEq/L). The pH is stabilized by multiple buffer systems in the ECF, cells, and bone. The CO_2 tension (pCO_2), primarily under neurorespiratory control, and the serum bicarbonate concentration ([HCO_3^-]), primarily under kidney/metabolic regulation, are the most important variables in this complex system of buffers.

Currently, three different methodologic approaches are widely used to describe normal acid-base status and simple and mixed acid-base disorders.

1. The *physiologic method* uses measurements of arterial pH, pCO_2, and [HCO_3^-], together with an analysis of the anion gap (AG) and a set of compensation rules.
2. The *base excess (BE) method* uses measurements of arterial pH and pCO_2 and calculation of the BE and the AG.
3. The *physicochemical method* uses measurements of arterial pH and pCO_2 together with the calculated apparent (SIDa) and effective (SIDe) "Strong Ion Difference," the "Strong Ion Gap" (SIG = SIDa – SIDe), and the total concentration of plasma weak acids (Atot).

Each of these approaches can be effectively used to characterize acid-base disorders, each has its vocal proponents and detractors, and each has certain unique characteristics that may be particularly helpful under certain conditions. We believe the physiologic method is the most straightforward and the easiest model to understand and use. It is generally acceptable in most clinical circumstances and will be the method we use in this chapter.

The physiologic method to elucidate acid-base disorders uses the following information:
1. Recognition of diagnostic clues provided by the patient's history and physical examination
2. Analysis of the serum [HCO_3^-], arterial pH, and pCO_2 (Although a blood gas analysis is not always necessary to make a diagnosis, it is generally required for complicated cases.)
3. Knowledge of the predicted compensatory response to simple acid-base disorders
4. Calculation of the AG, with consideration of the expected "baseline" AG for each patient
5. Analysis of the degree of change (Δ) in AG and the degree of Δ in [HCO_3^-] to see if the magnitude of these respective changes is reciprocal. This has been dubbed the Δ[AG]/Δ[HCO_3^-] or Delta/Delta.

Acidemia, Alkalemia, Acidosis, and Alkalosis

The normal arterial blood pH range is between 7.36 and 7.44 ([H^+] between 44 and 36 nEq/L). Acidemia is defined as an arterial pH <7.36 ([H^+] >44 nEq/L) and may result from a primary elevation in pCO_2, a fall in [HCO_3^-], or both. Alkalemia is defined as an arterial pH >7.44 ([H^+] <36 nEq/L). Alkalemia may result from a primary increase in [HCO_3^-], a fall in pCO_2, or both.

The relationship among pH, pCO_2, and HCO_3^- concentrations is described by the familiar Henderson-Hasselbalch equation:

$$pH = 6.1 + \log\left([HCO_3^-]/(0.03 \times pCO_2)\right)$$

Acidosis and alkalosis are pathophysiologic processes that, if unopposed by therapy or complicating disorders, would cause acidemia or alkalemia, respectively.

Simple (Single) Acid-Base Disturbances and Compensation

The simple acid-base disorders are divided into primary metabolic and primary respiratory disturbances. Each of these simple, or single, acid-base disorders generates a compensatory response that acts to return the blood pH back toward the normal range. By convention, the physiologic approach to acid-base analysis considers the compensatory response to a simple acid-base disorder to be an integral component of that disorder. Hence, there are four primary simple acid-base disturbances (six, if each respiratory disorder is divided into an acute and chronic phase):

- *Metabolic acidosis:* The underlying pathophysiology reduces the serum bicarbonate concentration $[HCO_3^-]$. Although we refer to serum bicarbonate here, it is often directly measured as total CO_2, which includes bicarbonate (HCO_3^-), carbonic acid (H_2CO_3), and dissolved CO_2. The last two components account for a very small fraction of the total (roughly 1.2 mEq/L at normal pCO_2). Therefore, for clinical purposes, total CO_2 is equated to serum bicarbonate concentration. Causes of metabolic acidosis include excess generation of metabolic acids, excessive exogenous acid intake, reduced kidney excretion of acid, excessive exogenous loss of HCO_3^- (usually in stool or urine), or combinations of these abnormalities. Metabolic acidosis reduces the arterial plasma pH and generates a hyperventilatory compensatory response, which reduces the arterial pCO_2 and blunts the degree of acidemia.
- *Metabolic alkalosis:* The underlying pathophysiology tends to increase the $[HCO_3^-]$. Causes include exogenous intake of HCO_3^- salts (or salts that can be converted to HCO_3^-) and/or endogenous generation of HCO_3^-. Regardless of the origin of the HCO_3^-, the pathology must also include reduced or impaired kidney HCO_3^- excretion. Metabolic alkalosis increases the arterial plasma pH and generates a hypoventilatory compensatory response, which increases the arterial pCO_2 and blunts the degree of alkalemia.
- *Respiratory acidosis:* The underlying pathophysiology increases the arterial pCO_2. The compensatory response is an increase of the plasma $[HCO_3^-]$ due to rapid generation from buffers and, over a period of days, kidney HCO_3^- generation and retention.
- *Respiratory alkalosis:* The underlying pathophysiology decreases the arterial pCO_2. The compensatory response reduces the plasma $[HCO_3^-]$. This occurs acutely as H^+ is released from buffers and chronically, over a period of days, as the kidneys excrete HCO_3^- and/or retain acid.

The magnitude of each compensatory response is proportional to the severity of the primary disturbance. Generally, respiratory responses to primary metabolic acid-base disorders occur rapidly (within an hour) and are fully developed within 12 to 36 hours. In contrast, the compensatory metabolic alterations triggered by the primary respiratory disorders are divided into two phases. A chemical buffering response occurs within minutes (acute), whereas the quantitatively more significant kidney response takes several days (chronic) to develop fully. Hence, each primary respiratory disorder is subdivided into an acute and a chronic disorder to differentiate the expected compensatory response.

The expected degree of compensation for each simple disorder has been determined by studying patients with isolated simple disorders and normal subjects with experimentally induced acid-base disorders. These data have been used to create various graphic acid-base nomograms, simple mathematical relationships, and a number of mnemonic methods for predicting expected compensation ranges. Fig. 12.1 and Table 12.1 provide some of these "compensation rules." Appropriate compensation should generally be present in all patients with an acid-base disorder, and when it is not identified, a complex, or mixed, acid-base disorder must be considered.

In general, with one exception, compensatory responses return the pH toward the normal range but do not completely normalize the pH. The exception is chronic respiratory alkalosis, wherein compensation results in a pH that is normal. With all other disorders, some degree of acidemia or alkalemia remains, even after full compensation. Compensatory responses result in the pCO_2 moving in the same direction as the primary $[HCO_3^-]$ change in case of metabolic acid-base disorder and the $[HCO_3^-]$ moving in the same direction as the primary pCO_2 change in case of respiratory acid-base disorder (see Table 12.1). If the pCO_2 and $[HCO_3^-]$ are deranged in the opposite directions (i.e., the pCO_2 or $[HCO_3^-]$ is increased and the other variable is decreased), then a mixed disturbance must exist.

Anion Gap

The ion profile of normal serum is depicted in Fig. 12.2A. In any solution, the total cation charge concentration must be equal to the total anion charge concentration (all measured in units of electrical charge concentration, i.e., mEq/L). Now consider only the three serum electrolytes that are at the highest concentration: Na^+, Cl^-, and HCO_3^-. The cation charge concentration $[Na^+]$ normally exceeds the sum of the anion charge concentrations $[Cl^-]$ and $[HCO_3^-]$. If the sum of the two anions is subtracted from $[Na^+]$, an "AG" is noted (see Fig. 12.2B):

$$AG = [Na^+] - ([Cl^-] + [HCO_3^-])$$

This AG is, of course, a function of the decision to consider only the three major serum electrolytes and not other ions that normally exist in serum. Nevertheless, the AG, as defined in this fashion, is a very useful diagnostic tool.

The normal value of the AG varies among laboratories as a result of the wide variety of analyte measurement technologies and unique normal ranges for each instrument. Typically, the normal AG range is considered to be 8 to 12 mEq/L. The normal AG is primarily composed of anionic albumin and, to a lesser degree, other proteins, sulfate, phosphate, urate, and various organic acid anions such as lactate. In general, if the concentration of these "unmeasured" anions increases, the AG increases. Conversely, the AG falls when the concentration of unmeasured anions is reduced. For example, hypoalbuminemia is a common cause of a reduced AG, with the AG falling about 2.5 mEq/L for each 1 g/dL reduction of albumin below the normal range.

The disorders that produce metabolic acidosis can be subdivided on the basis of an increased or normal AG. An examination of the AG equation reveals that the only way the $[HCO_3^-]$ can fall while the AG remains normal is for the $[Cl^-]$ to increase relative to the $[Na^+]$. Consequently, all "non-AG" metabolic acidoses must be hyperchloremic metabolic acidoses. This is shown graphically in Fig. 12.3.

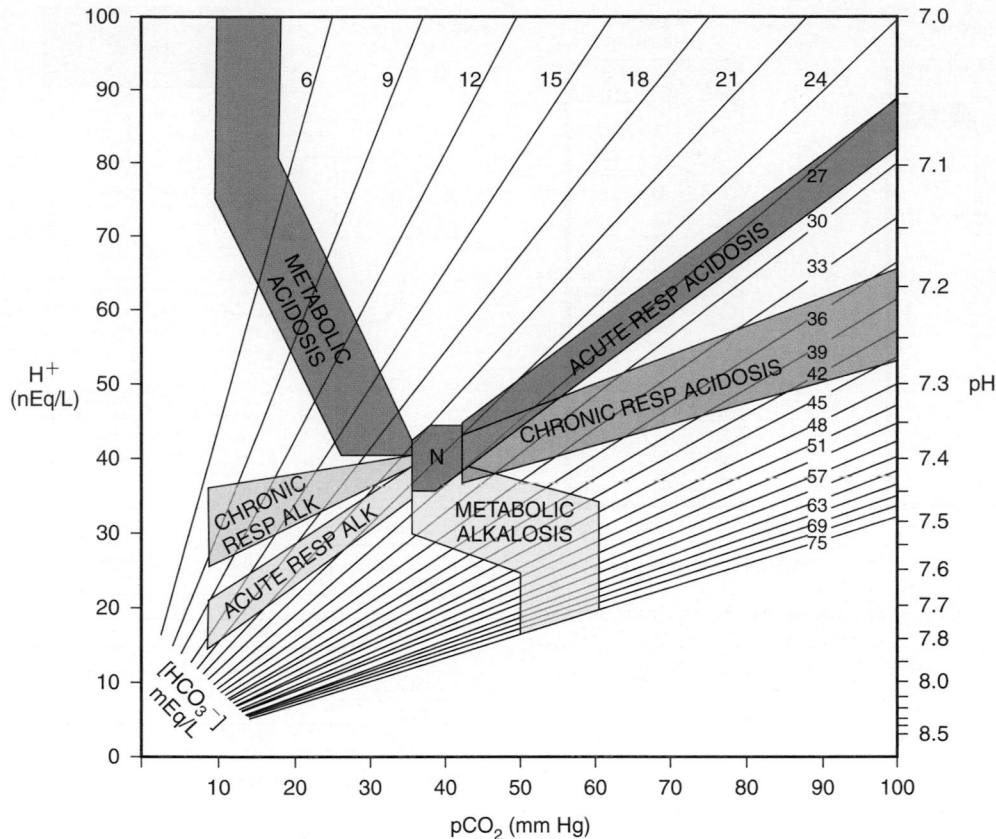

• **Fig. 12.1 The acid-base map.** Shaded areas represent the 95% confidence limits for zones of compensation for the simple acid-base disorders. Numbered diagonal lines represent isopleths of plasma bicarbonate concentration ([HCO$_3^-$]). Laboratory values that fall within a colored zone are consistent with the simple acid-base disorder, as shown. If the values fall outside a colored zone, a mixed acid-base disorder is likely. *ALK*, Alkalosis; *N*, normal range; *RESP*, respiratory. (Modified and updated from Goldberg M, Green SB, Moss ML, Marhacli MS, Garfinkel D. Computer-based instruction and diagnosis of acid-base disorders. *JAMA*. 1973;223:269–275.)

TABLE 12.1	Acid-Base Rules: Changes in pH, pCO$_2$, and [HCO$_3^-$] and Expected Compensatory Responses in Simple Disturbances			
Primary Disorder	**pH**	**Initial Chemical Change**	**Compensatory Response**	**Expected Compensation**
Metabolic acidosis	Low	↓ [HCO$_3^-$]	↓ pCO$_2$	PCO$_2$ = (1.5 × [HCO$_3^-$]) + 8 ± 2 PCO$_2$ = [HCO$_3^-$] + 15 PCO$_2$ = decimal digits of pH
Metabolic alkalosis[a]	High	↑ [HCO$_3^-$]	↑ PCO$_2$	PCO$_2$ variably increased PCO$_2$ = (0.9 × [HCO$_3^-$]) + 9 PCO$_2$ = (0.7 × [HCO$_3^-$]) + 20
Respiratory Acidosis				
Acute	Low	↑ PCO$_2$	↑ [HCO$_3^-$]	[HCO$_3^-$] increases 1 mEq/L for every 10 mm Hg increase in PCO$_2$
Chronic	Low	↑ PCO$_2$	Further ↑ [HCO$_3^-$]	[HCO$_3^-$] increases 3 to 4 mEq/L for every 10 mm Hg increase in PCO$_2$
Respiratory Alkalosis				
Acute	High	↓ PCO$_2$	↓ [HCO$_3^-$]	[HCO$_3^-$] decreases 2 mEq/L for every 10 mm Hg decrease in PCO$_2$
Chronic	High	↓ PCO$_2$	Further ↓ [HCO$_3^-$]	[HCO$_3^-$] decreases 5 mEq/L for every 10 mm Hg decrease in PCO$_2$

[a]Compensation formulas for metabolic alkalosis have wide confidence limits because the PCO$_2$ of individuals with this disorder varies greatly at any given [HCO$_3^-$].

[HCO$_3^-$], Serum bicarbonate concentration; *PCO$_2$*, arterial partial pressure of carbon dioxide.

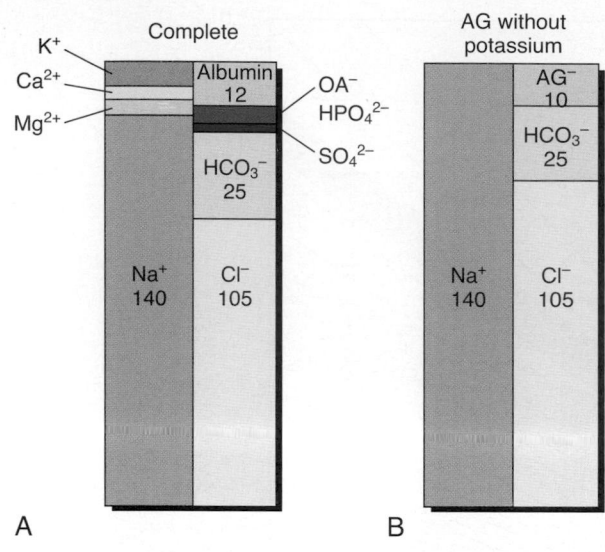

A   B

$$AG = Na^+ - (Cl^- + HCO_3^-)$$

• **Fig. 12.2** **The ionic anatomy of plasma.** All units are milliequivalents per liter (mEq/L). (A) Ion profile of normal serum. (B) Calculation of the anion gap *(AG)* using the concentrations of sodium, chloride, and bicarbonate concentrations only. *OA,* Organic acid.

Most often, an elevated AG indicates the presence of a metabolic acidosis. Several mnemonics have been published as guides to the most common clinically relevant etiologies of high AG metabolic acidosis. We suggest the mnemonic "GOLDMARK" for this purpose (Glycols [ethylene, propylene, and diethylene], Oxoproline [acetaminophen], L-Lactate, D-Lactate, Methanol, Aspirin, Renal failure, Ketoacidosis). However, a high AG can sometimes occur in the absence of metabolic acidosis. Exceptions include:

• Dehydration, as the loss of water in excess of salts, increases the concentration of all electrolytes, including albumin and other unmeasured ions, thereby increasing the AG.
• Rapid infusion, and transient accumulation, of metabolizable sodium salts such as lactate, acetate, citrate, and so on. To the extent these salts are metabolized, they generate $NaHCO_3$, and the AG does not increase; if metabolic conversion is delayed, the AG increases.
• Infusion of nonmetabolizable sodium salts, other than sodium chloride or bicarbonate. For example, anionic antibiotics such as carbenicillin and penicillin G may be infused as sodium (or potassium) salts and, to the extent that they accumulate, increase the AG.
• Metabolic alkalosis causes a small increase in AG (usually less than 3 to 4 mEq/L) as a result of (1) increased concentrations of the anions of organic acids (mainly lactate), which accumulate because of metabolic stimulation of production, and (2) increased concentration of albumin, due to ECF volume contraction.
• Laboratory error, or measurement artifact, of one or more analytes.

Mixed Acid-Base Disturbances

A mixed acid-base disturbance is the simultaneous existence of two or more simple acid-base disturbances. Mixed acid-base disorders may develop concurrently or sequentially. The disorders may be additive, with each process having a similar directional

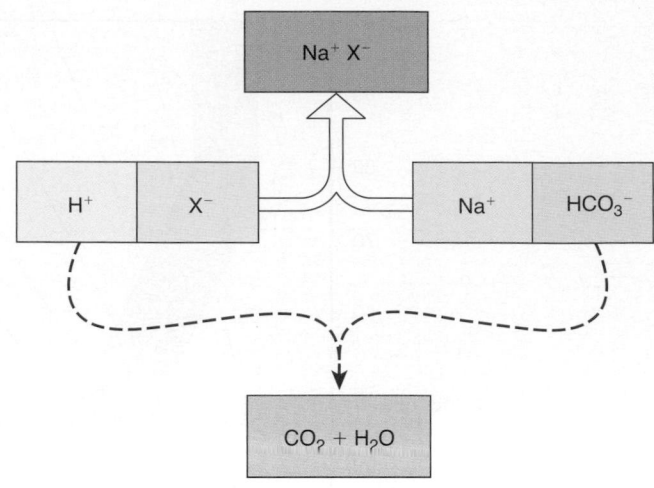

		METABOLIC ACIDOSIS	
	Normal	Hyperchloremic	High AG
Na^+	140	140	140
Cl^-	105	115	105
HCO_3^-	25	15	15
AG	10	10	20
ΔHCO_3^-	0	−10	−10
ΔAG	0	0	+10
Lactate	1	1	11

• **Fig. 12.3** **Pathogenesis of a metabolic acidosis.** If any relatively strong acid, HX (where X^- is an anion), is added to a solution containing $NaHCO_3$, there is decomposition of some HCO_3^- and an equivalent increase of the X^- concentration. If HX is HCl, then a hyperchloremic, or normal anion-gap, acidosis develops. If HX is any acid other than HCl, such as lactic acid or a keto acid, then a high anion-gap acidosis develops.

effect on pH. Alternatively, they may oppose each other, having offsetting effects on pH. Sometimes three simultaneous acid-base disorders, or a triple acid-base disturbance, can be identified.

Recognition of mixed acid-base disorders is important for several reasons. First, when these disorders are additive (i.e., coexisting metabolic and respiratory acidoses or coexisting metabolic and respiratory alkaloses), the pH excursions may become severe, with toxic consequences. When offsetting disorders coexist, the pH may be normal or near normal. Nonetheless, their identification serves as an important diagnostic clue to the underlying pathophysiology. Mixed disorders often suggest specific clinical derangements. For example, concurrent high AG metabolic acidosis and respiratory alkalosis are typical of salicylate poisoning, whereas patients with diabetic ketoacidosis often vomit and may present with concurrent high AG metabolic acidosis and metabolic alkalosis.

Inadequate or "Excessive" Compensation

The expected compensatory responses shown in the acid-base nomogram (see Fig. 12.1) and described in Table 12.1 are used to determine whether respiratory compensation for a metabolic disorder, or metabolic compensation for a respiratory disorder, is quantitatively appropriate, inadequate, or excessive. The arterial pH, pCO_2, and $[HCO_3^-]$ values are required for this determination; therefore, an arterial blood gas analysis is necessary for complete characterization of the acid-base disturbance. If a patient with a metabolic acidosis has a pCO_2 that is lower than the expected compensatory response, a respiratory alkalosis also exists; conversely, a pCO_2 that is too high indicates a complicating respiratory acidosis. Analogously, if a primary respiratory acid-base disorder is identified, then the measured $[HCO_3^-]$ should be in the range predicted by the nomogram or compensation rules (see Fig. 12.1 and Table 12.1). It should be noted that the determination of the appropriate compensation range for any primary respiratory disorder also requires the classification of that disorder as acute (from minutes to 1 to 2 days) or chronic (>2 days), a decision that is usually based on the patient's history and physical exam. If the measured $[HCO_3^-]$ is higher than the compensatory range expected with a respiratory acidosis, then a coexistent metabolic alkalosis should be considered; conversely, if the $[HCO_3^-]$ is too low, a coexistent metabolic acidosis should be considered. Examples of such mixed acid-base disorders are provided in Tables 12.2–12.5 and they are discussed later in this chapter (see the "Clinical Examples" section).

The Delta/Delta($\Delta AG/\Delta HCO_3^-$)

Whenever an AG metabolic acidosis exists as a single acid-base disorder, the magnitude of the increase in AG should be quantitatively similar to the magnitude of reduction in $[HCO_3^-]$. If the AG increases by 10 mEq/L as a result of an accumulation of keto acids that have titrated the serum bicarbonate, then the $[HCO_3^-]$ should also decrease by about 10 mEq/L (see Fig. 12.3). The absolute value of each change should be equivalent, such that $\Delta[AG] = \Delta[HCO_3^-]$.

If the increase in AG above its baseline (the ΔAG) exceeds the fall in $[HCO_3^-]$ from its baseline of 24 mEq/L (the ΔHCO_3^-), then the presence of an additional acid-base disorder that has elevated the $[HCO_3^-]$ is suggested. Two situations usually cause this discrepancy. Most often, it is the result of a coexistent metabolic alkalosis (Table 12.6 and *Clinical Example 5*). Another possibility is a coexistent chronic respiratory acidosis for which compensation has increased the $[HCO_3^-]$ to a value greater than the normal range (Fig. 12.4). The resulting arterial pH and pCO_2 should allow the clinician to readily distinguish between these possibilities.

Conversely, if the increase of the AG is smaller than the fall in $[HCO_3^-]$ from a normal baseline of about 24 mEq/L (i.e., $\Delta AG < \Delta HCO_3^-$), the $[Cl^-]$ must be increased relative to $[Na^+]$. The presence of relative hyperchloremia usually indicates the existence of a hyperchloremic metabolic acidosis, or compensation for chronic respiratory alkalosis. Again, the history, physical exam, and the resulting arterial pH and pCO_2 should readily distinguish between these possibilities.

These $\Delta AG/\Delta HCO_3^-$ comparisons usually assume that the AG has started in the normal range. If the initial AG is abnormally

TABLE 12.2 Mixed Metabolic Acidosis and Respiratory Acidosis (Clinical Example 1)

Analyte	Normal Concentration	High AG Metabolic Acidosis With Appropriate Compensation	MIXED HIGH AG METABOLIC ACIDOSIS AND RESPIRATORY ACIDOSIS	
			Mixed High AG Metabolic Acidosis and Mild Respiratory Acidosis	Mixed High AG Metabolic Acidosis and Severe Respiratory Acidosis
Na^+	140	140	140	140
K^+	4.0	5.0	5.0	5.0
Cl^-	105	105	105	105
HCO_3^-	25	15	15	15
AG	10	20	20	20
PCO_2	40	30	40	50
pH	7.42	7.32	7.20	7.10

AG, Anion gap; *PCO₂*, arterial carbon dioxide tension.

TABLE 12.3 Mixed Metabolic Alkalosis and Chronic Respiratory Acidosis (Clinical Example 2)

Analyte	Normal Concentration	Chronic Respiratory Acidosis With Appropriate Compensation	Metabolic Alkalosis With Appropriate Compensation	Mixed Chronic Respiratory Acidosis and Metabolic Alkalosis
Na^+	140	140	140	140
K^+	4.0	5.0	3.4	3.5
Cl^-	105	98	98	90
HCO_3^-	25	32	31	37
AG	10	10	12	13
PCO_2	40	60	43	60
pH	7.42	7.35	7.47	7.41

low to begin with (e.g., if the patient has a very low albumin concentration), then the excursion (or Δ) must begin from this lower baseline.

Clinical Examples

Clinical Example 1

A patient becomes septic and develops a lactic acidosis. If that same patient also develops acute respiratory distress syndrome (ARDS), then mild or severe respiratory acidosis may occur as well (see Table 12.2).

Clinical Example 2

A patient with chronic obstructive pulmonary disease (COPD) may show a pattern of chronic respiratory acidosis, as depicted in the "Chronic Respiratory Acidosis with Appropriate Compensation" column of Table 12.3, whereas a patient receiving loop diuretic therapy may develop metabolic alkalosis, as shown in the "Metabolic Alkalosis with Appropriate Compensation" column of Table 12.3. If a patient with COPD is treated with a loop diuretic, the pattern in the last column of the table may develop. Note that a chronic pCO_2 of 55 mm Hg should raise the $[HCO_3^-]$ to about 31 mEq/L, so the $[HCO_3^-]$ of 34 mEq/L is higher than a simple respiratory acidosis could account. Also, note that this has resulted in a pH of 7.41, which is too high. Patients with chronic respiratory acidosis should continue to have a slightly acidic pH, even after full compensation.

Clinical Example 3

Patients with uncomplicated AG metabolic acidosis will have a reduced $[HCO_3^-]$, an appropriately reduced pCO_2, and an acidic pH. Superimposed respiratory alkalosis will further reduce the PCO_2 and raise the pH toward normal or even enough to generate alkalemia (see Table 12.4). Patients with aspirin overdose will often present with this mixed acid-base pattern. Inhibition

TABLE 12.4 Mixed Metabolic Acidosis and Respiratory Alkalosis (Clinical Example 3)

Analyte	Normal Concentration	High AG Metabolic Acidosis With Appropriate Compensation	MIXED METABOLIC ACIDOSIS AND RESPIRATORY ALKALOSIS	
			Mild Respiratory Alkalosis	Severe Respiratory Alkalosis
Na^+	140	140	140	140
K^+	4.0	5.0	5.0	5.0
Cl^-	105	105	105	105
HCO_3^-	25	15	15	15
AG	10	20	20	20
PCO_2	40	30	25	20
pH	7.42	7.32	7.4	7.5

AG, Anion gap; *PCO₂*, arterial carbon dioxide tension.

TABLE 12.5 Simple and Mixed Metabolic and Respiratory Alkalosis (Clinical Example 4)

Analyte	Normal Concentration	SIMPLE ALKALOSIS		MIXED METABOLIC AND CHRONIC RESPIRATORY ALKALOSIS	
		Metabolic Alkalosis With Appropriate Compensation	Chronic Respiratory Alkalosis With Appropriate Compensation	Mild Metabolic Alkalosis	Severe Metabolic Alkalosis
Na^+	140	140	140	140	140
K^+	4.0	3.2	3.4	3.1	2.9
Cl^-	105	96	108	103	96
HCO_3^-	25	32	19	23[a]	29
AG	10	12	12	14	15
PCO_2	40	44	30	30	30
pH	7.42	7.48	7.42	7.51	7.61

[a]Note that a lack of metabolic compensation—the serum $[HCO_3^-]$ has not decreased—in the presence of chronic respiratory alkalosis is consistent with coexisting metabolic alkalosis. This pattern could also exist in simple *acute* respiratory alkalosis.

AG, Anion gap; *PCO₂*, arterial carbon dioxide tension.

TABLE 12.6 **Mixed Metabolic Acidosis and Metabolic Alkalosis (Clinical Example 5)**

				MIXED METABOLIC ALKALOSIS AND METABOLIC ACIDOSIS	
Analyte	Normal Concentration	High AG Metabolic Acidosis With Appropriate Compensation	Normal AG Metabolic Acidosis With Appropriate Compensation	High AG Metabolic Acidosis and Metabolic Alkalosis	Normal AG Metabolic Acidosis and Metabolic Alkalosis
Na^+	140	140	140	140	140
K^+	4.0	5.0	3.8	4.0	4.0
Cl^-	105	105	115	95	105
HCO_3^-	25	15	15	25	25
AG	10	20	10	20	10
PCO_2	40	30	30	40	40
pH	7.42	7.32	7.32	7.42	7.42

AG, Anion gap; *PCO_2*, arterial carbon dioxide tension.

of normal oxidative metabolic reactions causes an accumulation of multiple organic acids and, hence, the AG metabolic acidosis. Acetylsalicylic acid also directly contributes to the large AG. Simultaneously, the toxic levels of salicylate stimulate central hyperventilation. The pattern in the last column of Table 12.4 is typically seen in adults with this disorder. Infants with salicylate poisoning more typically present with less marked respiratory alkalosis, so their arterial pH is generally acidic.

Clinical Example 4

Metabolic alkalosis occurs with elevation of the $[HCO_3^-]$, and compensation should increase the pCO_2. Respiratory alkalosis reduces the pCO_2, and compensation should decrease the $[HCO_3^-]$.

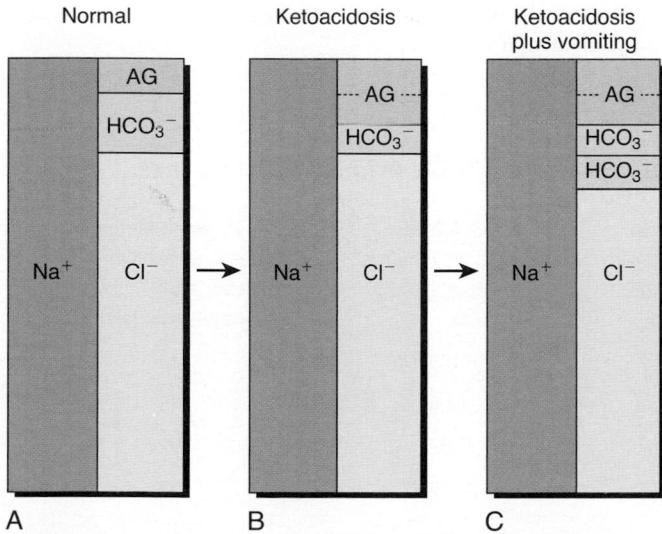

• **Fig. 12.4 The effect of ketoacidosis plus vomiting on the ionic profile of blood.** (A) The normal electrolyte pattern. (B) The development of a typical anion gap *(AG)* metabolic acidosis. (C) The superimposed effect of vomiting, which causes proton loss without the loss of any organic acid anions. This results in a decrease in the serum chloride concentration and an increase in the bicarbonate concentration. The latter normalizes the $[HCO_3^-]$, but the AG remains large because the keto acid concentration is unchanged by the vomiting.

Hence, in simple alkaloses, both components should deviate in the same direction. If the $[HCO_3^-]$ is increased and the pCO_2 is decreased, then metabolic alkalosis and respiratory alkalosis coexist (see Table 12.5). This mixed acid-base disorder is often seen in patients with severe liver disease. Chronic respiratory alkalosis is extremely common as a result of diaphragmatic elevation, A-V shunting, and a deranged hormonal milieu that stimulates ventilation. Nausea and vomiting occur frequently, nasogastric suction is often employed, and diuretics are commonly prescribed. These disorders and treatments generate metabolic alkalosis, which complicates the chronic respiratory alkalosis. Combined, these disorders can generate extreme alkalemia.

Clinical Example 5

The combination of mixed metabolic acidosis with high AG and metabolic alkalosis can develop in different ways.
1. A large AG metabolic acidosis may develop in a patient with pre-existing metabolic alkalosis. In this situation, the $[HCO_3^-]$ falls from a supranormal level as the AG increases (see Table 12.6).
2. Metabolic alkalosis may develop in a patient with a large AG metabolic acidosis. The metabolic alkalosis raises the $[HCO_3^-]$, while the AG remains large because the chloride concentration falls.
3. AG metabolic acidosis and metabolic alkalosis can develop simultaneously.

In each of these scenarios, the elevated AG remains as a residual marker of the metabolic acidosis. However, the magnitude of increase of the AG is greater than the $[HCO_3^-]$ fall from its baseline. This relationship can be expressed as the Delta/Delta or $\Delta[AG]/\Delta[HCO_3^-]$, which will be increased above 1 (the $\Delta[AG] > \Delta[HCO_3^-]$).

Patients with diabetic ketoacidosis have metabolic acidosis with a large AG. If nausea and vomiting occur, they generate a simultaneous or sequential metabolic alkalosis through loss of acidic gastric fluids. Although the final arterial pH is typically acidic, it may sometimes become normal or even alkaline if the alkalosis is more severe than the acidosis. Regardless of the resultant pH and $[HCO_3^-]$, the large AG remains a major chemical clue to the presence of a metabolic acidosis. A similar pattern is seen when uremic patients develop nausea and vomiting.

Other Mixed Acid-Base Disorders

The combination of a hyperchloremic metabolic acidosis and metabolic alkalosis may be more difficult to diagnose. In these patients, there is no persisting AG increase to indicate that an underlying metabolic acidosis exists. Instead, the hyperchloremic acidosis reduces the [HCO$_3^-$] and increases the [Cl$^-$], whereas the metabolic alkalosis increases the [HCO$_3^-$] and decreases the [Cl$^-$] (see Table 12.6). If the two disorders are of similar intensity, the final [HCO$_3^-$] and [Cl$^-$] may be restored to their normal ranges with a normal AG. This mixed disorder can be suspected on the basis of the history, clinical setting, and physical exam. For example, a patient with gastroenteritis who has a history of both watery diarrhea and vomiting may have this mixed acid-base disorder, despite a normal pH, pCO$_2$, [HCO$_3^-$], AG, and [Cl$^-$]. Marked hypokalemia may be present. If the vomiting improves but the diarrhea continues, overt hyperchloremic metabolic acidosis and acidemia may be revealed.

Other forms of mixed acid-base disorders are combinations of different metabolic acidosis disorders or, much less commonly, metabolic alkalosis disorders. For example, it is not uncommon for ketoacidosis to coexist with lactic acidosis; similarly, hyperchloremic acidosis caused by diarrhea or renal tubular acidosis may present in conjunction with lactic acidosis or uremic acidosis. Some patients with nausea and vomiting may medicate themselves with baking soda. The vomiting generates HCO$_3^-$, and the baking soda is a form of exogenous alkali (sodium bicarbonate).

Mixed respiratory acid-base disorders can also develop and are usually suspected on the basis of the history and clinical setting rather than any specific laboratory results. The patient with chronic obstructive lung disease who presents with recent pulmonary deterioration caused by a mucus plug or pneumonia may have chronic respiratory acidosis and a superimposed acute respiratory acidosis. A pregnant woman with underlying physiologic hyperventilation who ingests an overdose of sedating drugs and develops respiratory depression will have chronic respiratory alkalosis and a superimposed acute respiratory acidosis.

Triple Acid-Base Disturbances

The most readily diagnosed type of triple acid-base disturbance is due to the combination of an elevated AG metabolic acidosis, metabolic alkalosis, and either respiratory acidosis or respiratory alkalosis. The offsetting effects of the coexistent metabolic acidosis and alkalosis result in a low, normal, or elevated [HCO$_3^-$]. Regardless of the [HCO$_3^-$], there is a large ΔAG, which exceeds the Δ[HCO$_3^-$]. This is the clue to the double disorder of metabolic acidosis and metabolic alkalosis. The final [HCO$_3^-$] from these two disorders is the parameter that should determine the degree of respiratory compensation and pCO$_2$. If the pCO$_2$ is lower than expected, a third disorder, respiratory alkalosis, exists. If the pCO$_2$ is higher than expected, the third disorder is respiratory acidosis.

A clinical example is shown in Table 12.7. Case 1 is a patient who vomits and develops metabolic alkalosis. The [HCO$_3^-$] increases to 38 mEq/L, the pCO$_2$ increases to 46 mm Hg, and the AG increases slightly. Case 2 illustrates the findings expected with high AG metabolic acidosis, such as lactic acidosis. The [HCO$_3^-$] has fallen by 13 mEq/L, and the AG has increased by the same amount. If the patient represented by Case 1 develops severe ECF volume depletion, then lactic acidosis may ensue (Case 3). Accordingly, the [HCO$_3^-$] falls, in this example from 38 to 25 mEq/L (a HCO$_3^-$ of 13 mEq/L), and the AG also increases to 23 mEq/L. The chemistries in Case 3 show a normal [HCO$_3^-$], despite an AG of 23 mEq/L. The discrepancy between the normal [HCO$_3^-$] and the large AG is the major clue to this mixed acid-base disorder. The normal [HCO$_3^-$], which is the result of equally severe degrees of metabolic acidosis and metabolic alkalosis, should be associated with a normal pCO$_2$. The last column (Case 4) shows an example of a pCO$_2$ that is too low, indicating that a third disorder, respiratory alkalosis, is also present. If the pCO$_2$ had been 50 mm Hg, then respiratory acidosis, metabolic alkalosis, and metabolic acidosis would be the triple disturbance.

The flow charts in Figs. 12.5 and 12.6 show one general approach to the diagnostic work-up of a patient with either acidemia or alkalemia.

TABLE 12.7 Metabolic Acidosis, Metabolic Alkalosis, and Respiratory Alkalosis: A Triple Acid-Base Disturbance

Analyte	Normal Concentrations	Case 1: Metabolic Alkalosis With Appropriate Compensation	Case 2: High AG Metabolic Acidosis With Appropriate Compensation	Case 3: Mixed Metabolic Acidosis and Metabolic Alkalosis	Case 4: Mixed Metabolic Acidosis, Metabolic Alkalosis, and Respiratory Alkalosis
Na$^+$	140	140	140	140	140
K$^+$	4.0	3.4	4.5	4.5	4.5
Cl$^-$	105	89	105	92	92
HCO$_3^-$	25	38	12	25	25
AG	10	13	23	23	23
PCO$_2$	40	46	26	40	30
pH	7.42	7.54	7.29	7.42	7.54

AG, Anion gap; *PCO$_2$*, arterial carbon dioxide tension.

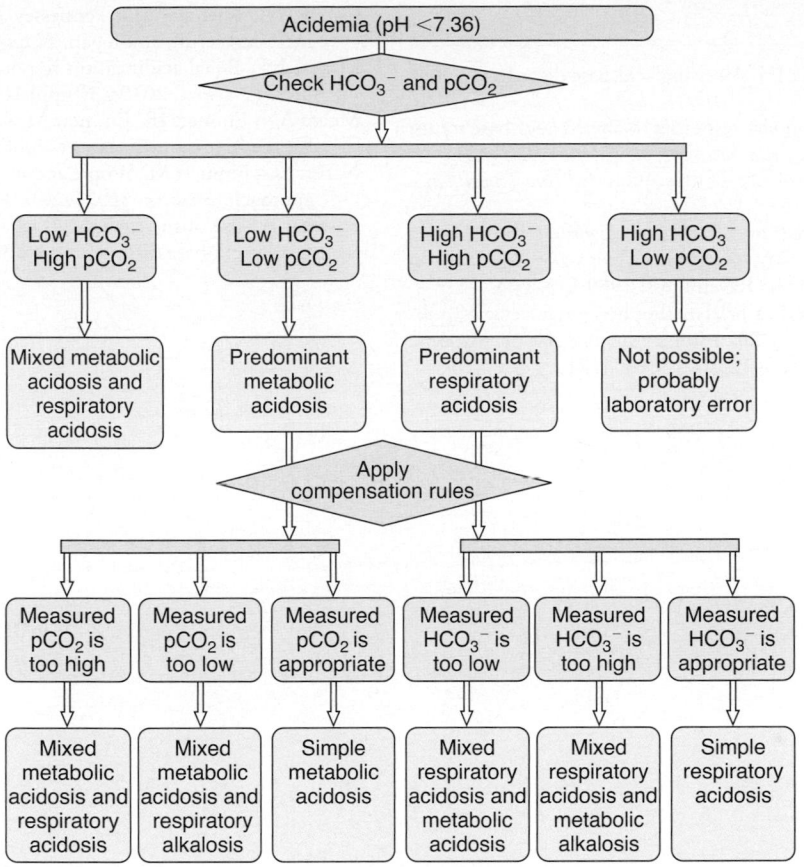

• **Fig. 12.5** A flowchart showing one approach to the diagnostic work-up of a patient with acidemia.

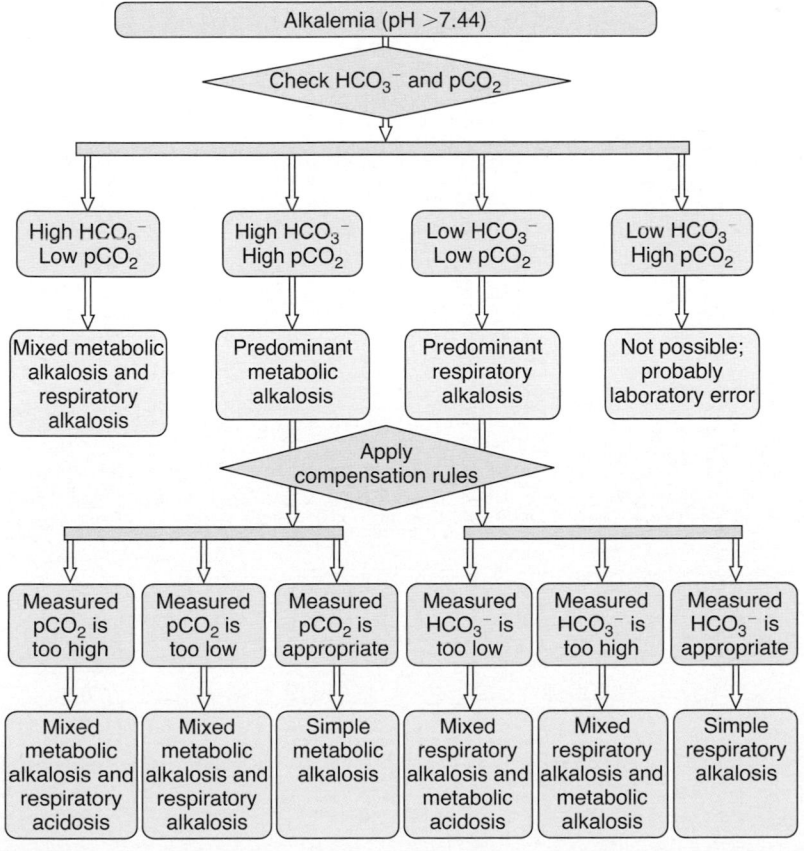

• **Fig. 12.6** A flowchart showing one approach to the diagnostic work-up of a patient with alkalemia.

Bibliography

Adrogué HJ, Gennari FJ, Galla JH. Assessing acid-base disorders. *Kidney Int*. 2009;76:1239–1247.

Adrogué HJ, Madias NE. Secondary responses to altered acid-base status: The rules of engagement. *J Am Soc Nephrol*. 2010;21:920–923.

Emmett M, Narins R. Clinical use of the AG. *Medicine (Baltimore)*. 1977;56:38–54.

Emmett M, Seldin DW. Evaluation of acid-base disorders from plasma composition. In: Seldin DW, Giebisch G, eds. *The Regulation of Acid-Base Balance*. New York: Raven Press; 1989:213–263.

Emmett M. Metabolic alkalosis: a brief pathophysiologic review [published online ahead of print, 2020 Jun 25]. *Clin J Am Soc Nephrol*. 2020. doi:10.2215/CJN.16041219 CJN.16041219.

Gabow PA, Kaehny WD, Fennessey PV. Diagnostic importance of an increased serum anion gap. *N Engl J Med*. 1980;303:854–858.

Madias NE. Renal acidification responses to respiratory acid-base disorders. *J Nephrol*. 2010;23(suppl 16):S85–S91.

Mehta AN, Emmett JB, Emmett M. GOLD MARK: an AG mnemonic for the 21st century. *Lancet*. 2008;372:892.

Narins RG, Emmett M. Simple and mixed acid-base disorders: a practical approach. *Medicine (Baltimore)*. 1980;59:161–187.

Rastegar A. Use of the DeltaAG/DeltaHCO3– ratio in the diagnosis of mixed acid-base disorders. *J Am Soc Nephrol*. 2007;18:2429–2431.

13

Metabolic Acidosis

HAROLD M. SZERLIP

Metabolic acidosis describes a process in which nonvolatile acids accumulate in the body. For practical purposes, this can result from either the addition of protons or the loss of base. The consequence of this process is a decline in the major extracellular buffer, bicarbonate, and, if unopposed, a decrease in extracellular pH. Depending on the existence and the magnitude of other acid-base disturbances, however, the extracellular pH may be low, normal, or even high. Normal blood pH is between 7.36 and 7.44, corresponding to a hydrogen ion concentration of 44 to 36 nmol/L.

Because the body tightly defends against changes in pH, a decreased pH sensitizes both peripheral and central chemoreceptors, which triggers an increase in minute ventilation. This compensatory respiratory alkalosis helps offset a marked fall in pH. Because increased ventilation is a compensatory mechanism stimulated by the acidemia, it never returns the pH to normal. The expected partial pressure of carbon dioxide (pCO_2) for any given degree of metabolic acidosis can be estimated by adding 15 back to the bicarbonate,

$$pCO_2 = 15 + HCO_3$$

or by using Winters' formula:

$$pCO_2 = (1.5 \times [HCO_3]) + 8 \pm 2$$

Overview of Acid-Base Balance

To maintain extracellular pH within the normal range, the daily production of acid must be excreted from the body (Fig. 13.1). The vast majority of acid production results from the metabolism of dietary carbohydrates and fats. Complete oxidation of these metabolic substrates produces CO_2 and water. The 15,000 mmoles of CO_2 produced daily are efficiently exhaled by the lungs and are therefore known as *volatile acid*. As long as ventilatory function remains normal, this volatile acid does not contribute to changes in acid-base balance. Nonvolatile or fixed acids are produced by the metabolism of sulfate-containing and phosphate-containing amino acids. In addition, incomplete oxidation of fats and carbohydrates results in the production of small quantities of lactate and other organic anions, which when excreted in the urine represent a loss of base. Individuals consuming a typical meat-based diet produce approximately 1 mmol/kg/day of hydrogen ions, which are buffered by HCO_3^- resulting in a decrease in serum HCO_3^- concentration. Fecal excretion of a small amount of base also contributes to total daily acid production.

The kidney is responsible not only for the regeneration of HCO_3^- lost in the buffering process but also for the reclamation of the approximately 4000 mmol of bicarbonate filtered daily. Bicarbonate reclamation occurs predominantly in the proximal tubule, mainly through the Na^+-H^+ exchanger. Active transporters in the distal tubule secrete hydrogen ion against a concentration gradient. Although urinary pH can fall to as low as 4.5, if there were no urinary buffers, this would account for very little acid excretion. For example, to excrete 100 mmoles of H^+ into unbuffered urine at a minimum urine pH of 4.5 ($[H^+] = 32$ mmol/L) would require a daily urine volume of 3000 L. Fortunately, urinary phosphate and creatinine help buffer these protons, allowing the kidney to excrete approximately 40% to 50% of the daily fixed acid load as titratable acid (TA), so called because they are quantitated by titrating the urine pH back to that of plasma, 7.4. In addition to TA, kidney excretion of acid is supported by ammoniagenesis. NH_3 is generated in the proximal tubule by the deamidation of glutamine to glutamate, which is subsequently deaminated to yield α-ketoglutarate. The enzymes responsible for these reactions are upregulated by acidosis and hypokalemia. Hyperkalemia, on the other hand, reduces ammoniagenesis. NH_3 builds up in the medullary interstitium and enters the tubule lumen along the length of the collecting duct by both passive diffusion and active transport, where it is trapped by H^+ as ammonium (NH_4^+).

Under conditions of increased acid production, the normal kidney can increase acid excretion primarily by augmenting NH_3 production. Kidney acid excretion varies directly with the rate of acid production. Net kidney acid excretion (NAE) is equal to the sum of TA and NH_4^+, minus any secreted HCO_3^- [NAE = (TA + NH_4^+) – HCO_3^-]. Thus, the etiology of a metabolic acidosis can be divided into four broad categories: (1) overproduction of fixed acids, (2) increased extrarenal loss of base, (3) decrease in the kidney's ability to secrete hydrogen ions, and (4) inability of the kidney to reclaim the filtered bicarbonate (Fig. 13.2).

Evaluation of Urinary Acidification

The cause of metabolic acidosis often is evident from the clinical situation. However, because the kidney is responsible for both the reclamation of filtered HCO_3^- and the excretion of the daily production of fixed acid, to evaluate a metabolic acidosis it may be necessary to assess whether the kidney is appropriately able to reabsorb HCO_3^-, secrete H^+ against a gradient, and excrete NH_4^+ (Table 13.1). The simplest test is to measure the urine pH. Although urine pH can be measured using a dipstick, the lack of precision of this technique prevents it from being useful in making

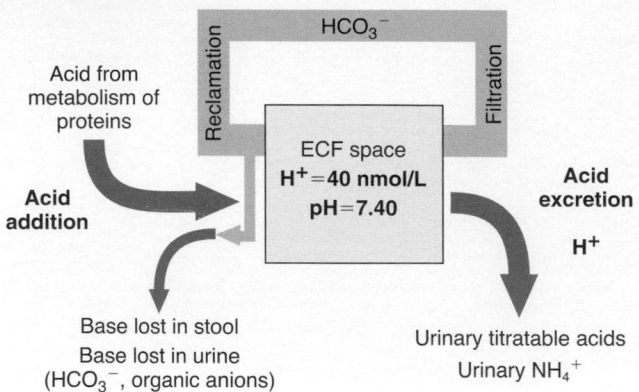

• **Fig. 13.1** Maintenance of acid-base homeostasis requires that the addition of acid to the body is balanced by excretion of acid. Production of fixed nonvolatile acid occurs mainly through the metabolism of proteins. A small quantity of base also is lost in the stool and urine. Acid excretion occurs in the kidney through the secretion of H^+ buffered by titratable acids and NH_3. Bicarbonate filtration and reclamation by the kidney are normally a neutral process.

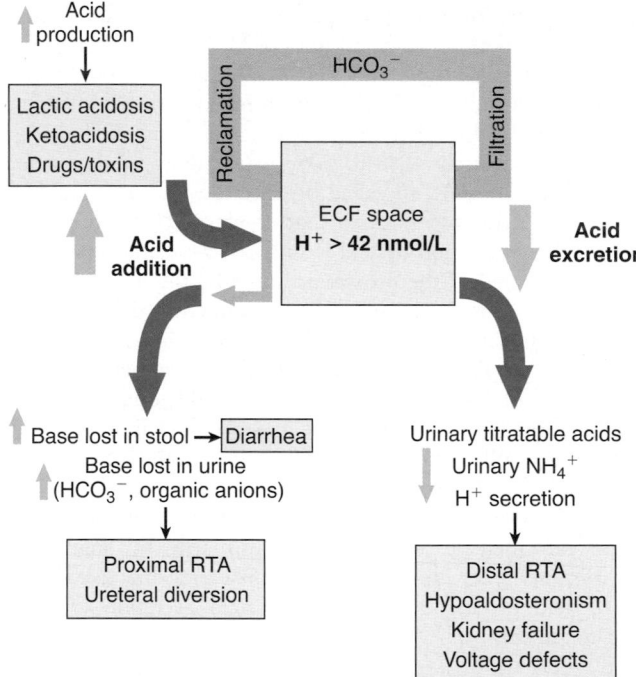

• **Fig. 13.2** Metabolic acidosis can result from increased acid production, increased loss of base in stool or urine, or decreased H^+ secretion in the distal tubule. The causes of these processes are shown. *RTA*, Renal tubular acidosis.

TABLE 13.1	Tests of Kidney Acid Excretion

Urine pH (enhanced by furosemide)
NH_4^+ excretion
- Urine NH_4^+
- Urine anion gap
- Urine osmolal gap

Urine pCO_2 with bicarbonate loading
Fractional excretion of HCO_3^-

clinical decisions. Although it has been suggested that urine be collected under oil and the pH measured using a pH electrode to prevent the loss of CO_2, in fact when the urine pH is less than 6.0, the amount of dissolved CO_2 is minimal and the use of oil is unnecessary. Under conditions of acid loading, urine pH should be below 5.5. A pH of higher than 5.5 usually reflects impaired distal hydrogen ion secretion. Measuring the pH after challenging the patient with the loop diuretic furosemide will increase the sensitivity of this test by providing Na^+ to the distal tubule for reabsorption. The reabsorption of Na^+ creates a negative electrical potential in the lumen and enhances H^+ secretion. It is important, however, to rule out urinary infections with urea-splitting organisms, which will increase pH. An elevated urine pH may also be misleading in conditions associated with volume depletion and hypokalemia, as can occur in diarrhea. In contradistinction to furosemide, volume depletion with decreased sodium delivery to the distal tubule impairs distal H^+ secretion. Furthermore, hypokalemia, by enhancing ammoniagenesis, raises the urine pH.

Because kidney excretion of NH_4^+ accounts for the majority of acid excretion, measurement of urine NH_4^+ can provide important information. Urinary NH_4^+ excretion can be decreased by a variety of mechanisms, including a primary decrease in ammoniagenesis by the proximal tubule, as seen in chronic kidney disease (CKD), or decreased trapping in the distal tubule either secondary to decreased H^+ secretion or an increased delivery of HCO_3^-, which will preferentially buffer H^+ and make it unavailable to form NH_4^+. Although direct measurement of NH_4^+ is becoming more readily available in clinical laboratories and is the gold standard, many laboratories still do not perform this assay. An estimate of NH_4^+ excretion, however, can be obtained by calculating the urine anion gap (UAG) or urine osmole gap. If, as is usual, the anion balancing the charge of the NH_4^+ is Cl^-, the UAG $[(Na^+ + K^+) - Cl^-]$ should be negative because the chloride is greater than the sum of Na^+ and K^+ (Fig. 13.3). The use of the urine anion gap as a surrogate marker of NH_4^+ excretion is less reliable in chronic kidney disease and in the presence of anions other than Cl^- (such as keto anions or hippurate). In the presence of these non-chloride anions, the urine osmole gap (see Fig. 13.3) may be helpful. The urine osmole gap is calculated as follows: [measured urine osmolality – calculated urine osmolality], where calculated urine osmolality is $[2(Na^+ + K^+) + (urea \ nitrogen/2.8) + (glucose/18)]$. The osmole gap is made up primarily of NH_4^+ salts. Thus, half of the gap represents NH_4^+. An osmole gap of greater than 100 mmol/L signifies normal NH_4^+ excretion.

Another test of distal H^+ ion secretory ability is measurement of urine pCO_2 during bicarbonate loading. Distal delivery of HCO_3^- in the presence of normal H^+ secretory capacity results in elevated pCO_2 in the urine. When there is a secretory defect, urine pCO_2 does not increase. In this case, accurate measurement of urine pCO_2 requires that the urine be collected under oil to prevent the loss of CO_2 into the air.

Complications of Acidosis

Although it has been accepted that a decrease in extracellular pH has detrimental effects on numerous physiologic parameters and should be aggressively treated, this dogma has been challenged. The proponents of treatment argue that acidemia depresses cardiac contractility, blocks activation of adrenergic receptors, and inhibits the action of key enzymes. Uncontrolled clinical studies are not easy to interpret because of the difficulties in separating the effects of the acidosis from the effects of the underlying illness. Most controlled

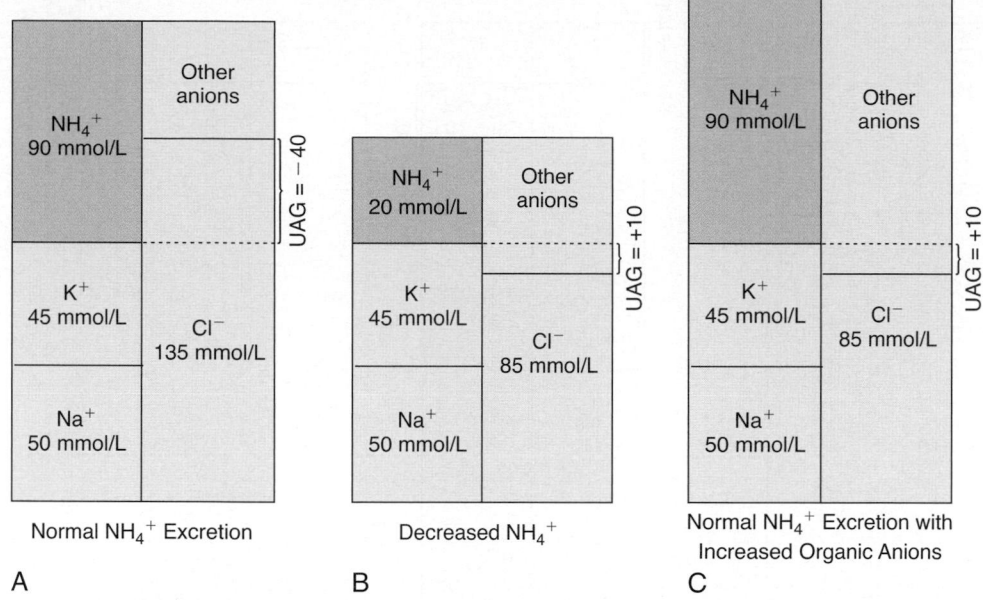

• **Fig. 13.3** In the presence of acidemia, the kidney increases NH_4^+ excretion. The urine anion gap *(UAG)* is an indirect method for estimating urine NH_4^+. (A) If the accompanying anion is chloride, the UAG ($Na^+ + K^+ - Cl^-$) will be negative, reflecting the large quantity of NH_4^+ in the urine. (B) A decrease in NH_4^+ secretion occurs when ammoniagenesis is diminished, H^+ secretion is impaired, or there is delivery of HCO_3^- to the distal tubule. In these cases, the UAG will be inappropriately positive. (C) If anions other than Cl^- are excreted (e.g., ketones, hippurate), the UAG will be positive despite increased NH_4^+ excretion, because these anions are not used in calculation of the gap.

studies investigating the role of acidosis on cellular processes have been done in isolated cells or organs; therefore, the effects of acidemia on whole-body physiology and their applicability to humans are unclear. In addition, it is often not possible to distinguish the effects of acidemia from those of the underlying pathology associated with the cause of the decrease in pH (e.g., sepsis).

The effect of pH on cardiac function has been strongly debated. Cardiac output is determined by multiple components, and it is the sum of the effects on these individual components that determines the net effect of acidemia on cardiac function. Myocardial contractile strength and changes in vascular tone determine cardiovascular performance, and the relative contributions of each in the context of acidemia remain to be clarified. Because of differing effects of acidemia on contractile force, vascular tone, and sympathetic discharge, it is difficult to predict what happens to cardiac output from studies using isolated myocytes or perfused hearts.

During continuous infusion of lactic acid, it has been shown that cardiac output and the rate of development of left ventricular force increase. In addition, fractional shortening of the left ventricle as assessed by transthoracic echocardiography appears to be normal, even in cases of severe acidemia. The pH at which cardiac output and blood pressure fall remains unclear.

Approach to Metabolic Acidosis

Complete evaluation of acid-base status requires a routine electrolyte panel, measurement of serum albumin, and arterial blood gas analysis (see Chapter 12). The traditional approach to metabolic acidosis relies on the calculation of the anion gap (AG) and the subsequent separation of metabolic acidosis into those with an elevated AG and those in which the AG is normal, or so-called *hyperchloremic metabolic acidosis* (HCMA; Fig. 13.4). The AG is defined as the difference between the concentration of sodium, the

major cation, and the sum of the concentrations of chloride and bicarbonate, the major anions: $Na^+-[Cl^- + HCO_3^-]$. Because the concentration of potassium changes minimally, its contribution is ignored for convenience. Obviously, electrical neutrality must exist, and the sum of the anions must equal the sum of the cations. The gap results from the unmeasured anions, such as sulfate, phosphate, organic anions, and especially the weak acid proteins, exceeding the unmeasured cations (i.e., calcium, magnesium, iron). Thus, it would seem upon examination of a basic chemistry panel that cations exceed anions, creating an AG. The normal AG is 10 ± 2 mEq/L. Any increase in the AG, even in the face of a normal or frankly alkalemic pH, represents the accumulation of acids and the presence of an acidosis. In many cases, the anions that make up the gap are not easily identifiable.

The one caveat in using the AG is to recognize that the normal gap is predominantly composed of the negative charge on albumin. When hypoalbuminemia is present, the AG must be corrected for the serum albumin. For each 1 g/dL decrease in the serum albumin, the calculated AG should be increased by 2.5 mEq/L. Thus, the corrected AG can be estimated as AGc = AG + 2.5 (4 − serum albumin). If the AG is not corrected, the presence of a metabolic acidosis may be masked. This is especially true in critically ill patients, who are catabolic or malnourished and typically have decreased serum albumin.

Anion Gap Acidosis

As previously described, an increased AG represents the accumulation of nonchloride acids. The mnemonic GOLDMARK is a useful tool that helps identify the causes of an AG acidosis (Fig. 13.5). AG acidosis can be divided into four major categories (Table 13.2): (1) lactic acidosis, (2) ketoacidosis, (3) toxin/drugs, and (4) severe kidney failure. In all but kidney failure, the accumulation

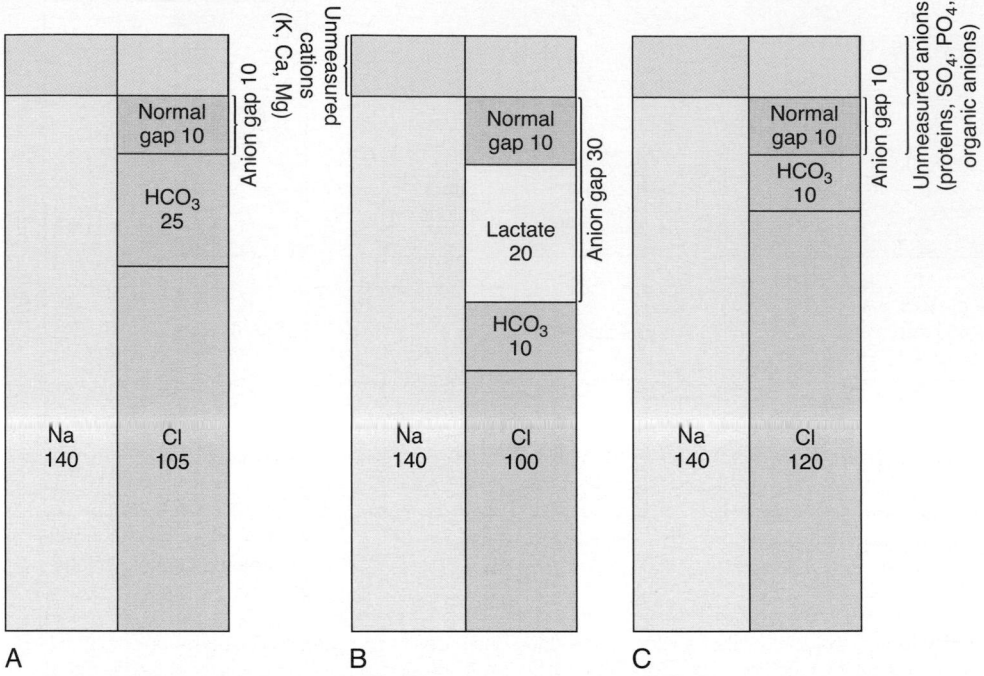

• **Fig. 13.4** The anion gap (AG) is equal to [Na⁺] + ([Cl⁻] + [HCO₃⁻], which is equal to the unmeasured anions minus the unmeasured cations. **(A)** The normal anion gap is 10 ± 2. **(B)** In an AG acidosis there is a decrease in [HCO₃⁻] and an increase in organic anions (e.g., lactate), which results in an elevated anion gap. **(C)** In a hyperchloremic acidosis, there is a decrease in [HCO₃⁻] and an increase in [Cl], with no change in anion gap.

• Glycols
• Oxoproline (pyroglutamic acid – acetaminophen)
• L-lactate
• D-lactate

• Methanol
• Aspirin
• Renal failure
• Ketoacidosis

• **Fig. 13.5** GOLDMARK is a useful mnemonic to remember the common causes of an anion gap metabolic acidosis.

TABLE 13.2 **Causes of Anion Gap Acidosis**

Lactic acidosis
• Type A
• Type B
• D-Lactic acidosis
Ketoacidosis
• Diabetic ketoacidosis
• Alcoholic ketoacidosis
• Starvation ketosis
Toxins/drugs
• Methanol
• Ethylene glycol
• Acetaminophen
• Salicylate
Kidney failure (with severe reductions in glomerular filtration rate)

---

of acids is caused by their overproduction. These acids dissociate into protons, which are quickly buffered by HCO_3^-, and into their respective conjugate bases, the unmeasured anions. As long as these anions are retained in the body and not excreted, they contribute to the elevation in the AG.

Lactic Acidosis

Lactic acidosis is a common AG acidosis and by far the most serious of all high-AG acidoses. Anaerobic metabolism of glucose (glycolysis) occurs in the extramitochondrial cytoplasm and produces pyruvate as an intermediary. If this were the end of the glycolytic process, there would be a net production of two protons and a metabolically unsatisfactory reduction of NAD to NADH. Fortunately, pyruvate rapidly undergoes one of two metabolic fates: (1) under anaerobic conditions, because of the high NADH/NAD ratio, pyruvate is quickly reduced by lactate dehydrogenase to lactate, releasing energy, consuming a proton, and decreasing the NADH/NAD ratio, thus allowing for continued glycolysis; or (2) in the presence of oxygen, pyruvate diffuses into the mitochondria and, after oxidation by the pyruvate dehydrogenase (PDH) complex, enters the tricarboxylic acid cycle, where it is completely oxidized to CO_2 and water. Neither of these pathways results in the production of H⁺. During glycolysis, glucose metabolism produces two molecules of lactate and two molecules of adenosine triphosphate (ATP). It is the hydrolysis of ATP (ATP = ADP + H⁺ + Pi) that releases protons. Therefore, the acidosis does not occur because of the production of lactate but because under hypoxic conditions the hydrolysis of ATP is greater than ATP production. Thus, the buildup of lactate is a surrogate marker for ATP consumption during hypoxic states.

Although lactate production averages about 1300 mmol/day, serum lactate levels are typically less than 1 mmol/L because lactate is either reoxidized to pyruvate and enters the tricarboxylic acid cycle or is used by the liver and kidney via the Cori cycle for gluconeogenesis. Increased concentration of lactate can, therefore, result from decreased oxidative phosphorylation, increased glycolysis, or decreased gluconeogenesis. Lactate levels between 2 and 3 mmol/L are frequently found in hospitalized patients. Some of these patients will go on to develop frank acidosis, but others will have no adverse events. Lactic acidosis is defined as the presence of a lactate level of greater than 5 mmol/L.

There is a poor correlation among arterial pH, uncorrected AG, and serum lactate levels, even in those patients with a serum lactic acid level greater than 5 mmol/L. Approximately 25% of patients with serum lactate levels between 5 and 9.9 mmol/L have a pH greater than 7.35, and as many as half have AGs of less than 12.

Lactic acidosis has been traditionally divided into types A and B (Table 13.3). Type A, or hypoxic lactic acidosis, results from an imbalance between oxygen supply and oxygen demand. In type B lactic acidosis, oxygen delivery is normal, but oxidative phosphorylation is impaired. This is seen in patients who have inborn errors of metabolism or who have ingested drugs or toxins. It has become increasingly clear, however, that lactic acidosis is

TABLE 13.3	Lactic Acidosis

Type A
- Generalized seizure
- Extreme exercise
- Shock
- Cardiac arrest
- Low cardiac output
- Severe anemia
- Severe hypoxemia
- Carbon monoxide poisoning

Type B
- Sepsis
- Thiamine deficiency
- Uncontrolled diabetes mellitus
- Malignancy
- Hypoglycemia
- Drugs/toxins
  - Ethanol
  - Metformin
  - Zidovudine
  - Didanosine
  - Stavudine
  - Lamivudine
  - Zalcitabine
  - Salicylate
  - Linezolid
  - Propofol
  - Niacin
  - Isoniazid
  - Nitroprusside
  - Cyanide
  - Catecholamines
  - Cocaine
  - Acetaminophen
  - Streptozotocin
  - Pheochromocytoma
  - Sorbitol/fructose
  - Malaria
- Inborn errors of metabolism

Other
- Liver failure
- Respiratory or metabolic alkalosis
- Propylene glycol
- D-Lactic acidosis

often caused by the simultaneous existence of both hypoxic and nonhypoxic factors, and, in many cases, it is difficult to separate one from the other. For example, hereditary partial defects in mitochondrial metabolism, as well as age-related declines in cytochrome IV complex activity, may result in lactic acidosis with a lesser degree of hypoxia than in patients without such defects. Even in cases of shock, in which tissue oxygen delivery is obviously inadequate, decreased portal blood flow and reduced hepatic clearance of lactate contribute to the acidosis. Similarly, in sepsis there is a decrease in both tissue perfusion and in the ability to use oxygen. Therefore, this division based solely on cause is largely of historic and conceptual interest.

The presence of lactic acidosis is considered a poor prognostic sign. Studies have found that as lactate levels increase above 4 mmol/L, the probability of survival decreases precipitously; however, it is unclear whether the blood lactate level is an independent contributor to mortality or whether it represents an epiphenomenon confounded by the severity of the patient's illness. Just as important to prognosis is the body's ability to metabolize lactate after the restoration of tissue perfusion. Patients able to reduce their lactate by half within 18 hours of resuscitation have a significantly greater chance of survival. In all likelihood, the inability to metabolize lactate is a surrogate marker for organ dysfunction.

Type A Lactic Acidosis

Lactic acidosis is commonly observed in conditions associated with inadequate oxygen delivery, such as low cardiac output, hypotension, severe anemia, and carbon monoxide poisoning. States of hypoperfusion are more prone to the accumulation of lactate than hypoxemic states. In the latter, tissue oxygenation is often preserved due to compensatory mechanisms such as increased cardiac output, augmented red blood cell production, and a reduced affinity of hemoglobin for oxygen. In all cases of type A lactic acidosis, oxygen is unavailable to the mitochondria, and pyruvate, unable to enter the tricarboxylic acid cycle, is reduced to lactate.

Type B Lactic Acidosis

Sepsis

Although sepsis is frequently associated with hypotension and, thus, type A lactic acidosis, lactic acidosis also may develop during sepsis even when oxygen delivery and tissue perfusion appear to be unimpeded. In fact, in the right clinical setting, a lactate level greater than 4 mmol/L has become a surrogate marker for severe sepsis independent of hypotension—so-called *compensated shock*. It has been postulated that in sepsis there is both an overproduction of pyruvate and an inhibition of PDH activity (the rate-limiting state in oxidative phosphorylation). Because of the increased NADH/NAD ratio, pyruvate is rapidly reduced to lactate. In septic patients with lactic acidosis, dichloroacetate, an activator of the PDH complex, lowers lactate levels significantly, suggesting that tissue oxygenation is adequate to support oxidative phosphorylation and, therefore, not the limiting factor.

Drugs

Numerous drugs and toxins can cause lactic acidosis. The biguanide derivatives phenformin and metformin are recognized causes of lactic acidosis. Phenformin was withdrawn from the US market in 1976 because of the high frequency of lactic acidosis associated with its use. Both of these agents bind to complex 1 of the mitochondrial respiratory chain, inhibiting its activity. Metformin, a newer biguanide, has a markedly lower incidence of lactic acidosis than phenformin, possibly because it is less lipid soluble and, thus, has limited ability to cross the mitochondrial membrane and bind to the mitochondrial complex. Although the incidence of lactic acidosis is rare with metformin, metformin has been shown in isolated mitochondria to inhibit the respiratory chain. Almost all reported cases of metformin-associated lactic acidosis have occurred in patients with underlying CKD due to reduced kidney clearance. Lactic acidosis is extremely uncommon when the drug is prescribed according to recommendations.

Lactic acidosis may occur in patients with human immunodeficiency virus infection who are taking earlier nucleoside reverse-transcriptase inhibitors. These agents, particularly stavudine, but also zidovudine, didanosine, and lamivudine, have been associated with severe lactic acidosis, often with concomitant hepatic steatosis. Nucleoside analogues inhibit mitochondrial DNA polymerase-γ. This causes mitochondrial toxicity and a decrease in oxidative phosphorylation, resulting in lipid accumulation within the liver and in decreased oxidation of pyruvate. Of note, hyperlactatemia without frank lactic acidosis is often present in patients on these medications. What converts these mild elevations in lactate levels into frank lactic acidosis is not known.

Salicylate intoxication often produces lactic acidosis. This occurs both because the salicylate-induced respiratory alkalosis stimulates lactate production and because of the inhibitory effects of salicylates on oxidative metabolism. Ethanol ingestion may cause mild elevations in lactate levels from impaired hepatic conversion of lactate to glucose. In addition, the metabolism of ethanol increases the NADH/NAD ratio, favoring the conversion of pyruvate to lactate. Concomitant thiamine deficiency, as is often seen in alcohol abusers, may exacerbate the acidosis.

Linezolid, an oxazolidinone antibiotic approved for use against methicillin- and vancomycin-resistant gram-positive organisms, has been reported to be associated with lactic acidosis. The presumed mechanism is mitochondrial toxicity. Infusions of high-dose propofol have also been associated with lactic acidosis.

Vitamin Deficiencies

Deficiency of thiamine, a cofactor for PDH, can also result in lactic acidosis. Patients requiring total parenteral nutrition may develop thiamine deficiency if not supplemented with this vitamin. During a national shortage of parenteral vitamin preparations, numerous cases of lactic acidosis were reported from inadequate thiamine supplementation.

Systemic Disease

Diabetes is often associated with lactic acidosis. Even under basal conditions, patients with diabetes have mildly elevated lactate levels. This is thought to be secondary to decreased PDH activity caused by free fatty acid oxidation by liver and muscle. Lactate increases even more during diabetic ketoacidosis (DKA), possibly secondary to decreased hepatic clearance. This accumulation of lactate contributes to the elevated AG present in ketoacidosis.

Malignancy

Lactic acidosis has been detected in patients with a variety of aggressive malignancies. Lactate levels usually parallel disease activity. Rapidly proliferating cells have a high rate of anaerobic glycolysis (so-called *Warburg effect*) producing excessive amounts of lactate. In addition, tumors often outgrow their blood supply, necessitating these under-perfused cells to rely on anaerobic metabolism for energy. Another cause of lactic acidosis with

malignancies is a decrease in hepatic lactate metabolism secondary to liver dysfunction from metastases.

Alternate Sugars

The use of sorbitol or fructose as irrigants during prostate surgery or in tube feedings can cause lactic acidosis. The metabolism of these sugars consumes ATP, inhibiting gluconeogenesis and stimulating glycolysis, leading to the accumulation of excess lactate.

Propylene Glycol

Propylene glycol is a common vehicle for many drugs, including topical silver sulfadiazine and intravenous preparations of nitroglycerin, diazepam, lorazepam, phenytoin, etomidate, and trimethoprim-sulfamethoxazole, among others. In addition, because of its better safety profile, newer formulations of antifreeze also contain propylene glycol. Although it is considered relatively safe, many case reports indicate toxicity. Approximately 40% to 50% of administered propylene glycol is oxidized by alcohol dehydrogenase to both D-lactic acid and L-lactic acid. Toxic patients commonly develop an unexplained AG acidosis with increased serum osmolality. Considering that patients receiving many of the medications solubilized with propylene glycol frequently have other possible causes for their acidosis, it is important to be aware of this iatrogenic cause for the acidosis. Correction of the metabolic abnormalities quickly occurs following discontinuation of the medication.

D-Lactic Acidosis

This unusual form of AG acidosis is the result of the accumulation of the D-isomer of lactate. Unlike the lactate produced by glycolysis in animals, which is the L-isomer, colonic bacteria produce both the L-isomer and the D-isomer. Overproduction of D-lactate occurs in patients with short-bowel syndrome and is usually precipitated by a high carbohydrate intake. Increased delivery of carbohydrates due to the shortened bowel and an overgrowth of bacteria is responsible for this overproduction. Mammalian clearance of D-lactate is far less efficient than that of L-lactate, and, with increased production within the gut, D-lactate accumulates within the blood. Because D-lactate is not detected on the routine assay that measures only L-lactate, diagnosis requires a high clinical suspicion. Patients typically present with mental status changes, ataxia, and nystagmus. Treatment consists of an oral fast with intravenous nutrition and restoration of gut flora to normal through the administration of oral antibiotics. In severe cases, hemodialysis can decrease the concentration of D-lactate.

Treatment of Lactic Acidosis

The treatment of lactic acidosis is fraught with controversy. The most important step is addressing the underlying cause. In sepsis, restoring oxygenation with mechanical ventilation and perfusion with intravenous fluids and vasopressors or inotropes are of paramount importance, although these interventions do not always improve the lactic acidosis. In some patients with medication-induced lactic acidosis, withdrawal of the offending agent may be sufficient. There are anecdotal case reports of successful use of riboflavin or L-carnitine to treat lactic acidosis associated with nucleoside analogues.

Often these measures fail, and clinicians are faced with the decision of whether to give sodium bicarbonate in an effort to increase serum pH. There are several potential problems with this approach. First, as previously discussed, it is not clear to what extent acidosis is deleterious and, therefore, whether normalizing pH is of any benefit. Also, increasing pH may actually increase lactic acid production. Sodium bicarbonate is often given as a hypertonic solution, which can lead to hypernatremia and cellular dehydration. Perhaps most important is the possibility that the administration of HCO_3^- can cause a paradoxic decrease in intracellular pH despite an increase in extracellular pH. Bicarbonate combines with hydrogen, forming carbonic acid, which is then converted to CO_2 and water. pCO_2 increases with the titration of acid by bicarbonate and rapidly diffuses into cells, causing acidification, while bicarbonate remains extracellular.

In a study of critically ill patients with metabolic acidosis and a pH < 7.20, increasing the pH to > 7.3 with a sodium bicarbonate infusion did not improve survival. However, in a subgroup of subjects with stage 2 or 3 acute kidney injury (AKI), raising the pH improved both survival and decreased the need for kidney replacement therapy. Thus, except possibly in patients with stage 2 or 3 AKI, it is difficult to recommend the use of bicarbonate for the treatment of a low serum pH alone. If the serum pH is less than 7.1, however, many clinicians, despite the lack of supporting data, opt for treatment because a further small decline in serum bicarbonate can have a profound effect on serum pH.

Other buffers may be better tolerated insofar as they buffer hydrogen ions without increasing CO_2. One such buffer is trishydroxymethyl aminomethane (THAM), a biologically inert amino acid that can buffer both CO_2 and protons. It does not lead to production of CO_2 and, thus, works well in a closed system. Because of side effects including hyperkalemia, hypoglycemia, ventilatory depression, and hepatic necrosis in neonates and no clear evidence of benefit, THAM is no longer available in the US.

Dichloroacetate has also been used in the treatment of lactic acidosis. This agent stimulates the activity of PDH, increasing the rate of pyruvate oxidation and thereby decreasing lactate levels. A large multicenter trial in humans showed a reduction in serum lactate, an increase in pH, and an increase in the number of patients able to resolve their hyperlactatemia. Despite these favorable changes, no improvement in hemodynamic parameters or mortality was found.

Various modes of kidney replacement therapy have been used in the treatment of lactic acidosis. Standard bicarbonate hemodialysis treats acidosis primarily by diffusion of bicarbonate from the bath into the blood and is, thus, another form of bicarbonate administration, albeit with several advantages. Hypernatremia and volume overload are not a concern with bicarbonate administered via hemodialysis. Unfortunately, there are no randomized, prospective trials demonstrating the benefit of dialysis in lactic acidosis, and its use in the absence of other indications cannot be routinely recommended.

Several studies have shown that high-volume hemofiltration using either lactate or bicarbonate-buffered replacement fluid can rapidly correct metabolic acidosis. These studies have been small, and the degree and type of acidosis have been poorly characterized. In addition, other treatment measures have usually been instituted, making it difficult to draw conclusions about the effectiveness of this treatment. Nevertheless, hemofiltration remains a potential therapeutic option.

Peritoneal dialysis has also been used in the treatment of metabolic acidosis. Although there are case reports of success using this modality, a randomized study comparing lactate-buffered peritoneal dialysis with continuous hemofiltration showed that hemofiltration corrected acidosis more quickly and more effectively than peritoneal dialysis. Whether newer bicarbonate-buffered peritoneal dialysis solutions will be more efficacious remains unknown.

Diabetic Ketoacidosis

DKA is another common cause of an AG acidosis. Although DKA may be the initial presentation of diabetes mellitus, more commonly patients have a known diagnosis of diabetes and either have been nonadherent with their insulin regimen or have a precipitating factor such as infection. Patients generally have polyuria and polydipsia, but polyuria may not be seen if volume depletion becomes severe enough. Although DKA is classically seen in type 1 diabetes, it can also occur in patients with type 2 diabetes. DKA results from insulin deficiency and concomitant increase in counterregulatory hormones such as glucagon, epinephrine, and cortisol. This hormonal milieu leads to an inability of cells to use glucose, causing them to oxidize fatty acids as fuel and produce large amounts of keto acids. A diagnosis of DKA requires a pH less than 7.35, elevated AG, positive serum ketones of at least 1:2 dilutions, and decreased serum bicarbonate. However, not all patients with DKA meet these criteria. If kidney perfusion and glomerular filtration rate (GFR) are well maintained, ketones (anions) are rapidly excreted by the kidney in place of chloride. With the loss of these anions in the urine, the AG acidosis may be replaced by a mixed AG/hyperchloremic acidosis or even a pure hyperchloremic acidosis. Furthermore, an increase in the NADH/NAD ratio, which frequently occurs during DKA, causes ketones to shift from acetoacetate to β-hydroxybutyrate, which is not detected on the standard nitroprusside test used to identify serum and urinary ketones. If this occurs, serum ketones may appear to be negative or only trace positive. Finally, vomiting may result in a metabolic alkalosis, which would raise the serum bicarbonate toward the normal range. In this case, the serum AG would almost certainly be elevated, and the astute clinician will not be fooled.

In addition, although glucose levels are usually elevated in patients with DKA, patients with DKA on sodium-glucose transport-2 inhibitors may present with glucose levels below 200 mg/dL.

Treatment

The treatment of DKA consists of three parts: fluid resuscitation, insulin administration, and correction of potassium deficits. Patients with DKA often have profound deficits of both sodium and free water. Hypovolemia, as demonstrated by hemodynamic compromise, should always be treated first. Patients should rapidly receive 0.9% saline or a balanced salt solution until their blood pressure is stabilized. Thereafter, hypotonic fluids in the form of 0.45% saline should be administered to correct free water deficits while continuing to provide volume. Insulin should be administered only after fluid resuscitation is well under way. If insulin is given precipitously, the rapid uptake of glucose by the cells will cause water to follow because of the fall in extracellular osmolality, potentially resulting in cardiovascular collapse. A continuous regular insulin infusion of 0.1 units/kg/h is given; use of an initial bolus of 0.1 unit/kg is controversial. If the glucose does not decline by 50 to 100 mg/dL/h, the infusion should be increased by 50%. As tissue perfusion improves, β-hydroxybutyrate is converted to acetoacetate, and serum ketones paradoxically increase before then decreasing. Serum glucose usually approaches normal before ketosis is resolved. When the serum glucose concentration is less than 250 mg/dL, 5% dextrose should be added to the intravenous fluids to avoid hypoglycemia while awaiting resolution of ketosis.

The insulin infusion should be continued until the AG closes, the HCO_3^- rises above 14 mmol/L, and the patient is taking food orally. Although the ADA recommends continuing the insulin infusion until the HCO_3^- is greater than 18 mmol/L, regeneration of HCO_3^- may take up to 24 hours after the termination of ketogenesis, and this is not hastened by insulin. A subcutaneous insulin dose should be given at least 1 hour before stopping the drip to avoid rebound ketosis.

Most patients with DKA have total-body potassium depletion. Nevertheless, their serum potassium may be normal to high because of a shift out of the cells caused by the hyperglycemia-induced hyperosmolality and the insulinopenia. When insulin is restored, extracellular potassium is rapidly taken up by cells and severe hypokalemia may ensue. Therefore, the addition of potassium to the intravenous fluids is recommended at a concentration of 10 to 20 mEq/L as soon as serum potassium falls below 4.5 mEq/L. Needless to say, this management algorithm requires frequent laboratory tests.

Although bicarbonate therapy has been used in severe DKA, this use is not supported by the literature. In fact, bicarbonate administration, even in patients with pH less than 7.0, has not been shown to be advantageous. In almost all cases, the acidosis rapidly improves with appropriate management without the use of bicarbonate. Thus, the administration of sodium bicarbonate to patients with DKA cannot be routinely recommended. It is important, however, that these patients be monitored in a setting where they can be closely observed and where frequent analyses of their arterial blood gases and electrolytes can be obtained.

Alcoholic Ketoacidosis

Alcoholic ketoacidosis (AKA) usually presents with an AG acidosis and ketonemia but without significant hyperglycemia. The classic presentation is that of a patient who has been on an alcohol binge, develops nausea and vomiting, and stops eating. The patient typically presents 24 to 48 hours after the cessation of oral intake and may complain of abdominal pain and shortness of breath. Alcohol levels are low or even unmeasurable by the time AKA develops. AKA is similar to DKA in that it is a state of insulinopenia and increased counterregulatory hormones; in fact, the levels of these hormones are similar in both disorders. In AKA, normoglycemia to hypoglycemia is usually observed despite a hormonal milieu favoring hyperglycemia, because decreased NAD curtails hepatic gluconeogenesis and starvation depletes glycogen stores. Patients with AKA, however, can occasionally present with hyperglycemia, and distinguishing it from DKA in those cases can be difficult. AKA almost always presents with an expanded AG, but acidemia is less universal. Patients often have concurrent metabolic alkalosis from vomiting or respiratory alkalosis from liver disease. Thus, patients with AKA may not be acidemic and rarely do they have a simple metabolic acidosis. Because of the increased NADH/NAD ratio, the primary keto acid present is β-hydroxybutyrate; therefore, serum ketones may be reported as negative. This ratio also favors the formation of lactic acid. Finally, electrolyte disorders, including hypokalemia, hypophosphatemia, and hypomagnesemia, are common.

Treatment

Therapy of AKA is straightforward and consists of volume repletion, provision of glucose (except in those patients with hyperglycemia), and correction of any electrolyte abnormalities. Patients are often volume depleted from vomiting combined with poor oral intake. Thiamine must be provided before or concurrently with glucose to avoid precipitating Wernicke encephalopathy. Acidosis resolves as insulin increases, and counterregulatory hormones are turned off in response to glucose infusion. The clinician must maintain a high degree of suspicion for AKA, as the acid-base disturbance may be subtle on routine laboratory analyses, with patients often demonstrating an elevated AG as the only abnormality. Chronic alcoholics often have hypoalbuminemia, which can further obscure the interpretation of the AG. Any patient with nausea and vomiting with a recent history of alcohol abuse should probably be treated for presumptive AKA until the diagnosis is clearly ruled out.

Starvation Ketosis

During prolonged fasting, insulin levels are suppressed, whereas glucagon, epinephrine, growth hormone, and cortisol levels are increased. This hormonal milieu results in increased lipolysis, with release of free fatty acids into the blood and stimulation of hepatic ketogenesis. The concentrations of both β-hydroxybutyrate and acetoacetate increase over the course of several weeks, resulting in a mild AG metabolic acidosis.

Toxins and Drugs

Ethylene Glycol

Ingestion of various toxins can cause severe metabolic acidosis with an increased AG and should always be suspected in these cases. Ethylene glycol is a sweet liquid often found in antifreeze. Ingestion of 100 mL or more can be fatal. Ethylene glycol is metabolized by alcohol dehydrogenase into glycolic acid and, subsequently, oxalic acid. This generates NADH, which encourages the formation of lactic acid. The AG acidosis results from the accumulation of the various acid metabolites of ethylene glycol as well as a lactic acidosis. Diagnosis can be difficult because ethylene glycol is not detected on routine toxicology assays. It should be suspected in anyone who presents with intoxication, a low blood alcohol, and a markedly increased AG metabolic acidosis without ketonemia. The serum osmolar gap may help detect ethylene glycol. The serum osmolar gap is the difference between the calculated serum osmolarity $[([Na^+] \times 2) + (glucose/18) + (BUN/2.8)]$ and the actual serum osmolality as measured by the laboratory. A difference of greater than 10 to 15 mOsm/kg suggests the presence of an unmeasured, osmotically active substance, which, in the right clinical setting, could be a toxin. However, it is important to understand the limitations of this approach. Some laboratories measure serum osmolality using the vapor pressure method rather than the freezing point depression, and volatile substances such as alcohols may not be detected. As the osmotically active alcohol is metabolized into the various acids, the osmolar gap disappears. Thus, early after ingestion, the osmolar gap is elevated without a significant increase in the AG. As the alcohol is metabolized, the osmolar gap decreases while the AG increases. Examination of the urine may reveal calcium oxalate crystals, a finding that can be considered pathognomonic. However, the absence of these crystals does not rule out the ingestion of ethylene glycol. Precipitation of calcium oxalate may occasionally cause hypocalcemia. Because fluorescein is added as a colorant to antifreeze, the urine of a patient with antifreeze ingestion may fluoresce under a Wood lamp.

Methanol

Methanol is an alcohol often found in solvents or as an adulterant in alcoholic beverages. Toxicity is usually caused by ingestion of as little as 30 mL but has also been reported after inhalation. Methanol is metabolized by alcohol dehydrogenase to formaldehyde and then to formic acid, resulting in an elevated AG acidosis. As with ingestions of other alcohols, NAD depletion favors the production of lactate. Methanol is less intoxicating than either ethanol or ethylene glycol. The most characteristic symptom of methanol toxicity is blurry vision. Blindness may occur due to optic nerve involvement, and pancreatitis may be seen in up to two-thirds of patients. As described previously, early after ingestion an osmolar gap may be found. The diagnosis of both ethylene glycol and methanol poisoning can be confirmed by specific toxicologic assays, but treatment should never be delayed while awaiting these results.

Treatment of Toxic Alcohol Ingestions

Treatment of both ethylene glycol and methanol toxicity is based on the fact that it is the metabolites of these alcohols that are actually harmful. Both substances are metabolized by alcohol dehydrogenase. Blocking the activity of this enzyme will prevent the metabolic acidosis and allow the alcohol to be excreted by the kidneys or removed by dialysis. Because alcohol dehydrogenase has a much higher affinity for ethanol than for either ethylene glycol or methanol, use of ethanol as a competitive inhibitor was the traditional treatment but is now rarely used. Fomepizole (4-methylpyrazole), a competitive inhibitor of alcohol dehydrogenase, has replaced ethanol as the treatment of choice. Fomepizole is a more potent inhibitor of alcohol dehydrogenase than ethanol and does not lead to central nervous system (CNS) depression. An initial loading dose of 15 mg/kg body weight is followed by 10 mg/kg every 12 hours for four doses, and then 15 mg/kg every 12 hours for four more doses. Although fomepizole, because of its potency, has begun to call into question the need for dialysis, until more studies are available it is recommended that dialysis be instituted in all patients with suspected ingestions of ethylene glycol or methanol who have end organ damage (kidney failure or visual impairment) and whose pH is less than 7.2. Both compounds can be rapidly removed by hemodialysis. Hemodialysis can also help improve the acidosis by providing a source of bicarbonate. It is important to increase the dose of fomepizole while a patient is receiving hemodialysis. For either ingestion, gastric lavage with charcoal should be performed when ingestion has occurred within the preceding 2 to 3 hours.

Salicylate Toxicity

The ingestion of salicylates is an important cause of mixed acid-base disturbances, producing both a respiratory alkalosis (salicylate is a direct respiratory stimulant) and a metabolic acidosis. Metabolic acidosis results from the accumulation of both lactic and keto acids. Salicylic acid, by itself, accounts for only a small quantity of the acid load. The common presenting sign of salicylate toxicity is tachypnea. The patient may also complain of tinnitus with serum concentrations of salicylic acid of 20 to 45 mg/dL or higher. Other CNS manifestations are agitation, seizures, and even coma. Both noncardiogenic pulmonary edema and upper gastrointestinal bleeding may occur. Hypoglycemia occurs in children but is rare in adults. Other symptoms include nausea, vomiting, and hyperpyrexia.

In the setting of salicylate overdose, peak serum concentrations are achieved 4 to 6 hours after ingestion. The severity of the ingestion can be predicted by the Done nomogram, which plots the toxic salicylate level at varying time points following ingestion. This nomogram cannot be used with chronic ingestions or with the ingestion of enteric-coated aspirin. The treatment of salicylate toxicity consists of supportive care, removal of unabsorbed compounds using charcoal lavage, administration of bicarbonate, and, if necessary, hemodialysis. Because the dissociation constant (pK) of salicylic acid is 3.0, alkalinization keeps the drug in its polar dissociated form, preventing diffusion into the CNS. In addition, because tissue salicylic acid is in equilibrium with the nondissociated compound in the plasma, alkalinization also decreases tissue levels. Concurrent alkalinization of the urine traps salicylate in the tubule, promoting its excretion. Hemodialysis is indicated in all patients with altered mental status, kidney failure that causes a decrease in kidney excretion, volume overload that prevents the administration of bicarbonate, or salicylate levels greater than 100 mg/dL.

Pyroglutamic Acidosis

It is increasingly recognized that glutathione depletion can cause an AG acidosis. This underreported acidosis occurs in patients who often have underlying infections and are treated with acetaminophen, even at therapeutic doses. Glutathione depletion decreases the negative feedback inhibition on γ-glutamylcysteine synthetase, resulting in an increase in pyroglutamic acid (5-oxoproline). Measurement of urine 5-oxoproline levels will confirm the diagnosis. Treatment is aimed at the underlying disease and discontinuation of the acetaminophen. In severe cases, N-acetylcysteine can be considered.

Kidney Failure

Kidney failure is a well-recognized cause of metabolic acidosis. With the reduction in nephron mass that occurs in CKD, there is decreased ammoniagenesis in the proximal tubule. Many patients with diminished kidney function may also have specific acidification defects in the form of a renal tubular acidosis (RTA). As the GFR declines, the kidney is unable to excrete the daily production of fixed acid. Serum bicarbonate may begin to decline when the GFR falls below 40 mL/min/1.73 m^2.

The acidosis of kidney failure is associated with either a normal AG or an elevated AG. With mild to moderate reductions in GFR, the anions that comprise the gap are excreted normally, and the acidosis reflects decreased ammoniagenesis and is, therefore, hyperchloremic. As kidney failure worsens, the kidney loses its ability to filter and excrete various anions, and the accumulation of sulfate, phosphate, urate, and other anions produces an elevated AG. With better control of phosphorus and more intensive dietary modifications, many patients initiating kidney replacement therapy may not manifest an AG.

Despite daily net positive acid balance, it is unusual for HCO_3^- to fall below 15 mmol/L. Why the acidosis of CKD is rarely severe is unclear. Whether this lack of severity is secondary to buffering of the retained protons in bone or retention of organic anions usually lost in the urine that are instead subsequently converted to HCO_3^- is controversial. The buffering of protons by bone results in the loss of calcium and negative calcium balance. In addition, chronic acidosis causes protein breakdown, muscle wasting, and negative nitrogen balance. In addition to improving muscle and bone health, several studies have shown that maintaining HCO_3^- levels at 22 mEq/L or higher also slows the progression of chronic kidney disease.

The metabolic acidosis commonly found in patients with CKD can easily be corrected with oral bicarbonate. Usually two 650-mg (7.8 mEq) tablets 3 times a day will keep the serum bicarbonate in the normal range. Although not yet approved for use, veverimer, a polymer that binds protons, can increase HCO_3^- without supplying a sodium load. It is rare that hemodialysis has to be initiated solely for the purpose of correcting acidosis.

Hyperchloremic Metabolic Acidosis

Acidosis associated with a normal AG, HCMA, has a limited number of causes (Fig. 13.6). HCMA can occur in CKD when reduced ammoniagenesis impairs the kidney's ability to excrete the daily acid load. In individuals with normal or near-normal kidney function, it can be divided into cases caused by the kidney's failure to reabsorb HCO_3^- or secrete the daily fixed load of H^+, commonly known as *RTA*, and cases in which kidney acid-base handling is normal. In contrast to AG acidosis, most cases of HCMA are easily treated with supplemental base.

Kidney Causes of Hyperchloremic Metabolic Acidosis

RTAs represent a heterogeneous cause of HCMA in which the kidney is unable to maintain acid-base balance, despite normal or near-normal GFR. There is often confusion regarding the RTAs because no standard nomenclature exists, numerous diverse transport defects have been identified, and the literature often presents contradictory information. A grasp of the underlying pathophysiology makes the approach to these disorders more comprehensible. The RTAs can be divided into four major categories: (1) primary defects in ammoniagenesis, (2) hypoaldosteronism, (3) disorders of the proximal tubule, and (4) disorders of the distal tubule (see Fig. 13.6). The distal tubule defects can be further divided into those with hypokalemia and those with hyperkalemia (Fig. 13.7).

Defective Ammoniagenesis

One of the most common causes of an HCMA is the inability of the kidney to generate ammonia because of CKD. By definition, *RTA* refers to a specific acid excretory defect occurring despite the

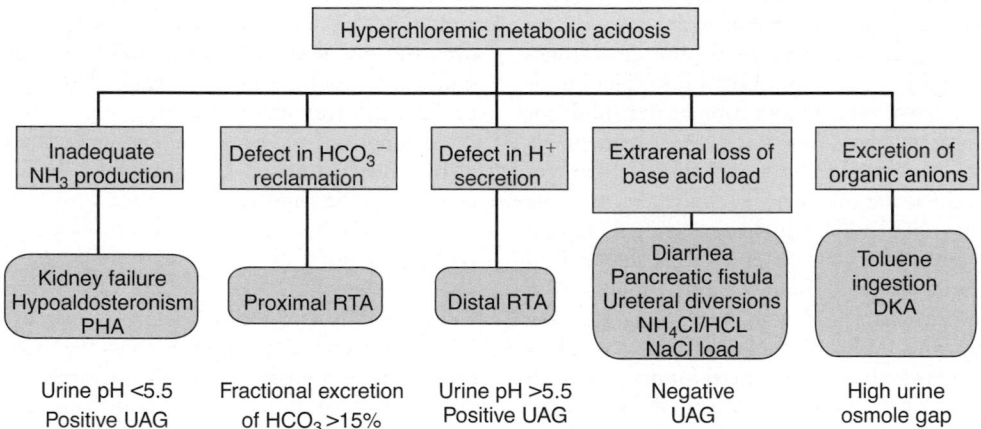

• **Fig. 13.6** The etiology of hyperchloremic metabolic acidosis. Shown at the bottom are useful diagnostic tools. *DKA,* Diabetic ketoacidosis; *PHA,* pseudohypoaldosteronism; *RTA,* renal tubular acidosis; *UAG,* urine anion gap.

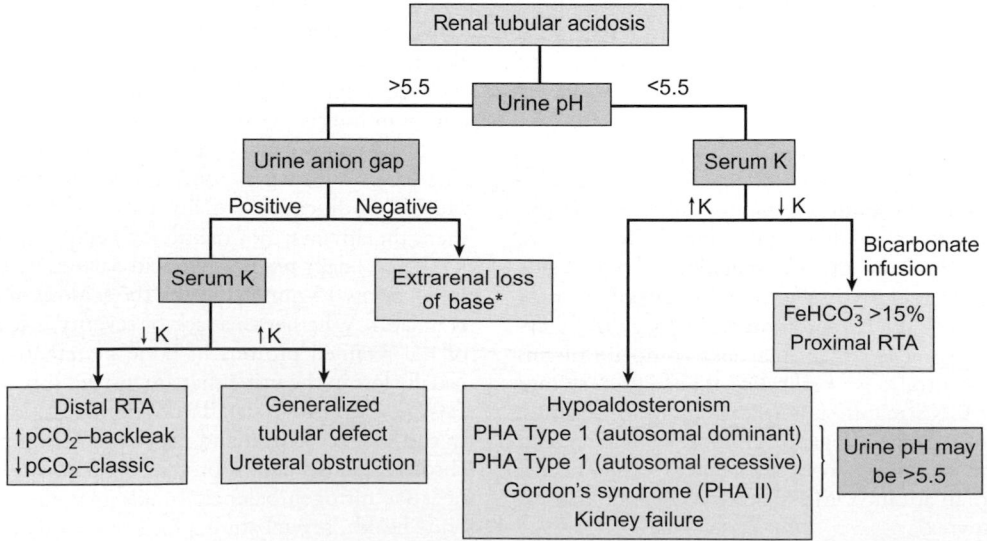

• **Fig. 13.7** Evaluation of renal tubular acidosis. *FeHCO3⁻,* Fractional excretion of bicarbonate; *PHA,* pseudohypoaldosteronism; *RTA,* renal tubular acidosis. Note that extrarenal loss of base is not a form of renal tubular acidosis.

presence of normal or near-normal kidney function. Thus, it bears emphasis that the HCMA of CKD is not classified as an RTA. As the number of nephrons decreases with CKD, there is a proportional decrease in the production of ammonia. As mentioned previously, when GFR falls below 40 mL/min/1.73 m^2, the kidney is less able to excrete the daily acid load and HCO$_3^-$ begins to decline with a concomitant increase in the serum Cl$^-$, producing HCMA. Only when the GFR falls below 15 to 20 mL/min/1.73 m^2 does the kidney lose the ability to excrete anions, thus converting this HCMA into an AG acidosis. It must be stressed that the acidosis in kidney failure, whether manifested by hyperchloremia or an AG, is primarily caused by defective ammoniagenesis. As such, the UAG will be positive because of the decrease in ammonia excretion, while urine pH will be less than 5.5.

Hypoaldosteronism

Primary and secondary hypoaldosteronism are common disorders causing hyperkalemia and metabolic acidosis (Table 13.4). Hyporeninemic hypoaldosteronism (type IV RTA) is the most frequently encountered variety of this disorder. This disorder is usually seen in patients with diabetes and mild CKD. The precise cause of hyporeninemia has not been clearly defined. The finding that hypertension is frequently present and that the disorder may be partly reversed with chronic furosemide use suggests that renin suppression may be secondary to chronic volume overload. The cause of the hypoaldosteronism has also not been fully explained. Renin suppression alone should not cause hypoaldosteronism, because hyperkalemia is an independent potent stimulus of aldosterone secretion, and anephric individuals still secrete aldosterone. The acidosis is primarily caused by decreased ammoniagenesis as a result of the associated hyperkalemia induced by the aldosterone deficiency. Hypoaldosteronism, by diminishing distal sodium reabsorption, also results in a less negative lumen potential, thus decreasing the rate of H$^+$ secretion but not the electromotive force of the pump. Because the hydrogen pump is not defective, urine pH is usually less than 5.5.

Patients with type IV RTA are usually asymptomatic, with only minor laboratory abnormalities (mild hyperkalemia and decreased HCO$_3^-$). However, when kidney potassium handling is further perturbed by various stressors (including sodium depletion, which decreases the delivery of sodium to the distal tubule; a high-potassium diet; and potassium-sparing diuretics or medications that further decrease renin and aldosterone levels, such as angiotensin-converting enzyme inhibitors, angiotensin receptor blockers, nonsteroidal antiinflammatory drugs, or heparin), marked hyperkalemia ensues with a decline in ammoniagenesis. Most patients can be treated by removing the insult to potassium homeostasis, restricting potassium intake, increasing potassium excretion using

a diuretic, and, if necessary, providing supplemental bicarbonate. Proving that type IV RTA is present requires the demonstration of low renin and aldosterone levels after sodium depletion. Because of practical considerations, these tests are rarely ordered and most patients are treated empirically.

Autosomal dominant pseudohypoaldosteronism (PHA) type I is an uncommon disorder caused by a mutation in the kidney mineralocorticoid receptor, resulting in decreased affinity for aldosterone. This genetic disorder presents in childhood with hyperaldosteronism, hyperkalemia, metabolic acidosis, salt wasting, and hypotension. Autosomal dominant PHA type I becomes less severe with age. Carbenoxolone and glycyrrhizic acid (found in true licorice) both inhibit 11-β-hydroxysteroid dehydrogenase, the enzyme in the kidney that converts cortisol, which binds the mineralocorticoid receptor, to cortisone, which does not bind. They can be used to treat this disorder by increasing the intrarenal supply of mineralocorticoid.

Proximal Renal Tubular Acidosis

Proximal RTA, often called *type II RTA* (because it was the second type described), is a defect in the ability of the proximal tubule to reclaim filtered HCO$_3^-$ (Table 13.5). In type II RTA, the proximal tubule has a diminished threshold (approximately 15 mmol/L instead of the normal 24 mmol/L) for HCO$_3^-$ reabsorption. When plasma HCO$_3^-$ falls below this threshold, complete reabsorption occurs. Proximal RTA can be congenital or acquired and may exist as an isolated defect in HCO$_3^-$ reabsorption or as part of a more generalized transport defect known as *Fanconi syndrome,* in which there is diminished reabsorption of other solutes across the proximal tubule. Patients with Fanconi syndrome, in addition to the loss of HCO$_3^-$, inappropriately excrete amino acids, glucose, phosphorus, and uric acid in their urine.

As would be expected, mutations in the Na$^+$-H$^+$ exchanger on the luminal membrane, the Na$^+$-HCO$_3^-$ cotransporter on the basolateral membrane, and cytosolic carbonic anhydrase have all been implicated in the isolated hereditary and sporadic forms of proximal RTA. Several drugs that block carbonic anhydrase, including the diuretic acetazolamide and the anticonvulsant topiramate, also cause isolated HCO$_3^-$ wasting. Proximal RTA with Fanconi syndrome is frequently found in patients with cystinosis,

---

TABLE 13.4 Hypoaldosteronism

Primary
- Addison disease
- Congenital enzyme defects
- Drugs
  - Heparin
  - Angiotensin converting enzyme inhibitors
  - Angiotensin receptor blockers

Hyporeninemic hypoaldosteronism (type IV RTA)

Pseudohypoaldosteronism I (autosomal dominant)—mineralocorticoid resistance

---

TABLE 13.5 Causes of Proximal Renal Tubular Acidosis

Isolated defects in HCO$_3^-$ reabsorption
- Carbonic anhydrase inhibitors
  - Acetazolamide
  - Topiramate
  - Sulfamylon
- Carbonic anhydrase deficiency

Generalized defects in proximal tubular transport
- Cystinosis
- Wilson disease
- Lowe syndrome
- Galactosemia
- Multiple myeloma
- Light chain disease
- Amyloidosis
- Vitamin D deficiency
- Ifosfamide
- Cidofovir
- Lead
- Aminoglycosides

Wilson disease, Lowe syndrome, multiple myeloma, and light chain disease, among others. A decrease in ATP production, which reduces basolateral Na^+/K^+-ATPase activity, is the presumed etiology of this global transport defect. Drugs, particularly the cyclophosphamide analogue ifosfamide and cidofovir, used in the treatment of cytomegalovirus, are associated with a generalized proximal tubulopathy.

Because distal H^+ excretion is normal, urine pH during steady state, when the HCO_3^- is below the lowered threshold and bicarbonaturia is absent, will be less than 5.5. At this time, the serum HCO_3^- will be between 15 and 18 mEq/L. It is important to recognize that whenever the HCO_3^- increases above the reabsorptive threshold, HCO_3^- will appear in the urine and the pH will be greater than 6.5. Although ammoniagenesis is preserved in proximal RTA, direct or indirect measurement of urine NH_4^+ may reveal an inappropriately low excretion. This can occur because HCO_3^-, which escapes proximal reabsorption, serves as a buffer sink for secreted H^+, thus reducing the trapping of NH_4^+. The diagnosis of proximal RTA is established by demonstrating a fractional excretion of HCO_3^- greater than 15% while supplemental bicarbonate is administered in an attempt to increase the serum bicarbonate to normal.

Treatment of proximal RTA is difficult because the administered base is rapidly excreted in the urine, and extremely large amounts of base (10 to 15 mmol/kg/day) are frequently required. The increased delivery of HCO_3^- to the distal nephron induces or exacerbates hypokalemia. It is recommended that frequent doses of a mixture of Na^+ and K^+ salts of bicarbonate and citrate be used.

Distal Renal Tubular Acidosis

Classic Distal Renal Tubular Acidosis With Hypokalemia

Distal RTA, also known as *type I RTA,* represents the inability of the distal tubule to acidify the urine (Table 13.6). As with proximal RTA, the distal variety can be congenital or acquired. Abnormalities have been identified in both the luminal H^+-ATPase and the basolateral Cl^--HCO_3^- exchanger. The acquired form is associated with autoimmune diseases, especially systemic lupus and Sjögren syndrome, dysproteinemia, and kidney transplant rejection. Immunocytochemical studies have revealed decreased staining of the H^+-ATPase and Cl^--HCO_3^- exchanger in patients with the acquired form of distal RTA. Ifosfamide, which is also

associated with a proximal RTA, can cause a distal defect. Amphotericin, which creates pores in membranes forming ion channels, causes a distal RTA by allowing the back leak of protons across the luminal membrane. The classic finding in type I RTA is an inappropriately high urine pH (greater than 5.5).

Because H^+ secretion is defective in distal RTA, less NH_4^+ can be trapped in the lumen of the tubule, and the UAG will be positive, reflecting this decrease in NH_4^+ excretion. Besides having an inappropriately high urine pH and a positive UAG, distal RTA can be further characterized by measuring urine pCO_2 during an HCO_3^- infusion. Distal delivery of HCO_3^- in the presence of a normal H^+ secretory capacity results in elevated pCO_2 in the urine. When there is a H^+ secretory defect, urine pCO_2 will not increase. As would be expected, in amphotericin-induced RTA when H^+ ion secretion is unaffected, urine pCO_2 increases normally. Occasionally, it may be difficult to distinguish HCMA induced by diarrhea from a distal RTA. Diarrhea results in HCMA and hypokalemia. Because the hypokalemia increases kidney ammoniagenesis, urine pH may be inappropriately elevated. Thus, on the surface, both forms of acidosis appear similar. Measurement of the UAG will easily distinguish the markedly elevated urine NH_4^+ with its negative UAG found in diarrheal illness from the low NH_4^+ excretion and positive UAG found with distal RTA. The one caveat is that sodium must be delivered to the distal tubule, as shown by urine Na^+ above 20 mmol/L.

Classic distal RTA is associated with hypokalemia (due to augmented distal K^+ secretion in lieu of H^+ secretion in exchange for Na^+ reabsorption), hypocitraturia (from augmented proximal tubule cell reabsorption), hypercalciuria (from the buffering of H^+ in bone and loss of calcium), and nephrocalcinosis. The treatment of distal RTA is simply to supply enough base (2 to 3 mmol/kg/day) to counter the daily fixed production of acid. This can be administered as a mixture of sodium and potassium salts of either bicarbonate or citrate.

Distal Renal Tubular Acidosis With Hyperkalemia

Although many textbooks place distal RTA with hyperkalemia under the rubric of type IV RTA (hyporenin-hypoaldosteronism), it is more appropriate to call it distal RTA with hyperkalemia because it has a pathophysiology that differs from type IV RTA. This disorder can be further divided into two broad, general categories: (1) a generalized defect of both distal tubular H^+ and K^+ secretion or (2) a primary defect in Na^+ transport, often called a "voltage defect" (Table 13.7).

TABLE 13.6	**Causes of Distal Renal Tubular Acidosis With Hypokalemia**

Familial
- Defective HCO_3^--Cl^- exchanger (autosomal dominant)
- Defective H^+-ATPase (autosomal recessive)

Endemic
- Thai endemic distal renal tubular acidosis

Drugs
- Amphotericin
- Toluene
- Lithium
- Ifosfamide
- Foscarnet
- Vanadium

Systemic disorder
Sjögren syndrome
Cryoglobulinemia
Systemic lupus erythematosus
Kidney transplant rejection

TABLE 13.7	**Causes of Distal Renal Tubular Acidosis With Hyperkalemia**

Lupus nephritis
Obstructive nephropathy
Sickle cell anemia
Voltage defects
Familial
- Pseudohypoaldosteronism type I (autosomal recessive)
- Pseudohypoaldosteronism type II (autosomal recessive)—Gordon syndrome

Drugs
- Amiloride
- Triamterene
- Trimethoprim
- Pentamidine

Generalized Distal Tubule Defect. Unlike classic distal RTA, a more generalized distal tubule defect can occur in which both H^+ and K^+ secretion is impaired. This has been best identified in cases of urinary obstruction and in patients with interstitial kidney disease resulting from sickle cell anemia or systemic lupus erythematosus. In animals with urinary obstruction, immunocytochemical staining has revealed loss of the apical H^+-ATPase. Why hyperkalemia occurs is less clear. Because K^+ excretion cannot be augmented by diuretics, a primary defect in K^+ transport is likely. Similar to classic distal RTA, urine pH is greater than 5.5.

Distal Sodium Transport Defects. Several disorders have been characterized by defective sodium transport in the distal tubule. The reabsorption of Na^+ by the distal tubule generates a lumen-negative potential. This electrical negativity helps promote the secretion of K^+ and H^+. Any drug or disorder that interferes with this lumen-negative potential will diminish both K^+ and H^+ secretion. These are commonly classified as voltage defects. Autosomal recessive PHA type I is a syndrome in which there is loss of function of the epithelial sodium channel (ENaC) in the distal tubule. Numerous mutations have been described in various subunits of this channel. This disease manifests in childhood with marked hyperkalemia, metabolic acidosis, hyperaldosteronism, and salt wasting. Because the ENaC also exists in other tissue, including lung, colon, and sweat glands, patients with this disorder often have symptoms related to these organs. Treatment consists of providing a high salt intake. Drugs that block ENaC produce a similar metabolic picture. These include the potassium-sparing diuretics amiloride and triamterene, as well as trimethoprim and pentamidine.

Another well-recognized disorder of distal transport is PHA type II, also known as *Gordon syndrome* (see Chapters 37 and 65). Individuals with this condition have mild volume overload with suppressed renin and aldosterone, hypertension, hyperkalemia, and metabolic acidosis. Mutations in two members of a family of serine-threonine kinases, WNK1 and WNK4 (*With No K* [K = lysine]), cause this syndrome. These kinases appear to have an important role in the regulation of Cl^- transport in various tissues. It appears that defects in these kinases result in an increase in the number of neutral NaCl transporters (NCCT) and, thus, increase NaCl transport across the distal convoluted tubule. Less sodium is delivered to the more distal tubule segments for reabsorption, which curtails the generation of the lumen-negative potential. This results in decreased H^+ and K^+ secretion. Supporting this hypothesis is the fact that Gordon syndrome can be treated with thiazide diuretics, which block the NCCT.

The acidosis in all of these sodium transport disorders is secondary to decreased H^+ secretion caused by an unfavorable electrical gradient in the distal tubule and the decreased ammoniagenesis caused by the hyperkalemia. Whether the urine pH is less than 5.5 depends on how severely H^+ secretion is affected.

Combined Proximal and Distal Renal Tubular Acidosis

This is a very rare disorder, previously called *type III RTA*. As would be expected, both proximal HCO_3^- reabsorption and distal H^+ secretion are impaired. Mutations in the gene for cytosolic carbonic anhydrase can cause such a defect. As already discussed, ifosfamide can also cause a combined defect.

Incomplete Distal Renal Tubular Acidosis

Patients with incomplete distal RTA will come to medical attention because of calcium stone disease and nephrocalcinosis. Serum HCO_3^- is normal, but urine pH never falls below 5.5, even after acid loading with NH_4Cl or $CaCl_2$. This disorder likely represents a milder form of distal RTA. Frank metabolic acidosis may become evident when patients are stressed by diarrhea or other conditions that require compensation by augmented kidney proton secretion.

Extrarenal Causes of Hyperchloremic Metabolic Acidosis

Extrarenal Bicarbonate Loss

The loss of base during episodes of diarrhea or with the overzealous use of laxatives is associated with HCMA. Loss of HCO_3^- can also occur with pancreatic fistulae or with pancreas transplants if drainage of the pancreatic duct is into the bladder. Ureteral diversions using an isolated sigmoid loop were frequently associated with bicarbonate loss because of $Cl-HCO_3^-$ exchange across bowel mucosa. These ureteral-sigmoidostomies have largely been replaced with ureteral diversions using ileal conduits, which have less surface area and contact time for loss of HCO_3^- to occur. If these become obstructed, however, HCMA can still develop.

Acid Load

An obvious cause of an HCMA is ingestion or infusion of a chloride salt of an acid. Both NH_4Cl and $CaCl_2$ can result in a metabolic acidosis and can be used as a provocative test to assess urinary acidification. In addition, total parenteral nutrition using hydrochloric acid salts of various amino acids can produce a metabolic acidosis if an insufficient quantity of base (usually acetate) is added to the infusion mixture. Another form of acid load is NaCl. Volume resuscitation with 0.9% NaCl will often produce an HCMA. This occurs because of "dilution" of the plasma HCO_3^- by the more acidic saline solution (pH 7.0) and because volume expansion diminishes proximal HCO_3^- reabsorption.

Urinary Loss of Anions

As previously discussed, if organic anions are excreted in the urine, they represent a source of base lost from the body. Although involving the kidney, this cannot be viewed as being caused by an intrinsic kidney defect. Because of the low kidney threshold for the excretion of keto acids, patients with DKA, if able to maintain their intravascular volume or if volume resuscitated, will excrete these anions in place of Cl^-, resulting in HCMA. A similar metabolic disturbance exists after toluene exposure. Toluene is a common solvent found in paint products and glues. Exposure is generally by inhalation, either accidental or intentional. Toluene is rapidly absorbed through the skin and mucous membranes and metabolized to hippuric acid. Hippurate is quickly excreted by the kidney, leaving behind an HCMA. Although hippurate is not a base, its rapid excretion into the urine conceals the AG origins of this disturbance. Both of these disorders are usually easily discovered after taking an adequate history.

Complete bibliography is available at Elsevier eBooks for Practicing Clinicians.

Key Bibliography

Alper SL. Genetic diseases of acid-base transporters. *Annu Rev Physiol.* 2002;64:899–923.

Adrogue HJ, Madias NE. Management of life-threatening acid-base disorders. *N Engl J Med.* 1998;338:107–111 26-34.

Bonny O, Rossier B. Disturbances of Na/K balance: pseudohypoaldosteronism revisited. *J Am Soc Nephrol.* 2002;13:2399–2414.

Brent J, McMartin K, Phillips S, et al. Fomepizole for the treatment of methanol poisoning. *N Engl J Med.* 2001;344:424–429.

Carlisle EJ, Donnelly SM, Vasuvattakul S, et al. Glue-sniffing and distal renal tubular acidosis: sticking to the facts. *J Am Soc Nephrol.* 1991;1:1019–1027.

Chang CT, Chen YC, Fang JT, Huang CC. Metformin-associated lactic acidosis: case reports and literature review. *J Nephrol.* 2002;15:398–402.

Claessens YE, Cariou A, Monchi M, et al. Detecting life-threatening lactic acidosis related to nucleoside-analog treatment of human immunodeficiency virus-infected patients, and treatment with l-carnitine. *Crit Care Med.* 2003;31:1042–1047.

Dargan PI, Wallace CI, Jones AL. An evidence based flowchart to guide the management of acute salicylate (aspirin) overdose. *Emerg Med J.* 2002;19:206–209.

DuBose Jr TD, Mcdonald GA. Renal tubular acidosis. In: Dubose TD, Hamm LL Jr, eds. *Acid-Base and Electrolyte Disorders: A Companion to Brenner and Rector's The Kidney.* Philadelphia: WB Saunders; 2002:189–206.

Figge J, Jabor A, Kazda A. Anion gap and hypoalbuminemia. *Crit Care Med.* 1998;26:1807–1810.

Fraser AD. Clinical toxicologic implications of ethylene glycol and glycolic acid poisoning. *Ther Drug Monit.* 2002;24:232–238.

Han J, Kim G-H, Kim J, et al. Secretory-defect distal renal tubular acidosis is associated with transporter defect in H+-ATPase and anion exchanger-1. *J Am Soc Nephrol.* 2002;13:1425–1432.

Hood VL, Tannen RL. Protection of acid-base balance by pH regulation of acid production. *N Engl J Med.* 1998;339:819–826.

Igarashi T, Sekine T, Inatomi J, Seki G. Unraveling the molecular pathogenesis of isolated proximal renal tubular acidosis. *J Am Soc Nephrol.* 2002;13:2171–2177.

Ishihara K, Szerlip HM. Anion gap acidosis. *Semin Nephrol.* 1998;18:83–89.

Izzedine H, Launay-Vacher V, Isnard-Bagnis C, Derray G. Drug-induced Fanconi's syndrome. *Am J Kid Dis.* 2003;41:292–309.

Jaber S, Paugam C, Futier E, et al. Sodium bicarbonate therapy for patients with severe metabolic acidemia in the intensive care unit (BICAR-ICU): a multicenter, open-labeled, randomized controlled phase 3 trial. *Lancet.* 2018;392:31–40.

Karet FE. Inherited distal renal tubular acidosis. *J Am Soc Nephrol.* 2002;13:2178–2184.

Kirschbaum B, Sica D, Anderson F. Urine electrolytes and the urine anion and osmolar gaps. *J Lab Clin Med.* 1999;133:597–604.

Lemann Jr J, Bushinsky DA, Hamm LL. Bone buffering of acid and base in humans. *Am J Physiol Renal Physiol.* 2003;285:F811–F832.

Levraut J, Grimaud D. Treatment of metabolic acidosis. *Curr Opin Crit Care.* 2003;9:260–265.

14

Metabolic Alkalosis

THOMAS D. DUBOSE JR., MITCHELL H. ROSNER

Pathogenesis

The pathogenesis of metabolic alkalosis requires two processes: (1) generation and (2) maintenance. Generation occurs by net gain of bicarbonate ions (HCO_3^-) or net loss of nonvolatile acid (usually HCl by vomiting) from the extracellular fluid. Although the kidneys have an impressive capacity to excrete HCO_3^- under normal circumstances, in the maintenance stage of metabolic alkalosis the kidneys fail to excrete HCO_3^-. The failure to appropriately excrete HCO_3^- is due to volume contraction, a low glomerular filtration rate (GFR), or depletion of chloride (Cl^-) or potassium (K^+). Retention, rather than excretion, of excess alkali by the kidney is also promoted by (1) volume and Cl^- depletion in combination with a reduced GFR or (2) hypokalemia from unregulated mineralocorticoid. In the first example, alkalosis is corrected by administration of sodium chloride (such as normal saline) and potassium chloride, whereas, in the latter example, it is necessary to treat the alkalosis by pharmacologic or surgical intervention (such as adrenalectomy) rather than saline administration.

In assessing a patient with metabolic alkalosis, two questions should be considered: (1) What is the source of alkali gain (or acid loss) that generated the alkalosis? and (2) What kidney mechanisms are operating to prevent excretion of excess HCO_3^-, thereby maintaining, rather than correcting, the alkalosis?

Differential Diagnosis

To establish the cause of metabolic alkalosis (Box 14.1), it is necessary to assess the extracellular fluid volume (ECV) status and the plasma electrolytes with attention to the serum potassium concentration ($[K^+]$). In hypertensive patients with chronic hypokalemia, it is also helpful to evaluate the renin-angiotensin-aldosterone system. For example, the presence of chronic hypertension and chronic hypokalemia in an alkalotic patient suggests either mineralocorticoid excess or a hypertensive patient receiving diuretics. Low plasma renin activity and urine sodium concentration ($[Na^+]$) and chloride concentration ($[Cl^-]$) values greater than 20 mEq/L in a hypertensive patient not taking diuretics are consistent with primary mineralocorticoid excess.

The combination of hypokalemia and alkalosis in a non-edematous patient with a low or normal BP can pose a challenging diagnostic problem. Possible causes include Bartter or Gitelman syndromes, magnesium deficiency, vomiting, exogenous alkali, and diuretic ingestion. Determination of urine electrolytes (especially $[Cl^-]$) and screening of the urine for diuretics (surreptitious use) may be helpful. When the urine $[Cl^-]$ is measured (Table 14.1), it should be considered in context with assessment of the ECV status of the patient. A low urine $[Cl^-]$ (i.e., <10 mEq/L) indicates avid Cl^- retention by the kidney and denotes ECV depletion even if the urine Na^+ is high (i.e., >20 mEq/L), whereas a high urine $[Cl^-]$ in the absence of concurrent diuretic use suggests inappropriate chloruresis resulting from a kidney tubular defect or mineralocorticoid excess. If the urine is alkaline, with an elevated $[Na^+]$ and $[K^+]$ but a urine $[Cl^-]$ is lower than 10 mEq/L, the diagnosis is usually either vomiting (overt or surreptitious) or alkali ingestion. If the urine is relatively acid and has low concentrations of Na^+, K^+, and Cl^-, the most likely possibilities are previous vomiting, a posthypercapnic state, or previous diuretic ingestion. If, on the other hand, neither the urine $[Na^+]$, $[K^+]$, nor $[Cl^-]$ is depressed, magnesium deficiency, Bartter or Gitelman syndromes, or active diuretic use should be considered. Gitelman syndrome is distinguished from Bartter syndrome by the presence of hypocalciuria. In addition, hypomagnesemia may be present in both, but is more common in Gitelman syndrome.

Metabolic Alkalosis Due to Exogenous Bicarbonate Loads

Alkali Administration

Administration of alkali to individuals with normal kidney function rarely causes alkalosis because the normal kidney has a high capacity for HCO_3^- excretion. Nevertheless, in patients with coexistent hemodynamic disturbances, alkalosis may develop because the normal capacity to excrete HCO_3^- has been exceeded. Examples include patients receiving oral or intravenous HCO_3^-, acetate loads such as with parenteral hyperalimentation solutions (acetate is converted on a 1:1 basis to bicarbonate by both the liver and skeletal muscle), citrate loads such as with transfusions, continuous kidney replacement therapy, or infant formula (citrate is metabolized to carbon dioxide and then bicarbonate on a 1:3 basis; thus, 1 mmol citrate yields 3 mmol carbon dioxide and then bicarbonate), or antacids plus cation-exchange resins (aluminum hydroxide and sodium polystyrene sulfonate). Moreover, metabolic alkalosis may develop when there is a coexisting problem that results in enhanced reabsorption of HCO_3^-, such as ECF depletion and a reduction in GFR, potassium depletion, or hypercapnia.

In patients with acute kidney injury or advanced chronic kidney disease, overt alkalosis can develop after alkali administration because the capacity to excrete HCO_3^- is exceeded or coexistent hemodynamic disturbances have caused enhanced HCO_3^- reabsorption. In this regard, alkali ingestion should be considered in

BOX 14.1

Causes of Metabolic Alkalosis

Exogenous HCO$_3^-$ Loads

Acute alkali administration
Milk-alkali syndrome
Use of NaOH in "free-basing" of crack cocaine
Street cocaine "cut" with baking soda
Baking soda pica in pregnancy
Bicarbonate precursors (citrate, acetate) in chronic or acute kidney disease
Skilled nursing home patients on nasogastric tube feeding

Effective ECV Contraction, Normotension, K$^+$ Deficiency, and Secondary Hyperreninemic Hyperaldosteronism

Gastrointestinal origin
  Vomiting
  Gastric aspiration
  Congenital chloridorrhea
  Villous adenoma
  Combined administration of sodium polystyrene sulfonate (Kayexalate) and aluminum hydroxide
  Cystic fibrosis and volume depletion
  Gastrocystoplasty
  Chronic laxative abuse
  Cl$^-$ deficient infant formula
Kidney origin
  Diuretics (remote use of thiazides or loop diuretics)
  Edematous states
  Posthypercapnic state
  Hypercalcemia–hypoparathyroidism
  Recovery from lactic acidosis or ketoacidosis
  Nonreabsorbable anions (e.g., IV penicillin derivatives such as carbenicillin or ticarcillin)
  Mg^{2+} deficiency
  K$^+$ depletion
  Bartter syndrome

Gitelman syndrome
Carbohydrate refeeding after starvation
Pendred syndrome (during thiazide diuretic use or intercurrent illness)

ECV Expansion, Hypertension, K$^+$ Deficiency, and Hypermineralocorticoidism

Associated with high renin levels
  Renal artery stenosis
  Accelerated hypertension
  Renin-secreting tumor
  Estrogen therapy
Associated with low renin levels
  Primary aldosteronism
    • Adenoma
    • Hyperplasia
    • Carcinoma
    • Glucocorticoid suppressible
  Adrenal enzymatic defects
    • 11β-Hydroxylase deficiency
    • 17α-Hydroxylase deficiency
  Cushing syndrome or disease
    • Ectopic corticotropin
    • Adrenal carcinoma
    • Adrenal adenoma
    • Primary pituitary
  Other etiologies
    • Licorice
    • Carbenoxolone
    • Chewing tobacco (containing glycyrrhizinic acid)

Gain-of-Function Mutation of ENaC with ECV Expansion, Hypertension, K$^+$ Deficiency, and Hyporeninemic Hypoaldosteronism

Liddle syndrome

ECV, Extracellular fluid volume; *ENaC,* epithelial sodium channel.

CKD patients, especially when the alkali is used as a home remedy for dyspepsia. The use of tube feedings in elderly patients in long-term care facilities has been associated with metabolic alkalosis because tube feeding preparations are a common and underappreciated source of alkali loads. Plasma electrolytes should be monitored more frequently in these patients. Other examples of acute metabolic alkalosis resulting from alkali ingestion include the association of pica for alkali (baking soda) in pregnancy. Additionally, the use of crack cocaine has been described as a cause of severe alkalosis in patients undergoing hemodialysis, as "free-basing" involves the addition of alkali (NaOH, a component of household drain cleaner) to cocaine hydrochloride.

Milk-Alkali Syndrome

A long-standing history of excessive ingestion of milk and antacids, termed *milk-alkali syndrome,* is a historically important cause of metabolic alkalosis. Since ingestion of calcium carbonate and vitamin D has become common for the treatment of osteoporosis, there has been a resurgence of milk-alkali syndrome since the

1990s. The majority of patients with this form of milk-alkali syndrome are asymptomatic women with incidental hypercalcemia, previously unappreciated CKD, and hypophosphatemia. Older women on diuretics and angiotensin-converting enzyme (ACE) inhibitors or angiotensin receptor blockers (ARBs) appear to be at higher risk. Both hypercalcemia and vitamin D excess increase kidney HCO$_3^-$ reabsorption. A critical component of this syndrome is reduced GFR. Patients with this disorder are prone to developing nephrocalcinosis, progressive kidney function impairment, and metabolic alkalosis. Discontinuation of alkali ingestion is usually sufficient to correct the alkalosis, but the kidney disease may be irreversible if nephrocalcinosis is advanced.

Citrate-Based Continuous Kidney Replacement Therapy

If citrate is used for regional anticoagulation in continuous kidney replacement therapy, metabolic alkalosis can occur, although recent studies using contemporary protocols demonstrate that this is not common and often mild. This is due to the metabolism of

TABLE 14.1 Diagnostic Evaluation of Metabolic Alkalosis	
Low Urinary [Cl⁻] ($<$10 mEq/L)	**High or Normal Urinary [Cl⁻]** ($>$15-20 mEq/L)
Normotensive	**Hypertensive**
Vomiting, nasogastric aspiration	Primary aldosteronism
Diuretics	Cushing syndrome
Posthypercapnia	Renal artery stenosis
K⁺ deficiency	Kidney failure plus alkali therapy
Bicarbonate treatment of organic acidosis	Liddle syndrome
	Normotensive or Hypotensive
	Mg^{2+} deficiency
	Severe K⁺ deficiency
	Bartter syndrome
	Gitelman syndrome
	Diuretics

citrate by the liver and skeletal muscle, which results in a net gain of HCO_3^-.

Metabolic Alkalosis Associated with Extracellular Fluid Volume Contraction, K⁺ Depletion, and Secondary Hyperreninemic Hyperaldosteronism

Metabolic Alkalosis of Gastrointestinal Origin

Gastrointestinal loss of H⁺, Cl⁻, Na⁺, and K⁺ from vomitus or gastric aspiration results in retention of HCO_3^-. The loss of fluid and electrolytes results in contraction of the ECV and stimulation of the renin-angiotensin-aldosterone system. Volume contraction causes a reduction in GFR and an enhanced capacity of the kidney tubule to reabsorb HCO_3^-. Excess angiotensin II stimulates Na⁺/H⁺ exchange in the proximal tubule. During active vomiting, there is continued addition of HCO_3^- to plasma in exchange for Cl⁻, and the plasma [HCO_3^-] exceeds the reabsorptive capacity of the proximal tubule. Aldosterone and endothelin also stimulate the proton-transporting adenosine triphosphatase (H⁺-ATPase) in the distal nephron, resulting in enhanced capacity for distal nephron HCO_3^- absorption and, paradoxically, aciduria. When the excess $NaHCO_3$ reaches the distal tubule, potassium secretion is enhanced by aldosterone and the delivery of the poorly reabsorbed anion, HCO_3^-. Thus, the predominant cause of the hypokalemia is kidney loss of K⁺, and not gastrointestinal potassium wasting.

Hypokalemia has selective effects on kidney bicarbonate absorption and ammonium production that are counterproductive to metabolic alkalosis. Hypokalemia dramatically increases the activity of the proton pump (H⁺,K⁺-ATPase) in the cortical and medullary collecting tubule for reabsorbing K⁺, but this occurs at the expense of both enhanced net acid excretion and HCO_3^- absorption. Hypokalemia also increases ammonium production independently of acid-base status, which, in the face of enhanced H⁺ secretion, results in increased ammonium production and excretion; this, in turn, adds new bicarbonate to the systemic circulation (increase in net acid excretion). Therefore,

hypokalemia plays an important role in the seemingly maladaptive response of the kidney to maintain the alkalosis. Because of contraction of the ECV and hypochloremia, Cl⁻ is avidly conserved by the kidney. This can be recognized clinically by a low urine [Cl⁻] (see Table 14.1). Correction of the contracted ECV with isotonic NaCl and repletion of the K⁺ deficit correct the acid-base disorder because such therapy restores the ability of the kidney to excrete the excess bicarbonate.

Congenital Chloridorrhea

Congenital chloridorrhea, a rare autosomal recessive disorder, causes metabolic alkalosis by an extrarenal mechanism of severe diarrhea, fecal acid loss, and HCO_3^- retention. The disease is the result of mutations in the *SLC26A3* gene that disrupt the ileal and colonic HCO_3^-/Cl⁻ anion exchange mechanism so that Cl⁻ cannot be reabsorbed in the gut. The parallel Na⁺/H⁺ ion exchanger remains functional, allowing Na⁺ to be reabsorbed and H⁺ to be secreted. Therefore, the stool has high concentrations of H⁺ and Cl⁻, causing Na⁺ and HCO_3^- retention in the extracellular fluid. The alkalosis is sustained by concomitant ECV contraction, hyperaldosteronism, and K⁺ deficiency. Delivery of Cl⁻ to the distal nephron is low because of volume contraction. As in cystic fibrosis, this low delivery of Cl⁻ results in impaired HCO_3^- secretion by the β-intercalated cell. Therapy consists of oral supplementation of sodium and potassium chloride. Administration of proton pump inhibitors may reduce chloride secretion by the parietal cells and improve the diarrhea. The long-term outcome is good with daily supplementation of sodium and potassium chloride.

Villous Adenoma

Metabolic alkalosis has been described in cases of villous adenomas. K⁺ depletion probably induces the alkalosis as colonic secretions are alkaline.

Gastrocystoplasty

Augmentation of the bladder by gastrocystoplasty, although uncommon, has been used as an alternative to enterocystoplasty. Implantation of a segment of vascularized stomach into the bladder in children with reduced bladder capacity has been associated with hypokalemia, hypochloremia, and metabolic alkalosis. Gastrointestinal complications have also been reported. Oral potassium chloride should be administered chronically to treat both hypokalemia and metabolic alkalosis.

Metabolic Alkalosis of Kidney Origin

The generation of metabolic alkalosis through kidney mechanisms involves three processes for increasing distal nephron H⁺ secretion and enhancing net acid (ammonium) excretion: (1) high delivery of Na⁺ salts to the distal nephron, (2) excessive elaboration of mineralocorticoids, and (3) K⁺ deficiency (Fig. 14.1).

Diuretics

Drugs that induce distal delivery of sodium salts, such as thiazides and loop diuretics (furosemide, bumetanide, torsemide, and ethacrynic acid), diminish ECV without altering total body bicarbonate content. Consequently, the serum [HCO_3^-] increases. The chronic administration of diuretics generates a metabolic alkalosis by increasing distal salt delivery that enhances the secretion of K⁺ and H⁺ by principal cells of the late distal tubule and collecting duct. The alkalosis is maintained by persistence of contraction of

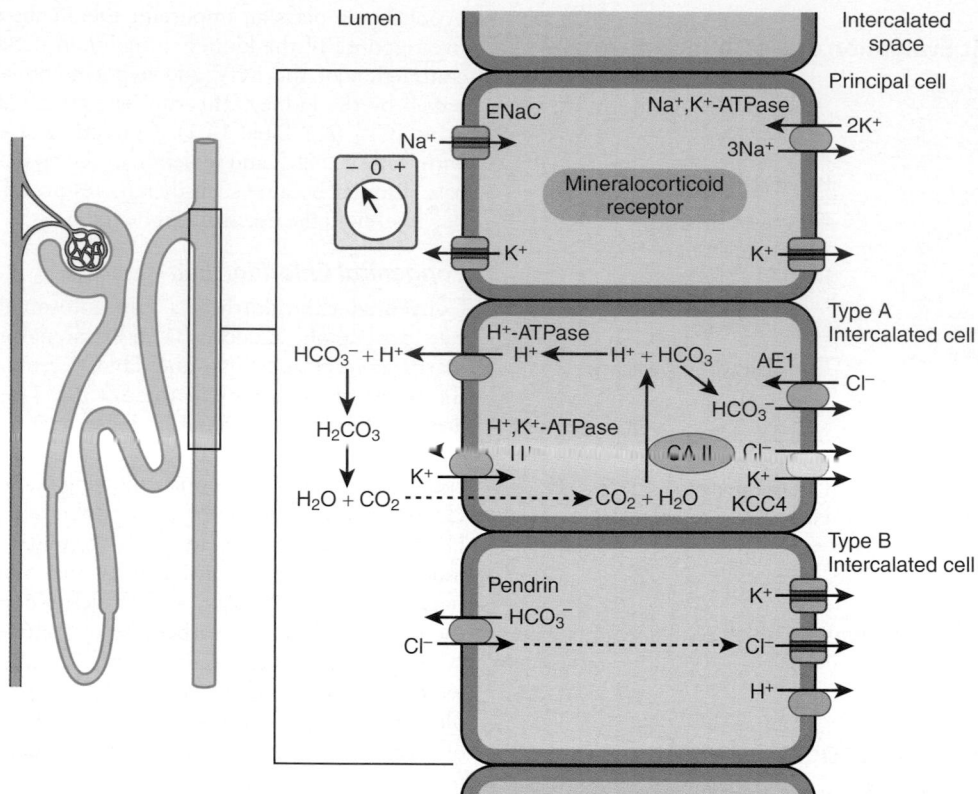

• **Fig. 14.1** Contribution of the distal nephron to maintenance of metabolic alkalosis. Extracellular volume depletion maintains metabolic alkalosis by increasing the activity of the epithelial sodium channel in principal cells (*top cell,* labeled ENaC) through enhanced elaboration of mineralocorticoid (secondary hyperaldosteronism), which further aggravates potassium wasting by increasing the negative transepithelial potential. Similarly, secondary hyperaldosteronism enhances H^+ secretion in Type A intercalated cells that inappropriately enhance absorption of HCO_3^- rather than its excretion. Correction of metabolic alkalosis with volume depletion requires correction of ECF and potassium deficits. When accomplished, the kidney can excrete HCO_3^- efficiently.

the ECV, secondary hyperaldosteronism, K^+ deficiency, and activation of the H^+,K^+-ATPase, as long as diuretic administration continues. The hypokalemia also enhances ammonium production and excretion. Repair of the alkalosis is achieved by withholding the diuretic, providing isotonic saline to correct the ECV deficit, and replacing the potassium deficit.

Bartter Syndrome

Classic Bartter syndrome is characterized by a milder clinical picture than the antenatal/infantile subtype and presents with failure to thrive, hypokalemic alkalosis, increased levels of plasma renin and aldosterone, low blood pressure, and vascular resistance to angiotensin II. Both classic Bartter syndrome and the antenatal type are inherited as autosomal recessive disorders that impair salt absorption in the thick ascending limb (TAL) of the loop of Henle; this results in salt wasting, volume depletion, and activation of the renin-angiotensin-aldosterone system. These manifestations are the result of loss-of-function mutations of one of the genes that encode three transporters involved in NaCl absorption in the TAL. The most prevalent disorder is a mutation of the gene *NKCC2,* which encodes the Na^+-K^+-$2Cl^-$ cotransporter on the apical membrane. A second mutation has been discovered in the gene *KCNJ1,* which encodes the ATP-sensitive apical K^+ conductance channel (ROMK) that operates in parallel with the Na^+-K^+-$2Cl^-$ cotransporter to recycle K^+. Both defects can be associated with antenatal Bartter syndrome or with classic Bartter syndrome. A mutation of the *CLCNKb*

gene encoding the voltage-gated basolateral chloride channel (ClC-Kb) is associated only with classic Bartter syndrome, is milder, and is rarely associated with nephrocalcinosis. All three defects have the same net effect: loss of Cl^- transport in the TAL with enhanced delivery of NaCl that stimulates K^+ and H^+ secretion by the collecting tubule, causing hypokalemia and metabolic alkalosis.

Antenatal Bartter syndrome is characterized by maternal polyhydramnios along with prematurity, postnatal polyuria, vomiting, failure to thrive, hypercalciuria, and, subsequently, nephrocalcinosis. Hypokalemia, metabolic alkalosis, secondary hyperaldosteronism, and hyperreninemia are other characteristic features that have been observed in consanguineous families in association with sensorineural deafness, a syndrome linked to chromosome 1p31. The responsible gene, *BSND,* encodes a subunit, barttin, that colocalizes with the ClC-Kb channel in the TAL and K^+-secreting epithelial cells in the inner ear. Barttin appears to be necessary for the function of the voltage-gated chloride channel. Expression of ClC-Kb is lost when coexpressed with mutant barttins. Therefore, mutations in *BSND* define a fourth category of patients with Bartter syndrome.

Such defects predictably lead to ECV contraction, hyperreninemic hyperaldosteronism, and increased delivery of NaCl to the distal nephron, with consequent alkalosis, kidney K^+ wasting, and hypokalemia. Secondary overproduction of prostaglandins, juxtaglomerular apparatus hypertrophy, and vascular pressor hyporesponsiveness ensue. Most patients have hypercalciuria and normal serum magnesium levels, distinguishing this disorder from Gitelman syndrome.

Bartter syndrome is inherited as an autosomal recessive defect. Most patients are homozygotes or compound heterozygotes for different mutations in one of these four genes, whereas a few patients with the clinical syndrome have no discernible mutation in any of these genes. Plausible explanations include unrecognized mutations in other genes, a dominant-negative effect of a heterozygous mutation, or other mechanisms. Patients with features of Bartter syndrome have been associated with autosomal dominant hypocalcemia and activating mutations in the calcium-sensing receptor, CaSR. Activation of CaSR on the basolateral cell surface of the TAL inhibits the function of ROMK; therefore, mutations in CaSR may represent a fifth gene associated with Bartter syndrome.

For diagnosis, Bartter syndrome must be distinguished from surreptitious vomiting, diuretic administration, and laxative abuse. The finding of a low urine [Cl⁻] is helpful in identifying the vomiting patient (see Table 14.1). The urine [Cl⁻] in a patient with Bartter syndrome would be expected to be normal or increased, rather than depressed.

The therapy for Bartter syndrome focuses on repair of the hypokalemia through inhibition of the renin-angiotensin-aldosterone system or the prostaglandin-kinin system, using propranolol, amiloride, spironolactone, eplerenone, prostaglandin inhibitors, and ACE inhibitors, as well as direct repletion of the deficits of potassium and magnesium.

Gitelman Syndrome

Patients with Gitelman syndrome resemble the Bartter syndrome phenotype in that an autosomal recessive metabolic alkalosis is associated with hypokalemia, a normal-to-low blood pressure, volume depletion with secondary hyperreninemic hyperaldosteronism, and juxtaglomerular hyperplasia. However, the consistent presence of hypocalciuria and the frequent presence of hypomagnesemia are useful in distinguishing Gitelman syndrome from Bartter syndrome on clinical grounds. These unique features mimic the effects of chronic thiazide diuretic administration. Missense mutations of the gene *SLC12A3*, which encodes the thiazide-sensitive sodium chloride cotransporter in the distal convoluted tubule (NCC), accounts for the clinical features, including the classic finding of hypocalciuria. However, it is not clear why these patients have pronounced hypomagnesemia. A study demonstrated that peripheral blood mononuclear cells from patients with Gitelman syndrome express mutated NCC messenger RNA (mRNA). In a large consanguineous Bedouin family, missense mutations were noted in *CLCNKb*, but the clinical features overlapped between Gitelman and Bartter syndromes.

Compared to Bartter syndrome, Gitelman syndrome becomes symptomatic later in life and is associated with milder salt wasting. A large study of adults with proven Gitelman syndrome and NCC mutations showed that salt craving, nocturia, cramps, and fatigue were more common than in sex-matched and age-matched controls. Women experience exacerbation of symptoms during menses and they may experience complicated pregnancies.

Treatment of Gitelman syndrome consists of a diet high in potassium and potassium salts, typically with the addition of magnesium supplementation. Amiloride is often more helpful than spironolactone or eplerenone, with dose escalation to as much as 10 mg twice daily. Amiloride may be used in combination with spironolactone or eplerenone. Importantly, almost all patients with Gitelman syndrome exhibit some degree of salt craving, which may be extreme in some cases. To the extent possible, offending foods high in salt should be identified and avoided because salt loading increases distal delivery of NaCl and greatly amplifies K⁺ secretion by the cortical collecting tubule. Careful questioning of dietary practices is necessary to expose unusual salt appetites. ACE inhibitors have been suggested in selected patients for which frank hypotension is not a complication.

Pendred Syndrome

Pendred syndrome consists of sensorineural deafness and goiter caused by impaired iodide uptake, and it is ascribed to a defect in pendrin (encoded by *SLC26A4*). Pendrin is expressed on the apical membrane of type B intercalated cells of the collecting tubule. Although these patients typically do not have acid-base disorders, two recent reports of severe metabolic alkalosis with hypokalemia (one was a patient prescribed a thiazide diuretic and another with alcoholism and severe vomiting after a cochlear implant) suggest that these patients are susceptible because of the inability of type B intercalated cells to secrete bicarbonate. These reports also underscore the importance of bicarbonate secretion during alkalotic challenges. Diuretics should not be prescribed to patients with Pendred syndrome, and clinicians should be aware that protracted vomiting may lead to severe metabolic alkalosis.

Non-Reabsorbable Anions and Magnesium Deficiency

Administration of large quantities of non-reabsorbable anions, such as penicillin derivatives (carbenicillin, ticarcillin) or bicarbonate, can enhance distal acidification and K⁺ secretion by increasing the negative transepithelial potential difference. Mg²⁺ deficiency frequently accompanies hypokalemia, and both electrolyte abnormalities must be corrected to ameliorate the metabolic alkalosis.

Metabolic Alkalosis Due to Potassium Depletion

Pure K⁺ depletion causes metabolic alkalosis, although usually of only modest severity. Hypokalemia independently enhances kidney ammoniagenesis, which increases net acid excretion and, thereby, the return of "new" bicarbonate to the systemic circulation. When access to salt and K⁺ is restricted, more severe alkalosis develops. Activation of the kidney H⁺,K⁺-ATPase in the collecting duct by chronic hypokalemia probably plays a major role in maintenance of the alkalosis. Specifically, chronic hypokalemia has been shown to increase markedly the abundance of the colonic H⁺,K⁺-ATPase mRNA and protein in the outer medullary collecting duct. Alkalosis associated with severe K⁺ depletion is resistant to salt administration, with repair of the K⁺ deficiency necessary to correct the alkalosis.

Posttreatment of Lactic Acidosis or Ketoacidosis

When an underlying stimulus for the endogenous generation of lactic acid or keto acid is removed rapidly, as with the repair of ineffective circulating volume or administration of insulin therapy, the lactate or ketones are metabolized to yield an equivalent amount of HCO₃⁻. Other sources of new HCO₃⁻ are additive to the original alkali generated by organic anion metabolism to create a surfeit of HCO₃⁻. Such sources include new HCO₃⁻ added to the blood by the kidneys as a result of enhanced acid excretion during the preexisting period of acidosis and exogenous alkali administered during the treatment phase of the acidosis. Acidosis-induced contraction of the ECV and K$^+$ deficiency act together to sustain the alkalosis.

Posthypercapnia

Prolonged CO$_2$ retention with chronic respiratory acidosis enhances kidney HCO$_3^-$ absorption and the generation of new HCO$_3^-$ (increased net acid excretion). If the partial pressure of carbon dioxide in arterial blood (Paco$_2$) is returned to normal by mechanical ventilation or other means, metabolic alkalosis results from the persistently elevated [HCO$_3^-$]. Associated ECV contraction does not allow complete repair of the alkalosis by correction of the Paco$_2$ alone, and alkalosis persists until isotonic saline is infused.

Metabolic Alkalosis Associated with Extracellular Fluid Volume Expansion, Hypertension, and Hyperaldosteronism

Mineralocorticoid administration or excess production (as a result of primary aldosteronism of Cushing syndrome or adrenal cortical enzyme defects) increases net acid excretion and may result in metabolic alkalosis, which is worsened by associated K$^+$ deficiency. ECV expansion from salt retention causes hypertension and antagonizes the reduction in GFR or increases tubule acidification induced by aldosterone and by K$^+$ deficiency through enhanced activity of the H$^+$-ATPase and H$^+$, K$^+$-ATPase, respectively. The kaliuresis worsens K$^+$ depletion, resulting in a urinary concentrating defect, polyuria, and polydipsia. Increased aldosterone levels may be the result of autonomous primary adrenal overproduction or secondary aldosterone release caused by kidney overproduction of renin. In both situations, the normal feedback of ECV on net aldosterone production is disrupted, and hypertension from volume retention can result.

Liddle Syndrome

Liddle syndrome is associated with severe hypertension presenting in childhood, accompanied by hypokalemic metabolic alkalosis. These features resemble those of primary hyperaldosteronism, but the renin and aldosterone levels are suppressed (pseudohyperaldosteronism). Liddle originally described patients with low renin and low aldosterone levels who did not respond to spironolactone. The defect is inherited as an autosomal dominant form of monogenic hypertension and is attributed to an abnormality in the gene that encodes the β or the γ subunit of the kidney epithelial Na$^+$ channel (ENaC) at the apical membrane of principal cells in the cortical collecting duct. This defect leads to constitutive activation of this channel. Either mutation results in deletion of the cytoplasmic tail (C-terminus) of the affected subunit. The C-termini contain a PY (proline-rich) amino acid motif that is highly conserved, and essentially all mutations in Liddle syndrome patients involve disruption or deletion of this motif. Such PY motifs are important in regulating the number of sodium channels in the luminal membrane by binding to the WW domains of the Nedd4-like family of ubiquitin protein ligases. Disruption of the PY motif dramatically increases the surface localization of the ENaC complex by failing to internalize or degrade (Nedd4 pathway) the channels from the cell surface. Ultimately, persistent Na$^+$ absorption results

in volume expansion, hypertension, hypokalemia, and metabolic alkalosis. Therefore, the urine [Na$^+$] is typically low and, while reasonable to assume that the urine [Cl$^-$] would also be low, there are no published reports of urine [Cl$^-$] in patients with documented Liddle syndrome.

Glucocorticoid-Remediable Hyperaldosteronism

Glucocorticoid-remediable hyperaldosteronism is an autosomal dominant form of hypertension, the features of which resemble primary aldosteronism (hypokalemic metabolic alkalosis and volume-dependent hypertension). However, in this disorder glucocorticoid administration corrects the hypertension as well as the excessive excretion of 18-hydroxysteroid in the urine. This disorder is due to an unequal crossover between two genes located in close proximity on chromosome 8. This results in the glucocorticoid-responsive promoter region of the gene encoding the 11-β-hydroxylase *(CYP11B1)* attaching to the structural portion of the *CYP11B2* gene encoding aldosterone synthase. The chimeric gene produces excess amounts of aldosterone synthase unresponsive to serum potassium or renin levels but can be suppressed by glucocorticoid administration. Although this syndrome is a rare cause of primary aldosteronism, it is important to diagnose, because the treatment is unique and the syndrome can be associated with severe hypertension and stroke, especially during pregnancy.

Cushing Disease and Cushing Syndrome

Abnormally high glucocorticoid production as a result of adrenal adenoma, carcinoma, or ectopic corticotropin production causes metabolic alkalosis. The alkalosis may be ascribed to coexisting mineralocorticoid (deoxycorticosterone and corticosterone) hypersecretion. Alternatively, glucocorticoids may have the capability of enhancing net acid secretion and NH$_4^+$ production, which may be caused by cross-reactivity with mineralocorticoid receptors.

Miscellaneous Conditions

Ingestion of authentic licorice or licorice-containing chewing tobacco can cause a typical pattern of mineralocorticoid excess. The glycyrrhizinic acid contained in authentic licorice inhibits 11β-hydroxysteroid dehydrogenase. This enzyme is responsible for converting cortisol to cortisone, an essential step in protecting the mineralocorticoid receptor from cortisol. When the enzyme is inactivated, cortisol can occupy type I kidney mineralocorticoid receptors, mimicking aldosterone. Genetic apparent mineralocorticoid excess (AME) resembles excessive ingestion of licorice, with volume expansion, low renin and aldosterone levels, and a salt-sensitive form of hypertension that may include metabolic alkalosis and hypokalemia. The hypertension responds to thiazides and spironolactone, but without abnormal steroid products in the urine. In genetic AME, 11β-hydroxysteroid dehydrogenase is defective and monogenic hypertension develops.

Symptoms of Metabolic Alkalosis

Patients with metabolic alkalosis experience changes in central and peripheral nervous system function similar to those of hypocalcemia. Symptoms may include mental confusion, obtundation, and a predisposition to seizures, paresthesia, muscular cramping, tetany, aggravation of arrhythmias, and hypoxemia in chronic obstructive pulmonary disease. Related electrolyte abnormalities include hypokalemia and hypophosphatemia.

Treatment of Metabolic Alkalosis

The maintenance of metabolic alkalosis represents a failure of the kidney to excrete bicarbonate efficiently because of chloride or potassium deficiency, continuous mineralocorticoid elaboration, or both. Treatment depends on the cause of the metabolic alkalosis and it is primarily directed at correcting the underlying stimulus for HCO_3^- generation and restoring the ability of the kidney to excrete the excess HCO_3^-. Assistance is gained in the diagnosis and treatment of metabolic alkalosis from measurement of a spot urine [Cl⁻] and correlation with arterial blood pressure and the ECV of the patient (particularly the presence or absence of orthostasis; see Box 14.1, Table 14.1). Helpful in the history is the presence or absence of vomiting, diuretic use, or alkali therapy.

A high urine [Cl⁻] and hypertension suggest that primary mineralocorticoid excess is present. If primary aldosteronism is diagnosed, correction of the underlying cause (adenoma, bilateral hyperplasia, Cushing syndrome) will reverse the alkalosis. Patients with bilateral adrenal hyperplasia may respond to spironolactone. Normotensive patients with a high urine chloride level may have Bartter or Gitelman syndrome if diuretic use or vomiting can be excluded. A low urine chloride level and relative hypotension suggest a chloride-responsive metabolic alkalosis such as vomiting or nasogastric suction. Loss of [H⁺] by the stomach or kidneys can be mitigated by the use of proton pump inhibitors or the discontinuation of diuretics. The second aspect of treatment is to remove the factors that sustain HCO_3^- reabsorption, such as ECV contraction or K⁺ deficiency. Although K⁺ deficits should be repleted, NaCl therapy is usually sufficient to reverse the alkalosis if ECV contraction is present as indicated by a low urine [Cl⁻].

Patients with congestive heart failure or unexplained volume expansion represent special challenges in the critical care setting. Patients with a low urine [Cl⁻], usually indicative of a "chloride-responsive" form of metabolic alkalosis, may not tolerate normal saline infusion. Kidney HCO_3^- loss can be accelerated by administration of the carbonic anhydrase inhibitor acetazolamide (250 mg intravenously) if associated conditions preclude infusion of saline (i.e., clinical evidence of congestive heart failure). Acetazolamide is usually effective in patients with adequate kidney function but can exacerbate urinary K⁺ losses (due to increases in distal tubular HCO_3^- delivery) and can cause hypokalemia. Dilute hydrochloric acid (0.1 N HCl) infused into a central vein is sometimes recommended. Several potentially serious complications, such as hemolysis, venous sclerosis, and imprecise dosing, result in a very high risk-to-benefit ratio. It is not recommended except in extreme metabolic alkalosis (pH > 7.6) in patients unresponsive or intolerant of isotonic saline infusion, acetazolamide, or ammonium chloride administration. Oral NH_4Cl is preferable to intravenous 0.1 N HCl except in patients with liver disease. Patients receiving continuous kidney replacement therapy in the intensive care unit may develop metabolic alkalosis with high-bicarbonate dialysate. Therapy should include reducing the bicarbonate concentration in the dialysate.

Bibliography

Birkenhager R, Otto E, Schurmann MJ, et al. Mutation of BSND causes Bartter syndrome with sensorineural deafness and kidney failure. *Nat Genet.* 2001;29:310–314.

Conn JW, Rovner DR, Cohen EL. Licorice-induced pseudoaldosteronism: hypertension, hypokalemia, aldosteronopenia, and suppressed plasma renin activity. *JAMA.* 1968;205:492.

Cruz DN, Shaer AJ, Bia MJ, et al. Gitelman's syndrome revisited: an evaluation of symptoms and health-related quality of life. *Kidney Int.* 2001;59:717–719.

Diskin CJ, Stokes TJ, Dansby M, et al. Recurrent metabolic alkalosis and elevated troponins after crack cocaine use in a hemodialysis patient. *Clin Exp Nephrol.* 2006;10:156–158.

DuBose Jr TD. Disorders of acid-base balance. In: Skorecki K, Chertow GM, Marsden PA, Taal MW, Yu SL, eds. *Brenner and Rector's The Kidney.* 10 Philadelphia: Elsevier; 2016:511–558.

Felsenfeld AJ, Levine BS. Milk alkali syndrome and the dynamics of calcium homeostasis. *Clin J Am Soc Nephrol.* 2006;4:641–654.

Fitzgibbons LJ, Snoey ER. Severe metabolic alkalosis due to baking soda ingestion: case reports of two patients with unsuspected antacid overdose. *J Emerg Med.* 1999;17(1):57–61.

Gennari JF. Pathophysiology of metabolic alkalosis: A new classification based on the centrality of stimulated collecting duct ion transport. *Am J Kidney Dis.* 2011;58:626–636.

Grotegut CA, Dandolu V, Katari S, et al. Baking soda pica: a case of hypokalemic metabolic alkalosis and rhabdomyolysis in pregnancy. *Obstet Gynecol.* 2006;107:484–486.

Hebert SC, Gullans SR. The molecular basis of inherited hypokalemic alkalosis: Bartter's and Gitelman's syndromes. *Am J Physiol.* 1996;271:F957–F959.

Hernandez R, Schambelan M, Cogan MG, et al. Dietary NaCl determines severity of potassium depletion-induced metabolic alkalosis. *Kidney Int.* 1987;31:1356.

Hihnala S, Kujala M, Toppari J, et al. Expression of SLC26A3, CFTR and NHE3 in the human male reproductive tract: role in male subfertility caused by congenital chloride diarrhea. *Mol Hum Reprod 12.* 2006:107–111.

Jamison RL, Ross JC, Kempson RL, et al. Surreptitious diuretic ingestion and pseudo-Bartter's syndrome. *Am J Med.* 1982;73:142.

Kamynina E, Staub O. Concerted action of ENaC, Nedd4-2, and Sgk1 in transepithelial Na⁺ transport. *Am J Physiol Renal Physiol.* 2002;283:F377.

Lifton RP, Dluhy RG, Powers M, et al. Hereditary hypertension caused by chimaeric gene duplications and ectopic expression of aldosterone synthase. *Nat Genet.* 1992;2:66–74.

Morgera S, Haase M, Ruckert M, et al. Regional citrate anticoagulation in continuous hemodialysis: acid-base and electrolyte balance at an increased dose of dialysis. *Nephron Clin Pract.* 2005;101(4):c211–c219.

Sanei-Moghaddam A, Wilson T, Kumar S, et al. An unfortunate case of Pendred syndrome. *J Laryngol Otol.* 2011;125(9):965–967.

Schroeder ET. Alkalosis resulting from combined administration of a "nonsystemic" antacid and a cation-exchange resin. *Gastroenterology.* 1969;56:868 1969.

Shimkets RA, Warnock DG, Bositis CM, et al. Liddle's syndrome: heritable human hypertension caused by mutations in the beta subunit of the epithelial sodium channel. *Cell.* 1994;79:407.

Yi JH, Han SW, Song JS, et al. Metabolic alkalosis from unsuspected ingestion: use of urine pH and anion gap. *Am J Kidney Dis.* 2012;59:577–581.

Zelikovic I, Szargel R, Hawash A, et al. A novel mutation in the chloride channel gene, CLCNKB, as a cause of Gitelman and Bartter syndromes. *Kidney Int.* 2003;63:24–32.

15

Respiratory Acidosis and Alkalosis

NICOLAOS E. MADIAS, HORACIO J. ADROGUÉ

Respiratory Acidosis

Respiratory acidosis, or primary hypercapnia, is the acid-base disturbance initiated by an increase in the carbon dioxide tension of body fluids and in whole-body CO_2 stores. Hypercapnia acidifies body fluids and elicits an adaptive increment in the plasma bicarbonate concentration ($[HCO_3^-]$) that should be viewed as an integral part of the respiratory acidosis. Arterial CO_2 tension (PCO_2), measured at rest and at sea level, is greater than 45 mm Hg in simple respiratory acidosis. Lower values of PCO_2 might still signify the presence of primary hypercapnia in the setting of mixed acid-base disorders (e.g., eucapnia, rather than the expected hypocapnia, in the presence of metabolic acidosis). Another special case of respiratory acidosis is the presence of arterial eucapnia, or even hypocapnia, in association with venous hypercapnia in patients who have an acute severe reduction in cardiac output but relative preservation of respiratory function (i.e., pseudorespiratory alkalosis).

Pathophysiology

The ventilatory system is responsible for maintaining PCO_2 within normal limits by adjusting minute ventilation ($\dot{V}_E$) to match the rate of CO_2 production. $\dot{V}_E$ consists of two components: ventilation distributed in the gas-exchange units of the lungs (alveolar ventilation, $\dot{V}_A$) and ventilation wasted in dead space ($\dot{V}_D$). Clinically important hypercapnia usually results from decreased $\dot{V}_A$ and only rarely from increased CO_2 production. Decreased $\dot{V}_A$ can occur from a reduction in $\dot{V}_E$, an increase in $\dot{V}_D$, or a combination of the two. An increase in $\dot{V}_D$ results from rapid and shallow ventilation or owing to an increase in "alveolar dead space" (ventilated alveoli with reduced perfusion). An increase in alveolar dead space is the main mechanism of hypercapnia in patients with parenchymal lung disease (asthma, pneumonia, COPD, cystic fibrosis, interstitial lung disease) and pulmonary vascular disease (thromboembolism, vasculitis).

Because the sum of PCO_2 and PO_2 in alveolar gas is constant in patients breathing room air (~150 mm Hg at sea level), development of substantial hypercapnia is necessarily accompanied by equivalent hypoxia. Estimation of the alveolar-arterial oxygen gradient (P_AO_2-P_aO_2) allows distinguishing hypercapnic respiratory failure due to decreased $\dot{V}_E$ from respiratory failure caused by intrinsic lung disease (hypercapnic and hypoxemic respiratory failure). The P_AO_2-P_aO_2 should be calculated from a room-air arterial blood gas (ABG) and remains normal (<20 mm Hg) in hypercapnic respiratory failure caused by global hypoventilation but increases in respiratory failure resulting from intrinsic lung disease (abnormal gas exchange).

The main elements of the ventilatory system are the respiratory pump, which generates a pressure gradient responsible for airflow, and the loads that oppose such action. The respiratory pump comprises the cerebrum, brainstem, spinal cord, phrenic and intercostal nerves, and the muscles of respiration. The respiratory loads include the ventilatory requirement (CO_2 production, O_2 consumption), airway resistance, lung elastic recoil, and chest wall/abdominal resistance. Most frequently, primary hypercapnia develops from an imbalance between the strength of the respiratory pump and the weight of the respiratory loads, thereby resulting in a decreased $\dot{V}_A$. Impairment of the respiratory pump can occur because of depressed central drive, abnormal neuromuscular transmission, or muscle dysfunction. Causes of augmented respiratory loads include ventilation/perfusion mismatch (increased $\dot{V}_D$), augmented airway flow resistance, lung/pleural/chest wall stiffness, impaired diaphragmatic function, and increased ventilatory demand. Overproduction of CO_2 is usually matched by increased excretion so that hypercapnia is prevented. However, patients with marked limitation in pulmonary reserve and those receiving constant mechanical ventilation might experience respiratory acidosis due to increased CO_2 production caused by increased muscle activity (agitation, myoclonus, shivering, and seizures), sepsis, fever, or hyperthyroidism. Increments in CO_2 production might also be imposed by the administration of large carbohydrate loads (>2000 kcal/day) to nutritionally bereft, critically ill patients or during the decomposition of bicarbonate infused in the course of treating metabolic acidosis.

The major threat to life from CO_2 retention in patients who are breathing room air is the associated obligatory hypoxemia (in accordance with the alveolar gas equation). In the absence of supplemental oxygen, patients in respiratory arrest develop critical hypoxemia within a few minutes, long before extreme hypercapnia ensues. Because of the constraints of the alveolar gas equation, it is not possible for PCO_2 to reach values much higher than 80 mm Hg while the level of PO_2 is still compatible with life. Extreme hypercapnia with PCO_2 values exceeding 100 mm Hg is occasionally seen in patients receiving oxygen therapy, and, in fact, it is often the result of unrestrained oxygen administration.

Secondary Physiologic Response

An immediate rise in plasma $[HCO_3^-]$ owing to titration of nonbicarbonate body buffers occurs in response to acute hypercapnia. This adaptation is complete within 5 to 10 minutes of the increase in PCO_2. On average, plasma $[HCO_3^-]$ increases by about 0.1 mEq/L for each 1 mm Hg acute increment in PCO_2; as a result, the plasma hydrogen ion concentration $[H^+]$ increases by about

0.75 nEq/L for each 1 mm Hg acute increment in P_{CO_2}. Therefore, the overall limit of adaptation of plasma $[HCO_3^-]$ in acute respiratory acidosis is quite small; even when P_{CO_2} increases to levels of 80 to 90 mm Hg, the increment in plasma $[HCO_3^-]$ does not exceed 3 to 4 mEq/L. Moderate hypoxemia does not alter the adaptive response to acute respiratory acidosis. On the other hand, preexisting hypobicarbonatemia (from metabolic acidosis or chronic respiratory alkalosis) enhances the magnitude of the bicarbonate response to acute hypercapnia, whereas this response is diminished in hyperbicarbonatemic states (from metabolic alkalosis or chronic respiratory acidosis). Other electrolyte changes observed in acute respiratory acidosis include mild increases in plasma sodium (1 to 4 mEq/L), potassium (0.1 mEq/L for each 0.1 unit decrease in pH), and phosphorus, as well as small decreases in plasma chloride and lactate concentrations (the latter effect originating from inhibition of the activity of 6-phosphofructokinase and, consequently, glycolysis by intracellular acidosis).

A small reduction in the plasma anion gap is also observed, reflecting the decline in plasma lactate and the acidic titration of plasma proteins. Acute respiratory acidosis induces glucose intolerance and insulin resistance that are not prevented by adrenergic blockade. These changes are likely mediated by direct effects of the low tissue pH on skeletal muscle.

The adaptive increase in plasma $[HCO_3^-]$ observed in the acute phase of hypercapnia is amplified markedly during chronic hypercapnia as a result of the generation of new bicarbonate by the kidneys. Both proximal and distal acidification mechanisms contribute to this adaptation, which requires 3 to 5 days for completion. The kidney response to chronic hypercapnia includes chloruresis and the generation of hypochloremia. Retrospective studies in the 1960s in hospitalized patients with hypercapnic respiratory failure estimated that, on average, plasma $[HCO_3^-]$ increases by approximately 0.35-0.4 mEq/L for each 1 mm Hg chronic increment in P_{CO_2}, while recent studies in outpatients with stable hypercapnic respiratory failure reported a substantially steeper slope for the change in plasma $[HCO_3^-]$ of 0.5 mEq/L for each 1 mm Hg chronic increase in P_{CO_2}. This slope is sufficient to maintain systemic acidity between the mid-normal range and mild acidemia, highlighting a remarkably effective secondary response to chronic hypercapnia. Thus, in uncomplicated steady-state chronic hypercapnia at a Pa_{CO_2} of 70 mm Hg, the 95% prediction interval for blood pH is 7.32–7.38. Empiric observations indicate a limit of adaptation of plasma $[HCO_3^-]$ on the order of 45 mEq/L.

The kidney response to chronic hypercapnia is not altered appreciably by dietary sodium or chloride restriction, moderate potassium depletion, alkali loading, or moderate hypoxemia. The extent to which chronic kidney disease of variable severity limits the kidney response to chronic hypercapnia remains unknown. Obviously, patients with end-stage kidney disease cannot mount a kidney response to chronic hypercapnia (i.e., generation of new bicarbonate by the kidneys), making them subject to severe acidemia. The degree of acidemia is more pronounced in patients who are receiving hemodialysis rather than peritoneal dialysis because the former treatment maintains, on average, lower plasma $[HCO_3^-]$. Recovery from chronic hypercapnia is crippled by a chloride-deficient diet. In this circumstance, despite correction of the level of P_{CO_2}, plasma $[HCO_3^-]$ remains elevated as long as the state of chloride deprivation persists, thus creating the entity of "posthypercapnic metabolic alkalosis." Chronic hypercapnia is not associated with appreciable changes in the anion gap or in plasma concentrations of sodium, potassium, or phosphorus.

Etiology

Primary hypercapnia can result from disease or malfunction within any element of the ventilatory system, including the central and peripheral nervous system, respiratory muscles, thoracic cage, pleural space, airways, and lung parenchyma. Commonly used clinical expressions are linked to certain etiologies: Patients with absent or depressed respiratory drive caused by CNS dysfunction "won't breathe"; those with abnormalities of the peripheral nervous system, respiratory muscles, chest wall and pleura, and upper airways exhibit respiratory effort and complain that they "can't breathe"; and patients with abnormal gas exchange owing to lung dysfunction report shortness of breath and that they "can't breathe enough". Tables 15.1 and 15.2 present causes of acute and chronic respiratory acidosis, respectively. This classification accounts for the usual mode of onset and duration of the various causes, and it emphasizes the biphasic time course that characterizes the secondary physiologic response to hypercapnia. Some conditions can cause acute, acute on chronic, or chronic hypercapnia. COPD, including emphysema, chronic bronchitis, and small-airway disease, is the most common cause of chronic hypercapnia. Importantly, certain causes of chronic respiratory acidosis (e.g., COPD) can superimpose an element of acute respiratory acidosis during periods of decompensation (e.g., pneumonia, major surgery, heart failure).

Clinical Manifestations

Because hypercapnia almost always occurs with some degree of hypoxemia, it is often difficult to determine whether a specific manifestation is the consequence of the elevated P_{CO_2} or the reduced P_{O_2}. Clinical manifestations of respiratory acidosis arising from the CNS are collectively known as *hypercapnic encephalopathy*. Mild to moderate hypercapnia (up to 70 mm Hg) is associated with irritability, inability to concentrate, headache, anorexia, mental cloudiness, apathy, and confusion. Higher P_{CO_2} values or rapidly developing hypercapnia is characterized by incoherence, combativeness, hallucinations, delirium, transient psychosis, seizures, and coma. Progressive narcosis develops at P_{CO_2} >75-80 mm Hg, but if chronic hypercapnia is present, levels >90-100 mm Hg are required. Neurological examination might reveal asterixis, myoclonus, and papilledema (pseudotumor cerebri). Severe hypercapnia can be misdiagnosed as a cerebral vascular accident or an intracranial tumor.

The hemodynamic consequences of respiratory acidosis include a direct depressing effect on myocardial contractility. An associated sympathetic surge, sometimes intense, leads to increases in plasma catecholamines; however, during severe acidemia (blood pH lower than approximately 7.20), receptor responsiveness to catecholamines is markedly blunted. Hypercapnia results in systemic vasodilatation via a direct action on vascular smooth muscle; this effect is most obvious in the cerebral circulation, where blood flow increases in direct relation to the level of P_{CO_2}. By contrast, CO_2 retention can produce vasoconstriction in the pulmonary circulation resulting in pulmonary hypertension and right-sided heart failure (cor pulmonale). Similarly, CO_2 retention can lead to vasoconstriction in the renal circulation that may be the result, at least in part, of enhanced sympathetic activity. Mild to moderate hypercapnia is usually associated with an increased cardiac output, normal or increased blood pressure, warm skin, a bounding pulse, and diaphoresis. However, if hypercapnia is severe or considerable hypoxemia is present, decreases in both cardiac output and blood pressure may be observed.

TABLE 15.1 Causes of Acute Respiratory Acidosis	
Normal Airways and Lungs	**Abnormal Airways and Lungs**
Central Nervous System Depression	**Upper Airway Obstruction**
General anesthesia Sedative overdose (opiates, benzodiazepines, tricyclic antidepressants, barbiturates) Head trauma Cerebrovascular accident Central sleep apnea Cerebral edema Brain tumor Encephalitis Hypothyroidism Hypothermia Starvation	Coma-induced hypopharyngeal obstruction Aspiration of foreign body or vomitus Laryngospasm Angioedema Epiglottitis Obstructive sleep apnea Inadequate laryngeal intubation Laryngeal obstruction post intubation
Neuromuscular Impairment	**Lower Airway Obstruction**
Cervical spine injury or disease (trauma, syringomyelia) Transverse myelitis (multiple sclerosis) Guillain-Barré syndrome Acute intermittent porphyria Tick paralysis Status epilepticus Botulism, tetanus Crisis in myasthenia gravis Electrolyte abnormalities (hyperkalemia, hypokalemia, hypophosphatemia, hypercalcemia, hypermagnesemia) Eaton-Lambert syndrome Hyperthyroidism Drugs or toxic agents (e.g., curare, succinylcholine, aminoglycosides, organophosphates, shellfish poisoning, ciguatera poisoning, procainamide myopathy)	Generalized bronchospasm Acute severe asthma Bronchiolitis of infancy and adult Disorders involving pulmonary alveoli Severe bilateral pneumonia Acute respiratory distress syndrome Severe pulmonary edema
	Pulmonary Perfusion Defect
	Cardiac arrest[a] Severe circulatory failure[a] Massive pulmonary thromboembolism Fat or air embolus
Ventilatory Restriction	
Rib fractures with flail chest Pneumothorax Hemothorax Impaired diaphragmatic function (e.g., peritoneal dialysis, ascites)	
Iatrogenic Events	
Misplacement or displacement of airway cannula during anesthesia or mechanical ventilation Bronchoscopy-associated hypoventilation or respiratory arrest Increased CO_2 production with constant mechanical ventilation (e.g., due to high-carbohydrate diet or sorbent-regenerative hemodialysis)	

[a]May produce "pseudorespiratory alkalosis."

Modified from Madias NE, Adrogué HJ. Respiratory alkalosis and acidosis. In: Alpern RJ, Moe OW, Kaplan M (eds). *Seldin and Giebisch's The Kidney: Physiology and Pathophysiology.* London: Academic Press; 2013: 2113–2138.

Concomitant therapy with vasoactive medications (e.g., β-adrenergic receptor blockers) or the presence of congestive heart failure may further impair the hemodynamic response. Cardiac arrhythmias, particularly supraventricular tachyarrhythmias not associated with major hemodynamic compromise, are common, especially in patients receiving digitalis. They do not result primarily from the hypercapnia but rather reflect the associated hypoxemia and sympathetic discharge, concomitant medication, other electrolyte abnormalities, and underlying cardiac disease. Cardiac arrhythmias are also observed after initiation of mechanical ventilation and likely result from sudden correction of acidemia. Retention of salt and water is commonly observed in sustained hypercapnia, especially in the presence of cor pulmonale. In addition to the effects of heart failure on the kidney, multiple other factors may be involved, including the prevailing stimulation of the sympathetic nervous system and the renin-angiotensin-aldosterone axis, increased renal vascular resistance, and elevated levels of antidiuretic hormone and cortisol.

Diagnosis

Respiratory acidosis is often not suspected and, if left untreated, may result in serious complications, including death. Therefore, even if there is a low clinical suspicion of CO_2 retention, ABGs should be obtained. Venous blood gases (VBGs) can be effectively used if ABGs cannot be obtained or frequent sampling is required. Notably, VBGs also provide information about the oxygenation of the tissues. If the acid-base profile of the patient reveals hypercapnia

TABLE 15.2 Causes of Chronic Respiratory Acidosis	
Normal Airways and Lungs	**Abnormal Airways and Lungs**
Central Nervous System Depression	**Upper Airway Obstruction**
Sedative overdose (narcotics, benzodiazepines, tricyclic antidepressants) Primary alveolar hypoventilation (Ondine's curse) Obesity-hypoventilation syndrome (pickwickian syndrome) Brain tumor Brainstem disease Bulbar poliomyelitis Hypothyroidism Hypothermia Starvation	Tonsillar and peritonsillar hypertrophy Retropharyngeal disorders Paralysis of vocal cords Severe laryngeal or tracheal disorders (stenosis, tumors, angioedema, tracheomalacia) Obstructive goiter Airway stenosis after prolonged intubation Thymoma, aortic aneurysm
Neuromuscular Impairment	**Lower Airway Obstruction**
Poliomyelitis Multiple sclerosis Muscular dystrophy Amyotrophic lateral sclerosis Diaphragmatic paralysis Myxedema Myopathic disease Hyperthyroidism Eaton-Lambert syndrome Glycogen storage and mitochondrial diseases	Chronic obstructive lung disease (bronchitis, bronchiolitis, bronchiectasis, emphysema)
	Disorders Involving Pulmonary Alveoli
	Severe chronic pneumonitis Diffuse infiltrative disease (e.g., alveolar proteinosis) End-stage interstitial lung disease Severe pulmonary vascular disease
Ventilatory Restriction	
Kyphoscoliosis, spinal arthritis Morbid obesity Pectus excavatum Thoracoplasty Ankylosing spondylitis Fibrothorax Hydrothorax Impaired diaphragmatic function	

Modified from Madias NE, Adrogué HJ. Respiratory alkalosis and acidosis. In: Alpern RJ, Moe OW, Kaplan M (eds). *Seldin and Giebisch's The Kidney: Physiology and Pathophysiology*. London: Academic Press; 2013: 2113–2138.

in association with acidemia, at least an element of respiratory acidosis must be present. However, hypercapnia can be associated with a normal or an alkaline pH because of the simultaneous presence of additional acid-base disorders (see Chapter 12). Information from the patient's history, physical examination, and ancillary laboratory data should be used for diagnosing respiratory acidosis and discerning whether the disorder is acute, acute on chronic, or chronic.

Therapeutic Principles

Treatment of acute respiratory acidosis should focus on four critical steps: (1) ensuring a patent airway, (2) restoring adequate oxygenation by delivering an oxygen-rich inspired mixture, (3) securing adequate ventilation to repair the abnormal blood gas composition, and (4) reversing or treating the underlying cause, if possible. For example, patients with suspected opiate or benzodiazepine overdose should receive antidote treatment (naloxone or flumazenil, respectively).

Once a patent airway is secured, patients with hypercapnic respiratory failure breathing spontaneously and likely to respond to conservative management (i.e., without ventilator assistance) are administered supplemental oxygen via nasal cannulas, venturi masks, or nonrebreathing masks. The target oxygen goal is Po_2 of 60-70 mm Hg and oxygen saturation of ≥90%-93%. Patients expected to require low levels of supplemental oxygen can be started at 1 to 2 L/min via nasal cannula or 24% to 28% Fio_2 via mask with gradual increases of 1 L/min or 4% to 7% Fio_2. Beyond standard oxygen therapy, which provides oxygen at <15 L/min, there is a growing application of high-flow oxygen supplementation via nasal cannula using 40-60 L/min; this modality has been associated with reduced mortality and may offer advantages compared to noninvasive ventilation (NIV) in some patients.

If the target Po_2 is not achieved with these measures, ventilator assistance must be initiated. Ventilator assistance comprises two general types: NIV and standard mechanical ventilation that requires airway intubation. NIV might be of benefit to patients with acute exacerbation of COPD, cardiogenic pulmonary edema, postextubation respiratory failure, obstructive sleep apnea, and neuromuscular diseases. Conversely, NIV is not suitable for patients with hemodynamic instability, severe cardiorespiratory distress, markedly impaired consciousness, inability to protect the airway, excessive bronchial secretions, and those following head, neck, esophageal, or gastric bypass surgery. Consensus has not been reached about the mode (pressure- or volume-controlled), type of mask (nasal, oro-nasal, full-face) and optimal settings of NIV, which can be modified according to patient comfort and underlying disease. Most frequently, NIV is started with an oro-nasal mask. Initial settings for pressure-control NIV can be bilevel positive airway pressure (BiPAP) with inspiratory pressure 8–12 cm H_2O and expiratory pressure 3-5 cm H_2O.

When ventilator assistance is required but NIV is contraindicated, endotracheal intubation followed by standard mechanical ventilation must be implemented. Large tidal volumes during mechanical ventilation often lead to alveolar overdistention, which results in hypotension and barotrauma, two life-threatening complications. To overcome these complications, prescription of tidal volumes of 6 mL/kg body weight (instead of the conventional level of 12 mL/kg body weight), to achieve plateau airway pressures of <30 cm H_2O, has been proposed. Because an increase in Pco_2 develops (but rarely exceeds 80 mm Hg), this approach is termed *permissive hypercapnia* or *controlled mechanical hypoventilation*. If the resultant hypercapnia reduces the blood pH to less than 7.20, many physicians would prescribe bicarbonate; however, this strategy is controversial, and others would intervene only for pH values closer to 7.00. Several studies indicate that permissive hypercapnia affords improved clinical outcomes. Heavy sedation and neuromuscular blockade are frequently needed with this therapy. After discontinuation of neuromuscular blockade, some patients develop prolonged weakness or paralysis. Contraindications to permissive hypercapnia include cerebrovascular disease, brain edema, increased intracranial pressure, and convulsions; depressed cardiac function and arrhythmias; and severe pulmonary hypertension. Notably, most of these entities can develop as adverse effects of permissive hypercapnia itself, especially in the presence of substantial acidemia.

Cardiopulmonary bypass represents a form of mechanical cardiopulmonary support that is often applied intraoperatively to facilitate cardiac surgery. A more prolonged type of extracorporeal life support, known as *extracorporeal membrane oxygenation* (ECMO), can be used in the intensive care unit in neonates, children, and adults. Application of ECMO involves either a venoarterial (VA) or venovenous (VV) vascular access. Both types provide respiratory support, but only VA ECMO provides hemodynamic support.

The presence of a concurrent *metabolic* acidosis is the primary indication for alkali therapy in patients with acute respiratory acidosis. Administration of sodium bicarbonate to the spontaneously breathing patient with simple respiratory acidosis is not only of questionable efficacy but also involves considerable risk. Concerns include pH-mediated depression of ventilation, enhanced CO_2 production because of bicarbonate decomposition, and volume expansion; however, alkali therapy may have a role in patients with severe bronchospasm by restoring the responsiveness of the bronchial musculature to β-adrenergic agonists. Successful management of intractable asthma in patients with blood pH lower than 7.00 by administering sufficient sodium bicarbonate to raise blood pH to greater than 7.20 has been reported.

Patients with chronic respiratory acidosis frequently develop episodes of acute decompensation that can be serious or life threatening. Common culprits include pulmonary infections, use of narcotics, and excessive oxygen therapy. In contrast to acute hypercapnia, injudicious use of oxygen therapy in patients with chronic respiratory acidosis can produce further reductions in alveolar ventilation. Respiratory decompensation superimposes an acute element of CO_2 retention and acidemia on the chronic baseline. Only rarely can one remove the underlying cause of chronic respiratory acidosis, but maximizing alveolar ventilation with relatively simple maneuvers is often successful in the management of respiratory decompensation. Such maneuvers include treatment with antibiotics, bronchodilators, or diuretics; avoid-

ance of irritant inhalants, tranquilizers, and sedatives; elimination of retained secretions; and gradual reduction of supplemental oxygen targeting a Po_2 of about 50 to 55 mm Hg. Administration of adequate quantities of chloride (usually as the potassium salt) prevents or corrects a complicating element of metabolic alkalosis (commonly diuretic-induced) that can further dampen the ventilatory drive. Acetazolamide may be used as an adjunctive measure, but care must be taken to avoid potassium depletion. Potassium and phosphate depletion should be corrected, as they can contribute to the development or maintenance of respiratory failure by impairing the function of skeletal muscles. Restoration of the Pco_2 of the patient to near its chronic baseline should proceed gradually, over a period of many hours to a few days. Overly rapid reduction in Pco_2 in such patients risks the development of sudden, posthypercapnic alkalemia with potentially serious consequences, including reduction in cardiac output and cerebral blood flow, cardiac arrhythmias (including predisposition to digitalis intoxication), and generalized seizures. In the absence of a complicating element of metabolic acidosis, and with the possible exception of the severely acidemic patient with intense generalized bronchoconstriction who is undergoing mechanical ventilation, there is no role for alkali administration in chronic respiratory acidosis.

Respiratory Alkalosis

Respiratory alkalosis, or primary hypocapnia, is the acid-base disturbance initiated by a reduction in carbon dioxide tension of body fluids and in whole-body CO_2 stores. Hypocapnia alkalinizes body fluids and elicits an adaptive decrement in plasma $[HCO_3]$ that should be viewed as an integral part of the respiratory alkalosis. The level of Pco_2 measured at rest and at sea level is lower than 35 mm Hg in simple respiratory alkalosis. Higher values of Pco_2 may still indicate the presence of an element of primary hypocapnia in the setting of mixed acid-base disorders (e.g., eucapnia, rather than the anticipated hypercapnia, in the presence of metabolic alkalosis).

Pathophysiology

Primary hypocapnia most commonly reflects pulmonary hyperventilation caused by increased ventilatory drive. The latter results from signals arising from the lung, from the peripheral (carotid and aortic) or brainstem chemoreceptors, or from influences originating in other centers of the brain. Hypoxemia is a major stimulus of alveolar ventilation, but Po_2 values lower than 60 mm Hg are required to elicit this effect consistently. Additional mechanisms for the generation of primary hypocapnia include maladjusted mechanical ventilators, extrapulmonary elimination of CO_2 by a dialysis device or ECMO, and decreased CO_2 production (e.g., sedation, skeletal muscle paralysis, hypothermia, hypothyroidism) in patients receiving constant mechanical ventilation.

A condition termed *pseudorespiratory alkalosis* occurs in patients who have profound depression of cardiac function and pulmonary perfusion but have relative preservation of alveolar ventilation, including patients with advanced circulatory failure and those undergoing cardiopulmonary resuscitation. In such patients, venous (and tissue) hypercapnia is present because of the severely reduced pulmonary blood flow that limits the amount of CO_2 delivered to the lungs for excretion. On the other hand, arterial blood reveals hypocapnia because of the increased ventilation-to-perfusion ratio ($\dot{V}_A/\dot{Q}$), which causes a larger than normal removal of CO_2 per unit of blood traversing the pulmonary circulation. However, absolute CO_2 excretion is decreased and the body CO_2 balance is positive. Therefore, respiratory acidosis, rather than respiratory alkalosis, is present. Such patients may have severe venous acidemia (often resulting from mixed respiratory and metabolic acidosis) accompanied by an arterial pH that ranges from mild acidemia to frank alkalemia. In addition, arterial blood may show normoxemia or hyperoxemia, despite the presence of severe hypoxemia in venous blood. Therefore, both arterial and mixed (or central) venous blood sampling is needed to assess the acid-base status and oxygenation of patients with critical hemodynamic compromise.

Secondary Physiologic Response

Adaptation to acute hypocapnia is characterized by an immediate drop in plasma $[HCO_3^-]$, principally as a result of titration of nonbicarbonate body buffers. This adaptation is completed within 5 to 10 minutes after the onset of hypocapnia. Plasma $[HCO_3^-]$ declines, on average, by approximately 0.2 mEq/L for each 1 mm Hg acute decrement in Pco_2; consequently, the plasma $[H^+]$ decreases by about 0.75 nEq/L for each 1 mm Hg acute reduction in Pco_2. The limit of this adaptation of plasma $[HCO_3^-]$ is on the order of 17 to 18 mEq/L. Concomitant small increases in plasma chloride, lactate, and other unmeasured anions balance the decline in plasma $[HCO_3^-]$, each of these components accounting for about one-third of the bicarbonate decrement. Small decreases in plasma sodium (1 to 3 mEq/L) and potassium (0.2 mEq/L for each 0.1 unit increase in pH) may be observed. Severe hypophosphatemia can occur in acute hypocapnia because of the translocation of phosphorus into the cells.

A larger decrement in plasma $[HCO_3^-]$ occurs in chronic hypocapnia as a result of kidney adaptation to the disorder, which involves suppression of both proximal and distal acidification mechanisms. Completion of this adaptation requires 2 to 3 days. Plasma $[HCO_3^-]$ decreases, on average, by about 0.4 mEq/L for each 1 mm Hg chronic decrement in Pco_2; as a consequence, plasma $[H^+]$ decreases by approximately 0.4 nEq/L for each 1 mm Hg chronic reduction in Pco_2. The limit of this adaptation of plasma $[HCO_3^-]$ is on the order of 12 to 15 mEq/L. About two-thirds of the decline in plasma $[HCO_3^-]$ is balanced by an increase in plasma chloride concentration, and the remainder reflects an increase in plasma unmeasured anions; part of the remainder results from the alkaline titration of plasma proteins, but most remains undefined. Plasma lactate does not increase in chronic hypocapnia, even in the presence of moderate hypoxemia. Similarly, no appreciable change in the plasma concentration of sodium occurs. In sharp contrast with acute hypocapnia, the plasma concentration of phosphorus remains essentially unchanged in chronic hypocapnia. Although plasma potassium is in the normal range in patients with chronic hypocapnia at sea level, hypokalemia and kidney potassium wasting have been described in subjects in whom sustained hypocapnia was induced by exposure to high altitude. Patients with end-stage kidney disease maintained on dialysis are obviously at risk for development of severe alkalemia in response to chronic hypocapnia because the damaged kidneys cannot generate a secondary decrease in plasma $[HCO_3^-]$. For example, this situation arises when such a patient develops marked hyperventilation because of severe pneumonia. This risk is somewhat higher in patients undergoing peritoneal dialysis rather than hemodialysis because the former treatment maintains, on average, higher plasma $[HCO_3^-]$.

Etiology

Primary hypocapnia is the most frequent acid-base disturbance encountered; it occurs in normal pregnancy and with high-altitude residence. Table 15.3 lists the major causes of respiratory alkalosis. Most are associated with the abrupt appearance of hypocapnia, but in many instances the process is sufficiently prolonged to permit full chronic adaptation. Consequently, no attempt has been made to separate these conditions into acute and chronic categories. Some of the major causes of respiratory alkalosis are benign, whereas others are life threatening. The *hyperventilation syndrome* refers to a condition characterized by episodes of acute hyperventilation associated with fear, anxiety, and sense of impending doom in the absence of significant cardiopulmonary disease. Primary hypocap-

TABLE 15.3	Causes of Respiratory Alkalosis
Hypoxemia or Tissue Hypoxia	**Central Nervous System Stimulation**
Decreased inspired O_2 tension	
High altitude	Voluntary
Bacterial or viral pneumonia	Pain
Aspiration of food, foreign body, or vomitus	Anxiety, hyperventilation syndrome
Laryngospasm, Angioedema	Psychosis
Drowning	Fever
Cyanotic heart disease	Subarachnoid hemorrhage
Severe anemia	Cerebrovascular accident
Left shift deviation of the HbO_2 curve	Meningoencephalitis
Hypotension[a]	Tumor
Severe circulatory failure[a]	Trauma
Pulmonary edema	
	Drugs or Hormones
Stimulation of Chest Receptors	Nikethamide, ethamivan
	Doxapram
Pneumonia	Xanthines
Acute asthma	Salicylates
Pneumothorax	Catecholamines
Hemothorax	Angiotensin II
Flail chest	Vasopressor agents
Acute respiratory distress syndrome	Progesterone
Cardiac failure	Medroxyprogesterone
Mechanical hyperventilation	Dinitrophenol
Noncardiogenic pulmonary edema	Nicotine
Pulmonary embolism	**Miscellaneous**
Interstitial lung disease	
	Exercise
	Pregnancy
	Hyperthyroidism
	Sepsis
	Chronic liver disease
	Heat exposure
	Heart-lung machine
	ECMO
	Heat exposure
	Recovery from metabolic acidosis

[a]May produce "pseudorespiratory alkalosis."

ECMO, Extracorporeal membrane oxygenation; *HbO₂*, oxyhemoglobin.

Modified from Madias NE, Adrogué HJ. Respiratory alkalosis and acidosis. In: Alpern RJ, Moe OW, Kaplan M (eds). *Seldin and Giebisch's The Kidney: Physiology and Pathophysiology.* London: Academic Press; 2013: 2113–2138.

nia is particularly common among the critically ill, occurring either as the simple disorder or as a component of mixed disturbances. Its presence constitutes an ominous prognostic sign, with mortality increasing in direct proportion to the severity of the hypocapnia.

Clinical Manifestations

Rapid decrements in Pco_2 to half the normal values or lower are typically accompanied by paresthesias of the extremities, chest discomfort (especially in patients manifesting increased airway resistance), circumoral numbness, lightheadedness, confusion, and, rarely, tetany or generalized seizures. These manifestations are common in patients with the hyperventilation syndrome. These patients also report dyspnea at rest; they need to sigh frequently, and minimal exertion may result in significant dyspnea. These manifestations are seldom present in the chronic phase. Episodes of acute hyperventilation may occasionally lead to posthyperventilation apnea caused by the depletion of CO_2 stores; the resulting hypoxemia can have serious consequences.

Acute hypocapnia decreases cerebral blood flow, which, in severe cases, may reach values less than 50% of normal, resulting in cerebral hypoxia. This hypoperfusion has been implicated in the pathogenesis of the neurologic manifestations of acute respiratory alkalosis along with other factors, including hypocapnia, alkalemia, pH-induced shift of the oxyhemoglobin dissociation curve, and decrements in the levels of ionized calcium and potassium. Some evidence indicates that cerebral blood flow returns to normal in chronic respiratory alkalosis.

Patients who are actively hyperventilating manifest no appreciable changes in cardiac output or systemic blood pressure. By contrast, acute hypocapnia in the course of passive hyperventilation, as typically observed during mechanical ventilation in patients with a depressed central nervous system or receiving general anesthesia, frequently results in a major reduction in cardiac output and systemic blood pressure, increased peripheral vascular resistance, and substantial hyperlactatemia. This discrepant response probably reflects the decline in venous return caused by mechanical ventilation in passive hyperventilation. Although acute hypocapnia does not lead to cardiac arrhythmias in normal volunteers, it may contribute to the generation of both atrial and ventricular tachyarrhythmias in patients with ischemic heart disease. Chest pain and ischemic ST-T wave changes have been observed in acutely hyperventilating subjects with or without coronary artery disease. Coronary vasospasm and Prinzmetal angina can be precipitated by acute hypocapnia in susceptible subjects. The pathogenesis of these manifestations has been attributed to the same factors that are incriminated in the neurologic manifestations of acute hypocapnia.

Diagnosis

Careful observation can detect abnormal patterns of breathing in some patients, yet marked hypocapnia may be present without a clinically evident increase in respiratory effort. Therefore, an ABG analysis should be obtained whenever hyperventilation is suspected. In fact, the diagnosis of respiratory alkalosis, especially the chronic form, is frequently missed; physicians often misinterpret the electrolyte pattern of hyperchloremic hypobicarbonatemia as indicative of a normal anion gap metabolic acidosis. If the acid-base profile of the patient reveals hypocapnia in association with alkalemia, at least an element of respiratory alkalosis must be present. Primary hypocapnia, however, may be associated with a

normal or an acidic pH as a result of the concomitant presence of other acid-base disorders. Notably, mild degrees of chronic hypocapnia commonly leave blood pH within the high-normal range. As always, proper evaluation of the acid-base status of the patient requires careful assessment of the history, physical examination, and ancillary laboratory data (see Chapter 12). After the diagnosis of respiratory alkalosis has been made, a search for its cause should ensue. The diagnosis of respiratory alkalosis can have important clinical implications, often providing a clue to the presence of an unrecognized, serious disorder (e.g., sepsis) or indicating the severity of a known underlying disease.

Therapeutic Principles

Management of respiratory alkalosis must be directed whenever possible toward correction of the underlying cause. Respiratory alkalosis resulting from severe hypoxemia requires oxygen therapy. The widely held view that hypocapnia, even if severe, poses little risk to health is inaccurate. In fact, transient or permanent damage to the brain, heart, and lungs can result from substantial hypocapnia. In addition, rapid correction of severe hypocapnia can lead to reperfusion injury in the brain and lung. Therefore, severe hypocapnia in hospitalized patients must be prevented whenever possible and, if it is present, a slow correction is most appropriate.

The long-term management of the hyperventilation syndrome centers on education regarding the nature of the underlying condition and cognitive-behavioral therapy. Other measures may include breathing retraining, β-blockers, benzodiazepines, and serotonin reuptake inhibitors. Rebreathing into a closed system (e.g., a paper bag) is not recommended, because of the potential of hypoxemia in patients with underlying respiratory or cardiovascular disease. Administration of 250 to 500 mg acetazolamide can be beneficial in the management of signs and symptoms of high-altitude sickness, a syndrome characterized by hypoxemia and respiratory alkalosis. Considering the risks of severe alkalemia, sedation or, in rare cases, skeletal muscle paralysis and mechanical ventilation may be required temporarily to correct marked respiratory alkalosis. Patients maintained on chronic hemodialysis who develop an acute illness resulting in marked hyperventilation may require dialysis against a low-bicarbonate bath. Management of pseudorespiratory alkalosis must be directed at optimizing systemic hemodynamics.

Complete bibliography is available at Elsevier eBooks for Practicing Clinicians.

Key Bibliography

Adrogué HJ, Chap Z, Okuda Y, et al. Acidosis-induced glucose intolerance is not prevented by adrenergic blockade. *Am J Physiol*. 1988;255:E812–E823.

Adrogué HJ, Madias NE. Alkali therapy for respiratory acidosis: A medical controversy. *Am J Kidney Dis*. 2019;75:265–271.

Adrogué HJ, Madias NE. Management of life-threatening acid-base disorders. *N Engl J Med*. 1998;338:26-34.

Adrogué HJ, Madias NE. Respiratory acidosis. In: Gennari FJ, Adrogué HJ, Galla JH, Madias NE, eds. *Acid-Base Disorders and Their Treatment*. Boca Raton: Taylor & Francis Group; 2005:597–639.

Adrogué HJ, Madias NE. Secondary responses to altered acid-base status: the rules of engagement. *J Am Soc Nephrol*. 2010;21:920–923.

Adrogué HJ, Rashad MN, Gorin AB, et al. Assessing acid-base status in circulatory failure. Differences between arterial and central venous blood. *N Engl J Med*. 1989;320:1312–1316.

Aoyama H, Uchida K, Aoyama K, et al. Assessment of therapeutic interventions and lung protective ventilation in patients with moderate to severe acute respiratory distress syndrome: A systematic review and network meta-analysis. *JAMA Netw Open*. 2019;2:e198116.

Arbus GS, Hebert LA, Levesque PR, et al. Characterization and clinical application of the "significance band" for acute respiratory alkalosis. *N Engl J Med*. 1969;280:117–123.

Boulding R, Stacey R, Niven R, Fowler SJ. Dysfunctional breathing: a review of the literature and proposal for classification. *Eur Respir Rev*. 2016;25:287–294.

Brackett Jr NC, Cohen JJ, Schwartz WB. Carbon dioxide titration curve of normal man: Effect of increasing degrees of acute hypercapnia on acid-base equilibrium. *N Engl J Med*. 1965;272:6–12.

Brackett Jr NC, Wingo CF, Muren O, Solano JT. Acid-base response to chronic hypercapnia in man. *N Engl J Med*. 1969;280:124–130.

Davidson AC, Banham S, Elliott M, et al. BTS/ICS guidelines for the ventilator management of acute hypercapnic respiratory failure in adults. *Thorax*. 2016;71:1–35.

Girardis M, Busani S, Damiani E, et al. Effect of conservative vs conventional oxygen therapy on mortality among patients in an intensive care unit. The oxygen-ICU randomized clinical trial. *JAMA*. 2016;316:1583–1589.

Goligher EC, Slutsky AS. Not just oxygen? Mechanisms of benefit from high-flow nasal cannula in hypoxemic respiratory failure. *Am J Respir Crit Care Med*. 2017;195:1128–1131.

González SB, Menga G, Raimondi GA, et al. Secondary response to chronic respiratory acidosis in humans: A prospective study. *Kidney Int Rep*. 2018;5:1163–1170.

Krapf R, Beeler I, Hertner D, Hulter HN. Chronic respiratory alkalosis: The effect of sustained hyperventilation on renal regulation of acid-base equilibrium. *N Engl J Med*. 1991;324:1394–1401.

Madias NE, Adrogué HJ. Respiratory alkalosis and acidosis. In: Alpern RJ, Moe OW, Kaplan M, eds. *Seldin and Giebisch's The Kidney: Physiology and Pathophysiology*. 5th ed. London: Academic Press; 2013:2113–2138.

Madias NE, Wolf CJ, Cohen JJ. Regulation of acid-base equilibrium in chronic hypercapnia. *Kidney Int*. 1985;27:538–543.

Martinu T, Menzies D, Dial S. Re-evaluation of acid-base prediction rules in patients with chronic respiratory acidosis. *Can Respir J*. 2003;10:311–315.

Palmer BF. Evaluation and treatment of respiratory alkalosis. *Am J Kidney Dis*. 2012;60:834–838.

PART 3

Glomerular Diseases

16

Glomerular Clinicopathologic Syndromes

SHANE A. BOBART, SANJEEV SETHI

Introduction

Glomerular disease is the third most common cause of end-stage kidney disease worldwide. Glomerulonephritis (GN) has diverse presentations and work-up requires serum chemistry, serology, urinalysis with microscopy, and quantification of proteinuria. Patients present with several clinicopathological syndromes that can have various etiologies. These syndromes share similar characteristics in terms of findings on urinalysis, degree of proteinuria, presence of reduced glomerular filtration rate, edema, and hypertension, among others. Kidney pathology identifies several patterns of injury that can overlap among the causes of GN and, as a result, an etiological-based classification of these disorders is preferred. In this chapter, we will describe nephrotic syndrome, nephritic syndrome, rapidly progressive glomerulonephritis, and pulmonary-renal syndrome and highlight glomerular diseases associated with systemic disorders such as lupus nephritis, monoclonal immunoglobulin associated glomerulonephritis, and thrombotic microangiopathies.

Nephrotic Syndrome

Nephrotic syndrome is defined as more than 3.5 g of proteinuria in 24 hours, with serum albumin level less than 3.5 g/dL accompanied by hyperlipidemia and clinically apparent edema. The most common glomerular diseases manifesting as nephrotic syndrome (NS) are minimal change disease (MCD), focal segmental glomerulosclerosis (FSGS pattern of injury), and membranous nephropathy (MN). These lesions share the clinical characteristic of nephrotic-range proteinuria and the pathological finding of extensive podocyte foot process effacement on electron microscopy. Systemic causes of NS include diabetic kidney disease (DKD) and amyloidosis (Fig. 16.1), among others. Demographic characteristics, clinical history, and laboratory and serological findings, in addition to kidney pathology, aid in obtaining an accurate diagnosis, etiology, and management.

The most common clinical characteristics include edema, lipiduria, and hyperlipidemia but are not necessary for diagnosis. Complications may arise due to urinary protein loss, including iron deficiency anemia due to the loss of transferrin, vitamin D deficiency due to loss of vitamin D-binding protein, and hypo-gammaglobulinemia predisposing to sepsis and concurrent acute kidney injury (AKI). An important clinical complication to recognize is hypercoagulability, which occurs due to the urinary loss

of protein C, protein S, plasminogen, and anti-thrombin III. Renal vein thrombosis can occur when there is severe proteinuria (>10 g/24 hr) and severe hypoalbuminemia (<2 g/dL). Hypercoagulability is more common in NS due to membranous nephropathy and amyloidosis. Due to low oncotic pressure, low effective circulating volume can also be present resulting in AKI.

The goals of management in nephrotic syndrome should be focused on addressing complications and a comprehensive anti-proteinuric strategy. A low-salt, protein-restricted diet (0.8 to 1 g/kg/day), in conjunction with ACE inhibitor or ARB therapy, is a cornerstone of non-disease-specific management. Diuretics can be used to address edema, statin therapy for hyperlipidemia, and anticoagulation for those at high risk for thrombotic complications.

Minimal Change Disease

Minimal change disease (MCD) accounts for approximately 15% of adult nephrotic syndrome, increasing to over 70%-90% in the pediatric population. The pathogenic mechanism of MCD is unknown. However, there are well-known associations with NSAID use, thymoma and Hodgkin lymphoma, the last being suggestive of a T-cell-mediated mechanism.

In children, the presence of nephrotic syndrome without additional findings such as hematuria and reduced glomerular filtration rate (GFR) is considered MCD until proven otherwise and is often diagnosed and managed without a kidney biopsy. However, in adults, biopsy is important as there can be other diagnoses associated with this presentation. In support of its nomenclature, there are minimal/absent changes on light microscopy, but extensive foot process effacement on electron microscopy. The mainstay of therapy is corticosteroids; however, some forms may be considered steroid resistant. Additional therapies such as anti-CD20 monoclonal antibodies have been promising. MCD is discussed in detail in Chapter 18.

Focal Segmental Glomerulosclerosis

Focal segmental glomerulosclerosis (FSGS) is a histopathological lesion that commonly presents with nephrotic-range proteinuria as a result of podocyte injury and glomerular scarring. This clinicopathological syndrome is less common in children (<15%) but contributes as much as 25% of adult nephrotic syndrome and is the most common cause of idiopathic nephrotic syndrome among those of African descent. Compared to MCD, in addition

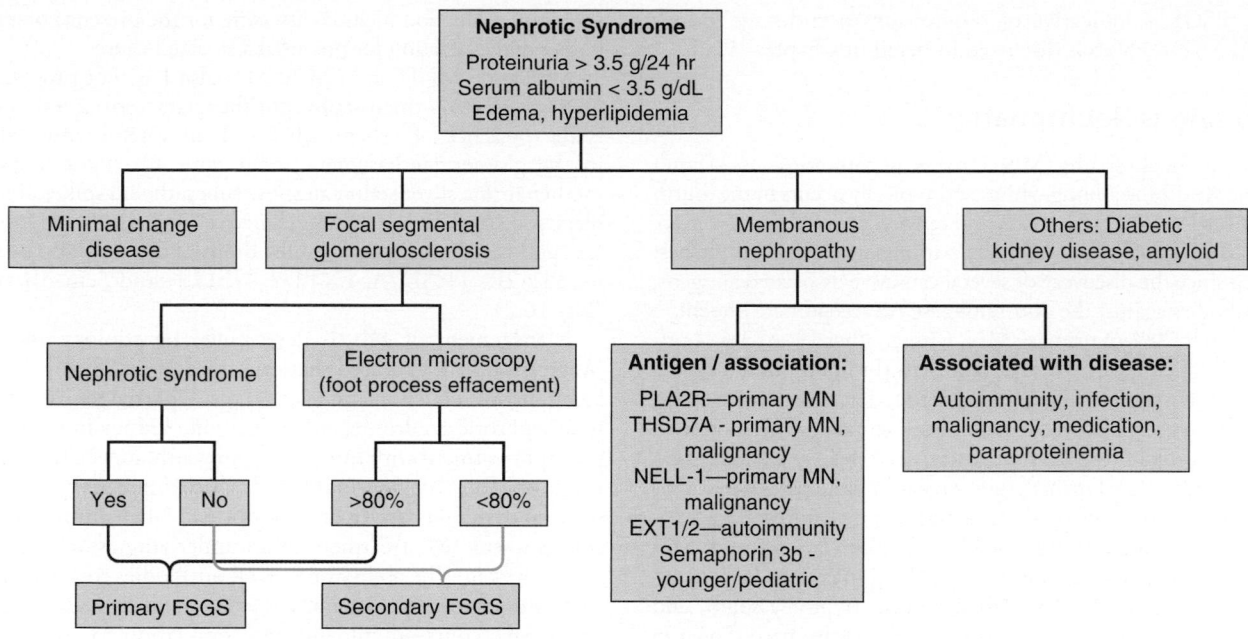

• **Fig. 16.1** Schematic showing the most common etiologies of nephrotic syndrome.

to having glomerular scarring, patients with FSGS can also have concomitant hypertension, reduced GFR, and even microscopic hematuria.

FSGS is currently classified as primary, due to a yet-to-be-discovered circulating podocyte permeability factor, versus secondary, due to maladaptive, drug, and viral causes and genetic etiologies (Table 16.1). As the name suggests, this histological lesion on light microscopy is focal, affecting only a portion of glomeruli, and segmental, involving a segment of the affected glomerulus. However, the lesion is not truly focal or segmental, as the name suggests, because on electron microscopy varying degrees of foot process effacement can be seen even in glomeruli

TABLE 16.1 Causes of FSGS

Primary FSGS

Attributed to a circulating podocyte permeability factor

Secondary FSGS

Viral: HIV-associated nephropathy, parvovirus B19, cytomegalovirus, COVID-19. Drug induced: heroin, interferon (α, β, γ), pamidronate, sirolimus, calcineurin inhibitors, anabolic steroids, direct-acting antiviral therapy (ledipasvir, sofosbuvir)

Adaptive: reduced nephron mass or glomerular adaptation, low birth weight, partial nephrectomy, unilateral renal agenesis, obesity-related glomerulopathy, basement membrane defects healing phase of focal proliferative glomerulonephritis, body building, sickle cell anemia, hypertensive nephrosclerosis, thrombotic microangiopathy, aging kidney

Genetic FSGS

Genetic mutations in podocyte genes: NPHS1(nephrin), NPHS2(podocin), PLCE1(phospholipase C epsilon), INF2(inverted formin), ACTN4 (α-actinin-alpha 4), APOL1

Adapted from De Vriese A, Sethi S, Nath K, et al. Differentiating Primary, Genetic, and Secondary FSGS in Adults: A Clinicopathologic Approach. *J Am Soc Nephrol.* 2018;29(3):759–774.

that appear normal on light microscopy. There are five variants that are distinguished on light microscopy: cellular, tip, perihilar, collapsing, and not otherwise specified (NOS). The five variants do not help in distinguishing primary from secondary causes of FSGS. Of these, collapsing FSGS is strongly associated with viral etiologies such as HIV infection and typically presents with the abrupt onset of severe nephrotic syndrome with high-risk, progressive loss of kidney function.

Since there is no discriminatory laboratory test to differentiate primary from secondary FSGS, a thorough history, combined with serum and urine studies and kidney biopsy, can help classify the lesion. Primary FSGS will typically have an acute onset of nephrotic syndrome with low serum albumin and >3.5 g/day of proteinuria. Electron microscopy can demonstrate varying degrees of foot process effacement, with >80% generally considered diffuse and favoring primary FSGS versus <80% considered segmental and favoring secondary FSGS (see Fig. 16.1).

The clinical course is dependent on the response to immunosuppressive therapy such as corticosteroids, calcineurin inhibitors, and mycophenolate mofetil. Primary FSGS typically recurs shortly after kidney transplant, supporting its pathogenic circulating factor hypothesis. In contrast, secondary FSGS can gradually develop proteinuria of varying degrees and typically has a slowly progressive disease course. Management of secondary FSGS should be focused on the underlying etiology with a comprehensive antiproteinuric strategy and avoidance of unnecessary immunosuppression. This algorithm, however, does not apply to collapsing FSGS, given its easily distinguishable clinicopathological features and genetic causes with variable degrees of foot process effacement (see Fig. 16.1). Genetic causes can be suggested by a family history of nephrotic syndrome or other congenital findings, as well as a history of poor response to immunosuppression. The presence of APOL1 risk alleles, which is associated with increased risk of FSGS lesions and advanced kidney disease in patients of African descent, is an increasingly recognized form of genetic FSGS. From a prognostic perspective, patients with non-nephrotic-range proteinuria have the best outcomes; conversely, persistent hematuria or poor response to immunosuppression in primary FSGS is indicative of progression to end-stage kidney disease (ESKD). FSGS is discussed in detail in Chapter 19.

Membranous Nephropathy

Membranous nephropathy (MN) is the most common cause of adult nephrotic syndrome among whites and typically occurs in the fourth to fifth decade of life, with males and females affected in a 2:1 ratio. Among MCD, FSGS, and MN, the pathogenesis of MN is the best described since the discovery of several causative/associated antigens. Autoantibodies against the phospholipase A2 receptor are present in approximately 70% of primary MN, with another 1% to 3% of primary MN patients with autoantibodies to thrombospondin type 1 domain containing 7a (THSD7A). More recently, additional target antigens have been discovered including Neural epidermal growth factor-like 1 protein (NELL-1), Exostosin1/2 (EXT1/2), and Semaphorin 3B (Sema3b). Further studies regarding the pathogenic ability and characterization of these antigens are required. However, several associations are already established. Secondary forms of MN are associated with autoimmunity (e.g., SLE), infections (e.g., hepatitis B), drugs (e.g., NSAIDs), malignancies (typically solid), and even paraproteinemias (see Fig. 16.1). EXT1/2 have been shown to be associated with MN in the setting of autoimmune diseases. As such, apart from recognizing the presence of nephrotic syndrome, a thorough evaluation includes assessing for the presence of autoantibodies and evaluation for potential associated causes.

Similar to MCD and FSGS, MN also has foot process effacement on electron microscopy, but the characteristic lesion of MN is the presence of subepithelial and intramembranous deposits in the glomerular basement membrane. On light microscopy, methenamine silver stain can show subepithelial spikes along capillary walls and immunofluorescence shows granular deposition of IgG and C3 along capillary walls. Biopsies can now also be stained for PLA2R, THSD7A, EXT1/2, NELL1, and Sema3B antigens (Fig. 16.2).

Management of MN is determined by etiology and risk of progression. It is expected that one-third of patients will undergo spontaneous remission and another third, partial remission. Persistent nephrotic syndrome and or declining kidney function should prompt treatment with immunosuppression, especially in primary forms of MN. Calcineurin inhibitors, rituximab, or cyclophosphamide and steroids are treatment options when immunosuppression is warranted. Treatment of an underlying associated cause is key, if present. The ability of PLA2R antibodies to guide response to immunosuppressive therapy is well established. Patients with a progressive course should undergo evaluation for superimposed disease such as crescentic GN, or acute interstitial nephritis. MN is discussed in detail in Chapter 20.

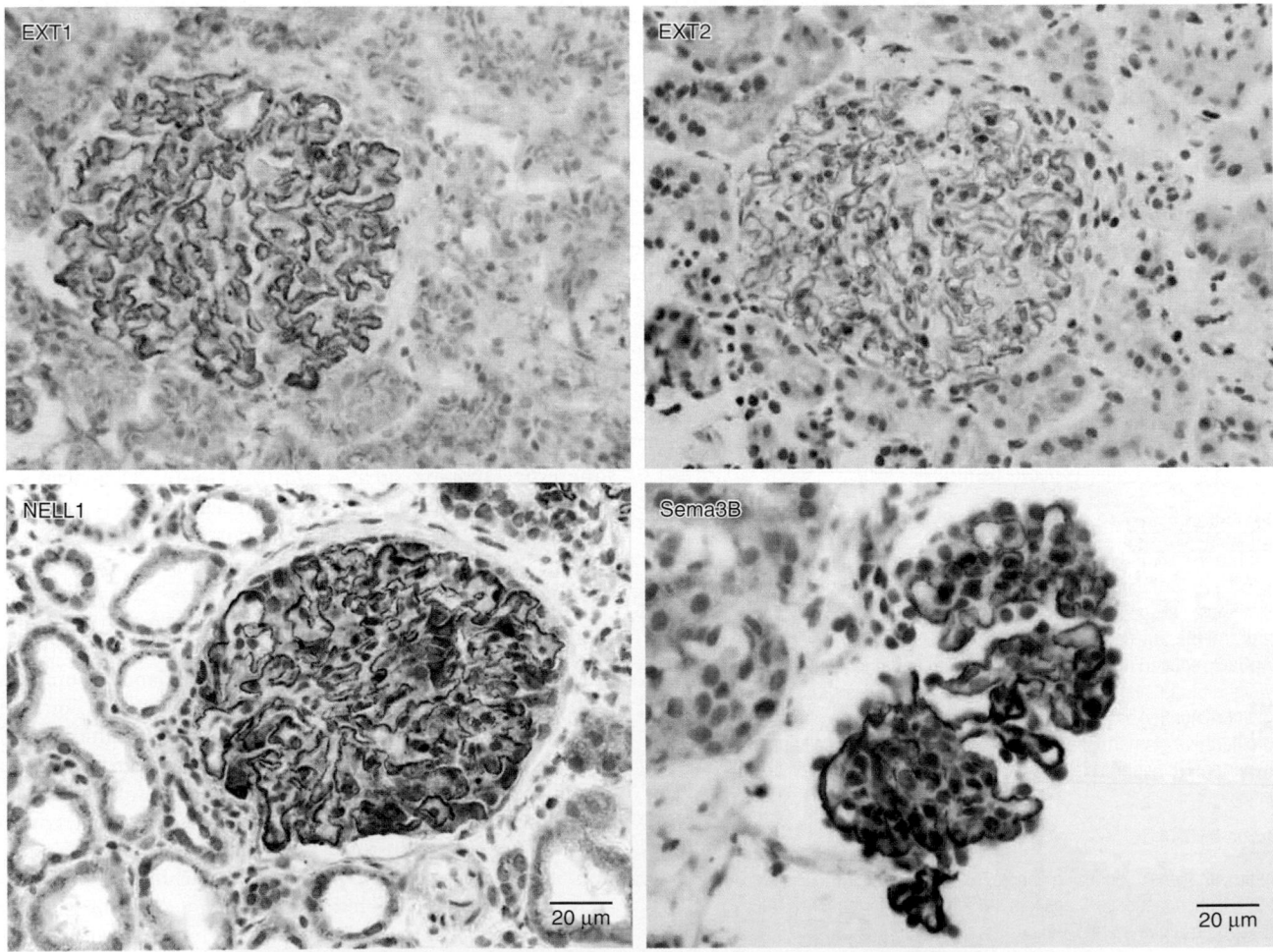

• **Fig. 16.2** New antigens in MN: immunohistochemistry showing granular staining for EXT1, EXT2, NELL1, and Sema3 along the capillary wall. EXT1 and EXT2 are from the same case; NELL1 and Sema3B represent one case each (all ×40).

Diabetic Kidney Disease

Diabetic kidney disease (DKD), discussed in more detail in Chapter 26, is the most common cause of kidney failure in the United States, with diabetic kidney disease often initially manifesting 10 to 15 years after diagnosis of diabetes. The presence of diabetic retinopathy also correlates strongly with the presence of DKD. Risk factors for kidney disease in people with diabetes include obesity, hypertension, ethnicity, and the degree of glycemic control.

DKD occurs as hyperglycemia results in glycosylation end products that accumulate in the glomeruli. The result is the development of moderately elevated albuminuria (30 to <300 mg/24hr) in the early phase of disease, which then progresses to severely elevated albuminuria (≥300 mg/24hr). As with most glomerular disorders, the extent of proteinuria correlates with prognosis. As proteinuria progresses, kidney failure is the end result.

Kidney biopsy is not always performed, as individuals with long standing diabetes who present with albuminuria and no other evidence of concomitant disease are presumed to have DKD. However, abnormal serology, dysmorphic RBCs, or rapid kidney function decline should prompt kidney biopsy. Kidney biopsy findings in DKD include thickening of the GBM, glomerular hypertrophy, and arteriolar hyalinosis. The classic finding is mesangial expansion and Kimmelstiel-Wilson nodules.

The mainstay of treatment is with ACEi or ARB to reduce albuminuria, controlling hypertension, which is often co-existent, strict glucose control, and weight loss. More recently, sodium glucose co-transporter-2 (SGLT-2) inhibitors have shown great promise for DKD (see Chapter 26).

Nephritic Syndrome

Nephritic syndrome is defined as the presence of glomerular hematuria in the form of dysmorphic red blood cells (RBCs) or RBC casts, in combination with hypertension, edema, reduced GFR with or without oliguria (depending on acuity), and non-nephrotic-range proteinuria. There are several forms of glomerulonephritis that can present with nephritic syndrome. They can be classified based on the etiology as immune complex-mediated, pauci-immune/ANCA-associated, anti-glomerular basement membrane (anti-GBM) antibody-mediated, or monoclonal gammopathy-associated, or linked to complement abnormalities (C3 glomerulonephritis) (Fig. 16.3).

Rapidly Progressive Glomerulonephritis

Rapidly progressive glomerulonephritis (RPGN) is a clinicopathologic syndrome that is defined by the rapid loss of kidney function over days to weeks in the context of nephritic syndrome. Many of the etiologies in immune complex-mediated, pauci-immune/ANCA-associated, and anti-GBM-mediated GN can present as an RPGN. In addition, several of the causes of RPGN can also present with concomitant pulmonary hemorrhage as a pulmonary renal syndrome, including ANCA-associated pauci-immune GN and anti-GBM glomerulonephritis (Goodpasture syndrome).

IgA Nephropathy

IgA nephropathy (IgAN) is the most common primary glomerulopathy worldwide. In the primary form, its pathogenesis is related to the deposition of immune complexes of anti-gliadin antibodies (IgG or IgA) and galactose deficient IgA1 in the mesangium of the glomerulus, resulting in an inflammatory cascade. This "primary form" is likely triggered by an inciting event such as an ongoing upper respiratory tract infection resulting in macroscopic ("synpharyngitic") hematuria. Patients can also present with asymptomatic or microscopic hematuria detected on urinalysis, which may or may not be accompanied by proteinuria. The proteinuria in IgAN is usually in the non-nephrotic range; when present, nephrotic-range proteinuria should prompt the search for an underlying podocytopathy as well. IgAN can also present as a systemic vasculitis in the form of Henoch-Schönlein purpura (HSP) or IgA vasculitis, with classic skin, joint, and intestinal manifestations that seem to have a more favorable prognosis in children compared to adults. Secondary forms of IgAN occur in the setting of inflammatory bowel disease, advanced liver disease, ankylosing spondylitis, and dermatitis herpetiformis.

On light microscopy, typical findings are mesangial proliferation (M), endocapillary proliferation (E), segmental sclerosis (S), tubulointerstitial fibrosis (T), and crescents (C). These five findings comprise the MEST-C score and, while each lesion is not pathognomonic for IgAN, they guide prognosis at the time of biopsy. On immunofluorescence, mesangial IgA deposition is noted, which corresponds to mesangial electron dense deposits on electron microscopy.

As many as 60% of patients with IgAN can have a benign course; however, progression to kidney failure occurs in up to 40% of patients over 10-20 years from diagnosis. Allograft recurrence, although common, does not often result in allograft loss. There are three well-studied clinical predictors of progression, namely, renal insufficiency, hypertension, and >1 g/24 hr of proteinuria at biopsy diagnosis. Although the hallmark finding is hematuria, studies assessing its role in prognosis have produced mixed results. IgAN is unique from a pathology standpoint as the MEST-C score is a reliable method of prognostication with T score providing the most consistent guide for progression to ESKD across studies. IgAN is discussed in detail in Chapter 21.

Infection-Related Glomerulonephritis

Infection-related glomerulonephritis, also referred to as *infection-associated glomerulonephritis,* can be classified as postinfectious glomerulonephritis (PIGN) or as GN related to an active infection. PIGN typically presents as nephritic syndrome 1 to 4 weeks after the onset of an infection; the infection has already resolved and, regardless of antibiotic therapy, the patient has developed a GN. In GN of active infection, the patient develops GN in the setting of an ongoing and often untreated infection. The two are indistinguishable by kidney biopsy; hence, an accurate medical history is key in this setting. PIGN was previously categorized as poststreptococcal glomerulonephritis (PSGN) due to group A beta-hemolytic streptococcal skin or pharyngitic infection; however, this current nomenclature has expanded to include various etiologies of this clinicopathological syndrome including several bacteria, especially staphylococci.

Non-invasive clues to the diagnosis include the presence of anti-streptolysin (ASO), anti-deoxyribonuclease (anti-DNAase B) antibodies, and hypocomplementemia. Other glomerulonephritides associated with hypocomplementemia include lupus nephritis (typically classes III, IV, V), cryoglobulinemia, cholesterol emboli, atypical hemolytic uremic syndrome, monoclonal Ig deposition disease, and C3 glomerulopathy.

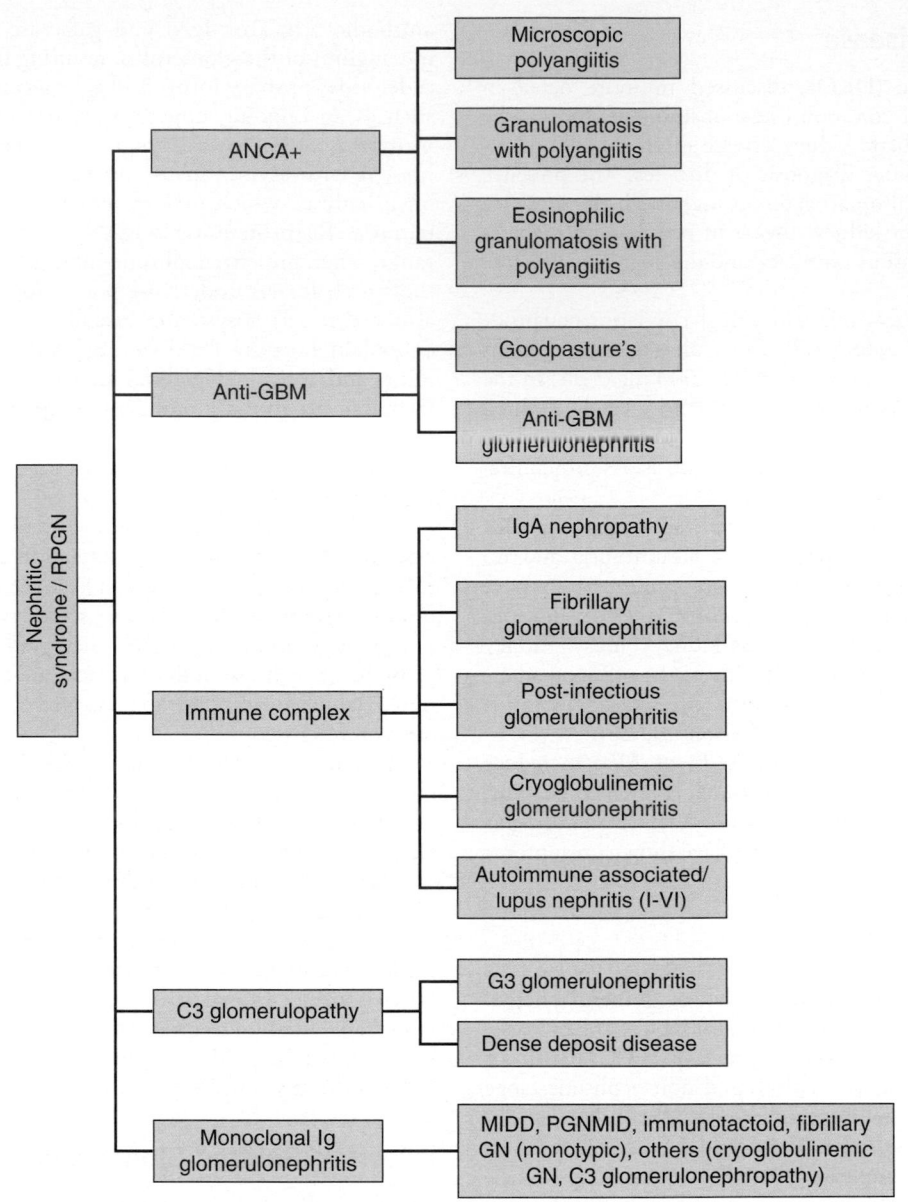

• **Fig. 16.3** Schematic of an etiology-based classification of glomerulonephritis. (Modified from Sethi S, Haas M, Markowitz GS, et al. Mayo Clinic/Renal Pathology Society Consensus report on pathologic classification, diagnosis, and reporting of GN. J Am Soc Nephrol. 2016;27:1278–1287.)

Typically, diffuse endocapillary proliferative glomerulonephritis is found on light microscopy and can often reveal neutrophils in the glomerular capillaries. In a resolving infection-related GN, diffuse proliferative features may be replaced by mesangial proliferative features. Immunofluorescence shows granular IgG and C3 deposition in capillary walls. Electron microscopy shows the classic "subepithelial humps" and can also show subendothelial deposits.

Given that the pathogenesis is an infection, treatment is supportive and centered around adequate treatment of the underlying infection. Prognosis appears more favorable in children versus adults. When patients initially present with PIGN but have persistent reduction in GFR and active urine sediment without ongoing infection, it should alert the clinician to test for alternative complement pathway abnormalities. Infection and hepatitis-related GN are discussed in detail in Chapters 23 and 24.

Fibrillary Glomerulonephritis

Fibrillary glomerulonephritis (FGN) is a rare form of immune complex GN that is defined by the presence of randomly oriented fibrillary deposits. It contributes less than 1% of all forms of GN; however, there has been a recent discovery of these fibrils containing DNA-J heat-shock protein family member B9 (DNAJB9), leading to a better diagnosis and understanding of the pathogenesis.

Fibrillary GN typically affects whites in the sixth decade of life, with a female predominance. The presentation is variable, with reduced GFR being common, and urine spanning from nephritic to nephrotic syndrome. It is questionable whether DNAJB9 is a potential autoantigen or a chaperone protein to which Ig can become attached. DNAJB9 has been identified in FGN patients but absent in amyloidosis, other forms of GN, and healthy kidneys. It has also been identified in serum of patients with FGN and its role is currently limited to aiding with diagnosis at this time. There are several conditions associated with FGN including hepatitis C infection, autoimmunity, diabetes mellitus, and malignancy. It was previously thought that monotypic FGN was strongly associated with the presence of a dysproteinemia and, thus, classified as a monoclonal gammopathy of renal significance (MGRS) lesion; however, a recent study has shown that performing paraffin IF studies often unmasks monotypic staining/restriction. In this study, only 1 of 11 patients had a circulating monoclonal protein, suggesting that over 90% of patients with FGN do not have an associated dysproteinemia.

The most common lesion on light microscopy is that of an MPGN or a diffuse proliferative pattern; however, one can find a mesangial proliferative, diffuse sclerosing, or, rarely, a membranous pattern. Immunofluorescence shows IgG, C3, kappa, and lambda. The characteristic finding on EM is non-branching, randomly oriented fibrils with average diameter of 20 nm (Fig. 16.4). Staining of the biopsy for DNAJB9 is useful to aid diagnosis in both native kidney and transplanted kidney biopsies. The prognosis is generally poor as there are limited options for treatment.

Membranoproliferative Glomerulonephritis

Membranoproliferative glomerulonephritis is not a distinct disease entity; rather, it is a kidney histopathological pattern that occurs as a result of various disease processes that typically present with nephritic syndrome. On light microscopy the classic finding is lobular accentuation of the glomerular tufts, double contouring of the capillary walls, mesangial expansion, and endocapillary proliferation. Electron microscopy usually demonstrates double contouring and subendothelial deposits. IF can help classify and determine the underlying etiology: immunoglobulin-mediated or complement-mediated. Depending on the type of immunoglobulins detected on IF, the underlying etiology can be traced to chronic infections, autoimmune diseases, or monoclonal gammopathy-associated kidney diseases. On the other hand, if there is dominant staining for complement with minimal or no immunoglobulins, then complement-mediated GN such as C3G is likely and work-up for dysregulation of the alternative complement pathway (e.g., mutations and/or autoantibodies to complement factors and proteins) should be pursued. However, if there is absence of immunoglobulin or complement on IF, then vascular phenomena such as thrombotic microangiopathy, malignant hypertension, and anti-phospholipid syndrome should be considered.

Lupus Nephritis

Over 50% of patients with systemic lupus erythematosus (SLE) develop some form of kidney involvement. This can manifest as microscopic hematuria, subnephrotic-range proteinuria, nephrotic or nephritic syndrome, and even RPGN. Laboratory testing often reveals a positive, double-stranded DNA antibody and low complement levels, especially when the disease is active, but this is non-specific for LN. It is important for patients with SLE to have frequent monitoring of kidney function and urinalyses as there are diverse histological findings that guide treatment decisions. Often, the findings on urinalysis do not correlate with the severity of disease, which is why kidney biopsy is the most important diagnostic tool in this form of glomerulonephritis. The International Society of Nephrology/Renal Pathology Society

(ISN/RPS) classification of lupus nephritis describes six classes/categories of lupus nephritis based primarily on the findings on LM (Table 16.2). The classic finding on immunofluorescence is that of a "full-house" pattern, meaning there is glomerular deposition of IgG, IgA, IgM, C3, and C1q. Electron microscopy can demonstrate deposits in the mesangial, subepithelial, or subendothelial regions, in addition to tubuloreticular inclusions in glomerular and endothelial cells. Recently, the antigen Exostosin 1/2 has been associated with Class V membranous LN. Throughout the course of this systemic disease, patients can switch between classes and severity of renal disease (see Table 16.2). Lupus can also manifest in the kidney as tubulointerstitial nephritis, thrombotic microangiopathy, or vasculitis. Lupus nephritis is discussed in detail in Chapter 25.

Cryoglobulinemic Glomerulonephritis

Cryoglobulinemia is characterized by immunoglobulins that precipitate at low temperatures. These cryoglobulinemic immune complexes cause a systemic syndrome of arthralgias, palpable purpura, and neuropathy via a small to medial vessel vasculitis. Apart from detectable cryoglobulins, patients typically have low complement (C4) and there is a strong association with hepatitis C infection. Kidney involvement is not uncommon and can present as reduced GFR, microscopic hematuria, proteinuria, nephrotic/nephritic syndrome, or a combination thereof. Cryoglobulinemic GN typically manifests with an MPGN pattern on light microscopy, with diffuse, dense subendothelial deposits with a microtubular substructure that can often occlude capillary loops. There are three types of cryoglobulins, each with different etiologies that ultimately help guide treatment. Type I cryoglobulins are monoclonal immunoglobulin and typically occur in the setting of multiple myeloma. Type II or mixed cryoglobulinemia with monoclonal immunoglobulins can occur in the setting of Waldenström macroglobulinemia (also type I), hepatitis C, Sjögren syndrome, or lymphoma. Type III or mixed polyclonal cryoglobulinemia is associated with autoimmunity (SLE), infection, and malignancy. Treatment is targeted toward the underlying etiology of the circulating cryoglobulin.

Antineutrophil Cytoplasmic Antibody-Associated Vasculitis

ANCA-associated vasculitis (AAV) is the most common cause of RPGN among those over 60 years old and is a common cause of the pulmonary renal syndrome. It is characterized by the presence of antibodies against antigens found in the cytoplasm of neutrophils: proteinase 3 (PR3) and myeloperoxidase (MPO). These antibodies are present in most cases but are not uniformly specific for three phenotypic syndromes: microscopic polyangiitis (MPA, 60% MPO), granulomatosis with polyangiitis (GPA, 75% PR3), and eosinophilic granulomatosis with polyangiitis (EPGA, 45% MPO). The initial screening test is by indirect immunofluorescence assay (IIF) as either a perinuclear (p-ANCA) or cytoplasmic (C-ANCA) pattern of staining of neutrophils. Once the IIF is positive, a confirmatory antigen-specific ELISA is performed. MPO is typically associated with p-ANCA while PR3 is typically associated with c-ANCA. There is also a subset of vasculitis that tests negative but shares all the systemic and clinical characteristics of AAV and is categorized as ANCA-negative vasculitis. There are also drug-induced forms of AAV associated with minocycline, allopurinol, hydralazine, anti-TNF agents, propylthiouracil, cocaine

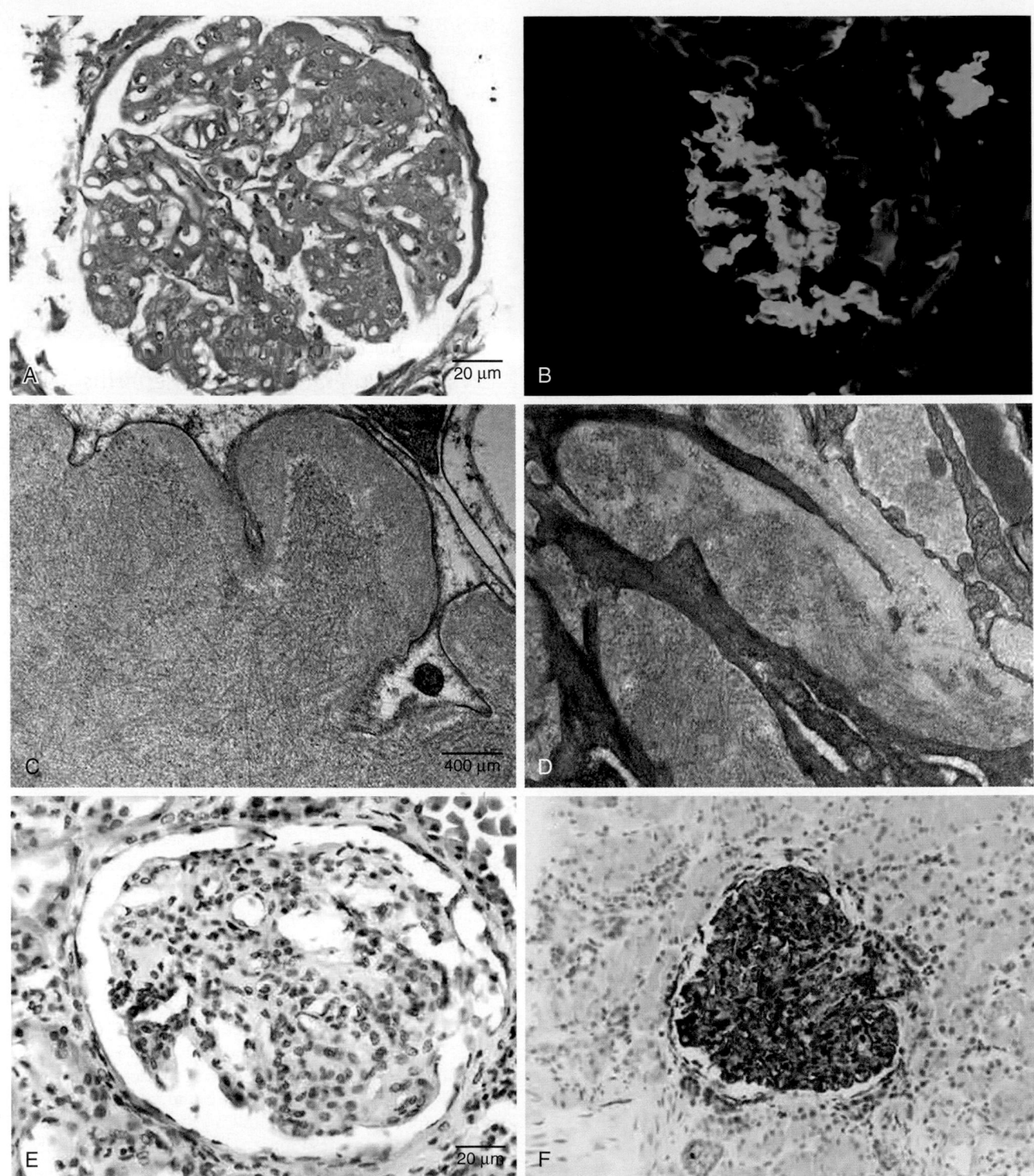

• **Fig. 16.4 Fibrillary GN.** (A) Light microscopy showing a membranoproliferative pattern of injury with mesangial expansion, endocapillary hypercellularity, and thickened capillary walls (PAS × 40). (B) Immunofluorescence microscopy showing IgG along the capillary walls. (C, D) Electron microscopy showing mesangial and capillary wall fibrillary deposits. (E) Congo red; the fibrillary deposits are Congo red negative. (F) The fibrillary deposits are strongly DNAJB9 positive.

(laced with levamisole), and other agents. ANCA can also be detected in SLE and inflammatory bowel disease, which is why kidney biopsy is important for diagnosis.

The pattern of kidney injury is that of necrotizing, crescentic, sclerosing, or mixed pattern, with the paucity of immune complex deposition (pauci-immune) on IF. This is uniform across all three phenotypes of AAV, but they can be differentiated by the absence of granulomas in MPA, presence of necrotizing granulomatous inflammation of the upper and lower airways in GPA, and asthma and eosinophilia in EGPA.

Initial treatment consists of a combination of pulse-dose corticosteroids with cyclophosphamide or rituximab. MPO-ANCA

TABLE 16.2	Abbreviated International Society of Nephrology/Renal Pathology Society 2003 Classification of Lupus Nephritis			
Class	Morphologic Type	Clinical Presentation	Location of Deposits	Management
I	Minimal mesangial	Bland urinalysis, preserved renal function	Mesangial (no mesangial proliferation)	Supportive
II	Mesangial proliferative	Microscopic hematuria +/− non-nephrotic-range proteinuria, preserved renal function	Mesangial (mesangial proliferation)	Nephrotic—corticosteroids or CNI Non-nephrotic—treat based on non-renal manifestations
III	Focal lupus nephritis	Active urinalysis, nephritic syndrome	Subendothelial (<50% w of gloms)	Corticosteroids plus MMF/ Cyclophosphamide
IV	Diffuse lupus nephritis	Nephritic/nephrotic syndrome, RPGN	Subendothelial (>50% of gloms)	Corticosteroids plus MMF/ Cyclophosphamide
V	Membranous lupus nephritis	Nephrotic syndrome	Subepithelial and intramembranous	Initially conservative; corticosteroids and MMF/CNI
VI	Advanced sclerosing lupus nephritis	Advanced kidney disease	>90% Global glomerulosclerosis	Prepare for kidney replacement therapy

Modified from Weening JJ, D'Agati VD, Schwartz MM, et al. The classification of glomerulonephritis in systemic lupus erythematosus revisited, *J Am Soc Nephrol.* 2004;15:241–250.

tends to have a more chronic course in an older population, compared to PR3-ANCA disease that has a more acute presentation and a higher risk of relapse. Previously, plasma exchange was recommended if patients presented with severe kidney failure (serum creatinine 5.8 mg/dL); however, the results of the PEXIVAS trial did not demonstrate any benefit in this group. Overall prognosis varies, relapses are common, and those with marked reductions in GFR at presentation often do poorly. AAV is discussed in detail in Chapter 17.

Anti-Glomerular Basement Membrane Antibody-Mediated Glomerulonephritis

Anti-glomerular basement antibodies can typically cause a severe necrotizing and crescentic GN. It often presents as RPGN but is differentiated from AAV by the detection of anti-GBM antibodies in the serum with the additional characteristic finding of linear IgG staining along the GBM for antibodies against the alpha 3 chain of type IV collagen (COL4A3). It can also present as a pulmonary-renal syndrome with concomitant pulmonary hemorrhage, which then classifies it as Goodpasture disease.

Prompt recognition and diagnosis of this syndrome is important, as those who present with a serum creatinine less than 5.0 mg/dL have a more favorable prognosis (90% chance of kidney survival at 5 years) compared to those who require dialysis at presentation and those with 100% circumferential crescents on kidney biopsy. The latter typically do not have kidney recovery and, in this scenario, immunosuppression is only recommended when there is concomitant pulmonary hemorrhage. Treatment of anti-GBM-mediated disease is similar to AAV with high-dose pulse corticosteroids combined with age- and kidney function-adjusted cyclophosphamide. In contrast to AAV, plasma exchange is a vital part of treatment, especially in the setting of pulmonary hemorrhage. Those who progress to ESKD should be referred for transplantation after the antibody has disappeared, as recurrence is rare.

Monoclonal Immunoglobulin-Associated Kidney Disease

Monoclonal gammopathy is a result of overproduction of a monoclonal Ig (MIg) that is detected in the tissue, serum, or urine due to clonal proliferation of immunoglobulin (Ig)-producing B lymphocytes or plasma cells. Specific etiologies are hematologic malignancies, such as multiple myeloma (MM), Waldenström macroglobulinemia (WM), B cell lymphoproliferative neoplasm, or a non-malignant small clonal proliferation of B lymphocytes or plasma cells. The resulting MIg due to the malignant or premalignant/non-malignant disease may then be the reason for the kidney disease. Monoclonal gammopathy of undetermined significance (MGUS) refers to when a MIg is found without evidence of plasma cell or lymphoid malignancy or end-organ damage and, therefore, is considered a "benign" condition. However, the term *monoclonal gammopathy of renal significance* (MGRS) acknowledges the presence of a clonal B cell or plasma cell population causing a kidney lesion, in the absence of a hematologic malignancy or other myeloma-defining events (MGRS = MIg-related kidney disease + MGUS). The resulting kidney lesion is due to the MIg, with major implications for prognosis and management. MGRS has been updated to note that some clonal plasma or B cell proliferative disorders do not require immediate treatment for the clonal disease such as smoldering myeloma and some low-grade lymphomas (e.g., CLL).

Testing for MIg-associated kidney disease involves serum and urine electrophoresis with immunofixation (SPEP/IFE, UPEP/IFE) and free light chains (FLCs); when used simultaneously, these tests are 97% sensitive for detecting amyloidosis or myeloma. Tissue diagnosis with bone marrow biopsy helps with determining the percent of clonal plasma cells present. Kidney biopsy diagnoses the kidney lesion, and the M-protein is considered to have a direct mechanism of action when Ig is found on IF, as noted in amyloidosis, monoclonal immunoglobulin deposition disease (MIDD), proliferative GN with monoclonal Ig deposits (PGNMID), immunotactoid GN, fibrillary GN (monotypic), cast nephropathy, or light chain proximal tubulopathy (LCPT). The M-protein can also have an indirect effect when Ig is absent on IF, as in C3 glomerulopathy and thrombotic microangiopathy. When reporting these lesions, the underlying MGRS lesions should be listed as the primary diagnosis, followed by the pattern of injury, additional findings such as chronicity, and, finally, if any ancillary studies are performed (e.g., Congo red staining, IgG subtypes, pronase digestion).

The clinical presentation is variable for these diseases (Fig. 16.5). MIg can also affect specific kidney compartments. Glomerular lesions are amyloidosis (can also be vascular and tubulointerstitial), MIDD, PGNMID, immunotactoid GN, monotypic fibrillary GN, cryoglobulinemic GN, and C3 glomerulopathy. Tubular lesions are cast nephropathy and LCPT, while there are other lesions such as crystal-storing histiocytosis and even parenchymal involvement of the kidney by the underlying malignancy. Amyloidosis is discussed briefly here, and other Monoclonal Ig-associated kidney diseases will each be discussed in detail in Chapter 28.

Amyloidosis

Amyloidosis is a systemic disorder that affects multiple organ systems; kidney involvement in amyloid often manifests as nephrotic syndrome and kidney failure. It is characterized by the extracellular deposition of amyloidogenic protein in multiple tissues. Amyloid protein deposition on light microscopy is periodic acid-Schiff (PAS) and methenamine silver stain negative and amorphous in appearance. On electron microscopy these deposits demonstrate randomly arranged fibrils, 8 to 12 nm in diameter. Congo red staining is pathognomonic (apple green birefringence on polarized light). Once amyloid is noted on a kidney biopsy specimen, amyloid typing should be performed as it yields the likely etiology and guides treatment decisions. Amyloid light chain (AL) amyloidosis is the most common form in approximately 85% of patients. Secondary (AA) amyloid comprises approximately 7% of cases and is often due to chronic inflammatory conditions such as inflammatory bowel disease, rheumatoid

arthritis, familial Mediterranean fever, or infections. A further 3% can be due to leukocyte chemotactic factor 2 (ALECT2). Mass spectrometry is a useful tool to identify the type of amyloid in up to 97% of cases.

C3 Glomerulopathy

C3 Glomerulopathy (C3G) is a disease that occurs due to dysfunctional regulation of the complement cascade. The result is uncontrolled activation and deposition of C3 in the glomerulus. Defects typically occur at the level of the C3 convertase of the alternative complement pathway and can be modulated by acquired and/or genetic abnormalities. Serum levels of C3 are low in approximately 75% of cases. Kidney biopsy is essential to diagnose C3G with LM findings being non-specific and IF findings of C3 dominant staining (characterized by an intensity two orders greater than Ig). While this pattern is common to both subtypes, C3GN can be distinguished based on electron microscopy. C3GN shows deposits in mesangial, paramesangial, subepithelial, or subendothelial regions, while DDD shows dense osmiophilic intramembranous and mesangial deposits. The findings of C3GN can often be mimicked by PIGN, making the diagnosis challenging. As such, extrarenal manifestations of C3G such as retinal drusen and acquired partial lipodystrophy, in addition to a chronic course progressing to kidney failure, can help distinguish between the two. C3G can be acquired or genetic. Genetic testing should encompass the genes that encode for complement pathway proteins (CFH, CFB, CFI, CFHR1-5, C3). These genetic mutations can potentially be causal or make patients susceptible to acquired etiologies such as infection or monoclonal gammopathy (in older populations). Acquired autoantibodies such a C3 nephritic factor and factor H autoantibody testing should be performed. As many as 50% of patients with C3G developed ESKD by 10 years. There is no established treatment strategy for C3G, although there have been several clinical studies looking at various forms of immunosuppressive therapy such as mycophenolate mofetil and eculizumab, with varying results. C3G is discussed further in Chapter 22.

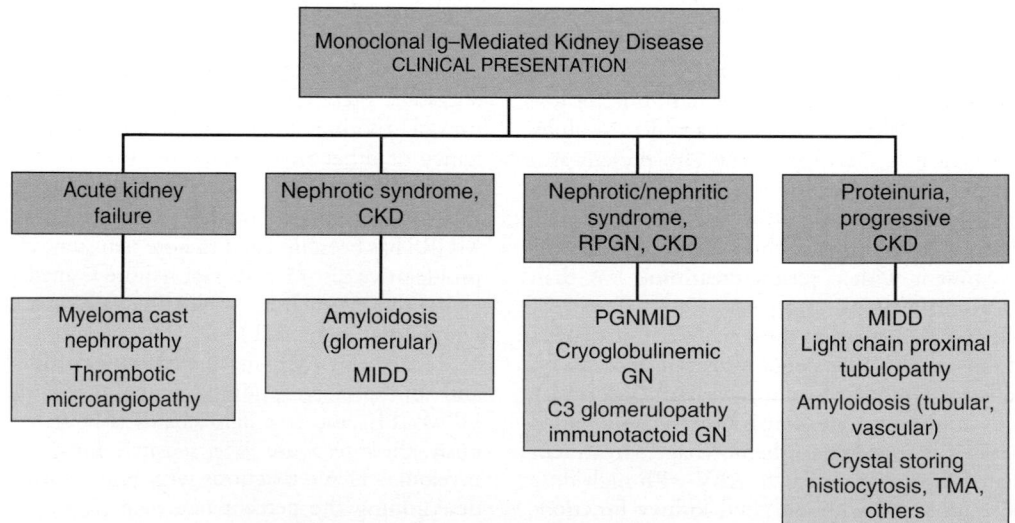

• **Fig. 16.5** **Clinical presentation of monoclonal Ig–mediated renal disease.** MIDD, monoclonal Ig deposition disease; PGNMID, proliferative GN with monoclonal Ig deposits; RPGN, rapidly progressive GN. (Adapted from Sethi S, Rajkumar V, D'Agati V. The complexity and heterogeneity of monoclonal immunoglobulin–associated renal diseases. JASN July 2018, 29 (7) 1810-1823; DOI: https://doi.org/10.1681/ASN.2017121319.)

Thrombotic Microangiopathies

Thrombotic microangiopathy (TMA) is a clinicopathological syndrome consisting of thrombocytopenia, microangiopathic hemolytic anemia evidenced by schistocytes on peripheral smear, elevated lactate dehydrogenase and reticulocyte count, and suppressed haptoglobin. The result is microvascular occlusion resulting in multi-organ dysfunction including kidney failure. Two major conditions in this category are Shiga toxin-associated hemolytic uremic syndrome (STEC-HUS) and thrombotic thrombocytopenic purpura (TTP). Other secondary etiologies of TMA include autoimmune diseases (SLE, anti-phospholipid antibody syndrome, scleroderma), malignant hypertension, malignancy, antibody-mediated rejection of the kidney allograft, drugs such as cocaine, and HIV. When none of these disorders are found, then the diagnosis is atypical HUS via exclusion (Fig. 16.6). Kidney biopsy reveals microthrombi in the glomerular capillaries and arterioles. Other findings include mesangiolysis (mesangial expansion with loose material), endothelial swelling, and double contour formation. Immunofluorescence microscopy is negative for Ig, although some fibrinogen and complement staining may be present. It is difficult to differentiate the various causes of TMA based on pathology alone. TMA is discussed further in Chapter 22.

Hemolytic Uremic Syndrome

Hemolytic uremic syndrome can be classified as typical when diarrhea is present. Diarrhea caused by the bacteria, Enterohemorrhagic *Escherichia coli*, produces a Shiga-like toxin that results in endothelial damage. Children are more commonly affected. Treatment is supportive and prognosis worsens with age.

Thrombotic Thrombocytopenic Purpura

When neurological involvement is present, TTP is the most likely diagnosis. Mutations in, autoantibodies against, or a deficiency (<10%) of ADAMTS13, the von Willebrand factor (vWF)-cleaving protease, are the cause of TTP. Since ADAMTS13 cleaves vWF, in its absence, large vWF multimers form microthrombi that deposit in the vasculature. If the clinical scenario fits, and no other etiology is found, treatment with plasma infusion/exchange should not be delayed while awaiting ADAMTS13 levels.

Atypical Hemolytic Uremic Syndrome

Atypical HUS is often seen in adults and is due to autoantibodies or mutations involving complement factors or their regulating proteins. This results in a defect in the control or regulation of the activity of C3 convertase in the alternative complement pathway. Unchecked activation of the complement cascade occurs. As a result, eculizumab, a complement (C5) inhibitor, is approved for treating atypical HUS.

Inherited Glomerular Disorders with Basement Membrane Abnormalities

Thin Basement Membrane Nephropathy

Thin basement membrane nephropathy is an autosomal dominant inherited disorder of the glomerular basement membrane occurring in the setting of heterozygous mutations of the *COL4A3* and *COL4A4* genes. It commonly presents as isolated glomerular hematuria with the characteristic finding on electron microscopy of GBM thickness less than 250 nm. Light microscopy and IF are both normal. Because thin basement membrane nephropathy rarely progresses to ESKD and otherwise has a benign clinical course, it is also known as *benign familial hematuria*.

Alport Syndrome

Alport syndrome (AS) is another inherited disorder of the GBM which, in contrast to thin basement membrane nephropathy, has extra-renal manifestations and often progresses to ESKD. The most common mutation is that of the *COL4A5* gene, which produces the alpha 5 chain of type IV collagen. The result is a clinicopathological syndrome with a friable renal GBM with concomitant sensorineural hearing loss and potential ocular abnormalities (lenticonus). On urinalysis, patients present with intermittent hematuria with varying degrees of proteinuria.

The main form of inheritance is X-linked but, less commonly, it can be autosomal dominant or recessive. Light microscopy is non-specific, while immunohistochemistry (IHC) shows diagnostic findings of absent alpha 3, 4, and 5 chains from the TBM and GBM. Depending on the time of biopsy, early on the GBM findings may appear similar to that of thin basement membrane

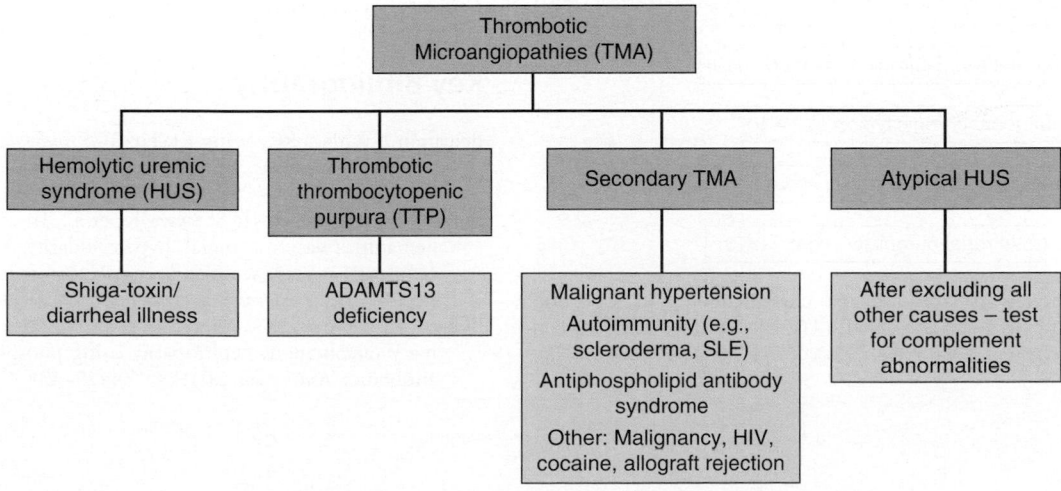

• **Fig. 16.6** Schematic of etiologies of thrombotic microangiopathy.

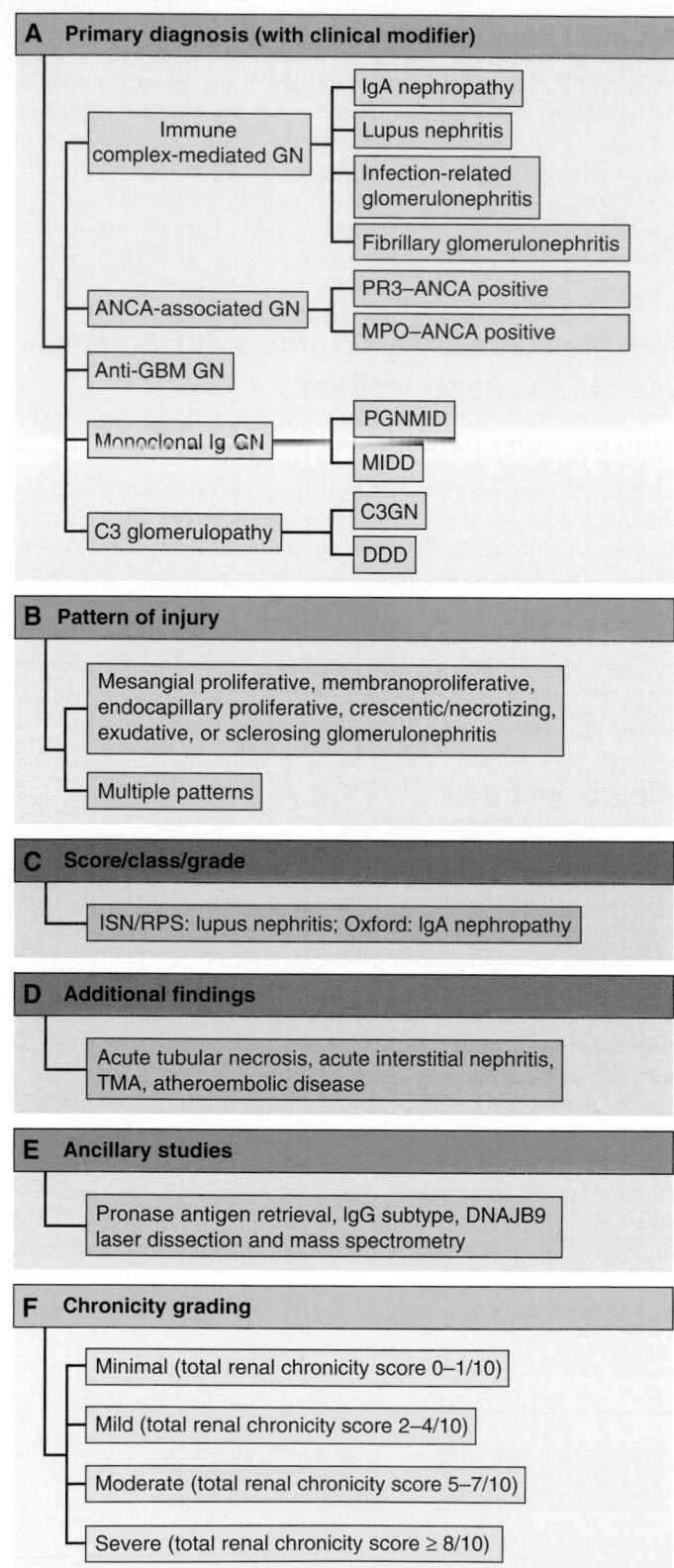

A Primary diagnosis (with clinical modifier)

Immune complex-mediated GN
- IgA nephropathy
- Lupus nephritis
- Infection-related glomerulonephritis
- Fibrillary glomerulonephritis

ANCA-associated GN
- PR3–ANCA positive
- MPO–ANCA positive

Anti-GBM GN

Monoclonal Ig GN
- PGNMID
- MIDD

C3 glomerulopathy
- C3GN
- DDD

B Pattern of injury

Mesangial proliferative, membranoproliferative, endocapillary proliferative, crescentic/necrotizing, exudative, or sclerosing glomerulonephritis

Multiple patterns

C Score/class/grade

ISN/RPS: lupus nephritis; Oxford: IgA nephropathy

D Additional findings

Acute tubular necrosis, acute interstitial nephritis, TMA, atheroembolic disease

E Ancillary studies

Pronase antigen retrieval, IgG subtype, DNAJB9 laser dissection and mass spectrometry

F Chronicity grading

Minimal (total renal chronicity score 0–1/10)

Mild (total renal chronicity score 2–4/10)

Moderate (total renal chronicity score 5–7/10)

Severe (total renal chronicity score ≥ 8/10)

• **Fig. 16.7** Overview of standardized classification and reporting of GN. (Adapted from Sethi S, Fervenza FC. Standardized classification and reporting of glomerulonephritis. *Nephrol Dial Transplant* 2019;34(2): 193–199.)

nephropathy, but subsequently thicken, often into several irregular layers, resulting in the classic "basket weave" appearance. Treatment is supportive, and the X-linked form in males almost always progresses to ESKD often by the fourth decade of life. Transplantation is a viable option but comes with a risk of anti-GBM disease in approximately 5%-10%. Hereditary kidney diseases are discussed further in Chapters 36-42.

Kidney Biopsy

Kidney biopsy is the gold standard for the diagnosis of most glomerular disorders. A kidney biopsy is indicated when the clinical scenario suggests parenchymal disease and the differential diagnosis includes disorders with different treatments/prognosis that cannot be adequately predicted by non invasive means. Therefore, all clinicopathological syndromes outlined in this chapter warrant a kidney biopsy, with the possible exception of pediatric nephrotic syndrome, which is MCD until proven otherwise. A more recent example of controversy as to whether a biopsy is essential is PLA2R-positive MN. It has been shown that in the setting of preserved kidney function (eGFR >60 mL/min/1.73 m^2) and negative work-up for secondary causes or diabetes, a positive PLA2R antibody test by simultaneous ELISA and IFA is MN until proven otherwise. However, additional studies are required to validate this finding.

Percutaneous kidney biopsy carries inherent risk of bleeding requiring surgery in less than 1%, intra-renal arteriovenous fistula in less than 1%, and death in less than 0.1%. Perinephric hematomas and gross hematuria are more common complications. Several contraindications include bleeding diathesis, ongoing or recent use of anticoagulant and anti-platelet agents, uncontrolled hypertension, severe anemia, solitary native kidney, hydronephrosis, kidney aneurysms, active kidney infection, the uncooperative patient, and chronic kidney failure with a low likelihood of recovery. Therefore, those performing kidney biopsy must be well trained to do so.

Once a kidney biopsy has been performed, light microscopy, IF, and EM together provide the best opportunity for an accurate diagnosis. Furthermore, classification should be standardized to include the primary diagnosis, pattern of injury, any associated scores/grades based on the primary diagnosis, additional findings, ancillary studies (e.g., Congo red, antigen staining), and chronicity grading, thus maximizing the information obtained from this costly and invasive procedure (Fig. 16.7).

Complete bibliography is available at Elsevier eBooks for Practicing Clinicians.

Key Bibliography

Benjamin IJ, Griggs RC, Wing EJ, Fitz JG. *Andreoli and Carpenter's Cecil Essentials of Medicine.* 9th edition Philadelphia, PA: Elsevier/Saunders; 2016.

Bobart SA, Alexander MP, Shawwa K, et al. The association of microhematuria with mesangial hypercellularity, endocapillary hypercellularity, crescent score and renal outcomes in immunoglobulin A nephropathy. *Nephrol Dial Transplant.* 2019.

Bobart SA, De Vriese AS, Pawar AS, et al. Noninvasive diagnosis of primary membranous nephropathy using phospholipase A2 receptor antibodies. *Kidney Int.* 2019;95(2):429–438.

Bridoux F, Leung N, Hutchison CA, et al. Diagnosis of monoclonal gammopathy of renal significance. *Kidney Int.* 2015; 87(4):698–711.

Couser WG. Primary membranous nephropathy. *Clin J Am Soc Nephrol.* 2017;12(6):983–997.

De Vriese AS, Glassock RJ, Nath KA, Sethi S, Fervenza FC. A Proposal for a serology-based approach to membranous nephropathy. *J Am Soc Nephrol.* 2017;28(2):421–430.

De Vriese AS, Sethi S, Nath KA, Glassock RJ, Fervenza FC. Differentiating primary, genetic, and secondary FSGS in adults: a clinicopathologic approach. *J Am Soc Nephrol.* 2018;29(3):759–774.

El Ters M, Bobart SA, Cornell LD, et al. Recurrence of DNAJB9-positive fibrillary glomerulonephritis after kidney transplantation: a case series. *Am J Kidney Dis.* 2020.

Fervenza FC, Appel GB, Barbour SJ, et al. Rituximab or cyclosporine in the treatment of membranous nephropathy. *N Engl J Med.* 2019;381(1):36–46.

Floege J, Barbour SJ, Cattran DC, et al. Management and treatment of glomerular diseases (part 1): conclusions from a Kidney Disease: Improving Global Outcomes (KDIGO) Controversies Conference. *Kidney Int.* 2019;95(2):268–280.

Rovin BH, Caster DJ, Cattran DC, et al. Management and treatment of glomerular diseases (part 2): conclusions from a Kidney Disease: Improving Global Outcomes (KDIGO) Controversies Conference. *Kidney Int.* 2019;95(2):281–295.

Sethi S, Debiec H, Madden B, et al. Neural epidermal growth factor-like 1 protein (NELL-1) associated membranous nephropathy. *Kidney Int.* 2020;97(1):163–174.

Sethi S, Fervenza FC. Standardized classification and reporting of glomerulonephritis. *Nephrol Dial Transplant.* 2019;34(2):193–199.

Sethi S, Fervenza FC. Pathology of renal diseases associated with dysfunction of the alternative pathway of complement: C3 glomerulopathy and atypical hemolytic uremic syndrome (aHUS). *Semin Thromb Hemost.* 2014;40(4):416–421.

Sethi S, Fervenza FC. Membranoproliferative glomerulonephritis–a new look at an old entity. *N Engl J Med.* 2012;366(12):1119–1131.

Sethi S, Glassock RJ, Fervenza FC. Focal segmental glomerulosclerosis: towards a better understanding for the practicing nephrologist. *Nephrol Dial Transplant.* 2015;30(3):375–384.

Sethi S, Nast CC, D'Agati VD, et al. Standardized reporting of monoclonal immunoglobulin-associated renal diseases: recommendations from a Mayo Clinic/Renal Pathology Society Working Group. *Kidney Int.* 2020;98(2):310–313. doi:10.1016/j.kint.2020.03.025.

Sethi S, Rajkumar SV, VD D'Agati. The complexity and heterogeneity of monoclonal immunoglobulin-associated renal diseases. *J Am Soc Nephrol.* 2018;29(7):1810–1823.

Thurman JM. Complement in kidney disease: core curriculum 2015. *Am J Kidney Dis.* 2015;65(1):156–168.

Vivarelli M, Massella L, Ruggiero B, Emma F. Minimal change disease. *Clin J Am Soc Nephrol.* 2017;12(2):332–345.

17

ANCA-Associated Kidney Disease and Vasculitis

FRANK B. CORTAZAR

Antineutrophil cytoplasmic antibody (ANCA)-associated vasculitis (AAV) is a predominantly small-vessel vasculitis with a predilection for the kidney and respiratory tract. In the majority of cases, the disease is associated with autoantibodies (i.e., ANCAs) directed against one of two proteins located within the azurophilic granules of neutrophils: proteinase 3 (PR3) or myeloperoxidase (MPO). ANCAs have a central role in the pathogenesis and diagnosis of AAV. AAV has a wide spectrum of protean manifestations and is the most common cause of rapidly progressive glomerulonephritis. Early diagnosis and rapid initiation of immunosuppressive therapy are essential to prevent irreversible organ damage.

Classification of AAV

Clinicopathologic Classification

The recognition of AAV as a clinical entity predated the discovery of ANCAs. Hence, AAV was initially classified based on clinical manifestations and pathologic findings. Three subtypes of AAV have been historically defined: (1) granulomatosis with polyangiitis (previously known as *Wegener's granulomatosis*), (2) microscopic polyangiitis, and (3) eosinophilic granulomatosis with polyangiitis (previously known as *Churg-Strauss syndrome*). All forms of AAV cause necrotizing small-vessel vasculitis and the same pathologic lesion in the kidney: a pauci-immune, necrotizing (and often crescentic) glomerulonephritis.

Granulomatosis with polyangiitis (GPA) is distinguished from MPA by the presence of extravascular granulomatous inflammation. Common clinical features of GPA include sinusitis, destructive nasal lesions, cavitary lung masses, and necrotizing glomerulonephritis. GPA is more commonly associated with PR3-ANCA than MPO-ANCA. Microscopic polyangiitis (MPA) is characterized by the absence of granulomatous inflammation and often presents with pauci-immune necrotizing glomerulonephritis and pulmonary hemorrhage. A subset of patients with isolated pauci-immune necrotizing vasculitis and no extrarenal manifestations (i.e., renal-limited vasculitis) is sometimes designated as MPA. MPA is more commonly associated with MPO-ANCA than PR3-ANCA.

Eosinophilic granulomatosis with polyangiitis (EGPA) is distinguished from other forms of AAV by the presence of asthma and eosinophilia in addition to extravascular granulomatous inflammation. Only approximately 40% of cases of EGPA are associated with ANCA, with MPO-ANCA being more common than PR3-ANCA. Clinical manifestations differ between ANCA-positive and ANCA-negative patients, and these subsets likely have a different underlying pathogenesis. Patients with EGPA and ANCA positivity are more likely to have vasculitic manifestations including glomerulonephritis and mononeuritis multiplex.

A clinicopathologic definition of disease can be limited in that granulomatous inflammation may be missed by sampling error or may not be present in the organ biopsied. Therefore, the decision to designate a patient with AAV as GPA or MPA is often inferred on the basis of clinical findings rather than confirmed by histopathology. This subjectivity can lead to variation across individual centers and specialties.

Serologic Classification

Another system for classifying AAV is based on ANCA serotype (MPO vs. PR3) rather than clinicopathologic features. Classification by ANCA serotype has several advantages including an inherent link to disease pathogenesis and a superior ability to predict clinically important outcomes. In genome-wide association studies, genetic variants associated with AAV correlate more strongly with ANCA serotype (MPO vs. PR3) than clinical phenotype (GPA vs. MPA). Certain disease manifestations are also closely linked with ANCA specificity. For example, renal-limited vasculitis and ANCA-associated interstitial lung disease predominantly occur in the setting of MPO-ANCA. Drug-associated AAV is uniformly associated with MPO-ANCA positivity, with dual positivity for MPO- and PR3-ANCA present in some cases, but essentially never PR3-ANCA alone.

ANCA serotype is also a predictor of clinically relevant outcomes, particularly relapse. In multiple retrospective series and clinical trials, PR3-ANCA consistently associates with a greater probability of relapse than MPO-ANCA. Moreover, ANCA serotype is a better predictor of relapse in most studies than the clinicopathologic designation of MPA or GPA. Clinical trials now routinely stratify randomization by ANCA serotype, and some future clinical trials are likely to enroll only patients with a single ANCA specificity.

Pathogenesis

The Pathogenic Role of ANCAs

There is substantial evidence that ANCAs are pathogenic and not merely biomarkers of AAV. Under normal conditions, the MPO and PR3 enzymes are sequestered in the cytoplasm of neutrophils in azurophilic (primary) granules. Priming of neutrophils by pro-inflammatory stimuli, such as tumor necrosis factor and complement factor C5a, leads to translocation of MPO and PR3 to the cell surface, where they can interact with circulating ANCAs. It has been hypothesized that infection can precipitate disease flare by leading to the priming of neutrophils in a patient with preexisting circulating ANCA.

In vitro, both MPO- and PR3-ANCA are able to activate primed neutrophils via binding of the target antigen at or near the cell surface and signaling through the Fcγ receptor. Activation of neutrophils by ANCA leads to the release of reactive oxygen species and lytic enzymes that mediate tissue damage. More recently, it has been appreciated that ANCA activation can promote the generation of neutrophil extracellular traps (NETs). NETosis is a unique form of cell death, whereby decondensed chromatin and associated granule proteins (including MPO and PR3) are released into the extracellular space, forming a web-like structure that can trap and kill invading pathogens. Components of NETs, predominantly histones and matrix metalloproteases, are toxic to the vascular endothelium and are thought to contribute to tissue injury in AAV. Moreover, NET formation increases exposure to MPO and PR3 antigens, which may further promote autoimmunity.

Strong evidence for the pathogenicity of ANCAs is also derived from animal models of AAV. In a classic experiment, passive transfer of MPO-ANCA into a recombinase-activating gene 2 (RAG-2)-deficient mouse, which lacks functioning B and T cells, was sufficient to reproduce the lesion of pauci-immune necrotizing glomerulonephritis seen in man. The pathogenic role of MPO-ANCA was substantiated in a natural human model, whereby placental transfer of MPO-ANCA from a mother with AAV resulted in pulmonary hemorrhage and RPGN in the neonate.

Given the central role of ANCA in the pathogenesis of AAV, it has been difficult to reconcile the observation that some patients with clinicopathologic features consistent with AAV do not have detectable ANCA. At least in some cases, this may be due to assay sensitivity. It has been demonstrated that ANCAs directed against specific epitopes on the MPO molecule are not detectable using commercially available assays. In other cases, particularly in those with predominantly granulomatous manifestations of disease, alternative pathogenic mechanisms not involving ANCA may predominate.

Development of ANCAs

The underlying mechanisms culminating in the production of autoantibodies targeting MPO or PR3 are not fully known; however, genetic studies and specific exposures that have been linked with ANCA production provide some insight. Antigens are presented to the adaptive immune system via human leukocyte antigen (HLA) class II molecules expressed on antigen-presenting cells. Given the central role of antigen presentation in the development of the adaptive immune response, it is not surprising that certain HLA variants have been linked to the development of autoimmunity. Indeed, specific HLA associations exist for a wide array of autoimmune diseases, including AAV. In two separate genome-wide association studies, the development of MPO-ANCA vasculitis was associated with HLA-DQ while PR3-ANCA vasculitis was associated with HLA-DP.

In addition to HLA variants, factors influencing the autoantigens themselves are also associated with the development of ANCAs.

Variants in SERPINA1, the gene encoding alpha-1 antitrypsin, have been associated with the development of PR3-ANCA. Alpha-1 antitrypsin is a protease inhibitor that targets PR3, and genetic polymorphisms that result in attenuated activity of the protein translate into reduced PR3 clearance. This finding is consistent with the observation that patients with alpha-1 antitrypsin deficiency are at increased risk for developing PR3-ANCA. A variant in the gene encoding PR3 itself, which leads to increased PR3 expression, has also been linked to the development of PR3-ANCA in genome-wide association studies.

ANCA production can also be stimulated by a number of medications including propylthiouracil, methimazole, hydralazine, and minocycline. The exact mechanisms remain unclear, although a number of plausible hypotheses have been proposed. Patients on long-term propylthiouracil develop seropositivity for MPO-ANCA at a rate of close to 30% in some series, although only a small fraction of these patients develop clinical vasculitis. Propylthiouracil accumulates in neutrophils, where it interacts with MPO, thereby resulting in structural alterations that may increase antigenicity. In addition, propylthiouracil promotes the development of NETs that are resistant to degradation by DNase I, resulting in extended durations of antigen exposure.

Hydralazine has also been demonstrated to induce NETosis. Moreover, in addition to its role as a vasodilator, hydralazine is an inhibitor of DNA methylation. This property may prevent the epigenetic silencing of certain genes, including *MPO* and *PR3*, which are important in the development of ANCA. Indeed, patients with active AAV exhibit hypomethylation at the *MPO* or *PR3* genes relative to healthy controls and patients with AAV who are in remission.

Role of Complement

Patients with AAV generally exhibit normal levels of serum complement and a paucity of C3 and C1q deposition on kidney biopsy. These observations have obscured the important role of complement in the pathogenesis of AAV. The alternative complement pathway, however, has recently been identified as a central and necessary mediator of the inflammatory cascade in AAV.

Experiments conducted with animal models provide the framework for the current understanding of complement in AAV. In a passive anti-MPO IgG transfer model, C4 knockout mice developed pauci-immune necrotizing and crescentic glomerulonephritis akin to that observed with wild-type mice, indicating ANCA-mediated injury can occur independently of the classical and alternative lectin pathways. Conversely, knockout of complement factor B, which is necessary for alternative pathway activation, resulted in complete abrogation of disease activity. Subsequent experiments revealed C5a, and not the membrane attack complex, is the key mediator of disease activity. Indeed, treatment of mice with a C5a receptor antagonist attenuated MPO-ANCA-induced injury in a dose-dependent fashion.

Studies conducted in vitro demonstrate that neutrophil activation by MPO-ANCA or PR3-ANCA results in the release of factors that activate the alternative complement pathway. The generated C5a then recruits and primes additional neutrophils, resulting in increased autoantigen migration to the cell surface and, hence, a greater propensity for interaction with ANCA. This interplay results in a positive feedback loop that propagates the inflammatory cascade in AAV (Fig. 17.1). Given the pivotal role of C5a, new therapies targeting this pathway are currently under investigation.

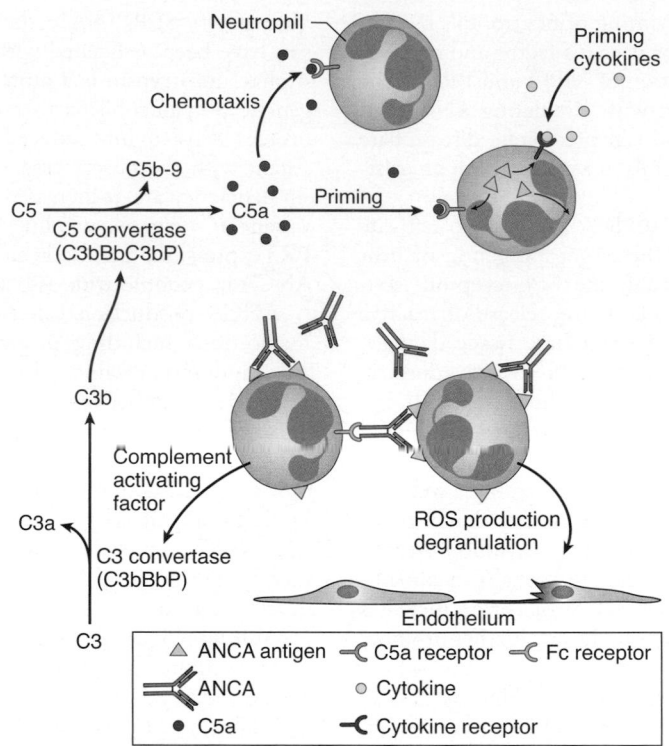

• **Fig. 17.1 The role of complement in AAV.** Priming of neutrophils by inflammatory mediators causes translocation of myeloperoxidase (MPO) and proteinase 3 (PR3) myeloperoxidase to the cell surface, where they can interact with antineutrophil cytoplasmic antibody (ANCA). Binding of ANCA to its target antigen results in neutrophil activation, leading to the release of reactive oxygen species and lytic enzymes that cause tissue damage. In addition, ANCA-induced neutrophil activation releases mediators that activate the alternative complement pathway, thereby leading to C5a generation. C5a is a chemoattractant that recruits and primes additional neutrophils, creating a positive feedback loop that drives disease activity.

Epidemiology

The incidence of AAV is approximately 20 per million/year with a slight male predominance. Although the disease can occur at any age, it predominantly affects older adults with a peak incidence in the seventh and eighth decades of life. Among patients older than 60, pauci-immune necrotizing glomerulonephritis is the most common cause of nephritic syndrome identified on kidney biopsy.

The distribution of PR3-ANCA and MPO-ANCA differs by geography. PR3-ANCA is more common in the United Kingdom and northern Europe. Conversely, MPO-ANCA is more common in southern parts of the world including southern Europe and Asia. This difference in distribution has been attributed to both genetic and environmental factors.

Clinical Features

AAV is heterogeneous in presentation, often leading to delays in diagnosis. Organ-specific manifestations of AAV are provided in Table 17.1. While some patients have an explosive presentation with little or no prodrome, many initially have a smoldering and protracted course. In this latter subgroup, the disease often first manifests with constitutional symptoms including fatigue, weight loss, and arthralgias, which may be present for months before more specific features become evident. Patients seeking care at this stage are often diagnosed with a viral or "postviral" syndrome. In the AAV patient presenting with sinusitis, otitis, or pulmonary symptoms, an infectious etiology is initially suspected in most cases. It is, therefore, common for yet undiagnosed AAV patients to be treated with multiple rounds of antibiotics without significant clinical improvement. Failure of appropriate antibiotic therapy for suspected ENT and pulmonary infections should raise suspicion for AAV. A major clue to the diagnosis is often the recognition of unexplained hematuria or abnormal kidney function in the context of other unexplained systemic disease manifestations. As with other causes of the nephritic syndrome, patients with AAV who have kidney involvement generally present with glomerular hematuria and subnephrotic proteinuria. The hematuria is microscopic in most patients, although gross hematuria can occur.

The tempo and severity of kidney involvement in AAV is highly variable. Patients often present with the syndrome of rapidly progressive glomerulonephritis, which generally leads to rapid evaluation and diagnosis. Other patients, however, can develop isolated hematuria followed by an insidious decline in kidney function. Such individuals may initially be thought to have IgA nephropathy or thin basement membrane disease. This is particularly true among a subset of patients with MPO-ANCA who have renal-limited disease and are often asymptomatic. It is important to evaluate for AAV in these cases to prevent the development of kidney and, potentially, subsequent extrarenal damage.

Diagnosis

ANCA Testing

An ANCA test should be conducted on all patients suspected of having AAV. In most laboratories, ANCA testing incorporates two different assays: indirect immunofluorescence and enzyme-linked

TABLE 17.1	Manifestations of ANCA-Associated Vasculitis
Organ	**Disease Manifestation**
Nose	Nasal crusting/discharge, nasal ulcers, saddle nose deformity, septal perforation
Paranasal sinuses	Sinusitis
Ear	Otitis media, conductive hearing loss, sensorineural hearing loss, polychondritis
Eye	Scleritis, episcleritis, conjunctivitis, uveitis, retinal vasculitis, retro-orbital pseudotumor
Skin	Purpura, cutaneous ulcers, nodules
Oral mucosa	Oral ulcers
Heart	Pericarditis, myocarditis
Trachea	Tracheal stenosis (typically subglottic)
Lung	Pulmonary nodules/masses, pulmonary hemorrhage, interstitial fibrosis, bronchial stenosis
Kidney	Pauci-immune necrotizing (and often crescentic) glomerulonephritis, interstitial nephritis (almost always associated with glomerulonephritis)
Nervous system	Mononeuritis multiplex, peripheral sensory neuropathy, pachymeningitis, CNS vasculitis
Gastrointestinal system	Mesenteric ischemia, ischemic colitis

immunosorbent assay (ELISA). In the indirect immunofluorescence assay, the serum of the patient being tested is incubated with ethanol-fixed human neutrophils. Under normal conditions, MPO and PR3 are located in azurophilic granules in the cytoplasm of neutrophils. It is the process of ethanol fixation that causes MPO and other strongly positive cationic granule components to migrate to the negatively charged nuclear envelope, while the more neutral PR3 molecule remains in the cytoplasm. This technical artifact is the reason patients with autoantibodies against MPO have a perinuclear ANCA (pANCA) staining pattern while patients with autoantibodies against PR3 have a cytoplasmic ANCA (cANCA) staining pattern (Fig. 17.2).

While sensitive, the indirect immunofluorescence assay lacks specificity. This is particularly true with the pANCA staining pattern.

Autoantibodies against other cationic proteins including cathepsin G, elastase, lactoferrin, and lysozyme can also lead to a pANCA staining pattern. Antibodies to these alternative antigens, which produce a pANCA pattern, often referred to as "atypical ANCAs," have no clear relation to vasculitis. Moreover, it is possible for antinuclear antibodies to be mistaken for a pANCA pattern. For these reasons, a positive result on indirect immunofluorescence should always be confirmed with ELISA.

Testing with ELISA evaluates for antibodies only against the antigens of interest (i.e., PR3 and MPO) and is, therefore, highly specific. Improvements in ELISA technology have resulted in assays with sensitivities that rival that of indirect immunofluorescence. This has led some experts to propose ANCA testing now be performed with ELISA alone.

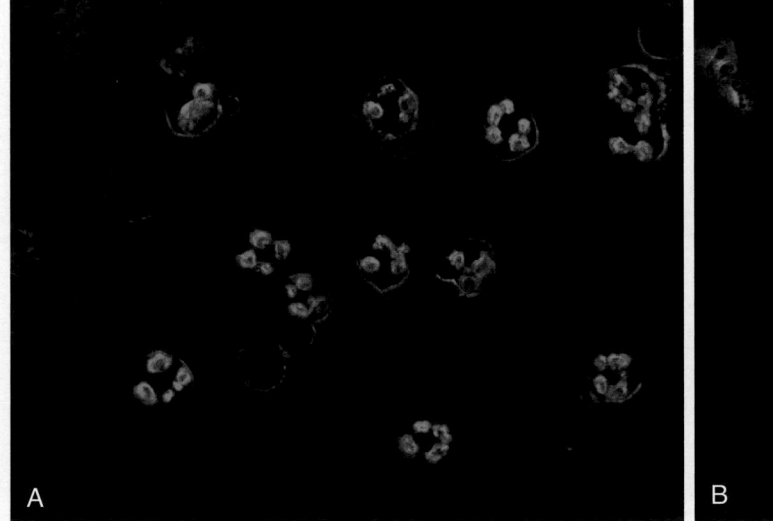
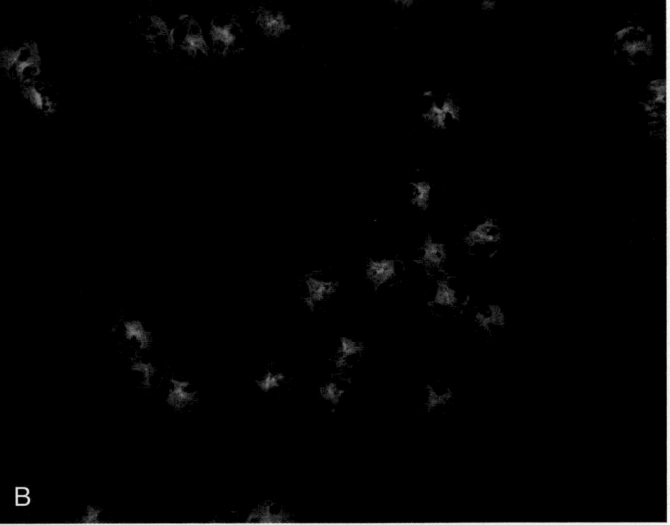

• **Fig. 17.2** Indirect immunofluorescence demonstrating a perinuclear antineutrophil cytoplasmic antibody (pANCA) (A) and cytoplasmic antineutrophil cytoplasmic antibody (cANCA) (B) staining pattern. (Courtesy John L. Niles, MD.)

Interpretation of ANCA Testing

Most patients with active AAV will test positive for MPO- or PR3-ANCA. Among patients with glomerulonephritis and those with widespread organ involvement, the sensitivity of ANCA testing is greater than 90%. Notably, the sensitivity is significantly lower in certain AAV populations. In patients with organ-limited GPA and predominantly granulomatous inflammation, such as patients with isolated sinusitis or tracheal stenosis, the sensitivity of ANCA testing falls to less than 80%. Repeat ANCA testing should be considered in patients with limited disease who subsequently develop more generalized features, as a subset will develop detectable ANCA. Only approximately 50% of patients with EGPA are ANCA-positive. However, based on differences in clinical manifestations and genetic risk variants, it is likely ANCA-positive EGPA and ANCA-negative EGPA represent different disease processes. Therefore, a negative ANCA test alone cannot exclude a diagnosis of AAV. In ANCA-negative cases, the diagnosis is based upon clinical features and biopsy of the affected organ.

A positive ANCA test is highly specific, with a specificity for AAV of >95%. As with any diagnostic test, however, the positive predictive value (i.e., percentage of patients with a positive test who actually have the disease) is dependent on the prevalence of the disease in the population being tested. For example, an adult patient presenting with rapidly progressive glomerulonephritis has a pretest probability of AAV of approximately 50%. In this setting, a positive ANCA has a positive predictive value of 99% and is essentially diagnostic. Conversely, in a patient presenting with isolated sinusitis, the pretest probability of AAV is significantly lower at approximately 1%. The positive predicative value of a positive ANCA test in this patient would be close to 40%. While this patient merits a meticulous evaluation for AAV, other etiologies of sinusitis would also need to be considered.

The results of an ANCA test are generally considered as binary, that is, either positive or negative. The cutoff point for a positive test is determined by each laboratory with the aim of optimizing the balance between sensitivity and specificity. In actuality, results lie along a continuum, and higher ANCA titers increase the probability that a patient has AAV.

Whether a diagnosis of AAV should be made with ANCA testing alone, or whether biopsy should be pursued in all cases, is debated. In patients with a low or moderate pretest probability of AAV and a positive ANCA test, biopsy should be obtained, if feasible, to secure the diagnosis. In a patient with a high pretest probability of AAV and an unequivocally positive ANCA test, the diagnosis is sometimes made without biopsy confirmation. The decision to pursue biopsy in these cases requires the clinician to assess the procedural risks of biopsy in an individual patient and how the results of the biopsy would change management.

Tissue Biopsy

In many cases, biopsy of an affected organ should be pursued to confirm the diagnosis of AAV. The most common organs biopsied are the skin and kidney. Biopsy of the skin reveals leukocytoclastic vasculitis, a nonspecific finding seen in other small-vessel vasculitides (Fig. 17.3). On immunofluorescence, there is minimal deposition of complement or immunoglobulins.

Less commonly, when the skin or kidney are not involved, lung biopsy may be pursued. An open or thoracoscopic lung biopsy is generally required to yield sufficient tissue for a diagnosis. In patients with alveolar hemorrhage, lung biopsy typically demonstrates pulmonary capillaritis. Conversely, biopsy of lung masses typically demonstrates necrotizing granulomatous inflammation and arteritis. In the latter case, it is important to evaluate for infectious processes, including fungal and mycobacterial infections, that have similar histopathologic findings. While less invasive, biopsy of sinonasal tissue typically demonstrates nonspecific inflammation and is rarely helpful in confirming the diagnosis.

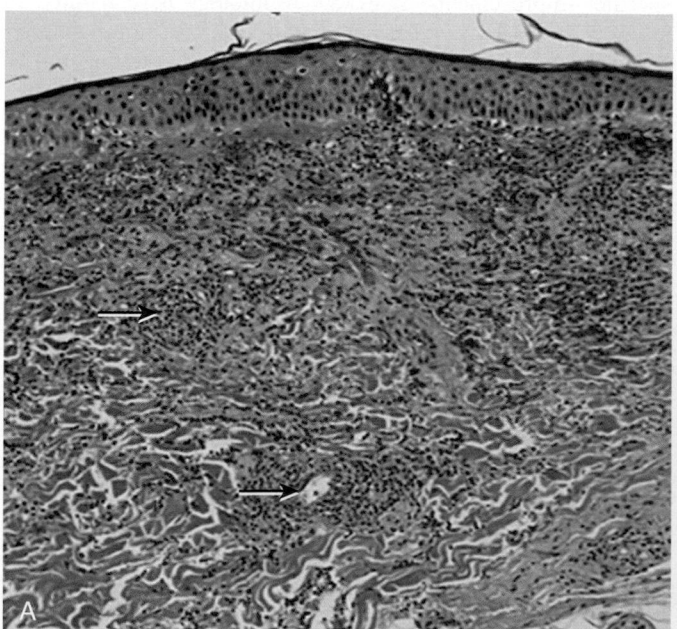 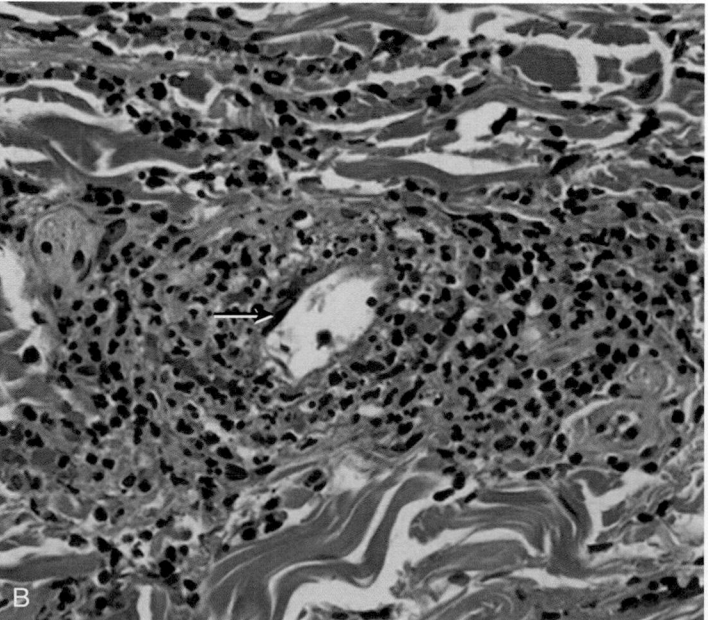

• **Fig. 17.3** Skin biopsy in a patient with AAV and palpable purpura. **(A)** Skin with underlying leukocytoclastic vasculitis (*arrows*) (H&E, ×20). **(B)** Leukocytoclastic vasculitis demonstrating an angiocentric neutrophilic infiltrate with fibrinoid necrosis and fragmented neutrophilic nuclei (*arrow*, endothelial cell) (H&E, ×200). (Courtesy Jacqueline M. Cortazar, MD.)

Kidney Pathology

Kidney biopsy reveals the same pathologic lesion in all forms of AAV: pauci-immune necrotizing (and often crescentic) glomerulonephritis. Light microscopy shows segmental fibrinoid necrosis and, in the majority of cases, crescent formation (Fig. 17.4). Unaffected portions of glomeruli generally appear normal without significant cellular proliferation. Crescents are often simultaneously present in different stages of chronicity (i.e., cellular, fibrocellular, and fibrous), providing a pathologic correlate of waxing and waning disease activity over time (Fig. 17.5). This contrasts with antiglomerular basement membrane disease, where crescents are more uniform in their temporal stage of development. Glomerulonephritis in AAV is often accompanied by an interstitial infiltrate predominantly comprised of mononuclear cells. Rarely, isolated tubulointerstitial nephritis can occur.

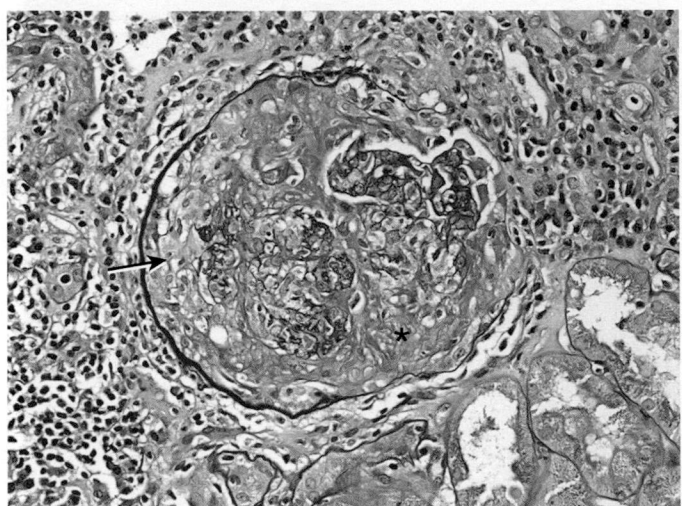

• **Fig. 17.4** Glomerulus in a patient with AAV and rapidly progressive glomerulonephritis demonstrating a prominent cellular crescent (*arrow*) and necrosis (*asterisk*). An inflammatory infiltrate involves the surrounding interstitium (PAS, ×400). (Courtesy Ivy Rosales, MD.)

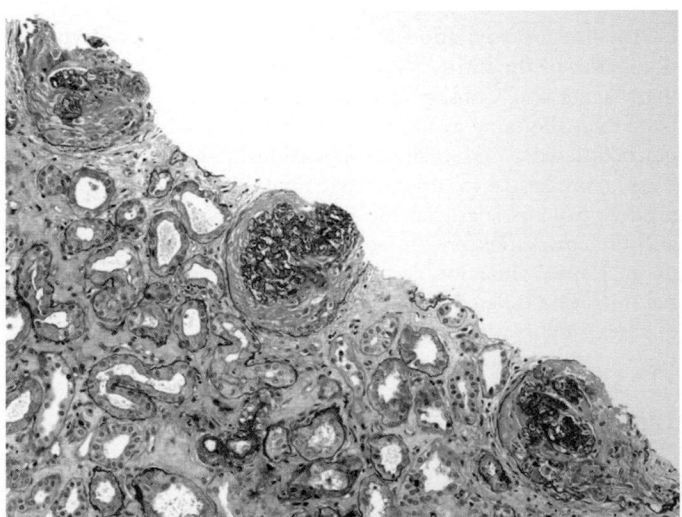

• **Fig. 17.5** Crescents in evolution in a case of chronic AAV. A cellular crescent is present in one glomerulus (*top left*) while two other glomeruli show fibrocellular to fibrous crescents, with sclerosis of the glomerular tuft (*bottom right*) (PAS, ×200). (Courtesy Ivy Rosales, MD.)

The key finding on immunofluorescence is the minimal amount of immunoglobulin and complement deposition, hence, the term "pauci-immune" (Fig. 17.6). This distinguishes AAV from both immune-complex diseases (e.g., lupus nephritis and IgA nephropathy) and anti-GBM disease. Consistent with the immunofluorescence findings, electron microscopy in AAV is marked by the absence of significant electron dense deposits. It should be noted that pauci-immune does not imply the complete absence of immunoglobulin and complement components. This is particularly true in drug-induced AAV, where the presence of other autoantibodies (e.g., ANA) may lead to a proportionally greater amount of immune deposition on immunofluorescence than in idiopathic cases.

On a population level, there are quantifiable histopathologic differences between patients with MPO-ANCA and PR3-ANCA. On average, patients with MPO-ANCA have more chronic damage as evidenced by greater degrees of interstitial fibrosis, a greater percentage of fibrous as opposed to cellular crescents, and a greater percentage of completely obliterated glomeruli. This may reflect greater delays in diagnosis in patients with MPO-ANCA, particularly among the subset of patients with kidney-limited disease who are often relatively asymptomatic until the development of kidney failure. It is also possible that there are underlying differences in pathogenesis, with MPO-ANCA leading to a more fibrotic pattern of injury. This latter hypothesis is supported by the recognition that MPO-ANCA can be associated with pulmonary fibrosis.

Drug-Induced AAV

While most cases of AAV are idiopathic, certain drugs induce ANCA production and, in some patients, overt disease. These drugs include hydralazine, minocycline, propylthiouracil, methimazole, and levamisole-adulterated cocaine. Allopurinol has also been postulated as a potential culprit, but a causal link is less well established. The initial evaluation of any patient with AAV should include a meticulous review of the medication list and discontinuation of implicated agents. In addition, patients should be questioned about cocaine use and tested for cocaine and levamisole exposure, if appropriate.

In some patients, the results of ANCA testing can provide a clue to the presence of drug-induced disease. Essentially, all patients with drug-induced disease have MPO-ANCA, often at a markedly elevated titer. In one study, the titer of MPO-ANCA in drug-induced cases was more than 12 times higher than the median titer observed in idiopathic cases. Even more suggestive of drug-induced disease is the presence of dual positivity for both MPO-ANCA and PR3-ANCA. This pattern is most commonly seen in patients using levamisole-adulterated cocaine, but can also be observed in the context of other drug culprits. Finally, patients with drug-induced AAV often have other autoantibodies including ANA and anti-histone antibodies.

While there is substantial overlap, certain causes of drug-induced ANCA have characteristic manifestations. Hydralazine-induced AAV often causes severe disease with rapidly progressive glomerulonephritis and pulmonary hemorrhage. Cases associated with levamisole-adulterated cocaine typically present with constitutional symptoms, neutropenia, and necrotic skin lesions. The high prevalence of antiphospholipid antibodies in these patients may explain the prominent cutaneous manifestations. Finally, cases due to propylthiouracil and minocycline often have arthralgias/arthritis and rash as the most prominent features.

The treatment of drug-induced AAV is dependent on the severity of the disease. In mild cases with only constitutional symptoms, discontinuation of the drug with close monitoring may be sufficient.

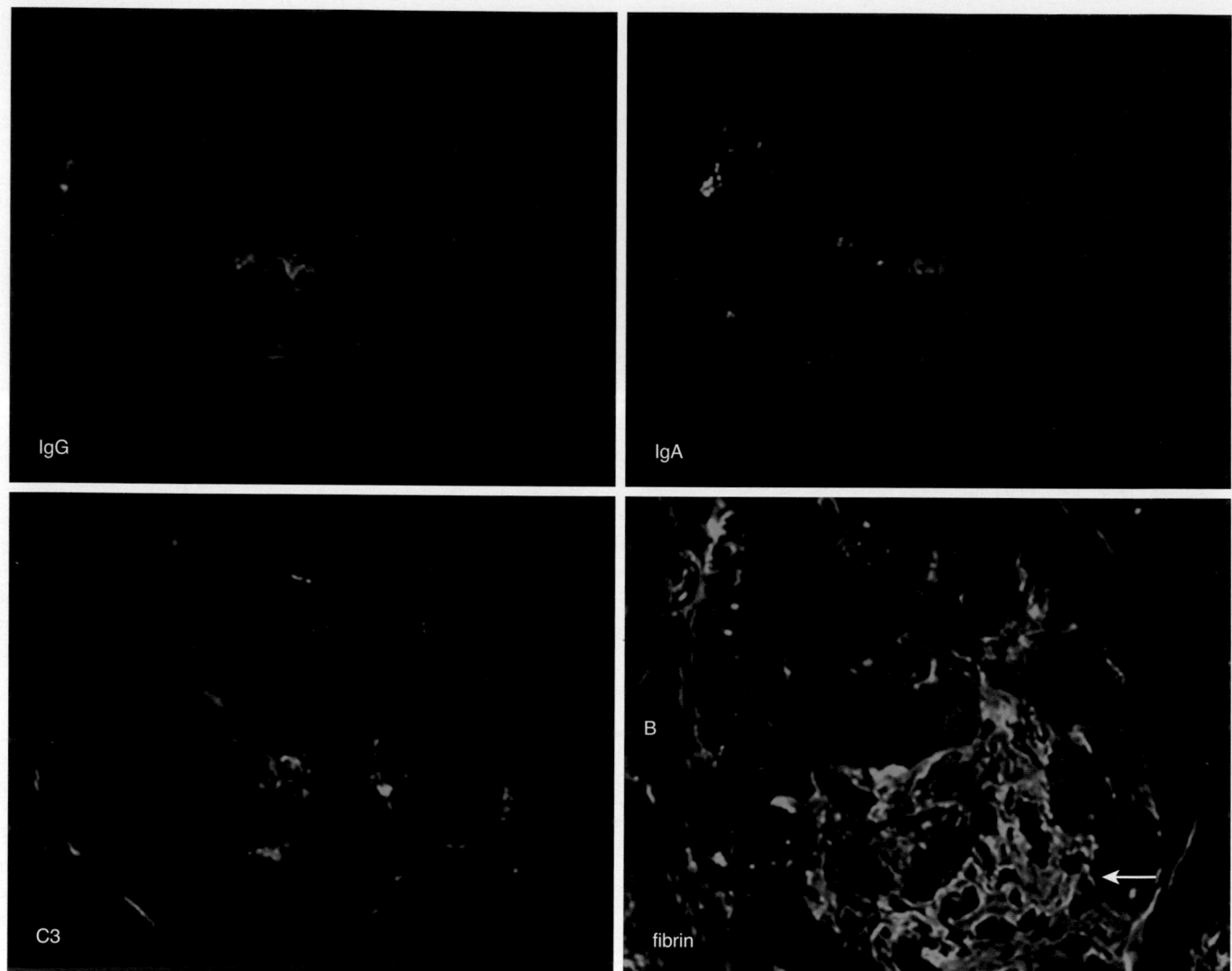

• **Fig. 17.6** Direct immunofluorescence microscopy images from a case of AAV showing minimal staining for immunoglobulins and complement. A crescent (*arrow*) stains positive for fibrin. (Courtesy Ivy Rosales, MD.)

Conversely, in patients with organ- or life-threatening disease, induction immunosuppression akin to that used for idiopathic disease is indicated.

Concurrent Anti-Glomerular Basement Membrane Disease

The simultaneous occurrence of ANCA and anti-glomerular basement membrane (anti-GBM) autoantibodies is a well-described phenomenon that occurs more commonly than would be expected by chance alone. Indeed, ANCA is detected in approximately one-third of patients with anti-GBM antibodies, with MPO-ANCA occurring more commonly than PR3-ANCA in double-positive patients. The mechanism responsible for concomitant ANCA and anti-GBM antibodies is unclear, but it appears ANCA predates anti-GBM antibodies in most cases. Injury to the glomerular basement membrane mediated by ANCA may lead to exposure of the normally sequestered Goodpasture antigen (NC1 domain of the alpha-3 chain of type IV collagen), thereby promoting the subsequent development of anti-GBM antibodies.

The initial presentation of double-positive patients is typically dominated by the anti-GBM component, which tends to be particularly aggressive. Consequently, initial therapy for double-positive patients is the same as for isolated anti-GBM disease: high-dose glucocorticoids, oral cyclophosphamide, and plasma exchange. Despite similarities in early management, identification of double-positive patients is crucial for appropriate long-term monitoring and therapy. Patients with isolated anti-GBM disease essentially never relapse, while double-positive patients have a relapse potential mirroring isolated AAV. Therefore, unlike isolated anti-GBM disease, patients with double-positive disease require maintenance therapy and monitoring for relapse, as is done for AAV.

Treatment

Treatment of AAV is conceptually divided into two phases: induction of remission and maintenance of remission. Induction therapy is intended to eradicate ongoing vasculitis activity and prevent or mitigate irreversible organ injury. Maintenance therapy is less aggressive treatment intended to prevent relapse once remission has been achieved.

Induction of Remission

Standard induction therapy for severe AAV consists of glucocorticoids combined with either cyclophosphamide or rituximab. The RAVE trial compared daily oral cyclophosphamide and glucocorticoids (followed by azathioprine maintenance) with rituximab and glucocorticoids in patients with severe AAV. At 6 months, there was no difference in the rate of disease remission or adverse events.

Certain factors may favor cyclophosphamide or rituximab in a given patient. Rituximab is the preferred agent in patients concerned about fertility and in those with high prior cumulative cyclophosphamide exposure. In addition, data from the RAVE trial suggest rituximab may be superior in patients with PR3-ANCA, particularly those with relapsing disease. In some settings, cyclophosphamide may be preferred due to cost considerations. In addition, there is a paucity of high-quality evidence for using rituximab induction in patients with RPGN and a serum creatinine >4 mg/dL, leading some experts to prefer cyclophosphamide in this context.

Regardless of which regimen is chosen, a key tenet of treating AAV is rapid initiation of therapy to prevent progressive disease, irreversible organ damage, and potentially death. In cases of organ- or life-threatening disease with a high clinical suspicion for AAV, treatment with high-dose glucocorticoids should commence before biopsy or even serologic confirmation.

Cyclophosphamide

Cyclophosphamide can be administered orally or intravenously. The CYCLOPs trial compared daily oral cyclophosphamide with intravenous pulse cyclophosphamide administered every 2-3 weeks, both with glucocorticoids. Remission rates were statistically equivalent in the two groups. Patients receiving intermittent pulse cyclophosphamide had lower cumulative cyclophosphamide exposure and lower rates of leukopenia. Conversely, patients receiving daily oral cyclophosphamide had a lower rate of subsequent relapse. It should be noted that patients in CYCLOPS received azathioprine maintenance, and the lower rate of relapse observed with oral cyclophosphamide induction may not apply to patients receiving rituximab maintenance.

If oral cyclophosphamide is used, it is initiated at 1.5-2 mg/kg daily. A complete blood count should be checked every 1-2 weeks while the patient is on therapy, and the dose should be temporarily held and/or reduced as needed to maintain the white blood cell count above 3500/μL. Although there are no standardized guidelines, it is important to reduce the cyclophosphamide dose for kidney function to avoid the development of significant leukopenia and the attendant infectious risks.

If intravenous pulse cyclophosphamide is chosen, the regimen from the CYCLOPS trial is commonly used: 15 mg/kg fortnightly for three doses, then every 3 weeks for 3 to 6 months. The dose in CYCLOPS was reduced by 2.5 mg/kg for patients older than 60, 5 mg/kg for patients older than 70, and 2.5 mg/kg for patients with a serum creatinine >3.3 mg/dL. Patients receiving pulse cyclophosphamide should have a complete blood count checked 2 weeks after each infusion to monitor the nadir white blood cell count. If the nadir white count is <3000/μL, the next dose should be reduced by 25% or more depending on the severity of leukopenia.

For both oral and intravenous cyclophosphamide, therapy is typically continued for 3 months before transitioning to maintenance therapy. In the minority of patients with ongoing disease activity after 3 months of therapy, cyclophosphamide may be continued for up to 6 months.

Rituximab

Two rituximab dosing regimens can be used for induction of remission. The standard approach is to use the regimen from the RAVE trial: 375 mg/m^2 weekly for 4 weeks. Alternatively, rituximab may be administered as two 1000-mg doses separated by 2 weeks, as is done for rheumatoid arthritis. Rituximab dosing should be modified in cases where plasma exchange is used, as the procedure removes the drug from circulation. A common approach is to delay the ensuing plasma exchange session for 48 hours after a rituximab dose and to administer at least one rituximab dose after the final plasma exchange session is completed.

Glucocorticoids

In patients with significant kidney involvement, glucocorticoids are typically initiated as pulse intravenous methylprednisolone (500-1000 mg daily) for 3 days. Thereafter, prednisone is initiated at approximately 60 mg/day and tapered over months to discontinuation or a low maintenance dose (e.g., 5 mg daily). Given the association of glucocorticoids with adverse events and reduced quality of life, a major goal in the treatment of AAV has been to reduce glucocorticoid exposure while preserving treatment efficacy. The recently completed PEXIVAS trial provides evidence that in patients with severe AAV, a "lower-dose" glucocorticoid regimen is non-inferior to a "higher-dose" glucocorticoid regimen for achieving remission (Table 17.2). Moreover, the "lower-dose" regimen had statistically fewer serious infections in the first year of treatment.

Given the results of the PEXIVAS trial, the "lower-dose" glucocorticoid regimen should be the default strategy used for induction of remission. It must be noted, however, that the trial regimen

TABLE 17.2 Prednisone Tapering in PEXIVAS Trial*

Week	50-75 kg Lower-dose PEXIVAS	50-75 kg Higher-dose PEXIVAS	> 75 kg Lower-dose PEXIVAS	> 75 kg Higher-dose PEXIVAS
1	60	60	75	75
2	30	60	40	75
3-4	25	50	30	60
5-6	20	40	25	50
7-8	15	30	20	40
9-10	12.5	25	15	30
11-12	10	20	12.5	25
13-14	7.5	15	10	20
15-16	5	10	7.5	15
17-18	5	10	7.5	15
19-20	5	7.5	5	10
21-22	5	7.5	5	7.5
23-52	5	5	5	5

*All patients received 3 days of intravenous pulse glucocorticoids before initiating the oral regimen. Doses are provided as mg of prednisone per day.

only provides an initial approach that may need to be modified by the treating clinician based upon careful longitudinal assessments of disease activity and side effects.

Infection Prophylaxis

Prophylaxis against Pneumocystis jiroveci pneumonia (PCP) is indicated in patients receiving induction immunosuppression. Trimethoprim-sulfamethoxazole is the agent of choice at most centers. In patients with an allergy to sulfonamide antibiotics, atovaquone or another alternative agent can be used. PCP prophylaxis is generally continued until the prednisone dose is tapered to less than 10 mg/day.

Plasma Exchange

The rationale for plasma exchange in AAV is predicated upon the pathogenic role of ANCA and the hypothesis that rapid removal of ANCA hastens resolution of disease activity. The addition of plasma exchange to induction immunosuppression is generally reserved for severe RPGN or pulmonary hemorrhage. In the MEPEX trial, the addition of plasma exchange in patients presenting with severe RPGN (Cr > 5.8 mg/dL) resulted in a decreased risk of dialysis dependence at 1 year. A subsequent metanalysis including 387 patients also found a benefit to plasma exchange on kidney outcomes. The recently completed PEXIVAS trial, however, failed to show a benefit of plasma exchange on the risk of dialysis dependence or mortality despite enrolling 704 patients. Notably, PEXIVAS included patients with less severe kidney involvement than prior studies (eGFR < 50 mL/min/1.73 m^2) and did not require kidney biopsy for enrollment. Consequently, it is possible a proportion of patients in PEXIVAS had mild disease or advanced fibrosis, subgroups that would not be expected to benefit from plasma exchange.

Given the results of the PEXIVAS trial, most patients with kidney involvement should not receive plasma exchange. There are certain patient subgroups, however, that may still derive benefit. At this time, plasma exchange can be considered for patients with severe and acute glomerulonephritis who are approaching or require kidney replacement therapy. Moreover, plasma exchange should be strongly considered in patients with severe pulmonary hemorrhage, as PEXIVAS was not adequately powered to exclude a benefit in this population. Ongoing analysis of the PEXIVAS trial is forthcoming and will likely further refine the optimal use of plasma exchange in AAV.

Patients with AAV selected for plasma exchange generally receive seven sessions over 14 days using an exchange volume of 60 mL/kg for each treatment. The default replacement fluid is albumin. For patients with a recent kidney biopsy or pulmonary hemorrhage, a proportion of the replacement fluid is administered as fresh frozen plasma to avoid coagulopathy.

Novel Induction of Remission Strategies

Despite significant improvements in patient outcomes, there is a need for therapeutic strategies with improved efficacy and fewer treatment-related side effects. Recognition of the importance of the alternative complement pathway in AAV, particularly C5a, provides new therapeutic targets. In the phase II CLEAR trial, the C5a receptor antagonist avacopan was able to effectively replace glucocorticoids in patients with active AAV receiving induction therapy with either cyclophosphamide or rituximab. Patients receiving avacopan had more rapid resolution of albuminuria and improved health-related quality of life. The ability of avacopan to replace glucocorticoids is being further evaluated in the phase III ADVOCATE trial.

In an attempt to minimize glucocorticoid exposure and obtain rapid disease control, some centers routinely combine cyclophosphamide with rituximab for induction of remission. Multiple case series have reported encouraging results with this strategy, including a significant reduction in glucocorticoid exposure compared with standard regimens. Randomized controlled trials are needed before combination therapy can be broadly recommended.

Maintenance of Remission

Disease relapse is common in AAV, particularly in the 12-18 months following discontinuation of immunosuppression. Consequently, maintenance therapy to prevent disease relapse is recommended in the vast majority of patients. For patients receiving induction with cyclophosphamide, maintenance therapy commences following the last cyclophosphamide dose and normalization of the white blood cell count. Patients who received induction therapy with rituximab start maintenance therapy 4-6 months after the last rituximab dose.

The optimal duration of maintenance therapy is unknown and should be individualized based upon the risk of relapse. For most patients, maintenance therapy should be continued for a minimum of approximately 2 years. Longer duration maintenance therapy is appropriate in some patients at high risk for relapse, including those with (1) history of prior disease relapse, (2) PR3-ANCA, (3) persistent ANCA positivity following induction therapy, and (4) lung or upper airway involvement. Rising ANCA titers correlate with impending relapse in certain patients but do not associate with disease activity in others. The positive predictive value of a rising ANCA titer is greater for kidney relapses than for non-kidney relapses. A rising ANCA titer in isolation should not lead to escalation of therapy, buy may lead to closer monitoring and continuance of maintenance therapy.

Extension of maintenance therapy should also be considered in patients who tolerated induction therapy poorly (e.g., significant glucocorticoid toxicity) and in those with advanced organ damage for whom a relapse would likely have deleterious consequences. A common example of the latter is a patient with advanced CKD who may become dialysis dependent following a relapse. Conversely, maintenance therapy may need to be abridged in patients with recurrent infections or other evidence of treatment-related toxicity.

First-line maintenance of remission agents used in AAV are azathioprine and rituximab. Mycophenolate mofetil was found to be inferior to azathioprine at preventing relapse in the IMPROVE trial and should generally be limited to patients unable to take either rituximab or azathioprine.

Recent clinical trials demonstrated superiority of rituximab compared with azathioprine at preventing disease relapse in AAV. The MAINRITSAN trial randomized patients to azathioprine or rituximab maintenance following induction with cyclophosphamide. At 28 months, the major relapse rate was significantly higher in the azathioprine arm (29%) compared with the rituximab arm (5%), with no difference in adverse events. Of note, the majority of patients enrolled in MAINRITSAN had PR3-ANCA, making the findings potentially less applicable to patients with MPO-ANCA. Another randomized trial, RITAZAREM, compared rituximab and azathioprine maintenance in relapsing patients following induction with rituximab, and initial reports indicate a lower relapse rate in the rituximab arm.

Based on the above results, rituximab is the preferred agent for most patients when available. The relative benefit of rituximab is greatest among patients with PR3-ANCA and in patients with a history of relapsing disease. In addition, as opposed to azathioprine, rituximab maintenance allows for complete discontinuation of glucocorticoids in most patients. Some experts use azathioprine as first-line therapy in specific subgroups with a lower risk of relapse, such as MPO-ANCA patients with renal-limited disease and no prior history of relapse. Azathioprine may also be preferred in patients with significant hypogammaglobulinemia (IgG level <300-400 mg/dL) and in patients with a history of hepatitis B exposure, given the risk of reactivation with rituximab. Finally, azathioprine is considered safe in pregnancy and is often used in this setting given the paucity of data with rituximab.

Rituximab

In patients receiving maintenance rituximab, a variety of dosing strategies can be used. The MAINRITSAN and RITZAREM trials used a fixed-schedule regimen, administering 500 or 1000 mg of rituximab every 4-6 months. Alternatively, after the initial maintenance dose, some centers use "B cell-triggered dosing." With this approach, peripheral B cells are monitored approximately every 3 months via flow cytometry (as the number of CD19+ cells), and rituximab is not re-dosed until peripheral B cell reconstitution occurs. The MAINRITSAN II trial compared a fixed-schedule regimen with dosing based upon B cell reconstitution or an increase in ANCA level (tailored therapy). There was no significant difference in the rate of relapse, but the tailored arm required fewer rituximab infusions than the fixed-schedule arm. The results of ongoing clinical trials will assist in refining rituximab dosing during maintenance.

Azathioprine

Azathioprine is generally initiated at 50 mg daily and uptitrated to a target dose of 1.5-2 mg/kg daily (maximum 200 mg daily) over the ensuing weeks, if tolerated. Although not routinely performed, if testing for thiopurine methyltransferase deficiency is negative, azathioprine can be initiated at the target dose. The rate of relapse is lower when azathioprine is combined with low-dose maintenance prednisone. Thus, some centers routinely continue low-dose prednisone (e.g., 7.5 mg daily) for extended periods in patients receiving maintenance azathioprine.

Management of Patients with Advanced Kidney Disease

Patients with Advanced Histologic Changes on Kidney Biopsy

A subset of patients with AAV, particularly those with MPO-ANCA and kidney-limited disease, have extensive global glomerulosclerosis and interstitial fibrosis on biopsy at the time of diagnosis. In contrast to other glomerular diseases (e.g., IgA nephropathy), patients with AAV have the potential for significant kidney recovery with treatment, despite the presence of advanced chronic histologic changes. Even among patients who become dialysis dependent around the time of diagnosis, no futility point with regard to histologic chronicity has been demonstrated. Therefore, induction immunosuppression should not be withheld on account of advanced histologic changes and/or initial dialysis dependence. Patients who recover sufficient kidney function to discontinue dialysis generally do so within 4 months of initiating treatment. Thereafter, recovery is unlikely, and continued induction therapy is not indicated in the absence of active extrarenal vasculitis.

Maintenance Therapy for Dialysis-Dependent Patients

Patients with AAV who remain dialysis dependent following induction therapy are at a significantly lower risk of disease relapse than their non-dialysis counterparts. Moreover, the risk of infectious complications is substantially greater in dialysis patients. This recognition has led many centers to abridge the duration of maintenance therapy to approximately 6 months in patients who are dialysis dependent with no evidence of active extrarenal disease. The ongoing MASTER-ANCA trial is formally evaluating the risks and benefits of maintenance therapy in patients with ESRD. Although the relapse risk is lower among dialysis patients, extrarenal flares have the potential to occur at any time, and patients should have indefinite longitudinal monitoring for disease activity.

Transplantation in AAV

All patients with AAV and chronic kidney failure should be evaluated for kidney transplant; overall, kidney transplant is associated with better survival in this population. Remission should be attained for a minimum of 6-12 months before transplantation is pursued. A positive ANCA titer in the absence of disease activity is not a contraindication to transplant, although patients with rising ANCA titers require close monitoring. The relapse rate of AAV following kidney transplant is low (0.02 relapses per patient year) due to the ongoing immunosuppressive treatment to prevent allograft rejection. Nonetheless, ongoing monitoring of AAV activity following transplant is needed to allow for early initiation of treatment should relapse occur.

Side Effects of Immunosuppressive Therapy

As treatment regimens have allowed for greater control of vasculitis activity, treatment-related toxicity has become a major driver of morbidity and mortality in AAV. Infections, many attributable to immunosuppressive therapy, are the most common cause of mortality in the first year of treatment. Although confounded by the presence of active vasculitis, infections are particularly correlated with exposure to high-dose glucocorticoids. In addition to the infectious risk common to all immunosuppressants, physicians treating AAV should be familiar with the unique side effects of each agent. These are summarized in Table 17.3.

TABLE 17.3 Side Effects of Immunosuppressants

Immunosuppressant	Key Side Effects
Glucocorticoids	Hyperglycemia, weight gain, hypertension, fluid retention, mood disturbances, skin thinning, easy bruising, cataracts, increased intraocular pressure, osteoporosis, myopathy
Cyclophosphamide	Leukopenia, hemorrhagic cystitis; dose-dependent risk of infertility and secondary malignancies
Rituximab	Infusion reactions, hypogammaglobulinemia, late-onset neutropenia (LON)
Azathioprine	Leukopenia, increase in MCV, nausea/anorexia, pancreatitis, hepatitis, hypersensitivity reaction; significant interaction with xanthine oxidase inhibitors

Bibliography

Bossuyt X, Cohen Tervaert JW, Arimura Y, et al. Position paper: Revised 2017 international consensus on testing of ANCAs in granulomatosis with polyangiitis and microscopic polyangiitis. *Nat Rev Rheumatol*. 2017;13(11):683–692.

Charles P, Terrier B, Perrodeau E, et al. Comparison of individually tailored versus fixed-schedule rituximab regimen to maintain ANCA-associated vasculitis remission: results of a multicentre, randomised controlled, phase III trial (MAINRITSAN2). *Ann Rheum Dis*. 2018;77(8):1143–1149.

Choi HK, Liu S, Merkel PA, Colditz GA, Niles JL. Diagnostic performance of antineutrophil cytoplasmic antibody tests for idiopathic vasculitides: metaanalysis with a focus on antimyeloperoxidase antibodies. *J Rheumatol*. 2001;28(7):1584–1590.

de Groot K, Harper L, Jayne DR, et al. Pulse versus daily oral cyclophosphamide for induction of remission in antineutrophil cytoplasmic antibody-associated vasculitis: a randomized trial. *Ann Intern Med*. 2009;150(10):670–680.

Guillevin L, Pagnoux C, Karras A, et al. Rituximab versus azathioprine for maintenance in ANCA-associated vasculitis. *N Engl J Med*. 2014;371(19):1771–1780.

Harper L, Morgan MD, Walsh M, et al. Pulse versus daily oral cyclophosphamide for induction of remission in ANCA-associated vasculitis: long-term follow-up. *Ann Rheum Dis*. 2012;71(6):955–960.

Hilhorst M, van Paassen P, Tervaert JW, Limburg Renal R. Proteinase 3-ANCA Vasculitis versus Myeloperoxidase-ANCA Vasculitis. *J Am Soc Nephrol*. 2015;26(10):2314–2327.

Jayne DR, Bruchfeld AN, Harper L, et al. Randomized Trial of C5a Receptor Inhibitor Avacopan in ANCA-Associated Vasculitis. *J Am Soc Nephrol*. 2017;28(9):2756–2767.

Jayne DR, Gaskin G, Rasmussen N, et al. Randomized trial of plasma exchange or high-dosage methylprednisolone as adjunctive therapy for severe renal vasculitis. *J Am Soc Nephrol*. 2007;18(7):2180–2188.

Jennette JC, Falk RJ, Bacon PA, et al. 2012 revised International Chapel Hill Consensus Conference Nomenclature of Vasculitides. *Arthritis Rheum*. 2013;65(1):1–11.

Lee T, Gasim A, Derebail VK, et al. Predictors of treatment outcomes in ANCA-associated vasculitis with severe kidney failure. *Clin J Am Soc Nephrol*. 2014;9(5):905–913.

Lyons PA, Rayner TF, Trivedi S, et al. Genetically distinct subsets within ANCA-associated vasculitis. *N Engl J Med*. 2012;367(3):214–223.

McAdoo SP, Tanna A, Hruskova Z, et al. Patients double-seropositive for ANCA and anti-GBM antibodies have varied renal survival, frequency of relapse, and outcomes compared to single-seropositive patients. *Kidney Int*. 2017;92(3):693–702.

Merkel PA, Xie G, Monach PA, et al. Identification of functional and expression polymorphisms associated with risk for antineutrophil cytoplasmic autoantibody-associated vasculitis. *Arthritis Rheumatol*. 2017;69(5):1054–1066.

Pendergraft WF, 3rd Niles JL. Trojan horses: drug culprits associated with antineutrophil cytoplasmic autoantibody (ANCA) vasculitis. *Curr Opin Rheumatol*. 2014;26(1):42–49.

Schreiber A, Xiao H, Jennette JC, Schneider W, Luft FC, Kettritz R. C5a receptor mediates neutrophil activation and ANCA-induced glomerulonephritis. *J Am Soc Nephrol*. 2009;20(2):289–298.

Specks U, Merkel PA, Seo P, et al. Efficacy of remission-induction regimens for ANCA-associated vasculitis. *N Engl J Med*. 2013;369(5):417–427.

Stone JH, Merkel PA, Spiera R, et al. Rituximab versus cyclophosphamide for ANCA-associated vasculitis. *N Engl J Med*. 2010;363(3):221–232.

Walsh M, Merkel PA, Peh CA, et al. Plasma exchange and glucocorticoids in severe ANCA-associated vasculitis. *N Engl J Med*. 2020;382(7):622–631.

Xiao H, Schreiber A, Heeringa P, Falk RJ, Jennette JC. Alternative complement pathway in the pathogenesis of disease mediated by anti-neutrophil cytoplasmic autoantibodies. *Am J Pathol*. 2007;170(1):52–64.

18

Minimal Change Disease

HOWARD TRACHTMAN, JONATHAN HOGAN, JAI RADHAKRISHNAN

Terminology and Histopathology

Minimal change disease (MCD) is a common cause of nephrotic syndrome (NS). Also known as *lipoid nephrosis, nil disease,* and *minimal change nephropathy*, the kidney histology on light microscopy in MCD is relatively normal and lacks the significant glomerular cell proliferation, infiltration by circulating immunoeffector cells, immune deposits, tubulointerstitial changes, or alterations in the glomerular basement membrane (GBM) that characterize other glomerular diseases. The defining features of MCD are ostensibly normal histological appearance on light microscopy and diffuse effacement and fusion of the majority of podocyte foot processes without electron-dense deposits on electron microscopy. There are variants of MCD that are characterized by diffuse mesangial hypercellularity. Immunofluorescence is typically negative or may show low-level focal staining for C3 and IgM.

Although MCD is histologically defined by the previously mentioned criteria, it can also be diagnosed clinically by exhibiting responsiveness to corticosteroid treatment. In children, because MCD is the cause of up to 90% of cases of idiopathic NS, a kidney biopsy is only warranted if the clinical and laboratory evidence, including disease onset before 6–9 months of age or following adolescence, unexpected systemic manifestations, or a low serum C3 level, suggests an alternative diagnosis. Children who do not exhibit these characteristics will typically have MCD and will consequently respond to steroids. The nomenclature "steroid-sensitive nephrotic syndrome (SSNS)" is also used to describe such children. Steroid responsiveness is a marker of a favorable long-term prognosis. In contrast, children with steroid-resistant nephrotic syndrome (SRNS), whether it occurs at the time of initial presentation or later in course of disease, are more likely on subsequent kidney biopsies to show focal segmental glomerulosclerosis (FSGS), a disease that is associated with a worse prognosis.

The causes of the NS in adults are more varied and include a higher percentage of cases with other histologies such as membranous nephropathy (MN), FSGS, and membranoproliferative glomerulonephritis (MPGN). Because MCD only accounts for approximately 10% to 15% of cases, a kidney biopsy is usually warranted to establish the etiology of nephrotic syndrome and guide management.

Pathophysiology

The pathogenesis of MCD is not well understood, but likely represents a fascinating instance of organ dysfunction caused by a variable interaction between intrinsic structural defects and immunologic disturbances. MCD, along with FSGS, is considered a podocytopathy, indicting the pivotal role of the visceral glomerular epithelial cell in the development of the disease. Various intracellular signaling pathways may mediate the effacement of podocyte foot processes that are a hallmark of MCD. For example, it has been demonstrated that markers of focal adhesion complex–mediated Crk-dependent signaling are enhanced in MCD but not FSGS. Moreover, increased production of proteins such as CD80 and angiopoietin-like protein 4 by podocytes in MCD models supports the central role of podocyte damage in the pathogenesis of MCD. It has been thought that proteinuria occurs solely because of a defect in glomerular permselectivity, although alterations in tubular reabsorption may contribute.

An assortment of clinical findings, namely, an association between MCD and atopic disease and Hodgkin lymphoma, measles-associated remission of MCD, and the beneficial effect of immunosuppressive drugs provides indirect evidence for an immunological basis for MCD. A link between abnormal T-cell function and MCD was initially proposed almost 50 years ago by Shalhoub, and many studies since then have documented altered subtype distribution and activity of lymphocytes in children with MCD. The efficacy of rituximab, a monoclonal antibody to CD20 on B-cells, suggests an important role of these antibody-producing cells in the development of MCD. The pivotal role of the immune system in MCD pathogenesis is underscored by a study in which albuminuria and podocyte foot process effacement were induced by injection of CD34+ stem cells isolated from patients with MCD or FSGS into immunodeficient NOD/SCID mice. This role is also supported by the finding of a higher Th17/Treg cell ratio in children with MCD. Genetic linkage between HLA-DQA1 and PLCG2 supports a role for adaptive and autoimmunity in the pathogenesis of MCD. Even stronger evidence was obtained in a transethnic meta-analysis involving 385 children that identified three SSNS-associated, single-nucleotide polymorphisms (SNP) within the HLA locus. These findings were confirmed in a similar studying involving 440 Japanese children with NS. Recent findings indicate that common genetic variants in TNF superfamily member 15 are also associated with increased risk of SSNS. Finally, two non-HLA loci in the calcium homeostasis modulating factor member 6 (CALHM6) gene have been linked to SSNS and result from inhibitory effects on the immune response.

Immunoeffector cells may elaborate soluble molecules, such as vascular endothelial growth factor, that directly increase GBM permeability to protein. It is likely that the molecular identity of circulating permeability factors that cause proteinuria will differ in patients with MCD and FSGS.

MCD is unique in that it predominantly reflects a decrease in the negative charge present in endothelial cells, the GBM, and podocytes, thereby causing selective proteinuria. The reduction in negative charge appears to be a diffuse abnormality that is manifest in capillaries throughout the body with leakage of albumin in the peripheral circulation and accumulation of interstitial fluid. The cause of the diminished negative charge density may reflect immune-mediated defects that inhibit sulfate incorporation into the GBM rather than a genetic mutation in a podocyte protein.

Although MCD can occur in familial clusters with both vertical (parent-child) and horizontal (sibling) patterns of inheritance, it has not been linked to mutations in any of the well-recognized proteins associated with FSGS, such as Wilms tumor-1, TRPC6, or α-actinin-4. Interestingly, there have been observations linking frequently relapsing childhood MCD to allelic heterogeneity in the gene for nephrin, a key component of the slit diaphragm and a major genetic locus for congenital NS. In addition, in a study of 214 Chinese patients with MCD, variants in the podocin gene were more common than in healthy controls and they correlated with the level of urinary protein excretion. Alterations in histone H3 lysine 4 trimethylation in children with MCD raise the possibility that epigenetic changes may contribute to the occurrence of MCD. Polymorphisms in the multi-drug resistance-1 gene may influence responsiveness to steroids in patients with MCD.

MCD also is associated with various "secondary" causes (Box 18.1), including medications, infections, toxins, and malignancies. The pathophysiologic link between these secondary causes and the resulting MCD is not understood.

MCD may be associated with significant short-term morbidity and can manifest with a chronic relapsing course with long-term adverse consequences well into adulthood. Patient-reported outcomes in children and adolescents with MCD reveal worse function in the domains of peer relationship, social functioning, school performance, and pain interference. Both first-line treatment and secondary therapeutic options for more difficult cases can lead to serious toxicity. Therefore, although the long-term prognosis is excellent, optimal management of MCD requires clinical acumen to balance the risks of untreated disease activity against the potential irreversible hazards of available pharmacologic choices.

Incidence

The overall incidence of primary or idiopathic NS comprised of MCD and its variants, FSGS, MN, and MPGN, is approximately three to five cases/100,000 population/year in children and adults. This rate is fairly constant throughout the world and in most racial and ethnic groups. Recent data suggest that the incidence of MCD is rising in India and Southeast Asia while FSGS may be increasingly prevalent throughout the world. The contribution of MCD to this general category varies tremendously with the age of the patient. Thus, in prepubertal patients more than 6 months of age, MCD accounts for nearly 90% of all cases of idiopathic NS, whereas in adults the percentage of cases attributable to MCD falls to 10% to 15%. Adolescence represents the transition period between the two ends of the spectrum. In a study of 1523 consecutive Chinese patients who underwent biopsy performed during the evaluation of NS, in those aged 14 to 24 years, MCD was documented in 33% of the subgroup. Similarly, in a report by Mubarak of biopsy findings in 538 pediatric patients in Pakistan, among whom 365 were younger children (mean age 7.3 years) and 173 were adolescents (mean age 15.1 years), approximately one-third of the older group had FSGS and only one-fourth had MCD. The incidence of MN

and MPGN was significantly higher in the older group than in the younger group. These findings suggest that adolescents correspond more closely to adults than they do to younger children and school-age pediatric patients.

Clinical Presentation

MCD causes the NS with nephrotic-range proteinuria, edema, hypoalbuminemia, and hypercholesterolemia. A hypercoagulable state secondary to the NS is much more common in adult versus pediatric patients. The pathogenesis of edema in NS is complex and represents an interplay between underfill and overfill mechanisms. Thus, hypoalbuminemia and reduced effective circulating blood volume can activate the renin-angiotensin-aldosterone axis. In addition, the NS is characterized by increased sodium reabsorption linked to plasmin-related degradation of corin, an inhibitor of the epithelial sodium channel.

BOX 18.1

Secondary Causes of Minimal Change Disease

Hematologic Tumors
Hodgkin lymphoma
Non-Hodgkin lymphoma
Leukemia

Solid Tumors
Thymoma
Renal cell carcinoma
Lung carcinoma
Mesothelioma

Infection
Syphilis
Mycoplasma
Ehrlichiosis
Strongyloidiasis
Echinococcus
Tuberculosis
HIV
Hepatitis C virus

Drugs
NSAIDs, including COX-2 inhibitors
Antimicrobials (ampicillin, rifampicin, cephalosporins)
Lithium
D-penicillamine
Bisphosphonates (Pamidronate)
Sulfasalazines (mesalazine and salazopyrine)
Trimethadione
Immunizations
Interferon-γ

Other Kidney and Systemic Diseases
SLE
Fabry disease
Polycystic kidney disease
IPEX syndrome

HIV, Human immunodeficiency virus; *IPEX,* immune dysregulation polyendocrinopathy, enteropathy, X-linked; *NSAIDs,* nonsteroidal antiinflammatory drugs; *SLE,* systemic lupus erythematosus.

Edema is the most common presenting symptom of MCD, and the onset may be acute.

Antecedent infections, typically respiratory, are often associated with the onset of MCD. Infections may also trigger subsequent relapses of MCD. The rapidity of the appearance of edema is characteristic of MCD compared to other etiologies of NS. In children, edema can occur anywhere in the body, including the periorbital region, scrotum, or abdomen.

Less frequent presenting complaints include infections such as cellulitis secondary to localized accumulation of fluid and skin breakdown, or bacterial peritonitis in patients with ascites. Hypercholesterolemia arises from alterations in lipoprotein lipase activity, and recent data support an important role for derangements in PCKS9 activity in mediating hypercholesterolemia in MCD. Thromboembolic events, including renal vein thrombosis and pulmonary emboli, may occur with MCD and correlate with severe hypoalbuminemia.

Urinalysis reveals microscopic hematuria in 10% to 30% of adults and children with MCD, but gross hematuria is rare. Microscopic examination of the urine may also show waxy casts and oval, fat bodies. In one series, acute kidney injury (AKI) occurred in 17.8% of adult patients who presented with NS and were subsequently diagnosed with MCD. These patients tended to be older, male, hypertensive, and had more severe proteinuria and hypoalbuminemia than patients who did not develop AKI. Kidney biopsies of these patients showed a variety of histologic patterns of injury including tubular atrophy, interstitial inflammation and fibrosis, and atherosclerotic disease. The cause of the AKI is not entirely clear and may reflect primary changes in glomerular permeability, the reason for which is not entirely clear. Serum levels of C3 and C4 are typically normal, and antinuclear antibodies and cryoglobulins are usually absent. AKI may complicate the course in nearly 50% of children with MCD who require hospitalization.

Initial Treatment

Corticosteroids represent the time-honored initial therapy for presumed and biopsy-confirmed MCD. As mentioned, the sensitivity of MCD to steroid treatment prompts many physicians to empirically treat nephrotic patients with glucocorticoids without a kidney biopsy, particularly children. Prednisone is the usual agent prescribed, and the standard dose in pediatric patients is 60 mg/m^2 or 2 mg/kg daily for 4 to 6 weeks followed by 40 mg/m^2 or 1.5 mg/kg every other day for 4 to 6 weeks. In children, 70% will achieve remission after 10 to 14 days of treatment and the vast majority will no longer have proteinuria after 4 weeks of therapy. There are conflicting data in the literature as to whether lengthening the course of the initial treatment from 8 to 12 weeks delays the time to first relapse and reduces overall exposure to steroids. Two recent controlled clinical trials indicated that a longer initial course of steroids had no beneficial impact on the development of a frequently relapsing course compared to a standard 8-week course. Efficacy may vary depending on the patient population, and the precise treatment should be guided by the experience at each center.

Adults are treated with oral prednisone 1 mg/kg/day or alternate-day prednisone at 2 mg/kg per every other day. However, unlike children, responses in adults may take up to 24 weeks before the patient is designated "steroid responsive" or "steroid resistant." In adults, up to 20% of patients with an initial diagnosis of MCD may be refractory to steroids at the end of 24 weeks.

Treatment of relapse involves similar corticosteroid doses, but usually for a shorter period of time. Various modifications in corticosteroid dosing such as extended tapering schedules, avoidance of every other day administration, and prolonged low-dose hydrocortisone to prevent adrenal insufficiency have been prescribed to prevent relapses and to minimize side effects. Different formulations of steroids such a deflazacort have also been tried with mixed results. Adults do not tolerate relapsing disease as well as children as a consequence of the intrinsic morbidity of MCD and the toxicity related to repeated exposures to corticosteroids. Therefore, these patients are often candidates for prompt implementation of second-line immunosuppressive therapy.

Short-Term Course

MCD is usually a chronic relapsing disease (Fig. 18.1). Less than 10% of cases will remain completely free of relapses after the initial episode. The remaining patients can be divided into three

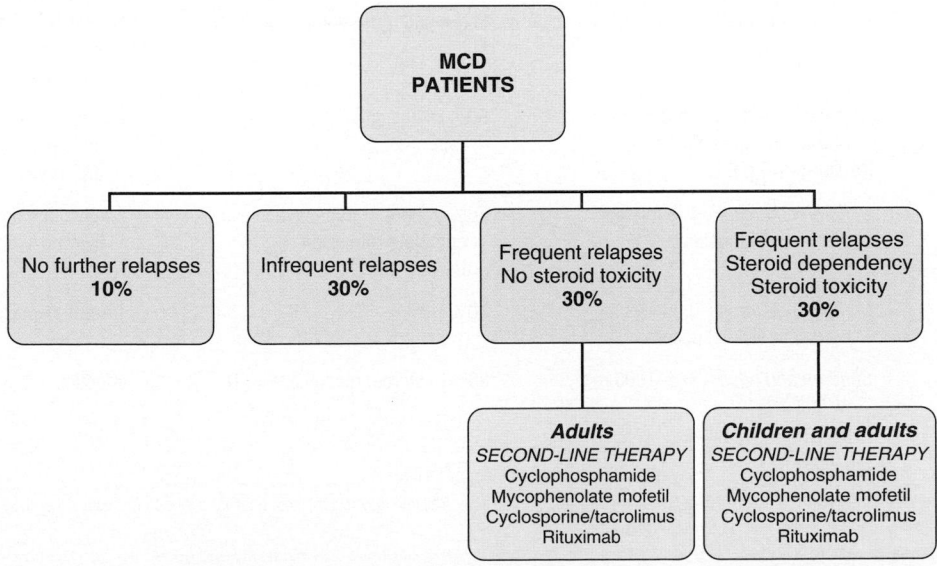

• **Fig. 18.1** Minimal change disease (MCD): short-term natural history.

categories based on clinical course. One-third will have infrequent relapses that are easily managed by intermittent administration of courses of corticosteroids. Another third will have frequent relapses defined by ≥2 relapses in a 6-month period; however, they, too, are successfully managed with intermittent administration of courses of corticosteroids and they do not manifest significant steroid-induced side effects. The remaining third are frequently relapsing patients or those with steroid dependence defined as relapse occurring on alternate-day steroid treatment or within 2 weeks of discontinuing corticosteroids. It has proved difficult to predict the short-term, that is, ≤2 years after disease onset, prognosis in individual patients. In children, those who go into remission during the first week of corticosteroid treatment and who have no hematuria are more likely to be infrequent relapsers, defined as <2 episodes in 6 months or <3 in 1 year. The presence of small, involuted glomeruli, which can be distinguished from other causes of global glomerulosclerosis by the presence of vital podocytes and parietal epithelial cells, may be a marker of frequently relapsing MCD in children. Extending the duration of the initial course of corticosteroids or implementing a prolonged tapering schedule do not seem to impact the likelihood of developing frequently relapsing or steroid-dependent MCD.

Children are generally treated with an 8-week course of steroids—4 weeks of daily and 4 weeks of every other day medication. There does not appear to be any substantial benefit to prolonging the initial course of steroids to 12 weeks or slowly tapering the steroids. Adults with MCD may be prescribed every other day steroids for up to 6 months because of poor tolerance of the drug.

Patients who experience frequent relapses/steroid dependence usually experience steroid toxicity, and they are candidates for second-line treatments to alleviate the steroid burden. The options are outlined below. Key steroid-induced side effects in children are impaired linear growth, obesity, behavioral changes, and cosmetic changes. In addition to these clinical effects, children with MCD also experience altered quality of life and psychosocial adjustment that are related both to illness-related variables and to alterations in the family climate. In adults, additional evidence of steroid toxicity includes cataracts and altered bone density. Hypertension and hyperlipidemia occur across the age spectrum. It is the last category of patients that most requires careful nephrologist attention for ongoing management and care.

Long-Term Treatment

Immunosuppressive Therapy

Second-line therapy is used in patients with frequently relapsing, steroid-dependent MCD, as well as those who experience, or are at risk from, steroid-related side effects (Table 18.1). The first class of drugs that was used under these circumstances was alkylating agents such as cyclophosphamide and chlorambucil. A prolonged remission of at least 1 year was achieved in 70% of patients. With cyclophosphamide, most patients require at least 12 weeks of therapy, and they should be monitored carefully for side effects including leukopenia, infection, hemorrhagic cystitis, gonadal toxicity, and malignancy. However, more than 25% of patients with MCD who were treated with cyclophosphamide were not in sustained remission after puberty and they required prolonged immunosuppressive treatment. Thus, because of the serious toxicity associated with the alkylating agents including gonadal injury in males, the reluctance to prescribe a second course, and the guarded long-term effect, there has been greater reliance on alternative medications to alkylating agents for frequently relapsing or steroid-dependent patients with MCD.

Antimetabolites such as azathioprine and mycophenolate mofetil can reduce the relapse rate by approximately 50%, although they are not as effective as alkylating agents in inducing a permanent remission. They are useful because they have a more favorable side-effect profile, can be administered for an extended period, and require less intensive monitoring.

TABLE 18.1 Second-Line Treatments of Minimal Change Disease

Drug	Dose	Efficacy	Side Effects
Cyclophosphamide	*Children and adults:* 2–2.5 mg/kg/day × 8–12 wk*	Prolonged remission (>1 yr) in 70%	Leukopenia, hemorrhagic cystitis, alopecia, seizures, gonadal toxicity, malignancy
Mycophenolate mofetil	*Children:* 24–36 mg/kg/day or 600 mg/m²/dose BID *Adults:* 1–1.5 g BID	50% reduction in overall relapse rate	Gastrointestinal complaints, leukopenia, elevated liver enzymes
Cyclosporine	*Children and adults:* 4–5 mg/kg/day in divided doses†	70% to 80% of patients achieve complete remission on treatment	Gingival hyperplasia, tremor, elevated liver enzymes, nephrotoxicity
Tacrolimus	*Children and adults:* 0.05–0.3 mg/kg/day in divided doses†	70%-80%	Tremor, nephrotoxicity, alopecia
Rituximab	*Children and adults:* 375–1000 mg/m²/dose 1–4 doses, 2 wk apart	80% in steroid responsive MCD	Infection

*It is recommended that the duration of therapy be extended to 12 weeks in patients with steroid-dependent disease.

†Target trough levels for cyclosporine and tacrolimus are 100–200 ng/mL and 4–8 ng/mL, respectively. Children may require more frequent dosing to maintain a therapeutic drug level. After achieving remission, reduce doses to the lowest dose compatible with staying in remission.

BID, Twice daily; *SSNS,* steroid-sensitive nephrotic syndrome.

A third option is calcineurin inhibitors such as cyclosporine and tacrolimus. These agents induce a prolonged remission in nearly 80% to 90% of patients while the patient is taking the drug; however, relapses frequently occur shortly after stopping the drug and there is a suggestion that use of these drugs may delay the spontaneous resolution of MCD. In addition, calcineurin inhibitors can cause undesirable cosmetic changes (hair growth and gingival hyperplasia with cyclosporine, alopecia with tacrolimus), hepatoxicity, hypertension, and nephrotoxicity. Therefore, patients taking calcineurin inhibitors for more than 1 year may require periodic blood tests to monitor drug levels and serial kidney biopsies to ensure that irreversible kidney injury does not occur.

Adrenocorticotropic hormone (ACTH), which was widely used in the past, has been reintroduced for the management of MCD. This hormone may act, in part, as a steroid substitute. In addition, it may act directly on the podocyte to restore functional integrity and normalize proteinuria. However, the results of the ATLANTIS trial suggest that ACTH is not an effective agent to reduce the relapse rate in children with difficult-to-treat MCD.

Finally, the newest agent used to treat children with frequently relapsing or steroid-dependent MCD and clinical evidence of steroid-induced side effects is rituximab. Administration of this anti-CD20 monoclonal antibody on B cells is likely to achieve remission in up to 80% of steroid-sensitive cases when used in combination with calcineurin inhibitors. This was confirmed in a study of 54 children (mean age 11 years) in which open-label administration of rituximab plus low-dose steroids and tacrolimus was as effective as treatment with standard doses of the last two drugs. The efficacy of rituximab has been confirmed in several randomized clinical trials that enrolled diverse populations of children and adolescents. In addition, in a head-to-head comparison with tacrolimus, rituximab was more effective at preventing relapses and reducing exposure to corticosteroids and was well tolerated in children with steroid-dependent MCD. Thus, this therapy is costly and the long-term risks are unknown. Therefore, it is advisable that ongoing surveillance be maintained to gain perspective on the proper place of this biologic agent in the therapeutic management of children with difficult-to-treat MCD.

The decision to recommend a second-line agent in an effort to alleviate the adverse consequences of steroids must be weighed on an individual basis and must take into account the patient's age, sex, and likely compliance with treatment. There is no consensus on the optimal sequence of agents for an individual child with MCD. Consideration should be given to the severity of the side effect, the likelihood of reversal of the complication, and the odds that the MCD will spontaneously resolve. Although a number of other immunomodulatory agents have been tried in the past in patients with MCD, the data have been collected in relatively small studies that hinder broad generalizations about efficacy. In addition, drugs such as levamisole are generally not available in the United States for use in patients with MCD. This underscores the need to develop newer agents that can be used to control proteinuria in patients with MCD, especially in children with steroid toxicity and adults with relapsing disease.

Supportive Care

After the initial diagnosis, patients with MCD are usually monitored with daily dipstick testing for proteinuria. In most patients, relapses are detected by the onset of proteinuria 3 to 4 days before edema ensues. In those patients who develop edema before a relapse is recognized or who respond slowly to prednisone, edema can be controlled by prescribing a low-salt (2 g sodium) diet and oral diuretics. Options include loop diuretics, such as furosemide 1 to 2 mg/kg administered once or twice daily or a thiazide diuretic. In patients who are refractory to standard diuretics, addition of metolazone, an agent that acts primarily in the cortical collecting duct and to a lesser extent in the proximal tubule, may improve urine output. Close monitoring is warranted to ensure that the patients do not develop severe hypokalemia, metabolic alkalosis, or intravascular volume contraction. The duration of action of diuretic agents may be diminished secondary to hypoalbuminemia and enhanced renal clearance, but this is rarely clinically significant because the medications are only needed for 1 to 2 weeks until treatment response occurs and proteinuria resolves.

Children who have frequent relapses and persistent edema are at risk for bacterial peritonitis and can be given prophylactic penicillin. Immunization with the pneumococcal vaccine is also helpful under these circumstances. If feasible, the timing of vaccine administration should be delayed for at least 2 weeks after administration of prednisone to ensure maximal immunologic response.

Prognosis

The prognosis for patients with MCD is excellent and, according to the literature, the disease eventually resolves without further relapses in >95% of patients. However, this presumed benign course is based on scarce data of patients followed into adulthood. A recent study of 42 adult patients, median age 28 years, who were monitored for a median of 22 years after the diagnosis of MCD, demonstrated that 33% were still relapsing in adulthood. Children who had a relapsing course and/or required immunosuppressive medications were more likely to have persistent disease in adulthood. Moreover, although final height was normal, nearly half of adult patients with relapsing MCD had excess weight gain, hypertension, cataracts, osteoporosis, and sperm abnormalities. Whether MCD has any long-term effect on the incidence or age at onset of cardiovascular disease in adults remains unclear. Clinical outcomes in patients enrolled in large health maintenance organizations indicate that persistent NS is associated with an increased incidence of atherosclerotic disease, and the relative risk in patients with MCD versus more refractory forms of idiopathic NS requires further study. Based on the persistence beyond childhood of relapsing disease and the development of serious side effects, transition from a pediatric to an adult nephrologist is warranted in patients with relapsing MCD or a history of prolonged steroid or immunosuppressive drug use for MCD as they reach adulthood.

The overwhelming majority of children with MCD have no evidence of progressive chronic kidney disease. Recognizing that the diagnosis of FSGS can be difficult to establish if a kidney biopsy specimen does not include the few abnormal glomeruli originating at the corticomedullary junction, it is conceivable that the rare cases of presumed MCD with a poor outcome and progressive GFR loss may represent unidentified FSGS.

Conclusion

Although MCD is not a common illness, it causes short-term morbidity related to edema and infection. Initial treatment with corticosteroids results in remission of proteinuria in nearly all patients; however, up to 40% of patients will manifest a frequently relapsing or steroid-dependent course with steroid toxicity. These patients are candidates for treatment with second-line agents such as alkylating agents, mycophenolate mofetil, calcineurin inhibitors, or rituximab. The choice of drug will vary from center to center and reflect local experience and preferences of the individual physician. The disease can persist into adulthood and can lead to chronic sequelae such as bone demineralization, atherosclerosis, and obesity. Therefore, long-term follow-up is warranted in those patients who continue to relapse and require immunosuppressive medication. Further research is needed to define better the cause of MCD, that is, the immunologic basis, the permeability factor(s) released by immunoeffector cells, and the role of podocyte protein abnormalities. This will lead to the development of more targeted treatments that can effectively achieve long-term remission without the side effects associated with current therapeutic options.

Complete bibliography is available at Elsevier eBooks for Practicing Clinicians.

Key Bibliography

Basu B, Sander A, Roy B, et al. Efficacy of rituximab vs tacrolimus in pediatric corticosteroid-dependent nephrotic syndrome: a randomized clinical trial. *JAMA Pediatr.* 2018;172(8):757–764.

Boumediene A, Vachin P, Sendeyo K, et al. NEPHRUTIX: a randomized, double-blind, placebo vs rituximab-controlled trial assessing t-cell subset changes in minimal change nephrotic syndrome. *J Autoimmun.* 2018;88:91–102.

Clement LC, Avila-Casado C, Macé C, et al. Podocyte-secreted angiopoietin-like-4 mediates proteinuria in glucocorticoid-sensitive nephrotic syndrome. *Nat Med.* 2011;17:117–122.

Constantinescu AR, Shah HB, Foote EF, et al. Predicting first-year relapses in children with nephrotic syndrome. *J Pediatr.* 2000;105:492–495.

Debiec H, Dossier C, Letouze E, et al. Transethnic, genome-wide analysis reveals immune-related risk alleles and phenotypic correlates in pediatric steroid-sensitive nephrotic syndrome. *J Am Soc Nephrol.* 2018;29(7):2000–2013.

Fakhouri F, Bocqueret N, Taupin P, et al. Children with steroid-sensitive nephrotic syndrome come of age: long-term outcome. *J Pediatr.* 2005;147:202–207.

Garin EH, Diaz LN, Mu W, et al. Urinary CD80 excretion increases in idiopathic minimal-change disease. *J Am Soc Nephrol.* 2009;20:260–266.

Gulati A, Sinha A, Jordan SC, et al. Efficacy and safety of treatment with rituximab for difficult steroid-resistant and -dependent nephrotic syndrome: multicentric report. *Clin J Am Soc Nephrol.* 2010;5:2207–2212.

Jia X, Horinouchi T, Hitomi Y, et al. Strong association of the HLA-DR/DQ locus with childhood steroid-sensitive nephrotic syndrome in the Japanese population. *J Am Soc Nephrol.* 2018;29(8):2189–2199.

Jia X, Yamamura T, Gbadegesin R, et al. Common risk variants in NPHS1 and TNFSF15 are associated with childhood steroid-sensitive nephrotic syndrome. *Kidney Int.* 2020.

Li X, Liu Z, Wang L, et al. Tacrolimus monotherapy after intravenous methylprednisolone in adults with minimal change nephrotic syndrome. *J Am Soc Nephrol.* 2017;28(4):1286–1295.

Medjeral-Thomas NR, Lawrence C, Condon M, et al. Randomized, controlled trial of tacrolimus and prednisolone monotherapy for adults with de novo minimal change disease: a multicenter, randomized, controlled trial. *Clin J Am Soc Nephrol.* 2020;15(2):209–218.

Polzin D, Kaminski HJ, Kastner C, et al. Decreased renal corin expression contributes to sodium retention in proteinuric kidney diseases. *Kidney Int.* 2010;78(7):650–659.

Rheault MN, Zhang L, Selewski DT, et al. AKI in children hospitalized with nephrotic syndrome. *Clin J Am Soc Nephrol.* 2015;10(12):2110–2118.

Selewski DT, Troost JP, Massengill SF, et al. The impact of disease duration on quality of life in children with nephrotic syndrome: a Midwest Pediatric Nephrology Consortium study. *Pediatr Nephrol.* 2015;30(9):1467–1476.

Sellier-Leclerc AL, Macher MA, Loirat C, et al. Rituximab efficiency in children with steroid-dependent nephrotic syndrome. *Pediatr Nephrol.* 2010;25:1109–1115.

Sinha A, Puraswani M, Kalaivani M, Goyal P, Hari P, Bagga A. Efficacy and safety of mycophenolate mofetil versus levamisole in frequently relapsing nephrotic syndrome: an open-label randomized controlled trial. *Kidney Int.* 2019;95(1):210–218.

Waldman M, Crew RJ, Valeri A, et al. Adult minimal-change disease: clinical characteristics, treatment, and outcomes. *Clin J Am Soc Nephrol.* 2007;2:445–453.

Webb NJA, Woolley RL, Lambe T, et al. Long term tapering versus standard prednisolone treatment for first episode of childhood nephrotic syndrome: phase III randomised controlled trial and economic evaluation. *BMJ.* 2019;365:l1800.

Zhu L, Yu L, Wang CD, et al. Genetic effect of the NPHS2 gene variants on proteinuria in minimal change disease and immunoglobulin a nephropathy. *Nephrology.* 2009;14:728–734.

19

Focal Segmental Glomerulosclerosis

JEFFREY B. KOPP, AVI Z. ROSENBERG, H. WILLIAM SCHNAPER

Focal segmental glomerulosclerosis (FSGS) is neither a disease nor a syndrome, but rather a set of clinicopathologic syndromes. The shared histopathologic findings include segmental glomerular scars, often with global glomerular tubulointerstitial scarring, no immunostaining or staining for immunoglobulin M (IgM) and C3, and no or minimal inflammatory cells in glomeruli or blood vessels. FSGS accounts for approximately 20% of cases of idiopathic nephrotic syndrome in children and as many as 35% of cases in adults. FSGS can present as nephrotic syndrome, nephrotic-range proteinuria without other features of nephrotic syndrome, or subnephrotic proteinuria. FSGS is the most common histopathologic pattern of injury in idiopathic nephrotic syndrome among individuals of sub-Saharan African descent and, in some published series, the most common pattern among all races. Studies in North America have documented increasing prevalence of FSGS in biopsy series over the past several decades. Spontaneous remission of FSGS is rare, and both untreated and treatment-resistant FSGS frequently progress to end-stage kidney disease.

Clinical Features and Diagnosis

Proteinuria in FSGS is typically nonselective, consisting of both small and large proteins, including albumin and, to a lesser extent, immunoglobulins. Edema, hypoalbuminemia, and hyperlipidemia are typically present in primary FSGS while less common in other forms. Hypertension is common. Decreased glomerular filtration rate (GFR) is noted in approximately one-third of patients at presentation. Microscopic hematuria may be present but is not typical.

Various nosologies of FSGS have been presented over the years; all are somewhat arbitrary and depend on judgment about where to split or combine categories. We have suggested that FSGS can be usefully classified into six forms and that making these distinctions can have clinical relevance (Table 19.1). These forms are primary, postadaptive FSGS, APOL1 FSGS, high-penetrance genetic FSGS, virus-associated FSGS, and medication-associated FSGS. Not listed here are cases that show a pattern of focal and segmental glomerular scarring that can result from a variety of inflammatory, proliferative, thrombotic, and hereditary conditions. There are situations where the proper diagnostic approach is unclear, including the case of an individual with diabetes with both classic changes of diabetic nephropathy and focal and segmental glomerular scars. We avoid the term "secondary FSGS" in this chapter, as it serves chiefly to distinguish primary disease (unknown cause) from other forms with known cause, although

we recognize that this term may have utility. Upon receiving a diagnosis of FSGS based on kidney biopsy findings, we believe that it is essential for clinicians to determine which form of FSGS their patient might have and to carry out additional diagnostic testing for this purpose.

The Six Focal Segmental Glomerulosclerosis Clinical Syndromes

Three FSGS syndromes are most common, with each of these perhaps accounting for approximately one-third of FSGS cases in the United States; the distribution will differ in other countries. Distinction among these forms involves collecting clinical history and laboratory data and evaluating kidney biopsy findings (Table 19.2).

Primary FSGS is the form whose pathogenesis is least well understood. Many patients have nephrotic proteinuria, often as part of nephrotic syndrome. Primary FSGS is believed to be due to circulating factor(s), with evidence that it may recur following kidney transplant. The causative factor remains elusive, with candidates that include soluble plasminogen activator urokinase-type receptor (suPAR) and cardiotrophin-like cytokine 1.

Post-adaptive FSGS arises from an imbalance between glomerular load (i.e., increased glomerular blood flow, arising from diverse factors) and glomerular capacity (i.e., the maximal effective glomerular capillary surface area), resulting in increased glomerular capillary pressures and, thus, placing podocytes under mechanical stress. Consequent to this maladaptation, glomerular hemodynamic alterations can arise through (1) a reduction in the number of functioning nephrons (such as after unilateral renal agenesis, surgical ablation, oligomeganephronia, or any advanced primary kidney disease) or (2) mechanisms that place hemodynamic stress on an initially normal nephron population (as in morbid obesity, cyanotic congenital heart disease, and sickle cell anemia). In postadaptive FSGS, proteinuria may be nephrotic range but is more typically subnephrotic. Plasma albumin concentration may be normal, even in the presence of nephrotic range proteinuria. Edema may be absent. Renin-angiotensin-aldosterone system (RAAS) antagonism, particularly when coupled with a diuretic and dietary sodium restriction (ideally to 1 g sodium per day), may have a particularly dramatic effect in reducing proteinuria in postadaptive FSGS, and such a response may help confirm the diagnosis of the form of FSGS.

APOL1 FSGS is due to coding-region variants in the apolipoprotein L1 gene. These variants are termed *G1* and *G2* and are seen

TABLE 19.1 Six Forms of Focal Segmental Glomerulosclerosis

	Mechanism	Setting	Therapy
Primary FSGS	Presumed circulating molecule(s)	Most common in children and young adults	Immunosuppression
Postadaptive FSGS	Mismatch between glomerular load and capacity	Premature birth, small for gestational age obesity, hypermuscularity (androgens)	RAAS antagonism, thiazide diuretic, sodium restriction, weight loss if obese
APOL1 FSGS	APOL1 risk alleles	Sub-Saharan African ancestry	Depends on phenotype
High-penetrance genetic FSGS	>50 genes, nuclear and mitochondrial		Most forms, treatment as for postadaptive FSGS
Virus-associated FSGS	HIV, possibly EBV, parvovirus B19		Antiviral therapy or reduced immunosuppression
Medication–associated FSGS	Interferon (APOL1), bisphosphonate, androgens, lithium		Stop the offending agent

APOL1, Apolipoprotein L1; EBV, Epstein-Barr virus; FSGS, focal segmental glomerulosclerosis; RAAS, renin-angiotensin-aldosterone system.

TABLE 19.2 Data Relevant in Evaluating a Patient with the Histologic Diagnosis of Focal Segmental Glomerulosclerosis

Relevant Clinical History	Laboratory Data	Kidney Biopsy Findings
Family history of kidney disease Birth weight Gestational age at birth Congenital cyanotic heart disease Sickle cell disease History consistent with reflux nephropathy or reduced kidney mass Peak and present body mass index: obesity, extreme muscular development Viral infection: HIV, parvovirus B19, Epstein-Barr virus Medication, past or present: interferon, lithium, bisphosphonate, androgen abuse, chronic use of nephrotoxic drugs	Serum albumin before therapy Urine PCR Percent change in urine PCR following maximal renin-angiotensin-aldosterone therapy and dietary sodium restriction Change in urine PCR following immunosuppressive therapy	FSGS histologic variant Glomerular size (glomerulomegaly) *Electron microscopy:* Extent of foot process effacement; podocyte microvillus transformation; tubuloreticular inclusions in glomerular endothelial cells (interferon effect)

FSGS, Focal segmental glomerulosclerosis; PCR, protein-to-creatinine ratio.
Adapted from Rosenberg A, Kopp J. Focal segmental glomerulosclerosis. *Clin J Am Soc Nephrol.* 2017;12:502–517.

exclusively in individuals of sub-Saharan African descent. While some have advocated calling this entity APOL1-associated FSGS, recent work adds important evidence that the APOL1 kidney risk variants cause glomerular injury, particularly impacting the podocytes. The clinical picture of APOL1 FSGS is diverse and can mimic that of other forms of FSGS, which provides the rationale for having its own category. APOL1 FSGS is a specific form of genetic FSGS; APOL1 FSGS subjects often have a family history of FSGS but, given the requirement for an additional provocative factor for kidney disease to manifest, the inheritance pattern of clinical disease is highly variable among families. Further, the high frequency of APOL1 FSGS (APOL1 variants are the cause of 72% of FSGS in African-descent individuals in the United States and South Africa) sets it apart from other forms of genetic FSGS.

The clinical picture of APOL1 FSGS can mimic that of primary FSGS or postadaptive FSGS, and it appears likely that the provocative factors that drive each of these two forms can also elicit and perhaps accelerate glomerular scarring in individuals with two *APOL1* risk alleles. APOL1 FSGS is also seen with virus-associated FSGS, augmenting risk for FSGS in this setting. Human immunodeficiency (HIV) infection is the most powerful interactor with APOL1 risk alleles, via virus-stimulated interferon expression driving *APOL1* gene expression. Carriage of a single *APOL1* risk allele poses a small increased risk for FSGS, but this association only reached statistical significance in a single study from South Africa. APOL1 FSGS can present as a form of medication-associated FSGS, as interferon increases *APOL1* gene expression and induces FSGS in genetically susceptible individuals. Finally, APOL1 FSGS can present in the setting of glomerulonephritides such as in lupus nephritis with collapsing glomerulopathy. At present, therapy for APOL1 FSGS should be based on whether the clinical presentation mimics primary FSGS, postadaptive FSGS, virus-associated FSGS, or medication-associated FSGS. For this reason, *APOL1* genetic testing is not clinically indicated at this time, but this may change once APOL1-specific therapies are developed. Indeed, a phase IIA study is in progress, testing the safety and efficacy of a small-molecule, oral medication directed against APOL1 protein (clinicaltrials.gov NCT04340362).

Three other forms of FSGS are less common. *High-penetrance genetic variants*, with *Mendelian or mitochondrial inheritance* patterns, manifest FSGS, often with a clinical picture that is not classic for primary FSGS and lacks risk factors for postadaptive FSGS. There are now over 50 genetic loci implicated in FSGS pathogenesis, and more are identified annually. Several *viruses* cause FSGS. Uncontrolled HIV-1 infection is associated with HIV-associated nephropathy, a form of collapsing FSGS. Infection with cytomegalovirus is a probable cause of FSGS, and parvovirus B19 and Epstein-Barr virus are possible causes. Certain medications also cause FSGS, including interferons (as mentioned above), anabolic androgenic steroids (likely a form of adaptive FSGS, although the mechanism is unknown, and possibly related to increased load on the kidney of increased muscle mass), bisphosphonates, and lithium.

Shared Pathways of Glomerular Injury

In health, the glomerular filtration barrier functions as a highly organized, semipermeable membrane, preventing the passage of large proteins into the urine (see Chapter 1). This barrier is composed of the fenestrated glomerular endothelium, the glomerular basement membrane, and the podocyte with slit diaphragms connecting adjacent podocyte foot processes (Fig. 19.1). Tubular function assists with the recycling of the small amount of proteins that cross the glomerular barrier, maintaining the normal urine protein excretion <0.2 g daily. In FSGS, particularly primary FSGS, podocytes lose their normal cytoarchitecture and ultrastructurally show foot process fusion, the degree of which is reported in routine kidney biopsy reports. This is relevant, as the extent of podocyte injury varies across the various forms of FSGS along a spectrum from limited to essentially complete foot process effacement.

With progressive glomerular injury, podocytes are lost from the glomerulus and excreted in the urine. The degree of podocyte depletion appears to correlate with glomerular sclerosis. When a loss of less than 40% is observed in animal models, limited scarring and mild proteinuria are observed; however, loss of more than 40% of podocytes is often associated with severe proteinuria and significant progressive kidney parenchymal scarring. In addition, initial podocyte injuries may be followed by a propagation of the injury to adjacent podocytes, augmenting frank podocyte loss, to cumulatively exceed these critical podocyte-loss thresholds.

The pathogenesis of the glomerular sclerosing lesions in FSGS is not completely understood, but, in recent years, the complexity of the podocyte and slit diaphragm has been partially elucidated and specific defects in the podocyte architectural and functional components have been identified in children and adults with defined genetic polymorphisms. To date, genetic mutations or polymorphisms in over 50 podocyte-expressed genes have been associated with FSGS. The gene products include proteins in the slit diaphragm, actin cytoskeleton, cell membrane, nucleus, lysosome, mitochondria, and cytosol that have been identified (see Fig. 19.1). The frequency of these polymorphisms varies by phenotype and by ancestry.

Another major potential contributor to glomerular disease is the role of circulating factors in plasma that directly or indirectly influence glomerular function in health and disease. In FSGS, the presence of a circulating factor that results in podocyte effacement and disruption of the glomerular filtration barrier has been postulated for decades. Evidence supporting the presence of a circulating factor is derived from clinical cases that have reported nearly immediate recurrence of massive proteinuria following kidney transplantation, as well as from studies with animal models that have demonstrated that plasma from patients with FSGS can increase glomerular permeability to albumin. Using an in vitro assay, Savin and colleagues were the first to demonstrate significantly increased albumin permeability of isolated glomeruli when

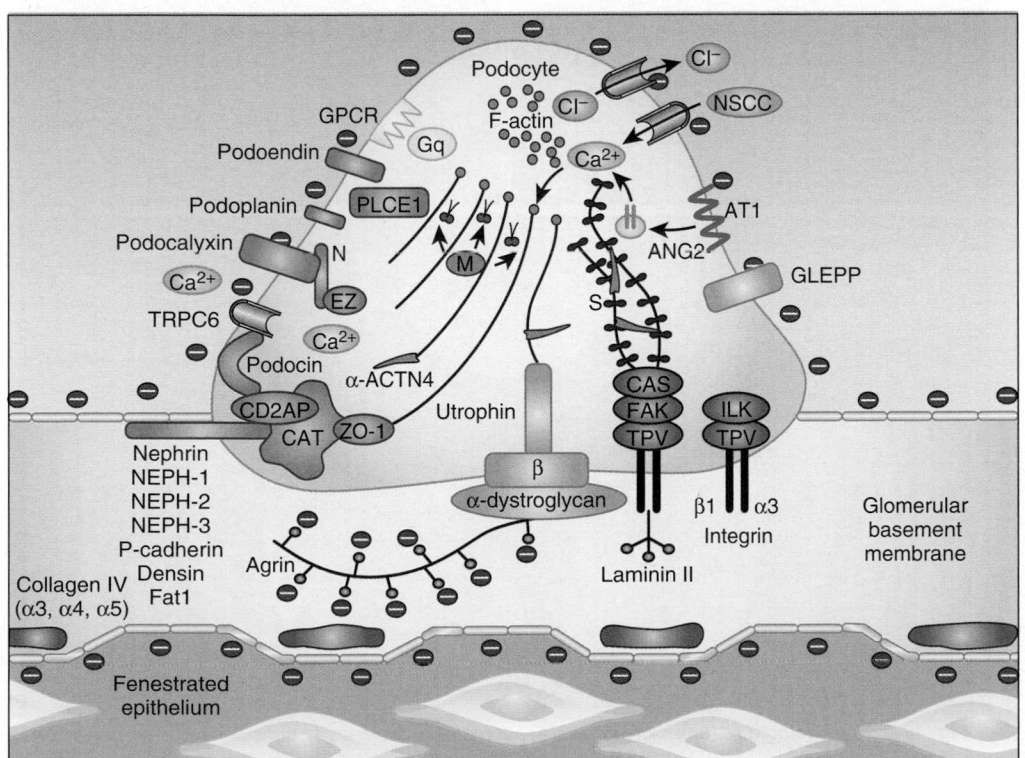

• **Fig. 19.1** Podocyte cytoarchitecture. (From Winn MP. 2007 Young Investigator Award: TRP'ing into a new era for glomerular disease. *J Am Soc Nephrol.* 2008;19:1071–1075.)

exposed to plasma from patients with FSGS and this group has identified the factor as cardiotrophin-like cytokine factor-1. Soluble urokinase-type plasminogen activator receptor (suPAR) has been proposed as a recurrent FSGS factor, but other groups have challenged this finding; if suPAR does contribute to FSGS recurrence, its role is more complicated than initially believed and it may be contributory but not sufficient.

A single, circulating permeability factor may be inadequate to disrupt the filtration barrier. Accordingly, others have hypothesized that a large number of circulating proteins have pro- or antiproteinuric effects on normal glomeruli and that changes in the relative ratio of these circulating proteins may be the major determinant of proteinuria in disease states. In fact, it may be more unlikely that any single protein would cause any specific disease. It is worth considering whether some particular glomerular diseases have characteristic circulating proteomes that influence pathogenesis. Other potential soluble proteins implicated in glomerular disease include angiopoietin-like-4, vascular endothelial growth factor, and hemopexin.

Pathology

The kidney biopsy may provide additional pathologic clues that allow for differentiation of primary FSGS from other forms. Fundamentally, FSGS is a segmental solidification of the glomerular tuft with loss of capillary lumens in the sclerosed segment. Early in the disease process, the pattern of glomerular sclerosis is *focal*, involving a subset of glomeruli, and *segmental*, involving a portion of the glomerular tuft, so it may be missed in superficial samples. A more diffuse and global pattern of scarring is usually seen as the disease progresses, which can make it difficult to label the underlying process as FSGS. The actual histologic spectrum of FSGS, however, is diverse. The ultrastructural findings are of importance as well. In FSGS there is glomerular podocyte damage and foot process effacement, which may be patchy in non-primary forms of FSGS and diffuse in primary FSGS. It is likely that the podocyte injury pattern of FSGS represents a common pathway for the various forms of FSGS. Because areas of segmental scarring can be observed in a variety of other forms of primary glomerulonephritis, assessing the biopsy for an absence of immune complexes in glomeruli and correlation with systemic findings is critical. In primary FSGS, effacement of the podocytes is typically diffuse and extensive. In HIV-associated nephropathy and other forms of viral FSGS, there is often a collapsing variant of glomerulosclerosis with global rather than segmental involvement along with tubuloreticular inclusions noted on electron microscopy. In patients with remnant kidneys or other forms of adaptive FSGS, glomerular enlargement, perihilar location of segmental scars, arteriolar hyalinosis, and incomplete effacement of the foot processes are often noted (Fig. 19.2).

In an effort to classify the histologic spectrum of glomerular lesions associated with FSGS, Dr. D'Agati proposed the Columbia

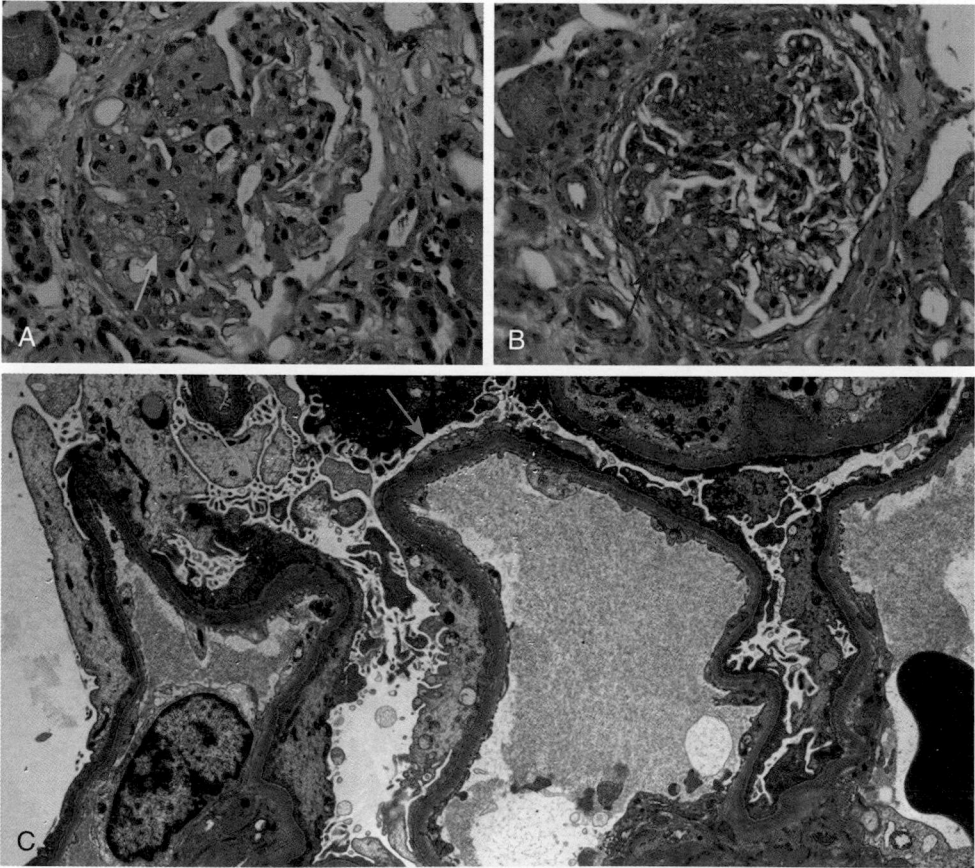

• **Fig. 19.2** Morphologic features of FSGS. **(A)** Glomerulus segmentally consolidated with endocapillary foam cells (*arrow*, H&E). **(B)** Hypertrophied podocytes cap segmental consolidated area (*arrow*, PAS). **(C)** Podocyte foot processes are fused *(orange arrow)*, and there is focal microvillous transformation (*green arrow*, electron microscopy).

classification for FSGS. In this system, the five histologic patterns of FSGS include the perihilar variant, cellular variant, glomerular tip lesion, collapsing variant, and not otherwise specified (NOS) if none of the features of the other four is present. Several of these patterns may occur in the same biopsy; the pattern with the most adverse prognosis is considered the principal diagnosis, as will be discussed shortly. Although the appearance of the glomerular tuft differs in these forms, all share the common feature of podocyte alterations at the ultrastructural level. New insights point toward the conclusion that these morphologic variants may reflect pathogenetic differences and, to some degree, different causes of podocyte injury.

The Columbia morphologic classification of FSGS variants provides useful prognostic information (Box 19.1). For example, collapsing FSGS exhibits a more aggressive clinical course, with fewer remissions, more rapid and more frequent progression to kidney failure, and recurrence in the allograft following kidney transplantation. By contrast, the tip lesion identifies a subset of FSGS that usually responds to glucocorticoids and rarely progresses to kidney failure. The cellular lesion is the least common variant of FSGS, identified in only 3% of cases of adult idiopathic FSGS, and the condition is similarly rare in children. This variant is a challenging histopathologic diagnosis to render, and the prognostic significance of cellular FSGS remains unclear. The cellular, collapsing, and tip lesions all share clinical presenting features of heavier proteinuria and more frequent nephrotic syndrome compared with FSGS NOS, suggesting that these three morphologic variants may reflect acute glomerular injury or possibly a response to heavy proteinuria. However, the prognostic value of morphologic classification of FSGS is not universally acknowledged, reflecting the inherent difficulty of accurately classifying focal patterns of injury based on pathologic examination of limited biopsy tissue and the potential for different types of lesions to coexist in individual biopsy samples.

Clinical Course

Spontaneous remissions are rare in primary FSGS, occurring in fewer than 5% of patients. If untreated and/or unresponsive, the disease course is typically one of progressive proteinuria and loss of kidney function. Primary and APOL1 FSGS often progresses to end-stage kidney disease over a period of 5 to 10 years in perhaps 50% of patients; prognosis appears similar among children and adults. Furthermore, these forms of FSGS may recur after transplantation, contributing significantly to loss of graft function. A rapidly progressive course to kidney failure in the native kidneys predicts a greater risk for recurrence following kidney transplant. The presence of high-penetrance genetic polymorphisms is associated with a lower risk for posttransplant recurrence compared with primary FSGS but is also suggestive of a reduced opportunity for response to immunomodulating therapy. However, partial responses to immunosuppression have been described in children and adults with FSGS-associated genetic polymorphisms. Furthermore, particular forms of genetic FSGS are amenable to targeted therapy, such as coenzyme Q10 supplementation for mitochondrial disorders associated with FSGS.

Several clinical and histologic features can be informative with respect to predicting disease course. Female sex appears to be protective and is associated with both slower progression as well as a higher likelihood of a partial or complete remission as compared with men. In contrast, APOL1 FSGS often has an aggressive course, sometimes despite an apparent response to therapy, as demonstrated by a reduction in proteinuria. Severe

BOX 19.1

Morphologic Classification of Focal Segmental Glomerulosclerosis

Perihilar Variant
Perihilar sclerosis and hyalinosis in more than 50% of segmentally sclerotic glomeruli

Tip Lesion
At least one segmental, either cellular or sclerosing, lesion involving the outer 25% of the glomerulus next to the origin of the proximal tubule

Collapsing Variant
At least one glomerulus with segmental or global collapse and overlying podocyte hyperplasia

Cellular Variant
At least one glomerulus with segmental endocapillary hypercellularity occluding lumina with or without foam cells and karyorrhexis

Not Otherwise Specified
At least one glomerulus with segmental increase in matrix-obliterating capillary lumina (excludes other variants)

Modified from D'Agati VD, Fogo AB, Bruijn AJ, Jennette JC. Pathologic classification of focal segmental glomerulosclerosis: a working proposal. *Am J Kidney Dis.* 2004;43:368–382.

nephrotic-range proteinuria (>10 g/24 hr), reduced glomerular filtration rate, and increased tubulointerstitial damage on kidney biopsy at the time of presentation are features that portend a poor prognosis. The collapsing variant is also associated with more rapid progression, whereas the tip lesion, which tends to be responsive to immunosuppression, has a better prognosis. During treatment of FSGS, absence of any response to immunosuppressive therapy is the strongest predictor of a poor prognosis, whereas complete remission of the nephrotic syndrome with normalization of urine protein excretion confers the best prognosis. However, even a partial response to treatment is associated with a significant delay in kidney disease progression and is, therefore, an acceptable treatment goal. Relapse is common (>50%) and is subsequently associated with more rapid progression and poor kidney survival.

Therapy

The treatment of primary FSGS is controversial because of the paucity of randomized, controlled trials and the lack of effective, well-tolerated treatment options, although this is now changing with increased interest in testing new therapies by pharmaceutical companies, both large and small (Table 19.3). In patients with nephrotic syndrome, immunosuppression may improve proteinuria and slow progression to kidney failure, but side effects associated with current treatment options, including high doses and prolonged courses of glucocorticoids, cytotoxic agents, calcineurin inhibitors, and mycophenolate mofetil, are significant and treatment failure and relapses are common. Immunosuppression typically is not used in primary FSGS with subnephrotic-range proteinuria or in FSGS with a suspected secondary cause.

Prednisone is the first line of therapy in children and many adults with primary FSGS, largely based on data from observational cohorts. The optimal dose and duration of therapy remain

TABLE 19.3	Overview of Treatment Options for Focal Segmental Glomerulosclerosis	
Setting	Therapy	Comment
Nephrotic forms of primary FSGS,* APOL1 FSGS, certain steroid-sensitive FSGS	Prednisone, initially daily or alternate day*; pulse oral dexamethasone	Alternatives for patients at high risk for steroid complications include calcineurin inhibitors, mycophenolate mofetil
Glucocorticoid-resistant FSGS with nephrotic syndrome*	Calcineurin inhibitor* (cyclosporine and possibly tacrolimus)	—
Refractory FSGS with nephrotic syndrome*	Mycophenolate mofetil ± high-dose dexamethasone*	—
All forms of FSGS with subnephrotic proteinuria	ACE inhibitor or angiotensin receptor blocker, possibly combined with aldosterone antagonist, and dietary sodium restriction	Thiazide diuretic may potentiate the antiproteinuric of RAAS antagonism

Recommendations from the Kidney Disease Improving Outcomes Global Initiatives for idiopathic FSGS with nephrotic syndrome are marked with asterisks (*) and are extended here to other forms of FSGS, as shown. Cyclosporine has been shown effective in randomized, controlled trials of FSGS, while tacrolimus has not. These recommendations would apply, when nephrotic syndrome is present, to primary FSGS, APOL1 FSGS, and certain rare forms of genetic FSGS that may be steroid sensitive.

FSGS, Focal segmental glomerulosclerosis, *RAAS,* renin-angiotensin-aldosterone system.

Adapted from Rosenberg A, Kopp J. Focal segmental glomerulosclerosis. *Clin J Am Soc Nephrol.* 2017;12:502–517.

uncertain and, therefore, vary widely across clinical centers. Daily steroid regimens as well as alternate-day regimens have been used. On average, if a patient is glucocorticoid-responsive, a response will be seen within 1 to 3 months, although adults may take longer to respond than children. Thus, although the minimum requirement of glucocorticoid exposure to define lack of response and resistance remains unclear, many practitioners would define steroid resistance as having received at least 8 to 16 weeks of therapy without substantial improvement in urine protein.

Among children, 20% to 25% experience a complete remission with glucocorticoids. Response rates in adults are lower and intolerance to steroid therapy tends to be more significant, especially in the presence of advanced age and comorbid conditions such as obesity and diabetes. Glucocorticoid resistance, even with prolonged treatment, occurs in more than 50% of adult patients. Prolonged courses of high-dose glucocorticoids can result in troubling side effects including, but not limited to, cataracts, skin thinning, acne, diabetes, osteoporosis/osteonecrosis, and weight gain, regardless of age.

Cytotoxic agents such as cyclophosphamide have been used with success in children with relapsing and remitting disease and in adults who have demonstrated at least a partial response to prednisone therapy; however, these agents carry significant immediate and long-term risks including infection, infertility, and propensity to late-onset malignancy. Thus, in patients with glucocorticoid resistance or intolerance, calcineurin inhibitors are generally second-line therapies and are first-line therapies for subjects with primary FSGS who are at increased risk for glucocorticoid-associated adverse events. In one randomized, controlled trial in glucocorticoid-resistant FSGS, patients were randomized to continue on low-dose prednisone either alone or in combination with cyclosporine. The therapy was continued for 26 weeks and then tapered over 4 weeks. The response rate in the cyclosporine-treated patients exceeded 70%, but relapses after discontinuation of therapy were common, exceeding 50%. In a larger randomized trial conducted over 12 months, only 46% of participants experienced a combined complete and partial remission in response to cyclosporine, and 33% relapsed following discontinuation of cyclosporine. In smaller studies, similar rates of complete and partial remission in patients with glucocorticoid-resistant or

glucocorticoid-dependent nephrotic syndrome are seen for tacrolimus and cyclosporine; accordingly, tacrolimus can be considered an alternative calcineurin inhibitor. Calcineurin inhibitors should be used with caution in patients with significant vascular or interstitial disease noted on kidney biopsy and in patients who have an estimated GFR of less than 40 mL/min/1.73 m^2 due to the greater potential to cause nephrotoxicity, hyperkalemia, and hypertension in this population.

Other therapeutic options include mycophenolate mofetil (MMF) or rituximab. A randomized, controlled trial of children and adults with steroid-resistant FSGS showed that the combination of a 12-month course of MMF with high-dose dexamethasone induced a 33% combined partial and complete remission. Following discontinuation of MMF and dexamethasone, 18% relapsed, demonstrating only a modest improvement with prolonged dexamethasone exposure and MMF. In two randomized, controlled trials involving Italian children, rituximab reduced proteinuria in treatment-dependent nephrotic syndrome but did not reduce proteinuria in children with treatment-resistant nephrotic syndrome. A randomized trial involving Indian adults compared prednisolone versus MMF plus low-dose prednisolone and found the latter reach remission faster, with reduced glucocorticoid dose. In kidney allografts, plasma exchange has been successful in treating some patients with recurrent FSGS.

The cornerstone of treatment for adaptive and genetic FSGS is RAAS antagonism, which reduces intraglomerular capillary hydrostatic pressure by reducing tone in the efferent glomerular arteriole; this approach should benefit all forms of FSGS (see Table 19.3). The ACE Inhibition in Progressive Renal Disease analysis examined prior studies of proteinuria, excluding studies of diabetes, and showed a benefit to slow progression. In the Effect of Strict Blood Pressure Control and ACE Inhibition on Progression of Chronic Renal Failure in Pediatric Patients (ESCAPE) trial involving children with proteinuric kidney disease, use of an angiotensin-converting enzyme inhibitor (ACEi) was associated with slowed progression of GFR loss, and the effect was greatest in those with hypertension, reduced GFR, and proteinuria.

A single RAAS agent may be sufficient. Dual blockage with an ACE inhibitor and an angiotensin receptor blocker (ARB) has been associated with inferior outcomes in older patients with vascular disease or diabetes in the ONTARGET (Ongoing Telmisartan Alone and in conjunction with Ramipril Global Endpoint Trial) study, but these results may be irrelevant for the child or young adult with FSGS. Another approach would be to combine an angiotensin-converting enzyme inhibitor (ACEi) or angiotensin receptor blocker (ARB) with an aldosterone antagonist (spironolactone or eplerenone), together with a low-dose thiazide diuretic and dietary sodium restriction, both of which potentiate the antiproteinuric effects of an ACEi or ARB, although there are no published data to support this regimen in FSGS. For those with obesity, weight loss may be beneficial.

There are no studies in FSGS addressing the optimal blood pressure target. Current blood pressure targets for adults with chronic kidney disease (CKD) are below 130/80 mm Hg according to the 2017 American College of Cardiology guidelines. Data from the African American Study of Kidney Disease and Hypertension (AASK) study suggest a target of 130/70 mm Hg, although this result is based on a subgroup analysis of AASK participants with proteinuria. The recent Systolic Blood Pressure Intervention Trial (SPRINT trial), enrolling hypertensive adults with additional cardiovascular risk factors, found cardiovascular benefit from a systolic blood pressure target of 120 mm Hg but excluded patients with heavy proteinuria. For children with CKD, blood pressure reduction to the 50th percentile for age is associated with slower disease progression.

Control of dyslipidemia with diet and pharmacologic therapy is recommended, and fluid retention and edema may be improved with salt restriction and diuretics. Although the risk of venous thromboembolism is highest in patients with membranous nephropathy, patients with FSGS are also at an increased risk of venous thromboembolism; risk factors include higher hematocrit and relapse of nephrotic syndrome.

The past few years have seen rapid advances in understanding FSGS mechanisms, particularly genetic factors, and there is new interest in developing and testing new drugs for this set of disorders. The research and the development communities, working together, have made great strides toward defining and implementing a personalized medicine approach to the diagnosis and treatment of FSGS, and more progress is expected.

Acknowledgment

This work was supported in part by the NIDDK Intramural Research Program, NIH, Bethesda, MD (JBK) and NCATS grant TL1 TR001423 (HWS).

Bibliography

Brown EJ, Pollak MR, Barua M. Genetic testing for nephrotic syndrome and FSGS in the era of next-generation sequencing. *Kidney Int.* 2014;85:1030–1038.

Cattran DC, Appel GB, Hebert LA, et al. A randomized trial of cyclosporine in patients with steroid-resistant focal segmental glomerulosclerosis. North America Nephrotic syndrome study group. *Kidney Int.* 1999;56:2220–2226.

Chandra P, Kopp JB. Viruses and collapsing glomerulopathy: a brief critical review. *Clin Kidney J.* 2013;6:1–5.

Cravedi P, Kopp JB, Remuzzi G. Recent progress in the pathophysiology and treatment of FSGS recurrence. *Am J Transplant.* 2013;13:266–274.

D'Agati VD. Pathobiology of focal segmental glomerulosclerosis: new developments. *Curr Opin Nephrol Hypertens.* 2012;21:243–250.

D'Agati VD, Kaskel FJ, Falk RJ. Focal segmental glomerulosclerosis. *N Engl J Med.* 2011;365:2398–2411.

Fogo AB. Causes and pathogenesis of focal segmental glomerulosclerosis. *Nat Rev Nephrol.* 2015;11:76–87.

Gipson DS, Trachtman H, Kaskel FJ, et al. Clinical trial of focal segmental glomerulosclerosis in children and young adults. *Kidney Int.* 2011;80:868–878.

Kashgary A, Sontrop JM, Li L, et al. The role of plasma exchange in treating post-transplant focal segmental glomerulosclerosis: a systematic review and meta-analysis of 77 case-reports and case-series. *BMC Nephrol.* 2016;17:104.

Konigshausen E, Sellin L. Circulating permeability factors in primary focal segmental glomerulosclerosis: a review of proposed candidates. *Biomed Res Int.* 2016;2016:3765608.

Kopp JB, Nelson GW, Sampath K, et al. APOL1 genetic variants in focal segmental glomerulosclerosis and HIV-associated nephropathy. *J Am Soc Nephrol.* 2011;22:2129–2137.

Lovric S, Ashraf S, Tan W, Hildebrandt F. Genetic testing in steroid-resistant nephrotic syndrome: when and how? *Nephrol Dial Transplant.* 2016;31:1802–1813.

Meyrier A. Focal and segmental glomerulosclerosis: multiple pathways are involved. *Semin Nephrol.* 2011;31:326–332.

Mondini A, Messa P, Rastaldi MP. The sclerosing glomerulus in mice and man: novel insights. *Curr Opin Nephrol Hypertens.* 2014;23:239–244.

Rosenberg A, Kopp J. Focal segmental glomerulosclerosis. *Clin J Am Soc Nephrol.* 2017;12:502–517.

Rosenberg AZ, Naicker S, Winkler CA, Kopp JB. HIV-associated nephropathies: epidemiology, pathology, mechanisms and treatment. *Nat Rev Nephrol.* 2015;11:150–160.

Schell C, Huber TB. New players in the pathogenesis of focal segmental glomerulosclerosis. *Nephrol Dial Transplant.* 2012;27:3406–3412.

Sethna CB, Gipson DS. Treatment of FSGS in children. *Adv Chronic Kidney Dis.* 2014;21:194–199.

Thomas DB, Franceschini N, Hogan SL, et al. Clinical and pathologic characteristics of focal segmental glomerulosclerosis pathologic variants. *Kidney Int.* 2006;69:920–926.

Troyanov S, Wall CA, Miller JA, et al. Focal and segmental glomerulosclerosis: definition and relevance of a partial remission. *J Am Soc Nephrol.* 2005;16:1061–1068.

20

Membranous Nephropathy

DANIEL C. CATTRAN, AN S. DE VRIESE, FERNANDO C. FERVENZA

Membranous nephropathy (MN) is the most common cause of adult-onset nephrotic syndrome in the white population. It is characterized by deposition of immunoglobulin G and complement components in the glomerular capillary wall and attendant new basement membrane synthesis. This histologic pattern is more properly called *nephropathy* than nephritis because there is rarely any inflammatory response in the glomeruli or interstitium.

Primary MN is a kidney-limited auto-immune disease and accounts for about 80% of cases. The immune deposits consist of immune complexes formed in situ by circulating autoantibodies and the endogenous podocyte surface antigen against which they are directed. The target antigen has been identified as the M-type phospholipase–A2-receptor 1 (PLA2R) in 70% to 80% and thrombospondin type 1 domain-containing 7a (THSD7A) in 2% to 5% of patients with primary MN. Neural epidermal growth factor-like 1 protein (NELL-1) is a recently discovered target antigen in 5% to 10% of patients. In the remaining cases, the target podocyte antigens have not yet been identified but concerted efforts are ongoing to elucidate their identity.

In 20% of patients, the disease is secondary to a variety of disorders (Table 20.1) and is therefore termed *secondary MN*. The list of known secondary causes of MN in Box 20.1 is not complete but provides an indication of the wide array of conditions associated with this histologic pattern. In some, such as hepatitis B or thyroiditis, the specific antigen has been identified as part of the immune complex within the deposits in the glomeruli. In others, the association is less well defined, but the designation remains, because treatment of the underlying condition or removal of the putative agent results in resolution of the clinical and histologic features of the disease. Recently, exostosin 1/exostosin 2 (EXT1/EXT2) were found to be the target antigens in a series of PLA2R- and THSD7A-negative patients. The large majority had active SLE or another systemic autoimmune disease and were therefore categorized as having secondary MN. In older patients, neoplasms are the most common cause of secondary MN. Recent studies show an association between the presence of anti-THSD7A and anti-NELL1 antibodies and malignancy-associated MN. As such, patients with anti-THSD7A– and NELL1-associated MN should be carefully screened for malignancy.

Primary MN is rare in children. In pediatric MN cases, a careful screening for other types of immunologically mediated disorders, especially systemic lupus erythematosus (SLE), is necessary. Antineutral endopeptidase (NEP) antibody-associated MN is an extremely rare form of MN in neonates. In very young children, the diagnosis of MN should raise the possibility of bovine serum albumin (BSA)–induced MN. More recently, semaphorin 3D-associated MN appears to be a distinct type of MN that is more likely to be present in pediatric patients.

Clinical Features

MN presents in 60% to 70% of cases with features associated with the nephrotic syndrome, such as edema, proteinuria greater than 3.5 g/day, hypoalbuminemia, and hyperlipidemia. The other 30% to 40% of cases present with asymptomatic proteinuria, usually in the subnephrotic range (≤3.5 g/day). The majority of patients present with normal glomerular filtration rate (GFR), but about 10% have diminished kidney function. The urine sediment is often bland, although microscopic hematuria may be present. Hypertension is uncommon at presentation, occurring in only 10% to 20% of cases. The clinical features associated with nephrotic-range proteinuria in MN can be severe: Patients with MN almost always have ankle swelling, and ascites, pleural effusions, and rarely pericardial effusions may be present. This pattern is particularly common in the elderly, and, unless a urinalysis is performed, these symptoms may be incorrectly labeled as signs of primary cardiac failure. Complications of MN include thromboembolic events and cardiovascular events. A recent study showed that clinically apparent venous thromboembolic events affect about 8% of MN patients, with renal vein thrombosis accounting for 30% of the thromboembolic events. This frequency is substantially lower than that previously reported in studies that used systematic screening for thromboembolic events. Secondary hyperlipidemia is common and characterized by an increase in total and low-density lipoprotein (LDL) cholesterol and often a decrease in high-density lipoproteins (HDLs), a profile associated with increased atherogenic risk.

Pathology

In early MN, glomeruli appear normal by light microscopy. Increasing size and number of immune complexes in the subepithelial space produces a thickening as well as a rigid appearance of the normally lacy-looking glomerular basement membrane (GBM) on light microscopy (Fig. 20.1). Over time, new basement membrane is formed around the immune complexes (deposits do not stain), producing the spikes along the epithelial side of the basement membrane; these are particularly well visualized when using the silver methenamine stains (Fig. 20.2). In contrast, on immunofluorescence microscopy, these immune complexes do stain, most commonly with antihuman immunoglobulin G (IgG) and complement C3 (Fig. 20.3). This produces a beaded appearance

TABLE 20.1 Secondary Causes of Membranous Nephropathy	
Etiology	**Examples**
Neoplasm	Carcinomas, especially solid organ (tumors of the lung, colon, breast, and kidney), leukemia, and non-Hodgkin lymphoma
Infections	Malaria, hepatitis B and C, secondary or congenital syphilis, leprosy
Drugs	Penicillamine, gold
Immunologic	Systemic lupus erythematosus, mixed connective tissue disease, thyroiditis, dermatitis herpetiformis, sarcoidosis
Post kidney transplant	Recurrent disease, de novo membranous nephropathy
Miscellaneous	Sickle cell anemia, bovine serum albumin in children

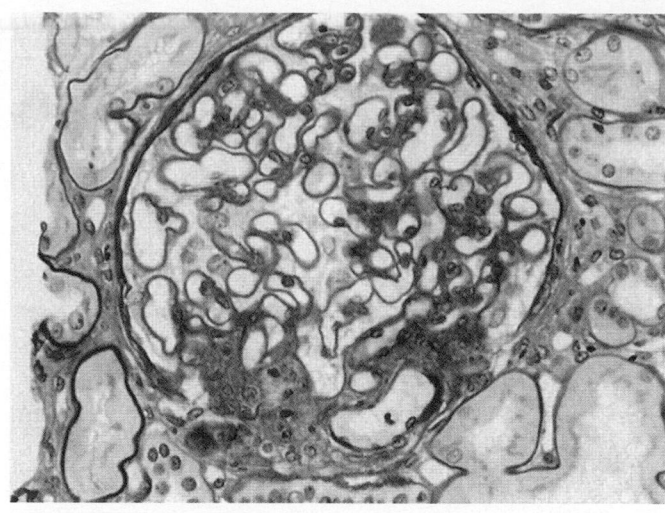

• **Fig. 20.1** Glomerulus from a patient with membranous nephropathy. Capillary walls are diffusely thickened, and there is no increase in mesangial cells or matrix (periodic acid–Schiff, original magnification ×250).

BOX 20.1

Risk for Progression Based on Proteinuria

Low Risk

Patients with normal serum creatinine/creatinine clearance and proteinuria consistently ≤4 g/24 hr over a 6-mo observation period have an excellent long-term kidney prognosis.

Medium Risk

Patients with normal and stable kidney function and with proteinuria >4 g but <8 g/24 hr during 6 mo of observation have a 55% probability of developing end-stage kidney disease within 10 yr.

High Risk

Patients with persistent proteinuria >8 g/24 hr independent of the degree of kidney function impairment, have a 66%–80% probability of progression to end-stage kidney disease within 10 yr.

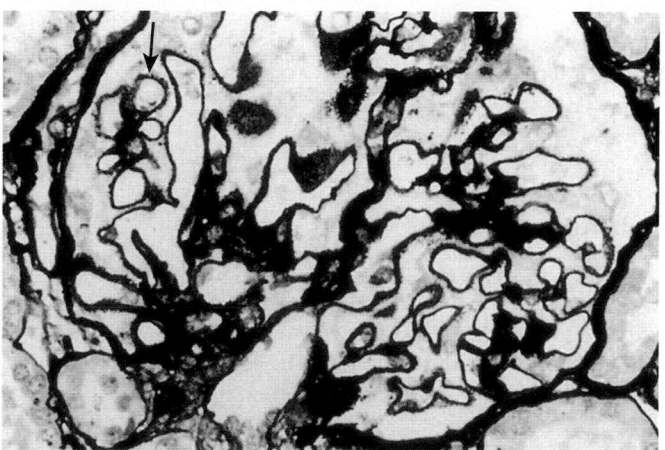

• **Fig. 20.2** Classic spike pattern along glomerular basement membrane as it grows around deposits (*arrow*; periodic acid–Schiff, original magnification ×400).

along the GBM (capillary wall), a pattern that is pathognomonic of MN on immunofluorescence. In the most extreme cases, this beading can become so dense that careful examination is required to distinguish it from a linear pattern. On electron microscopy, the majority of cases show extensive podocyte foot process effacement, even at the early stages (Fig. 20.4).

Features that favor a secondary cause of MN, in particular an autoimmune disease, include (1) proliferative features (mesangial or endocapillary); (2) full-house pattern of Ig staining (G, M, and A), including staining for C1q on immunofluorescence microscopy; (3) electron dense deposits in the subendothelial location of the capillary wall and mesangium or along the tubular basement membrane and vessel walls; and (4) endothelial tubuloreticular inclusions on electron microscopy. Electron microscopy showing only a few superficial scattered subepithelial deposits may suggest a drug-induced secondary MN. Additional diagnostic value may be obtained by staining kidney biopsies for IgG subclasses. IgG1,

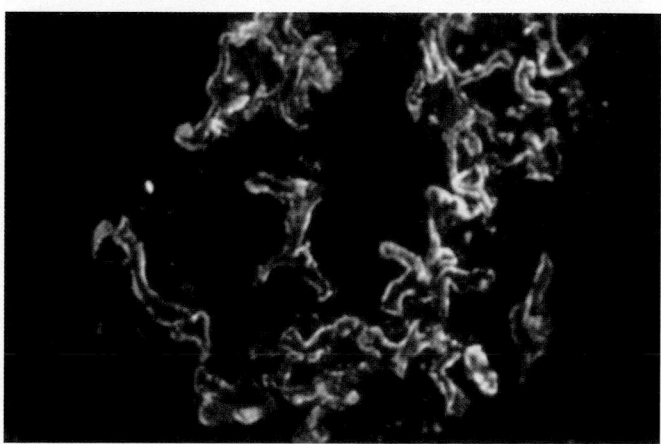

• **Fig. 20.3** Glomerulus with diffuse granular capillary wall staining with antiimmunoglobulin G antibody (immunofluorescence microscopy, original magnification ×250).

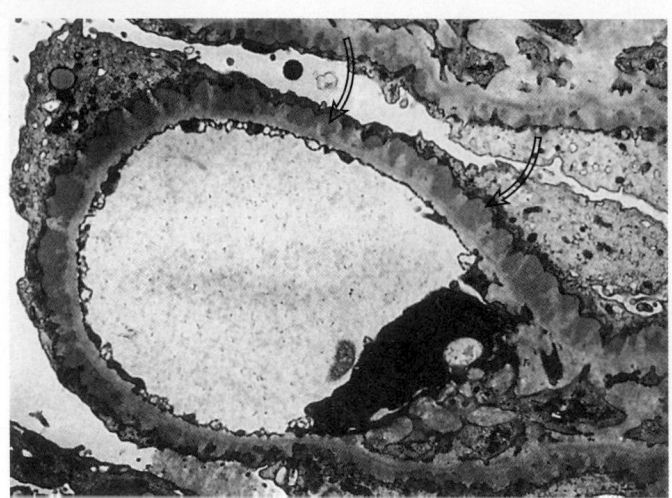

• **Fig. 20.4** Electron photomicrograph of capillary loop with multiple electron-dense deposits along the subepithelial side of the glomerular basement membrane (*arrows*; original magnification ×7500).

IgG2, and IgG3 tend to be expressed in lupus MN. IgG4 tends to be more commonly expressed in primary MN and absent in MN secondary to malignancy.

Pathogenesis

Over the past decade, major advances have been made in our understanding of the pathogenesis of human MN.

Neutral Endopeptidase

The first breakthrough involved a case report of a patient with neonatal MN caused by transplacental transfer of circulating anti-neutral endopeptidase antibodies. Neutral endopeptidase (NEP) is a membrane-bound enzyme that is able to digest biologically active peptides. Mothers with truncating mutations of the metallomembrane endopeptidase (MME) gene fail to express NEP on cell membranes. NEP-deficient mothers, who were immunized during pregnancy, were able to transplacentally transfer nephritogenic antibodies against NEP to their children, causing MN in the newborns. Rabbits injected with the maternal IgG from these mothers also developed MN, providing additional proof that the disease is related to circulating anti-NEP antibodies.

Bovine Serum Albumin

High levels of circulating anti-BSA antibodies of both IgG1 and IgG4 subclasses have been reported as a cause of secondary MN in children and adults. BSA immunopurified from the serum of children migrated in the basic range of pH, whereas the BSA from adult patients migrated in the neutral region as native BSA. BSA staining colocalized with IgG immune deposits only in four children with circulating cationic BSA but in none of the adults with MN for whom biopsy specimens were available, implying that only cationic BSA can induce MN.

M-Type Phospholipase A2 Receptor

The M (muscle)-type phospholipase A2-receptor 1 (PLA2R) is a member of the mannose receptor family and is composed of an N-terminal cysteine-rich domain, a fibronectin-like II domain,

eight C-type lectin-like domains (CTLD), a transmembrane region, and a short cytoplasmic tail containing motifs used in endocytic recycling. Anti-PLA2R antibodies are present in 70% to 80% of adult patients with primary MN and a lesser proportion of affected children. These antibodies are not present in the serum of healthy controls or in patients with other kidney or systemic diseases, yielding a 100% specificity for the lesion of MN. In some studies, small numbers of patients with various forms of secondary MN tested positive for anti-PLA2R antibodies. Whether these cases represent true secondary MN, or rather PLA2R-associated MN with coincident secondary disease, requires further investigation.

A growing body of evidence has documented that PLA2R Ab titer tightly correlates with disease activity in MN. In one study, 75% of patients with active disease were positive for anti-PLA2R antibodies. This contrasted with positivity in only 37% of patients in partial remission and 10% of patients in complete remission. Remission is reported to occur in 50% of patients with low titers but in only 30% of patients with high titers of anti-PLA2R antibodies at the time of diagnosis. High titers of anti-PLA2R antibody are associated with lower response rates to therapy and longer time to remission. Antibody titers at the time of clinical remission correlate with the rate of relapse: Patients who become anti-PLA2R negative after immunosuppressive treatment have lower relapse rates than patients who remain positive at the end of treatment. Anti-PLA2R levels may indicate which patients presenting with subnephrotic-range proteinuria are likely to progress to full nephrotic syndrome. Moreover, high anti-PLA2R antibodies levels are associated with a high risk of kidney failure over time. In one study, more than 50% of patients with high anti-PLA2R levels had a doubling of serum creatinine over 5-year follow-up. The evolution of PLA2R antibody levels in response to immunosuppression reliably predicts outcome. A decline in levels consistently precedes a decline in proteinuria. Generally, antibody levels decrease rapidly in the first 3 months of treatment and disappear over 6 to 9 months, followed by a remission of proteinuria over 12 to 24 months (or longer, as discussed later), independently of the type of immunosuppressive agent used.

Taken together, these observations strongly suggest that serial quantification of anti-PLA2R antibody levels can help in monitoring disease activity and response to immunosuppressive therapy. When taken in concert with follow-up of proteinuria, antibody testing may allow early intervention and earlier stopping of potent immunosuppressive agents. Pending more evidence from prospective studies, anti-PLA2R antibody levels (measured by the commercially available ELISA method) are currently arbitrarily defined as low when <50 RU/mL, intermediate when 50-150 RU/mL, and high when >150 RU/mL.

Immunofluorescence staining for PLA2R can now be performed on kidney biopsy material. Positive staining, mirroring the distribution of immune deposits that are detected on electron microscopy examination, strongly favors primary MN over a secondary form of disease. Some patients may be negative in terms of circulating anti-PLA2R autoantibody at the time of kidney biopsy but still exhibit positive glomerular PLA2R staining. This state could represent completely different phases of the disease, either indicating that PLA2R-associated MN has gone into an immune remission while leaving footprints of the previous immunologic activity or indicating that early disease is present, with the very high affinity between anti-PLA2R autoantibodies and the podocyte antigen, leading to such a rapid depletion of antibodies from the circulation and deposition in the kidney that antibody is not measurable despite active disease.

Thrombospondin Type 1 Domain Containing 7A

THSD7A is a transmembrane protein initially described in human endothelial vein cells but also expressed in many organs, including the kidney. The function of THSD7A may relate to binding to extracellular matrix, especially to glycosaminoglycan chains present on matrix proteoglycans. Immunogold electron microscopy has localized the protein within podocytes to the foot process near the slit diaphragm and in endosomal structures. Antibodies against THSD7A, predominantly of the IgG4 subclass, are reported in 2% to 5% of patients with primary MN. So far, anti-THSD7A antibodies have not been detected in healthy controls or in patients with other kidney and systemic diseases, yielding 100% specificity for MN. Limited evidence suggests that, as in the case of PLA2R antibodies, circulating anti-THSD7A antibodies correlate with disease activity and may be used to monitor disease activity in patients with THSD7A-associated disease. A genetic link to the THSD7A locus has not yet been established, possibly because of the small number of cases identified so far. Initially, it appeared that anti-PLA2R and anti-THSD7A autoantibodies were mutually exclusive, but several cases of dual antibody positivity have been described more recently. Tissue staining for the THSD7A antigen in kidney biopsies is technically more difficult than the "on or off" pattern described for the PLA2R antigen because a linear staining pattern for THSD7A is seen in normal biopsies and other types of glomerular disease.

In the initial series, a high proportion of patients with THSD7A-associated MN were diagnosed with a malignancy within 3 months of MN diagnosis. Furthermore, several cases of THSD7A-associated MN had a concomitantly diagnosed malignant tumor that overexpressed THSD7A, and remission of the MN was observed after treatment of the malignancy alone, as typically occurs in secondary MN. On the other hand, the majority of THSD7A-associated MN cases are diagnosed without coincidental malignancy and respond to immunosuppression. Recent case reports suggest a link between THSD7A-associated MN and conditions associated with eosinophilia. In sum, the link between THSD7A and malignancy-associated MN needs further exploration, but the presence of THSD7A antibodies should elicit a thorough screening for malignancy.

Neural Epidermal Growth Factor-Like 1 Protein

Neural epidermal growth factor-like 1 protein (NELL-1) is a recently discovered target antigen in 5% to 10% of patients with MN. This protein was initially identified by laser microdissection and mass spectrometry of glomeruli in six of 35 cases of PLA2R-negative primary MN. Immunohistochemistry for NELL-1 showed positive staining and colocalization with IgG along the GBM in all cases of NELL-1-positive MN while no staining was observed in patients with PLA2R-associated MN or other glomerular diseases. Circulating anti-NELL-1 antibodies were detected in all of five patients with NELL-1-positive MN for whom serum was available, but none of the control patients with PLA2R-associated MN, minimal change disease, or IgA nephropathy. Mass spectrometry data and limited characterization of the circulating anti-NELL-1 antibodies suggest IgG1 as the predominant IgG subclass in this disease. Additional studies are required to determine the role of this protein in the pathogenesis of MN. Most patients with NELL-1-associated MN presented with kidney-limited disease, but in a few cases a close temporal association with a malignancy was reported.

Semaphorin 3B

More recently, semaphorin 3B was identified in 11 cases of PLA2R-negative MN. Semaphorin 3B localized as granular deposits along the GBM by immunohistochemistry. In four of 11 cases, kidney biopsy also showed tubular basement membrane deposits of IgG on frozen sections. Western blot analysis in five available sera showed reactivity to reduced semaphorin 3B in four of four patients with active disease and no reactivity in one patient in clinical remission. Eight (73%) of the 11 cases of semaphorin 3B-associated MN were pediatric cases, and in five cases, the disease started at or below the age of 2 years. These observations suggest that semaphorin 3B-associated MN appears to be a distinct type of MN that is more likely to be present in pediatric patients.

Exostosin 1 (EXT1) and Exostosin 2 (EXT2)

Recently, positive immunostaining for the proteins exostosin 1 (EXT1) and exostosin 2 (EXT2) helped identify a subset of patients with class V lupus nephritis or another autoimmune disease such as Sjögren syndrome resembling lupus nephritis. EXT1- and EXT2-positive staining in MN may also help to identify a PLA2R-negative patient who subsequently may develop SLE. So far, no circulating anti-exostosin antibodies have been identified. At the present time, the diagnosis of EXT1/EXT2-associated MN can only be made by special studies of kidney biopsy material. The available data suggest that EXT1 and EXT2 may represent target antigens or biomarker proteins of systemic autoimmune MN.

Genetic Associations

Single-nucleotide polymorphisms (SNPs) in the genes encoding M-type PLA2R and HLA complex class II HLA-DQ alpha chain 1 (HLA-DQA1) have been reported in white and Asian populations with MN. The risk for primary MN was significantly higher when both the HLA-DQ1 allele and the PLA2R1 allele were present. Patients carrying one or two alleles for HLA DQA1*05:01 or for DQB1*02:01 have higher anti-PLA2R titers than those with neither of these HLA alleles. A theory has been proposed that the rare confluence of several relatively common factors triggers the development of MN: a particular isoform of HLA-DQA1 that confers increased susceptibility to autoimmunity, polymorphisms in PLA2R1 that alter expression, and/or create a unique conformation identified by HLA class II on antigen-presenting cells, and other environmental factors. Genetic analysis has also been proposed as a disease predictor that could enhance a non-invasive diagnosis of MN.

Diagnosis

Tests for anti-PLA2R antibodies and anti-THSD7A antibodies are commercially available and a test for anti-NELL-1 antibodies is currently being developed.

The gold standard for the diagnosis of MN is a kidney biopsy. However, kidney biopsy is costly and carries a risk for major complications. A recent study showed that a positive serum PLA2R antibody titer is a useful and non-invasive method for the diagnosis of primary MN in the setting of preserved kidney function and negative work-up for secondary causes of nephrotic syndrome. In this setting, a kidney biopsy may not be necessary to make treatment decisions, especially for patients at high risk of complications or in whom a kidney biopsy may be contraindicated.

However, if kidney function is significantly impaired, a biopsy allows exclusion of concomitant kidney disease and may provide useful information to guide management.

Primary/idiopathic and secondary forms of MN have similar clinical presentations. As such, secondary MN should be ruled out by careful history, physical, and laboratory examinations, aided by features on pathology. Investigations should include a complement profile, assays for antinuclear antibodies, rheumatoid factor, hepatitis B surface antigen and hepatitis C antibody, thyroid antibodies, and cryoglobulins. Malignancy is associated with MN in approximately 20% of cases in people above 60 years old. More recent epidemiologic data suggest that the standardized incidence ratio of malignancy in MN is in the range of 2 to 3 in all age groups; however, because the absolute incidence of malignancies in younger people is lower, extensive testing for malignancy is not usually performed unless there are clinical clues. In contrast, older patients who present with MN should receive a history and physical examination focused on possible evidence of occult malignancy, especially if they are anti-THSD7A or anti-NELL1 antibody positive. The role of malignancy in anti-PLA2R antibody-positive patients is controversial. Positive anti-PLA2R testing has been reported in a minority of patients with MN associated with solid tumors, but oncologic treatment was not accompanied by remission of proteinuria, suggesting that the two processes were not causally related but rather coincidental. The evaluation should consist of most age-appropriate screening tests, including colon cancer screening, mammography, a prostate-specific antigen assay in men, and a chest radiograph (or, in high-risk patients, a chest computed tomography). The cost-benefit ratio of this additional screening in the absence of symptoms remains unknown, but, given the dramatic difference in management and outcome, it seems prudent to perform these investigations. Ongoing vigilance is also necessary, because the causative agent may not be obvious for months or even years after presentation. For example, in about 45% of malignancy-associated MN, kidney disease antedates the diagnosis of malignancy; in 40%, there is a simultaneous presentation; and in the remaining 10%, MN appears after the diagnosis of malignancy.

Prognosis of Primary Membranous Nephropathy

Natural History

The natural history of primary MN must be understood before considering specific treatment. Spontaneous, complete remission, defined as a reduction in proteinuria to less than 0.3 g/day, occurs in 20% to 30% of patients with primary MN, whereas progressive kidney failure develops in 20% to 40% of cases after more than 5 to 15 years of observation. In the remaining patients, mild to moderate proteinuria persists. A summary review of 11 large studies demonstrated a 10-year kidney survival rate of 65% to 85%, whereas a more recently pooled analysis of 32 reports indicated a 15-year kidney survival rate of 60%. Complicating the understanding of the natural history is the fact that primary MN often follows a spontaneous remitting and relapsing course. Spontaneous, complete remission rates have been reported in 20% to 30% of long-term (>10 years) follow-up studies, with 20% to 50% of these cases exhibiting at least one relapse. A complete remission and a lower relapse rate are more common in patients with persistent, low-grade (subnephrotic) proteinuria and in women. In contrast, male gender, age greater than 50 years, high levels of proteinuria

(more than 6 g/day), abnormal kidney function at presentation, tubulointerstitial disease, and focal and segmental lesions on biopsy are all associated with poorer kidney survival rates.

Predicting Outcome

Prior predictive models for outcomes in MN incorporated the initial creatinine clearance (CrCl), the slope of the CrCl, and the lowest level of proteinuria during a 6-month observation period. The predictive value of the risk score was much greater than that of presence of nephrotic-range proteinuria at presentation alone when proteinuria values during 6-month time frames were monitored. When proteinuria was consistently ≥4 g/day, its overall accuracy was 71%; when ≥6 g/day, 79%; and when ≥8 g/day, 84% (see Box 20.1). The advantages of this algorithm are that it only requires assessing kidney function and proteinuria, and the risk can be calculated repeatedly during the period of follow-up. Age, sex, degree of nephrosclerosis, and presence of hypertension are relevant but do not add to the predictive ability of this model. This model has ongoing utility, particularly when anti-PLA2R testing is unavailable or negative.

Importantly, proteinuria and kidney function may not accurately reflect disease activity. Proteinuria and kidney function do not discriminate between immunologically active disease and irreversible structural damage to podocytes and the basement membrane, and a change in proteinuria typically lags behind a change in anti-PLA2R levels by several months. Patients may be judged to be at high risk and exposed to potentially toxic immunosuppressive therapy but could still develop a spontaneous remission. In addition, the observation period required to assess the risk of progression may delay treatment, resulting in significant residual kidney damage. As discussed earlier, the ability to monitor PLA2R antibodies has added a new marker that can be used to predict clinical outcomes. Patients with low levels of anti-PLA2R antibodies are more likely to undergo spontaneous remission, suggesting that immunosuppressive treatment may be withheld. On the other hand, persistently elevated or increasing levels of anti-PLA2R antibodies are associated with lower rates of spontaneous remission and an increased risk of progressive loss of kidney function, such that earlier initiation of immunosuppressive treatment should be considered. A serology-based assessment of prognosis for patients with PLA2R-associated MN, which takes into consideration the degree of proteinuria, has been proposed (Fig. 20.5). The hope is that such an approach will improve diagnostic and prognostic accuracy and provide for an individualized treatment of patients with PLA2R-associated MN that will limit unnecessary exposure to immunosuppression. A randomized controlled trial (RCT) comparing the serology-based versus the traditional prognostic approach is needed.

Management of patients with primary MN who are antibody negative is uncertain. Considering that a high proportion of PLA2R- and THSD7A-negative patients develop a spontaneous remission, maximizing conservative therapy (discussed later) may be a reasonable initial approach. Studies that have included both anti-PLA2R-positive and -negative cases seem to indicate a similar natural history and response to treatment for both groups.

Response Goals

The treatment target in MN has been debated for some time. Obviously, the best target would be sustained complete remission (<0.3 g/day of proteinuria), but this presently occurs in only

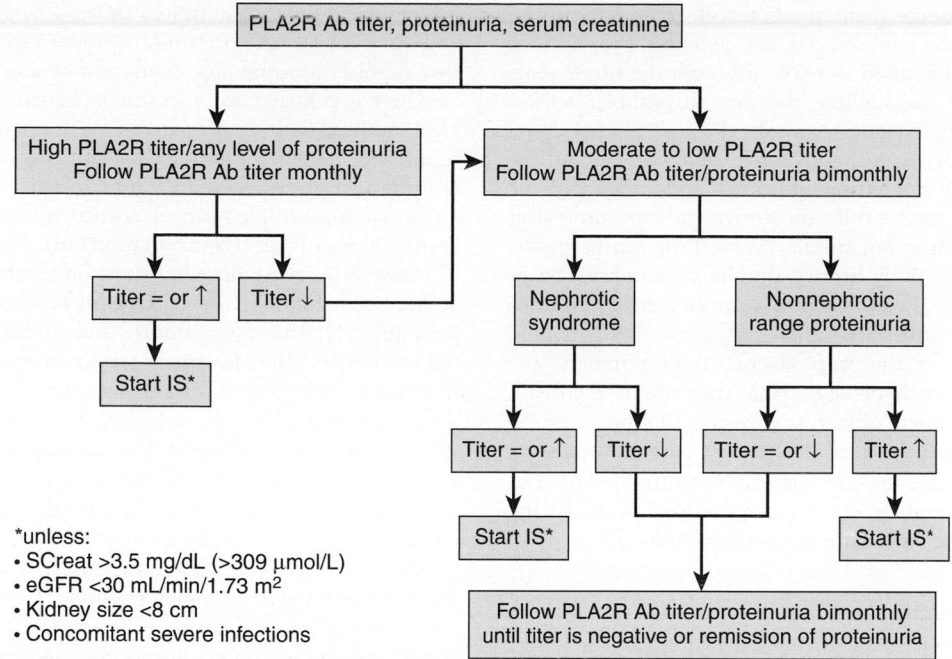

• **Fig. 20.5** A proposal for a serologic approach to the treatment of antibody-positive membranous nephropathy. *eGFR*, Estimated glomerular filtration rate; *IS*, immunosuppression; *PLA2R*, phospholipase A2 receptor; *SCreat*, serum creatinine.

30% to 50% of cases, even when combining spontaneous and drug-induced remissions. However, there is now good evidence that partial remission (<3.5 g/day and a 50% reduction from peak proteinuria) is an appropriate and valid target. Achieving a partial remission is associated with a significant slowing of the decline in kidney function at 10 years when compared with patients who do not experience remission. Most patients experience partial remission, suggesting that the process of remodeling of the GBM may take years to complete and does not necessarily reflect immunologic activity. Repeat biopsy studies in patients who have been successfully treated with rituximab in recurrent MN post kidney transplant showed persistence of deposits containing IgG and complement components for a significant amount of time despite disappearance of circulating anti-PLA2R antibodies. In patients with a history of positive anti-PLA2R or anti-THSD7A antibodies, monitoring these antibodies may help reveal if proteinuria reflects residual damage to the GBM or persistent immunologic disease.

Treatment

Nonspecific Non-Immunosuppressive Therapy

Nonspecific, non-immunosuppressive treatment involves restricting dietary sodium to less than 2 g/day, restricting protein intake, and controlling blood pressure, hyperlipidemia, and edema; this treatment is applicable to all patients with MN. Blood pressure reduction has been shown to reduce proteinuria and should be part of the management from the time of diagnosis. Blockade of the renin-angiotensin aldosterone system (RAAS), either with angiotensin-converting enzyme (ACE) inhibitors or angiotensin receptor blockers (ARBs), yields improvement in proteinuria beyond that expected by their antihypertensive action alone and, unless there is a specific contraindication, should be a first-line therapy in all cases, even when the blood pressure is not significantly elevated.

However, evidence that such therapy is beneficial in patients with MN is weak, and the antiproteinuric effect of ACE inhibitors and ARBs in these patients, for example, in comparison to their use in IgA nephropathy, is modest (<30% decrease from baseline). Although dietary protein restriction has never been associated with a complete remission of the nephrotic syndrome, it does result in lower levels of proteinuria; however, this needs to be balanced with the risk of malnutrition. Sodium restriction is much more critical, as poor adherence can lead to both an increase in proteinuria and escape from the benefits of RAAS blockade.

Treatment Focused on the Secondary Effects of Membranous Nephropathy

Patients with nephrotic syndrome have elevated total cholesterol and triglycerides, normal or low HDL, and increased LDL. This dyslipidemia probably plays a role in the increased risk for cardiovascular disease in patients with prolonged high-grade proteinuria. Although no trial has been conducted to determine if cholesterol lowering reduces the risk for cardiovascular disease in such patients, most clinicians apply evidence from patients without kidney disease to promote the use of statins in patients with primary MN and persistent high-grade proteinuria. A recent meta-analysis showed a small benefit on proteinuria reduction but no beneficial effect on GFR with statins in these proteinuric conditions.

Studies of the risk for thrombotic disease in primary MN demonstrate wide variation and are largely either retrospective or derived from small, uncontrolled trials, with variable inclusion criteria (all patients versus inclusion of high-risk patients only) and variable criteria for ascertainment of thrombosis. A retrospective study showed that clinically apparent venous thromboembolic events occurred in approximately 7% of patients with primary MN. In this study, a serum albumin level below 2.8 g/dL was the most significant independent predictor of venous thrombo-embolism. No consensus has emerged as to whether prophylactic anticoagulation should be used in MN, although the first 2 years of presentation show the highest risk for thromboembolism. One approach uses prophylactic acetylsalicylic acid (81 mg daily) when the albumin is between 2 and 3 g/L, reserving full anticoagulation to those with presenting albumin <2 g/L. Notably, the majority of physicians reserve full-dose anticoagulation until after documentation of a thromboembolic event. Proteinuria greater than 10 g/day, positive family history, previous thrombotic event before the patient was known to have MN, prolonged serum albumin levels less than 2 g/dL, bedridden status, or obesity should prompt consideration for the prophylactic anticoagulation. The precise mechanism of the hypercoagulable state observed in MN is unclear, although a variety of factors converge that heighten the thrombotic risk, including a local decrease in perfusion pressure in the renal vein from the lowered oncotic pressure, loss of clotting factors in the urine, increased hepatic production of clotting factors, and perhaps even a genetic predisposition to clot.

Immunosuppression

As discussed previously, a serology-based approach that takes into consideration anti-PLA2R levels together with the degree of proteinuria monitored over time currently is the best way to define prognosis in patients with primary MN. This approach will probably also apply to patients with other associated autoantibodies such as anti-THSD7A–associated MN but the evidence for this remains much weaker. Because many of the studies evaluating immunosuppression in MN were conducted at a time when no MN-specific antibody testing was available, much of the evidence supporting therapy relied on sustained proteinuria as a risk marker for disease progression. However, given the subsequent finding that approximately 70% of MN cases are anti-PLA2R-positive cases, the treatment risk/benefits seen today are unlikely to be dramatically different.

Low Risk for Progression

The prognosis for patients with proteinuria ≤4 g/day and with normal kidney function is excellent. In a series of more than 300 cases from three distinct geographic regions followed for more than 5 years, fewer than 8% developed a measurable decrease in kidney function. Normalization of blood pressure and reduction of protein excretion with ACE inhibitors or ARBs should be implemented. Because some patients do progress, long-term follow-up should include regular measurements of blood pressure, kidney function, and proteinuria as well as monitoring for anti-PLA2R antibodies. Immunosuppression is not recommended as long as the patient remains in the low-risk-for-progression category. Approximately 50% of patients who present with non-nephrotic-range proteinuria in MN will eventually progress to nephrotic-range proteinuria—most commonly those with high anti-PLA2R levels at presentation. In most cases (70%), this increase in proteinuria will occur within the first year after diagnosis. Their subsequent prognosis is then dictated by the course of their proteinuria and anti-PLA2R level.

Moderate Risk for Progression

Corticosteroid monotherapy has been ineffective in inducing remission of proteinuria in all controlled trials conducted to date and in preventing progression in all but one study. Although the

follow-up periods were limited to less than 4 years, and the dose and duration of corticosteroid treatment varied, it is generally held that steroid monotherapy should not be used in primary MN.

There is evidence for a treatment benefit when corticosteroids are combined with a cytotoxic agent. In a series of RCTs in Italy, a significant increase in both partial and complete remission of proteinuria and preserved kidney function at 10 years was seen after an initial 6-month course of corticosteroids and the alkylating agent, chlorambucil (Ponticelli protocol). Therapy consisted of 1 g of intravenous methylprednisolone on the first 3 days of months 1, 3, and 5, followed by 27 days of oral methylprednisolone at 0.4 mg/kg, alternating in months 2, 4, and 6 with chlorambucil at 0.2 mg/kg/day. This therapeutic regimen was superior to either no treatment or methylprednisolone monotherapy. The original regimen was remarkably safe, and all adverse events were reversed after stopping the drugs. When 2.5 mg/kg/day oral cyclophosphamide was substituted for chlorambucil and compared with the original regimen, similar complete and partial remission rates of proteinuria were seen. A relapse rate of approximately 30% was seen within 2 years in these studies, regardless of whether the treatment was chlorambucil or cyclophosphamide. Fewer patients had to discontinue cyclophosphamide (5%) compared with chlorambucil (14%) because of adverse events, and cyclophosphamide remains the favored cytotoxic agent when this regimen is used. More recently, this regimen showed similar long-term positive results in an East Asian population (India). Regimens using longer-term (1 year) cyclophosphamide and lower-dose prednisone have also demonstrated a similar outcome but compared only to historical controls. The cumulative dose of cyclophosphamide using this regimen exceeded the total dose used in the Ponticelli protocol and had significantly higher early adverse effects during the treatment and, years later, a higher incidence of cancer.

An alternative immunosuppressive agent is rituximab, a chimeric monoclonal antibody to B cells carrying the CD 20 epitope. Several prospective but nonrandomized pilot studies using rituximab monotherapy demonstrated complete or partial remission in proteinuria in 60% to 80% of patients by the end of the trial. The first RCT of rituximab versus conservative therapy showed no significant difference in remission rate at 6 months, but by 17 months the rituximab remission was twice that of the controls. Adverse events were low and similar to the control population. Changes in PLA2R titer were noted to precede or to parallel proteinuria response. The great majority of these patients remained in long-term remission. The most recent RCT tested the efficacy of rituximab versus cyclosporine in patients with high-grade proteinuria (>5g/d) and found no significant difference in PR and CR rates after 12 months of treatment, approximately 60% in both groups, but preservation of remission in virtually all the rituximab patients versus a 60% relapse rate in the cyclosporine arm at 24 months. In PLA2R-positive participants at trial entry (70%), those with the highest antibody titers at presentation were most resistant to treatment and those with complete immunologic response (complete depletion of antibody) at 12 months were least likely to relapse post-therapy.

The ideal treatment regimen using rituximab is still unclear. A recent retrospective study compared a low-dose to a high-dose regimen and found substantially lower early remission rates and less suppression of anti-PLA2R antibodies at 6 months with a lower dose. Other single- center studies have shown remission rates as high as 60% but as low as 38% with rituximab given as a single dose. It has also been noted that lower antibody levels at baseline and full antibody depletion at 6 months after rituximab treatment were strong predictors of remission. All 12 PLA2R-positive patients with complete remission at 12 months in the MENTOR trial had complete immunological remission at that time. A B-cell-titrated protocol using a single dose of 375 mg/m² rituximab has been proposed to be as effective as the four-dose protocol, at a lower cost, but recent reports have challenged the success of this regimen. Reemergence of circulating antibodies may predict clinical disease relapse. The response to rituximab is independent of patients receiving it as first- or second-line therapy. An important recent small pilot study found that PR with rituximab was achieved in nine of 13 in PLA2R-positive patients with low GFR (< 30 mL/min) and was associated with complete immunological remission. Four serious adverse events were reported, suggesting a higher than average infectious risk may exist in this population. Rituximab has also allowed successful CNI withdrawal in patients previously dependent on this treatment. Taken in sum, these results suggest that rituximab is effective for inducing remission of proteinuria in 60%–70% of patients with MN, either as initial treatment or in patients refractory to previous therapeutic regimens.

In the most recent trial, serious adverse events were also numerically fewer in the rituximab arm compared to cyclosporine therapy. Early concerns about the long-term effects of rare but fatal complications, including reports of progressive multifocal leukoencephalitis, potentially related to B-cell depletion, remain, although no such cases have been reported in MN patients treated with rituximab monotherapy. The short-term, favorable side-effect profile, equal efficacy and guaranteed adherence given its required intravenous administration, supports the opinion of many nephrologists that this therapy, where available and affordable, should be the first immunosuppressive treatment for primary MN.

Cyclosporine has also shown results similar to the cytotoxic/steroid regimen in terms of improving proteinuria in the medium-risk-for-progression group. MN patients who remained nephrotic after a minimum of 6 months of observation and remained nephrotic were given 6 months of cyclosporine (3 to 5 mg/kg/day) plus low-dose prednisone (maximum 10 mg/day) and were compared with a prednisone-alone/placebo group. Complete or partial remission in proteinuria was seen in 70% of the cyclosporine group compared with 24% of the control group. The relapse rate (40% to 50% within 2 years of discontinuing the drug) was higher than that seen in the cyclophosphamide/glucocorticoids trials. A study using a longer duration of cyclosporine treatment at a dose of 2 to 4 mg/kg/day for 12 months, followed by a reduction in the cyclosporine therapy to the range of 1.5 mg/kg/day, showed a much lower relapse rate of approximately 20% within the 2-year period. A 12-month RCT using tacrolimus monotherapy confirmed the benefit of the CNI but without supplemental steroid, achieving a partial or complete remission in proteinuria in 75% to 80% of the treated group, as well as a significant slowing of kidney disease progression compared with a control group; however, nephrotic syndrome reappeared in almost half the patients after tacrolimus withdrawal. In a recent RCT of severe nephrotic MN patients, the efficacy of cyclosporine was similar to rituximab, but in the 12 months following, the relapse rate was in the range of 60%. In a large retrospective review of MN patients, the subgroup analysis of those treated long-term with either a CNI or cyclophosphamide only and followed for up to 10 years found no difference in complete and partial remissions or relapse rates between regimens, but serum creatinine was substantially higher at study termination in the CNI cohort.

Although the incidence of MN in children, both PLA2R-positive and -negative, is low, case reports suggest that treatment with CNIs and rituximab have a response rate similar to adults. Cytotoxic therapy is not warranted as first line in this age group given the potential effect on fertility and long-term risk of cancer.

Initial results of combined use of mycophenolate mofetil (MMF) with high-dose corticosteroids were similar to cyclophosphamide therapy but with a significantly higher relapse rate after the drug was discontinued (>70% by 3 years post-treatment). Monotherapy with MMF appears ineffective in primary MN.

An additional therapeutic option is the subcutaneous administration of synthetic adrenocorticotrophic hormone (ACTH). There have been two small RCTs with this agent, showing short-term benefits similar to the results seen with the cytotoxic/steroid regimen, with quite a different rate of adverse effects. A retrospective case series of 11 patients with nephrotic syndrome resistant to previous immunosuppression treated with a natural, highly purified ACTH gel formulation reported similar encouraging results. Most patients were treated for a minimum of 6 months, with the longest treatment period being 14 months. Nine of the 11 patients achieved a complete or partial remission. In a more recent study, 20 patients with MN were randomly treated with this ACTH gel formulation, either 40 or 80 IU twice weekly for 120 days. ACTH therapy resulted in a significant reduction in median proteinuria from 9.0 ± 3.3 g/day at baseline to 3.7 ± 4.2 g/day at 12 months. A clear dose-response relationship was also reported, with 80 IU units twice weekly for at least 4 months appearing necessary for maximal effect. The reduction in anti-PLA2R antibodies and the decline in proteinuria correlated in some but not all patients, suggesting a possible direct effect on the podocyte of the drug as well as its immunosuppressive action. No serious adverse effects were reported. Although promising, evidence for the efficacy of ACTH in improving long-term kidney outcomes in patients with MN is lacking. It has been suggested that ACTH may mediate its effects via melanocortin receptor 1 on podocytes, and this unique interaction may explain why patients who are resistant to previous immunosuppressive therapies may respond to ACTH.

High Risk for Progression

In patients who are at high risk of progression, we recommend treatment with immunosuppressive therapy in addition to general supportive measures. Immunosuppression should be started promptly rather than observing the patient during a 3-to-6-month period first. In patients who are classified as high risk but have a stable kidney function, rituximab should be the first-line therapy. In patients who are classified as high risk because of abnormal or declining kidney function, we suggest combination treatment with glucocorticoids and cyclophosphamide rather than rituximab or other therapies. Such patients have a higher urgency for initiating treatment, and cytotoxic therapy appears to provide the best protection against progressive kidney disease. In patients who wish to avoid cytotoxic therapy, treatment with rituximab may be a reasonable alternative. The rationale for treatment in high-risk patients is based primarily upon the results of the Membranous Nephropathy Trial of Rituximab (MENTOR) and the United Kingdom Membranous Trial. In the

MENTOR trial, which included patients with primary MN who had average proteinuria that was >10 g/d but mostly preserved kidney function, treatment with rituximab was more effective than cyclosporine at maintaining complete or partial remission of proteinuria at 24 months. The United Kingdom Membranous Trial, which specifically enrolled patients with primary MN who had deteriorating kidney function, found that the combination of glucocorticoids and chlorambucil therapy was superior to cyclosporine and to supportive therapy alone at preventing further loss of kidney function and end-stage kidney disease. Significantly more serious adverse events (particularly hematologic issues) were reported in the chlorambucil group. It should be noted that the starting dose of 5 mg/kg/day of cyclosporine used in this study is higher than currently recommended, particularly in patients who already have reduced kidney function, potentially prompting acute GFR decline and subsequent high failure rate in this arm. An earlier small RCT using lower-dose cyclosporine studied a group of high-risk MN patients, defined by a substantial decline in kidney function in the year prior to randomization, and noted improvement in proteinuria and better preservation of kidney function after 1 year of therapy in comparison to the placebo group, and this improvement in rate of kidney function decline and proteinuria persisted over a 20-month follow-up in the great majority of these patients. Calcineurin inhibitors have substantial nephrotoxic potential, and monitoring for this and other adverse events must be part of any treatment routine that includes this class of agent.

The algorithm for management of high-risk patients (Fig. 20.6) lists the option of rituximab or a cytotoxic agent plus prednisone regimen as initial options, but cyclosporine should also be considered if there are contraindications to the above choices. Additionally, when the GFR is below 30 mL/min, the dose of cyclophosphamide must be adjusted downward to avoid the risk of significant bone marrow toxicity. If the GFR is low and deteriorating rapidly and/or if the biopsy shows extensive tubular interstitial disease and/or severe vascular changes, calcineurin inhibitors should either be avoided or given with great caution. Overall, the decision to treat this group of patients is not to be undertaken without carefully weighing the risks and benefits, and often a second opinion is warranted. A repeat biopsy to confirm adequate viable tissue and/or new subepithelial deposits on EM and/or increasing PLA2R titer, suggesting ongoing activity, should be considered before further immunosuppressive treatment is warranted.

Patients with MN who experience a rapid decline in kidney function should be evaluated for other potential causes of worsening kidney function, such as crescentic glomerulonephritis, acute hypersensitivity interstitial nephritis, or acute bilateral renal vein thrombosis. Further, immunosuppressive therapy should be avoided if there is evidence of severe and irreversible kidney damage (e.g., history of chronic kidney disease with a serum creatinine >3.5 mg/dL or eGFR <30 mL/min/1.73 m^2 for >3 months; kidney size less than 8 cm on kidney ultrasound; or evidence of severe interstitial fibrosis, tubular atrophy, or glomerulosclerosis on kidney biopsy), since immunosuppressive therapy is not likely to be effective in such patients. Finally, we do not give immunosuppressive therapy to patients with concomitant severe or potentially life-threatening infections.

Newer Therapies

Combination treatments with either rituximab or cytotoxic therapies combined with CNIs are ongoing. Several small studies have suggested that plasma exchange treatment or immune absorption in combination with rituximab may lower autoantibody faster than immunosuppression alone. Newer, fully humanized biologics of anti-CD20 monoclonal antibodies are available and small studies already completed have shown success. The rapid development of complement inhibitors acting at different stages of activation are also potentially promising therapies for MN and are already in early phase I and II trials.

Complications of Therapy

Many large studies in the kidney transplantation field and in postmenopausal women indicate that agents such as bisphosphonates or supplemental oral calcium and vitamin D reduce bone loss during long-term use of corticosteroids. The use of such agents in primary MN should be considered when a course of therapy includes prednisone treatment. Trimethoprim-sulfamethoxazole reduces the incidence of *Pneumocystis jirovecii* infection in patients on prolonged immunosuppressive therapy in both the transplantation field and in certain autoimmune diseases. Its use, when the patients with primary MN are exposed to prolonged glucocorticoid treatment, cytotoxic agents, calcineurin inhibitors, or rituximab, seems prudent. Appropriate vaccinations against hepatitis and pneumococcal pneumonia should be initiated pre-immunosuppression and annual influenza vaccination should occur.

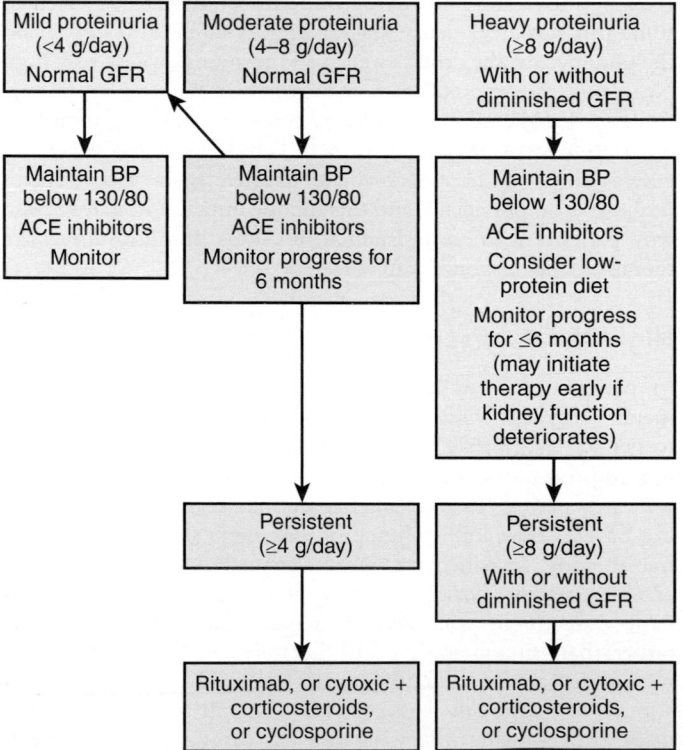

• **Fig. 20.6** Guideline for the treatment of antibody-negative primary membranous nephropathy. Patients may change from one category to another during the course of follow-up. *ACE,* Angiotensin-converting enzyme; *BP,* blood pressure; *GFR,* glomerular filtration rate.

Management Plan for Primary Membranous Nephropathy

Fig. 20.6 shows a treatment framework for patients with primary MN. In addition, the following general rules should be applied:

1. Establish whether the disease is primary (anti-PLA2R, anti-THSD7A, anti-NELL-1 –associated MN) or secondary MN.
2. Patients who are seronegative for anti-PLA2R antibodies, kidney biopsy negative for PLA2R antigen, and negative for anti-THSD7A antibodies and the newer autoantibodies may have MN due to still-unidentified autoantibodies or may have secondary MN.
3. Antibodies against PLA2R, and possibly antibodies against THSD7A, closely correlate with disease activity. Low baseline and decreasing anti-PLA2R antibody levels strongly predict spontaneous remission, thus favoring conservative therapy.
4. High baseline or increasing anti-PLA2R antibody levels are associated with nephrotic syndrome, lower probability of spontaneous remission, and progressive loss of kidney function, thereby encouraging early initiation of immunosuppressive therapy.
5. Changes in serum anti-PLA2R antibody levels reliably predict response to therapy, and levels at completion of therapy may forecast long-term outcomes.
6. Reemergence of or increase in anti-PLA2R antibody levels may predict clinical relapse, but the timing of these increases is currently largely unknown.
7. For patients who have anti-PLA2R–associated MN, we suggest monitoring proteinuria and antibody levels to guide immunosuppressive therapy (see Fig. 20.5).
8. For patients who are anti-PLA2R negative, we recommend monitoring kidney function during a 6-month period (3 months for the high-risk category patient), establishing a risk-for-progression score based on the traditional levels of proteinuria and kidney function algorithm, and tailoring therapy accordingly.
9. Treatment of secondary MN depends on the underlying cause.
10. The first-choice, specific therapies for patients with a medium risk for progression are either cyclophosphamide alternating monthly with prednisone for 6 months or rituximab. Rituximab, at least over the short term (3-5 years), seems equally effective and has less adverse events, has no apparent fertility implications, and has a definite adherence advantage compared to cytotoxic based regimens. Calcineurin inhibitors (cyclosporine and tacrolimus) are also effective but often require prolonged therapy to maintain remission.
11. The first choice for high-risk patients, defined by high-grade proteinuria but preserved kidney function, is rituximab or cyclosporine for 6 to 12 months. The most recent RCTs favor rituximab, given its greater remission durability. If the proteinuria is accompanied by deteriorating kidney function or low GFR or if both of these regimens fail, a course of cyclophosphamide combined with corticosteroids may be considered if there are other indicators of ongoing immunologic activity and the assessed risk-benefit warrants further treatment.
12. ACTH can be considered if all of the above have failed or created intolerable side effects.
13. A significant proportion of patients who achieve either a partial or complete remission will relapse, especially if they remain anti-PLA2R positive at the time immunosuppression is discontinued. Retreatment with the previously successful regimen (or with one of the other proven regimens if toxicity is a major concern) should be undertaken, but cumulative cyclophosphamide dose should not exceed 36 g (~2 courses of the Ponticelli protocol). This should replace labeling the patient as a treatment failure, because even a partial remission is associated with significantly improved kidney survival.

Treatment of Secondary Membranous Nephropathy

In the secondary types of MN, attention should be focused on removing the putative agent or treating the underlying cause. If this can be done successfully, both the histopathology and the clinical manifestations typically resolve with time.

Complete bibliography is available at Elsevier eBooks for Practicing Clinicians.

Key Bibliography

Beck LH Jr, Bonegio RG, Lambeau G, et al. M-type phospholipase A2 receptor as target antigen in idiopathic membranous nephropathy. *N Engl J Med.* 2009;361:11–21.

Beck LH Jr, Fervenza FC, Beck DM, et al. Rituximab-induced depletion of anti-PLA2R autoantibodies predicts response in membranous nephropathy. *J Am Soc Nephrol.* 2011;22:1543–1550.

Bobart SA, Pawar A, De Vriese AS, et al. Non-invasive diagnosis of primary membranous nephropathy using phospholipase A2 receptor antibodies. *Kidney Int.* 2019;95(2):429–438.

Cattran DC, Appel GB, Hebert LA, et al. Cyclosporine in patients with steroid resistant membranous nephropathy: a randomized trial. *Kidney Int.* 2001;59:1484–1490.

Cattran DC, Greenwood C, Ritchie S, et al. A controlled trial of cyclosporine in patients with progressive membranous nephropathy. Canadian Glomerulonephritis Study Group. *Kidney Int.* 1995;47:1130–1135.

Cattran DC, Kim ED, Reich H, Hladunewich M, Kim SJ. Membranous nephropathy: quantifying remission duration on outcome. Toronto Glomerulonephritis Registry group. *J Am Soc Nephrol.* 2017;28:995–1003.

Dahan K, Debiec H, Plaisier E, et al. Rituximab for severe membranous nephropathy: a 6-month trial with extended follow-up. *J Am Soc Nephrol.* 2017;28:348–358.

De Vriese AS, Glassock RJ, Nath KA, Sethi S, Fervenza FC. A proposal for a serology-based approach to membranous nephropathy. *J Am Soc Nephrol.* 2017;28:421–430.

Fervenza FC, Appel GB, Barbour SJ, et al. Rituximab or cyclosporine in the treatment of membranous nephropathy. *N Engl J Med.* 2019;381(1):36–46.

Howman A, Chapman TL, Langdon MM, et al. Immunosuppression for progressive membranous nephropathy: a UK randomised controlled trial. *Lancet.* 2013;381:744–751.

Hofstra JM, Fervenza FC, Wetzels JF. Treatment of idiopathic membranous nephropathy. *Nat Rev Nephrol.* 2013;9:443–458.

Kanigicherla D, Gummadova J, McKenzie EA, et al. Anti-PLA2R antibodies measured by ELISA predict long-term outcome in a prevalent population of patients with idiopathic membranous nephropathy. *Kidney Int.* 2013;83:940–948.

Ponticelli C, Zucchelli P, Passerini P, et al. A 10-year follow-up of a randomized study with methylprednisolone and chlorambucil in membranous nephropathy. *Kidney Int.* 1995;48:1600–1604.

Ruggenenti P, Debiec H, Ruggiero B, et al. Anti-phospholipase A2 receptor antibody titer predicts post-rituximab outcome of membranous nephropathy. *J Am Soc Nephrol.* 2015;26:2545–2558.

Ruggenenti P, Fervenza FC, Remuzzi G. Treatment of membranous nephropathy: time for a paradigm shift. *Nat Rev Nephrol.* 2017;13:563–579. doi:10.1038/nrneph.2017.92.

Seitz-Polski B, Debiec H, Rousseau A, et al. Phospholipase A2 receptor 1 epitope spreading at baseline predicts reduced likelihood of remission of membranous nephropathy. *J Am Soc Nephrol.* 2018;29:401–408.

Sethi S, Madden B, Charlesworth C, et al. Exostosin 1 and Exostosin 2-associated Membranous nephropathy. *J Am Soc Nephrol.* 2019;30(6):1123–1136.

Sethi S, Debiec H, Madden B, et al. Neural epidermal growth factor-like1 protein (NELL-1) associated membranous nephropathy. *Kidney Int.* 2020 Jan; 97(1):163–174.

Sethi S, Debiec H, Madden B, et al. Semaphorin 3B-associated membranous nephropathy. *Kidney Int.* 2020;98(5):1253–1264.

Tomas NM, Hoxha E, Reinicke AT, et al. Autoantibodies against thrombospondin type 1 domain-containing 7A induce membranous nephropathy. *J Clin Invest.* 2016;126:2519–2532.

21

Immunoglobulin A Nephropathy and Related Disorders

SEE CHENG YEO, JONATHAN BARRATT

Immunoglobulin A nephropathy (IgAN) was first described in 1968 by the Parisian pathologist Jean Berger, and at one time it was known as *Berger's disease*. It is the most common pattern of glomerulonephritis (GN) identified in areas of the world where kidney biopsy is widely performed. IgAN is defined by mesangial IgA deposition often accompanied by a mesangial proliferative GN, and it is an important cause of kidney failure. Recurrent visible hematuria is the hallmark of the disease. Closely related to IgAN is Henoch-Schönlein purpura, now referred to as *IgA vasculitis* (IgAV), and this less common disease is more frequently found in children. IgAV is a small vessel systemic vasculitis characterized by IgA deposition in affected blood vessels, with kidney biopsy findings indistinguishable from IgAN.

Epidemiology

IgAN is most common in Asian populations and is extremely uncommon in people of African descent. The highest worldwide incidence is in Southeast Asia; however, reported incidence is likely influenced by different approaches to evaluation of kidney disease and different thresholds for kidney biopsy. Peak incidence of IgAN is in the second and third decades of life, and there is a 2:1 male to female predominance in North American and Western European populations that is not seen in Asian populations. Subclinical IgAN is estimated to occur in up to 16% of the general Asian population and up to 3% of the Caucasian population. IgAN is occasionally familial, but the vast majority of cases are sporadic.

Clinical Presentation

Episodic Visible Hematuria

Episodic visible hematuria most frequently occurs in the second or third decades of life and is the presenting complaint in 40% to 50% of patients. The urine is usually brown rather than red and will often be described by the patient as looking like "tea without milk" or "cola-colored." The passage of clots is very unusual. There may be bilateral loin pain accompanying these episodes, which may be due to renal capsular swelling. Hematuria usually follows intercurrent mucosal infection, most commonly in the upper respiratory tract, but it is occasionally seen following gastrointestinal infection and may be provoked by heavy physical exercise. Spontaneous episodes occur as well. The time course is

characteristic, with hematuria appearing within 24 hours of the onset of the symptoms of infection. This differentiates it from the 2- to 3-week delay between infection and subsequent hematuria characteristic of poststreptococcal GN. Visible hematuria resolves spontaneously over a few days in nearly all cases, but nonvisible (microscopic) hematuria may persist between attacks. Most patients only experience a few episodes of visible hematuria, and such episodes typically recur for a few years at most. These episodes are infrequently associated with acute kidney injury (AKI).

Asymptomatic Nonvisible (Microscopic) Hematuria

Asymptomatic nonvisible hematuria is usually detected during routine health screening and identifies 30% to 40% of patients with IgAN in most series. Hematuria may occur alone or with proteinuria. It is rare for proteinuria to occur without hematuria in IgAN.

Nephrotic Syndrome

Nephrotic syndrome is uncommon, occurring in fewer than 5% of patients with IgAN, but it is more common in children and adolescents. Nephrotic-range proteinuria is principally seen in patients with advanced glomerulosclerosis. In children and adults presenting with concurrent nephrotic syndrome, nonvisible hematuria, and mesangial IgA deposition, one should always consider the possibility of the coincidence of the two most common glomerular diseases of young adults: minimal change disease and IgAN. A number of case series have reported patients who, on kidney biopsy, have normal light microscopy, foot process effacement on electron microscopy, and electron-dense mesangial IgA deposits and in whom proteinuria resolved completely in response to corticosteroid therapy. Typically, in these cases, following resolution of proteinuria, both nonvisible hematuria and IgA deposits persist.

Acute Kidney Injury

AKI is uncommon in IgAN (less than 5% of all cases) and develops by two distinct mechanisms. The first is in association with heavy visible glomerular hematuria, which leads to tubular occlusion by red cell casts. This is a reversible phenomenon and recovery of kidney function occurs with supportive measures. The second is a rapidly progressive GN (RPGN) associated with a nephritic presentation and kidney biopsy that shows acute, severe immune and inflammatory injury with fibrinoid necrosis and crescent formation. This may be the initial presentation of the disease or can occur superimposed on known mild IgAN.

Other Presentations

Other presentations of IgAN include hypertension, very occasionally malignant hypertension, and chronic kidney disease (CKD).

Secondary Immunoglobulin A Nephropathy

Mesangial IgA deposition may occur in a number of other diseases, and kidney biopsy findings are often indistinguishable from primary IgAN. Although some associations are well established, other anecdotal observations based on single case reports should be interpreted with caution. The most common form of secondary IgAN is associated with chronic liver disease, particularly with alcoholic cirrhosis. It is thought to be a consequence of impaired hepatic clearance of IgA. Mesangial IgA is a common autopsy finding in patients with chronic liver disease; however, few patients have clinical manifestations of kidney disease other than nonvisible hematuria. IgAN is also reported in association with HIV infection and AIDS. The polyclonal increase in serum IgA, which is a feature of AIDS, has been cited as a predisposing factor for the disease. The closeness of this association has been controversial, as autopsy studies have indicated a prevalence of IgAN between 0% and 8%. Other secondary causes of IgAN include inflammatory bowel disease and autoimmune disease. Some patients with infection-related GN may also demonstrate IgA dominance on kidney biopsy. Treatment of secondary IgAN should target the primary disease.

Pathology

Elevated serum IgA levels are found in 30% to 50% of adult patients with IgAN. Serum IgA levels do not correlate with disease activity or severity. Likewise, measurement of poorly *O*-galactosylated IgA1 *O*-glycoform levels is neither sensitive nor specific enough to be used as a diagnostic test in IgAN, although there are a number of studies that report an association between high levels of poorly *O*-galactosylated IgA1 *O*-glycoforms and a worse prognosis. The diagnosis of IgAN requires a kidney biopsy.

Light Microscopy

Light microscopic abnormalities may be minimal, but the most frequent finding is mesangial hypercellularity (Fig. 21.1). This is most commonly diffuse and global, but focal segmental hypercellularity is also seen. Focal segmental glomerulosclerosis is also described, and crescents may be superimposed on diffuse mesangial proliferation with or without associated segmental necrosis. Crescents are a common finding in biopsies performed during episodes of visible hematuria with reduced glomerular filtration rate (GFR).

Tubulointerstitial changes do not differ from those seen in other forms of progressive GN, reflecting the final common pathway of parenchymal kidney disease. Mononuclear cell infiltration is associated with tubular atrophy and interstitial fibrosis, ultimately leading to a widening of the cortical interstitium. This finding correlates with a poor prognosis.

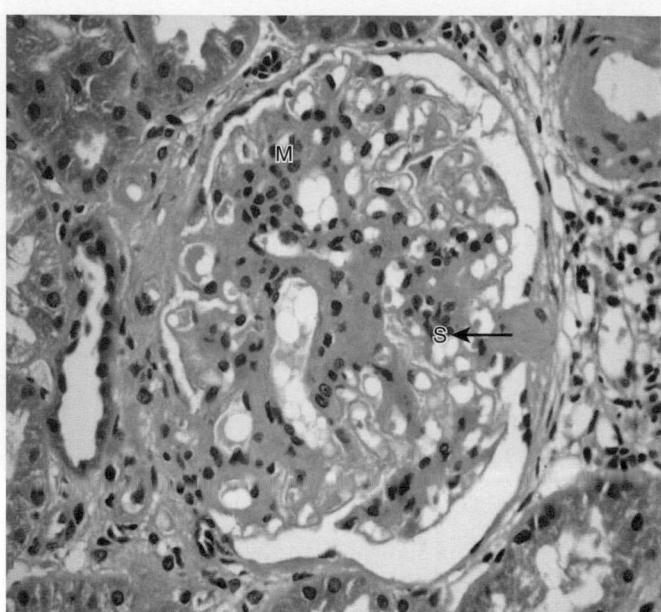

• **Fig. 21.1** Kidney biopsy showing mesangial proliferation *(M)* and expansion of the mesangial extracellular matrix *(S)* in a patient with immunoglobulin A (IgA) nephropathy. A capsular adhesion can also be seen *(arrow)*.

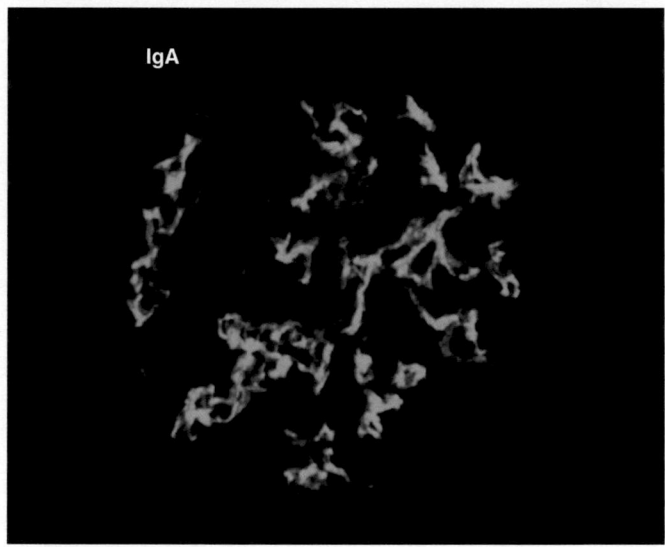

• **Fig. 21.2** Kidney biopsy showing immunofluorescent staining for mesangial immunoglobulin A *(IgA)*.

Immunohistology

The presence of dominant or codominant IgA deposits in the mesangium is the defining feature of IgAN. This is detected in kidney biopsy specimens by immunofluorescence or immunohistochemistry (Fig. 21.2). IgA deposition is diffuse and global. In 15% of cases, IgA is the only deposited immunoglobulin. Other immunoglobulins are also frequently detectable (IgG in 50% to 70%, IgM in 31% to 66%), but their presence does not appear to correlate with clinical outcomes. The complement component C3 is commonly present, but C1q staining is almost universally absent, arguing against a role for the classical pathway in IgAN. However, there is evidence for both lectin and alternative pathway activation in IgAN, and activation of both pathways has been associated with a worse prognosis.

Electron Microscopy

Electron microscopy shows mesangial and paramesangial electron-dense deposits corresponding to IgA immune complexes (Fig. 21.3). The size, shape, quantity, and density of the deposits vary between glomeruli. Glomerular capillary wall deposits may also be seen in the subepithelial or, more commonly, subendothelial space. Capillary loop deposits are associated with disease that is more severe. Glomerular basement membrane abnormalities are seen in 15% to 40% of cases and are associated with heavy proteinuria, more severe glomerular changes, and crescent formation. A group of patients have thinning of the glomerular basement

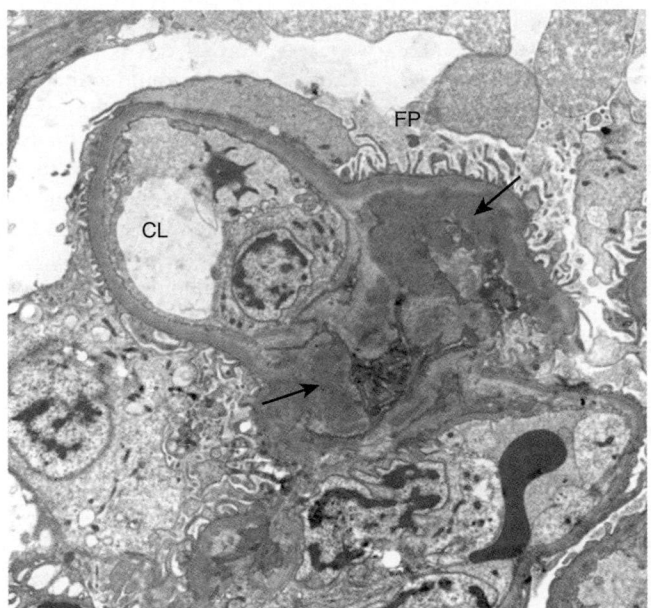

• **Fig. 21.3** Electron micrograph showing immunoglobulin A immune complex deposition within the mesangium and paramesangium *(arrows)*. *CL*, Capillary loops; *FP*, normal podocyte foot processes.

membrane indistinguishable from thin membrane disease. It is unclear whether the clinical course of these patients is different.

The Oxford Classification of IgAN

The Oxford Classification, published in 2009, is an international scoring system for evaluating pathologic features of IgAN on kidney biopsy. Four variables were identified that correlated most strongly with clinical outcome, independent of known clinical indicators of disease severity at the time of diagnosis, including the presence of hypertension, reduced GFR, and degree of proteinuria. These four variables included the presence of mesangial hypercellularity (M), segmental glomerulosclerosis (S) and tubular atrophy/interstitial fibrosis (T), and endocapillary hypercellularity (E) (Table 21.1). The first three of these (M, S, and T) were independent predictors of rate of GFR decline and the composite of kidney failure or a 50% decline in GFR. A similar association was seen with endocapillary hypercellularity (E) in patients who had not received immunosuppression; this difference was not observed in patients who received immunosuppression, suggesting that endocapillary lesions may be responsive to immunosuppressive treatment. The presence of multiple pathologic features (M, E, S, and/or T) in combination results in additive risk of kidney disease progression. Among the four predictors, studies have consistently demonstrated that the degree of interstitial fibrosis/tubular atrophy is the strongest predictor of kidney survival. The predictive value of these biopsy features was similar in both adults and children. Since its publication, the Oxford Classification of IgAN has been validated in different patient populations from North America, Europe, and Asia, and it is now widely accepted as the histopathologic scoring system of choice for IgAN.

In the original 2009 Oxford Classification, the presence of crescents did not independently predict clinical outcomes in IgAN. However, the Oxford study excluded patients with advanced CKD at presentation as well as those with rapid progression to kidney failure. A working subgroup of the IgAN Classification Working Group subsequently demonstrated that crescents were independent predictors of kidney outcomes in a pooled cohort of 3096 patients, leading to the 2016 addition to the Oxford Classification of a crescent score (MEST-C): C0 (no crescents),

TABLE 21.1	Oxford Classification of Immunoglobulin A Nephropathy, 2016 Update	
Histologic Variable	**Definition**	**Score**
Mesangial hypercellularity	Mesangial hypercellularity score defined by the proportion of glomeruli with mesangial hypercellularity	M0 ≤0.5 M1 >0.5
Endocapillary hypercellularity	Hypercellularity because of increased number of cells within glomerular capillary lumina, causing narrowing of the lumina	E0 absent E1 present
Segmental glomerulosclerosis	Any amount of the tuft involved in sclerosis but not involving the whole tuft or the presence of an adhesion	S0 absent S1 present
Tubular atrophy/interstitial fibrosis	Percentage of cortical area involved by the tubular atrophy or interstitial fibrosis, whichever is greater	T0 0%–25% T1 26%–50% T2 >50%
Crescents	Percentage of glomeruli with cellular or fibrocellular crescents	C0: absent C1: 0–25% of glomeruli C2: >25% of glomeruli

Note: Scoring should be assessed on period acid-Schiff-stained sections and there must be a minimum of eight glomeruli in the section.

C1 (crescents in less than 25% of glomeruli), and C2 (crescents in over 25% of glomeruli). A score of C1 identifies a group of patients with significantly higher risk of poor kidney outcomes if not treated with immunosuppression, although outcomes were similar to C0 if these patients were treated with immunosuppressive therapy. Notably, these observational data are not sufficient to extrapolate to a recommendation that those with C1 lesions should be treated with immunosuppression. A score of C2 identifies patients at risk of a poor kidney outcome even if treated with immunosuppression.

Pathogenesis

Although considerable progress has been made in characterizing a number of pathogenic pathways operating in IgAN, there remains a great deal that is not understood. In particular, it is uncertain whether IgAN is a single entity or whether mesangial IgA deposition is simply the final common pathway for a number of distinct kidney diseases.

Immunoglobulin A in IgAN

In humans, IgA is the most abundant antibody. It is predominantly present at mucosal surfaces and in secretions such as saliva and tears, where it protects against mucosal pathogens. The IgA molecule exists as two isoforms, IgA1 and IgA2, with each existing as monomers (single molecules) or polymers (most commonly dimeric IgA). It is predominantly polymeric IgA1 that is found in mesangial IgA deposits in IgAN. The major difference between IgA1 and IgA2 is that IgA1 includes a hinge region that carries a variable complement of O-linked carbohydrates (Fig. 21.4). Changes in the composition of these O-linked sugars is the most consistent finding in

patients with IgAN across the world, with identical changes seen in patient cohorts from North America, Europe, and Asia.

The key change is an increase in the serum of IgA1 O-glycoforms that contain less galactose. This increase in poorly O-galactosylated IgA1 O-glycoforms is believed to play a central role in the pathogenesis of IgAN. Poorly O-galactosylated IgA1 O-glycoforms form high-molecular-weight circulating immune complexes, either through self-aggregation, aggregation with soluble CD89, or through the generation of IgG and IgA hinge region-specific autoantibodies ("antiglycan" antibodies). These high-molecular-weight immune complexes are prone to mesangial deposition, resulting ultimately in mesangial cell proliferation, release of proinflammatory mediators, and glomerular injury.

Origins of Mesangial Immunoglobulin A

Many of the features of mesangial IgA are those typically seen in IgA secreted at mucosal surfaces. Mucosal IgA is polymeric, low affinity, and poorly O-galactosylated and is found at increased concentrations in the serum in IgAN. In addition, a number of studies report elevated levels of IgA antibodies specific for food antigens, mucosal vaccines, and gut-associated bacteria in the serum in IgAN. There are also intriguing data suggesting that gut bacteria may themselves be capable of modulating IgA class switching, the amount of mucosal IgA production, and IgA1 O-galactosylation in the gut-associated lymphoid tissue through activation of lymphoid toll-like receptors. Additionally, pathway analysis based on a large meta-analysis of genome-wide association studies identified the intestinal immune network for IgA production as the most enriched Kyoto Encyclopedia of Genes and Genomes (KEGG) pathway in IgAN. Most of the identified risk alleles are either directly associated with risk of inflammatory

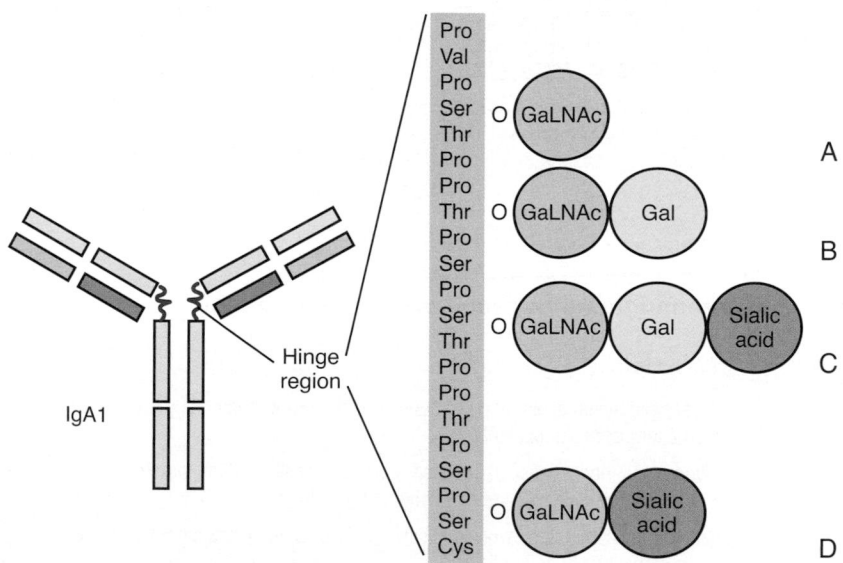

• **Fig. 21.4** O-glycosylation of IgA1 hinge region. IgA1 contains a 17-amino-acid hinge region that undergoes co/posttranslational modification by the addition of ≤6 O-glycan chains. (A) These chains comprise N-acetylgalactosamine (GaLNAc) in O-linkage with either serine or threonine residues. (B) Galactose can be β1,3-linked to GaLNAc by the enzyme Core 1 β-3 galactosyltransferase (C1GaLT1) and its molecular chaperone Core 1 β-3 galactosyltransferase molecular chaperone (Cosmc), which ensures its correct folding and stability. (C) Galactose may also be sialylated. (D) In addition, sialic acid (N-acetylneuraminic acid, NeuNAc) may be attached directly to GaLNAc by α-2,6 linkage to prevent further addition of galactose. *Cys*, Cysteine; *Pro*, proline; *Ser*, serine; *Thr*, threonine; *Val*, valine.

bowel disease or maintenance of the intestinal epithelial barrier, as well as response to mucosal pathogens. These genetic observations are also entirely consistent with known secondary causes of IgAN, which include a range of gastrointestinal disorders including inflammatory bowel disease and celiac disease.

Key Events in the Development of Kidney Scarring in Immunoglobulin A Nephropathy

The Oxford Classification of IgAN identified key pathologic consequences of IgA deposition that independently determine the risk of developing progressive kidney disease: mesangial cell proliferation (M), endocapillary proliferation (E), segmental glomerulosclerosis (S), tubulointerstitial scarring (T), and crescent formation (C). There is increasing evidence, predominantly from *in vitro* models, that circulating IgA immune complexes containing poorly *O*-galactosylated polymeric IgA1 are key drivers for all of these processes.

Exposure to IgA immune complexes triggers mesangial cell activation, proliferation (M), and release of proinflammatory and profibrotic mediators. These mediators, along with the direct effects of exposure to IgA immune complexes, recruit inflammatory cells into the glomerular endothelial space (E); cause podocyte injury, a process fundamental to segmental glomerular scarring (S); and cause proximal tubule cell activation, which drives tubulointerstitial scarring (T). If unregulated, this inflammatory response in the glomeruli leads to crescent formation (C).

Genetics of Immunoglobulin A Nephropathy

Genetic factors heavily influence the composition of circulating IgA1 *O*-glycoforms in the serum, and it is apparent that first-degree unaffected relatives of patients with IgAN often also display high levels of poorly *O*-galactosylated IgA1, supporting the hypothesis that changes in the composition of serum IgA1 *O*-glycoforms are only one part of the pathogenic process.

Several susceptibility loci have been identified from genomewide association studies, and one region that has gained particular interest is the major histocompatibility complex (MHC). Polymorphisms within the MHC have been associated with several autoimmune diseases, and an association in IgAN is consistent with an autoimmune component to IgAN. This could be mediated through production of autoantibodies with specificity for the poorly *O*-galactosylated IgA1 hinge region. Other identified susceptibility risk loci implicate pathways involving mucosal immunity and complement activation, further suggesting a pathogenic role for these molecular pathways in the pathogenesis of the disease.

Natural History and Prognosis

Fewer than 10% of all patients with IgAN have complete resolution of urinary abnormalities. IgAN has the potential for slowly progressive CKD leading eventually to kidney failure. Approximately 25% to 30% of any cohort will require kidney replacement therapy within 20 to 25 years of presentation.

TABLE 21.2	Data Elements Included in the International IgAN Prediction Tool*	
Estimated GFR at biopsy (mL/min/1.73m²)		MEST M-score
Systolic blood pressure at biopsy (mm Hg)		0
Diastolic blood pressure at biopsy (mm Hg)		1
Proteinuria at biopsy (g/day)		MEST E-score
Age at biopsy (years)		0
Race		1
Caucasian		MEST S-score
Chinese		0
Japanese		1
Other		MEST T-score
Use of ACE inhibitor or ARB at the time of biopsy		0
No		1
Yes		2
		Immunosuppression use at or before biopsy
		No
		Yes

*Using clinical and histologic data at biopsy, users can determine a 50% decline in eGFR or kidney failure at selected time intervals. The tool is not validated for use with data obtained remotely from the time of biopsy.
ACE, Angiotensin-converting enzyme; *ARB,* angiotensin receptor blocker; *GFR,* glomerular filtration rate.

Many studies have identified clinical, laboratory, and histopathologic features at presentation that mark a poor prognosis. In 2019 a new IgAN risk prediction tool was published by the International IgA Nephropathy Network (IIGANN). This tool incorporates 12 parameters, including the MEST-C histologic scores and clinical variables measured at the time of kidney biopsy and allows calculation of individual risk of progression to a combined endpoint of 50% decline in eGFR or ESKD up to 5 years from diagnosis (Table 21.2). The tool is available as an online calculator and should be regarded as the current gold standard for predicting individualized risk in IgAN.

Treatment of Immunoglobulin A Nephropathy

Management of patients with IgAN is currently limited to generic strategies applicable to all chronic glomerulonephritides: reduction of proteinuria, use of renin-angiotensin blockade, and control of hypertension (Table 21.3). As with all other causes of CKD, cardiovascular risk factors should be addressed and advice provided, when necessary, regarding weight reduction, smoking cessation, a healthy diet with specific recommendations on sodium consumption, and exercise.

TABLE 21.3	Treatment Recommendations for Immunoglobulin A Nephropathy According to Clinical Features	
Clinical Presentation	**Recommended Treatment**	
Recurrent visible hematuria	No specific treatment—no role for antibiotics or tonsillectomy	
Proteinuria <0.5 g/24 h ± nonvisible hematuria	No specific treatment—no role for tonsillectomy	
Proteinuria >0.5 g/24 h ± nonvisible hematuria	Maximal supportive care, which must include:	
	1. Advice where necessary on optimal weight, smoking cessation, a healthy diet with specific recommendations on sodium consumption, and exercise	
	2. Control of hypertension (Target BP 125/75 mm Hg: ACE inhibitors/ARB first-choice agents)	
	3. Address cardiovascular risk factors	
	4. Commencement of an ACE inhibitor or ARB (even if normotensive) with the dose increased to either the maximal approved dose or the maximally tolerated dose to reduce proteinuria to <0.5 g/day	
Proteinuria >1 g/24 h despite maximal supportive care	Consider a 6-month course of corticosteroids based on an individualized risk-benefit assessment	
Acute kidney injury	Acute tubular necrosis	
	• Supportive measures for acute tubular necrosis	
	Rapidly progressive IgAN (with little or no chronic damage)	
	• Induction (~8 weeks)	
	• Prednisolone (or similar) 0.5–1 mg/kg/day	
	• Cyclophosphamide 2 mg/kg/day	
	• Maintenance	
	• Prednisolone in reducing dosage	
	• Azathioprine 2.5 mg/kg/day	
Nephrotic syndrome	With minimal change on light microscopy	
	• Prednisolone (or similar) 0.5–1 mg/kg/day for ≤8 weeks	
	With structural glomerular changes	
	• No specific treatment	

Note: Treatment of rapidly progressive IgAN mirrors that of systemic vasculitides with rapidly progressive GN (see Chapter 24).
ACE, Angiotensin-converting enzyme; *ARB,* angiotensin receptor blocker; *BP,* blood pressure; *CKD,* chronic kidney disease; *GN,* glomerulonephritis; *IgAN,* immunoglobulin A nephropathy.

Nonvisible Hematuria and Less Than 0.5 g/Day Proteinuria

No specific therapy is advised for these patients, although long-term follow-up is recommended to monitor for increasing proteinuria, declining GFR, and hypertension.

Recurrent Visible Hematuria

No specific treatment is required for patients with recurrent visible hematuria, and there is no role for prophylactic antibiotics. Tonsillectomy reduces the frequency of acute episodes of visible hematuria when tonsillitis is the provoking factor, and tonsillectomy has its advocates, especially in Japan, as a treatment to reduce kidney disease progression. However, data from clinical trials are conflicting, and larger studies are needed before any conclusion can be drawn regarding the role of tonsillectomy in preserving long-term kidney function in IgAN.

Above 0.5 g/Day Proteinuria

Several randomized controlled trials have shown that renin-angiotensin blockade, with an angiotensin-converting enzyme (ACE) inhibitor or angiotensin II receptor blocker (ARB) to reduce proteinuria is beneficial in slowing progression of proteinuric IgAN, regardless of whether hypertension is present. Therefore, an ACE inhibitor or ARB should be introduced and the dose increased to either the maximally approved or the maximally tolerated dose. Although the combination of ACE inhibitor and ARB reduces proteinuria in IgAN, long-term beneficial effects on kidney survival have not been demonstrated and the safety of this approach has been questioned.

Above 1g/Day Proteinuria Despite Maximal Supportive Care

There are a number of patients who will continue to experience proteinuria in excess of 1 g/day despite maximal supportive care, including maximally tolerated doses of ACE inhibitor or ARB. These patients are at significant risk of declining kidney function. In these patients, current evidence regarding additional therapy is controversial. For those patients with proteinuria between 0.5 g/day and 1 g/day, the risk-to-benefit ratio of additional therapies is even more uncertain and, therefore, the therapies discussed below should at this time be avoided in this patient group.

Corticosteroids

The efficacy of corticosteroids in IgAN has been tested in several studies. Overall results are equivocal, and reports showing positive outcomes have been criticized for inadequate trial design and the presence of multiple confounding factors. The risks of high-dose corticosteroid use must also be considered, particularly in patients with a low GFR. The 2012 Kidney Disease Improving Global

Outcomes (KDIGO) Clinical Practice Guideline suggests that a 6-month course of corticosteroids may slow progression of GFR loss in patients with persistent proteinuria greater than 1 g/day despite renin-angiotensin blockade and preserved kidney function (eGFR greater than 50 mL/min).

Since publication of the KDIGO Guidelines, two important clinical trials have questioned this approach. In the STOP-IgAN trial, patients with persistent proteinuria greater than 0.75 g/day following optimized supportive therapy for 6 months were randomized to continued supportive therapy or additional immunosuppressive therapy (corticosteroids if eGFR ≥60 mL/min, corticosteroids plus cyclophosphamide/azathioprine if eGFR <60 mL/min). There was no difference in kidney disease progression for patients who received immunosuppression in addition to optimized intensive supportive therapy, compared with patients receiving optimized intensive supportive therapy alone; this has subsequently been confirmed in a long-term follow-up study. The prematurely halted TESTING trial (Therapeutic Evaluation of STeroids in IgA Nephropathy Global study) reported its results in 2016. While there was a suggestion of efficacy, the high-dose oral steroid therapy was associated with significantly higher rates of serious adverse outcomes in participants and was stopped by the data safety monitoring committee due to an excess of deaths, primarily from opportunistic infection, in the steroid treatment arm.

Fish Oil

Fish oil is widely prescribed in IgAN and appears safe, although tolerability is a major issue because of a fishy odor to the breath and sweat and increased flatulence. A meta-analysis of available clinical trial data, however, failed to detect a benefit of fish oils on kidney outcomes in IgAN.

Other Immunosuppressive Agents

There is currently insufficient evidence to support the routine use of cyclophosphamide and azathioprine in IgAN outside of those rare cases presenting with an RPGN. Mycophenolate mofetil (MMF) has been studied in a number of small, randomized, controlled trials, but results have been inconsistent, and a recent meta-analysis of these trials concluded that there is no significant benefit of MMF in reducing proteinuria in IgAN. A single study from China reported efficacy of MMF as a steroid-sparing agent in Chinese patients presenting with marked inflammation in their kidney biopsy. There is no convincing data to support the use of MMF in Caucasian patients. In the only RCT of rituximab in IgAN, no treatment efficacy was observed despite adequate peripheral CD20+ B cell depletion.

Emerging Therapies

A greater understanding of the key molecular pathways operating in IgAN (mucosal IgA synthesis, B-cell activation, and complement activation) has stimulated a number of phase II and III clinical trials of novel therapies in IgAN. In 2020, therapies being evaluated included lectin (MASP-2), alternative (Factor B) and final common (C5) complement pathway inhibitors, combined angiotensin and endothelin receptor blockade, inhibition of BAFF and APRIL signaling to B cells, and modulation of enteric IgA synthesis.

IgAN with Acute Kidney Injury

In patients with IgAN who develop AKI and fail to respond to simple, supportive measures, a kidney biopsy is required to differentiate between the two most common causes of AKI in IgAN:

1. *Acute tubular necrosis with intratubular erythrocyte casts.* This requires supportive care only, and recovery to baseline GFR is usual.
2. *RPGN.* Patients with rapidly progressive loss of kidney function, active and severe glomerular inflammation with crescents on kidney biopsy, and no significant chronic damage are treated similarly to other forms of RPGN. Evidence for treatment of a rapidly progressive IgAN is derived from small case-series and retrospective data. Response to treatment is worse in rapidly progressive IgAN than in other causes of RPGN, and kidney survival is estimated to be only 50% at 1 year and 20% at 5 years.

Nephrotic Syndrome

Nephrotic syndrome in association with mesangial IgA deposition may be a result of advanced glomerular scarring because of longstanding IgAN or occasionally a second distinct coincident GN such as minimal change disease. A kidney biopsy, including electron microscopy, is key to distinguishing between these two extremes. Patients with IgAN, nephrotic syndrome, minimal glomerular scarring, and podocyte effacement typical of minimal change disease should be treated as having minimal change disease.

Follow-Up

Patients with IgAN and CKD stages 1 to 3 should have kidney function, quantification of proteinuria, and blood pressure monitoring at least annually or more frequently if higher risk features are present. Patients with more advanced CKD or high-risk features such as nephrotic-range proteinuria require nephrology follow-up.

Kidney Transplant

Recurrence of IgA deposition following kidney transplant is common, affecting up to 50% of grafts within 5 years. However, graft failure due to recurrence of IgAN is relatively rare, most often occurring in patients who had a rapidly progressive course in their native kidneys. There is little evidence that the choice of posttransplant immunosuppression modifies the risk of recurrence, although an analysis of the Australia and New Zealand Dialysis and Transplant Registry (ANZDATA) suggests that recurrent disease is more common in patients who undergo steroid withdrawal. There is no evidence to support any specific treatment regimen after recurrent IgAN has been diagnosed, although a single-center retrospective analysis has suggested that ACE inhibitor/ARB treatment may reduce the rate of decline in allograft function in recurrent IgAN.

Immunoglobulin A Vasculitis (Henoch-Schönlein Purpura)

IgAV is the most common form of systemic vasculitis in children and is characterized by IgA deposition in affected blood vessels. The kidney lesion is a mesangioproliferative GN with mesangial IgA deposition that is indistinguishable from IgAN.

Epidemiology

Although IgAV may occur at any age, it is most common during childhood between ages 3 and 15 years old. There is a slight male predominance. Most cases occur in the winter, spring, and autumn months, which may be because of its association with preceding upper respiratory tract infections.

Etiology and Pathogenesis

The exact cause of IgAV remains unknown. There are, however, many factors that suggest a common pathogenic pathway operating in IgAV and IgAN. Identical twins have been reported where one presents with IgAN and the other with IgAV. IgAV developing on a background of IgAN is described in both adults and children. Both diseases share similar kidney biopsy findings and they also share changes in the complement of serum IgA1 *O*-glycoforms. There is a similar association between mucosal infection and presentation of disease.

Natural History

Kidney disease does not always develop in IgAV, but, when present, is often transient and self-limited in nature, with hematuria or proteinuria typically resolving within weeks of presentation. AKI due to rapidly progressive IgAV associated with severe inflammation on kidney biopsy is more common than RPGN in IgAN (although still uncommon), and AKI tends to occur early in the course of the disease. The prognosis of patients who have transient IgAV-associated nephritis is generally very good; however, up to 10% of patients with IgAV and nephritis will develop kidney failure.

Clinical Features

The classic tetrad of symptoms in IgAV is a palpable purpuric rash, arthritis/arthralgia, abdominal pain, and kidney disease. Symptoms appear in any order and can evolve over days to weeks, but it is important to appreciate many patients will not develop the complete tetrad.

The rash is classically distributed on extensor surfaces, with sparing of the trunk and face (Fig. 21.5). It typically appears in crops and is symmetrically distributed. Polyarthralgia is common and is usually transient and migratory. There is often swelling and tenderness but no chronic destructive damage. Gastrointestinal symptoms often appear after the rash. Abdominal pain is usually mild and transient, but it may be severe and lead to

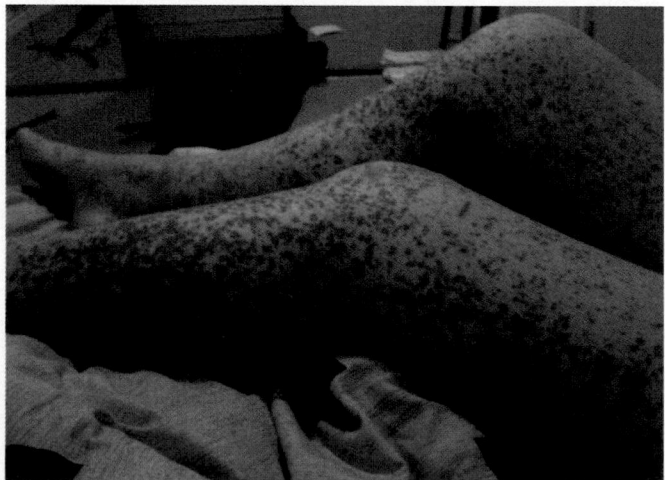

Fig. 21.5 Typical appearance of leukocytoclastic vasculitic rash of Henoch-Schönlein purpura.

gastrointestinal hemorrhage, bowel ischemia, intussusception, and perforation. Kidney involvement typically manifests as transient asymptomatic nonvisible hematuria and/or proteinuria. More severe complications, such as nephrotic syndrome or rapidly progressive deterioration of kidney function, occur less frequently and are more common in adults than in children.

Pathology

As in IgAN, elevated serum IgA levels are found in 30% to 50% of adult patients with IgAV. Serum IgA levels do not correlate with disease activity or severity. Similarly, changes in the levels of poorly *O*-galactosylated IgA1 *O*-glycoform levels are neither sensitive nor specific enough to be used as a diagnostic test in IgAV. Confirmation of the clinical diagnosis requires histologic evidence of IgA deposition in affected tissue, often the skin or kidney.

Skin Biopsy

Biopsy of the skin rash typically shows a leukocytoclastic vasculitis. IgA immune complex deposition can be seen using immunofluorescence staining, but detection of IgA in the skin is variable.

Kidney Biopsy

Kidney biopsy is usually reserved for adult cases of diagnostic uncertainty or when a child presents with more severe kidney involvement. Histologic features are the same as those in IgAN. Work is underway by the International IgAN Network to determine if the Oxford Classification is also valid in IgAV but at the time of writing there were no data to support its use in IgAV.

Management

There is little evidence to guide the treatment of IgAV with nephritis, and that which exists is derived from small, retrospective case series. What is clear from RCTs is that corticosteroids given at the time of presentation do not reduce the risk of subsequent development of an IgAV-associated nephritis. Patients with hematuria, proteinuria, and mildly reduced GFR do not require any specific treatment and the nephritis usually resolves spontaneously. In patients with an RPGN typified by a rapidly progressive loss of kidney function, there is limited evidence that high-dose corticosteroids are beneficial. Regimens include pulsed methylprednisolone followed by a 3-month course of oral prednisolone. There is currently no conclusive evidence that other immunosuppressive agents, including cyclophosphamide or azathioprine, or other interventions, such as plasmapheresis, have any beneficial effect on outcome.

Follow-Up

Patients should be monitored in the same way as described for IgAN. Those with persistent proteinuria are at highest risk of developing progressive CKD.

Transplantation

Kidney transplant is the treatment of choice in patients with kidney failure due to IgAV. As with IgAN, recurrence of mesangial IgA deposition may occur, although loss of the graft to IgAV is less common and tends to occur in patients who had a rapidly progressive original disease. Kidney transplant traditionally is delayed for 12 months from date of presentation.

Pregnancy

Evidence from cohort studies of children with IgAV suggests that all women with a history of IgAV should be carefully monitored during pregnancy, even if they had no evidence of kidney disease at the time of diagnosis. These women are at increased risk of developing hypertension and proteinuria during pregnancy.

Bibliography

Immunoglobulin A Nephropathy

Natural History, Epidemiology, and Diagnosis

Barbour SJ, Coppo R, Zhang H, et al. Evaluating a New International Risk-Prediction Tool in IgA nephropathy. *JAMA Intern Med.* 2019;179(7):942–952.

Berger J, Hinglais N. Les depots intercapillaries d'IgA-IgG. *J Urol Nephrol (Paris).*

Pouria S, Barratt J. Secondary IgA nephropathy. *Semin Nephrol.* 2008;28:27–37.

Schena FP, Nistor I. Epidemiology of IgA nephropathy: a global perspective. *Semin Nephrol.* 2018 Sep;38(5):435–442.

Trimarchi H, Barratt J, Cattran DC, et al. IgAN Classification Working Group of the International IgA Nephropathy Network and the Renal Pathology Society; Conference Participants. Oxford Classification of IgA nephropathy 2016: an update from the IgA Nephropathy Classification Working Group. *Kidney Int.* 2017 May;91(5):1014–1021.

Pathogenesis

Coppo R. The gut-renal connection in IgA nephropathy. *Semin Nephrol.* 2018 Sep;38(5):504–512.

Novak J, Barratt J, Julian BA, Renfrow MB. Aberrant glycosylation of the IgA1 molecule in IgA nephropathy. *Semin Nephrol.* 2018 Sep;38(5):461–476.

Rizk DV, Maillard N, Julian BA, et al. The emerging role of complement proteins as a target for therapy of IgA nephropathy. *Front Immunol.* 2019 Mar;10:504.

Yeo SC, Cheung CK, Barratt J. New insights into the pathogenesis of IgA nephropathy. *Pediatr Nephrol.* 2018;33(5):763–777.

Genetics

Li M, Yu X. Genetic determinants of IgA nephropathy: eastern perspective. *Semin Nephrol.* 2018;38(5):455–460.

Neugut YD, Kiryluk K. Genetic determinants of iga nephropathy: western perspective. *Semin Nephrol.* 2018;38(5):443–454.

Treatment

Floege J, Barbour SJ, Cattran DC, et al. Management and treatment of glomerular diseases (part 1): conclusions from a Kidney Disease: Improving Global Outcomes (KDIGO) Controversies Conference. *Kidney Int.* 2019 Feb;95(2):268–280.

Lv J, Zhang H, Wong MG, et al. Effect of oral methylprednisolone on clinical outcomes in patients with IgA nephropathy: The TESTING randomized clinical trial. *JAMA.* 2017;318(5):432–442.

Rauen T, Eitner F, Fitzner C, et al. Intensive supportive care plus immunosuppression in IgA nephropathy. *N Engl J Med.* 2015;373:2225–2236.

Rauen T, Wied S, Fitzner C, et al. STOP-IgAN investigators. After ten years of follow-up, no difference between supportive care plus immunosuppression and supportive care alone in IgA nephropathy. *Kidney Int.* 2020 May 22S0085–2538(20)30549–4.

Selvaskandan H, Cheung CK, Muto M, Barratt J. New strategies and perspectives on managing IgA nephropathy. *Clin Exp Nephrol.* 2019 May;23(5):577–588.

IgA Vasculitis

Audemard-Verger A, Terrier B, Dechartres A, et al. Characteristics and management of IgA vasculitis (Henoch-Schönlein) in adults: data from 260 patients included in a French Multicenter Retrospective Survey. *Arthritis Rheumatol.* 2017 69(9):1862–1870.

Ozen S, Marks SD, Brogan P, et al. European consensus-based recommendations for diagnosis and treatment of immunoglobulin A vasculitis-the SHARE initiative. *Rheumatology (Oxford).* 2019 Sep;58(9):1607–1616.

Pillebout E, Thervet E, Hill G, Alberti C, Vanhille P, Nochy D. Henoch-Schönlein Purpura in adults: outcome and prognostic factors. *J Am Soc Nephrol.* 2002 May;13(5):1271–1278.

Ronkainen J, Nuutinen M, Koskimies O. The adult kidney 24 years after childhood Henoch-Schönlein purpura: a retrospective cohort study. *Lancet.* 2002;360:666–670.

Sanders JT, Wyatt RJ. IgA nephropathy and Henoch-Schönlein purpura nephritis. *Curr Opin Pediatr.* 2008;20:163–170.

PART 4

Kidney in Systemic Diseases

22

Complement-Mediated Glomerulonephritis and Thrombotic Microangiopathy

MARINA VIVARELLI, JOSHUA M. THURMAN

The complement system is a group of proteins that provide an important part of the immune defense against infection. Many components of the complement system circulate as inactive proteins in the plasma. Activation of the complement system generates peptide fragments that serve as ligands for several receptors and complete a multimeric complex (C5b-9) that forms pores in membranes resulting in cell lysis.

As with all components of the immune system, proper function of the complement system helps with the effective elimination of invasive pathogens while causing minimal inflammation or injury to host tissues. However, uncontrolled activation of the complement system can cause tissue injury, and there is clear evidence that the complement cascade is activated in many autoimmune and inflammatory diseases. The kidney is particularly susceptible to complement-mediated injury, and the complement system has been implicated in the pathogenesis of multiple kidney diseases. It is also evident that acquired and congenital defects in the complement system are important risk factors for several kidney diseases. For the most part, these disease-associated defects impair the body's ability to regulate the complement system, thereby permitting overactivation or "dysregulation" of the complement cascade.

Uncontrolled complement alternative pathway activation appears to be central to the development of two kidney diseases: atypical hemolytic uremic syndrome (aHUS) and C3 glomerulopathy (C3G). These diseases are clinically and histologically distinct yet share similar risk factors. Our understanding of the pathogenesis of these diseases has been significantly advanced by recent discoveries. Although aHUS and C3G are both rare diseases, greater understanding of these diseases as extreme examples of complement dysregulation have provided insight into more common forms of glomerulonephritis that also involve complement activation.

Brief Overview of the Complement System

The complement system is composed of soluble proteins, soluble regulatory proteins, cell surface regulatory proteins, and cell surface receptors. Activation proceeds through three different pathways: the classical pathway, the mannose-binding lectin (MBL) pathway, and the alternative pathway (Fig. 22.1). Each pathway is activated by multiple different molecules. IgM- and IgG-containing immune complexes (ICs) activate the classical pathway, for example, but C-reactive protein, beta-amyloid fibrils, and other molecules also activate this pathway. The MBL pathway is activated when several different types of proteins, including MBLs, collectins, and ficolins, bind to sugars displayed on the surface of bacteria or damaged cells. All three pathways result in the cleavage of C3, forming C3b that can be covalently fixed to tissue surfaces.

Full activation of the complement cascade generates C3a, C3b, C5a, and C5b-9. Receptors for C3a and C5a induce several different inflammatory responses. Leukocytes also express receptors for C3b and the C3b inactivation fragments (iC3b and C3d). C5b-9 is also called the *membrane attack complex* (MAC) or the *terminal complement complex* (TCC). The insertion of C5b-9 into cell membranes can result in cell activation or lysis.

Several features of the alternative pathway are notable and may explain the link between activation of this pathway and kidney disease. Like the classical and MBL pathways, some proteins, including IgA, directly activate the alternative pathway. Tissue-bound C3b can combine with a protein called factor B to form an alternative pathway-activating enzyme (C3bBb). Consequently, the deposition of C3b on tissue surfaces by the classical and MBL pathways can secondarily engage the alternative pathway, resulting in increased complement activation through an alternative pathway "amplification loop." Finally, C3 in plasma is hydrolyzed at a slow rate, forming an enzyme complex that cleaves more C3 and activates the alternative pathway unless adequately controlled. This spontaneous "tickover" process continuously generates C3b that can also bind to surfaces and be amplified through the alternative pathway.

Complement Regulatory Proteins

Because the alternative pathway of complement is continuously active in plasma and tends to self-amplify, it is crucial that the body adequately controls this process. Complement activation is controlled by a group of regulatory proteins expressed on the surface of cells or that circulate in plasma. The ability of a surface to regulate alternative pathway activation determines whether the process continues to self-amplify or is terminated (Fig. 22.2).

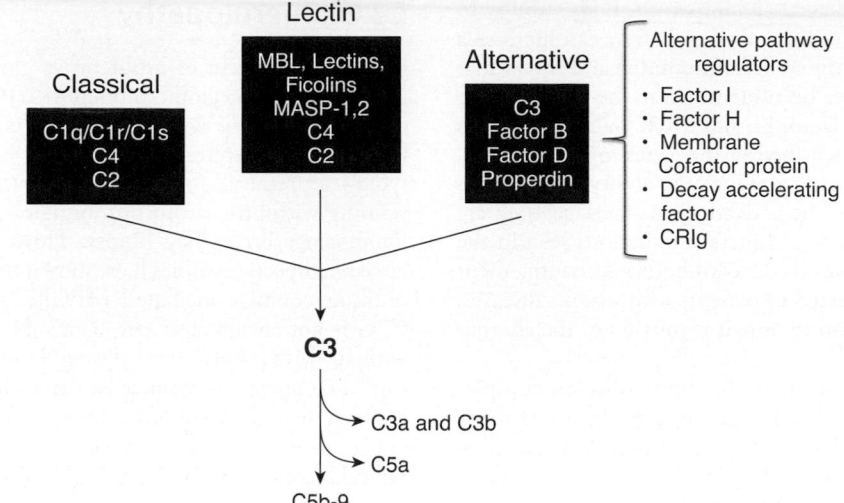

• **Fig. 22.1** **Overview of the complement cascade.** The complement cascade can be activated through the classical pathway, the alternative pathway, and the mannose-binding lectin (MBL) pathway. Activation through each of these pathways leads to the cleavage of C3. Full activation of the complement cascade generates several proinflammatory fragments: C3a, C3b, C5a, C5b-9 *(shown in red font)*. Proteins that regulate activation through the alternative pathway are shown. Of these regulators, defects in factor I, factor H, and membrane cofactor protein are associated with kidney disease.

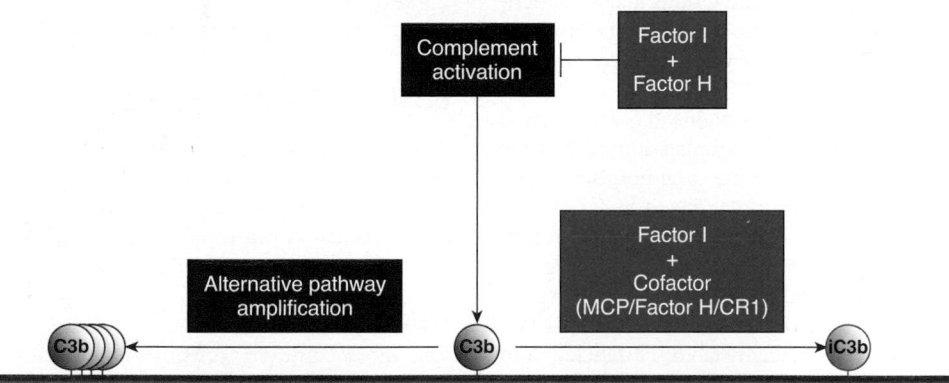

• **Fig. 22.2** **Activation and regulation of the alternative pathway on tissue surfaces.** The cleavage of C3 by any of the activation pathways causes deposition of C3b on tissue surfaces. C3b is part of the alternative pathway C3-convertase, and this enzyme generates additional C3b unless the convertase decays or C3b is inactivated by the plasma protease factor I, generating iC3b. To inactivate C3b, factor I requires cofactor proteins. Membrane cofactor protein (MCP) and complement receptor-1 (CR1) are cell surface cofactors. Factor H is a cofactor for inactivation of C3b in the fluid phase and on cell surfaces.

These regulatory proteins provide a shield that protects the host from complement-mediated injury. Pathogens do not express complement regulatory proteins, and expression of these proteins is decreased on damaged host cells.

Specific activating proteins can trigger complement activation on a particular cell or surface, but the degree of activation is also determined by the local expression of complement regulatory proteins. Impaired regulation may lower the threshold for activation within a particular tissue, and local impairments of regulation may even be sufficient to permit spontaneous activation. Endothelial cells and podocytes each express several of the complement regulatory proteins, and ordinarily there is little evident complement activation within the glomerular capillary wall.

Several different proteins can regulate the complement system. Factor I is a circulating protein that cleaves (inactivates)

C3b, forming iC3b (see Fig. 22.2). To function, however, factor I requires a "cofactor" protein. Several proteins with cofactor function are expressed on cell surfaces (e.g., membrane cofactor protein [MCP] and complement receptor-1 [CR1]). Factor H, a soluble alternative pathway inhibitor, also has cofactor activity. Other proteins regulate complement activation by reducing the half-life of the activating enzymes through a process termed *decay acceleration*. Decay-accelerating factor (DAF, or CD55) is a protein linked to the surface of cells that limits complement activation, and factor H also controls complement activation by this mechanism. Several additional proteins also control the complement system through other mechanisms. For example, carboxypeptidase N is a plasma enzyme that rapidly inactivates C3a and C5a, and CD59 is a protein that is linked to cell membranes to prevent the addition of C9 during formation of C5b-9.

Congenital or acquired defects can impair the body's ability to regulate the complement system, and these defects can increase a patient's risk of developing different autoimmune and inflammatory diseases. Mutations have been identified in the genes for the regulatory proteins factor I, factor H, and MCP. Gain-of-function mutations have also been identified in the genes for C3 and factor B. These mutations appear to reduce the ability of the regulatory proteins to inactivate the activating enzymes, so they are functionally similar to the loss-of-function mutations seen in the complement regulatory proteins. Autoantibodies to complement proteins have also been detected in patients with various diseases, and these autoantibodies tend to impair regulation of the alternative pathway.

Defects in factor H function are the most common complement abnormalities seen in aHUS, and impaired factor H function is also seen in some patients with C3G. Factor H is a soluble protein that is primarily produced by the liver and circulates in plasma at a concentration of 300 to 500 µg/mL. Factor H is made of up 20 repeating structures called *short consensus repeats*, or *SCRs*. Regulation of the alternative pathway is performed at the amino terminus of the protein in the first four SCRs, whereas the last two SCRs (19 and 20) mediate binding of factor H to molecules displayed on tissue surfaces such as glycosaminoglycans (GAGs) and sialic acid. Although it is not known why impairments in factor H so frequently manifest as injury within the glomerulus, one possibility is that the glomerular basement membrane (GBM) does not contain the other regulatory proteins and is completely dependent on factor H to control the alternative pathway.

The complement factor H–related proteins (CFHRs) are a group of five proteins that arose through reduplication of the gene for factor H with which they have high structural homology. The CFHRs all contain regions that are homologous to SCRs 19 and 20 of factor H, suggesting that they can bind similar molecules and surfaces. Various deletions and mutations in the CFHR genes have been identified in patients with aHUS and C3G. Experiments suggest that the mutant CFHRs competitively inhibit factor H. This can render patients functionally factor H deficient and cause complement dysregulation.

Complement in Immune-Complex Glomerulonephritis

IgG and IgM containing ICs are activators of the classical pathway of complement, and there is strong evidence that the complement system is an important mediator of injury in diseases associated with glomerular IC deposition. The interaction between the complement system and ICs is complex. Some isotypes of IgG activate complement more efficiently than other isotypes. Also, the complement system helps solubilize ICs, mediating the downstream effects of ICs but also reducing their deposition in tissues. Moreover, complement activation fragments affect the adaptive immune response, so the complement system may also influence disease upstream of antibody formation.

In addition to the involvement of the classical pathway, evidence from studies examining large cohorts of patients with immune-complex glomerulonephritis have revealed in a substantial proportion of cases a dysregulation (both genetic and serological) of the alternative pathway of complement. This indicates that the presence of glomerular immune complexes does not rule out this pathway as a mediator of kidney injury.

C3 Glomerulopathy

C3G is a rare form of proliferative glomerulonephritis comprising two forms: C3 glomerulonephritis (C3GN) and dense-deposit disease (DDD; previously known as type II membranoproliferative glomerulonephritis [MPGN] or MPGN type II). The unifying feature of all forms of C3G is the presence of intense C3 staining with little or no immunoglobulin staining by immunofluorescence on kidney biopsy. However, as mentioned above, large retrospective studies have shown that the distinction between immune-complex mediated MPGN (so-called IC-MPGN) and C3G is not always clear cut, as a substantial number of patients with IC-MPGN also have dysregulation of the alternative pathway of complement. Clinically, these forms of primary alternative pathway-driven IC-MPGN are recognizable by low circulating C3 levels with normal circulating C4, setting them apart from typical secondary forms of MPGN in which C4 is also reduced.

Epidemiology

Incidence of C3G is reported as one to two per million per total population. The age of onset is highly variable. The youngest reported patient was 1 year old, and about 40% of patients presented before 16 years of age in one large cohort. There was a slight prevalence of men in this series (60%), and a family history of glomerulonephritis was reported in about 11% of cases.

Etiology and Pathogenesis

A large number of molecular causes of alternative pathway complement dysregulation have been identified in patients with C3G, including autoantibodies and genetic variants that encode dysfunctional complement proteins (Table 22.1). Patients with monoclonal gammopathies can also develop C3G.

Autoantibodies

The most common autoantibody associated with C3G is C3 nephritic factor (C3Nef). C3Nef can be detected in approximately 70% to 80% of patients with C3G. It is more common in DDD than in C3GN and correlates with lower levels of C3. The presence of C3Nef does not correlate with clinical outcomes, however, and can be detected in healthy control subjects.

A monoclonal immunoglobulin light chain that inhibited factor H was identified in a C3G patient. This antibody blocked the regulatory function of factor H, thereby impairing regulation of the alternative pathway. A similar mechanism may cause complement dysregulation in some patients over the age of 40 years with monoclonal gammopathies. Anti-factor H IgG antibodies have also been identified in additional patients with C3G. These antibodies bind to the amino terminus of the protein and block its regulatory function. Antibodies reactive to factor B and C3b have also been reported. These different autoantibodies are associated with increased alternative pathway activation, lending further support to the concept that alternative pathway activation is central to the pathogenesis of C3G. Recently, antibodies directed against factor B have been detected in a majority of children with acute postinfectious glomerulonephritis, suggesting that alternative pathway dysregulation plays a central but transient role in this acute form of glomerulonephritis. The detection of antibodies specific for the complement proteins is currently only performed in research labs and is not widely available.

TABLE 22.1	Complement Abnormalities Associated With C3 Glomerulopathy
Complement Protein	**Abnormality**
C3 convertase (C3bBb)	Autoantibody • C3Nef (70%–80% of patients). Stabilizes C3 convertase; resistance to inactivation by factor H
Factor H	Protein • Levels low in some patients Autoantibody • Mini-autoantibody to factor H (light chain dimer) blocks regulatory function • Antibodies to factor H block regulatory function Mutations • Heterozygous mutation • Homozygous mutations • Compound heterozygous mutation
Factor B	Protein • Levels low in some patients Autoantibody • Binds factor B and stabilizes C3 convertase (C3bBb) Mutations • Gain of function mutation in factor B reported
Factor I	Protein • Levels low in some patients Mutations • Associated with reduced levels and activity
C3	Protein • Levels low in 50%–60% of patients. C4 levels are low in only ~2% of patients. Autoantibody • Binds C3b and stabilizes C3 convertase (C3bBb) Mutations • Heterozygous C3 mutation. C3 convertases resistant to inactivation by factor H
CFHR1	Mutations • Heterozygous internal duplication in SCR • Heterozygous hybrid CFHR1-3 gene
CHFR2	Mutations • Heterozygous hybrid CFHR2-5 gene
CHFR3	Mutations • Heterozygous hybrid CFHR1-3 gene
CFHR5	Mutations • Heterozygous internal duplication in SCR1-2 • Heterozygous internal duplication of SCR1-2 with deletion of CFHR1 and 3 in one affected subject

C3Nef, C3 nephritic factor; *CFHR*, complement factor H–related protein; *CFH*, complement factor H; *SCR*, short consensus repeat.

formation of a hybrid CFHR2-CFHR5 protein was found in two related patients with C3G.

The different molecular causes of C3G increase alternative pathway activation or make this system resistant to regulation. It is not known, however, whether the disease is primarily caused by systemic complement activation in the plasma or local activation directly on the mesangium and glomerular capillary wall. Complement activation in the plasma could lead to deposition of complement proteins within the glomeruli as plasma is filtered by the kidney. The GBM may be dependent upon factor H for regulating the alternative pathway. Bruch's membrane in the eye may be similarly dependent upon factor H, and patients with C3G develop retinal lesions and visual impairments.

Pathology

The identification of C3G is based on pathology, and particularly on immunofluorescence (Fig. 22.3). The presence of intense C3 staining is necessary for diagnosis. A commonly used criterion for the diagnosis is C3 predominance, with at least twofold greater intensity of C3 staining compared to other immune proteins (in particular IgG, IgA, IgM, C1q). However, this has become increasingly controversial. Discrimination between C3G and IC-mediated forms of proliferative glomerulonephritis may be much less relevant than was previously thought, as many forms of primary IC-MPGN have been found to have either genetic or autoantibody-driven alterations of the alternative pathway of complement. In the presence of persistently low circulating C3 with normal C4 and lack of secondary causes (i.e., systemic autoimmune diseases such as lupus, infections such as HCV, HIV, monoclonal gammopathy), a complete genetic and serological work-up for alternative pathway dysregulation is warranted.

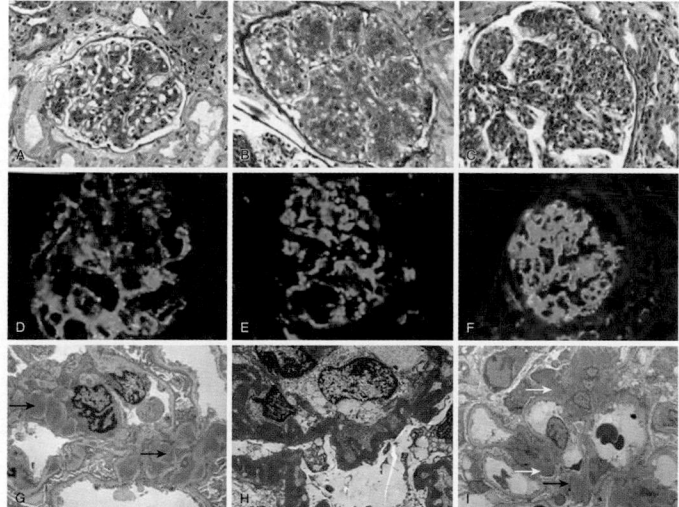

• **Fig. 22.3** Histologic appearance of the kidney in C3 glomerulopathy. (A) Mesangial proliferation. (B) Membranoproliferative glomerulonephritis. (C) Diffuse endocapillary proliferation by light microscopy. (D–F) C3 immunofluorescence. (G–I) Electron microscopy. (H) A typical dense-deposit disease aspect. (G, I) A typical C3GN with *black arrows* showing mesangial deposits and *white arrows* showing subepithelial deposits or "humps." (A–G, I from Sethi S, Fervenza FC, Zhang Y, et al. C3 glomerulopathy: clinicopathological findings, complement abnormalities, glomerular proteomic profile, treatment, and follow-up. *Kidney Int.* 2012;82:465–473; H courtesy Dr. Francesca Diomedi-Camassei.)

Genetic Causes

Disease-associated mutations and rare variants have been identified in the genes for factor H, factor I, factor B, C3, and CFHRs 1, 2, 3, and 5 (see Table 22.1). An internal reduplication of a region in CFHR5 is associated with C3G, and a deletion causing

The features of C3G by light microscopy are extremely heterogeneous. It most frequently presents with a membranoproliferative pattern, although mesangial proliferation, diffuse proliferation, and, more rarely, necrotizing lesions with extracapillary proliferation may be observed. Different patterns may coexist in the same kidney biopsy, and there may be an evolution of the lesion from mesangial proliferation to MPGN. Pathologists rely on the immunofluorescence pattern, therefore, to distinguish forms of C3G from other glomerular diseases that may appear similar by light microscopy. The other causes of MPGN can be idiopathic or secondary to viral infections, autoimmune diseases such as systemic lupus erythematosus, malignancies, and monoclonal gammopathies. Immunofluorescence in these forms of MPGN typically shows intense immunoglobulin staining and positive staining for C4d. Positive IF staining for C4d in equal or greater magnitude than C3 suggests activation of the classical and/or lectin pathways of complement, and it has been proposed as a metric to rule out C3 glomerulopathies. However, these findings have not been confirmed in subsequent studies, particularly in a pediatric setting where glomerular C4d staining has been found also in children with C3G.

Two subtypes of C3G have been identified: DDD and C3GN. The distinction of these subtypes relies on electron microscopy (see Fig. 22.3). In DDD, deposits are dense, intensely osmiophilic sausage-like ribbons located within the GBM (intramembranous). The GBM becomes altered and thickened to an extent that may be visible by light microscopy. Discrete, intensely C3-positive granular deposits are also located within the mesangium. In C3GN, the C3-positive deposits are less dense, less discrete, and more diffusely located, mostly within the mesangium and on the subendothelial side of the GBM, but also in the subepithelial and intramembranous portions of the GBM. Subepithelial deposits may closely resemble the "humps" that in the past were considered pathognomonic of acute postinfectious glomerulonephritis (PIGN).

Laser microdissection of the deposits visible by electron microscopy in C3GN and DDD and proteomic analysis of their content have shown similar profiles, with no immunoglobulin but abundant components of the alternative pathway of complement. Analysis by immunofluorescence of different components of the complement pathway in kidney biopsies from patients with C3GN and DDD has also not revealed significant differences. These results confirm that these two forms of nephropathy have a shared pathogenesis and are, therefore, correctly classified under the common definition of C3G.

Clinical and Laboratory Features

The clinical features of C3G are extremely heterogeneous, reflecting the frequently subtle and unpredictable disease course. In one series, 41% of patients had nephrotic-range proteinuria (>3 g/day) at presentation and 61% had microscopic hematuria. The frequency of gross hematuria was around 16% in another report. High blood pressure was present in 30.5% of patients and reduced kidney function at diagnosis in 45.5% of cases, with a mean eGFR of 69.3 mL/min/1.73 m^2.

The clinical presentation of disease is frequently concomitant with an infectious episode. Upper respiratory tract infection was reported in 57% of children with DDD. The first manifestation of disease may be gross hematuria, with recurrent episodes of gross hematuria during intercurrent infections. These patients often have persistent proteinuria and microscopic hematuria with dysmorphic red blood cells between acute episodes. This clinical picture can resemble IgA nephropathy (IgAN) and is typical but not exclusive to C3G associated with genetic alterations of CFHR5, initially described in a cluster of families from Cyprus. C3G can also resemble classic acute PIGN in which the urinary alterations appear 2 to 3 weeks after an infectious episode, frequently accompanied by hypertension and some degree of GFR loss. The associated illness is typically an upper respiratory tract infection, and the low circulating C3 with normal C4 may lead to a clinical diagnosis of PIGN. Persistently low complement levels without resolution of hematuria and proteinuria within 3 to 6 months of infection suggest a variant of C3G (sometimes called *atypical postinfectious GN*).

Patients can also present with nephrotic syndrome and kidney failure. Hypertension is very frequent and may be severe, as is glomerular hematuria. The forms of C3G that present with nephrotic syndrome tend to have more intensely proliferative lesions at kidney biopsy, more severe kidney failure at onset, and poorer outcomes. More frequently, though, C3G has a subtle and remitting disease course, with no overt clinical symptoms. In such patients, microscopic hematuria and low-grade proteinuria are usually detected during routine urinalysis. In these cases, age at presentation is highly variable, and disease diagnosis may be very distant from actual disease onset. In about 10% of patients, the family history is positive for glomerulonephritis or for kidney failure of unknown origin.

Laboratory features mainly consist of low circulating C3 with normal C4 levels, reflecting activation of the alternative pathway of complement. This feature, however, is not always present and may be more frequent and intense in DDD compared with C3GN. In a French cohort, low C3 plasma levels were present in 46% of all patients and 60% of those with DDD, in whom C3 levels were, on average, also lower. Low C4 was rare (only about 2% of cases). Therefore, normal circulating C3 levels do not rule out a diagnosis of C3G. However, persistently low C3 levels with normal C4, if present, are suggestive of alternative pathway dysregulation and C3G.

A diagnosis of C3G, particularly in familial forms, warrants investigation of the alternative pathway of complement with assessment of circulating levels of different factors, measurement of C3Nef, and genetic analysis of mutations in genes coding for an alternative pathway of complement proteins or regulators (Table 22.2; see also Table 22.1). The majority of patients older than 50 years old have a detectable paraprotein, and adults with C3G should be tested for evidence of an underlying monoclonal gammopathy.

The outcome of C3G is variable but is unfavorable in a majority of patients. In both DDD and C3GN, most reports indicate that 40% to 50% of patients will reach end-stage kidney disease (ESKD) within 10 years of disease onset. Factors negatively influencing outcome are the degree of proteinuria, especially the presence of nephrotic syndrome at onset, kidney failure at onset, severe hypertension at onset, older age, the presence of crescents, and tubular atrophy/interstitial fibrosis on the kidney biopsy. In the CFHR5-related forms of C3G, men have a markedly poorer outcome. Forms of C3G with the clinical picture of so-called atypical PIGN generally have a favorable outcome. In general, the impression of clinicians is that DDD is more severe than C3GN, although recent studies show that the outcomes are similar.

Extrarenal Features

Because C3G is caused by systemic defects in regulation of the alternative pathway of complement, extrarenal manifestations of disease can occur. Accumulation of C3 in the retina can give rise

TABLE 22.2	Evaluation of Patients Suspected of Having C3 Glomerulopathy
History	Family history of hematuria, glomerulonephritis, kidney failure
	Gross hematuria (if yes, concomitant or 15–20 days subsequent to infection and number of episodes)
	Infection (especially upper respiratory tract) in the preceding 2–3 weeks
	Previous urinalysis results
Clinical examination	Signs of nephrotic syndrome (peripheral edema)
	Blood pressure
	Urine dipstick, presence of frothy urine, reduction in urinary output
	Extrarenal features: partial lipodystrophy, retinal drusen
Laboratory workup	Urinalysis, 24-hour proteinuria
	Complete blood count, urea, creatinine, protein, IgG, IgA, IgM
	Serum C3, C4
	Autoantibodies (ANA, anti-dsDNA), serology for HCV and HBV, serum protein electrophoresis

to drusen, an ocular abnormality visible as white or yellow dots between the retinal pigment epithelium and Bruch's membrane. Drusen is detected by electroretinogram, and patients with kidney features of C3G should be screened for their presence. Drusen may partially impair vision and is similar to the alterations seen in age-related macular degeneration, another complement-related disorder that is limited to the eye.

Another systemic feature that has been reported in patients with C3G is acquired partial lipodystrophy. This manifestation is secondary to complement-mediated destruction of adipocytes. It has a cranio-caudal distribution usually limited to the upper body, starting with the face and progressing to the neck, thorax, arms, and abdomen. Acquired partial lipodystrophy usually precedes the development of kidney symptoms.

Differential Diagnosis

The various clinical presentations of C3G can overlap with other glomerular diseases. The differential diagnosis, especially in young women, includes lupus nephritis, although a low C3 level in lupus nephritis is usually accompanied by low C4 due to activation of the classical pathway of complement (see Fig. 22.1). Intrainfectious recurrent gross hematuria, as seen in C3G associated with genetic mutations in CFHR5, can simulate IgAN, but IgAN is readily distinguished by IgA predominance with immunofluorescence. The kidney biopsy is less useful to distinguish PIGN from C3G, as light microscopy can be very similar, and electron microscopy can show subepithelial deposits ("humps") in both diseases. Immunofluorescence in PIGN may show more IgG than in C3G, although a recent review of 23 cases shows that this distinction may not be accurate. C4d staining is present in only about 50% of patients with PIGN, so it is of limited use in distinguishing between this disease and C3G. Clinical features suggestive of PIGN include a normalization of circulating C3 within 8 to 12 weeks from onset and the absence of disease recurrence (gross hematuria, proteinuria). Given that C3 levels may be normal in some patients with C3G, we recommend that all patients with a diagnosis of PIGN,

however classic, undergo periodic urinalysis for 2 years after disease resolution.

If immunoglobulin is present in the glomeruli, even when not predominant, it is prudent to exclude immune-mediated, infection-associated, and malignancy-related causes of MPGN.

Treatment

The treatment of C3G is not standardized, as there is no solid evidence of effective therapeutic options. Moreover, the extremely variable clinical picture and the often unpredictable, spontaneously remitting and relapsing natural history of the disease render the evaluation of responses to different therapeutic approaches difficult. Lastly, the fact that C3G is a recently defined disease makes analysis of long-term outcomes under different therapeutic regimens impossible.

Immunosuppression has been attempted with various approaches, but very few trials are available to guide treatment. In general, when the kidney biopsy shows abundant inflammation and proliferation with moderate or little sclerosis, immunosuppression appears reasonable even though most of these agents do not block activation of the complement alternative pathway. Prednisone is frequently used although no studies are available to confirm its effectiveness. Current guidelines based on expert opinion, but not on results of clinical trials, suggest that a reasonable approach may be to use alternate day 40 mg/m² prednisone for 6 to 12 months in patients with intense proteinuria or kidney failure, tapering and discontinuing treatment if there is no sign of improvement after 3 to 4 months.

Some studies show a favorable response to mycophenolate mofetil in C3G. This therapeutic approach is warranted in forms with intense proliferation and inflammation. Other immunosuppressants, such as calcineurin inhibitors, appear successful in some forms of C3G. Rituximab has been proposed for forms with demonstrated C3Nef, but results have been mostly unsatisfactory. Therefore, at the present time, these therapies cannot be recommended and must be judged on a case-by-case basis.

Plasmapheresis or plasma infusions allow the removal of excess fluid-phase complement factors and the substitution of insufficient factors by fresh plasma. However, reports on the effectiveness of this approach are discordant. Its use may be recommended only for forms with rapid progression where other options seem ineffective or in the presence of CFH mutations or anti-CFH antibodies as these forms of disease seem to be most responsive to this approach.

Based on our understanding of disease pathogenesis, complement inhibition is a rational therapeutic option. However, the only complement inhibitors currently available are eculizumab and ravulizumab, monoclonal antibodies that bind C5 and block formation of the MAC, clearly acting downstream of the disease-initiating process. Published reports of small groups of patients or case reports have shown the clear benefit of eculizumab for reducing proteinuria in some but not all patients. A reduction in the degree of mesangial proliferation and inflammation detected by kidney biopsy has also been reported in keeping with the proinflammatory role played by C5a, while discordant results have been reported on its effect on C3 deposition. Interestingly, patients with high circulating levels of sC5b-9 appear to be more responsive to this therapeutic approach. Moreover, eculizumab appears more clearly beneficial in patients with intense proteinuria and a relatively brief disease history, and treatment seems to have little or no impact on chronic lesions. However, treatment with eculizumab is expensive, requires chronic intravenous administration, and puts patients at increased risk of meningococcal infection. Furthermore, the only available clinical trial assessing this therapeutic agent for C3G failed to show significant benefit in most patients. A variety of other complement inhibitors are becoming available and are currently being assessed in clinical trials.

In patients with an underlying monoclonal gammopathy, it is believed that the paraprotein causes complement dysregulation and drives the disease. Some patients with C3G and a monoclonal gammopathy do not have an underlying malignancy, but they still develop kidney injury as a result of the excess paraprotein ("monoclonal gammopathy of kidney significance"). In patients who do have an underlying malignancy, treatment is usually dictated by the nature of malignant process. Treatment may also be beneficial in patients who do not have a malignancy but who have C3G, even though these patients might otherwise not be treated. A study of 50 adult patients with C3g and a detectable monoclonal spike, for example, demonstrated that B cell- or plasma cell-targeted treatments improved the kidney disease, and those patients with a hematologic response were the ones most likely to have an improvement in their kidney disease.

Transplantation

The rate of recurrence after transplantation is 60% to 85% for patients with DDD, and the risk of allograft failure is about 45% to 50% at 5 years. For C3GN, reports are scantier, but studies have shown recurrence in approximately two-thirds of recipients, with approximately one-third losing their allograft within 5 years of transplantation. Of note, patients with C3G in their native kidneys have developed thrombotic microangiopathy in their allografts after transplantation.

Published reports have shown the benefit of complement inhibition with eculizumab in treating posttransplant recurrences of disease. In general, the therapeutic approach to posttransplant recurrences should mirror the approach to native kidney disease, with a more aggressive attitude, due to the fact that these are usually rapidly progressive forms and promptly detected with routine monitoring. Plasmapheresis or complement inhibition may be considered early, particularly due to the fact that all patients are already receiving transplant-related immunosuppression.

Complement-Mediated Thrombotic Microangiopathy

The thrombotic microangiopathies (TMAs) refer to a group of diseases that are characterized by microangiopathic hemolytic anemia, thrombocytopenia, and kidney injury. Multiple systemic diseases, infections, and drugs are associated with the development of TMA. The clinical presentation can also vary among patients, making TMAs challenging to diagnose and classify.

Over time there has been debate as to whether thrombotic thrombocytopenic purpura (TTP) and HUS are the same disease or distinct entities. The discovery that TTP is usually associated with a deficiency of ADAMTS13 lent support to the distinction of these two diseases. HUS was first identified as a distinct entity in children, and it was recognized that affected patients develop particularly severe kidney failure. The majority of cases of HUS occur in pediatric patients after infections with bacteria that produce Shiga-like toxin (Stx). Over time, HUS that is not associated with Stx-producing bacteria has been termed *diarrhea negative* and

atypical HUS. A large body of evidence now demonstrates that the majority of these HUS patients have defects in regulation of the alternative pathway, and some experts refer to this subset of patients as having complement-mediated TMA.

There are several systemic diseases, drugs, and infections that are associated with TMAs (Table 22.3). It is not yet clear to what extent TMAs in these different settings share a common pathophysiology, but there is some overlap. In patients with complement-mediated HUS, for example, disease is often triggered by systemic illness. Conversely, only a small proportion of the patients exposed to the events that can trigger TMAs go on to develop the disease, indicating that other predisposing or mitigating factors must be present. For these reasons, it can be difficult to identify which patients have complement-mediated TMA. Furthermore, complement activation may be important in the pathogenesis of TMA caused by other clinical triggers. For example, underlying complement defects may be present in the majority of women who develop postpartum HUS. In this chapter, we use the term *Stx-HUS* for disease caused by Stx-producing bacteria, *secondary HUS* for patients with known causes of the disease, and *aHUS* for patients with complement-mediated disease and no identifiable cause of secondary disease. The classification of individual patients can be challenging, however, and the diagnosis and classification of

TABLE 22.3	Secondary Causes of Hemolytic Uremic Syndrome
Metabolic	Cobalamin deficiency (homozygous deficiency)
	Diacylglycerol kinase ε mutation (homozygous or compound heterozygous)
Infections	Shiga-like toxin producing bacteria (primarily *Escherichia coli* serotypes 0157:H7, 0111:H8, 0103:H2, 0123, 026 or *Shigella dysenteriae*)
	Neuraminidase producing *Streptococcus pneumoniae*
	Human immunodeficiency virus
	Hepatitis A, B, and C
	Parvovirus B19
	Cytomegalovirus
	Coxsackie B virus
	Influenza H1/N1
Autoimmune diseases	Systemic lupus erythematosus
	Scleroderma
	Antiphospholipid syndrome
	Dermatomyositis
Drugs	Calcineurin inhibitors
	Quinine
	Mitomycin
	Clopidogrel
	VEGF inhibitors
	Vincristine
	Gemcitabine
	Alemtuzumab
	Cocaine
Other systemic clinical conditions	Pregnancy
	Cancer
	Bone marrow transplantation
	Malignant hypertension
	Antibody-mediated rejection of a kidney transplant

the different types of TMA will undoubtedly evolve as additional studies improve our understanding of these diseases.

Epidemiology

The incidence of aHUS is extremely low and has been estimated at approximately 3.3 cases per million children and 0.5 to 2 cases per million adults. Onset of TMA in the first 6 months of life is extremely suggestive of aHUS. Most patients present before 40 years of age, but patients have presented in their 80s. The two most critical ages for development of the disease are early childhood (before 5 years of age) and after pregnancy for women. In general, atypical complement-mediated HUS represents the majority of adult HUS cases and 5% to 10% of HUS cases in children, where Stx-HUS is predominant. Approximately 20% of patients have familial disease, and these patients are more likely to present as children. Men and women are affected equally overall, but among adults, the disease is more common in women. Approximately 40% of patients with aHUS will have a relapse, the majority of which occur within the first year after disease onset.

Etiology and Pathogenesis

An underlying complement defect can be identified in approximately 70% of patients with aHUS. The majority of complement defects are genetic mutations or rare variants in the genes of complement factors, but autoantibodies to complement proteins are seen in some patients (Table 22.4). Similar to C3G, these various molecular defects are usually associated with defective regulation or enhanced activity of the alternative pathway of complement.

Genetic Causes

Mutations in the genes for many different complement proteins have been identified in patients with aHUS, including factor H, factor I, MCP, C3, the CFHRs, and factor B (see Table 22.4). Mutations in non-complement genes have also been identified in patients with aHUS. For example, thrombomodulin mutations have been found in approximately 3% of patients. Although this protein is not usually regarded as part of the complement system, there is evidence that it has complement regulatory functions that are impaired by these mutations. Mutations in the gene for diacylglycerol kinase ε *(DGKE)* have been identified in infants with HUS. It is not known whether *DGKE* mutations affect complement regulation or whether these patients have a distinct pathophysiology.

Functionally, most complement mutations associated with aHUS cause impaired regulation of the alternative pathway. In most patients, the mutations are heterozygous, causing only a partial defect in regulation. The mutations also tend to affect complement regulation on cell and tissue surfaces. MCP, for example, is expressed on the plasma membrane of cells. The underlying complement defects affect disease severity, and the prognosis is better for patients with *MCP* mutations than for patients with mutations in other complement genes. Even without treatment, most patients with *MCP* mutations will have self-limited disease, whereas the majority of patients with mutations in other complement genes will reach ESKD or death without treatment. Because MCP is a cell surface protein, kidney transplantation effectively corrects this molecular defect. Approximately 3% of patients have combined mutations in multiple complement genes, and the presence of multiple complement mutations increases disease penetrance.

TABLE 22.4	Complement Defects Associated With Atypical Hemolytic Uremic Syndrome	
Complement Protein	**Defect**
Factor H	Protein • Levels low in some patients Autoantibody • Present in ~5%–10% of patients. Usually binds carboxy terminus Mutations • Most commonly affected gene in aHUS. Majority of mutations are heterozygous. More than 150 variants described, and most affect SCR19-20 region.
Membrane cofactor protein	Protein • Levels low in some patients with mutations. Can be measured by flow cytometry Mutations • Majority of mutations are heterozygous. Present in 8%–10% of patients.
Factor I	Mutations • Majority of mutations are heterozygous. Present in 4%–8% of patients.
C3	Protein • Levels low in ~50% of patients Mutations • Present in 4%–8% of patients. Can increase binding to factor B or decrease binding to regulatory proteins.
Factor B	Mutations • Present in 1%–4% of patients. Mutations cause gain of function
CFHR1	Mutations • Hybrid *CFH/CFHR1* gene may be present in 3%–5% of patients with aHUS
CFHR3	Mutation • Hybrid *CFH/CFHR3* gene
CHFR1-3 deletion	Deletion of CFHR1 in 90% of patients with anti-factor H autoantibodies

aHUS, Atypical hemolytic uremic syndrome; *CFHR*, complement factor H–related protein; *CFH*, complement factor H; *SCR*, short consensus repeat.

Mutations and variants in the gene for factor H *(CFH)* are seen in more than 20% of patients with aHUS, and *CFH* is the most commonly affected complement gene. Most of the mutations in the gene for factor H that are associated with aHUS affect the carboxy terminus of the protein, a region of the protein that binds GAGs and sialic acid moieties on cell surfaces but does not directly contribute to the complement regulatory function of the protein. Consequently, mutations in this region of factor H specifically limit the ability of the protein to regulate the alternative pathway on tissue surfaces. *CFH* and the complement factor H–related *(CFHR 1–5)* genes are located next to each other on chromosome 1q32. Various hybrid genes caused by nonallelic homologous recombination of the *CFH* and *CFHR* genes have been identified. Some of the identified mutations in the CFHRs affect the tendency of these proteins to form multimers, which are believed to have increased affinity for surfaces and competitively reduce the binding of factor H. Thus, mutations and deletions of the *CFHRs* may affect the availability of factor H, indirectly affecting alternative pathway activation.

Autoantibodies

Approximately 10% of patients with aHUS have autoantibodies to factor H. The antibodies usually bind the carboxy terminus of factor H, the region where most of the aHUS-associated mutations are found. Interestingly, more than 90% of the patients who develop these antibodies have deletions in the *CFHR1* and *CFHR3* genes.

Triggers

Disease penetrance is approximately 50% for patients carrying disease-associated complement mutations. Furthermore, many patients with congenital complement mutations present in adulthood. These observations indicate that additional factors contribute to the development of disease, even in patients with underlying impairments in their ability to regulate the alternative pathway. Approximately 30% of aHUS episodes are preceded by diarrhea, and this is the most common trigger in children. Pregnancy is the most common trigger in adults. Disease recurrence is frequent in patients following kidney transplantation, likely because the recipients have an impaired ability to control alternative pathway activation on the ischemic allograft.

Pathology

Kidney biopsy is seldom performed at disease onset, as severe hypertension and very low platelet counts make this procedure too dangerous. However, due to the importance of establishing a correct diagnosis for treatment and prognosis, a biopsy is warranted as soon as clinical conditions allow.

TMA is characterized by (1) endothelial damage with swelling and, as the lesion progresses toward chronicity, formation of double contours along the glomerular capillary walls; (2) thrombi with schistocytes in glomerular capillaries, arterioles, and small arteries; and (3) mesangiolysis (Fig. 22.4). Glomeruli can appear shrunken and ischemic, with wrinkling of the basement membrane corresponding to the injured glomerular capillaries. Obstruction of the microcirculation due to thrombi can lead to acute cortical ischemia with cortical necrosis, which is irreversible and correlates with the degree of chronic kidney damage. Involvement of arteries is accompanied by severe hypertension. Immunofluorescence is negative for immunoglobulin and complement factors and positive for fibrinogen within blood vessels. The endothelium of arterioles and small arteries can be positive for complement activation products. Electron microscopy shows intracapillary fibrin and platelet aggregates, lucent subendothelial expansion with deposition of fluffy material and reduplication of the GBM, and no electron-dense deposits. These features are common to all forms of TMA, including TTP and Stx-HUS. Although the TMA in HUS by definition involves primarily the kidney microvasculature, other organs can be involved. The brain is the next most frequently involved organ (70%), followed by the heart, intestine, lungs, and pancreas in about 20% of patients.

Clinical and Laboratory Features

Clinical onset of aHUS is usually sudden, with pallor, fatigue, general malaise, drowsiness, vomiting, and sometimes edema. Triggering events are very common. In children, these events are most frequently infections (80% of pediatric cases, 50% of cases in adults), usually involving the respiratory or gastrointestinal tracts. Other triggers of HUS in adults include pregnancy (80% of these cases occur in the postpartum period), malignancies, autoimmune diseases, transplantation or other surgical procedures, trauma, and drugs (calcineurin inhibitors, sirolimus, anti-vascular endothelial growth factor agents; see Table 22.3).

The clinical picture is characterized by the triad of (1) anemia with hemoglobin less than 10 g/dL, (2) thrombocytopenia with platelets less than 150,000/μL, and (3) reduced kidney function with oligoanuria and hypertension. If urinary output is present, proteinuria and hematuria are observed with red blood cell casts and cellular debris in the sediment.

Anemia is caused by intravascular hemolysis with platelet consumption due to formation of microthrombi, primarily in the blood vessels of the kidney and less frequently in other organs, including the brain. Schistocytes are present in the peripheral blood smear, lactate dehydrogenase is markedly elevated, and haptoglobin is severely reduced or undetectable. Coombs test is negative as the hemolysis is of mechanical origin, not immune-mediated. Low circulating complement, particularly C3, may be present but is not required.

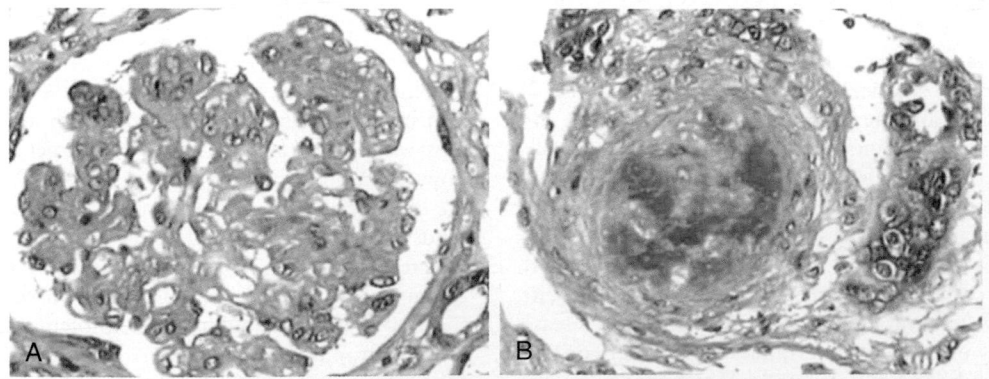

• **Fig. 22.4** Histologic appearance of the kidney in atypical hemolytic uremic syndrome. (A) A typical glomerular lesion with microthrombi within the glomerular capillary lumen. (B) A small artery nearly entirely occluded by thrombotic material and erythrocytes and showing myointimal proliferation. (From Noris M, Remuzzi G. Glomerular diseases dependent on complement activation, including atypical hemolytic uremic syndrome, membranoproliferative glomerulonephritis, and C3 glomerulopathy: core curriculum 2015. *Am J Kidney Dis*. 2015;66:359–375.)

Arterial hypertension is generally severe due to fluid overload when oligoanuria is present and to increased renin secretion due to arterial TMA. However, if the clinical condition is severe, the blood pressure can be low due to infection, hypovolemia, or critical illness. Frequently, electrolyte abnormalities (hyperkalemia, hyponatremia) and metabolic acidosis are present, and about half of children and 80% of adults require dialysis at presentation.

Extrarenal symptoms are present in about 20% of patients. Patients may seek attention for neurologic symptoms of variable intensity, ranging from mild findings in approximately 10% of cases (drowsiness, slight confusion, and irritability) to more severe signs such as seizures and profound loss of conscience with stupor and coma. Diplopia or cortical blindness, hemiparesis, and hemiplegia have also been reported. Heart failure from cardiac involvement and fluid overload can be present and severe, leading to sudden death.

Stool must be checked for intestinal bleeding, and an abdominal ultrasound looking at the integrity of intestinal walls should be performed. Some patients (about 5%) present with fulminant multiorgan involvement, with kidney failure, seizures, intestinal bleeding, heart failure, pulmonary hemorrhage, hepatic cytolysis, and pancreatitis. Some cases present with a less acute, more indolent presentation, and fluctuating progression may be observed with mild GFR loss, proteinuria, microscopic hematuria, moderate hematologic abnormalities, and some degree of arterial hypertension. This is characteristic of HUS associated with transplantation, both of solid organ and of bone marrow. Rarely, hematologic abnormalities can be absent, with kidney findings of proteinuria, occasionally in the nephrotic range, microscopic hematuria, some degree of GFR loss, and arterial hypertension predominating.

All efforts must be made to rapidly make the correct diagnosis as aHUS is a life-threatening disease in which kidney biopsy is frequently not possible. Screening for Shiga toxin must be performed by stool or rectal swab culture and polymerase chain reaction and serologies for antilipopolysaccharides should be sent in all children, even if diarrhea is not reported, as Stx-HUS is by far the most common form of HUS in children. Other infectious causes (*Streptococcus pneumoniae*, HIV, other viruses, etc.) must be investigated based on the presenting features and clinical history. The diagnosis of TTP is based on measurement of ADAMTS13 activity, keeping in mind that, especially in the pediatric setting, this value may be lower than the normal range, and it is considered indicative of TTP only if activity is less than 10%. In children, especially infants younger than 6 months of age, serum homocysteine levels and urinary organic acids should be measured to search for cyanocobalamin C deficiency leading to methylmalonic aciduria, a rare metabolic disorder that can cause HUS. Infants or small children, especially with concomitant nephrotic syndrome, must also be screened for DGKE mutations.

When typical HUS, TTP, and secondary forms of HUS have been excluded or appear unlikely, patients should be screened for complement abnormalities. This is particularly true in patients with reduced circulating C3 levels or a family history of kidney failure, sudden unexplained death, coagulopathies, hypertension, or glomerulopathies. Complement analysis includes measurement of circulating complement factors, anti-factor H antibodies, and screening for genetic mutations of CFH, CFI, MCP (or CD46), C3, CFB, and thrombomodulin (see Table 22.4). The age of onset, circulating C3 levels, and clinical features can be useful indicators of which complement gene or abnormality to screen first. For example, age greater than 1 year and relatively mild phenotype with a normal C3 level suggest MCP mutations, whereas a low C3 level suggests fluid phase abnormalities such as CFH, CFI, or C3 mutations. Concomitant coagulopathy or pulmonary hypertension suggests thrombomodulin mutations. Children older than 7 years with a low C3 level suggests anti-factor H antibodies.

Untreated, the natural history of the full-blown clinical syndrome is severe, with 2% to 10% of patients dying and one-third of patients progressing to ESKD. Nearly half of patients experience disease relapses. Moreover, except for patients with MCP mutations, all others have a high risk of posttransplant recurrence.

Treatment

Many patients with a full clinical picture of HUS are critically ill and require intensive care and hemodialysis. Every effort should be made to manage them in a setting with expertise in emergent dialysis. Infusion of platelets is contraindicated, unless there is a hemorrhagic event or a high-risk procedure is necessary. Before 2010, the use of intensive and early plasma exchange was advocated to replenish missing or malfunctioning factors and to curb the complement alternative pathway dysregulation. This approach was accompanied by significant side effects, especially in children, and it was only partially effective.

The use of the monoclonal anti-C5 antibody eculizumab, which inhibits the terminal complement pathway, has dramatically changed the natural history of this disease from a dismal prognosis to a severe but manageable condition. Eculizumab acts by binding C5 and blocking formation of C5b-9. Several clinical trials and a vast number of case reports have shown that its use is effective at all ages, both in normalizing hematologic parameters and improving kidney function in primary disease, and in allowing successful kidney transplantation in patients who have already reached ESKD. A longer acting anti-C5 antibody (ravulizumab) is also effective for treating aHUS. Although it was not compared side-by-side with eculizumab, the response to treatment was similar to previously reported results, and the drug only needs to be re-dosed every 8 weeks.

The availability of eculizumab makes rapid diagnosis of aHUS crucial, as early initiation of therapy is essential for optimal outcome. Therefore, aHUS must be considered the primary diagnosis, and eculizumab therapy, if available, must be initiated if (1) secondary HUS has been excluded (no drugs, malignancies, autoimmune diseases, etc.), especially in adults; (2) Stx-HUS has been excluded, especially in children; and (3) ADAMTS13 activity is greater than 10% and TTP has been excluded. When these criteria are established, a complete workup of complement proteins, alternative pathway genes, and anticomplement factor H autoantibodies should be performed.

Because eculizumab blocks the terminal complement pathway, the drug makes patients more susceptible to infections by encapsulated bacteria—mainly *Neisseria meningitidis*. Therefore, when possible, all patients should receive anti-meningococcal vaccination (both serotype A, C, Y, W, and serotype B) 15 days before first infusion. In critically ill patients, treatment should start under antibiotic prophylaxis (with methylpenicillin or a macrolide), and vaccination should be performed when possible. Vaccination against *S. pneumoniae* and *Haemophilus influenzae* is also prudent. Moreover, in immunocompromised patients, children, and individuals at increased risk (e.g., young adults living in communities), it may be advisable to maintain antibiotic prophylaxis as long as the patient is on eculizumab therapy.

Therapy with eculizumab is not disease modifying, and treatment discontinuation entails a nonquantifiable risk of disease relapse. During therapy, a simple way to evaluate effective complement inhibition is measurement of CH50, which must be less than 10%. The issue of if and when to discontinue eculizumab is much debated and beyond the scope of this chapter but must be assessed on a case-by-case basis, depending on age, type of mutation, risk of relapse, kidney function, and vascular access.

Of note, when anti-factor H autoantibodies are present, therapy with plasma exchange combined with immunosuppression (steroids plus azathioprine, mycophenolate mofetil, cyclophosphamide, or rituximab) is effective, though not standardized. The response to therapy can be monitored by measuring anti-factor H antibodies, which correlate closely with the risk of disease relapse.

When eculizumab is not available or ADAMTS13 activity is not readily available, plasma exchange therapy can be started at 1.5 plasma volumes (about 65 to 70 mL/kg), exchanging with fresh frozen plasma. If plasma exchange therapy is not available, plasma infusion can be considered if the patient does not present with fluid overload, heart failure, or severe hypertension. Of note, if HUS is secondary to *S. pneumoniae* infection, therapy with plasma must be avoided as it worsens the disease. In other forms of HUS, lack of improvement of hemolysis parameters and kidney function after 3 to 5 days of daily plasma exchange or plasma infusion indicates a failure of this therapeutic approach.

Kidney Transplantation

The risk of aHUS recurrence after transplantation varies according to the mutation type, but most experts currently agree that all patients with aHUS, with or without a known mutation, should be transplanted under eculizumab therapy. An alternative option is a combined liver-kidney transplant, as liver transplantation in aHUS due to mutations in the genes for factor H, factor I, C3, or factor B can restore the malfunctioning complement regulator. This is currently the only disease-modifying definitive cure, but plasma exchange or eculizumab should be used at the time of transplantation to protect the transplanted liver from complement-mediated injury until it can replenish these proteins.

Comparison of the Underlying Mechanisms of C3 Glomerulopathy and Atypical Hemolytic Uremic Syndrome

C3G and aHUS are both associated with defects in the regulation of the alternative pathway of complement, and it is striking that the kidney is the target of complement-mediated injury in patients with such a large number of different congenital and acquired complement defects. Yet aHUS and C3G are clinically distinct diseases—C3G typically presents as a proliferative glomerulonephritis, whereas aHUS presents as a TMA (Table 22.5). There is heterogeneity in both diseases, however. For example, the histologic patterns of injury can vary among patients with C3G. In general, the molecular complement defects in patients with aHUS tend to affect complement regulation on surfaces. Most of the mutations in *CFH*, for example, affect SCRs 19 and 20. Complement defects in patients with C3G, on the other hand, tend to affect complement regulation in the fluid phase. These differences are not absolute, however, and some of the mutations found in patients with C3G (e.g., mutations in *CFHR5*) are believed to reduce binding of factor H to tissue surfaces. Furthermore, some complement gene mutations have been identified in patients with both diseases, and C3G patients have developed TMA in their kidney allografts after transplantation.

It is not yet known why patients with similar defects in alternative pathway regulation manifest at different ages and with distinct clinical syndromes. It is possible that variations in other genes modify the exact location and nature of these diseases or that disease triggers or associated illnesses influence how the diseases manifest. Future work will hopefully answer these questions and improve our understanding of how best to predict, diagnose, and treat these kidney diseases.

Complete bibliography is available at Elsevier eBooks for Practicing Clinicians.

TABLE 22.5	Comparison of Findings in C3 Glomerulopathy and Atypical Hemolytic Uremic Syndrome	
	C3 Glomerulopathy	**Atypical Hemolytic Uremic Syndrome**
Membranoproliferative pattern by light microscopy/C3 deposition	+++	±
Low C3	++	±
Mutations	CFH, C3, CFI, MCP, CFHR5	CFH, MCP, CFI, CFB, C3, THBD
Type of mutations	DDD: Homozyg > Heterozyg GN-C3: Heterozyg > Homozyg	Heterozyg > Homozyg
Common polymorphisms	CFH	CFH, MCP CFHR1/CFHR3
Common haplotypes	Maybe	Yes
Autoantibodies	C3Ne FAnti-FH Anti-C3b, factor B	Anti-FH
Activation of the alternative pathway	Fluid phase/?cell surfaces	Yes/cell surfaces
Activation of the terminal pathway	+	+++
Response to anti-C5	±	++++

CFHR, Complement factor H–related protein; *CFH*, complement factor H; *DDD*, dense-deposit disease; *MCP*, membrane cofactor protein.

Key Bibliography

Bomback AS, Santoriello D, Avasare RS, et al. C3 glomerulonephritis and dense deposit disease share a similar disease course in a large United States cohort of patients with C3 glomerulopathy. *Kidney Int.* 2018;93(4):977–985.

Chauvet S, Fremeaux-Bacchi V, Petitprez F, et al. Treatment of B-cell disorder improves renal outcome of patients with monoclonal gammopathy-associated C3 glomerulopathy. *Blood.* 2017;129(11):1437–1447.

Chen Q, Wiesener M, Eberhardt HU, et al. Complement factor H-related hybrid protein deregulates complement in dense deposit disease. *J Clin Invest.* 2014;124:145–155.

Dragon-Durey MA, Fremeaux-Bacchi V, Loirat C, et al. Heterozygous and homozygous factor H deficiencies associated with hemolytic uremic syndrome or membranoproliferative glomerulonephritis: report and genetic analysis of 16 cases. *J Am Soc Nephrol.* 2004;15:787–795.

Dragon-Durey MA, Sethi SK, Bagga A, et al. Clinical features of anti-factor H autoantibody-associated hemolytic uremic syndrome. *J Am Soc Nephrol.* 2010;21:2180–2187.

Fakhouri F, Le Quintrec M, Fremeaux-Bacchi V. Practical management of C3 glomerulopathy and immunoglobulin-mediated MPGN: facts and uncertainties. *Kidney Int.* 2020.

Fakhouri F, Roumenina L, Provot F, et al. Pregnancy-associated hemolytic uremic syndrome revisited in the era of complement gene mutations. *J Am Soc Nephrol.* 2010;21:859–867.

Fremeaux-Bacchi V, Fakhouri F, Garnier A, et al. Genetics and outcome of atypical hemolytic uremic syndrome: a nationwide French series comparing children and adults. *Clin J Am Soc Nephrol.* 2013;8:554–562.

Gale DP, de Jorge EG, Cook HT, et al. Identification of a mutation in complement factor H-related protein 5 in patients of Cypriot origin with glomerulonephritis. *Lancet.* 2010;376:794–801.

Loirat C, Fakhouri F, Ariceta G, et al. An international consensus approach to the management of atypical hemolytic uremic syndrome in children. *Pediatr Nephrol.* 2015;31:15–39.

Martinez-Barricarte R, Heurich M, Valdes-Canedo F, et al. Human C3 mutation reveals a mechanism of dense deposit disease pathogenesis and provides insights into complement activation and regulation. *J Clin Invest.* 2010;120:3702–3712.

Nasr SH, Valeri AM, Appel GB, et al. Dense deposit disease: clinicopathologic study of 32 pediatric and adult patients. *Clin J Am Soc Nephrol.* 2009;4:22–32.

Noris M, Caprioli J, Bresin E, et al. Relative role of genetic complement abnormalities in sporadic and familial aHUS and their impact on clinical phenotype. *Clin J Am Soc Nephrol.* 2010;5:1844–1859.

Pickering MC, D'Agati VD, Nester CM, et al. C3 glomerulopathy: consensus report. *Kidney Int.* 2013;84:1079–1089.

Rabasco C, Cavero T, Roman E, et al. Effectiveness of mycophenolate mofetil in C3 glomerulonephritis. *Kidney Int.* 2015;88:1153–1160.

Ruggenenti P, Daina E, Gennarini A, et al. C5 convertase blockade in membranoproliferative glomerulonephritis: a single-arm clinical trial. *Am J Kidney Dis.* 2019;74(2):224–238.

Servais A, Fremeaux-Bacchi V, Lequintrec M, et al. Primary glomerulonephritis with isolated C3 deposits: a new entity which shares common genetic risk factors with haemolytic uraemic syndrome. *J Med Genet.* 2007;44:193–199.

Servais A, Noel LH, Roumenina LT, et al. Acquired and genetic complement abnormalities play a critical role in dense deposit disease and other C3 glomerulopathies. *Kidney Int.* 2012;82:454–464.

Smith RJH, Appel GB, Blom AM, et al. C3 glomerulopathy - understanding a rare complement-driven renal disease. *Nature reviews Nephrology.* 2019;15(3):129–143.

23

Infection-Related Glomerulonephritis

LAURA FERREIRA PROVENZANO, LEAL HERLITZ

In previous editions, this chapter was titled "Post-infectious Glomerulonephritis," which aptly describes classic post-streptococcal glomerulonephritis (PSGN) but is a misnomer for the increasingly recognized forms of glomerulonephritis (GN) that are manifestations of ongoing infection. Indeed, infection has a much broader role in the development of GN, sometimes serving as a trigger for a variety of common autoimmune responses including lupus, antineutrophil cytoplasmic antibody (ANCA) vasculitis, and IgA nephropathy. This chapter addresses both classic PSGN as well as forms of GN resulting from active bacterial infections. Glomerular disease due to viral hepatitis and HIV are discussed elsewhere. The change in the title from "Post-infectious" to "Infection-Related Glomerulonephritis (IRGN)" is meant to draw attention to the changing epidemiology of IRGN and to emphasize that infection may be ongoing at the time of the development of GN, which is important for guiding therapy.

Clinical Features

The clinical presentation of IRGN is variable, ranging from asymptomatic, incidentally discovered urinary abnormalities to a rapidly progressive GN requiring kidney replacement therapy. Clinical findings include hematuria, which can be either microscopic or gross; proteinuria, which is usually subnephrotic but can be in the nephrotic range; and variable degrees of hypertension, edema, and glomerular filtration rate (GFR) loss. The presentation and outcomes in children are often different from those in adults (Table 23.1).

In classic PSGN, symptomatic children usually present with acute nephritic syndrome characterized by hematuria, proteinuria, hypertension, edema, oliguria, and variable elevation of the serum creatinine. The urinary sediment is usually active, with dysmorphic red blood cells, red blood cell casts, and leukocyturia. Hypocomplementemia is very common, with decreased C3 in up to 90% of cases and, to a lesser extent, depleted levels of C4. There is usually a "latent" period between the resolution of the streptococcal infection and the acute onset of the nephritic syndrome. This period is often 7 to 10 days after oropharyngeal infections and 2 to 4 weeks after skin infections. Serologic markers of a recent streptococcal infection include elevated antistreptolysin O (ASO), antistreptokinase, antihyaluronidase, and antideoxyribonuclease B (anti-DNase B) levels. Elevation of these four markers has a yield of approximately 80% in documenting recent streptococcal infection.

In adults, most cases of IRGN no longer follow streptococcal infection, and the GN often coexists with the triggering infection. In cases of ongoing active infection, other clinical manifestations related to the specific infectious disease are common. Sites of infection can include the upper and lower respiratory tract, skin/soft tissue, bone, teeth/oral mucosa, heart, deep abscesses, shunts, and indwelling catheters. GFR loss and the nephrotic syndrome are more common in adults than in children, whereas gross hematuria is less commonly seen. Hypocomplementemia is only seen in 30% to 80% of these patients. Adults more commonly present with kidney failure and with complications of hypervolemia, including decompensated heart failure. Up to 50% of adults with IRGN may require dialysis, and mortality may approach 20%.

Epidemiology

The incidence of PSGN has declined throughout most of the world over the past several decades due to improvements in hygiene, sanitation, and infection control, but still remains a health concern in many developing countries. An effort by Carpentis and colleagues to evaluate the incidence of PSGN using 11 population-based studies suggests that approximately 472,000 cases of PSGN occur worldwide annually, resulting in approximately 5000 deaths (1% of total cases). Approximately 97% of these cases of PSGN occur in less developed countries. Other estimates of the burden of PSGN in the developing world range between 9.5 and 28.5 cases of PSGN per 100,000 individuals per year.

In industrialized countries, much of the burden of IRGN has shifted to adults, with a lower proportion attributed to PSGN. IRGN associated with other microorganisms, including *Staphylococcus* species and gram-negative bacteria, are increasingly recognized, mainly in the adult population. In these cases, coexistence of the glomerular disease and the infection is common, and classic clinical findings of low complement levels may be absent. The clinical course and prognosis of these newly recognized forms are also different, with more patients developing progressive chronic kidney disease (CKD), sometimes to end-stage kidney disease (ESKD). Diabetes is the most commonly recognized comorbidity and is associated with poor outcomes. Other common comorbidities seen in patients with IRGN include malignancy, immunosuppression, AIDS, alcoholism, cirrhosis, malnutrition, and IV drug use. The elderly population is especially prone to IRGN, with patients over 65 years of age accounting for about 34% of IRGN cases in the developed world, increased from only 4% to 6% of recognized IRGN 40 years ago.

Histopathology

A spectrum of histologic findings can be seen in IRGN, and biopsy findings are influenced by the associated organism and site and duration of infection.

TABLE 23.1	Common Differences in Infection-Related Glomerulonephritis Between Children and Adults				
	Onset of Glomerulonephritis	Infection Site	Bacterial Organisms	Low C3	Prognosis
Children	After infection (typical latency 1–4 weeks)	Pharyngitis, skin (impetigo)	Predominantly streptococcal	≈90% of cases	Excellent (>90% make a full recovery)
Adults	During ongoing infection	Highly variable, including respiratory tract, skin, heart, urinary tract, bone, oral/dental	Staphylococcal ≥ streptococcal, gram-negative organisms	30%–80% of cases	Guarded, with residual chronic kidney disease common; elderly patients and those with diabetic nephropathy show full recovery in <25% of cases

Light microscopy can reveal a wide range of proliferative glomerular lesions (Fig. 23.1). The most common finding in acute IRGN, including PSGN, is that of diffuse endocapillary hypercellularity, with significant numbers of infiltrating neutrophils. While occasional cellular crescents may be seen with these diffuse proliferative GNs, crescent formation in >50% of glomeruli is uncommon. More subacute or remote cases of IRGN may show only focal endocapillary hypercellularity or simply mesangial hypercellularity. In longer-standing, ongoing infections such as shunt nephritis, a membranoproliferative pattern with large subendothelial deposits can be seen. Necrotizing and crescentic histology, similar to what can be seen in ANCA vasculitis, is increasingly recognized as a pattern of IRGN associated with endocarditis. In the adult population, acute GN may be superimposed on chronic conditions such as diabetic nephropathy, and this can alter the histologic appearance.

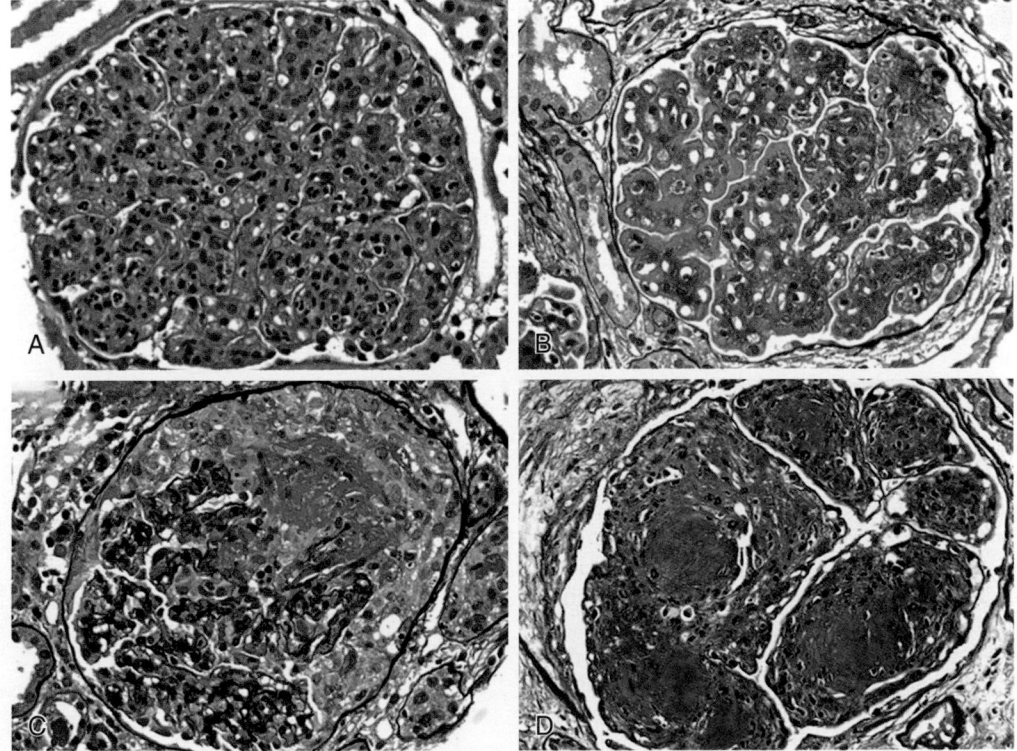

• **Fig. 23.1** Diverse light microscopic patterns of glomerular injury in infection-related glomerulonephritis. (A) Diffuse endocapillary hypercellularity and exudative (neutrophil-rich) glomerulonephritis (hematoxylin and eosin, 400× magnification) is the most common pathology encountered in infection-related glomerulonephritis. (B) A membranoproliferative pattern (Jones methenamine silver stain, 400× magnification) with large subendothelial immune deposits can be seen in cases where infection is long-standing, such as in shunt nephritis. (C) Intravascular infections such as endocarditis may display a necrotizing crescentic glomerulonephritis with few immune deposits (Jones methenamine silver stain, 400× magnification), strikingly similar to what is classically seen in ANCA vasculitis. (D) Underlying chronic diseases, such as diabetic nephropathy, may exist and modify the appearance of glomeruli. A glomerulus with large mesangial nodules due to diabetes, as well as an exudative endocapillary proliferative glomerulonephritis (periodic acid–Schiff, 400× magnification).

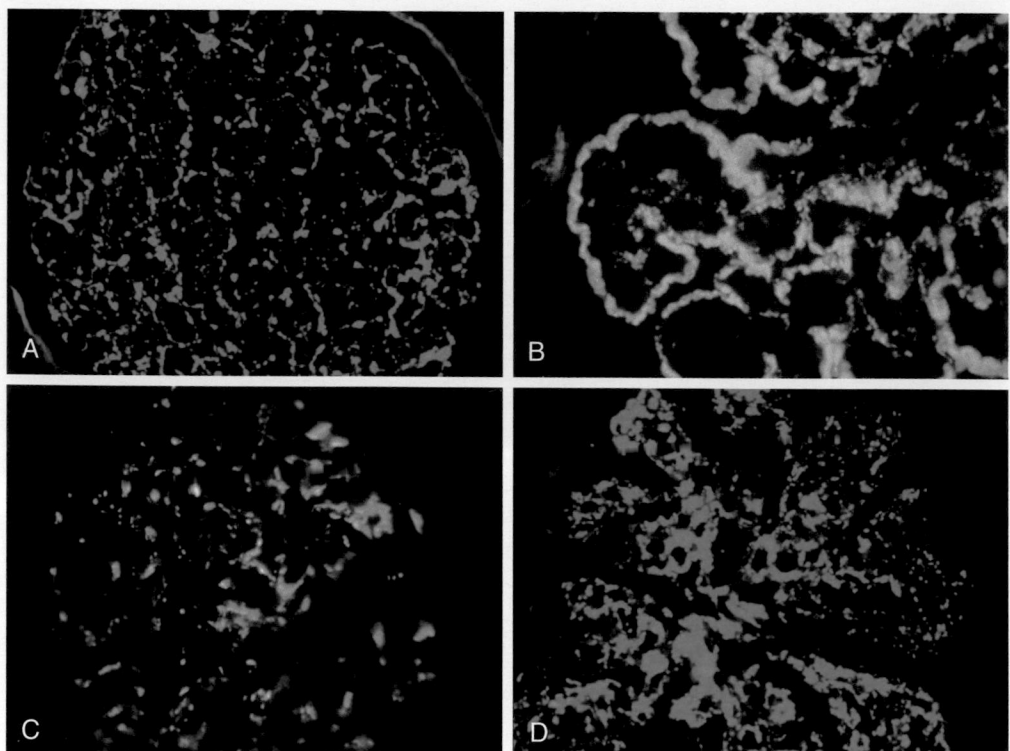

• **Fig. 23.2** Immunofluorescence findings in infection-related glomerulonephritis. Deposits are typically C3 dominant or co-dominant and accompanied by immunoglobulin staining of lesser intensity. (A) The classic "starry sky" appearance of C3 encountered in infection-related glomerulonephritis (IRGN), which results from the scattered combination of subepithelial, mesangial, and subendothelial deposits (400× magnification). The "garland pattern" of C3 staining is illustrated in (B) (600× magnification), and more clearly demonstrates the contour of the glomerular basement membrane, because subepithelial deposits are in abundance and nearly confluent. (C) Predominantly mesangial deposits of C3 with only rare peripheral capillary wall deposits (400× magnification). This pattern of staining is most commonly seen in the subacute and resolving stages of IRGN. The staining in (D) is for IgA (400× magnification), and a nodular, largely mesangial distribution of positive staining can be seen. This glomerulus is from a patient with a *Staphylococcus aureus*–associated IRGN superimposed on underlying diabetic nephropathy (for the corresponding light microscopic image, see Fig. 23.1D).

Immunofluorescence typically shows dominant or codominant staining for C3, usually accompanied by lesser degrees of immunoglobulin staining. In classic PSGN, IgG is typically seen in a similar distribution to C3. In staphylococcal infections, IgA may be the dominant immunoglobulin, and in up to 25% of cases the C3 is not associated with significant amounts of immunoglobulin staining. The distribution of the deposits in glomeruli can range from the classic "starry sky" appearance, reflecting an admixture of mesangial and peripheral capillary deposits, to the "garland" appearance, in which the subepithelial deposits are confluent, to a mesangial pattern often seen in the resolving stages (Fig. 23.2). A significant portion of endocarditis-associated IRGN may have a pauci-immune appearance on immunofluorescence studies.

The classic electron microscopic finding in PSGN is the hump-shaped subepithelial electron-dense deposit (Fig. 23.3). While often present, these subepithelial deposits are not required for the diagnosis of IRGN, and their presence alone does not constitute the diagnosis of IRGN. Subendothelial deposits, though often less pronounced, are largely responsible for the prominent endocapillary hypercellularity that is often seen. Mesangial deposits, while sometimes sparse, are almost universally encountered in IRGN.

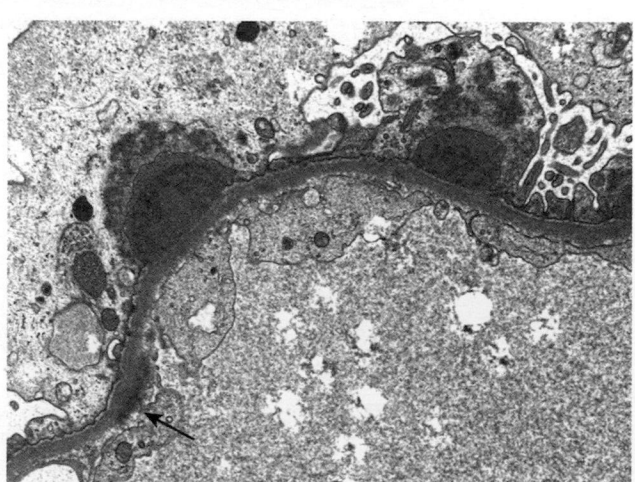

• **Fig. 23.3** Classic ultrastructural findings in infection-related glomerulonephritis. Subepithelial hump-shaped deposits pictured here (original magnification 9300×) are distinctive findings in many cases of infection-related glomerulonephritis (IRGN) but are neither required nor sufficient to make the diagnosis of IRGN. It is the typically smaller subendothelial deposits *(arrow)* that are likely responsible for producing much of the diffuse proliferative changes usually seen by light microscopy.

Differential Diagnosis

Given the highly variable clinical presentation, the differential diagnosis of IRGN is broad. Due to the association of IRGN with hypocomplementemia, diagnoses including lupus nephritis, C3 GN, and cryoglobulinemic GN are often considered. IgA nephropathy, because of its synpharyngitic presentation, is also frequently considered in the differential diagnosis. A combination of serologic testing and features on kidney biopsy can help distinguish these entities, but pitfalls exist. Serologic findings such as positive antinuclear antibody (ANA) and anti-DNA antibodies would typically favor the diagnosis of lupus nephritis, but it is important to remember that infections such as shunt nephritis can also be accompanied by a positive ANA. Cryoglobulinemic GN is most often characterized by disproportionate lowering of C4 rather than C3, and IgA nephropathy is usually associated with normocomplementemia.

In many cases, C3 GN can be difficult or impossible to distinguish from IRGN. Both C3GN and IRGN can present with very similar clinical, pathologic, and laboratory findings, including elevated ASO levels in more than 50% of cases of C3GN. C3GN should be strongly considered in cases that have been diagnosed as IRGN if there is persistence of low C3 levels after 8–12 weeks. In these cases, evaluation for abnormalities of the alternative complement pathway should be considered. The presence of anti-factor B autoantibodies has recently been demonstrated to be a sensitive and specific marker of PSGN in children, helping to differentiate PSGN from C3GN. These anti-factor B autoantibodies appear to be transient in the wake of infection and are correlated with the degree of hypocomplementemia. Histologically, C3GN is a consideration in the cases where immunoglobulin staining is sparse or absent, but sparse or absent immunoglobulin staining with prominent C3 staining is also a recognized immunofluorescence pattern in up to 25% of IRGN. One recent study proposes that C4d staining can help differentiate C3GN from IRGN, as prominent glomerular C4d positivity was detected in about half of the tested cases of IRGN but not in any of the C3GN cases, suggesting additional involvement of the classic or lectin complement pathways in IRGN. Importantly, the intensity of the C4d staining should be equal to or greater than that of C3 to be considered significant, as mild background C4d staining is routinely detected in mesangial areas of normal glomeruli.

Cases of IRGN with significant amounts of IgA deposition, as are commonly seen with IRGN due to staphylococcal organisms, can potentially be confused with IgA nephropathy or IgA vasculitis. In one series of culture-proven staphylococcal-associated GN, 22% had a vasculitic presentation, including a purpuric skin rash over the lower extremities.

IRGN with a pauci-immune phenotype by immunofluorescence can be encountered in conjunction with a necrotizing crescentic GN histologically indistinguishable from ANCA vasculitis. This variant of IRGN is most frequently encountered in patients with endocarditis or other intravascular infections. Further complicating attempts to distinguish endocarditis-associated IRGN from a more purely ANCA-driven vasculitis is the presence of positive ANCA serologies in approximately 25% of endocarditis-associated IRGN. Ultimately, the possibility of recent or active infection should be at least considered in the differential diagnosis of almost any proliferative GN.

Pathogenesis

The pathogenesis of IRGN is multifactorial and far from fully understood. The development of glomerular immune complexes in IRGN is likely due to both deposition of preformed circulating immune complexes and the binding of antibodies directed at bacterial antigens that are planted within glomeruli, resulting in *in situ* formation of immune complexes. Identification of nephritogenic streptococcal antigens has been pursued for decades, and streptococcal pyrogenic exotoxin B (SPEB) appears to be responsible for most cases of PSGN. SPEB is cationic and, therefore, can more easily penetrate the anionic glomerular basement membrane, resulting in the ability of SPEB to localize subepithelially. SPEB has been demonstrated to colocalize with IgG and C3 in the subepithelial humps of many patients with PSGN, supporting the theory that in situ immune complex formation is important in the development of PSGN. In addition, SPEB can directly activate the alternative complement pathway, helping explain the disproportionate consumption of C3 in PSGN.

Outside of PSGN, the search for nephritogenic antigens is in its infancy. Staphylococcal superantigens, which have the ability to cause massive T-cell activation and high levels of proinflammatory cytokines, have been proposed to play a role in staphylococcal IRGN. Potential nephritogenic antigens associated with gram-negative bacteria and other less common organisms responsible for IRGN are yet to be identified.

The development of IRGN is also likely largely dependent on host factors that significantly influence the susceptibility of a given patient to developing IRGN. IRGN can be caused by many types and strains of bacteria, but only a small percentage of people infected with these pathogens develop clinically significant GN. The presence of hypocomplementemia and the overlapping features of C3GN and IRGN suggest that differences in the way that the alternative complement pathway is regulated likely plays a role in the development of IRGN. The recent demonstration of transiently produced anti-factor B antibodies, and the normalization of complement once these antibodies disappear, suggests that these antibodies may be one factor driving activation of the alternative complement pathway in PSGN.

Treatment and Prognosis

Treatment in most instances of IRGN is supportive, focusing on managing the manifestations of kidney disease (hypervolemia, hypertension, uremia) and controlling active infections when they coexist with the GN. Hypervolemia usually responds to salt restriction and loop diuretics. Volume control is often sufficient to manage the new-onset hypertension, but in some cases the addition of antihypertensive medications is needed. Dialysis may be necessary, and the need for dialysis is more frequent in adults. In instances of epidemic PSGN, antibiotic prophylaxis of household or community members can help decrease the incidence of the disease. In select cases with aggressive crescentic disease and a rapidly progressive glomerulonephritis presentation, immunosuppressive therapy, typically with corticosteroids, may be of benefit, as long as the infection is controlled; however, there are no randomized clinical trials to support this approach. Plasmapheresis has also been reported to be of benefit as an adjunct therapy in some cases of infective endocarditis-related glomerulonephritis, when kidney function fails to improve despite appropriate antibiotic therapy.

Prognosis is usually excellent in children, with more than 95% experiencing complete recovery, though it may take 4 to 8 weeks for symptoms to resolve and kidney function to return to baseline. Hematuria often lasts up to 6 months and proteinuria might be present for years; however, only 1% will progress to ESKD. In children with an atypical presentation and limited recovery, the possibility of C3GN should be considered.

The prognosis of epidemic PSGN affecting adults is also good. In a recent 10-year follow-up study of the PSGN outbreak that occurred in Brazil after ingestion of contaminated dairy with *Streptococcus zooepidemicus*, there was no significant difference in the level of kidney function or proteinuria at 10 years compared with matched controls. However, cases had a higher incidence of hypertension compared with control subjects (45% vs. 20.8%).

The prognosis for adults with sporadic IRGN cases is notably worse, with only about half experiencing complete recovery. This is not surprising, as many adult patients affected by IRGN have comorbid conditions that are also risk factors for kidney disease. Diabetes imparts a particularly poor outcome and very high rates of progression to ESKD after IRGN (>50% in some reports). In a series focusing on elderly patients with IRGN, only 22% experienced a complete kidney recovery, 44% developed CKD, and 33% progressed to ESKD.

Complete bibliography is available at Elsevier eBooks for Practicing Clinicians.

Key Bibliography

Boils CL, Nasr SH, Walker PD, et al. Update on endocarditis-associated glomerulonephritis. *Kidney Int.* 2015;87:1241–1249.

Bratsford SR, Mezzano S, Mihatsch M, et al. Is the nephritogenic antigen in post-streptococcal glomerulonephritis pyrogenic exotoxin B (SPEB) or GAPDH? *Kidney Int.* 2005;68:1120–1129.

Carpentis JR, Steer AC, Mulholland EK, Weber M. The global burden of group A streptococcal diseases. *Lancet Infect Dis.* 2005;5:685–694.

Chamarthi G, Clapp W L, Bejjanki H, et al. Infection-related Glomerulonephritis and C3 glomerulopathy-Similar yet Dissimilar: A case report and brief review of current literature. *Cureus.* 2020;12(2):e7127.

Chauvet S, Berthaud R, Devriese M, et al. Anti-factor B antibodies and acute postinfectious GN in children. *J Am Soc Nephrol.* 2020;31:829–840.

Couser WG, Johnson RJ. The etiology of glomerulonephritis: roles of infection and autoimmunity. *Kidney Int.* 2014;86:905–914.

Dagan R, Cleper R, Davidovits M, et al. Post-infectious glomerulonephritis in pediatric patients over two decades: severity-associated features. *Isr Med Assoc J.* 2016;18:336–340.

Gaut JP, Mueller S, Liapis H. IgA dominant post-infectious glomerulonephritis update: pathology spectrum and disease mechanisms. *Diagnostic Histopathology.* 2017;23(3):126–132.

Glassock RJ, Alvarado A, Prosek J, et al. Staphylococcus-related glomerulonephritis and poststreptococcal glomerulonephritis: why defining "post" is important in understanding and treating infection-related glomerulonephritis. *Am J Kidney Dis.* 2015;65:826–832.

Halpin M, Kozyreva O, Bijol V, Jaber B. Plasmapheresis for treatment of immune complex-mediated glomerulonephritis in infective endocarditis: a case report and literature review. *Clinical Nephrology- Case studies.* 2017;5:26–31.

Hunt EAK, Somers MJG. Infection-related glomerulonephritis. *Pediatr Clin N Am.* 2019;66:59–72.

Khalighi MA, Wang S, Henriksen KJ, et al. Revisiting post-infectious glomerulonephritis in the emerging era of C3 glomerulopathy. *Clin Kidney J.* 2016;9:397–402.

Kidney Disease: Improving Global Outcomes (KDIGO) Glomerulonephritis Work Group. KDIGO clinical practice guideline for glomerulonephritis. Chapter 9: Infection-related glomerulonephritis. *Kidney Int Suppl.* 2012;2:200–208.

Malhotra K, Yerram P. Plasmapheresis and corticosteroids in infective endocarditis-related crescentic glomerulonephritis. *BMJ Case Rep.* 2019;12:e227672.

Nasr SH, Fidler ME, Valeri AM, et al. Post infectious glomerulonephritis in the elderly. *J Am Soc Nephrol.* 2011;22:187–195.

Nasr SH, Markowitz GS, Stokes MB, et al. Acute postinfectious glomerulonephritis in the modern era: experience with 86 adults and review of the literature. *Medicine (Baltimore).* 2008;87:21–32.

Nasr SH, Radhakrishnan J, D'Agati VD. Bacterial infection-related glomerulonephritis in adults. *Kidney Int.* 2013;83:792–803.

Nast CC. Infection-related glomerulonephritis: changing demographics and outcomes. *Adv Chronic Kidney Dis.* 2012;19:68–75.

Pinto SW, Mastroianni-Kirsztajn G, Sesso R. Ten-year follow-up of patients with epidemic post infectious glomerulonephritis. *PLoS One.* 2015;10:e0125313.

Rodriguez-Iturbe B, Bratsford S. Pathogenesis of poststreptococcal glomerulonephritis a century after Clemens con Pirquet. *Kidney Int.* 2007;71:1094–1104.

24

Viral Nephropathies: Human Immunodeficiency Virus, Hepatitis C Virus, Hepatitis B Virus, and SARS-CoV-2

MEGHAN E. SISE, IAN A. STROHBEHN, SARAH SCHRAUBEN, JEFFREY S. BERNS

Human immunodeficiency virus (HIV), hepatitis C virus (HCV), and hepatitis B virus (HBV) are the most important causes of viral-related kidney disease in the world. Several mechanisms are involved in the pathogenesis of virus-related kidney disease, including tropism of the virus in the kidney, direct cytopathic effects, and immune response to the virus including production of immune complexes. These lead to a spectrum of glomerular and tubulointerstitial diseases. Some of the most important features of the kidney diseases associated with these viruses are shown in Table 24.1.

Human Immunodeficiency Virus

Kidney disease is a frequent complication of HIV infection. The classic kidney disease caused by HIV is a form of collapsing focal segmental glomerulosclerosis (FSGS), referred to as *HIV-associated nephropathy* (HIVAN). Its pathophysiology is linked to viral gene replication within kidney cells. Immune complex-mediated glomerular diseases have been associated with HIV infection; however, the mechanistic link to HIV is undefined. Finally, the use of antiretroviral therapies (ARTs) has led to long-term survivorship and, thus, an increasing prevalence of diabetic nephropathy, hypertensive nephrosclerosis, and arteriopathy in patients with HIV, as well as chronic kidney disease (CKD) that result from chronic ART use.

Pathophysiology of HIVAN

In the setting of HIV infection, kidney disease is mediated by factors related to the virus, host genetic predisposition, host response to infection, and environmental factors. HIVAN typically occurs in patients of African ancestry. This predilection is associated with high frequencies of *APOL1* genetic polymorphisms on chromosome 22 in this population, specifically G1 (two missense mutations) and G2 (two base pair deletion). The G1 and G2 variants confer risk for HIVAN and an HIV-associated noncollapsing form of FSGS, as well as other glomerular diseases and arteriolar nephrosclerosis. The effect is largely recessive, in that homozygous

(G1/G1 or G2/G2) or compound heterozygous (G1/G2) individuals have the highest risk of HIVAN. The mechanisms by which the risk variant proteins alter kidney cell function and lead to CKD and end-stage kidney disease (ESKD) remain unclear and are a matter of considerable interest and ongoing research.

Evidence from clinical and animal studies supports a direct role of HIV infection of renal parenchymal cells in the pathogenesis of HIVAN. Although renal epithelial cells do not generally express viral receptors, uptake of HIV into renal epithelial cells is thought to be mediated by transfer from infected lymphocytes. Expression of HIV transgenes in podocytes and renal tubular epithelial cells results in de-differentiation and/or loss of expression of important proteins (e.g., nephrin), which leads to apoptosis, proliferation, and tubular microcyst formation. Expression of HIV regulatory and accessory proteins in HIV transgenic mice (Tg26 or TgFVB) produces the glomerular and tubular features of HIVAN-like pathology, even in the absence of intact virus, thereby supporting the direct effects of HIV transcript expression in glomerular (mesangial and epithelial) and tubular cells. The mechanism that drives aberrant expansion of podocyte stem cells, which are located in the parietal epithelium, remains unknown.

HIVAN Clinical Presentation and Kidney Biopsy Findings

The classic presentation of HIVAN is nephrotic syndrome, with rapid estimated glomerular filtration (eGFR) loss, relatively bland urinary sediment, and large, often densely echogenic kidneys on ultrasound. Most patients are normotensive and relatively edema free despite advanced CKD, possibly due to salt wasting from the prominent tubular abnormalities in HIVAN. HIVAN occurs predominantly in those of African ancestry with advanced HIV (high viral loads, CD4 counts less than 200 cells/μL), but HIVAN may also occur at the time of acute HIV seroconversion when viral load is often very high. Left untreated, HIVAN progresses rapidly to ESKD, often in a few months.

TABLE 24.1 **Important Clinical Features of Viral Nephropathies**

	HIV	HCV	HBV
Major risk groups	Infected individuals of African ancestry who are homozygous for *APOL*1 gene polymorphisms	Adults with longstanding untreated chronic HCV infection	Children and adults from HBV endemic areas
Presentation	Proteinuria, nephrotic syndrome, with rapid eGFR decline Large, echogenic kidneys on ultrasound Advanced HIV (if HIVAN)	Hematuria Proteinuria Hypocomplementemia Palpable purpura Systemic vasculitis Cryoglobulinemia	Proteinuria Nephrotic syndrome
Primary kidney pathology	Collapsing FSGS Microcystic dilation of tubules Interstitial inflammation/fibrosis	MPGN	MN
Pathogenesis	Direct HIV infection Host genetic factors Immune complex deposition	Direct HCV toxicity Cryoglobulinemia Immune-complex deposition	Antigen-antibody complex deposition causing membranous nephropathy or vasculitis
Therapy	ART ACE-I and ARBs	Direct-acting antiviral therapy Steroids and Rituximab Cyclophosphamide +/- Plasmapheresis in severe cases	Antiviral therapy

ACE-I, Angiotensin-converting enzyme inhibitor; *ARB,* angiotensin receptor blocker; *ART,* antiretroviral therapy; *eGFR,* estimated glomerular filtration rate; *FSGS,* focal segmental glomerulosclerosis; *HBV,* hepatitis B virus; *HCV,* hepatitis C virus; *HIV,* human immunodeficiency virus; *HIVAN,* HIV-associated nephropathy; *HIV-ICD,* HIV immune complex disease; *MN,* membranous nephropathy; *MPGN,* membranoproliferative glomerulonephritis.

The characteristic pathologic changes of HIVAN are observed along the full length of the nephron with glomerular and tubulointerstitial features. Light microscopy reveals a collapse of glomerular capillaries that typically involves the entire glomerulus (Fig. 24.1), visceral glomerular epitheliosis, podocyte hypertrophy and proliferation surrounding the shrunken glomerulus, and mesangial prominence and hypercellularity. Tubular injury is marked by microcystic tubular dilation, tubular atrophy, and proteinaceous casts (Fig. 24.2). Many patients have modest interstitial inflammation with lymphocytes, plasma cells, and monocytes. Immunofluorescence is generally nonspecific, and electron microscopy shows diffuse food process effacement with frequent endothelial tubuloreticular inclusions (TRIs) but no immune complex deposits (Fig. 24.3).

Treatment of HIVAN

ART is key to preventing and treating HIVAN. Previously, kidney disease was an important indication for early initiation of ART; however, current guidelines recommend initiating ART in all patients with HIV as soon as possible, regardless of CD4 count. The use of ART has been associated with a lower incidence of HIVAN, improved kidney function, and lower risk of ESKD. Control of blood pressure and proteinuria with angiotensin-converting enzyme (ACE) inhibitors and angiotensin receptor blockade (ARB) are important to slow progression of HIVAN. Immunosuppression is not recommended in patients with HIVAN; corticosteroids have not shown sufficient efficacy, and the risk of infectious complications is high.

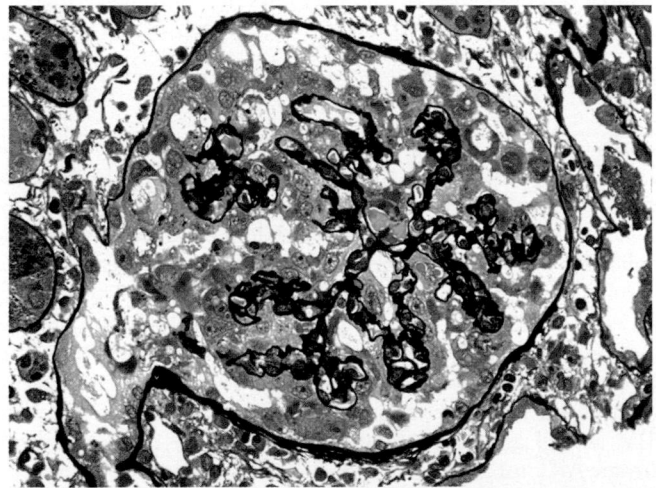

• **Fig. 24.1** Collapsing focal segmental glomerulonephritis in human immunodeficiency virus–associated nephropathy (Jones methenamine silver stain, ×400).

Patients with HIVAN may progress to ESKD despite ART. Mortality rates of HIV-infected dialysis patients are slightly higher than HIV-uninfected dialysis patients, particularly among non-Caucasian patients. The outcome of kidney transplantation in HIV-positive patients who receive organs from HIV-negative or HIV-positive donors is similar to the outcome of HIV-negative recipients and HIV-negative donors. There is a clear survival advantage for HIV-infected patients who undergo kidney transplantation

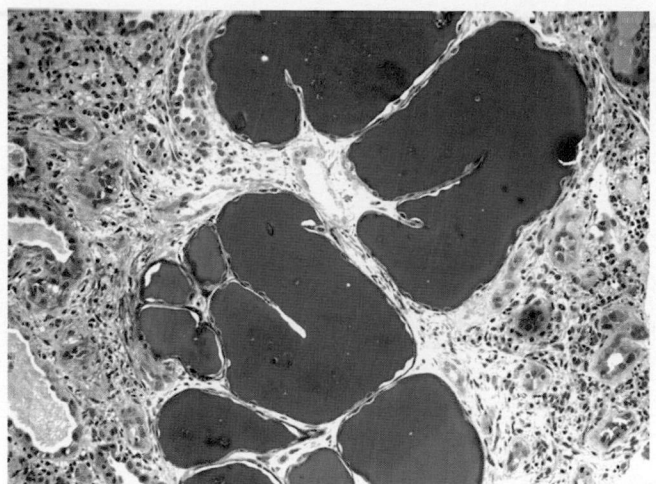

• **Fig. 24.2** Tubulointerstitial disease in human immunodeficiency virus–associated nephropathy, characterized by tubular atrophy, microcystic tubular dilation with proteinaceous casts, and mild interstitial inflammation (trichrome stain, ×200).

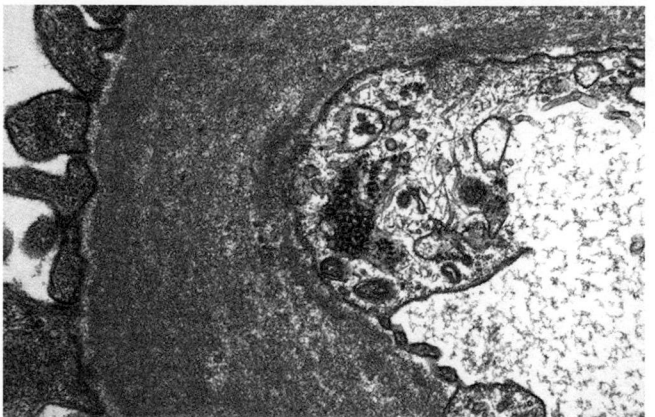

• **Fig. 24.3** Tubuloreticular inclusions in the endothelium classically seen on electron microscopy in human immunodeficiency virus–associated nephropathy (electron micrograph, ×50,000).

compared to remaining on dialysis. Classic HIVAN does not seem to recur in allografts, but other immune complex-related kidney diseases may. There are important interactions between antiretroviral drugs and posttransplant immunosuppressants. Ritonavir, an inhibitor of cytochrome P450 enzyme systems, decreases metabolism of tacrolimus, resulting in up to a fivefold increase in blood levels. In contrast, the NNRTIs efavirenz and nevirapine induce P450s and increase metabolism of tacrolimus, necessitating much higher doses to maintain adequate levels.

Immune Complex Diseases in Patients with HIV Infection

Immune complex-mediated glomerular diseases that have been associated with HIV infection include cryoglobulinemic glomerulonephritis (particularly in patients co-infected with HCV), IgA nephropathy, membranous glomerulopathy, and "lupus-like" glomerulonephritis (a proliferative glomerulonephritis with a "full-house" immunofluorescence, but without serologic or clinical evidence of systemic lupus erythematosus). These diseases are heterogenous, and the association with HIV is not well understood. Chronic HIV infection is associated with polyclonal expansion of immunoglobulins, and immune complex disease may result from deposition from the systemic circulation or from in situ binding of immunoglobulins to lodged HIV antigens; however, there is very limited understanding of the epidemiology and pathophysiology of immune complex-mediated glomerular disease in patients with HIV. Previous studies have shown there is no strong association with race or APOL1 genotype. A recently published KDIGO consensus guideline recommended that the terminology *HIV-associated immune complex kidney disease* ("HIVICK") be replaced with the specific description of the immune complex disease followed by "in the setting of HIV." There are three important reasons for this distinction: First, there is no clear mechanistic link between HIV and these glomerular lesions; second, patients should undergo a work-up searching for other potential causes for these kidney diseases; and, finally, ART therapy alone is unlikely to improve kidney function. Patients with well-controlled HIV infection should be strongly considered for immunosuppressive therapies using standard-of-care approaches to treat the underlying immune complex-mediated glomerular disease.

Finally, HIV-related thrombotic microangiopathy presents similarly to idiopathic forms of TMA with hypertension, acute kidney injury (AKI), microscopic hematuria, and non-nephrotic proteinuria, along with features of a microangiopathic hemolytic anemia. It is an uncommon presentation that typically occurs in patients with very advanced AIDS.

ART Nephrotoxicity

ART nephrotoxicity is an important cause of AKI and CKD in patients with HIV (Table 24.2). Common, currently used ARV such as tenofovir disoproxil fumarate, a nucleoside reverse transcriptase inhibitor (NRTI), may cause proximal tubular damage and Fanconi syndrome due to uptake of its active metabolite, tenofovir, into the proximal tubular cell where it can inhibit mitochondrial DNA synthesis. Tenofovir-induced nephrotoxicity causes proximal tubulopathy, which can result in hypophosphatemia, nonalbumin proteinuria, and, in its severe form, Fanconi syndrome or acute tubular necrosis (ATN). Dose adjustment of tenofovir according to eGFR is mandatory to minimize nephrotoxic effects. Tenofovir alafenamide is a newly approved NRTI pro-drug that may be less nephrotoxic.

Atazanavir is a protease inhibitor that can lead to AKI from intratubular crystal formation or nephrolithiasis. Atazanavir stones can be hard to diagnose even on computed tomography because they are radiolucent. Kidney stones occur in 1%-2% of atazanavir users, substantially lower than was seen with indinavir, a protease inhibitor no longer in use that was notorious for causing kidney stones. Darunavir, another protease inhibitor is also rarely associated with crystalluria, nephrolithiasis, and crystalline nephropathy.

Both dolutegravir, an integrase inhibitor, and cobicistat, a CYP inhibitor used to boost levels of certain protease inhibitors, may cause a slight rise in creatinine (0.2–0.3 mg/dL) due to inhibition of creatinine secretion, but neither is nephrotoxic. Cystatin c-based eGFR equations accurately reflect kidney function in patients on these agents. Patients with HIV may be commonly treated with other medications that can also cause nephrotoxicity (see Table 24.2). Additional material on kidney disease caused by therapeutic agents can be found in Chapter 34.

TABLE 24.2 Drug-Induced Nephrotoxicity in Patients With Human Immunodeficiency Virus-1 Infection

Class	Renal Abnormality
Nucleos(t)ide Reverse Transcriptase Inhibitors	
Abacavir	Lactic acidosis, AIN[a], Fanconi syndrome[a]
Didanosine	Lactic acidosis, AKI, proximal tubule dysfunction, Fanconi syndrome, nephrogenic diabetes insipidus
Lamivudine	Lactic acidosis, renal tubular acidosis, hypophosphatemia[a]
Stavudine	Lactic acidosis, renal tubular acidosis, hypophosphatemia[a]
Zidovudine	Lactic acidosis
Tenofovir	Proximal tubule dysfunction with Fanconi syndrome, nephrogenic diabetes insipidus, nonalbumin proteinuria, CKD, acute and chronic tubular injury, severe ATN
Adefovir	Proximal tubule dysfunction with Fanconi syndrome, AKI, nephrogenic diabetes insipidus, lactic acidosis
Non-Nucleoside Reverse Transcriptase Inhibitors	
Efavirenz	Nephrolithiasis
Protease Inhibitors	
Atazanavir	Nephrolithiasis, crystalline nephropathy, AIN[a]
Indinavir	Crystalluria, nephrolithiasis, interstitial nephritis (AKI, CKD), papillary necrosis, hypertension, renal atrophy
Nelfinavir	Nephrolithiasis[a]
Ritonavir	AKI, hyperuricemia
Saquinavir	AKI in association with ritonavir
Darunavir	Crystalluria, nephrolithiasis, crystalline nephropathy
Fusion or Entry Inhibitors	
Enfuvirtide	Membranoproliferative glomerulonephritis[a]
Integrase inhibitors	
Dolutegravir	Inhibition of creatinine secretion
Other Antimicrobials	
Acyclovir	AKI, crystalluria, obstructive nephropathy
Aminoglycosides	AKI, renal tubular acidosis
Amphotericin	AKI, hypokalemia, hypomagnesemia, renal tubular acidosis
Cidofovir	Proximal tubular damage, bicarbonate wasting, proteinuria, AKI
Foscarnet	AKI, hypocalcemia and hypercalcemia, hypophosphatemia and hyperphosphatemia, hypomagnesemia, nephrogenic diabetes insipidus
Pentamidine	AKI, hyperkalemia, hypocalcemia
Rifampin	Interstitial nephritis
Sulfadiazine	Proximal tubule dysfunction
Valacyclovir	Thrombotic microangiopathy

[a]Case reports.

AIN, Acute interstitial nephritis; *AKI,* acute kidney injury; *CKD,* chronic kidney disease; *ATN,* acute tubular necrosis

CKD in the Aging HIV-Infected Population

Increasing comorbidity burden among the aging HIV-infected population leads to high rates of CKD. The incidence of HIVAN has decreased due to the widespread use of ART, and the distribution of HIV-associated kidney disease has changed substantially over the last 30 years. Whereas in 1989 HIVAN was the most common lesion found on kidney biopsy, a recent biopsy series out of New York City shows that immune complex disease, diabetic nephropathy, HIVAN, tenofovir toxicity, and non-HIVAN FSGS each make up 12%-16% of kidney biopsy diagnoses. Though ART led to a decline in the incidence of HIVAN, with a corresponding reduction in ESKD attributed to HIVAN, the rates of ESKD are still higher in the HIV-infected population.

Prolonged use of ART and the corresponding increased life span of HIV-infected individuals have led to increasing comorbidity burden and higher prevalence of associated kidney disease in patients with HIV. Despite the suppression of HIV replication with ART, a state of chronic inflammation and dysmetabolism persists, which is linked to diabetic kidney disease, arteriolar nephrosclerosis, and possibly FSGS.

Hepatitis C Virus

Epidemiology

Globally, over 71 million individuals are living with chronic HCV infection. In the United States, approximately 1% of the population has chronic HCV infection. There are six major genotypes of HCV infection, and the prevalence of each genotype varies by region. In the United States, the majority (approximately 70%) are infected with genotype 1 (genotype 1a > genotype 1b); 15% to 20%, genotype 2; 10% to 12%, genotype 3; 1%, genotype 4; and less than 1%, genotype 5 or 6. Worldwide, genotype 1 is the most prevalent and genotype 3 is the next most common; together, genotypes 1 and 3 account for the majority of infections. The prevalent, long-term complications of chronic HCV infection result from chronic liver disease (cirrhosis, liver failure, hepatocellular carcinoma), but HCV can also lead to extrahepatic complications involving the blood lines, skin, and kidney. HCV infection is a major cause of mixed cryoglobulinemia syndrome (MCS), a systemic vasculitis characterized by involvement of small-to-medium-sized vessels, leading to clinical manifestations ranging from skin changes to more serious lesions with neurologic and kidney involvement. Kidney disease is considered a major cause of morbidity and mortality in MCS. Kidney disease typically occurs after longstanding infection, and the classic kidney lesion is cryoglobulinemic MPGN, but other glomerular lesions have been described. Screening for urinary abnormalities and eGFR in all HCV-positive patients is strongly recommended.

Pathophysiology and Clinical Presentation of Cryoglobulinemic Glomerulonephritis

HCV infection is implicated in 80% to 90% of the cases of MCS. HCV infection causes chronic stimulation of B lymphocytes with widespread autoantibody synthesis and production of cryoglobulins. Cryoglobulins are proteins that circulate in the serum, precipitate below core body temperature, and dissolve upon rewarming. MCS results from the production of polyclonal IgG and monoclonal (type II cryoglobulin) or polyclonal (type III cryoglobulin) IgM with rheumatoid factor (RF) activity. Cryoglobulinemic glomerulonephritis may result due to the affinity of IgM-RF for cellular fibronectin in the mesangial matrix. Cryoglobulins are deposited in the glomerular capillaries and mesangium, which can lead to complement activation, inflammatory cytokine release, vasculitis, fibrinoid necrosis, and crescent formation. MPGN may be found in patients with chronic HCV even without a circulating cryoglobulin.

Cryoglobulinemia often presents with a systemic vasculitis, with palpable purpura that most commonly involves the lower limbs, arthralgias, neuropathy, and nonspecific symptoms of fever, fatigue, and malaise. However, many patients with cryoglobulinemia are asymptomatic or have mild, nonspecific symptoms. Patients with HCV-associated cryoglobulinemic glomerulonephritis experience asymptomatic non-nephrotic proteinuria, nephrotic syndrome, or acute glomerulonephritis with GFR loss. Most patients (80%) have severe hypertension. Laboratory evaluation demonstrates marked hypocomplementemia, with a greater reduction in C4 than C3, as well as positive anti-HCV antibodies and HCV RNA. The majority of patients are RF positive, almost invariably IgMκ. The natural history of this disease can be variable, with some patients having an indolent course, while others develop progressive kidney failure. ESKD requiring dialysis is relatively uncommon (10% of cases). In about 10% of patients, acute oliguric AKI is the first indicator of kidney disease. Risk factors for ESKD included older age, male sex, higher serum creatinine, and greater degrees of proteinuria at diagnosis.

Other Kidney Lesions Associated with HCV

Various other histologic types of kidney diseases are reported in association with HCV infection, including membranous nephropathy (MN), FSGS, fibrillary glomerulonephritis, immunotactoid glomerulonephritis, IgA nephropathy, thrombotic microangiopathy, renal vasculitis, and interstitial nephritis. The histologic findings of HCV-associated MN are similar to that of idiopathic MN, and data are conflicting as to whether there is a real pathophysiologic link between HCV and MN. Future studies testing for antibodies to the phospholipase A2 receptor may be useful in this regard. Polyarteritis nodosa (PAN), although classically associated with hepatitis B infection, has also been observed in patients with chronic HCV infection.

Direct cytopathic effects of HCV play a role in HCV-related kidney disease. HCV is able to bind and penetrate into renal parenchymal cells. HCV RNA has been found in mesangial cells, tubular epithelial cells, and endothelial cells of the glomerulus and peritubular capillaries. In one study, the presence of HCV-related proteins in the mesangium was associated with greater proteinuria.

HCV-Associated CKD Progression

In addition to causing cryoglobulinemic glomerulonephritis, HCV may speed progression to ESKD even in patients with other forms of kidney disease, such as diabetic kidney disease. The adverse effects of chronic HCV infection on eGFR decline and ESKD risk has been shown in large population studies. This may be particularly dramatic in patients with HIV and HCV co-infection. In patients with CKD, the risks of other adverse outcomes are also significantly higher in HCV-infected patients than those without infection, including progression to cirrhosis, hepatocellular carcinoma, and liver-related mortality. HCV-infected dialysis patients also experience higher rates of morbidity and mortality and lower quality of life. The association of HCV and glomerular disease has been observed in both native and transplanted kidneys. Recent data suggest that direct-acting antiretroviral (DAA) therapy may slow eGFR decline in patients with CKD.

Pathology

A kidney biopsy is recommended to determine the histologic pattern of glomerular injury in those with proteinuria and/or hematuria and remains the gold standard for diagnosis of HCV-associated glomerular disease. The most common HCV-associated glomerular disease is cryoglobulinemic glomerulonephritis. Light

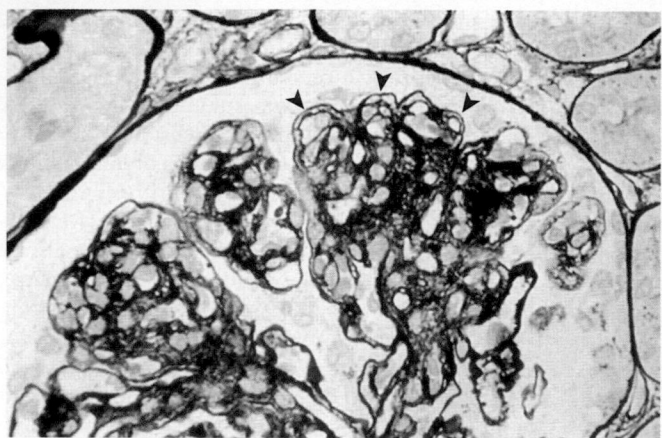

• **Fig. 24.4** Membranoproliferative glomerulonephritis seen in hepatitis C virus infection with typical glomerular basement membrane double contours (*arrowheads*; Jones methenamine silver stain).

microscopy demonstrates a membranoproliferative pattern of injury with expanded and hypercellular mesangium, endocapillary proliferation, monocytic infiltration, thickened capillary loops, and large eosinophilic and PAS-positive intraluminal deposits, with or without vasculitis of small- and medium-sized renal arteries. Silver staining shows double contours of the glomerular basement membranes (GBMs) resulting from immune complex deposition and mesangial cell matrix interposition between the GBM and endothelial cell, with a new basement membrane forming around these deposits (Fig. 24.4). Immunofluorescence may reveal C3, IgM, and IgG granular deposits in the capillary wall and mesangium. On electron microscopy, subendothelial deposits are usually present and may have tubular and crystalline patterns similar to that of cryoglobulins. Cryoglobulins may be associated with histologic signs of vasculitis and downstream fibrinoid necrosis. One-third of these patients may have vasculitis of small renal arteries. Distinctive features of cryoglobulinemic glomerulonephritis, especially in patients with rapid deterioration of kidney function, are the presence of "pseudo-thrombi," which include large intraglomerular immune deposits, commonly observed in a subendothelial location, that can fill the capillary lumen.

Treatment

The management of HCV-associated glomerular disease depends on the severity of the clinical presentation, with consideration of the level of kidney function and the degree of proteinuria. Three approaches can be considered for HCV-associated glomerulopathies and cryoglobulinemic kidney disease: (1) antiviral therapy to prevent further direct HCV damage to kidneys and the synthesis of immune complexes, (2) B-cell depletion therapy to prevent the formation of immune complexes and cryoglobulins, and (3) nonspecific immunosuppressive therapy targeting inflammatory cells to prevent the synthesis of immune complexes and to treat cryoglobulin-associated vasculitis. In patients with moderate proteinuria and stable kidney function, initiating antiviral therapy for HCV alone is advised while closely monitoring kidney function and proteinuria. Though DAAs are first-line treatment for patients with cryoglobulinemic glomerulonephritis who had stable eGFR, it is important to note that approximately one-third of patients with cryoglobulinemic glomerulonephritis did not achieve remission with DAAs alone; those who do not enter

clinical remission within 3 months of completing treatment with DAAs should receive immunosuppressive therapy. In patients with nephrotic-range proteinuria and/or progressive kidney injury and other serious extrarenal manifestations (such as CNS vasculitis or pulmonary hemorrhage), immunosuppressive therapy with rituximab, corticosteroids, and plasmapheresis should be considered. Antiviral therapy should also be initiated.

Direct-Acting Antiviral Therapy for HCV Infection

Historically, HCV drug therapy depended on interferon-α (IFN-α), in standard form or pegylated form (PEG-IFN), and ribavirin. Patients required treatment for 6 to 12 months with suboptimal efficacy and often severe side effects. In 2013, the first direct-acting antiviral (DAA), sofosbuvir, was approved. DAAs target HCV's replicative machinery and do not rely on the host immune response to exert antiviral effects. DAAs target HCV's NS3/4A protease, NS5A protein, and NS5B polymerase. The newest combination DAAs are IFN free and provide outstanding efficacy (>95% sustained viral remission) with few side effects. According to the most recent guidelines issued by the American Association of the Study of Liver Disease (AASLD) and the Infectious Diseases Society of America (IDSA) (http://www.hcvguidelines.org), pan-genotypic therapies are preferred to treat HCV (summarized in Table 24.3). While there was initial concern about the safety of sofosbuvir in patients with eGFR < 30mL/min/1.73 m², as sofosbuvir and its active metabolite are renally eliminated, it is now generally recognized to be safe and the FDA label for sofosbuvir now includes use for all levels of kidney function. Other DAA combinations, including elbasvir/grazoprevir and glecaprevir/pibrentasvir, are hepatically eliminated and have also been studied and shown to be safe and effective in patients with eGFR < 30 or kidney failure on dialysis.

Immunosuppression

In the setting of nephrotic syndrome, rapidly progressive kidney failure, and/or acute flare of cryoglobulinemia, patients are typically treated with aggressive immunosuppressive therapy, which includes corticosteroids, cyclophosphamide or rituximab, and/or plasma exchange. Rituximab is a monoclonal antibody against CD-20 used to control severe vasculitis by rapidly depleting

TABLE 24.3	Currently Recommended Pan-Genotypic HCV Direct-Acting Antiviral Therapy		
Agent	**Genotypes**	**Kidney Considerations**	**Liver Considerations**
Glecaprevir-Pibrentasvir	1–6	No renal adjustment, approved for all levels of eGFR and ESRD	Should not be used in decompensated cirrhosis
Sofosbuvir-Velpatasvir	1–6	No renal adjustment, approved for all levels of eGFR and ESRD	Can be used in decompensated cirrhosis

eGFR, Estimated glomerular filtration; *ESRD*, end-stage renal disease; *HCV*, hepatitis C virus.
For the most recent updates to guidelines, please refer to https://www.hcvguidelines.org

circulating and tissue B cells, interfering with the synthesis of cryoglobulins, and reducing kidney deposition of immune complexes. Rituximab has been associated with reduction in proteinuria and cryoglobulin levels and increases in complement levels and is recommended by KDIGO guidelines for patients with biopsy-proven cryoglobulinemic glomerulonephritis who have severe manifestations at presentation. Alternatively, pulse intravenous steroids and oral cyclophosphamide can be used. Cyclophosphamide is effective in inhibiting B-lymphocyte proliferation and, thus, cryoglobulin production. Corticosteroids control the acute inflammatory response (e.g., prednisone 0.5 to 1.5 mg/kg/day or IV pulses of methylprednisolone 0.5 to 1.0 g/day for 3 days followed by oral prednisone). Plasma exchange is used in patients with rapidly progressive crescentic glomerulonephritis or other life-threatening manifestations of MCS. When plasmapheresis is used, it should be combined with immunosuppressive therapies to prevent the re-accumulation of immune complexes and cryoglobulins. DAAs should also begin promptly.

Dialysis and Transplantation

HCV positivity has been linked to lower graft and patient survival after kidney transplantation. HCV-associated liver disease increases the risk of graft rejection, proteinuria, infection, and diabetes. In addition, recurrent or de novo glomerulonephritis, thrombotic microangiopathy, acute rejection, and new onset diabetes after transplant may all be more common in HCV-infected kidney transplant recipients. However, it is important to note that these adverse outcomes are reported from a period when HCV was rarely treated in kidney transplant recipients. IFN-based therapies were largely avoided in the post-kidney transplantation setting as IFN can induce acute graft rejection. Fortunately, dedicated clinical trials have shown that DAAs can be used safely after kidney transplantation without significantly increasing the rate of acute rejection while leading to extremely high cure rates.

The opioid crisis has led to a rise in available HCV-infected donor kidneys, and many of these potential kidneys are discarded. Thus, HCV-infected ESKD patients willing to accept an organ from an HCV-infected donor may benefit from shorter waiting list times compared to HCV-uninfected patients. Due to the remarkable breakthrough of DAA therapy and the demonstrated safety after kidney transplantation, protocols to transplant HCV-infected donors into HCV-naïve transplant waitlist candidates followed by DAA therapy have been developed, and single- and multi-center trials have reported outstanding results. These efforts will increase the kidney donor pool and decrease discard of potentially viable organs.

Hepatitis B

Epidemiology

Approximately one-third of the world's population has serologic evidence of past or present infection with HBV, and more than 350 million are chronically infected. Kidney involvement is a common extrahepatic manifestation in those who have chronic HBV antigenemia; the most common pathologic manifestation being MN and membranoproliferative glomerulonephritis (MPGN). The reported prevalence of HBV-associated nephropathy, particularly MN, closely matches the geographic patterns of HBV prevalence. Other kidney manifestations, including PAN, FSGS, minimal change disease, lupus-like nephritis, and IgA nephropathy may be less commonly associated with HBV.

Clinical Presentation and Pathogenesis of HBV-Associated Glomerular Disease

Hepatitis B virus–associated MN or MPGN is more common in children than adults, with a male predominance, especially in children. MN typically presents with the full nephrotic syndrome of heavy proteinuria, hyperlipidemia, hypoalbuminemia, and lower extremity edema. Adults are more likely than children to have hypertension, reduced GFR, and clinical evidence of liver disease. Patients with nephrotic syndrome and abnormal liver function tests have a greater than 50% chance of progressing to ESKD. The natural history of HBV-related MN is not well defined. In children, there is a high spontaneous remission rate (up to 60%). In adults, MN is usually progressive, with up to one-third eventually developing kidney failure. CKD progression is seen more commonly in patients with MPGN.

The main pathogenic mechanism in HBV-related glomerular disease is through deposition of immune complexes in the glomerulus. The immune complexes consist of HBV antigens and host antibodies. It remains unknown if the complexes are formed in situ or are derived from circulating immune complexes. The immune complexes are predominantly deposited in the subepithelial region, where they activate complement and cause glomerular injury. The subepithelial deposits seen in this form of secondary MN are likely composed of HBe antigen (HBeAg) and anti-e antibody (anti-HBe) complex. This is supported by the clinical observation that this disease often remits if a patient undergoes clearance of the HBeAg and seroconversion to anti-HBe. In children who develop MN, there is a decreased cellular immune response to the HBV, resulting in reduced clearance of the antigen compared with chronic carriers who do not develop MN. MPGN in the setting of HBV is also likely caused by deposition of immune antigen-antibody complexes within the mesangium and subepithelial space. Deposits containing both HBeAg and hepatitis B surface antigen (HBsAG) have both been reported, along with IgG and C3.

Clinical Presentation and Pathogenesis of HBV-Associated Polyarteritis Nodosa

Patients with HBV-associated PAN present similarly to those with idiopathic PAN with features of hypertension, reduced eGFR, and systemic symptoms such as fatigue, malaise, and fever. Other organ system involvement, including the skin, the nervous system, and the gastrointestinal tract, may be present.

The pathogenesis of HBV-associated PAN has been attributed to antigen-antibody complex deposition in the walls of medium-sized vessels causing inflammation of the arterial walls leading to microaneurysm formation and necrosis that can lead to glomerular ischemia/infarcts and accelerated hypertension leading to AKI. Very small vascular beds (i.e., glomerular) are usually not involved.

Diagnosis

Kidney biopsy is the gold standard for diagnosing glomerular disease in the setting of HBV infection. Contrast angiography of the renal circulation showing microaneurysms is diagnostic of classic PAN.

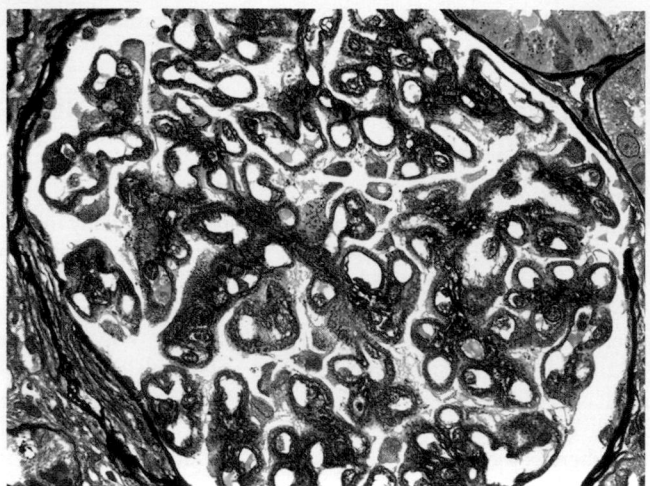

• **Fig. 24.5** Membranous glomerulonephritis seen in the setting of hepatitis B infection. Thickened glomerular basement membrane with spikes extending around immune deposits (Jones methenamine silver stain, ×400).

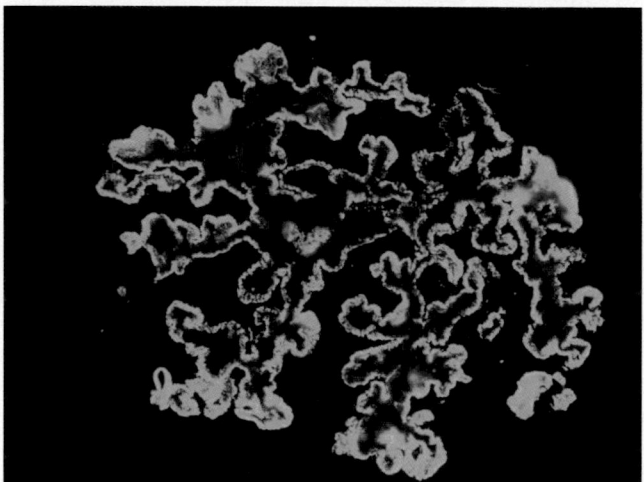

• **Fig. 24.6** Immunofluorescence with granular deposition of IgG in membranous glomerulonephritis resulting from hepatitis B infection (×400).

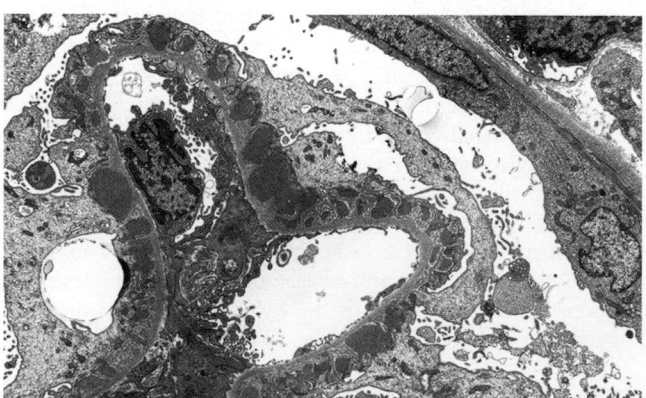

• **Fig. 24.7** Electron microscopy with subepithelial immune deposits in membranous glomerulonephritis resulting from hepatitis B infection (×6000).

Pathology

As stated earlier, MN and MPGN are most common. MN is characterized by thickened capillary walls and GBMs due to immune complex deposition. With silver or trichrome staining, characteristic spikes of the GBM can be seen extending around these deposits (Fig. 24.5). Immunofluorescence demonstrates granular IgG, C3, and some IgM staining in the subepithelial region (Fig. 24.6). Electron microscopy demonstrates classic intramembranous and subepithelial deposits (Fig. 24.7) and extensive effacement of the podocyte foot processes. In some cases, viral particles can be identified. MPGN is characterized by mesangial expansion and capillary wall thickening, resulting in a lobular appearance of the glomerular tuft, and the capillary walls demonstrate double contours and hypercellularity with interposition of cells. Immune deposits containing IgG, complement components, and IgM appear granular and are located in the subendothelial and mesangial areas.

Laboratory Data

Laboratory evaluation should include HBV DNA to confirm active replication as well as determination of antigen status, including HBeAg, HBsAg, and HBcAg. Other secondary causes of MN should be excluded, as well as common co-infections such as HCV and HIV. Unlike idiopathic MN, complement levels may be low in HBV-associated MN.

Treatment of HBV-Associated Glomerular Disease and PAN

Antiviral treatment can promote clearance of HBV; however, little is known about the treatment of HBV-associated glomerular disease. Corticosteroids and other immunosuppressive agents (e.g., mycophenolate mofetil and tacrolimus) have been used to treat those with nephrotic syndrome, but immunosuppression can lead to active replication of HBV with worsening of liver and/or kidney disease. Given these findings, immunosuppression is not recommended in HBV-related MN or MPGN.

Because severe cases of PAN can be life-threatening, corticosteroids and plasma exchange can be employed concurrently with antivirals to rapidly control the most severe manifestations. The current options of antiviral therapies include nucleoside/nucleotide analogues (lamivudine, entecavir, telbivudine, adefovir, and tenofovir) and IFN-α (conventional or PEG-IFN), which both decrease HBV DNA levels. Entecavir has replaced lamivudine as first-line therapy in the treatment of HBV infection in naïve subjects because of the propensity of drug resistance. In the treatment of HBV-mediated glomerular disease, only lamivudine and IFN-α have demonstrated benefit thus far, with reduced proteinuria, increased HBV clearance, and stabilization of kidney function. However, there is a need for high-quality, prospective, controlled studies to address the effects of antiviral therapy in patients with HBV-associated glomerular diseases. Nucleoside/nucleotide analogs such as entecavir and tenofovir disproxil fumarate must be dose adjusted by eGFR, while tenofovir alafenamide does not need dose adjustment but should not be administered to those with eGFR<15 mL/min/1.73 m² (unless on dialysis). Mild cases of PAN (those without severe skin ulceration, kidney disease, intestinal arteritis, or central nervous system, or cardiac involvement) may potentially be treated with antiviral therapy alone.

Dialysis and Transplantation

HBV infection confers a significantly negative impact on the clinical outcomes of kidney transplant recipients because of an increased risk of hepatic complications.

After transplant, patients should receive antiviral therapy regardless of their viral load, due to the risk of reactivation under induction immunosuppression. Before the availability of oral nucleoside/nucleotide analogues, chronic HBV infection was managed with IFN therapy. However, IFN should be avoided in kidney transplant recipients, as it commonly precipitates allograft dysfunction and rejection. The use of nucleoside/nucleotide analogues to effectively suppress HBV replication offers advantages of convenient administration and high tolerability, although they often require long-term use and could result in drug-resistant HBV strains. Among hepatitis B–infected transplant recipients, lamivudine therapy resulted in effective viral suppression, reduced liver complications, and improved patient survival, with patient survival rates comparable between kidney transplant recipients uninfected with HBV. A preventative approach is generally recommended to suppress reactivation of HBV. Entecavir is generally recommended because of its high resistance barrier and favorable safety profile, especially as several years of therapy may be indicated. Entecavir is effective in both treatment-naïve and lamivudine-resistant patients.

SARS-CoV-2

Coronavirus disease 2019 (COVID-19) is an infectious disease caused by severe acute respiratory syndrome coronavirus 2 (SARS-CoV-2) that has incited a global pandemic. Though SARS-CoV-2 mainly targets the respiratory system, it has been shown to affect virtually every other organ system in the human body, particularly highly vascularized ones such as the kidney. Given the lack of reliable COVID-19 testing data, the incidence of acute kidney injury (AKI) in patients with COVID-19 is variable. The first reports came from China, where AKI ranged from 0.5% to 39%. Later reports from the United States and United Kingdom described higher rates, ranging from 17.4% to 43%. The clearest data available are from critically ill patients, who have AKI rates greater than 50% and kidney replacement therapy (KRT) rates greater than 25%, according to multiple reports. The most common etiology of AKI in these patients seems to be acute tubular injury in the setting of multiorgan failure. The full pathologic spectrum of kidney injury resulting from COVID-19 has not yet been fully elucidated, but there are increasing pathological reports of thrombotic microangiopathy as well as APOL-1-mediated collapsing glomerulopathy in patients with COVID-19. Though it is established that ACE2, the receptor for SARS-CoV-2, is highly expressed in the kidney, it is yet to be determined whether SARS-CoV-2 directly infects the kidney. Additionally, some autopsy studies have detected viral RNA in kidney tissue while others have not. Both acute and chronic kidney disease are important risk factors for severe illness and death in COVID-19 patients.

Complete bibliography is available at Elsevier eBooks for Practicing Clinicians.

Key Bibliography

AASLD-IDSA. Recommendations for testing, managing, and treating hepatitis C. http://www.hcvguidelines.org. Accessed. July 23, 2020.

Elewa U, Sandri AM, Kim W, Fervenza F. Treatment of hepatitis B virus-associated nephropathy. *Nephron Clin Pract.* 2011;119:c41–c49.

Gane E, Lawitz E, Pugatch D, et al. Glecaprevir and Pibrentasvir in Patients with HCV and Severe Renal Impairment. *N Engl J Med.* 2017;377(15):1448–1455.

Goodkin DA, Bieber B, et al. Mortality, hospitalization, and quality of life among patients with hepatitis C infection on hemodialysis. *Clin J Am Soc Nephrol.* 2017;12(2):287–297 Feb 7.

Guillevin L, Mahr A, Callard P, et al. Hepatitis B virus-associated polyarteritis nodosa: clinical characteristics, outcome, and impact of treatment in 115 patients. *Medicine (Baltimore).* 2005;84(5):313–322.

Hirsch JS, Ng JH, Ross DW, et al. Northwell COVID-19 research consortium; Northwell Nephrology COVID-19 Research Consortium. Acute kidney injury in patients hospitalized with COVID-19. *Kidney Int.* 2020;98(1):209–218.

Jadoul M, Berenguer MC, et al. Executive summary of the 2018 KDIGO Hepatitis C in CKD Guideline: welcoming advances in evaluation and management. *Kidney Int.* 2018;94(4):P663–P673.

Kopp JB, Nelson GW, Sampath K, et al. APOL1 genetic variants in focal segmental glomerulosclerosis and HIV-associated nephropathy. *J Am Soc Nephrol.* 2011;22(11)2129–2137.

Kudose S, Santoriello D, et al. The spectrum of renal biopsy findings in HIV patients in the modern era. *Kidney Int.* 2020.

Lai KN, Li PK, Lui SF, et al. Membranous nephropathy related to hepatitis B virus in adults. *N Engl J Med.* 1991;324(21):1457–1463.

Lucas GM, Eustace JA, Sozio S, Mentari EK, Appiah KA, Moore RD. Highly active antiretroviral therapy and the incidence of HIV-1-associated nephropathy: a 12-year cohort study. *AIDS.* 2004;18(3):541–546.

Molnar MK, et al. Association of hepatitis C viral infection with incidence and progression of chronic kidney disease in a large cohort of US veterans. *Hepatology.* 2015;61(5):1495–1502 May.

Muller E, Barday Z, Mendelson M, Kahn D. HIV-positive-to-HIV-positive kidney transplantation—results at 3 to 5 years. *N Engl J Med.* 2015;372:613–620.

Reese PP, et al. Twelve-month outcomes after transplant of hepatitis C-infected kidneys into uninfected recipients: a single-group trial. *Ann Intern Med.* 2018;169(5):273–281.

Roth D, Nelson DR, Bruchfeld A, et al. Grazoprevir plus elbasvir in treatment-naive and treatment-experienced patients with hepatitis C virus genotype 1 infection and stage 4–5 chronic kidney disease (the C-SURFER study): a combination phase 3 study. *Lancet.* 2015;386(10003):1537–1545.

Sise ME, Chute DF, Oppong Y, et al. Direct-acting antiviral therapy slows kidney function decline in patients with hepatitis C virus infection and chronic kidney disease. *Kidney Int.* 2020;97(1):193–201.

Stock PG, Barin B, Murphy B, et al. Outcomes of kidney transplantation in HIV-infected recipients. *N Engl J Med.* 2010;363(21):2004–2014.

Swanepoel CR, Atta MG, et al. Kidney disease in the setting of HIV infection: conclusions from a Kidney Disease: Improving Global Outcomes (KDIGO) Controversies Conference. *Kidney Int.* 2018;93(3):545–559.

Wu H, Larsen CP, Hernandez-Arroyo CF, et al. AKI and collapsing glomerulopathy associated with COVID-19 and APOL 1 high-risk genotype. *J Am Soc Nephrol.* 2020.

25

Systemic Lupus Erythematosus and the Kidney

ANDREW S. BOMBACK, VIVETTE D. D'AGATI

Systemic lupus erythematosus (SLE) is a chronic autoimmune disease that can affect multiple organs, including the skin, joints, brain, peripheral nervous system, heart, gastrointestinal tract, and kidneys. Kidney involvement in SLE, generally termed *lupus nephritis (LN)*, is a major contributor to SLE-associated morbidity and mortality. Up to 50% of SLE patients have clinically evident kidney disease at presentation, and, during follow-up, kidney involvement occurs in up to 75% of patients, with an even greater representation among children and young adults. LN impacts clinical outcomes in SLE both directly via target organ damage and indirectly through complications of therapy.

Presentation

Most patients with SLE will develop laboratory evidence of kidney involvement at some point during the course of their disease. In about one-third of SLE patients, kidney involvement first manifests with proteinuria and/or microscopic hematuria; this eventually progresses to reduction in kidney function. However, early in the course of disease, it is unusual for patients to present with a low glomerular filtration rate (GFR), except in very aggressive cases of LN, some of which present as rapidly progressive glomerulonephritis. Instead, patients often present initially with evidence of non-kidney organ involvement, such as malar rash, arthritis, and oral ulcers. After a diagnosis of SLE is confirmed with appropriate laboratory tests, evidence of kidney disease, if present, usually emerges within the first 3 years of diagnosis.

Signs of kidney involvement tend to correlate with laboratory abnormalities. For example, patients with nephrotic-range proteinuria often present with edema of the lower extremities and, if proteinuria is severe, periorbital edema in the morning. When GFR falls, as is the case with progressive forms of LN, elevated blood pressure is common. The rare development of dark or tea-colored urine is a sign of gross hematuria. A number of tools, such as the SLE Disease Activity Index (SLEDAI) and the British Isles Lupus Assessment Group (BILAG) Index, have been developed to assess the systemic severity of lupus symptoms. Although these questionnaires are primarily used to codify symptoms for clinical trial settings, they also can be helpful to elicit a detailed history from a patient with SLE.

Evaluation

Laboratory Findings

The American College of Rheumatology (ACR) lists 11 diagnostic criteria for SLE: antinuclear antibodies (ANA), arthritis, immunologic disorders (including anti-double-stranded DNA [dsDNA] antibody, antiphospholipid antibody, or anti-Smith antibody), malar rash, discoid rash, photosensitivity, oral ulcers, serositis, hematologic disorder, neurologic disorder, and kidney disorder (Table 25.1). Ideally, four or more of these criteria should be present to diagnose SLE, including laboratory findings of a positive ANA and/or anti-dsDNA antibody. In addition to the ANA and dsDNA antibody, serum complement (C3, C4, CH50) should be checked whenever kidney involvement is suspected, because these are often low when disease is active, as is usually the case with any severe proliferative LN. Antiphospholipid and anticardiolipin antibodies are useful in gauging the risk for clotting abnormalities that can accompany SLE.

Laboratory testing is used both to diagnose kidney involvement and to assess response to therapy in patients with SLE. Traditional parameters, such as serum creatinine and urinary protein excretion (quantified by either 24-hour collection, urine protein-to-creatinine ratio, or urine albumin-to-creatinine ratio), are supplemented by serial review of microscopic urinary sediment, changes in serum complement levels, and titers of ANA and dsDNA antibodies. Because cytopenias are often seen in active SLE, complete blood counts should be checked regularly. A number of urine and serologic tests have been studied as biomarkers for SLE and, specifically, LN disease activity. These include molecules specific to lupus (e.g., anti-C1q antibodies), mediators of chronic inflammation (e.g., TNF-like weak inducer of apoptosis [TWEAK]), and generalized markers of kidney injury (urinary neutrophil gelatinase-associated lipocalin [uNGAL]). However, the clinical utility of this approach remains unproven, and no serum or urine disease markers are able to provide as much information as a kidney biopsy. Hence, virtually all patients with SLE with suspected kidney involvement undergo one or more kidney biopsies at some point during their care.

TABLE 25.1 American College of Rheumatology Criteria for the Diagnosis of Systemic Lupus Erythematosus

Criteria	Description
Malar rash	Flat or raised erythematous rash over the malar eminences
Discoid rash	Erythematous raised patches, usually circular, with adherent keratotic scaling; atrophic scarring may occur
Photosensitivity	Rash upon exposure to ultraviolet light
Oral ulcers	Oral and/or nasopharyngeal ulcerations
Arthritis	Nonerosive arthritis of at least two peripheral joints, with tenderness and/or swelling
Serositis	Pleuritis or pericarditis
Kidney disorder	Proteinuria, hematuria, and/or elevated creatinine
Neurologic disorder	Seizures or psychosis without other etiologies
Hematologic disorder	Anemia (hemolytic), leukopenia, or thrombocytopenia without other etiologies
Immunologic disorder	Anti-dsDNA, anti-Sm, and/or antiphospholipid antibodies
ANA	An abnormal ANA titer in the absence of drugs known to induce ANAs

Any combination of ≥4 criteria at any time during a patient's course suggests a diagnosis of systemic lupus erythematosus.
ANA, Antinuclear antibodies; *dsDNA,* double-stranded DNA.

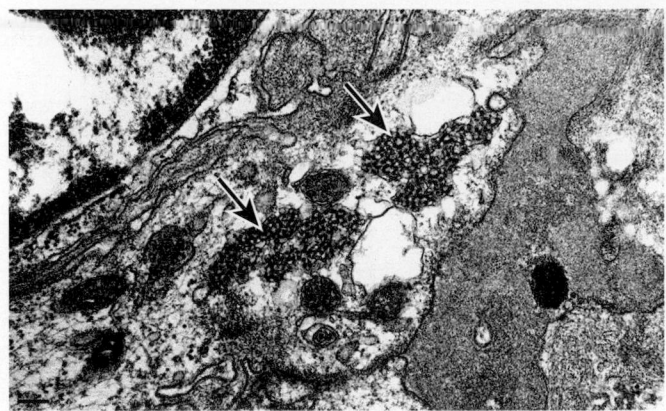

• **Fig. 25.1** Several large endothelial tubuloreticular inclusions *(arrows)* are located in dilated cisternae of the endoplasmic reticulum of this glomerular endothelial cell. These interanastomosing structures, which are commonly identified in systemic lupus erythematosus, are induced in endothelial cells by exposure to ambient interferon, earning them the name "interferon footprints" (electron micrograph, × 50,000).

Kidney Biopsy Findings

The classic pattern of LN is an immune complex–mediated glomerulonephritis; however, the pathology of LN can be varied and at times can cause confusion with other immune complex–mediated glomerulonephritides. Particular biopsy findings highly characteristic of LN include (1) glomerular deposits that stain dominantly for IgG with co-deposits of IgA, IgM, C3, and C1q, the so-called *full house immunofluorescence (IF) pattern*; (2) intense staining for C1q; (3) extraglomerular immune-type deposits within tubular basement membranes, the interstitium, and/or blood vessels; (4) the ultrastructural finding of coexistent mesangial, subendothelial, and subepithelial electron-dense deposits; and (5) the ultrastructural finding of tubuloreticular inclusions, which represent "interferon footprints" in the glomerular endothelial cell cytoplasm (Fig. 25.1).

Although lupus may affect all compartments of the kidney, including glomeruli, tubules, interstitium, and blood vessels, glomerular involvement is the best studied component and correlates well with presentation, course, and treatment response. Accordingly, disease classification is based largely on the glomerular alterations, as assessed by the combined modalities of light microscopy, IF, and electron microscopy (EM). Over the past 5 decades, there have been attempts by different societies, particularly the World

Health Organization (WHO), to classify the diverse glomerulopathies associated with SLE. Based on clinicopathologic correlations, a revised classification system of LN was developed by a working group of kidney pathologists, nephrologists, and rheumatologists under the joint auspices of the International Society of Nephrology (ISN) and the Renal Pathology Society (RPS) and was published in 2004 as the ISN/RPS classification. A minor revision of this classification was published in 2018. By refining and clarifying many of the deficiencies of the older WHO classification, this revised schema has eliminated ambiguities and has achieved greater reproducibility. The ISN/RPS classification recognizes six different classes of immune complex–mediated lupus glomerulonephritis based on biopsy findings (Table 25.2). These classes are not static entities but may transform from one class to another, both spontaneously and after therapy.

ISN/RPS class I represents the mildest possible glomerular lesion—immune deposits limited to the mesangium, without associated mesangial hypercellularity. In class II, the mesangial deposits detected by IF and/or EM are accompanied by mesangial hypercellularity of any degree. In class III, there is focal and predominantly segmental endocapillary proliferation and/or sclerosis, affecting less than 50% of glomeruli sampled. The active endocapillary lesions typically include infiltrating monocytes and neutrophils and may exhibit necrotizing features, including fibrinoid necrosis, rupture of glomerular basement membrane, and nuclear apoptosis, forming pyknotic or karyorrhectic debris. These segmental lesions often arise on a background of mesangial proliferation and immune deposits. In class IV, the endocapillary lesions involve ≥50% of glomeruli sampled, typically in a diffuse and global distribution (Fig. 25.2). Subendothelial immune deposits are a feature of the endocapillary lesion in class III and class IV, where they vary from focal and segmental (class III) to more diffuse and global (class IV; Fig. 25.3). Both class III and class IV may exhibit extracapillary proliferation in the form of cellular crescents, a feature that correlates best with a rapidly progressive clinical course. Subendothelial deposits that are large enough to be visible by light microscopy may form "wire loops," or intracapillary "hyaline thrombi" (Fig. 25.4). A pathognomonic, but uncommon, feature of active LN is glomerular "hematoxylin bodies," which consist of extruded nuclei from dying cells that have

TABLE 25.2	International Society of Nephrology/Renal Pathology Society 2004 Classification of Lupus Nephritis, Updated in 2018	
Designation	**Description**	**Characteristic Clinical Features**
Class I: minimal mesangial lupus nephritis	No LM abnormalities; isolated mesangial IC deposits on IF and/or EM	Normal urine or microscopic hematuria
Class II: mesangial proliferative lupus nephritis	Mesangial hypercellularity or matrix expansion with mesangial IC deposits on IF and/or EM	Microscopic hematuria and/or low-grade proteinuria
Class III: focal lupus nephritis[a]	<50% of glomeruli on LM display segmental (<50% of glomerular tuft) or global (>50% of glomerular tuft) endocapillary and/or extracapillary proliferation or sclerosis; mesangial and focal subendothelial IC deposits on IF and EM	Nephritic urine sediment and subnephrotic proteinuria
Class IV: diffuse lupus nephritis[a]	≥50% of glomeruli on LM display segmental or global endocapillary and/or extracapillary proliferation or sclerosis; mesangial and diffuse subendothelial IC deposits on IF and EM	Nephritic and nephrotic syndromes, hypertension, reduced kidney function
Class V: membranous lupus nephritis[b]	Diffuse thickening of the glomerular capillary walls on LM with subepithelial IC deposits on IF and EM, with or without mesangial IC deposits	Nephrotic syndrome
Class VI: advanced sclerosing lupus nephritis	>90% of glomeruli on LM are globally sclerosed with no residual activity	Markedly reduced kidney function, hypertension

[a]Both class III and class IV may have active (proliferative), chronic, inactive (sclerosing), or combined active and chronic lesions, which should be graded using modified NIH activity and chronicity indices.
[b]Class V may coexist with class III or class IV, in which case both classes are diagnosed.
EM, Electron microscopy; *IC,* immune complex; *IF,* immunofluorescence; *LM,* light microscopy.

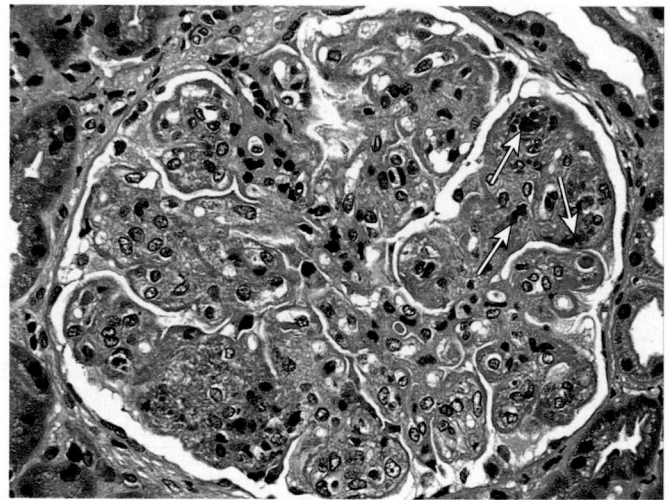

• **Fig. 25.2** Class IV lupus nephritis. A representative glomerulus shows global narrowing or obliteration of its capillary lumina by endocapillary hypercellularity, including infiltrating leukocytes. The glomerular capillary walls are thickened by eosinophilic material, forming wire loops. Rounded basophilic structures ("hematoxylin bodies," *arrows*) represent extruded nuclei altered by binding to antinuclear antibody (hematoxylin and eosin, ×400).

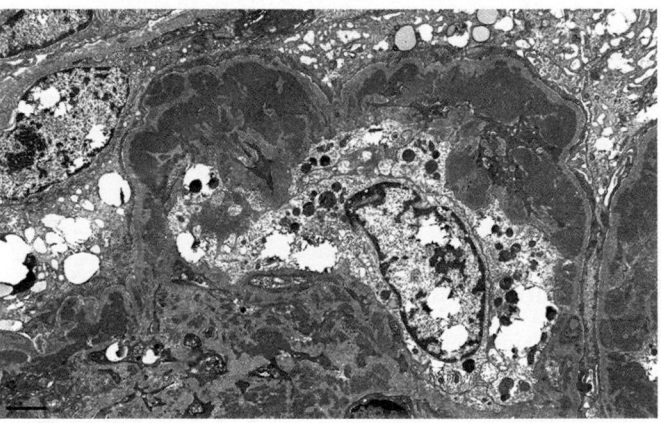

• **Fig. 25.3** Class IV lupus nephritis. There are large electron-dense deposits within the mesangium and in the subendothelial region. Podocyte foot processes are effaced (electron micrograph, ×6000).

bound to ambient ANA to form basophilic rounded bodies ("LE bodies"; see Fig. 25.2). Class V denotes membranous LN. Subepithelial deposits are the defining feature, usually superimposed on a base of mesangial hypercellularity and/or mesangial immune deposits. Well-developed examples of class V typically exhibit glomerular basement membrane spikes between the subepithelial deposits (Fig. 25.5). Class V may progress to glomerulosclerosis without the development of a superimposed proliferative lesion. In those patients with combined membranous and endocapillary lesions, a diagnosis of both class V and class III or IV is made. These mixed classes carry a worse prognosis than pure class V LN. Class VI identifies advanced chronic disease exhibiting greater than 90% sclerotic glomeruli, without residual activity.

Unusual kidney biopsy findings in SLE patients include "lupus podocytopathy," presenting as nephrotic syndrome with diffuse foot process effacement in the absence of peripheral capillary wall immune deposits. Mesangial immune deposits and variable mesangial hypercellularity (consistent with underlying class I or II LN) may accompany the podocyte alterations. Such cases resemble minimal change disease or focal segmental glomerulosclerosis

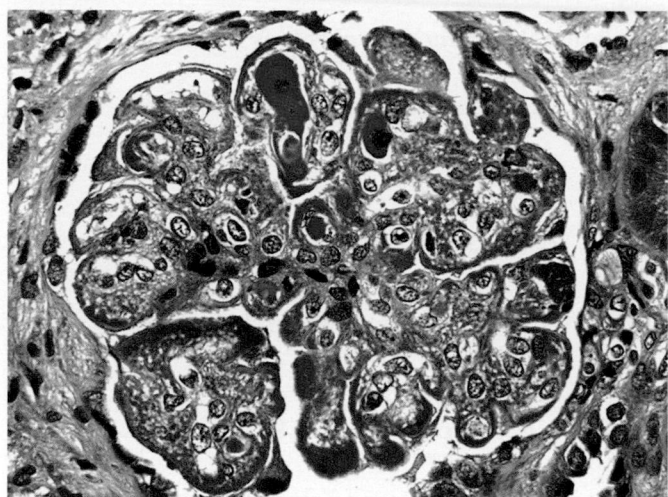

• **Fig. 25.4** Class IV lupus nephritis. Trichrome stain is useful to highlight fuchsinophilic *(red)* deposits against the blue-staining glomerular basement membrane and mesangial matrix. In this glomerulus, many subendothelial "wire loops" and intracapillary "hyaline thrombi" are seen (Masson trichrome, ×600).

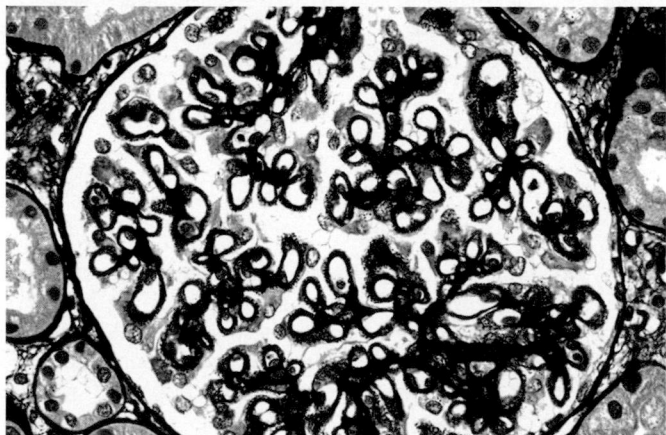

• **Fig. 25.5** Class V lupus nephritis. Membranous lupus nephritis has global thickening of glomerular capillary walls. Silver stain delineates the characteristic silver-positive spikes projecting from the glomerular basement membranes. These spikes form between silver-negative subepithelial deposits (Jones methenamine silver, ×600).

in their histopathologic findings and response to glucocorticoids. An altered systemic cytokine milieu, rather than immune complex deposition, is thought to mediate direct podocyte injury. Lupus podocytopathy with collapsing features has been associated with APOL1 high-risk genotype in patients of African descent and carries a poor prognosis. Rare cases of LN have predominant tubulointerstitial nephritis with abundant tubulointerstitial immune deposits in the absence of significant glomerular lesions. Some cases with necrotizing and crescentic features and a paucity of peripheral capillary wall immune deposits are associated with circulating antineutrophil cytoplasmic antibody (ANCA), in addition to ANA. This "pauci-immune" variant is particularly common in those cases of LN class IV with diffuse but segmental lesions of necrosis and crescent formation. In any patient with SLE who develops thrombotic microangiopathy affecting the glomeruli and/or vessels, the possibility of a circulating lupus anticoagulant or an antiphospholipid antibody should be investigated. Other

unusual vascular lesions include lupus vasculopathy (a noninflammatory narrowing of arterioles by a mixture of immune deposits and fibrin) and true inflammatory arteritis.

Kidney biopsy evaluation is not complete without an assessment of both histologic activity and chronicity as a guide to therapy. The use of modified National Institutes of Health (NIH) indices for activity and chronicity should be included in the kidney biopsy report. Active lesions include any combination of six features: glomerular endocapillary hypercellularity, neutrophil infiltration, fibrinoid necrosis, wire-loop deposits, cellular and/or fibrocellular crescents, and interstitial inflammation. Each component of activity is graded on a scale of 0 to 3+ based on the proportion of glomeruli or cortical area affected. Among features of activity, necrotizing lesions and cellular crescents carry the worst prognosis and are, therefore, accorded double weight. Thus, the total composite score for activity ranges from 0-24. Chronic changes include any combination of four features: global and/or segmental glomerular scarring (glomerulosclerosis), fibrous crescents, tubular atrophy, and interstitial fibrosis, each of which is graded on a scale of 0-3+ for a total composite score of 0-12. Because lesions of activity (A) and chronicity (C) can vary widely in a given biopsy, standard approaches to therapy weigh the extent and severity of active lesions (considered potentially responsive to immunosuppressive therapy) against the extent of chronic, irreversible disease.

Treatment

The current approach to treating LN, as well as studying new therapeutic modalities in clinical trials, has largely been guided by histologic findings (i.e., ISN/RPS class) with appropriate consideration of presenting clinical parameters and the degree of kidney function impairment (Table 25.3). Class I and class II LN, which represent purely mesangial disease, carry a better prognosis and do not require specific therapy directed to the kidney. Rather, conservative, non-immunomodulatory therapy is appropriate for patients with these findings on kidney biopsy. Optimal control of blood pressure through blockade of the renin-angiotensin-aldosterone system (RAAS) is a cornerstone of conservative therapy in LN. Epidemiologic studies have suggested that ACE inhibitor use delays the development of kidney involvement in SLE and reduces overall disease activity.

Classes III and IV Lupus Nephritis

The treatment of active class III and class IV LN is generally divided into induction and maintenance phases of immunosuppression. Most patients with active proliferative LN are treated initially with corticosteroids, traditionally a "pulse" of intravenous steroids (500 to 1000 mg/day of methylprednisolone for 3 days), followed by a high-dose oral regimen (usually prednisone at 1 mg/kg/day, not exceeding 60 mg daily) that begins to taper at 8 weeks.

Induction Therapy

Steroids should be used in conjunction with other immunosuppressive therapy. Currently, cyclophosphamide and mycophenolate mofetil (MMF) are the two main agents used for induction-phase immunosuppression. Intravenous, compared to oral, cyclophosphamide therapy involves a lower cumulative exposure to drug, less frequent cytopenias, enhanced bladder protection, and fewer problems with adherence. Several small, randomized controlled trials at the National Institutes of Health (NIH) in patients with

TABLE 25.3	Treatment Options for Lupus Nephritis, Stratified by International Society of Nephrology Classification and Phase of Therapy	
Class	**Induction Phase**[a]	**Maintenance Phase**[a]
I	Conservative, nonimmunomodulatory therapy (e.g., RAAS blockade)	Not applicable
II	Conservative, nonimmunomodulatory therapy	Not applicable
III, IV	Pulse IV steroids followed by tapering doses of oral steroids *and* IV cyclophosphamide 0.75–1.0 g/m^2 IV monthly for 6 doses *or* IV cyclophosphamide 500 mg IV every 2 weeks for 6 doses *or* MMF 2000–3000 mg/day for 6 months	Lowest tolerable amount of oral steroids *and* MMF 2000 mg/day for 6 months, then 1500 mg/day for 3–6 months, then 1000 mg/day afterward assuming stable disease *or* Azathioprine 2.0 mg/kg/day for 6 months, then 1.5 mg/kg/day for 3–6 months, then 1.0 mg/kg/day afterward assuming stable disease
V	Pulse IV steroids followed by tapering doses of oral steroids *and* IV cyclophosphamide 0.75–1.0 g/m^2 IV monthly for 6 doses *or* Cyclosporine (dose adjusted to goal trough level 125–200 mcg/L) *or* Tacrolimus (dose adjusted to goal trough level 5–10 mcg/L) *or* MMF 2000–3000 mg/day for 6 months	Lowest tolerable amount of oral steroids *and* MMF 2000 mg/day for 6 months, then 1500 mg/day for 3–6 months, then 1000 mg/day afterward assuming stable disease *or* Azathioprine 2.0 mg/kg/day for 6 months, then 1.5 mg/kg/day for 3–6 months, then 1.0 mg/kg/day afterward assuming stable disease
VI	Conservative, nonimmunomodulatory therapy (e.g., RAAS blockade) with preparation for kidney replacement therapy	Not applicable

[a]Doses listed as mg/day are appropriate for adults. See alternate source for pediatric dosing.
IV, Intravenous; *MMF,* mycophenolate mofetil; *RAAS,* renin-angiotensin-aldosterone system.

severe proliferative LN resulted in the induction regimen widely known as the "NIH protocol," which uses six pulses of intravenous cyclophosphamide (0.5 to 1 g/m^2) on consecutive months. A trial by the EuroLupus Group aimed to decrease the risk of side effects from cyclophosphamide therapy without sacrificing efficacy; their shorter treatment course (the "EuroLupus protocol") of 500 mg of intravenous cyclophosphamide every 2 weeks for six doses (total dose 3 g) was equally effective as the NIH protocol in various kidney and non-kidney outcomes, with less toxicity and fewer total infections. Although this trial was largely performed in white subjects and may not be applicable to populations at high risk for poor kidney outcomes, reports from this trial with up to 10 years of follow-up continue to show no differences in outcome among treatment groups.

MMF has emerged as an alternative first-choice agent for inducing a remission in severe active proliferative LN. An initial report from China compared oral MMF to oral cyclophosphamide and showed similar rates of remission with lower rates of infection and overall mortality in the MMF arm at 1 and 5 years of follow-up. A larger US induction trial in a more diverse population (more than 50% Black patients) of proliferative or membranous LN compared monthly intravenous cyclophosphamide pulses with oral MMF therapy, each in conjunction with a fixed tapering dose of corticosteroids, as induction therapy throughout 6 months. Although the study was powered as a non-inferiority trial, complete remissions and complete plus partial remissions at 6 months were significantly more common in the MMF arm (52%) than the cyclophosphamide arm (30%). Subsequently, a 370-patient, international multicenter trial of induction therapy with either MMF (goal 3 g/day) or monthly intravenous cyclophosphamide pulses

showed, after 6 months of therapy, virtually identical rates of complete and partial remission (56% of patients receiving MMF vs. 53% of patients receiving IV cyclophosphamide). A subgroup analysis of those presenting with significant kidney failure (defined as GFR <30 mL/min) showed no indication that MMF was less effective than cyclophosphamide in this setting.

Maintenance Therapy

After remission has been achieved, maintenance-phase therapy should focus on the long-term management of chronic disease. The goals of continued immunosuppressive therapy are to prevent relapses and flares of disease activity, to eliminate smoldering activity leading to kidney scarring, and to minimize long-term side effects of therapy. Azathioprine and MMF have replaced intravenous cyclophosphamide as the preferred immunosuppressive agents for maintenance therapy. Given the risk for long-term toxicities with all immunosuppressive agents, as well as their potential effect on fertility and risk for teratogenicity, the selection and dosage of maintenance therapy are important and modifiable choices that doctors and patients should make together. Although no clinical studies exclude the use of steroids in maintenance therapy, many clinicians will discontinue steroids within the first 1 to 6 months of maintenance therapy to minimize side effects, despite a lack of trial data for such a strategy. Early data suggested equivalence of MMF and azathioprine in sustaining remission during the maintenance phase. For example, in the MAINTAIN Nephritis trial, after standard induction therapy with steroids and cyclophosphamide, 105 subjects with class III (31%), IV (58%), or V (10%) LN underwent either azathioprine or MMF maintenance therapy. After at least 3 years of follow-up, both groups showed equal rates of remission, steroid withdrawal, and disease flares. However, results from the Aspreva Lupus Management Study maintenance study suggested that MMF is more effective than azathioprine as maintenance therapy. In this study of 227 patients who had responded to induction therapy with either MMF or intravenous cyclophosphamide, 36 months of maintenance therapy with MMF appeared to be superior to azathioprine with respect to time to treatment failure, time to renal flare, and time to rescue therapy, regardless of induction therapy. Withdrawals resulting from severe adverse events were significantly more common among patients who were administered azathioprine.

Class V Lupus Nephritis

The treatment of class V (membranous) LN is also divided into induction and maintenance phases of immunosuppression. As for proliferative LN, induction therapy options include cyclophosphamide and MMF; additionally, in class V, calcineurin inhibitors (cyclosporine or tacrolimus), which have emerged as a first-line therapy for primary membranous nephropathy, are another available treatment. Remission may occur more quickly with a calcineurin inhibitor than with cyclophosphamide or MMF, but these therapies include a higher rate of relapse after withdrawal, similar to the experience of using calcineurin inhibitors in other forms of nephrotic syndrome. One strategy, particularly when a class V lesion is superimposed on a proliferative class III or IV lesion, is to combine a calcineurin inhibitor with MMF. This multi-targeted regimen, akin to those used to protect kidney transplants, was tested in a multicenter randomized trial from China that compared induction therapy with MMF, tacrolimus, and steroids versus intravenous cyclophosphamide and steroids. Intention-to-treat analysis showed a higher rate of complete remission (45.9% in the multi-targeted group vs. 25.6% in the cyclophosphamide group) at 24 weeks, with no difference in adverse event rates.

Alternative and Future Therapies

Because of the unacceptably high rate of treatment failure (30% to 50%) of induction therapies as well as the high rate of relapsing disease, newer agents and treatment strategies are continuously sought for LN. Most of these therapies, when studied in a rigorous manner, are administered in addition to current standard treatment regimens of MMF or cyclophosphamide.

Rituximab, an anti-CD20 monoclonal antibody that depletes B cells, was studied in a placebo-controlled trial conducted in 140 patients with severe LN, all of whom were receiving concurrent MMF (up to 3 g/day) and tapering dose of corticosteroids. Although more individuals in the rituximab group achieved complete or partial remission, there was no statistically significant difference in the primary clinical endpoint at 1 year. A post-hoc analysis of this study, however, identified that participants who experienced a rapid and complete depletion of B cells showed statistically higher remission rates than those participants who did not deplete B cells completely. A phase II study of obinutuzumab, which has been shown to more effectively deplete B cells than rituximab, has now reported higher remission rates than placebo when added to standard induction therapy of MMF plus steroids. Belimumab, a humanized monoclonal antibody that targets the B cell growth factor B lymphocyte stimulator protein, has been approved for treatment of SLE and, in a recent trial encompassing

2 years of treatment, yielded higher kidney response rates than placebo when added to standard induction and maintenance therapies. Voclosporin, a new calcineurin inhibitor with more predictable pharmacokinetics, allowing for fixed dose administration, has also been shown in phase II and phase III studies to induce higher rates of remission than placebo when added to MMF-based induction therapy. Plasma exchange has been added to induction therapies in several trials, without any demonstrated clear benefit in kidney or patient survival; therefore, the routine use of plasma exchange is not justified in LN, although this procedure may be of value in unique individuals, such as those with a refractory antiphospholipid antibody and contraindications to anticoagulation or those with both positive lupus and ANCA serologies.

Prognosis

The proliferative forms of LN, specifically class III and class IV, as well as class V superimposed on class III or IV, are progressive diseases unless a remission is quickly achieved and sustained. In recent decades, the increasing armamentarium of immunosuppressive agents along with an improved knowledge, based on well-performed clinical trials, of how best to dose these agents has led to an improved prognosis for patients with LN. Whereas kidney survival at 5 years was as low as 20% before 1980, current treatment strategies have improved this rate to as high as 80% in the past decade. Risk factors for progressive disease include demographic variables, such as male sex, African lineage, Hispanic ethnicity, low socioeconomic status, and young age at presentation, as well as clinical and biopsy features, such as lower GFR at presentation, hypertension, anemia, higher percentage of glomeruli with necrosis or crescents, and degree of scarring or chronicity in the glomeruli and tubulointerstitium. Repeat kidney biopsy after 6 or more months to assess treatment response and evaluate ongoing activity and chronicity is a valuable tool to guide subsequent adjustments in therapy.

When LN does progress to end-stage kidney disease, most patients experience a gradual complete or partial resolution of their extrarenal manifestations of lupus, including lupus serologies. Furthermore, those patients who continue to experience active disease generally have only mild to moderate symptoms. The mechanisms responsible for this apparent remission of systemic lupus in kidney failure remain unclear. The recommendation that patients with end-stage kidney disease due to LN should be dialyzed for at least 3 to 6 months before kidney transplantation to allow for this "burning out" applies only for those patients with relatively rapid progression to kidney failure. This period allows for a potential further reduction in lupus activity before transplantation but also affords patients with acute kidney injury sufficient time to recover kidney function if therapy is effective. The majority of LN patients, however, will benefit from the earliest possible transplant date. The overall graft survival in patients with lupus who receive a kidney transplant is similar to those in patients with other kidney diseases, despite a recurrence rate of LN that ranges from 5% to 30%, depending on the indications for kidney allograft biopsy. Recurrence can occur as early as the first week and as late as 10 to 15 years after transplantation. Recurrent LN does not necessarily follow the pattern of the native disease but often takes the form of a milder, non-proliferative lesion.

Complete bibliography is available at Elsevier eBooks for Practicing Clinicians.

Key Bibliography

Almaani S, Meara A, Rovin BH. Update on lupus nephritis. *Clin J Am Soc Nephrol.* 2017;12(5):825–835.

Appel GB, Contreras G, Dooley MA, et al. Mycophenolate mofetil versus cyclophosphamide for induction treatment of lupus nephritis. *J Am Soc Nephrol.* 2009;20:1103–1112.

Austin HA 3rd, Illei GG, Braun MJ, et al. Randomized, controlled trial of prednisone, cyclophosphamide, and cyclosporine in lupus membranous nephropathy. *J Am Soc Nephrol.* 2009;20:901–911.

Bajema IM, Wilhelmus S, Alpers CE, et al. Revision of the International Society of Nephrology/Renal Pathology Society classification for lupus nephritis: clarification of definitions, and modified National Institutes of Health activity and chronicity indices. *Kidney Int.* 2018;93(4):789–796.

Dooley MA, Jayne D, Ginzler EM, et al. Mycophenolate versus azathioprine as maintenance therapy for lupus nephritis. *N Engl J Med.* 2011;365:1886–1895.

Ginzler EM, Dooley MA, Aranow C, et al. Mycophenolate mofetil or intravenous cyclophosphamide for lupus nephritis. *N Engl J Med.* 2005;353:2219–2228.

Gourley MF, Austin 3rd HA, Scott D, et al. Methylprednisolone and cyclophosphamide, alone or in combination, in patients with lupus nephritis. A randomized, controlled trial. *Ann Intern Med.* 1996;125:549–557.

Houssiau FA, D'Cruz D, Sangle S, et al. Azathioprine versus mycophenolate mofetil for long-term immunosuppression in lupus nephritis: results from the MAINTAIN nephritis trial. *Ann Rheum Dis.* 2010;69:2083–2089.

Hu W, Chen Y, Wang S, et al. Clinical-morphological features and outcomes of lupus podocytopathy. *Clin J Am Soc Nephrol.* 2016;11:585–592.

Illei GG, Austin HA, Crane M, et al. Combination therapy with pulse cyclophosphamide plus pulse methylprednisolone improves long-term renal outcome without adding toxicity in patients with lupus nephritis. *Ann Intern Med.* 2001;135:248–257.

Liu Z, Zhang H, Liu Z, et al. Multitarget therapy for induction treatment of lupus nephritis: a randomized trial. *Ann Intern Med.* 2015;162:18–26.

Miyasaka N, Kawai S, Hashimoto H. Efficacy and safety of tacrolimus for lupus nephritis: a placebo-controlled double-blind multicenter study. *Mod Rheumatol.* 2009;19:606–615.

Nasr SH, D'Agati VD, Park H-R, et al. Necrotizing and crescentic lupus nephritis with antineutrophil cytoplasmic antibody seropositivity. *Clin J Am Soc Nephrol.* 2008;3:682–690.

Ortega LM, Schultz DR, Lenz O, et al. Lupus nephritis: pathologic features, epidemiology and a guide to therapeutic decisions. *Lupus.* 2010;19:557–574.

Radhakrishnan J, Moutzouris DA, Ginzler EM, et al. Mycophenolate mofetil and intravenous cyclophosphamide are similar as induction therapy for class V lupus nephritis. *Kidney Int.* 2010;77:152–160.

Tunnicliffe DJ, Palmer SC, Henderson L, et al. Immunosuppressive treatment for proliferative lupus nephritis. *Cochrane Database Syst Rev.* 2018;6(6):CD002922.

Weening JJ, D'Agati VD, Schwartz MM, et al. The classification of glomerulonephritis in systemic lupus erythematosus revisited. *J Am Soc Nephrol.* 2004;15:241–250.

Wu LH, Yu F, Tan Y, et al. Inclusion of renal vascular lesions in the 2003 ISN/RPS system for classifying lupus nephritis improves renal outcome predictions. *Kidney Int.* 2013;83:715–723.

26

Pathogenesis, Pathophysiology, and Treatment of Diabetic Kidney Disease

LISA DUBROFSKY, DAVID Z. CHERNEY, PETTER BJORNSTAD

Diabetic kidney disease (DKD) is the leading cause of kidney failure in adults. In the United States, approximately half of patients initiating dialysis have diabetes mellitus, and most of these have type 2 diabetes; patients with youth-onset type 2 diabetes, as shown in the Treatment Options for Type 2 Diabetes in Adolescents and Youth (TODAY) study, exhibit a particularly high risk of progressive DKD after a relatively short duration of disease. Mortality among patients with DKD is high, with cardiovascular diseases predominating. Once overt DKD (as defined by the presence of proteinuria and/or impaired kidney function) is present, kidney failure can often be postponed, but, in most instances, not prevented, by effective antihypertensive treatment and careful glycemic control. Accordingly, there has been intensive research into pathophysiologic mechanisms of diabetic kidney injury, predictors of risk for DKD, and early intervention strategies.

The classic terminology used to describe different states of urinary albumin excretion include normoalbuminuria, moderately increased albuminuria (previously microalbuminuria), and severely increased albuminuria (previously macroalbuminuria or "overt proteinuria"). Normoalbuminuria is typically defined as urinary albumin excretion rate (UAER) <20 μg/min or urinary albumin-to-creatinine ratio (UACR) < 30 mg/g (or 30 mg/day), moderately increased albuminuria as UAER between 20–200 μg/min or UACR between 30–300 mg/g (30–300 mg/day), and severely increased albuminuria as UAER >200 μg/min or UACR >300 mg/g (>300 mg/day). This chapter refers to categories of albuminuria using the updated nomenclature, translating from the original studies.

Pathophysiology

The pathophysiology underlying DKD is complex and remains incompletely understood. Although other important modulating factors may contribute, the long-term deleterious impacts of hyperglycemia and insulin resistance are central to the development and progression of DKD. Studies in both type 1 and type 2 diabetes have shown that improved glycemic control can mitigate the risk of developing DKD. Moreover, the development of the earliest diabetic kidney lesions can be slowed or prevented by strict glycemic control, as was demonstrated in a randomized trial in type 1 diabetic kidney transplant recipients. Similarly, intensive insulin treatment decreases the progression rates of glomerular lesions in patients with type 1 diabetes and moderately increased albuminuria. Finally, established diabetic glomerular lesions in the native kidneys of patients with type 1 diabetes regress with prolonged normalization of glycemic levels after successful pancreas transplantation. In summary, these studies strongly suggest that hyperglycemia is necessary for the development and maintenance of DKD in type 1 diabetes, as correction of hyperglycemia allows expression of reparative mechanisms that facilitate healing of the original diabetic glomerular injury.

Intraglomerular hemodynamic mechanisms, including hyperfiltration, likely play a significant role in the pathogenesis of DKD through neurohormonal (e.g., renin-angiotensin-aldosterone system activation) and tubular (e.g., tubuloglomerular feedback) pathways. However, patients with other causes of glomerular hyperfiltration, such as unilateral nephrectomy, do not typically develop evidence of kidney disease. Furthermore, it is unlikely that all patients with diabetes and glomerular hyperfiltration develop DKD. Therefore, glomerular hyperfiltration alone cannot fully explain the genesis of the early lesions of DKD. However, previous studies and clinical observations suggest that hemodynamic factors are important in modulating the initiation of nephropathy, and the rate of progression of diabetic lesions that are already well established. Studies in adults with type 1 and type 2 diabetes have also demonstrated that glomerular hyperfiltration is associated with a greater risk of experiencing a rapid glomerular filtration rate (GFR) decline. However, these findings were not recapitulated by an analysis in the Diabetes Control and Complications Trial (DCCT) where no association was found between glomerular hyperfiltration and the development of stage 3 CKD. It is worth noting that the presence of impaired GFR in normoalbuminuric patients with type 1 diabetes is associated with more severe glomerular lesions of DKD, and these patients may be at magnified risk of further progression, possibly on the basis of ischemia and inflammation-related mechanisms.

Systemic hypertension and a lack of normal nocturnal blood-pressure dipping may both be implicated in the pathogenesis of DKD. Supporting this hypothesis is the association between intensive blood-pressure control and decreased rates of progression from normoalbuminuria to moderately increased albuminuria and from moderately to severely increased albuminuria in both normotensive and hypertensive patients with type 2 diabetes.

Studies on human genetics offer important mechanistic insights into complex traits such as DKD. A genetic predisposition to diabetic nephropathy is suggested in multiple cross-sectional studies in type 1 and type 2 diabetic siblings concordant for diabetes. Importantly, diabetic sibling pairs that are concordant for DKD risk are also highly concordant for diabetic glomerulopathy lesions, and this risk is in part independent of glycemia. Novel loci associated with albuminuria were identified by genome-wide association study (GWAS) meta-analysis of albuminuria traits in the general population. An association between protein coding gene for cubilin (CUBN) and albuminuria was demonstrated, and gene-by-diabetes interactions were detected and confirmed for variants in HS6ST1 and near RAB38/CTSC. One large GWAS found a common missense mutation encoding for the collagen type IV alpha 3 chain gene and associated with a thinner GBM to be protective against DKD in T1D, a paradoxical finding that may guide new research on the pathogenesis of the disease. Another large GWAS in African American patients with T2D identified eight associations in seven genetic loci for DKD-related ESKD; further studies are required to confirm replicability. Additionally, an integrated biological approach linking clinical phenotyping with histopathological and molecular phenotyping of kidney tissue can enhance our understanding of the molecular pathogenesis engendering DKD.

Diabetic kidney disease is characterized not only by glomerular disease but also by tubulointerstitial injury. While glomerular changes have received more attention than tubulointerstitial changes in DKD research, tubular injury may be more closely associated with kidney function than glomerular injury. Tubular proteinuria predates microalbuminuria in youths with type 1 diabetes, suggesting that tubular damage may occur earlier than glomerular injury in the course of diabetic nephropathy. Tubular changes associated with DKD include basement membrane thickening, tubular hypertrophy, epithelial–mesenchymal transition, glycogen accumulation, and interstitial inflammation. Basement membrane thickening and tubular hypertrophy are mainly related to extracellular matrix (ECM) accumulation, which reflects an imbalance between ECM synthesis and degradation, is the principal cause of mesangial expansion that also contributes to expansion of the interstitium late in the disease. Several mechanisms have been proposed to explain the link between hyperglycemia and ECM accumulation. These include higher levels of TGFβ; activation of protein kinase C, (which stimulates ECM production through the cyclic adenosine monophosphate (cAMP) pathway); increased advanced glycation end products; and increased activity of aldose reductase, leading to accumulation of sorbitol. There is also growing evidence that oxidative stress is increased in diabetes and is also related to DKD, mediated through altered nitric oxide production and action, and endothelial dysfunction. Importantly, many factors associated with DKD may act through both hemodynamic and non-hemodynamic pathways. For example, angiotensin II increases intraglomerular pressure and hyperfiltration and also increases the production of injurious mediators such as protein kinase C. Intraglomerular hypertension, whether a consequence of angiotensin II, other neurohormones, or tubular factors, is associated with increased glomerular wall tension and shear stress, leading to the activation of proinflammatory and profibrotic pathways.

Glycocalyx dysfunction has recently attracted attention as a potential mediator of both diabetic glomerulopathy and tubulopathy. The glycocalyx is a polysaccharide gel that covers the luminal surface of the endothelium, thereby acting as a filtration barrier and regulator of endothelial vascular function. Under exposure to hyperglycemic conditions, the glycocalyx is modified, leading to exposure of heparin sulfate domains that allow chemokine binding and inflammation and result in glycocalyx degradation. Albuminuria is likely to, at least in part, occur as a consequence disruption of the glycocalyx. The presence of overlapping and interrelated injurious pathways that promote diabetic nephropathy highlight the need for a multifaceted therapeutic approach, as outlined below.

Pathology

Type 1 Diabetes

In patients with type 1 diabetes, glomerular lesions can appear within a few years after diabetes onset. The same progression time frame occurs when a normal kidney is transplanted into a patient with diabetes. The changes in kidney structure caused by diabetes are specific, creating a pattern not seen in any other disease, and the severity of these diabetic lesions is related to the functional disturbances of the clinical kidney disease as well as to diabetes duration, glycemic control, and genetic factors. However, the relationship between the duration of type 1 diabetes and extent of glomerular pathology is not precise. This is consistent with the marked variability in susceptibility to this disorder, such that some patients may develop kidney failure after having diabetes for 15 years, whereas others escape kidney complications despite having type 1 diabetes for decades.

Light Microscopy

Kidney hypertrophy is the earliest structural change in type 1 diabetes but is not reflected in any specific light microscopic changes. In many patients, glomerular structure remains normal or near normal even after decades of diabetes, whereas others develop progressive diffuse mesangial expansion, seen mainly as increased periodic acid–Schiff (PAS)-positive ECM mesangial material. In about 40% to 50% of patients developing proteinuria, there are areas of extreme mesangial expansion called *Kimmelstiel-Wilson nodules* (nodular mesangial expansion). Mesangial cell nuclei in these nodules are palisaded around masses of mesangial matrix material with compression of surrounding capillary lumina. Nodules are thought to result from earlier glomerular capillary microaneurysm formation. Notably, about half of patients with severe diabetic nephropathy do not have these nodular lesions; therefore, although Kimmelstiel-Wilson nodules are diagnostic of diabetic nephropathy, they are not necessary for severe kidney disease to develop.

Early changes often include arteriolar hyalinosis lesions involving replacement of the smooth muscle cells of afferent and efferent arterioles with PAS-positive waxy, homogenous material (Fig. 26.1). The severity of these lesions is directly related to the frequency of global glomerulosclerosis, perhaps as the result of glomerular ischemia. GBM and TBM thickening may be seen with light microscopy, although they are more easily seen with electron microscopy. In addition, tubular glomeruli and glomerulotubular junction abnormalities are present in proteinuric patients with type 1 diabetes and may be important in the progressive loss of GFR in DKD. Finally, usually quite late in the disease, tubular atrophy and interstitial fibrosis occur.

Immunofluorescence

Diabetes is characterized by increased linear staining of the GBM, TBM, and Bowman capsule, especially for immunoglobulin G (mainly IgG4) and albumin. Although this staining is removed only by strong acid conditions, consistent with strong ionic binding, the intensity of staining is not related to the severity of the underlying lesions.

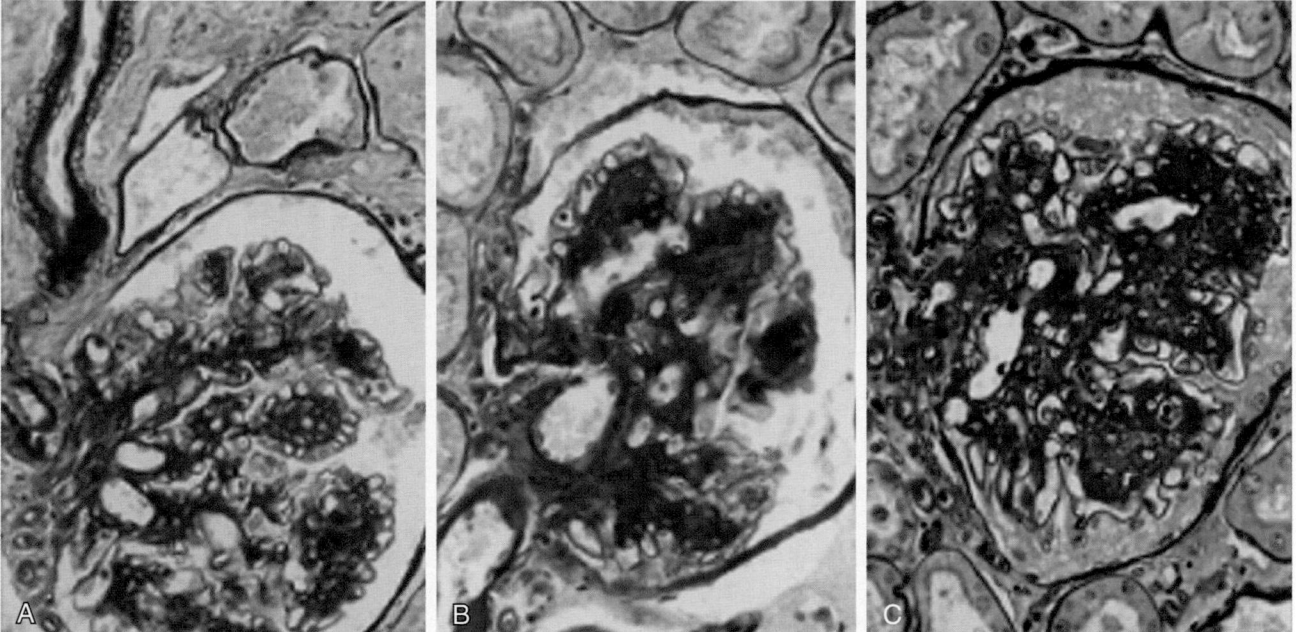

• **Fig. 26.1** Light microscopy photographs of glomeruli in sequential kidney biopsies performed at baseline and after 5 and 10 years of follow-up in a patient with long-standing normoalbuminuric type 1 diabetes with progressive mesangial expansion and kidney function deterioration. (A) Diffuse and nodular mesangial expansion and arteriolar hyalinosis in this glomerulus from a patient who was normotensive and normo-albuminuric at the time of this baseline biopsy, 21 years after diabetes onset (periodic acid–Schiff [PAS] stain, original magnification ×400). (B) Five-year follow-up biopsy showing worsening of the diffuse and nodular mesangial expansion and arteriolar hyalinosis in this now microalbuminuric patient with declining glomerular filtration rate (GFR) (PAS stain, ×400). (C) Ten-year follow-up biopsy showing more advanced diabetic glomerulopathy in this now proteinuric patient with further reduced GFR. Note also the multiple small glomerular (probably efferent) arterioles in the hilar region of this glomerulus (PAS stain, ×400) and in the glomerulus shown in (A).

Electron Microscopy

The first measurable change observed in DKD is thickening of the GBM, which can be detected as early as 1.5 to 2.5 years after onset of type 1 diabetes (Fig. 26.2). TBM thickening is also seen and parallels GBM thickening. A measurable increase in the relative area of the mesangium begins by 4 to 5 years, with the proportion of the glomerular volume that is mesangium increasing from about 20% (normal) to about 40% when proteinuria begins and to 60% to 80% in patients with stage 3 chronic kidney disease (CKD). Immunohistochemical studies indicate that these changes in mesangium, GBM, and TBM represent expansion of the intrinsic ECM components at these sites, most likely including types IV and VI collagen, laminin, and fibronectin.

Qualitative and quantitative changes in the kidney interstitium are observed in patients with various kidney diseases. Interstitial fibrosis is characterized by an increase in ECM proteins and cellularity. Preliminary studies suggest that the pathogenesis of interstitial changes in diabetic nephropathy is different from the changes that occur in the mesangial matrix, GBM, and TBM. Whereas, for all but the later stages of DKD, GBM, TBM, and mesangial matrix changes represent the accumulation of basement membrane ECM material, early interstitial expansion is largely a result of cellular alterations and only later, when GFR is already compromised, is interstitial expansion associated with increased interstitial fibrillar collagen and peritubular capillary loss. Consistent with most kidney diseases affecting the glomeruli, the fraction of GBM covered by intact, non-detached foot processes is

lower in proteinuric patients with diabetes when compared with either control subjects or individuals with type 1 diabetes with low levels of albuminuria. Moreover, the fraction of the glomerular capillary luminal surface covered by fenestrated endothelium is reduced in all stages of DKD, with increasing severity in normoalbuminuria, moderately increased albuminuria, and severely increased albuminuria in patients with type 1 diabetes as compared with controls.

Type 2 Diabetes

Glomerular and tubular structures in type 2 diabetes are less well studied but overall seem to manifest in a more heterogeneous fashion than is observed in type 1 diabetes. Between 30% and 50% of patients with type 2 diabetes who have clinical features of DKD have typical pathology findings, including diffuse and nodular mesangial expansion and arteriolar hyalinosis (Fig. 26.3). Notably, some patients, despite the presence of albuminuria, have absent or only mild diabetic glomerulopathy, whereas others have disproportionately severe tubular and interstitial abnormalities and/or vascular lesions and/or an increased number of globally sclerosed glomeruli. Patients with type 2 diabetes with moderately increased albuminuria more frequently have morphometric glomerular structural measures in the normal range on electron microscopy and less severe lesions compared to patients with type 1 diabetes with moderately or severely increased albuminuria. Interestingly, Pima Indians with type 2 diabetes, a high-risk population

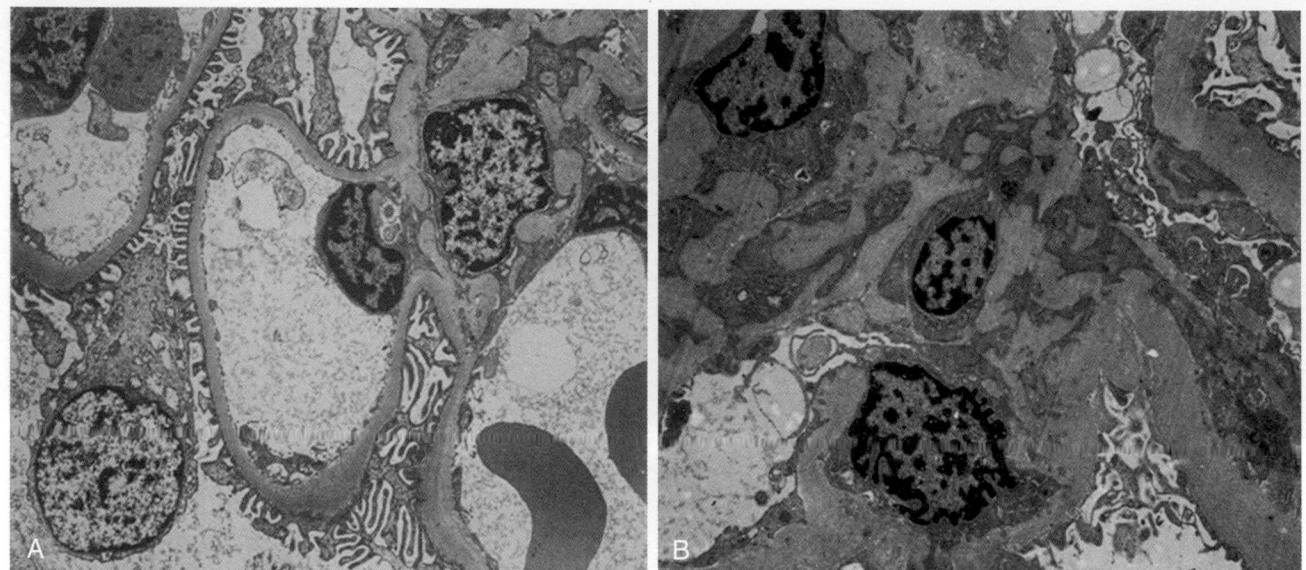

• **Fig. 26.2** Electron microscopy photographs of mesangial area in a normal control individual (A) and in an individual with type 1 diabetes (B) (original magnification ×3900). Note the increase in mesangial matrix and cell content, the glomerular basement membrane thickening, and the decrease in the capillary luminal space in the diabetic patient (B).

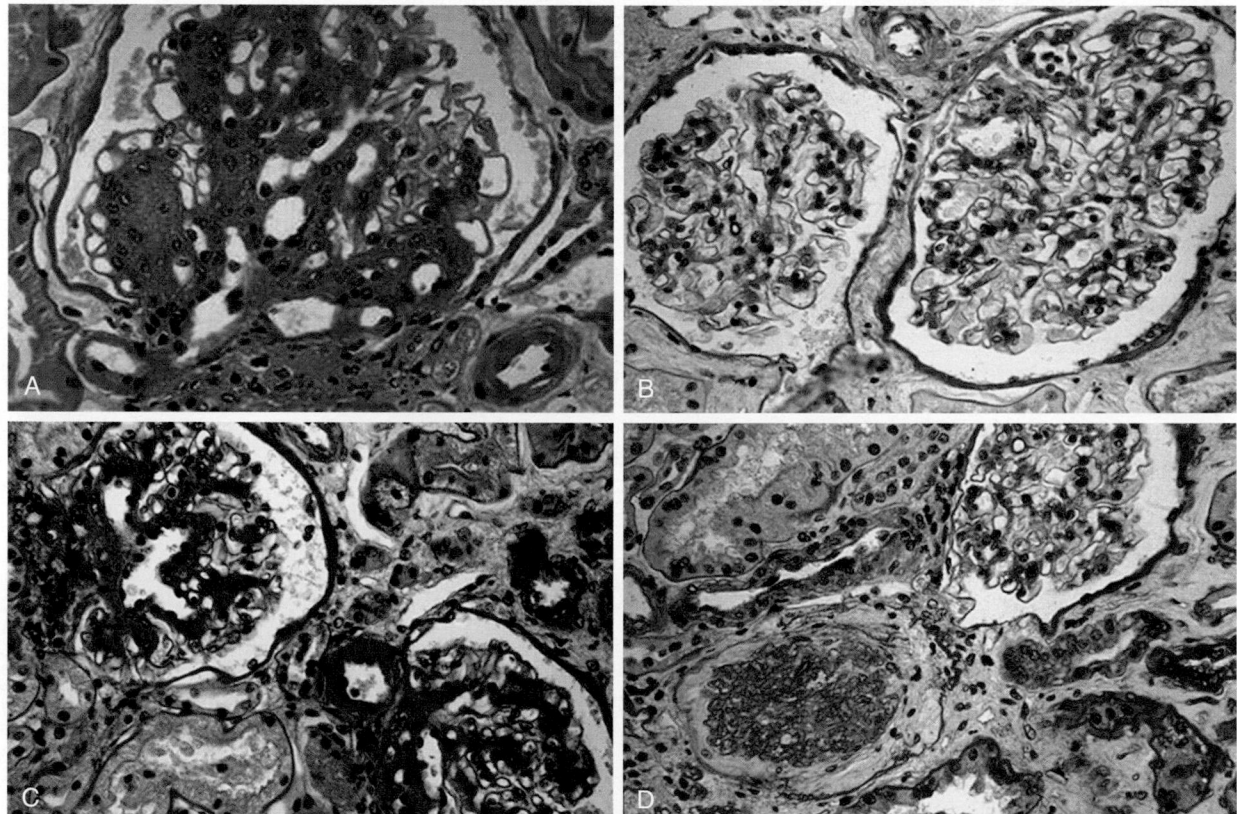

• **Fig. 26.3** **Light microscopy photographs of glomeruli from type 1 (A) and type 2 (B through D) diabetic patients.** (A) Diffuse and nodular mesangial expansion and arteriolar hyalinosis in a glomerulus from an individual with type 1 diabetes and moderately elevated albuminuria (periodic acid–Schiff [PAS] stain, original magnification ×400). (B) Normal or near-normal kidney structure in a glomerulus from an individual with type 2 diabetes and moderately elevated albuminuria (PAS stain, ×400). (C) Changes "typical" of diabetic kidney disease (glomerular, tubulointerstitial, and arteriolar changes occurring in parallel) in a kidney biopsy specimen from an individual with type 2 diabetes and moderately elevated albuminuria (PAS stain, ×400). (D) "Atypical" patterns of injury, with absent or only mild diabetic glomerular changes associated with disproportionately severe tubulointerstitial changes. Note also a glomerulus undergoing glomerular sclerosis (PAS stain, ×400) (B through D).

for kidney failure, have lesions more typical of those seen in type 1 diabetes and were found to have structural defects up to a decade prior to onset of impaired GFR.

It is unclear why some studies show more structural heterogeneity in type 2 than in type 1 diabetes whereas others do not. Regardless, the rate of kidney disease progression in type 2 diabetes is related, at least in part, to the severity of the classic changes of diabetic glomerulopathy. Although there are reports that patients with type 2 diabetes have an increased incidence of nondiabetic lesions, such as proliferative glomerulonephritis and membranous nephropathy, this likely reflects biopsies more often being performed in patients with atypical clinical features. When biopsies are performed for research purposes, the incidence of other definable kidney diseases is very low (<5%). It is also noteworthy that a significant proportion of patients with type 2 diabetes exhibit an accelerated GFR decline in the absence of albuminuria. Although this phenotype is not yet completely understood, it has been suggested that this may reflect a predominance of microvascular disease rather than glomerular disease, thereby attenuating albuminuria risk. GFR reduction in the absence of albuminuria highlights the need to identify alternate biomarkers that better capture early DKD risk.

Structural–Functional Relationships in Diabetic Kidney Disease

Kidney disease progression rates vary greatly among individuals with diabetes. Patients with type 1 diabetes and patients with proteinuria who are biopsied for research purposes always have advanced glomerular lesions and usually have vascular, tubular, and interstitial lesions as well. There is considerable overlap in glomerular structural changes between patients with long-standing normoalbuminuria and those with moderately increased albuminuria, as some normoalbuminuric patients with long-standing type 1 diabetes can have quite advanced kidney lesions, whereas many patients with long-standing diabetes and normoalbuminuria have structural measurements within the normal range.

Ultimately, expansion of the mesangium, mainly resulting from ECM accumulation, reduces or even obliterates the glomerular capillary luminal space, decreasing the glomerular filtration surface and, therefore, decreasing the GFR. Accordingly, the fraction of the glomerulus occupied by mesangium correlates with both GFR and albuminuria in patients with type 1 diabetes, reflecting in part the inverse relationship between mesangial expansion and total peripheral GBM filtration surface per glomerulus. GBM thickness is also directly related to the albumin excretion rate. Finally, the extent of global glomerulosclerosis and interstitial expansion are correlated with the clinical manifestations of DKD (proteinuria, hypertension, and declining GFR).

In patients with type 1 diabetes, glomerular, tubular, interstitial, and vascular lesions tend to progress more or less in parallel, whereas in patients with type 2 diabetes this often is not the case. Current evidence suggests that, among type 2 diabetes patients with moderately increased albuminuria, those patients with typical diabetic glomerulopathy have a higher risk of progressive GFR loss than those with lesser degrees of glomerular changes. A remarkably high frequency of glomerular tubular junction abnormalities can be observed in proteinuric type 1 diabetic patients. Most of these abnormalities are associated with tuft adhesions to Bowman capsule at or near the glomerular tubular junction (tip lesions). The frequency and severity of these lesions (as well as the presence of completely atubular glomeruli) predict GFR loss.

The data on structural–functional relationships in type 2 diabetes are less abundant. In several small studies, morphometric measures of diabetic glomerulopathy correlated with kidney function parameters similar to those observed in type 1 diabetes, although there seems to be a subset of patients who have normal glomerular structure despite persistent albuminuria. Overall, the relationships between kidney function and glomerular structure are less precise in patients with type 2 diabetes. Importantly the rate of GFR decline significantly correlates with the severity of diabetic glomerulopathy lesions. Thus, kidney lesions different from those typical of diabetic glomerulopathy should be considered when investigating the nature of abnormal levels of albuminuria in type 2 diabetes. These lesions include changes in the structure of renal tubules, interstitium, arterioles, and podocytes. For example, Pima Indians with type 2 diabetes and proteinuria have fewer podocytes per glomerulus than those without evidence of kidney disease, and, in this population, a lower number of podocytes per glomerulus at baseline was the strongest predictor of greater increases in albuminuria and of progression to overt DKD in individuals with moderately increased albuminuria. These results suggest that changes in podocyte structure and density occur early in DKD and might contribute to increasing albuminuria in these patients. More biopsy data are needed in people with type 1 and type 2 diabetes to better characterize DKD and rule out non-diabetes-related kidney disease. Data from genome-wide intrarenal gene expression profiling, morphometric analyses of protocol biopsies, and clinical outcomes were recently integrated to explore novel pathways of early DKD in T2D. This data linked genes associated with cortical interstitial fractional volume (a marker of tubule-interstitial damage) and long-term clinical outcomes of albuminuria and GFR, suggesting potential novel targets for markers of early DKD.

Reversal of Diabetic Kidney Disease Lesions

The lesions of DKD have long been considered irreversible. Theoretically, if reversal were possible, this would happen in the setting of long-term normoglycemia. Interestingly, in pancreas transplant recipients, the lesions of diabetic injury were unaffected after 5 years of normoglycemia but reversed in all patients by 10 years posttransplant, with a remarkable amelioration of glomerular structure abnormalities evident by light microscopy, including total disappearance of Kimmelstiel-Wilson nodular lesions. The latency needed for diabetic lesions to disappear is consistent with their slow rate of development. The understanding of the molecular and cellular mechanisms involved in these repair processes could provide new directions for the treatment of DKD.

Medical Management of Diabetes

Both kidney and cardiovascular morbidity and mortality are increased in patients with type 2 diabetes, particularly in those with DKD. Accordingly, treatment goals in these individuals focus on slowing the rate of GFR decline and delaying the onset of kidney failure as well as primary and secondary prevention of cardiovascular disease. This is mainly done by targeting multiple kidney and cardiovascular risk factors, such as hyperglycemia, hypertension, and dyslipidemia (Fig. 26.4). Multiple completed cardiovascular outcome trials with glucose-lowering agents have shown substantial cardiac and kidney benefits, altering the clinical approach to

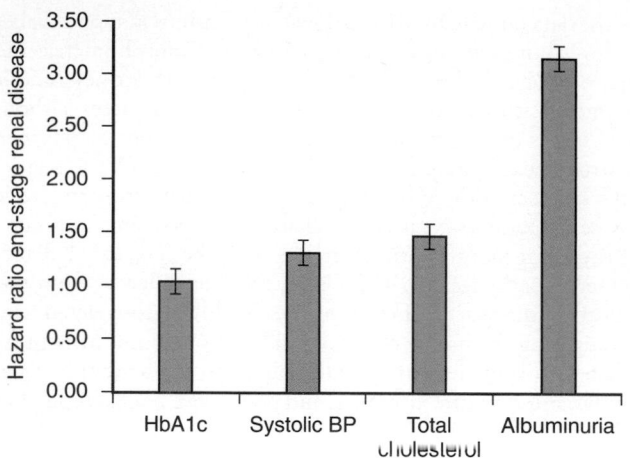

• **Fig. 26.4** Comparison of different risk markers for prediction of kidney failure in individuals with type 2 diabetes and nephropathy participating in the Trial to Reduce cardiovascular Events with Aranesp Therapy (TREAT). The kidney failure risk per standard deviation increment in the risk factor is shown. Per standard deviation increment in albuminuria, the risk of kidney failure markedly amplifies compared with the other kidney disease risk factors. (Adapted from Pfeffer MA, Burdmann EA, Chen CY, et al: A trial of darbepoetin alfa in type 2 diabetes and chronic kidney disease, *N Engl J Med* 361:2019-2032, 2009.)

anti-glycemic therapies in type 2 diabetes. The remainder of this chapter reviews the traditional and novel therapeutic options to decrease the risk of kidney and cardiovascular morbidity and mortality in patients with diabetes.

Traditional Therapeutic Strategies for Diabetic Kidney Disease

Glycemic Control

Rationale

Poor glycemic control, as reflected by higher hemoglobin A1c (HbA1c) levels, is associated with markedly worse kidney and cardiovascular outcomes in observational studies of patients with type 1 and type 2 diabetes, and targeting HbA1c values lower than 7% (53 mmol/mol) may delay the progression of DKD, including development of albuminuria. In patients with type 1 diabetes, the benefit of intensive glucose control in the prevention of microvascular complications (specifically retinopathy or moderately increased albuminuria) was demonstrated in the DCCT, where long-term follow-up showed a significant reduction in the risk of developing reduced GFR among individuals who were treated intensively earlier in the course of diabetes. In type 2 diabetes, the United Kingdom prospective diabetes study (UKPDS) and ADVANCE-ON documented benefit of intensive glucose targeting on microvascular complications. Of note, although most studies of type 2 diabetes have shown a benefit in kidney outcomes, multiple trials failed to show a benefit of intensive glycemic control on mortality and cardiovascular disease, with some trials actually showing higher mortality with intensive control. In contrast with this older literature, more recent trials with sodium-glucose cotransporter-2 inhibitors (SGLT-2 inhibitors) and glucagon-like peptide-1 (GLP-1) receptor agonists have shown reductions in cardiovascular risk (and kidney benefits in the case of SGLT-2 inhibitors), with only modest reductions in HbA1c. This highlights the importance of non-glycemic mechanisms leading to

cardiorenal damage, although the underlying pathways require further study. Accordingly, a careful, individualized approach is required when assigning glycemic targets in individuals with diabetes and kidney disease.

Medications of Choice

Kidney and cardiac risk should be considered when prescribing glucose-lowering therapies in patients with type 2 diabetes, given the increasing body of evidence for cardiac and kidney benefits with newer drug classes such as SGLT-2 inhibitors and GLP-1 receptor agonists. While dipeptidyl peptidase 4 (DPP-4) inhibitors are frequently prescribed in patients with kidney disease due to safety concerns around hypoglycemia at late stages of CKD with other classes of drugs such as insulin and sulfonylureas, DPP-4 inhibitors have shown cardiac neutrality with no benefit on primary cardiovascular or secondary kidney outcomes.

When prescribed for glycemic control, most drug classes may be used in patients with diabetes, including those with and without kidney function impairment until late stage 3 CKD (Table 26.1). Metformin is cleared by the kidney but is considered safe to use in patients with kidney disease and estimated glomerular filtration rate (eGFR) of ≥30 mL/min/1.73 m². Reduction in the doses of other oral hypoglycemic agents in later stages of CKD may be necessary, especially for some sulfonylurea compounds that are metabolized by the kidney. In many countries, SGLT-2 inhibitor initiation is currently approved until eGFR<30 mL/min/1.73 m², and similar approaches have been reflected in the KDIGO Clinical Practice Guidelines. An important caveat is that the DAPA-CKD trial enrolled participants with eGFR as low as 25 mL/min/1.73 m², resulting in US FDA approval for initiation at this GFR level. Of note, SGLT-2 inhibitors are authorized to be continued at lower eGFR levels, with these thresholds only for drug initiation. Some GLP-1 receptor agonists such as semaglutide and dulaglutide can be used until eGFR<15 mL/min/1.73 m². Most DPP4i require dose reduction in late stages of CKD, whereas linagliptin is not cleared by the kidney and, therefore, dose adjustment is not required. As insulin is degraded by the kidney, dose reduction of insulin may be needed to prevent hypoglycemia as GFR declines.

Sodium-Glucose Cotransporter-2 Inhibition

The role of the kidney in maintaining glucose homeostasis is increasingly appreciated. Glucose is filtered at the glomerulus and reclaimed via tubular reabsorption along with sodium through SGLT-2, which is located in the proximal tubule. The SGLT-2 transporter accounts for the reabsorption of approximately 90% of all filtered glucose, whereas the SGLT-1 transporter, located in the more distal proximal tubule, reabsorbs the remaining 10%. SGLT-2 inhibitors reversibly inhibit the SGLT-2 transporter, leading to enhanced glucose and sodium excretion and, in turn, to reductions in plasma glucose, HbA1c, and body weight (see Table 26.1).

In addition to improving glycemic control, SGLT-2 inhibitors have heart and kidney protective roles, although the mechanisms for cardiorenal protection remain to be fully elucidated. SGLT-2 inhibitors induce an acute diuretic effect due to both osmotic diuresis and natriuresis, leading to a sustained reduction in plasma volume of approximately 7%. These agents lower systolic and diastolic blood pressure by approximately 3–5/1–2 mm Hg, respectively. As a consequence, modest weight loss (2–3 kg) observed with SGLT-2 inhibitors typically includes both fluid and

TABLE 26.1 Currently Available Oral Hypoglycemic Agents for the Management of Hyperglycemia

Class	Mechanism of Action	Examples of Drugs	Renal Clearance	HbA1c Lowering (%)	Use in Non-Dialysis CKD	Use in Dialysis	Advantage	Disadvantage
Biguanides (European Union 1958; United States 1995[a])	Inhibits hepatic glucose production and increases insulin sensitivity	Metformin	Excreted unchanged in urine	1.5	Contraindicated in advanced CKD	Contraindicated	Long-term safety; low costs; weight neutral	Risk of lactic acidosis in CKD patients; gastrointestinal side effects
Sulfonylureas (1946[a])	Binds to SU receptor in β-cells and increases calcium influx followed by insulin release	Gliclazide, Glipizide, Glimepiride, Glyburide	More than 90% metabolized in liver to weakly active or inactive metabolites and excreted in urine and feces	1.5	May be used	Glipizide may be used; use Glimepiride and glyburide with caution	Long-term safety; low costs	Hypoglycemia; weight gain
Meglitinides (1997[a])	Binds to SU receptor (different from SU site) and increases calcium influx followed by insulin release	Nateglinide, Repaglinide	Metabolized by liver (100%) and excreted in urine (10%) and feces (90%)	1.0	May be used	No data for patients with creatinine clearance less than 20 mL/min	Rapid onset of action and short acting	Few long-term safety data; weight gain
Thiazolidinediones (1997[a])	Decreases peripheral insulin resistance, thus increasing insulin sensitivity	Pioglitazone	Metabolized by liver to weakly active metabolites; excreted in urine (15%) and feces (85%)	0.6 to 1.5	May be used; no dose adjustments necessary; caution around edema/heart failure	May be used; no dose adjustments necessary; caution around edema/heart failure	Low-risk hypoglycemia	Pioglitazone is associated with increased risk of bladder cancer; Rosiglitazone withdrawn from the market because of increased cardiovascular risk
GLP-1 receptor agonists (2005[a])	Binds to the pancreatic GLP-1 receptor and promotes insulin secretion, decreases glucagon secretion, gastric emptying, and appetite	Short acting: Exenatide, Lixisenatide; Long-acting: Liraglutide, Dulaglutide, Semaglutide, Exenatide long acting release	Metabolized by kidney, excreted in urine	0.7 to 1.2 on top of metformin or SU derivatives	Semaglutide, dulaglutide, and liraglutide may be used	Semaglutide and dulaglutide may be used with caution	Reduced rate of death from cardiovascular causes, nonfatal myocardial infarction, or nonfatal stroke (LEADER, SUSTAIN-6, REWIND trials), weight loss, low risk of hypoglycemia	Subcutaneous administration, cost
DPP-4 inhibitors (2006[a])	Blocks DPP-4, which inactivates endogenous incretins	Saxagliptin, Sitagliptin, Linagliptin, Alogliptin	Excreted mostly unchanged in urine and feces (Linagliptin metabolized and excreted in feces)	~0.8 (on top of metformin/SU derivatives)	Dose adjustments necessary for saxagliptin, sitagliptin, and alogliptin	Dose adjustments necessary for saxagliptin, sitagliptin, and alogliptin	Weight neutral; low risk of hypoglycemia	No proven cardiovascular benefits; possible risk of heart failure with saxagliptin and alogliptin

Continued

TABLE 26.1 Currently Available Oral Hypoglycemic Agents for the Management of Hyperglycemia—cont'd

Class	Mechanism of Action	Examples of Drugs	Renal Clearance	HbA1c Lowering (%)	Use in Non-Dialysis CKD	Use in Dialysis	Advantage	Disadvantage
SGLT-2 inhibitors (2013)	Inhibits proximal tubular glucose reabsorption	Empagliflozin Canagliflozin Dapagliflozin Ertugliflozin	Metabolized by liver to active metabolites; excreted in urine and feces	~0.8 (on top of metformin)	Less A1c lowering in CKD but kidney and cardiovascular benefits extended to patients with CKD Canagliflozin continued in CREDENCE and dapagliflozin in DAPA-CKD until dialysis	No clinical experience; not recommended	Reduced cardiac endpoints (death from cardiovascular causes, nonfatal myocardial infarction, or nonfatal stroke), renal endpoints (doubling of serum creatinine, ESRD and renal death) (EMPA-REG, CANVAS, CREDENCE, DAPA-CKD trials), and improved heart failure outcomes (cardiovascular death, HF presentation) (DAPA-HF, EMPORER-Reduced) weight loss, low risk of hypoglycemia	Cost, risk of euglycemic diabetic ketoacidosis

aYear drug became available for clinical us

CKD, Chronic kidney disease; DPP-4, dipeptidylpeptidase 4; GLP-1, glucagon-like peptide-1; SGLT-2, sodium–glucose cotransporter-2; SU, sulphonylurea; HF, heart failure adipose tissue loss. SGLT-2 inhibition also induces uricosuria via exchange of filtered glucose for uric acid in the kidney, resulting in a 10% to 15% reduction in plasma uric acid levels. While the glycosuric effect and, hence, HbA1c lowering of SGLT-2 is attenuated in patients with GFR <60 mL/min/1.73 m², the beneficial effects on blood pressure and body weight loss are generally preserved in patients with impaired GFR. Initiation of SGLT-2 inhibition is associated with an acute, initial "dip" in GFR of 3-4 mL/min/1.73 m², which reverses with cessation of therapy, likely reflecting intrarenal hemodynamic effects.

The acute effect of SGLT-2 on kidney function is likely to be primarily mediated by the tubuloglomerular feedback (TGF) mechanism (Fig. 26.5). Increased bioactivity of SGLT-2 in patients with diabetes leads to increased sodium reabsorption at the proximal tubule and decreased distal sodium delivery to the macula densa, which is sensed as a reduction in effective circulating volume by the juxtaglomerular apparatus. This leads to downregulation of the TGF, vasodilation of the afferent renal arteriole, and attenuated hyperfiltration, at least in the setting of early T1D. Aside from attenuating TGF-mediated hyperfiltration, other direct kidney effects of SGLT-2 inhibition are being investigated, including suppression of proinflammatory and pro-fibrotic pathways and protection against kidney ischemia.

Four recent trials with SGLT-2 inhibition have demonstrated important cardiac benefits in patients with type 2 diabetes. Empagliflozin, Cardiovascular Outcomes, and Mortality in Type 2 Diabetes (EMPA-REG OUTCOME) and Canagliflozin and Cardiovascular and Renal Events in Type 2 Diabetes (CANVAS Program) included patients with type 2 diabetes and known atherosclerotic cardiovascular disease (ASCVD) in 100% and 66% of patients, respectively; each trial demonstrated a 14% reduction in the primary endpoint of major adverse cardiac event (MACE)

outcome of cardiovascular death, non-fatal myocardial infarction, or non-fatal stroke in the group randomized to SGLT-2 inhibitors compared to placebo. Dapagliflozin and Cardiovascular Outcomes in Type 2 Diabetes (DECLARE TIMI-58) included patients with cardiac risk factors and only 40% of patients with a history of ASCVD, and demonstrated a 17% reduction in cardiovascular death or hospitalization for heart failure. Finally, in the Evaluation of Ertugliflozin Efficacy and Safety Cardiovascular Outcomes Trial (VERTIS CV), ertugliflozin demonstrated non-inferiority but did not impact MACE or CV death. Hospitalization for heart failure was, nevertheless, reduced by 30% in the cohort with established ASCVD, highlighting the consistency of the effect on this important clinical marker of benefit. Meta-analyzed data from the first three trials (excluding VERTIS CV) including over 34,000 patients revealed a reduction in the MACE outcome of 11% in patients with a history of ASCVD, and a 23% reduction in the risk of CV death or hospitalization for heart failure in patients with and without a history of ASCVD and heart failure.

The abovementioned cardiovascular outcome trials demonstrated a kidney-protective role of SGLT-2 inhibition on top of usual therapy, with 80% of participants on renin-angiotensin-aldosterone system (RAAS) blockers. Patients randomized to SGLT-2 inhibitors had a 45%, 40%, 47%, and 35% reduction in the secondary composite renal endpoint (doubling of serum creatinine, 40% eGFR decline, end-stage kidney disease (ESKD), or renal death) in the EMPA-REG OUTCOME, CANVAS Program, DECLARE TIMI-58, and VERTIS CV trials, respectively. In the Canagliflozin and Renal Outcomes in Type 2 Diabetes and Nephropathy (CREDENCE) trial, the first dedicated kidney outcome trial using an SGLT-2 inhibitor, the investigators focused on patients with type 2 diabetes on maximum tolerated RAAS blockade, with eGFR 30–90 mL/min/1.73 m² and albuminuria (urine

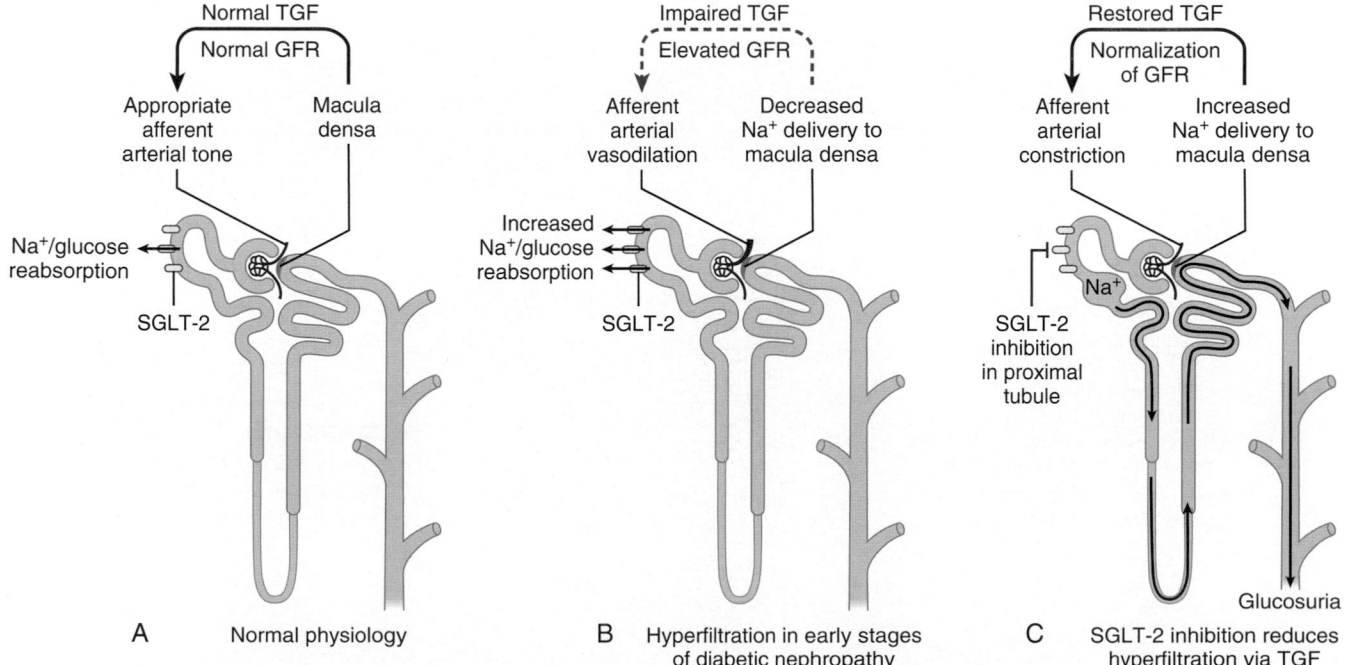

• **Fig. 26.5** Proposed tubuloglomerular feedback mechanisms in (A) normal physiology, (B) early stages of diabetic nephropathy, and (C) after sodium-glucose cotransporter 2 (SGLT-2) inhibition. *GFR,* Glomerular filtration rate; *TGF,* tubuloglomerular feedback; (Adapted from Cherney DZI, Perkins BA, Soleymanlou N, et al: The renal hemodynamic effect of sodium-glucose cotransporter 2 inhibition in patients with type 1 diabetes mellitus. *Circulation* 129(5):587–597, 2014.)

albumin-to-creatinine ratio 300 to 5000 mg/g). A 30% reduction in the primary outcome of ESKD, doubling of serum creatinine, or kidney or cardiovascular death was seen in the group randomized to canagliflozin 100 mg versus placebo. Meta-analyzed data from EMPA-REG OUTCOME, the CANVAS program, DECLARE TIMI-58, and CREDENCE included over 38,723 participants with 335 kidney failure events and demonstrated a consistent 35% reduction of kidney failure with SGLT-2 inhibition. Renal benefits were observed across all studied GFR subgroups, down to GFR of 30 mL/min/1.73 m² and across albuminuria levels.

The Dapagliflozin And Prevention of Adverse outcomes in Chronic Kidney Disease (DAPA-CKD) trial enrolled patients with eGFR between 25 and 75 mL/min/1.73 m² and albuminuria (urine albumin-to-creatinine ratio 200 – 5000 mg/g), including patients with and without type 2 diabetes. DAPA-CKD was stopped early in March of 2020 due to overwhelming efficacy in the primary composite outcome of time to 50% eGFR decline, ESRD, and kidney or CV death, with similar results seen in participants with and without diabetes. The Study of Heart and Kidney Protection With Empagliflozin (EMPA-KIDNEY) is enrolling patients with eGFR as low as 20 mL/min/1.73 m², with a range of albuminuria, who can be included depending on their baseline eGFR level (Fig. 26.6). As of late 2021, this trial is ongoing. Based on this body of literature, SGLT-2 inhibitors are now recommended in clinical practice guidelines for secondary prevention of cardiovascular and/or kidney disease in patients with type 2 diabetes and albuminuria, with eGFR>30 mL/min/1.73 m². There are currently limited data around the use of SGLT-2 inhibitors in individuals with type 1 diabetes, and approval varies with jurisdiction and depends on other factors such as BMI, with significant care required to mitigate the known risk of (euglycemic) diabetic ketoacidosis in this population.

Glucagon-Like Peptide-1 Receptor Agonists

Glucagon-like peptide-1 receptor agonists (GLP-1RA) bind to the pancreatic GLP-1 receptor and induce an incretin-like effect. GLP-1 RAs lower HbA1c by 0.55%–1.2% versus placebo in patients with T2D by promoting insulin secretion and by reducing glucagon secretion and hepatic gluconeogenesis (see Table 26.1). GLP-1RAs slow gastric emptying and increase satiety at the level of the central nervous system, inducing an average weight loss of 3 kg. This class is thought to have direct beneficial effects on the endothelium, resulting in a blood pressure lowering effect of 1.2–4.6 mm Hg systolic / 0 – 1.1 mm Hg diastolic.

There is increasing evidence for cardiovascular protection with GLP-1RA therapy, although the mechanisms behind the observed benefits remains elusive. Through early 2021, seven cardiovascular outcome trials of GLP-1RAs vs. placebo have been published, with

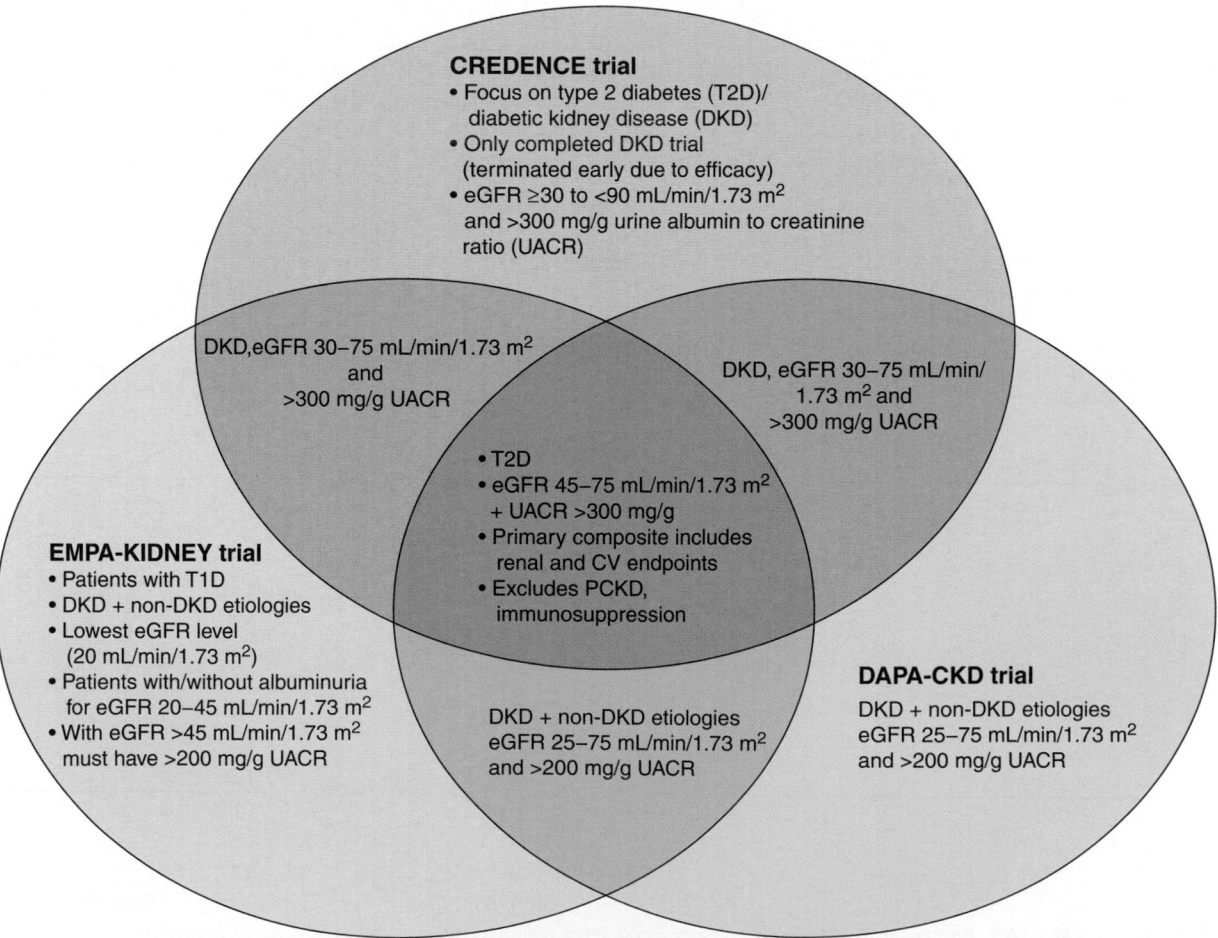

• Fig. 26.6 Study populations and areas of overlap for clinical trials with sodium-glucose cotransporter 2 inhibitors in patients with chronic kidney disease. (From Cherney DZ, Odutayo A, Aronson R, Ezekowitz J, Parker JD. Sodium Glucose Cotransporter-2 Inhibition and Cardiorenal Protection: JACC Review Topic of the Week. *J Am Coll Cardiol.* 2019;74(20):2511–2524.)

meta-analyzed data showing an overall 12% relative risk reduction for MACE with GLP-1RA therapy vs. placebo in patients with T2D. Several of these trials of GLP-1RAs show improvements in secondary kidney composite endpoints, largely driven by reductions in severely increased albuminuria, with less know about preservation of GFR over time. Based on these cardiovascular benefits, recent guidelines suggest prioritizing GLP-1 agonists for patients with T2D and known atherosclerotic cardiovascular disease to reduce the risk of MACE. Kidney benefits of GLP1-RAs on clinical outcomes including substantial loss of GFR and need for kidney replacement therapy is being assessed in ongoing dedicated trials, such as the Semaglutide on the Progression of Renal Impairment in Subjects with Type 2 Diabetes and Chronic Kidney Disease trial (FLOW, NCT03819153). Until the results of these trials are known, SGLT2 inhibitors should be favored in patients with T2D and kidney disease in order to reduce the risk of kidney disease progression. SGLT2 inhibitors are also favored in patients with T2D and heart failure, given the positive results of the Dapagliflozin in Patients with Heart Failure and Reduced Ejection Fraction (DAPA-HF) and Empagliflozin Outcome Trial in Patients With Chronic Heart Failure and a Reduced Ejection Fraction (EMPEROR-Reduced) trials, and the consistent HF benefits seen in several cardiovascular outcome trials and in DAPA-CKD and CREDENCE.

Blood-Pressure Control

Rationale

Treatment of high blood pressure is of paramount importance for preventing and delaying the progression of diabetic nephropathy. Blood pressure–lowering therapy is vital during any stage of CKD and is a mainstay of kidney protective therapy in all kidney diseases. In the UKPDS trial, where average blood pressure levels of 144/82 mm Hg were achieved, there was no threshold below which further blood pressure reduction did not reduce risk of progressive diabetic nephropathy and cardiovascular morbidity. The Hypertension Optimal Treatment (HOT) Study included an a priori-specified subgroup of patients with diabetes and showed a reduction in major adverse cardiovascular events targeting a diastolic blood pressure <80 mm Hg versus <85 or < 90 mm Hg. However, data from the Action to Control Cardiovascular Risk in Diabetes (ACCORD) trial showed that intensive (average 119 mm Hg) versus standard blood pressure (average 134 mm Hg) control conferred no benefit on kidney outcomes in type 2 diabetes patients. Critically, patients with more than 1 g of proteinuria per day were excluded from this trial, leaving the benefits of a lower blood pressure target (<120 mm Hg systolic) for patients with type 2 diabetes and more marked DKD untested. The effects of more aggressive blood pressure control on the development of DKD may differ in patients with type 1 versus type 2 diabetes. Long-term observational data in patients with T1D in DCCT-EDIC demonstrated an association between systolic blood pressure of <120 mm Hg compared to 130 to 140 mm Hg, and a lower risk of developing severely increased albuminuria and incident stage 3 CKD. Interventional trials of aggressive blood pressure control in patients with type 1 diabetes are warranted. Of note, patients with diabetes were excluded from the SPRINT trial, which showed a reduction in cardiovascular events and mortality in patients at high risk of cardiovascular disease who were randomized to a systolic blood pressure target of <120 mm Hg versus <140 mm Hg.

Overall, there remains insufficient evidence from randomized controlled trials to conclude that a lower target blood pressure actually reduces kidney or cardiovascular risk in people with diabetes and CKD, and this is reflected in discrepancies in clinical practice guideline recommendations. The American Heart Association and the Canadian Diabetes Association both recommend a blood pressure target of <130/80 mm Hg in patients with hypertension and diabetes, while the American Diabetes Association Guidelines suggest a target of less than 140/90 mm Hg for patients with diabetes and hypertension at low risk of cardiovascular disease (CVD), with consideration of a target of <130/80 mm Hg for patients with diabetes at high risk of CVD.

Medication of Choice

Any antihypertensive agent can be effectively used in the diabetic population, with agents that block the RAAS being the first choice in those with diabetes and hypertension as well as those with (normotensive) diabetes with moderate or severely increased albuminuria. Medication choice is further tailored to the need of the individual patient and the tolerability of the individual drugs. Patients with diabetic nephropathy are often volume overloaded; accordingly, diuretic therapy is often indicated. Increasing doses of loop diuretics, rather than thiazide diuretics, may become necessary to control fluid retention and accompanying hypertension at very low GFRs.

RAAS blocking agents lead to additional cardiovascular and kidney benefits beyond those expected with blood pressure reduction alone, leading many guidelines to advocate the use of angiotensin-converting enzyme (ACE) inhibitors or angiotensin receptor blockers (ARB) as first-choice antihypertensive therapy to achieve renoprotection. Notably, the degree of reduction in albuminuria induced by RAAS intervention in the first months of therapy is linearly associated with the magnitude of long-term kidney protection both in early and in late stages of diabetic kidney disease. The "blood-pressure independent" effect of RAAS kidney disease has been attributed to a reduction in intraglomerular hypertension and consequent decrease in urine albumin excretion. Interesting, and consistent with the concept of reduced intraglomerular pressure leading to kidney protection, is the observation that in patients with type 2 diabetes, the magnitude of the initial, acute decline in eGFR after ARB treatment is independently associated with better kidney function over time.

ACE Inhibitors

The captopril trial by the Collaborative Study Group was the first large trial to show definitively the benefit of ACE inhibitor therapy in delaying progression of overt DKD in patients with type 1 diabetes throughout a 4-year period of follow-up, with a nearly 50% reduction in the risk of doubling of serum creatinine concentration or in the combined endpoints of death, dialysis, and kidney transplantation, despite similarly achieved blood pressure between the captopril and non-captopril groups. Moreover, aggressive antihypertensive treatment with ACE inhibitors throughout a 7-year follow-up period in patients with type 1 diabetes and kidney disease was shown to induce regression or remission of nephrotic-range albuminuria, slow deterioration of kidney function, and substantially improve survival. Thus, ACE inhibitors should be used in type 1 diabetic patients as soon as persistent, moderately elevated albuminuria is documented, even if blood pressure is not elevated, to delay and/or prevent the development of overt nephropathy. In type 2 diabetes and normoalbuminuria, ACE inhibitors have consistently reduced the risk of development of moderately elevated albuminuria and reduced the rate of GFR decline. Furthermore, patients with type 2 diabetes who received ramipril in the Heart and Outcome Protection Evaluation (HOPE) trial had significantly fewer cardiovascular events. Consequently, RAAS inhibitors can be prescribed for cardioprotective indications in all patients with type 2 diabetes, regardless of the presence or absence of kidney disease.

Angiotensin Receptor Blockers

The merits of ARBs to protect the kidney and heart beyond blood pressure control have been demonstrated in numerous randomized, placebo-controlled trials, including the Irbesartan in Patients with Type 2 Diabetes and Microalbuminuria (IRMA2) and the Incipient to Overt: Angiotensin II Blocker Telmisartan Investigation on Type 2 Diabetic Nephropathy (INNOVATION) trials, where ARB-based regimens significantly reduced progression from moderately elevated to severely elevated albuminuria. Similarly, large-scale trials in patients with type 2 diabetes and overt nephropathy, including the Reduction in Endpoints in NIDDM with the Angiotensin-II Antagonist Losartan (RENAAL) and Irbesartan Diabetic Nephropathy Trial (IDNT) trials, showed that ARB-based therapy reduces the risk of a composite endpoint consisting of doubling of serum creatinine, dialysis, and all-cause death. IDNT also established the superiority of irbesartan over the calcium channel blocker (CCB) amlodipine in this setting. Apart from kidney protection, ARBs also afford cardiovascular protection in diabetic patients, as demonstrated in the Losartan Intervention for Endpoint Reduction in Hypertension (LIFE) trial. Contrary to the beneficial effects of RAAS blockers on GFR decline in patients with severely elevated albuminuria, in a trial including 6 years of randomization and 8 years of observational follow-up, there was no improvement on the outcome of GFR decline in patients with T2D and normo- or moderately elevated albuminuria who received the losartan versus placebo therapy during the trial period. ACE inhibitor use in the placebo group during the trial period may have contributed to the negative trial result.

Comparing ACE Inhibitors to ARBs

Data comparing the benefits of ACE inhibitors and ARBs for cardiovascular and/or kidney protection in patients with type 2 diabetic nephropathy are scarce. One small study directly compared the effects of telmisartan and enalapril on kidney function in type 2 diabetes and reported no difference between the two drugs. Similar results were noted in the Ongoing Telmisartan Alone and in Combination with Ramipril Trial (ONTARGET), where, in people at cardiovascular risk, there was no difference in the incidence of kidney or cardiovascular outcome in subjects treated with ACE inhibitor- or ARB-based regimens in either the overall population or in the one-third of participants with diabetes. Accordingly, there is no evidence of differential efficacy for ACE inhibitors over ARB in patients with type 2 diabetes, although the not-infrequent occurrence of cough and rare but serious risk of angioedema with ACE inhibitors have increased the popularity of ARB-based regimens despite higher cost.

Combinations of Blood Pressure–Lowering Drugs

Rationale

More than one medication is often required to control blood pressure, and patients with overt DKD often require three or four different antihypertensive drugs, including a diuretic. In addition, synergistic combinations may have the advantage that one can reduce the dose of individual components of the antihypertensive regimen, potentially retaining efficacy while reducing side effects.

Combinations of Choice

Logical combinations can be used, just as in uncomplicated hypertensive patients. Since RAAS blockade will typically be the first-line agent, clinicians should use other agents, in conjunction with RAAS blockade, that have proven efficacy for preventing both surrogate and hard clinical outcomes.

The combination of a diuretic plus ACE inhibitor or ARB effectively reduces both blood pressure and proteinuria in patients with and without diabetes; however, no studies with hard outcomes have been done to compare this combination with single therapies. The ADVANCE trial showed that the combination of an ACE inhibitor (perindopril) with a thiazide diuretic (indapamide) significantly reduces blood pressure and the risk of kidney and cardiovascular complications as compared with placebo in a broad range of patients with type 2 diabetes.

The combination of a calcium channel blocker (CCB) plus ACE inhibitor or ARB has been investigated in two large trials. The BENEDICT trial compared the combination of the non-dihydropyridine CCB verapamil and the ACE inhibitor trandolapril versus the single use of these agents in preventing the onset of microalbuminuria in type 2 diabetes, demonstrating that the combination of verapamil and trandolapril provided no advantage over trandolapril alone, whereas trandolapril was superior to verapamil. The ACCOMPLISH trial compared benazepril plus hydrochlorothiazide versus benazepril plus amlodipine in high-cardiovascular-risk patients and reported that the combination of benazepril and amlodipine was superior in preventing cardiovascular and kidney outcomes. Although a prespecified analysis in the diabetic population in ACCOMPLISH (60% of the overall population) showed results similar to the main study, the small number of kidney events in ACCOMPLISH renders the interpretation of this outcome difficult.

Combinations of RAAS-Interventions

ACE Inhibitor Plus ARB

The recognition of the importance of the RAAS in kidney and cardiovascular health has led to the idea that more stringent RAAS blockade by means of combination of ACE inhibitor and ARB therapy would afford additional protection. Indeed, combination therapy with ACE inhibitors and ARBs does result in additional blood pressure and albuminuria reduction. In 2013, the VA NEPHRON-D trial, which compared ARB alone to combination therapy in patients with diabetic nephropathy, was terminated early per recommendations of the Data Monitoring Committee, based on a greater number of observed acute kidney injury events and hyperkalemia in the combination therapy group. Similarly, the ONTARGET demonstrated that, despite additional blood pressure reduction and less progression of albuminuria, dual RAAS blockade did not reduce kidney or cardiovascular events in a lower-kidney-risk population.

ACE Inhibitor/ARB and Direct Renin Inhibition

Blockade of the RAAS by renin inhibition was considered an attractive target to prevent kidney and cardiovascular outcomes. The direct renin inhibitor aliskiren is a potent inhibitor of renin, and short-term studies demonstrated its efficacy as well as its safety; however, the ALTITUDE trial, which tested the combination of the direct renin inhibitor aliskiren plus ACE inhibitor or ARB treatment, demonstrated that aliskiren was associated with more adverse kidney and cardiovascular events in participants with type 2 diabetes at cardiovascular risk, leading to premature termination of the trial and recommendations from drug regulatory agencies that aliskiren is contraindicated in patients with diabetes and moderate or severe CKD who are taking ACE inhibitors or ARBs.

ACE Inhibitor/ARB and Mineralocorticoid Receptor Antagonists (MRA)

Adding aldosterone blockers to ACE inhibitors or ARBs is another strategy to block the deleterious effect of the RAAS in diabetic nephropathy. Because aldosterone promotes tissue fibrosis, and to counteract aldosterone breakthrough, a phenomenon defined by elevations of plasma aldosterone levels during chronic ACE inhibitor or ARB treatment that occurs in approximately 40% of patients receiving these agents, mineralocorticoid receptor blocking agents may be beneficial as add-on therapy to ACE inhibitors or ARBs. The widely available MRAs, spironolactone and eplerenone, reduce albuminuria in patients with DKD, but their use has been constrained by high rates of hyperkalemia. The novel, non-steroidal, selective MRA, finerenone, also attenuates albuminuria in patients with type 2 diabetes and DKD when used in addition to conventional ACE inhibitor or ARB treatment, with phase II data suggesting lower rates of adverse events, including hyperkalemia, with this agent.

In the Finerenone in Reducing Kidney Failure and Disease Progression in Diabetic Kidney Disease (FIDELIO-DKD, NCT02540993) trial, 5734 patients with type 2 diabetes, eGFR 25–75 mL/min/1.73 m² and albuminuria were randomized to finerenone vs. placebo to determine the effects on a primary composite kidney endpoint of time to first occurrence of kidney failure, sustained decrease of eGFR ≥40%, or kidney death. FIDELIO-DKD showed a significant 18% lower risk of the primary outcome as well as a 14% reduction in the secondary cardiovascular disease outcome, with 2.3% of participants randomized to finerenone as compared to 0.9% of those randomized to placebo discontinuing treatment due to hyperkalemia. Similarly, the Finerenone in Reducing Cardiovascular Mortality and Morbidity in Diabetic Kidney Disease trial (FIGARO-DKD, NCT02545049) is examining the effects of finerenone vs. placebo in 7437 patients with T2D and CKD on the primary composite CV endpoint of time to first occurrence of CV death, MI, stroke, or hospitalization for heart failure; results are expected in 2021.

Lipid Management

Rationale

Cholesterol lowering has contributed to improved cardiovascular outcomes in a range of patient populations; however, whether lipid management delays the progression of DKD and decreases the risk of kidney failure is debatable. Meta-analyses report that statin therapy may reduce proteinuria in CKD patients, but the lack of well-designed, long-term trials fueled uncertainty as to whether improved lipid management reduces kidney risk. The results of the Study of Heart and Renal Protection (SHARP) trial provided much needed insight into the long-term efficacy and safety of lipid management among kidney disease patients. The SHARP results, reviewed in greater detail in Chapter 55, showed that the combination of simvastatin and ezetimibe reduced the risk of major vascular events by 16% vs. placebo in individuals with advanced CKD. However, the compilation of available data suggests that the cardiovascular-protective effect of statins is attenuated at lower eGFR levels, and, unfortunately, the combination of simvastatin and ezetimibe in SHARP did not decrease the risk of progression to kidney failure.

Choice of Lipid-Lowering Therapy

Choosing among lipid-lowering strategies in CKD patients is challenging, given a lack of adequate data, with most studies focusing on statins. Several studies have assessed the comparative effects of statins on kidney or cardiovascular outcomes, with the results of the Prospective Evaluation of Proteinuria and Renal Function in Diabetic Patients with Progressive Renal Disease Trial (PLANET) suggesting a benefit for atorvastatin over rosuvastatin on kidney function. Further studies are needed to evaluate the long-term effects of lipid-lowering therapies, including PCSK9 inhibitors and omega-3 fatty acid derivatives on kidney function and the development of diabetic nephropathy.

Treatment of Type 2 Diabetes in Dialysis Patients

When a patient with diabetes approaches kidney failure, the various options for kidney replacement therapies should be offered: peritoneal dialysis, hemodialysis, or kidney transplantation. Survival with any kidney replacement modality is generally worse for patients with diabetes compared with nondiabetic patients, and cardiovascular complications markedly contribute to earlier deaths. In fact, more than 70% of deaths in the diabetic dialysis population are attributed to a cardiovascular cause.

Control of Hyperglycemia

While the HbA1c target associated with the best outcome among dialysis patients with type 2 diabetes has not been established, glycemic control in dialysis patients is important because (severe) hyperglycemia not only increases cardiovascular risk but also causes thirst and high fluid intake. A meta-analysis of observational studies demonstrated that a mean HbA1c ≥8.5% was associated with a moderate increase in mortality compared to mean HbA1c values between 6.5%–7.4% among patients on hemodialysis. Data suggest it is equally important to avoid hypoglycemia, which is also associated with increased mortality in dialysis.

The assessment of glycemic control in dialysis patients is complicated because interpretation of the commonly used assays for HbA1c is confounded by interference with uremic toxins. In addition, altered red blood cell survival, blood transfusion, and use of erythropoietin all impact the accuracy of HbA1c measurement. The pharmacologic management of hyperglycemia in dialysis patients must take into account that dialysis reverses insulin resistance so that the insulin requirement is generally lower than before dialysis. The glucose concentration in hemodialysate typically is 100 mg/dL (6.1 mmol/L) to minimize the risk of intradialytic hypoglycemic episodes.

Blood Pressure Control

The benefits and harms of blood pressure–lowering therapies in the dialysis population remain uncertain and likely do not differ from non-diabetic dialysis patients. Large-outcome trials are needed to evaluate this further.

Lipid Control

Based on 4D (Die Deutsche Diabetes Dialysis Study) and the AURORA (A Study to Evaluate the Use of Rosuvastatin in Subjects on Regular Hemodialysis: An Assessment of Survival and Cardiovascular Event) trial, patients treated with hemodialysis should not be started on a statin. Although the SHARP trial noted a benefit in a mixed CKD/ESRD population, meta-analyses of these studies have not demonstrated a substantial benefit in dialysis. Accordingly, the Kidney Disease Improving Global Outcomes guidelines recommend not initiating a statin in patients treated with dialysis but to continue statin treatment in those who are already receiving these agents at dialysis initiation.

Novel Strategies and Agents for Diabetic Kidney Disease

Optimizing glucose, blood pressure, and lipid control in CKD patients with diabetes has undoubtedly improved their prognosis; however, a considerable proportion of patients continue to develop DKD and progress to kidney failure. An overview of novel agents that target well-established or novel pathophysiologic pathways is provided in the next section. Many of these novel agents not only affect the target for which they are developed (on-target risk factor) but impact multiple other risk markers as well (off-target risk factors). Optimizing drug regimens to impact multiple parameters may lead to better drug use in the future.

Novel Blood Pressure- and Lipid-Lowering Agents

Endothelin Antagonists

Endothelin receptor blockers influence hemodynamics and endothelial function, and preclinical data suggest a role for these agents in the treatment of DKD. Murine diabetes models demonstrate that endothelin-1 signaling, as occurs in endothelial activation, induces heparanase expression in podocytes with resultant damage to the glycocalyx and subsequent albuminuria and kidney failure. The selective endothelin A receptor antagonist, atrasentan, has been shown to significantly reduce albuminuria and increase glycocalyx thickness in streptozotocin-induced diabetic mice. Furthermore, the restoration of glycocalyx with atrasentan was accompanied by increased renal nitric oxide levels and reduced expression of glomerular heparanase. Unfortunately, the first clinical trial demonstrated an increased incidence of edema and hospitalization for heart failure with avosentan, leading to the premature discontinuation of the trial.

Atrasentan, a more specific inhibitor of the endothelin-1A receptor than avosentan, has been shown to markedly lower albuminuria with fewer side effects in phase II studies. Atrasentan and Renal Events in Patents with Type 2 diabetes and Chronic Kidney Disease (SONAR) was a randomized, placebo-controlled study showing a 35% reduction with atrasentan versus placebo on a primary kidney outcome of doubling of serum kidney, ESRD, or kidney death. Of note, the study was stopped early due to low event rates. Importantly, SONAR utilized a novel study design in which all patients entered a 6-week enrichment period of open-label atrasentan and excluded patients with evidence of sodium retention during this period. Despite this, patients in the atrasentan group experienced more episodes of hypervolemia/fluid retention compared to placebo. The study also primarily enrolled patients who demonstrated a minimum of a 30% reduction in albuminuria during the enrichment period, potentially limiting the validity of the clinical findings to patients who demonstrate a biologic response to atrasentan.

Insulin Resistance and Lifestyle Modification

While insulin resistance is a key feature of type 2 diabetes, the role of insulin resistance in the development and progression of vascular complications in type 1 diabetes is increasingly recognized. A growing body of evidence suggests associations between insulin resistance and hemodynamic changes in the kidney, particularly elevation of glomerular hydrostatic pressure causing increased renal vascular permeability and ultimately glomerular hyperfiltration. Another possible mechanistic pathway linking insulin resistance to DKD is via effects on overall non-esterified fatty acid exposure and lipotoxicity, leading to the development of vascular disease.

Despite the BARI-2D study showing no benefit of insulin-sensitizing strategies compared to insulin therapy on diabetic nephropathy in older adults with type 2 diabetes and coronary artery disease, it is plausible that the long-standing vascular injury in older adults with type 2 diabetes, hypertension, and dyslipidemia may not be responsive to changes in insulin sensitivity. Early intervention prior to establishment of vascular lesions may result in significant delay of clinical pathology, as suggested by the concept of 'metabolic memory' in the DCCT-EDIC study. Also, clinical cardiovascular disease typically does not manifest until older ages; for example, it took 17 years of follow-up for the benefits of intensive management to manifest in DCCT. Ongoing research over the last decade has investigated the role of insulin sensitivity in the management of type 1 diabetes, with a focus on the role of metformin therapy in patients with T1D. The randomized, placebo-controlled trial Effects of Metformin on Cardiovascular Function in Adolescents With Type 1 Diabetes (EMERALD) demonstrated improved insulin sensitivity as well as aortic wall shear stress and pulse wave velocity in response to 3 months of metformin therapy. Additionally, several small, randomized, control trials of metformin versus placebo therapy in patients with T1D have suggested that, while metformin may limit the required insulin dose in T1D, there is little evidence in sustained improvement in HbA1c. The REMOVAL study examined the effect of metformin on markers of atherosclerosis in patients with T1D and demonstrated some evidence for benefit, but long-term studies on clinical atherosclerotic disease are lacking in this population.

Dietary sodium restriction enhances the blood pressure- and albuminuria-lowering effects of ACE inhibitors and ARBs, with both RENAAL and IDNT showing that the effects of ARBs on hard kidney and cardiovascular outcomes in patients with type 2 diabetes are greater in patients with moderately low dietary sodium intake. Dietary protein restriction has been shown in a meta-analysis of nine randomized controlled trials (seven in patients with type 1 diabetes, one in patients with type 2 diabetes, and one in patients with either type 1 or type 2 diabetes) to have a small, statistically non-significant, long-term beneficial effect in slowing the rate of decline in GFR without demonstrable evidence of malnutrition. Another recent meta-analysis showed a statistically significant reduction in both GFR and proteinuria with dietary protein restriction. Currently, the ADA recommends 0.8 g/kg/day of protein restriction for diabetic patients with increased albuminuria, which is a manageable and safe recommendation for most patients with challenging dietary prescriptions related to their diabetes and CKD. Dietary counseling by a nutritionist may be useful to assist CKD patients in safely implementing dietary changes (see Chapter 52).

Novel Targets

Despite recent success with agents such as GLP-1 receptor agonists and SGLT2 inhibitors, other therapeutic areas have been less successful. For example, two recent studies, PERL and CKD-FIX, examining uric acid-lowering therapies in people with T1D and T2D, respectively, failed to show kidney- or cardiovascular-protective effects. Nevertheless, other therapeutic areas have shown promising preliminary study results and merit further consideration, including agents that target inflammation.

Monocyte Chemoattractant Protein-1 Inhibitors

An increasing body of evidence demonstrates that the potent cytokine, monocyte chemoattractant protein-1 (MCP-1), also called *C-C chemokine ligand 2 (CCL2)*, plays an important role in initiating and sustaining chronic inflammation in the kidney. MCP-

1, secreted in response to high glucose concentrations, attracts blood monocytes and macrophages and facilitates inflammation. A 52-week prospective, randomized, controlled trial showed an 18% reduction in albuminuria with the CCL2 receptor antagonist CCX140-B vs. placebo in patients with DKD on top of usual therapy, but data on hard kidney outcomes are lacking.

Interleukin-1ß (1L-1ß) Antagonists
In the Canakinumab Anti-Inflammatory Thrombosis Outcome Study (CANTOS), the monoclonal antibody Canakinumab vs. placebo reduced the primary MACE endpoint in patients with a history of myocardial infarction and elevated C-reactive protein levels, including 40% with a history of T2D. A *post hoc* analysis demonstrated a similar benefit in the 1875 CANTOS participants with eGFR <60 mL/min/1.73 m². Canakinumab did not impact CKD progression in CANTOS, and future research is necessary to assess the safety and efficacy of IL-1ß antagonism in a high-risk renal cohort.

Uric Acid (UA) Lowering
The Preventing Early Renal Loss in Diabetes (PERL) study included patients with type 1 diabetes and evidence of DKD, and showed no benefit in GFR decline in the group randomized to allopurinol versus placebo. The Controlled Trial of Slowing of Kidney Disease Progression from the Inhibition of Xanthine Oxidase (CKD-FIX) included patients with stage 3 and 4 CKD, 58% of whom had diabetes, and again failed to show a benefit in eGFR decline in the group randomized to allopurinol. In sum, these data illustrate that uric acid-lowering therapy is not indicated in asymptomatic patients with diabetes, hyperuricemia, and chronic kidney disease.

Novel Biomarkers
Diabetic kidney disease clinically presents as albuminuria and, once significant kidney parenchymal damage has already occurred, GFR decline. Due to the presence of clinically silent disease over a long period of time, the identification of novel biomarkers of DKD may improve the ability of clinicians to target high-risk patients with earlier therapies prior to the development of albuminuria or GFR decline. Significant progress was achieved in developing a classifier based on 273 urinary peptides (CKD273), which likely reflects extracellular matrix turnover based on collagen peptide fragments. CKD273 is highly correlated with urine ACR and eGFR and has been validated in a number of trials for early detection of DKD in patients with type 1 and type 2 diabetes. Soluble tumor necrosis factor α receptors (TNFRs) are another potential biomarker at an early stage of development for diabetic nephropathy. TNFRs were shown to predict progression of CKD in patients with type 1 diabetes with normal eGFR at baseline and also to predict progression to kidney failure in proteinuric and non-proteinuric patients with type 2 diabetes. Recently, three other members of the TNF Receptor Superfamily, in addition to the previously recognized TNF receptors 1 and 2, were found to be associated with kidney failure in three separate cohorts of patients with type 1 and type 2 diabetes. Other non-TNF Receptor Superfamily proteins, most notably IL15RA, were also identified. Larger multicenter trials are needed to examine promising biomarkers prior to the transition into a clinical practice.

Conclusion

Diabetic kidney disease is a leading cause of morbidity and mortality in people with type 1 and type 2 diabetes (T2D). The 2020 US Renal Data System reported that diabetes accounted for 47% of all incident cases of end-stage kidney disease. Despite the successful use of glycemic, lipid, and blood pressure controls, including ACE inhibitor and ARB therapy, kidney risk in patients with diabetes remains very high. A focus on cardio-renal benefits in large clinical trials over the last 5 years has yielded impressive results for patients with T2D, including those with chronic kidney disease. Specifically, the CREDENCE (canagliflozin) and DAPA-CKD (dapagliflozin) trials and perhaps the ongoing EMPA-KIDNEY (empagliflozin) trial, the FIDELIO-DKD, and the FIGARO-DKD (finerenone) trials are rapidly changing the standard-of-care therapy in patients with DKD, providing nephrologists with new tools to slow the progression of kidney disease in patients with type 2 diabetes.

Complete bibliography is available at Elsevier eBooks for Practicing Clinicians.

Key Bibliography

Badve SV, Pascoe EM, Tiku A, et al. Effects of allopurinol on the progression of chronic kidney disease. *N Engl J Med*. 2020;382:2504–2513.

Barbosa J, Steffes MW, Sutherland DE, et al. Effect of glycemic control on early diabetic renal lesions: a 5-year randomized controlled clinical trial of insulin-dependent diabetic kidney transplant recipients. *JAMA*. 1994;272:600–606.

Bjornstad P, Snell-Bergeon JK, Rewers M, et al. Early diabetic nephropathy: a complication of reduced insulin sensitivity in type 1 diabetes. *Diabetes Care*. 2013;36(11):3678–3683.

Cherney DZ, Perkins BA, Soleymanlou N, et al. The renal hemodynamic effect of SGLT2 inhibition in patients with type 1 diabetes. *Circulation*. 2014;129(5):587–597.

Cho A, Noh JW, Kim JK, et al. Prevalence and prognosis of hypoglycemia in patients receiving maintenance dialysis. *Intern Med J*. 2016 Aug 23.

Cushman WC, Evans GW, Byington RP, et al. Effects of intensive blood-pressure control in type 2 diabetes mellitus. *N Engl J Med*. 2010;362:1575–1585.

de Boer IH, Rue TC, Cleary PA, et al. Long-term renal outcomes of patients with type 1 diabetes mellitus and microalbuminuria: an analysis of the Diabetes Control and Complications Trial/Epidemiology of Diabetes Interventions and Complications cohort. *Arch Intern Med*. 2011;171(5):412–420.

de Boer IH, Sun W, Cleary PA, et al. Intensive diabetes therapy and glomerular filtration rate in type 1 diabetes. *N Engl J Med*. 2011;365(25):2366–2376.

Gerstein HC, Miller ME, Byington RP, et al. Effects of intensive glucose lowering in type 2 diabetes. *N Engl J Med*. 2008;358:2545–2559.

Heerspink HJL, Parving HH, Andress DL, et al. Atrasentan and renal events in patients with type 2 diabetes and chronic kidney disease (SONAR): a double-blind, randomised, placebo-controlled trial. *Lancet*. 2019;393:1937–1947.

Heerspink HJL, Stefansson BV, Correa-Rotter R, et al. Dapagliflozin in patients with chronic kidney disease. *N Engl J Med*. 2020;383:1436–1446.

Kristensen SL, Rorth R, Jhund PS, et al. Cardiovascular, mortality, and kidney outcomes with GLP-1 receptor agonists in patients with type 2 diabetes: a systematic review and meta-analysis of cardiovascular outcome trials. *Lancet Diabetes Endocrinol*. 2019;7:776–785.

Lewis EJ, Hunsicker LG, Clarke WR, et al. Renoprotective effect of the angiotensin-receptor antagonist irbesartan in patients with nephropathy due to type 2 diabetes. *N Engl J Med*. 2001;345:851–860.

Nathan DM, Cleary PA, Backlund JY, et al. Intensive diabetes treatment and cardiovascular disease in patients with type 1 diabetes. *N Engl J Med*. 2005;353(25):2643–2653.

Neal B, Perkovic V, Mahaffey KW, et al. Canagliflozin and cardiovascular and renal events in type 2 diabetes. *N Engl J Med*. 2017;377:644–657.

Parving HH, Lehnert H, Brochner-Mortensen J, et al. The effect of irbesartan on the development of diabetic nephropathy in patients with type 2 diabetes. *N Engl J Med*. 2001;345:870–878.

Patel A, MacMahon S, Chalmers J, et al. Intensive blood glucose control and vascular outcomes in patients with type 2 diabetes. *N Engl J Med*. 2008;358:2560–2572.

The Diabetes Control and Complications Trial Research Group, Nathan DM, Genuth S, Lachin J, et al. The effect of intensive treatment of diabetes on the development and progression of long-term complications in insulin-dependent diabetes mellitus. *N Engl J Med*. 1993;329(14):977–986.

Wiviott SD, Raz I, Bonaca MP, et al. Dapagliflozin and cardiovascular outcomes in type 2 diabetes. *N Engl J Med*. 2019;380(4):347–357.

Zinman B, Wanner C, Lachin JM, et al. Empagliflozin, cardiovascular outcomes, and mortality in type 2 diabetes. *N Engl J Med*. 2015;373(22):2117–2128.

27

Onconephrology

JAYA KALA, KEVIN W. FINKEL

Onconephrology is a growing field within nephrology, with many malignancies and their treatments affecting the kidneys and kidney disease impacting the management of many cancers. Although patients with malignancy can develop kidney diseases similar to other acutely and chronically ill patients, they are also at risk for unique kidney syndromes because of either the cancer itself or its treatment. Understanding these unique disorders is a prerequisite to providing outstanding clinical care. In addition, because patient survival has improved, owing to advances in cancer treatment, chronic kidney disease (CKD) prevalence has also increased. Providing expert advice on the impact of CKD on patient survival; drug response, toxicity, and clearance; and clinical study eligibility are important considerations in onconephrology. Finally, patients with advanced malignancy can develop severe acute kidney injury (AKI) with multiple organ dysfunction syndrome. In these cases, the nephrologist is an essential partner in discussions about end-of-life issues and the appropriateness of initiating kidney replacement therapies.

This chapter provides an overview of kidney diseases either caused by cancer or its treatment, including AKI, CKD, electrolyte abnormalities, glomerular diseases, tumor lysis syndrome (TLS), anticancer drug nephrotoxicity, and hematopoietic stem cell-induced kidney injury. Multiple myeloma, amyloidosis, and other dysproteinemias are discussed in Chapter 28.

Acute Kidney Injury

In hospitalized cancer patients, AKI is associated with increased morbidity, mortality, length of stay, and costs. In a northern Denmark study with a 1.2 million population in the catchment area, incident cancer was found in 44,116 patients. The 1-year and 5-year risk of AKI in this population was 17.5% and 27.5%, respectively. The incidence of AKI was highest for kidney cancer (44%), multiple myeloma (33%), liver cancer (32%), and acute leukemia (28%).

Among critically ill patients, 20% have underlying malignancy with overall prognosis strongly dependent on the admitting diagnosis and the type of cancer. Patients with solid tumors have lower mortality (56%) than those with hematologic malignancies (67%). In the Sepsis Occurrence in Critically Ill Patients (SOAP) study, in the subset of patients with more than three failing organs, over 75% of patients with cancer died; this compares to 50% of those without cancer. In a retrospective analysis of 1009 critically ill patients with hematologic malignancies, Darmon and colleagues

reported an AKI incidence of 66.5%. After adjustment, factors associated with AKI development were older age, history of hypertension, TLS, multiple myeloma, exposure to nephrotoxins, and sequential organ failure assessment (SOFA) score.

The etiology of AKI in cancer patients is quite varied and is often multifactorial. Causes vary from those common to all hospitalized patients, such as exposure to various nephrotoxins (NSAIDs, antibiotics, and radiocontrast), sepsis, and volume depletion, and factors unique to the underlying malignancy or its treatment. Table 27.1 provides a comprehensive list of causes of AKI.

Chemotherapeutic Agents

Chemotherapeutic agents can cause a variety of kidney manifestations including AKI, tubulointerstitial nephritis (TIN), acid-base and electrolyte disturbances, hypertension, proteinuria/nephrotic syndrome, and thrombotic microangiopathy (TMA). One challenge for clinicians is the vast array of new agents with unique mechanisms of action; given potentially unknown adverse kidney effects, a great degree of vigilance is needed.

The adverse kidney effects of chemotherapy can be classified by the primary site of injury. For example, these include injury to the endothelium (hypertension and TMA), visceral podocyte (proteinuria and nephrotic syndrome), kidney tubules (AKI), and tubulointerstitium (renal tubular acidosis, Fanconi syndrome, and electrolyte wasting). A list of anticancer agents and their known associated kidney effects is found in Table 27.2. The nephrotoxic effects of specific anticancer drugs are reviewed in Chapter 34.

Tumor Lysis Syndrome

TLS is defined by laboratory criteria (any two of hyperuricemia, hyperphosphatemia, hypocalcemia, and hyperkalemia) and clinical criteria (one of three among AKI, seizures, arrhythmias, and death). TLS complicated by AKI often is a dramatic presentation, characterized by the development of hyperphosphatemia, hypocalcemia, hyperuricemia, and hyperkalemia of varying severity. TLS can occur spontaneously during the rapid growth phase of malignancies, such as bulky lymphoblastomas and Burkitt and non-Burkitt lymphomas that have extremely rapid cell turnover rates, or when cytotoxic chemotherapy induces lysis of malignant cells in patients with large tumor burdens.

The pathophysiology of AKI associated with TLS classically is attributed to two main factors: preexisting volume depletion and

TABLE 27.1	Causes of Acute Kidney Injury in Malignancy
Perfusion related	Sepsis Volume depletion (vomiting, diarrhea, mucositis, diuretics, GVHD of GI tract, increased gastric output) Sinusoidal occlusion syndrome Capillary leak (interleukin-2) Hypercalcemia (multifactorial including nephrogenic diabetes insipidus) CAR T cell therapy Cytokine release syndrome (inflammation, vasodilation, third spacing of fluids) • Acute cardiomyopathy (hypotension, hypoperfusion, cardiorenal syndrome) • High fever/nausea/vomiting • Tumor lysis syndrome • Acute uric acid nephropathy • Iodinated contrast agents • Drugs (NSAIDs, ACE inhibitors) • Tumor lysis syndrome
Intrinsic	Acute tubular necrosis • Ischemic • Nephrotoxic Tubulointerstitial nephritis • Tumor lysis syndrome • Infection (BK virus) • Pyelonephritis • Infiltration (lymphoma and leukemia) • Lysozymuria • Medications Vascular/thrombotic microangiopathy • Underlying malignancy (gastric cancer) • Drug induced (gemcitabine, mitomycin C, anti-VEGF, tyrosine kinase inhibitor) • Bone marrow/stem cell transplantation • Radiation Glomerular • Monoclonal gammopathy-associated proliferative GN • Rapidly progressive GN • Minimal change, focal segmental GN, membranoproliferative GN, membranous nephropathy
Obstruction	Intrarenal • Uric acid crystals • Methotrexate • Acyclovir Extrarenal • Retroperitoneal fibrosis • Lymphadenopathy • Direct invasion • Collecting system blood clots

ACE, Angiotensin-converting enzyme; *GN*, glomerulonephritis; *GVHD*, graft-versus-host disease; *NSAIDs*, nonsteroidal antiinflammatory drugs; *VEGF*, Vascular endothelial growth factor.

TABLE 27.2	Chemotherapy and Associated Kidney Manifestations
Chemotherapy and Miscellaneous	**Kidney Effects**
Cisplatin	Acute kidney injury Proximal tubulopathy Fanconi syndrome Nephrogenic diabetes insipidus Salt-wasting nephropathy Magnesium wasting
Ifosfamide	Acute kidney injury Proximal tubulopathy Fanconi syndrome Nephrogenic diabetes insipidus
Methotrexate	Acute kidney injury (crystalline nephropathy)
Pamidronate	Acute kidney injury Collapsing focal segmental glomerulosclerosis
Calcineurin inhibitors	Acute kidney injury Thrombotic microangiopathy Hypertension Hyperkalemia
Biologic Agents	
Interferon-α	Acute kidney injury Minimal change disease Focal segmental glomerulosclerosis
Interleukin-2	Acute kidney injury (perfusion-related) Capillary leak syndrome
Targeted Therapies	
Antivascular endothelial growth factor (e.g., bevacizumab, sorafenib)	Acute kidney injury Thrombotic microangiopathy Hypertension Proteinuria
Epidermal growth factor blockade (e.g., cetuximab, erlotinib)	Urinary magnesium wasting
BRAF inhibitors	Acute kidney injury Electrolyte disorders
ALK inhibitors	Acute kidney injury Electrolyte abnormalities Kidney microcysts
Immunotherapeutic Agents	
CTLA-4 inhibitors (cytotoxic T lymphocytic antigens)	Acute kidney injury Proteinuria Acute tubulointerstitial nephritis Glomerular disease
PD-1 (Programmed death) inhibitors	Acute kidney injury Proteinuria Acute tubulointerstitial nephritis Glomerular disease
Chimeric antigen receptor T cells	Capillary leak with perfusion-related acute kidney injury Ischemic acute tubular injury

the precipitation of uric acid and calcium phosphate complexes in the kidney tubules and tubulointerstitium. There is also a major contribution from a "cytokine release syndrome" associated with tumor cell lysis. This leads to kidney underperfusion and AKI. Volume depletion is multifactorial and may reflect anorexia, nausea and vomiting from the malignancy or its treatment, and increased insensible losses from fever or tachypnea.

Hyperuricemia may develop despite allopurinol prophylaxis in patients with spontaneous TLS or after therapy in very chemosensitive malignancies. Excess serum uric acid is filtered into the tubular space. In general, uric acid is nearly completely ionized at physiologic pH, but it becomes progressively more insoluble in the acidic environment of the renal tubules. Precipitation of uric acid causes intratubular obstruction, while hyperuricemia may also lead to increased renal vascular resistance and decreased glomerular filtration rate (GFR). In addition, a granulomatous reaction to intraluminal uric acid crystals and necrosis of tubular epithelium may occur, resulting in inflammation and further kidney injury. Hyperphosphatemia and hypocalcemia also occur in TLS. In patients who develop AKI but do not develop hyperuricemia, kidney injury has been attributed to metastatic intrarenal calcification or acute nephrocalcinosis. Tumor lysis with release of inorganic phosphate may promote both kidney and systemic metastatic calcification, which is complicated by acute hypocalcemia.

Optimal management of TLS can reduce the risk of developing AKI and symptomatic electrolyte abnormalities. Management includes ensuring a high urine output with intravenous fluids, reducing uric acid levels, and controlling serum phosphate levels. It is recommended that urine output be maintained at a rate of 200 mL/hr by infusion of isotonic crystalloid solutions. In the absence of significant hypervolemia, use of loop diuretics should be avoided because they acidify the urine and can lead to volume depletion.

A consensus statement on the treatment of TLS was published by the American Society of Clinical Oncology in 2008. In patients at low risk of TLS, allopurinol is administered to inhibit uric acid formation. Through its metabolite oxypurinol, allopurinol inhibits xanthine oxidase and thereby blocks the conversion of hypoxanthine and xanthine to uric acid. During massive tumor lysis, excessive uric acid production with increased uric acid excretion by the kidneys may occur despite allopurinol administration, making intravenous hydration necessary to prevent AKI. Because allopurinol and its metabolites are excreted by the kidneys, the starting dose should be lower in those with reduced GFR. Other limitations to allopurinol use include hypersensitivity reaction, drug interactions, and delayed time to lowering uric acid levels.

In the past, because uric acid is very soluble at physiologic pH, sodium bicarbonate was often added to intravenous fluids to achieve a urinary pH greater than 6.5. However, this therapy is no longer recommended for several reasons. First, systemic alkalosis from alkali administration can aggravate hypocalcemia, resulting in tetany and seizures. Second, an alkaline urine pH markedly decreases the urinary solubility of calcium phosphate, thereby promoting development of acute nephrocalcinosis from intratubular calcium-phosphate crystals.

Patients at high risk for TLS can be treated with rasburicase (recombinant urate oxidase). Risk factors for TLS include bulky lymphadenopathy, elevated lactate dehydrogenase (LDH) (>2 × normal), increased white blood cell count (>25,000/mm³), baseline creatinine greater than 1.4 mg/dL, and baseline uric acid greater than 7.5 mg/dL. Rasburicase converts uric acid to water-soluble allantoin, thereby decreasing serum uric acid levels and urinary uric acid excretion. Importantly, use of rasburicase obviates the need for urinary alkalinization and its complications. However, high urine flow rates achieved with normal saline are important given the probability of preexisting volume depletion and its consequences. Rasburicase treatment should be avoided in patients with glucose-6-phosphate dehydrogenase deficiency because hydrogen peroxide, a breakdown product of uric acid, can cause methemoglobinemia and, in severe cases, hemolytic anemia. Management of TLS is outlined in Fig. 27.1.

Thrombotic Microangiopathy

TMA is a disorder of multiple etiologies that manifests as nonimmune (microangiopathic) hemolytic anemia with thrombocytopenia and other organ dysfunction including AKI. In addition to anemia and thrombocytopenia, laboratory findings include elevated indirect bilirubin and LDH levels, depressed serum haptoglobin values, and schistocytes on peripheral blood smear. The characteristic kidney lesion consists of vessel wall thickening in capillaries and arterioles, with swelling and detachment of endothelial cells from the basement membranes and accumulation of subendothelial fluffy material. In the past, TMA was classified as either thrombotic thrombocytopenia purpura (TTP), diarrhea-associated (Shiga toxin) hemolytic uremic syndrome (HUS), HUS associated with an underlying condition (cancer, malignant

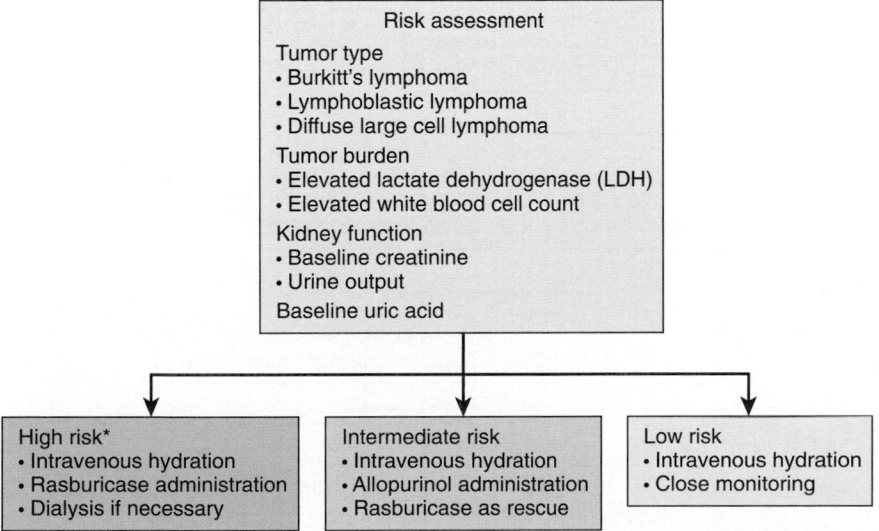

*High-risk features include: Bulky lymphadenopathy, LDH > 2x normal, White blood cell count > 25 K/mm³, Creatinine > 1.4 mg/dL, Uric acid > 7.5 mg/dL

• **Fig. 27.1** Management of tumor lysis syndrome.

hypertension, pregnancy), or atypical HUS. However, this classification is an oversimplification, as it is nearly impossible to differentiate these disorders based on phenotypic presentation. As such, the best approach uses classification based on pathophysiology, which ultimately will inform therapy. TTP is generally characterized by decreased enzymatic activity of the metalloprotease ADAMTS13 (a disintegrin and metalloproteinase with thrombospondin type 1 motif, member 13) and responds to therapeutic plasma exchange (TPE), whereas atypical HUS is due to dysregulated complement activity and responds to complement inhibition but not TPE. It is likely that there is overlap among these similar entities.

In cancer patients, malignancy itself, chemotherapy, radiation therapy, immunosuppressive agents, and stem cell transplantation all can induce endothelial injury leading to TMA and AKI. TMA is most commonly associated with gastric carcinoma, which accounts for more than half of cases, followed by breast and lung cancer. Chemotherapeutic agents are also associated with the development of TMA. Mitomycin C is the classic drug associated with TMA with an incidence as high as 10%. Bleomycin, cisplatin, and 5-fluorouracil are less frequently reported causes. Gemcitabine, a nucleoside analog, and the antivascular endothelial growth factor (VEGF) agents, such as bevacizumab and sunitinib, also are associated with TMA. Gemcitabine likely acts through direct, toxic endothelial injury, while the anti-VEGF agents deprive endothelial cells of VEGF, which is required to maintain endothelial health and modulate local inhibitory complement proteins (complement factor H), which prevents complement activation.

Treatment of AKI and TMA in cancer patients, regardless of etiology, is primarily supportive, with initiation of dialysis when indicated. Any offending agent associated with TMA should be discontinued. The role of plasma exchange is controversial for TMA unrelated to ADAMTS13 deficiency, reflecting a lack of trial data. If stopping the culprit drug or treating the underlying cause for TMA is unsuccessful and the patient continues to deteriorate, plasma exchange should be considered; however, it is mandatory that ADAMTS13 activity be measured. If there is a delay in ascertaining the ADAMTS13 activity, plasma exchange should be started empirically. A low activity level (<5%) confirms the diagnosis of TTP, and plasma exchange should continue. If activity level is normal and TTP is excluded as a diagnosis, plasma exchange can be discontinued. If the diagnosis of atypical HUS is likely, strong consideration should be given to administering eculizumab. This drug is a humanized monoclonal antibody that inhibits terminal complement activation by binding to complement C5 and preventing formation of the terminal membrane attack complex. The overall management of TMA is outlined in Fig. 27.2.

Hematopoietic Stem Cell Transplantation

Hematopoietic stem cell transplantation (HSCT) can cause both AKI and CKD. The incidence of AKI is approximately 10% in autologous transplants and ranges from approximately 50% (with reduced intensity conditioning) to 73% (with high-intensity conditioning) in those who receive allogeneic transplants. Causes of AKI include acute graft-versus-host disease (GVHD), sinusoidal obstruction syndrome (SOS), TMA, use of calcineurin inhibitors, viral infections, and sepsis (Table 27.3).

The incidence of CKD following HSCT varies from 7% to 48% and is clinically manifest anywhere from 6 months to 10 years after transplant. Risk factors for CKD are prior AKI, acute or chronic GVHD, age over 45 years at the time of transplant, hypertension, calcineurin inhibitor therapy, and exposure to total

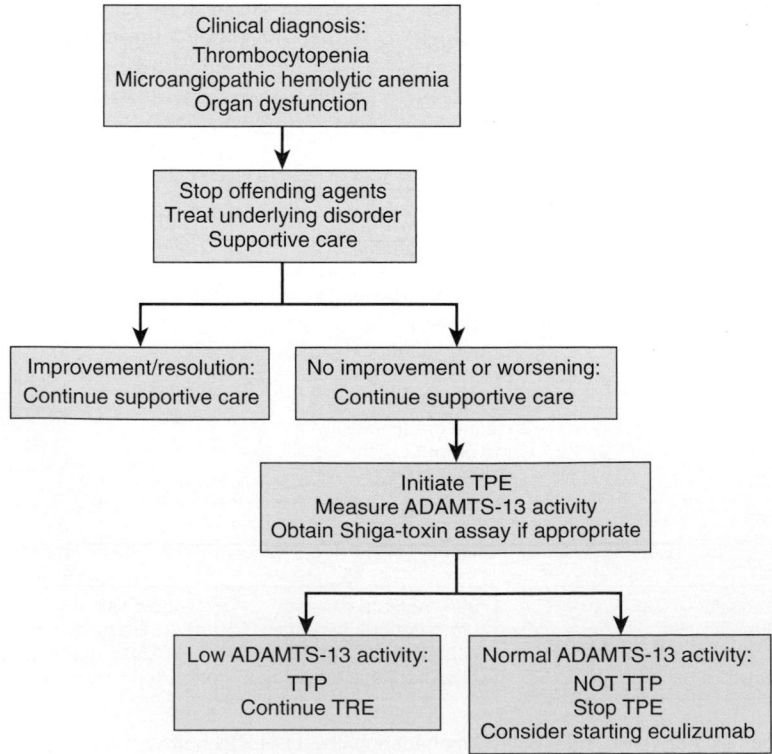

• **Fig. 27.2** Management of malignancy-associated thrombotic microangiopathy. *TPE*, Therapeutic plasma exchange; *TTP*, thrombotic thrombocytopenic purpura.

TABLE 27.3	Hematopoietic Stem Cell Transplantation Induced Acute Kidney Injury
Perfusion related	Sepsis
	Hypotension
	Capillary leak syndrome
	Engraftment syndrome
	Calcineurin inhibitor
	Contrast nephropathy
	Sinusoidal obstruction syndrome
Intrinsic	Tubular/interstitial
	Ischemic
	Toxic (marrow infusion syndrome → hemoglobin pigment nephropathy)
	Drugs (aminoglycosides, vancomycin, amphotericin-B, methotrexate, fludarabine)
	Infections (pyelonephritis, BK, CMV, parvovirus B19, adenovirus)
	Tumor lysis syndrome
	Vascular/thrombotic microangiopathy
	Calcineurin inhibitors
	mTOR inhibitors
	Acute graft-versus-host disease
	Viral-mediated
	Complement dysregulation
	Total body irradiation
Obstruction	BK-induced bladder disease
	Retroperitoneal fibrosis
	Adenovirus cystitis

CMV, Cytomegalovirus; *mTOR,* mammalian target of rapamycin.

body irradiation (TBI). Kidney biopsy is generally required to diagnose the cause of CKD.

Sinusoidal Obstruction Syndrome

SOS, formerly referred to as *venoocclusive disease of the liver,* is a unique form of AKI that occurs between 10 and 21 days after HSCT. It is characterized by tender hepatomegaly, fluid retention with ascites formation, and jaundice. It results from fibrous narrowing of small hepatic venules and sinusoids triggered by the pretransplant cytoreductive regimen and is more common after allogeneic than autologous HSCT. The development of SOS is most commonly associated with pretreatment with cyclophosphamide, busulfan, and/or TBI. AKI typically behaves similarly to hepatorenal syndrome with hyperdynamic vital signs, hyponatremia, oliguria, and low urinary sodium concentration. Urinalysis shows minimal proteinuria, and urine sediment examination reveals bile-stained renal tubular cells and granular casts possibly due to the toxicity of bile salts in the urine. Patients are usually resistant to diuretics, and spontaneous recovery is quite rare. Risk factors for the development of AKI include edema formation, hyperbilirubinemia, use of amphotericin B, vancomycin, or acyclovir, and higher pretransplant serum creatinine. AKI adversely affects survival, as seen in patients who require dialysis, where the mortality rate approaches 80%. Small trials using infusions of prostaglandin E, pentoxifylline, or low-dose heparin to prevent the development of SOS have been promising. Smaller trials with defibrotide, an antithrombotic and fibrinolytic agent, have shown benefit in patients with SOS; however, use of these agents is not commonplace because of the associated risk of bleeding.

Glomerular Diseases and Paraneoplastic Syndromes

Several solid and hematologic malignancies are associated with glomerular diseases, thought to be the result of abnormal tumor cell products. As discussed in Chapter 20, membranous nephropathy (MN) is associated with solid malignancies, including lung and gastric tumors. Because treatment may differ, with malignancy-associated MN often responding to treatment of the malignancy, it is essential to differentiate between primary MN and MN associated with solid tumors. Table 27.4 illustrates characteristics associated with paraneoplastic MN.

Minimal change disease (MCD) is classically associated with Hodgkin lymphoma. It usually occurs at the time the malignancy is diagnosed and is associated with a high rate of steroid and cyclosporine resistance. The most common glomerular disease seen with thymoma is also MCD. Focal segmental glomerulosclerosis is associated with solid malignancies, kidney cancer, and thymoma. Membranoproliferative glomerulonephritis (MPGN) is associated with lung, kidney, and stomach cancers, while immunoglobulin A nephropathy has been most frequently associated with kidney cell cancer and is also associated with T-cell lymphoma. Glomerular lesions associated with malignancy are noted in Table 27.5.

TABLE 27.4	Characteristics of Cancer-Associated Membranous Nephropathy

Age > 65 years
Smoking history
Absence of antiphospholipase A2 receptor antibody
Kidney biopsy findings:
- Presence of high IgG1 and IgG2 subtype deposits
- Less than eight inflammatory cells per glomerulus observed in kidney biopsy specimen

Regression of glomerular lesions and proteinuria upon remission of cancer
No other obvious cause

TABLE 27.5	Paraneoplastic Glomerulonephritis

Membranous Glomerulopathy

- Breast
- Colon
- Lung
- Prostate
- Graft-versus-host disease
- Others (case reports)

Minimal Change Disease

- Hodgkin lymphoma
- Non-Hodgkin lymphoma
- Graft-versus-host disease
- Others (case reports)

Glomerulopathies from Case Reports

- Rapidly progressive glomerulonephritis
- Immunoglobulin A nephropathy
- Focal segmental glomerulonephritis
- Membranoproliferative glomerulonephritis

Lymphoma and Leukemia

Although a variety of cancers can metastasize to the kidneys and invade the parenchyma, the most common to do so are lymphomas and leukemias. The true incidence of kidney involvement is unknown because kidney infiltration may not manifest with significantly abnormal kidney function. On autopsy, lymphomatous kidney infiltration is seen in approximately 30% of cases.

Lymphoma

Kidney involvement in lymphoma is often clinically silent, such that patients present with slowly progressive CKD often attributed to other etiologies. Therefore, a high index of suspicion is needed to make a diagnosis. Patients may present with AKI, but this is rare and is most commonly seen in highly malignant and disseminated disease. Other presentations include both nephrotic- and nonnephrotic-range proteinuria due to a variety of glomerular lesions including pauci-immune crescentic glomerulonephritis. Patients may also present with flank pain and hematuria, likely due to interstitial infiltration with lymphoma causing kidney capsule distention and hemorrhage of small capillaries.

Kidney involvement in lymphoma may be suspected from clinical features and imaging studies. Kidney imaging, including ultrasound or computed tomography, may reveal diffusely enlarged kidneys, multiple focal lesions, or retroperitoneal involvement with hydronephrosis. The following criteria support the diagnosis of kidney disease due to lymphomatous infiltration: (1) kidney enlargement without obstruction; (2) absence of other causes of kidney disease; and (3) rapid improvement of kidney function after radiotherapy or systemic chemotherapy. Kidney biopsy is often required to confirm the diagnosis, especially in patients with kidney-limited lymphoma.

Leukemia

Leukemic cells can infiltrate any organ, and the kidneys are the most frequent extramedullary site of infiltration, with autopsy studies revealing that 60% to 90% of patients with leukemia have kidney involvement. As with lymphoma, leukemic infiltration of the kidneys is often an indolent and clinically silent aspect of leukemia. Most often, leukemic kidney infiltration is incidentally noted after autopsy or by detection of kidney enlargement on imaging often performed for other indications. Although relatively uncommon, many cases of AKI attributable to leukemic infiltration have been described. Patients may also experience hematuria or proteinuria. Occasionally, kidney enlargement is accompanied by flank pain or fullness. Patients with significantly elevated white blood cell counts, especially those with leukemic blasts, can develop AKI from intrarenal leukostasis. Treatment is directed at the type of leukemia diagnosed. Although some patients do not recover, kidney function improves in the majority of cases as the leukemia responds to systemic treatment.

Radiation-Associated Kidney Injury

Radiation-associated kidney injury has a long latency period. With the exception of patients who undergo HSCT, there is no acute form that presents during or shortly after radiation therapy. Evidence of kidney dysfunction does not occur until at least 6 months following radiation, and it may take several years for progression to clinically apparent CKD.

Common symptoms of radiation-associated kidney injury include edema formation, fluid retention, increased weight, and malaise. In addition, symptoms can overlap with those of other kidney diseases such as malignant hypertension (headaches, vomiting, and blurry vision) and other end-organ damage (dyspnea and lethargy). It is important to recognize that these symptoms do not differentiate radiation nephropathy from many other causes of kidney failure. The complete blood count may reveal a microangiopathic hemolytic anemia with schistocytes on the peripheral smear. Thrombocytopenia may also be present. Proteinuria often is present although seldom reaches nephrotic range, while urine sediment examination reveals granular casts and red blood cells.

The diagnosis of radiation nephropathy is made clinically by identifying a syndrome of progressive CKD in a cancer patient who previously received radiation to the total body, spine, abdomen, or pelvis. A thorough history and physical examination should be performed, and the clinician should have a strong index of suspicion in such patients. A kidney biopsy does not necessarily need to be performed. Many of the histopathologic findings in radiation nephropathy are nonspecific and common to a large host of other causes of CKD; however, kidney biopsy may demonstrate TMA. Blockade of the renin-angiotensin-aldosterone system (RAAS) is useful once radiation-induced injury has developed, with several studies showing benefits associated with angiotensin-converting enzyme (ACE) inhibitors on the overall course of the disease.

Electrolyte Abnormalities

Hyponatremia

Hyponatremia is the most common electrolyte disorder in hospitalized patients with cancer, and is associated with higher mortality rates, longer hospital stays, and higher health care costs. In one report, the hazard ratio for 90-day mortality was 2.04 for patients with mild hyponatremia, 4.74 for moderate hyponatremia, and 3.46 for severe hyponatremia. The differential diagnosis for and evaluation and management of hyponatremia are similar to that in patients without malignancy (see Chapter 7).

The most common etiology of hyponatremia is the syndrome of inappropriate antidiuresis (SIAD). SIAD is particularly common in individuals with small-cell lung cancer, with an estimated incidence of 10% to 15%. Antineoplastic drugs such as cyclophosphamide, vinblastine, and vincristine also cause SIAD. Cisplatin-associated hyponatremia is due to both a salt-wasting nephropathy and SIAD. Other factors contributing to hyponatremia in cancer patients are pain, nausea and vomiting, edema formation with third spacing (liver and heart failure), adrenal insufficiency, and hypotonic intravenous fluid administration. Therapy is determined by the cause and the severity of hyponatremia. In patients with SIAD, fluid restriction is difficult, especially during administration of chemotherapy when increased hydration is often required. Hypertonic saline acutely and salt tablets chronically may be used, with indications similar to the treatment of hyponatremia in the noncancer population. Use of vasopressin receptor antagonists such as tolvaptan has been studied in a small, randomized, controlled trial treating hyponatremia in cancer patients, with 14 days of tolvaptan therapy correcting hyponatremia in 94% of patients compared with only 8% in the placebo group.

Hyperkalemia

Hyperkalemia in cancer patients is most commonly seen with AKI, TLS, or obstructive nephropathy (hyperkalemic or type 4 renal tubular acidosis). More rarely, elevated plasma potassium levels are due to pseudohyperkalemia as a result of marked leukocytosis or thrombocytosis. Transport of blood specimens to the laboratory in an icebox to prevent cell lysis or using plasma samples for correct potassium measurements is helpful in this circumstance. Less common causes of hyperkalemia in these patients include adrenal insufficiency due to metastatic disease and exposure to ketoconazole, calcineurin inhibitors, NSAIDs, renin-angiotensin-aldosterone system antagonists, trimethoprim, or heparin.

Hypokalemia

Hypokalemia is a common electrolyte abnormality seen in cancer patients. This disorder may result from poor oral intake, vomiting, diarrhea, ureteral diversions, diuretic use, hypercalcemia (kaliuretic effect), hypomagnesemia, various drugs, or mineralocorticoid excess. Medications such as cisplatin, ifosfamide, amphotericin B, and aminoglycosides cause hypokalemia via either proximal tubular damage or both gastrointestinal and kidney losses. Ectopic release of adrenocorticotropic hormone (ACTH) is an uncommon cause of hypokalemia. A significant association between hypokalemia and acute myelogenous leukemia has also been noted in 40% to 60% of patients. This is associated with other electrolyte abnormalities and acid-base disorders, indicating tubular injury from high concentrations of urinary lysozyme.

Hypophosphatemia

Dysregulation of phosphate levels is another electrolyte disorder seen with cancer, in particular, hypophosphatemia. Calcium and vitamin D deficiency are often due to malnutrition in these ill patients. Phosphaturia from proximal tubular damage develops from cisplatin use, multiple myeloma (light chain proximal tubular injury), and oncogenic osteomalacia, which is associated with increased FGF23 production. Evaluation includes a thorough medical history, review of medications and nutritional status assessment, serum free light chain and urine protein electrophoresis measurement, and evaluation for tumor-associated osteomalacia.

Hypercalcemia

Malignancy is the most common cause of severe hypercalcemia in hospitalized patients. In general, hypercalcemia is a late finding, occurring with very advanced cancer and carrying a poor prognosis. The major mechanisms involved in malignancy-associated hypercalcemia are (1) secretion of parathyroid hormone-related protein (PTHrP) by several solid tumors; (2) direct osteolytic metastases with release of local cytokines from multiple myeloma and breast cancer; and (3) secretion of 1,25-dihydroxy vitamin D from lymphoma.

Hypercalcemia induces a perfusion-related picture by causing volume depletion through renal sodium loss, water depletion through nephrogenic diabetes insipidus, and vasoconstriction; in addition, intratubular calcium-phosphate deposition (acute nephrocalcinosis) may result in direct tubular injury. When the serum calcium level is over 13 mg/dL, most patients will have some degree of intravascular volume depletion. In these cases, administration of isotonic saline will restore volume and increase renal cal-

cium excretion. Furosemide or other loop diuretics sometimes are used in hypervolemic patients to further promote calcium excretion, although the benefits of this approach remain uncertain, particularly given other effective calcium-lowering therapies. At a minimum, loop diuretics should be avoided early in the course of hypercalcemia management and likely should not be part of the armamentarium for use in hypercalcemia management in the absence of symptomatic volume overload.

Bisphosphonates, which are pyrophosphate analogs with a high affinity for hydroxyapatite, may be necessary to control serum calcium, particularly in severe hypercalcemia. Pamidronate and zoledronate, two second-generation bisphosphonates, are commonly used preparations. Pamidronate can be given as a single intravenous dose of 30 to 90 mg and may maintain normal serum calcium concentrations for several weeks. However, onset of action may be delayed with a mean time to achieve normocalcemia of 4 days. Therefore, other means of lowering the serum calcium level must be implemented in the immediate period. Bisphosphonates have been associated with AKI.

Calcitonin, derived from the thyroid C-cell, inhibits osteoclast activity. The onset of action of calcitonin is rapid, but this drug has a short half-life and is usually not given as a sole therapy. Tachyphylaxis to calcitonin may be seen at 48 hours because of downregulation of the calcitonin receptor. More often, calcitonin is combined with pamidronate. Concomitant administration of glucocorticoids can prolong the effective duration of action of calcitonin. Glucocorticoids are effective in the therapy of hypercalcemia in patients with hematologic malignancies or multiple myeloma. In these cases, glucocorticoids inhibit osteoclastic bone resorption by decreasing tumor production of locally active cytokines and reducing active vitamin D synthesis.

Denosumab is an agent increasingly being used to treat hypercalcemia of malignancy. It is a humanized monoclonal antibody directed against receptor of nuclear factor κB ligand (RANKL), thereby decreasing osteoclast differentiation and proliferation. Denosumab has been effective in lowering serum calcium levels in breast and prostate cancer and in multiple myeloma. Importantly, vitamin D levels should be checked and repleted if low to prevent post-therapy hypocalcemia. Finally, hemodialysis with a low calcium bath is the preferred method of reducing serum calcium levels in patients with severe symptomatic hypercalcemia and kidney failure.

Chronic Kidney Disease and Malignancy

It is well established that patients with CKD or those who have undergone kidney transplantation are at a higher risk of cancer. CKD patients are more prone to renal cell carcinoma (RCC) as well as cancers of the lips, thyroid, and urinary tract. Cohort studies highlight the risk of cancer in patients with estimated GFR (eGFR) of less than 55 mL/min/1.73 m². For every 10 mL/min/1.73 m² reduction in eGFR, there was a 29% increased risk of cancer independent of age and smoking. It is, therefore, essential for clinicians to be aware of the cancer risk in the CKD population and undertake prompt evaluations to detect cancers at earlier, treatable stages. Treating cancer in CKD patients is more difficult than in the general population. Mortality and morbidity due to the adverse effects of surgery and chemotherapy are higher in this group of patients. Drug dosing and toxicity also are problematic in CKD patients. A summary of key issues and proposed recommendations for cancer patients with CKD is highlighted in Table 27.6. In addition, most cancer trials

TABLE 27.6	Chronic Kidney Disease (CKD)- and End-Stage Kidney Disease (ESKD)-Related Concerns in Cancer Patients
Medication dose adjustments	**Dose reduction for GFR:** Alkylating agents: Carmustine, cyclophosphamide, ifosfamide, melphalan Anti-metabolites: Capecitabine, clofarabine, cytarabine, fludarabine, methotrexate, gemcitabine, pemetrexed, pentostatin, pralatrexate Anti-tumor agents: Bleomycin, daunorubicin, mitomycin Platinum agents: Carboplatin, cisplatin, oxaliplatin Topoisomerase inhibitors: Etoposide, topotecan Proteasome inhibitors: Carfilzomib, ixazomib Immunomodulators: Lenalidomide, pomalidomide Molecularly targeted agents: anti-VEGF- bevacizumab, TKI- imatinib, lenvatinib, sorafenib, vandetanib **Timing in relation to kidney replacement therapy:** Dosing after dialysis (especially for highly dialyzable drugs, e.g., cisplatin) **Medication interactions:** Methotrexate with NSAIDs, PPIs, antifungals, platinum-based agents
Erythropoiesis stimulating agents (ESA) for anemia	CKD: Hgb <10 and symptomatic; Hgb <9 and asymptomatic ESKD: Hgb <9.5 Chemotherapy-induced anemia: Goal Hgb 10, discontinue ESA 1 month after chemotherapy Avoid novel oral ESA (hypoxia-inducible factor prolyl hydroxylase inhibitors): possible increased angiogenesis/tumor progression
Mineral bone disorder (MBD)	Transplant recipients: Bisphosphonates slow bone loss CKD: Increased bone mineral density. Raloxifene may prevent vertebral fractures but not MBD. Teriparatide has no strong evidence of benefit with GFR < 50mL/min **Adverse drug effects:** *Bisphosphonates:-* ATN, collapsing focal glomerulosclerosis, adynamic bone disease, hypocalcemia, osteomalacia, contraindicated in GFR <30 mL/min *Denosumab:* Hypocalcemia *Raloxifene:* No reported adverse effects *Teriparatide:* Adynamic bone disease, hypocalcemia
Cancer screening	Screening: High-risk population, long expected survival, transplant candidate Tumor markers: Interpret cautiously **Impact of CKD on common tumor markers:** Unchanged: α-fetoprotein, total PSA Increased in CKD or states of volume overload: CA 19-9, CA 125, MUC I Tumor markers always increased: β2-microglobulin, CEA, free PSA
Dialysis modality, palliative care	Peritoneal dialysis and hemodialysis mortality Early palliative care referral

VEGF, Vascular endothelial growth factor; *TKI,* tyrosine kinase inhibitor, *NSAIDS,* nonsteroidal anti-inflammatory inhibitor drugs; *PPI,* proton pump inhibitor; *Hgb,* hemoglobin; *GFR,* glomerular infiltration rate; *CA,* cancer antigen; *CEA,* carcinoembryonic antigen; *MUC,* mucin; *PSA,* prostate-specific antigen

exclude advanced CKD patients, thereby denying them access to potentially beneficial therapies.

Cancer occurring after kidney transplantation is well described in the literature. There is a higher incidence of lymphoma and skin cancers. In the United States, the risk of skin cancers (excluding melanomas) was 7.4% at 3 years and that of nonskin cancers and melanomas was 7.5%. Several studies have shown that risk of death from certain cancers developing after solid organ transplant is increased as compared with the general population. Posttransplant malignancies are discussed in more detail in Chapter 61.

Kidney Cysts and Kidney Cancer

The rate of RCC varies globally and is more common in industrialized countries. Established risk factors for sporadic RCC are cigarette smoking, obesity, and hypertension. The overall odds ratio for cancer of ever-smokers to never-smokers is 1.38 for both sexes based on studies undertaken in North America, Europe, and Australia. Obesity, as defined by the World Health Organization (WHO) as body mass index above 30 kg/m^2, increases risk of RCC. In several observational trials, high blood pressure has had a dose-dependent association with RCC risk. The risk decreases with reduction in blood pressure, possibly suggesting that the risk for RCC can be modified with antihypertensive medications. Several angiogenic and other growth factors are elevated in hypertension and may be involved in renal carcinogenesis. In contrast, blood pressure control could mitigate their potential effects over time.

In patients with CKD, particularly among those receiving dialysis with acquired cystic kidney disease (ACKD), the risk of RCC is also increased. The frequency of ACKD increases with number of years on dialysis, and nearly 50% of patients on dialysis for more than 3 years will develop ACKD. As compared with the general population, there is 50-fold increased risk of developing RCC in patients with ACKD. ACKD is usually asymptomatic but can lead to complications such as bleeding, rupture, and infections. Occasionally, patients may develop erythrocytosis from cyst synthesis of erythropoietin, and, in patients undergoing dialysis, a lack of erythropoiesis stimulating agent requirement may be an important clue that triggers imaging for RCC.

Sensitive newer imaging techniques have increased detection of small renal masses (SRM) such as early-stage T1 RCC (<7 cm, confined to kidneys) and T1a RCC (<4 cm, confined to kidneys). Tissue sampling is crucial for diagnosis. This is achieved by either core biopsy or tumor removal. With the advent of coaxial biopsy techniques, no cases of tumor seeding of the needle tract have been reported. The removal of localized tumors is diagnostic as well as therapeutic.

The goal of treatment of SRM is toward kidney function preservation, cardiovascular risk reduction, and long-term CKD care. Preoperative optimization of glycemic and blood pressure control minimizes GFR decline after tumor resection. Nephron-sparing procedures, including partial nephrectomy and percutaneous ablative therapies, are emerging as mainstream treatment for SRM, rather than traditional radical nephrectomy. Radical nephrectomy remains the conventional therapy for larger renal masses and nonlocalized tumors. Concomitant assessment of nonneoplastic parenchyma in kidney resection specimens provides an opportunity to identify patients with glomerular, tubulointerstitial, or vascular diseases and helps expedite therapy.

Reassessment of kidney function with serum creatinine measurement, GFR assessment, and urine protein quantification should be performed following nephrectomy. Nephrology involvement is recommended before RCC treatment for patient at high risk of CKD development and with postsurgical, new-onset proteinuria, worsening kidney function, or hypertension. Systemic treatment for advanced RCC includes immunotherapy (checkpoint inhibitor immunotherapy, interleukin-2, interferon-α), molecular targeted therapy (antiangiogenic VEGF pathway, mTOR inhibitors), or combined angiogenic plus checkpoint inhibitor therapy. Although RCC is characterized as radioresistant tumor, conventional and stereotactic radiation therapy are frequently useful to treat single or limited number of metastases (painful bone, brain, painful recurrences in kidney bed).

Complete bibliography is available at Elsevier eBooks for Practicing Clinicians.

Key Bibliography

Cairo MS, Coiffier B, Reiter A, et al. Recommendations for the evaluation of risk and prophylaxis of tumour lysis syndrome (TLS) in adults and children with malignant diseases: an expert TLS panel consensus. *Br J Haematol*. 2010;149:578–586.

Cohen EP, Krzesinski M, Launay-Vacher V, et al. Onco-nephrology: core curriculum 2015. *Am J Kidney Dis*. 2015;66:869–883.

Darmon M, Vincent F, Canet E, et al. Acute kidney injury in critically ill patients with haematological malignancies: results of a multicentre cohort study from the Groupe de Recherche en Reanimation Respiratoire en Onco-Hematologie. *Nephrol Dial Transplant*. 2015;30:2006–2013.

Dawson LA, Kavanagh B, Paulino A, et al. Radiation-associated kidney injury. *Int J Radiat Oncol Biol Phys*. 2010;76:S108–S115.

Grill V, Martin TJ. Hypercalcemia of malignancy. *Rev Endocr Metab Disord*. 2000;1:253–263.

Hingorani S. Renal complications of hematopoietic-cell transplantation. *N Engl J Med*. 2016;374:2256–2267.

Howard SC, Jones DP, Pui CH, et al. The tumor lysis syndrome. *N Engl J Med*. 2011;364:1844–1854.

Hu SL, Chang A, Perazella MA, Okusa MD, Jaimes EA, Weiss RH. American Society of Nephrology Onco-Nephrology Forum. The Nephrologist's Tumor: Basic Biology and Management of Renal Cell Carcinoma. *J Am Soc Nephrol*. 2016;27(8):2227–2237.

Jhaveri KD, Shah H, Patel C, et al. Glomerular diseases associated with cancer, chemotherapy, and hematopoietic stem cell transplantation. *Adv Chronic Kidney Dis*. 2014;21:48–55.

Kala J. Radiation-induced kidney injury. *Journal of Onco-Nephrology*. 2019;3(3):160–167.

Lam AQ, Humphreys BD. Onco-nephrology: AKI in the cancer patient. *Clin J Am Soc Nephrol*. 2012;7:1692–1700.

Lameire N, Vanholder R, Van Biesen W, Benoit D. Acute kidney injury in critically ill cancer patients: an update. *Crit Care*. 2016;20:209.

Lynch MR, Hu SL. Onco-nephrology highlights: Chronic kidney disease, end-stage kidney disease, and cancer patients. *Journal of Onco-Nephrology*. 2020;4(1-2):7–14.

McDonald GB, Hinds M, Fisher L, et al. Veno-occlusive disease of the liver and multiorgan failure after bone marrow transplantation: a cohort study of 355 patients. *Ann Intern Med*. 1993;118:255–267.

Rosner MH, Perazella MA. Acute kidney injury in the cancer patient. *N Engl J Med*. 2017;376(18):1770–1781.

Rosner MH, Jhaveri KD, McMahon BA, Perazella MA. Onconephrology: the intersections between the kidney and cancer. *CA Cancer J Clin*. 2020. doi:10.3322/caac.21636.

Skinner R. Strategies to prevent nephrotoxicity of anticancer drugs. *Curr Opin Oncol*. 1995;7:310–315.

Stengel B. Chronic kidney disease and cancer: a troubling connection. *J Nephrol*. 2010;23:253–262.

Wanchoo R, Stotter BR, Bayer RL, Jhaveri KD. Acute kidney injury in hematopoietic stem cell transplantation. *Curr Opin Crit Care*. 2019;25(6):531–538.

Widakowich C, de Castro G, de Azambuja E, et al. Review: side effects of approved molecular targeted therapies in solid cancers. *Oncologist*. 2007;12:1443–1455.

28

Myeloma, Amyloid, and Other Dysproteinemias

ALA ABUDAYYEH, PAUL W. SANDERS

Paraproteinemic kidney diseases are typically the result of deposition of immunoglobulins or immunoglobulin fragments (heavy chains and light chains; Fig. 28.1) in specific parts of the nephron, and they can be divided generally into those diseases that manifest primarily as glomerular or as tubulointerstitial injury (Box 28.1). Glomerular diseases include AL-type amyloidosis (amyloid composed of light chains), AH-type amyloidosis (amyloid composed of heavy chains), monoclonal immunoglobulin deposition disease (MIDD, which includes light-chain deposition disease [LCDD], heavy-chain deposition disease, and light- and heavy-chain deposition disease), proliferative glomerulonephritis with monoclonal immunoglobulin deposition (PGMID), paraprotein-associated C3 glomerulopathy, immunotactoid glomerulopathy, and glomerulonephritis associated with type I cryoglobulinemia. In this review, AL-type amyloidosis, monoclonal LCDD, fibrillary glomerulonephritis, and immunotactoid glomerulopathy will be discussed. Patterns of tubular injury include Fanconi syndrome, proximal tubulopathy, and cast nephropathy (also known as "*myeloma kidney*"). In addition to these paraproteinemic kidney lesions, this chapter includes a discussion of Waldenström macroglobulinemia.

Aside from notable exceptions, such as AH-type amyloidosis and heavy-chain deposition disease, immunoglobulin light-chain deposition is directly responsible for most of the kidney pathologic alterations that occur with paraproteinemia. In one large study of multiple myeloma, kidney dysfunction was present in approximately 2% of patients who did not exhibit significant urinary free light-chain levels, while increasing urine free light-chain levels were strongly associated with kidney failure, with 48% of myeloma patients who had high urinary monoclonal free light chains having kidney failure and associated poor survival. The type of kidney lesion induced by light chains depends on the physicochemical properties of these proteins.

Immunoglobulin Light-Chain Metabolism and Clinical Detection

The original description of immunoglobulin light chains is attributed to Dr. Henry Bence Jones in 1847. He reported these unique proteins, that now bear his name, and correlated this early urine biomarker with the disease known as *multiple myeloma*. More than a century later, Edelman and Gally demonstrated that Bence Jones proteins were immunoglobulin light chains.

Plasma cells synthesize light chains that become part of the immunoglobulin molecule (see Fig. 28.1). In normal states, a slight excess production of light, compared to heavy, chains appears to be required for efficient immunoglobulin synthesis, but this excess results in the release of polyclonal free light chains into the circulation. After entering the bloodstream, light chains are handled similarly to other low-molecular-weight proteins, which are usually removed from the circulation by glomerular filtration. Monomeric (molecular weight ~22 kDa) and dimeric (~44 kDa) forms of light chains are filtered through the glomerulus and reabsorbed by the proximal tubule. Endocytosis of light chains into the proximal tubule occurs through a single class of heterodimeric, multiligand receptor that is composed of megalin and cubilin. After endocytosis, lysosomal enzymes hydrolyze the proteins, and the amino-acid components are returned to the circulation. The uptake and catabolism of these proteins are very efficient, with the kidney readily handling the approximately 500 mg of free light chains that are produced daily by the normal lymphoid system. However, in the setting of a monoclonal gammopathy, light chain production increases, and binding of light chains to the megalin-cubilin complex can become saturated, allowing light chains to be delivered to the distal nephron and to appear in the urine as Bence Jones proteins.

Light chains are modular proteins that possess two independent globular regions, termed *constant* (C_L) and *variable* (V_L) *domains* (see Fig. 28.1). Light chains can be isotyped as kappa (κ) or lambda (λ), based on sequence variations in the constant region of the protein. Within the globular V_L domain are four framework regions that consist of β sheets that develop a hydrophobic core. The framework regions separate three hypervariable segments that are known as *complementarity determining regions* (CDR1, CDR2, and CDR3; see Fig. 28.1). The CDR domains, which represent those regions of sequence variability among light chains, form loop structures that constitute part of the antigen-binding site of the immunoglobulin. Diversity among the CDR regions occurs because the V_L domain is synthesized through rearrangement of multiple gene segments. Thus, although possessing similar structures and biochemical properties, no two light chains are identical; however, there are enough sequence similarities among light chains to permit categorizing them into subgroups. There are four κ and 10 λ subgroups, although, of the λ subgroups, most patients (94%) with multiple myeloma express λI, λII, λIII, or λV subgroups. While the κ isotype is typically a monomer, the λ isotype often homodimerizes before secretion into the circulation and,

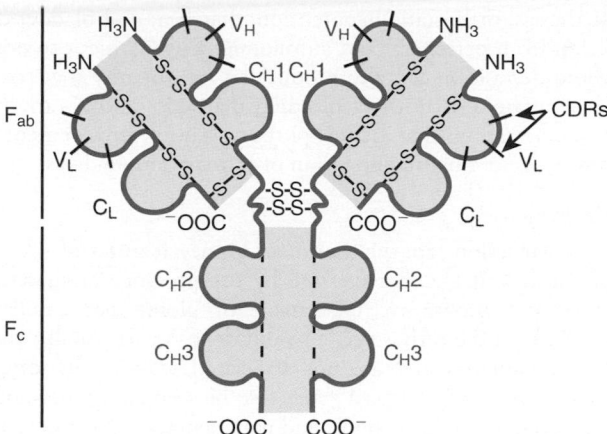

• **Fig. 28.1** Schematic of the immunoglobulin G molecule, which consists of two heavy chains and two light chains that are stabilized by inter- and intramolecular disulfide bonds. Light chains consist of two domains that are termed *constant* (C_L) and *variable* (V_L) *regions*. Within the V_L domain are the complementarity determining regions that are primarily responsible for variations in the amino-acid sequences among light chains. Heavy chains also consist of a variable domain (V_H) and three constant domains (C_H1, C_H2, C_H3). *CDRs*, Complementarity determining regions.

therefore, circulating levels of κ free light chains are more sensitive to changes in glomerular filtration rate than are λ free light chains.

The multiple kidney lesions from monoclonal light chain deposition affect virtually every compartment of the kidney (see Box 28.1) and may be explained by sequence variations, particularly in the V_L domain of the offending monoclonal light chain. Light chains that are responsible for monoclonal LCDD (a subset of MIDD) are frequently members of the κIV subfamily and appear to possess unusual hydrophobic amino-acid residues in CDR1. In AL-type amyloidosis, sequence variations in the V_L domain of the precursor light chain confer the propensity to polymerize to form amyloid. A classic kidney presentation of multiple myeloma is Fanconi syndrome, which is produced almost exclusively by members of the κI subfamily. Unusual nonpolar residues in the CDR1 region and absence of accessible side chains in the CDR3 loop of the variable domain of κI light chains result in homotypic crystallization of the light chain in this syndrome. In cast nephropathy, the secondary structure of CDR3 is a critical determinant of cast formation. In summary, sequence variations in the V_L domain appear to determine the type of kidney lesion that occurs with monoclonal light chain deposition.

Free light chains were originally detected with turbidimetric and heat tests. Because these tests lack sensitivity, they are no longer in use. The qualitative urine dipstick test for protein also has a low sensitivity for detection of light chains. Although some Bence Jones proteins react with the chemical impregnated onto the strip, other light chains cannot be detected; the net charge of the protein may be an important determinant of this interaction. Because of the relative insensitivity of routine serum protein electrophoresis (SPEP) and urinary protein electrophoresis (UPEP) for free light chains, these tests are not recommended as screening tools in the diagnostic evaluation of the underlying etiology of kidney disease. For example, SPEP is positive in 87.6% of multiple myelomas but only 73.8% of immunoglobulin light-chain (AL) amyloidosis and 55.6% of LCDD. The sensitivity of the UPEP is also low: Among a population of 2799 plasma cell dyscrasia patients, only 37.7% had a positive UPEP.

Highly sensitive and reliable immunoassays now are available to detect the presence of monoclonal light chains in the urine and serum and are adequate tests for screening when both urine and serum are examined. When a clone of plasma cells exists, significant amounts of monoclonal light chains may appear in the circulation and the urine. In healthy adults, the urinary concentration of polyclonal light chain proteins is about 2.5 mg/L. Causes of monoclonal light-chain proteinuria, a hallmark of plasma cell dyscrasias, are listed (Box 28.2). Urinary light chain concentration is generally between 0.02 g/L and 0.5 g/L in patients with monoclonal gammopathy of undetermined significance (MGUS) and is often much higher (range 0.02 g/L to 11.8 g/L) in patients with multiple myeloma or Waldenström macroglobulinemia. Immunofixation electrophoresis is sensitive and detects monoclonal light chains and immunoglobulins, even in very low concentrations, but it is a qualitative assay that may be limited by interobserver variation. A nephelometric assay that quantifies serum-free κ and λ light chains is also useful because most of the kidney lesions in paraproteinemias are caused by light chain overproduction and

---

BOX 28.1

Paraproteinemia-Associated Kidney Diseases

Glomerulopathies

AL-type and AH-type amyloidoses
Monoclonal immunoglobulin deposition disease
Proliferative glomerulonephritis with monoclonal immunoglobulin deposition
Paraprotein-associated C3 glomerulopathy
Paraprotein-associated fibrillary glomerulonephritis
Immunotactoid glomerulopathy
Cryoglobulinemia, type I

Tubulointerstitial Lesions

Cast nephropathy ("myeloma kidney")
Fanconi syndrome
Proximal tubulopathy
Tubulointerstitial nephritis (rare)

Vascular Lesions

Asymptomatic Bence Jones proteinuria
Hyperviscosity syndrome
Neoplastic cell infiltration (rare)

BOX 28.2

Potential Causes of Monoclonal Light-Chain Proteinuria

Multiple myeloma
AL-type amyloidosis
Monoclonal light-chain deposition disease
Waldenström macroglobulinemia
MGUS
POEMS syndrome (rare)
Heavy-chain (μ) disease (rare)
Lymphoproliferative disease (rare)

MGUS, Monoclonal gammopathy of undetermined significance; *POEMS,* syndrome consisting of polyneuropathy, organomegaly, endocrinopathy, M protein, and skin changes.

much less commonly by heavy chains or intact immunoglobulins. Because an excess of light chains, compared with heavy chains, is synthesized and released into the circulation, this sensitive assay detects small amounts of serum polyclonal free light chains in healthy individuals. This assay can also distinguish polyclonal from monoclonal light chains and further quantifies the free light chain level in the serum. Quantifying serum light chain levels may be of use clinically to monitor chemotherapy as well as to determine risk for development of kidney failure, as myeloma patients with baseline serum-free monoclonal light chain levels greater than 500 mg/L are more likely to have lower glomerular filtration rate (serum creatinine concentration ≥2 mg/dL) from cast nephropathy. In the evaluation of kidney disease, particularly if amyloidosis is suspected, perhaps the ideal screening tests for an associated plasma cell dyscrasia include immunofixation electrophoresis of serum and urine and quantification of serum free κ and λ light chains, which have been added as a diagnostic criterion for myeloma. The addition of serum free light chain assay to immunofixation increases detection of multiple myeloma, Waldenström macroglobulinemia, and smoldering multiple myeloma.

Glomerular Lesions of Plasma Cell Dyscrasias

AL-Type Amyloidosis

Amyloid proteins are characterized by a misfolding event that renders them insoluble and, therefore, deposit in organs as fibrils, leading to dysfunction. AL-type amyloidosis, which is also known as "*primary amyloidosis,*" represents a plasma cell dyscrasia that is characterized by organ dysfunction related to deposition of amyloid and usually only a mild increase in monoclonal plasma cells in the bone marrow. However, about 20% of patients with AL-type amyloidosis exhibit overt multiple myeloma or other lymphoproliferative disorders. It is important to note that more than 23 different amyloid proteins have been identified. The type of amyloid that is produced is named according to the precursor protein that polymerizes to produce amyloid. For example, in AL-type amyloidosis, the amyloid deposits are composed of immunoglobulin light chains versus AA-type amyloidosis, where the precursor protein (serum amyloid A protein) is an acute phase reactant. The identification of the type of amyloid protein is an essential first step in the management of these patients.

AL-type amyloidosis is a systemic disease that typically involves multiple organs (Table 28.1). Cardiac infiltration frequently produces congestive heart failure and is a relatively common presenting manifestation of primary amyloidosis. Infiltration of the lungs and gastrointestinal tract is also common but is generally asymptomatic.

Dysesthesias, orthostatic hypotension, diarrhea, and bladder dysfunction from peripheral and autonomic neuropathies can occur. Amyloid deposition can also produce an arthropathy that resembles rheumatoid arthritis, a bleeding diathesis, and a variety of skin manifestations that include purpura. Kidney involvement is a common presenting manifestation of primary amyloidosis.

Pathology

Glomerular lesions are the dominant kidney features of AL-type amyloidosis and are characterized by the presence of mesangial nodules and progressive effacement of glomerular capillaries (Fig. 28.2). In the early stage, amyloid deposits are usually found in the mesangium and are not associated with an increase in mesangial cellularity. Deposits may also be seen along the subepithelial space of capillary loops, and may penetrate the glomerular basement membrane in more advanced stages. Amyloid has characteristic tinctorial properties and stains with Congo red, which produces an apple-green birefringence when the tissue section is examined under polarized light and with thioflavins T and S. On electron microscopy, the deposits are characteristic, randomly oriented, nonbranching fibrils 7 to 10 nm in diameter. In some cases of early amyloidosis, glomeruli may appear normal on light microscopy; however, careful examination can identify scattered monotypic light chains on immunofluorescence microscopy.

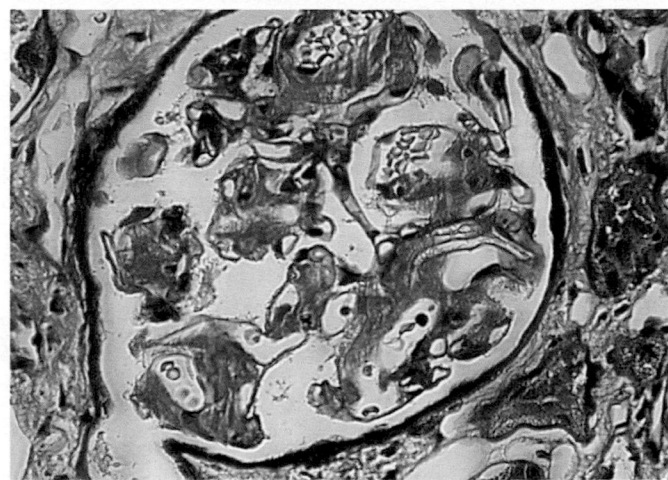

• **Fig. 28.2** Glomerulus from a patient with AL-type amyloidosis, showing segmentally variable accumulation of amorphous acidophilic material that is effacing portions of the glomerular architecture (PASH stain, magnification × 40).

TABLE 28.1	Relative Frequency of Organ Infiltration by Light Chains in AL-Type Amyloidosis and Light Chain Deposition Disease						
		ORGAN INVOLVEMENT					
	Isotype	Kidney	Heart	Liver	Neurologic	GI	Lung
AL-amyloid	λ > κ	+++	+++	+	+	+++	++++
LCDD	κ > λ	++++	+++	++	+	Rare	Rare

Note: From +, uncommon but can occur during the course of the disease, through ++++, extremely common during the course of the disease.
GI, Gastrointestinal; *LCDD*, monoclonal light-chain deposition disease.

Immunofluorescence microscopy is an essential component of the pathologic evaluation of these lesions and can demonstrate that the deposits consist of light chains, although the sensitivity of this test is not high. Ultrastructural and immunohistochemical examination of biopsies of other affected organs can also establish the diagnosis, although tissue diagnosis of AL-type amyloidosis can also be difficult, because commercially available antibodies may not detect the presence of the light chain in the tissue. For these reasons, in uncertain cases, the amyloid is extracted from tissue using sophisticated techniques such as laser capture microdissection followed by tandem mass spectrometry-based proteomic analysis, which determines the chemical composition of the amyloid. As the disease advances, mesangial deposits progressively enlarge to form nodules of amyloid protein that compress the filtering surfaces of the glomeruli and cause kidney failure. Epithelial proliferation and crescent formation are rare in AL-type amyloidosis.

Clinical Features

Proteinuria and reduced kidney function are the major kidney manifestations of AL-type amyloidosis. Proteinuria ranges from asymptomatic non-nephrotic proteinuria to nephrotic syndrome. Isolated microscopic hematuria and nephritic syndrome are not common in AL-type amyloidosis. More than 90% of patients have monoclonal light chains either in urine or blood, but occasionally even sensitive assays will not detect a circulating monoclonal light chain in patients with documented AL-type renal amyloidosis. Reduced kidney function is present in 58% to 70% of patients at the time of diagnosis. Scintigraphy using ^{123}I-labeled serum amyloid P component, which binds to amyloid, can assess the degree of organ involvement from amyloid infiltration, but this test is not currently widely available.

Pathogenesis

The pathogenesis of AL-type amyloidosis is incompletely understood. Presumably, intracellular oxidation or partial proteolysis of light chains by mesangial cells in the kidney, for example, allows formation of amyloid, which is then extruded into the extracellular space. With continued production of amyloid, the mesangium expands, compressing the filtering surface of the glomeruli and producing progressive kidney failure. Not all light chains are amyloidogenic. Members of the λ family are more commonly associated with AL-type amyloidosis, and sequence variations in the V_L domain confer the propensity to polymerize to form amyloid. Experimental evidence demonstrated that amyloidogenic light chains also have intrinsic biological activity that modulates cell function independently of amyloid formation. These properties may explain, for example, the striking proteinuria that occurs in many of these patients.

Treatment and Prognosis

Patients with both multiple myeloma and AL-type amyloidosis should be managed with treatment regimens that target myeloma. For patients who experience AL-type amyloidosis and lack the criteria for multiple myeloma, the initial approach is to ensure that the patient has AL-type amyloidosis and not amyloidosis related to a nonlymphoid-derived precursor protein, because the approaches to treatment are different. Because a randomized trial suggested improved survival in patients who received chemotherapy, more aggressive anti-plasma cell therapies have been undertaken in AL-type amyloidosis, including high-dose chemotherapy with autologous peripheral stem-cell transplantation (HDT/SCT). Although reduced kidney function may not be an exclusion criteria, because

of increased treatment-related mortality of HDT/SCT in higher-risk individuals, more conservative approaches should be considered for patients age ≥80 years or with decompensated heart failure, left ventricular ejection fraction below 40%, systolic blood pressure below 90 mm Hg, oxygen saturation less than 95% on room air, or significant overall functional impairment. Patients who have evidence of multiorgan system dysfunction, particularly cardiac disease, and are considered ineligible for HDT/SCT have an expected median survival of only 4 months, so delays in diagnosis and treatment can be costly. In contrast, one study reported a median survival of 4.6 years in 312 patients who underwent HDT/SCT. Almost half achieved a complete hematologic response, which portended improved long-term survival.

Patients with AL-type amyloidosis usually die from organ failure due to amyloid infiltration and not from tumor burden. An important observation from these studies is that survival and organ function can improve with successful reduction in the monoclonal plasma cell population and light chain production. Other novel chemotherapeutic regimens may be of benefit in AL-type amyloidosis and are being considered, particularly given the potential toxicity of chronic treatment with alkylating agents. The recent success of thalidomide as an alternative treatment of multiple myeloma has prompted treatment of AL-type amyloidosis with this agent, although thalidomide is not well tolerated in these patients and dosage reductions are often required. Lenalidomide, an analogue of thalidomide, is another potentially attractive therapy in AL-type amyloidosis. Bortezomib-based regimens have also provided promising results in AL-type amyloidosis.

There has been increasing interest in improving amyloid-associated end-organ damage that did not recover, despite an adequate hematologic response to therapy. Novel treatment approaches are being evaluated, including methods to target precursor protein production, administration of small molecules to prevent misfolding, and introduction of agents to increase amyloid degradation. For example, NEOD001, a monoclonal antibody directed against free light chains, was shown to specifically bind soluble and insoluble aggregated light chains and mediate antibody-dependent phagocytosis. VITAL phase III/NCT02312206 and PRONTO phase IIb are randomized, placebo-controlled, global trials that are under way to evaluate NEOD001 further.

Monoclonal Ig Deposition Disease

Monoclonal Ig deposition disease (MIDD) is defined as the deposition of nonamyloid monoclonal light and/or heavy chains in a nonorganized manner in the kidney. MIDD is further categorized into three subtypes that are based on the composition of the monoclonal protein in the deposits: light chain deposition disease (LCDD), light and heavy chain deposition disease (LHCDD), and heavy chain deposition disease (HCDD). LCDD is the most common and will be further discussed. MIDD is a systemic disease but typically presents as an isolated kidney injury related to nonamyloid electron-dense granular deposits of monoclonal light chains with or without heavy chains in the glomerulus. It may accompany other clinical features of multiple myeloma or another lymphoproliferative disorder or may be the sole manifestation of a plasma cell dyscrasia.

Pathology

Nodular glomerulopathy with distortion of the glomerular architecture by amorphous, eosinophilic material is the most common pathologic finding observed with light microscopy (Fig. 28.3).

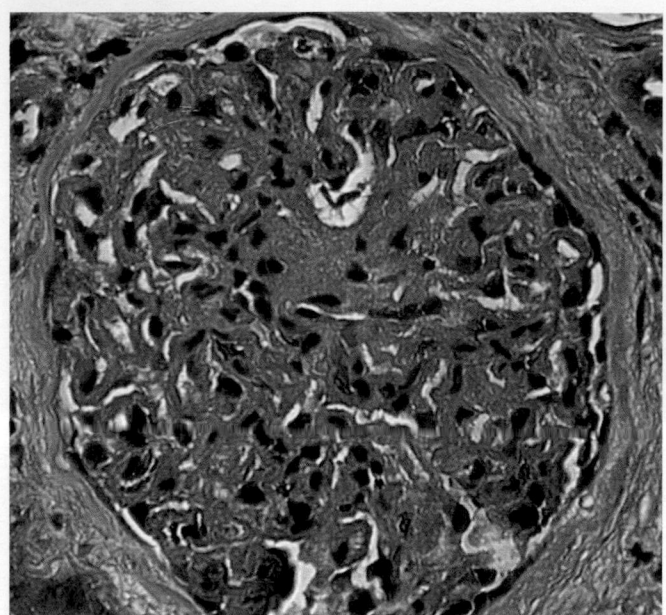

• **Fig. 28.3** Glomerulus from a patient with monoclonal κ light-chain deposition disease, showing expansion of the mesangium, related to matrix protein deposition, and associated compression of capillary lumens (hematoxylin-eosin stain, magnification ×40).

These nodules, which are composed of light chains and extracellular matrix proteins, begin in the mesangium. The appearance is reminiscent of diabetic nephropathy. Less commonly, other glomerular morphologic changes in addition to nodular glomerulopathy can be seen in LCDD. Immunofluorescence microscopy demonstrates the presence of monotypic light chains in the glomeruli. Under electron microscopy, deposits of light chain proteins are present as electron-dense deposits located in a subendothelial position along the glomerular capillary wall, along the outer aspect of tubular basement membranes, and in the mesangium.

There are significant differences between amyloidosis and LCDD. For amyloid deposition to occur, amyloid P glycoprotein must also be present. The amyloid P component is not part of the amyloid fibrils but binds them. This glycoprotein is a constituent of normal human glomerular basement membrane and elastic fibrils. In contrast to AL-type amyloid, in LCDD the light chain deposits are punctate, granular, and electron-dense and are identified in the mesangium and/or subendothelial space; amyloid P component is absent. Unlike amyloid, the granular light-chain deposits of LCDD do not stain with Congo red or thioflavin T and S. Another difference between these lesions is the tendency for κ light chains to compose the granular deposits of LCDD, whereas usually λ light chains constitute AL-amyloid. Both diseases can involve organs other than the kidney (see Table 28.1).

Clinical Features

The typical clinical presentation is reminiscent of a rapidly progressive glomerulonephritis. The major symptoms of LCDD include proteinuria, sometimes in the nephrotic range, microscopic hematuria, and kidney failure. Albumin and monoclonal free light chains are the dominant proteins in the urine. The presence of albuminuria and other findings of nephrotic syndrome are important clues to the presence of glomerular injury and not cast nephropathy. The amount of excreted light chain is usually less

than that found in cast nephropathy and can be difficult to detect in some patients. Progressive kidney failure in untreated patients is common. Because kidney manifestations generally predominate and are often the sole presenting features, it is not uncommon for nephrologists to diagnose the plasma cell dyscrasia. Kidney biopsy is necessary to confirm the diagnosis. Other organ dysfunction, especially in the liver and heart, can develop and is related to deposition of light chains in those organs. Although extrarenal manifestations of overt multiple myeloma can manifest at presentation or over time, a majority (~50% to 60%) of patients with LCDD will not develop myeloma or other malignant lymphoproliferative disease.

Pathogenesis

LCDD represents a prototypical model of progressive kidney disease that has a pathogenesis related to glomerulosclerosis from increased production of transforming growth factor-β (TGF-β). The response to monoclonal light chain deposition includes expansion of the mesangium by extracellular matrix proteins to form nodules and eventually glomerular sclerosis. Experimental studies have shown that mesangial cells exposed to light chains obtained from patients with biopsy-proven LCDD produce TGF-β, which serves as an autacoid to stimulate these same cells to produce matrix proteins, including type IV collagen, laminin, and fibronectin. Thus, TGF-β plays a central role in glomerular sclerosis from LCDD. As is true for AL-type amyloidosis, not all light chains can produce LCDD. Many offending light chains are κ, particularly the κIV subfamily, and appear to possess unusual hydrophobic amino-acid residues in the V_L domain.

Although deposition of light chains is the prominent feature of these glomerular lesions, both heavy chains and light chains can be identified in the deposits. In these specimens, the punctate electron-dense deposits appear larger and more extensive than deposits that contain only light chains, but it is unclear whether the clinical course of these patients differs from the course of isolated light chain deposition without heavy chain components, and the management is similar.

Treatment and Prognosis

For patients with both multiple myeloma and LCDD, therapy is directed toward the underlying myeloma. The treatment of LCDD without an associated malignant lymphoproliferative disorder is difficult because guidance from randomized controlled trials is unavailable. However, patients appear to benefit from the same therapeutic approach as that used for multiple myeloma. The serum creatinine concentration at presentation is an important predictor of subsequent outcome, so intervention should be early in the course of the disease.

Melphalan/prednisone therapy improves kidney prognosis, but the long-term toxicity of melphalan makes this approach less attractive. More aggressive anti-plasma cell therapy in the form of HDT/SCT has been used with some success in LCDD. In the small numbers of patients in whom HDT/SCT was performed, the procedure-related death rate was low, and when a complete hematologic response was observed, improvement in affected organ function with histologic evidence of regression of the light chain deposits occurred. This has been further confirmed in a recent study looking at overall survival and kidney outcomes in 88 patients with LCDD. Novel chemotherapeutic regimens that include thalidomide and bortezomib have efficacy in this setting.

The high incidence of progressive kidney disease in LCDD has prompted treatment with kidney transplantation, but the disease will recur in the allograft if the underlying plasma cell dyscrasia is not addressed. The study with the largest collection of patients (seven) concluded that LCDD recurred commonly in the kidney allograft, significantly impacting long-term graft survival; these findings emphasize the need to control monoclonal light chain production before kidney transplantation in LCDD.

Fibrillary Glomerulonephritis and Immunotactoid Glomerulopathy

Fibrillary glomerulonephritis is a rare disorder characterized ultra-structurally by the presence of amyloid-like, randomly arranged fibrillary deposits in the capillary wall (Fig. 28.4). Unlike amyloid, these fibrils are usually thicker (18 nm to 22 nm) and are not detected with Congo red and thioflavin T stains. Immuno-fluorescence microscopy typically shows IgG (usually IgG4) and C3. Most patients with fibrillary glomerulonephritis do not have a plasma cell dyscrasia; however, occasionally a plasma cell dyscrasia is present, so screening is advisable. Tests for cryoglobulins and hepatitis C infection should be obtained. Patients typically manifest nephrotic syndrome and varying degrees of kidney injury; progression to end-stage kidney failure is the rule. Fibrillary glomerulonephritis may recur in the kidney allograft following transplantation. Standardized treatment for the idiopathic fibrillary glomerulonephritis is currently unavailable.

Immunotactoid, or microtubular, glomerulopathy is even less common than fibrillary glomerulonephritis and is usually associated with a plasma cell dyscrasia or another lymphoproliferative disorder. The deposits in this lesion contain thick (greater than 30 nm), organized, microtubular structures that are located in the mesangium and along capillary walls. Cryoglobulinemia, which is also discussed in Chapter 24, should be considered in the differential diagnosis and should be ruled out clinically. Treatment of the underlying plasma cell dyscrasia is indicated for this rare disorder.

Tubulointerstitial Lesions of Plasma Cell Dyscrasias

Cast Nephropathy

Pathology

Cast nephropathy is an inflammatory tubulointerstitial kidney lesion. Characteristically, multiple intraluminal proteinaceous casts are identified mainly in the distal portion of the nephrons (Fig. 28.5). The casts are usually acellular, homogeneous, and eosinophilic with multiple fracture lines. Immunofluorescence and immunoelectron microscopy confirm that the casts contain light chains and Tamm-Horsfall glycoprotein, a protein produced exclusively in the kidney. Persistence of the casts produces the giant cell inflammation and tubular atrophy that typify myeloma kidney. Glomeruli are usually normal in appearance.

Clinical Features

Kidney failure from this lesion may present acutely or as a chronic progressive disease and may develop at any stage of myeloma. Diagnosis of multiple myeloma is usually evident when chronic bone pain, pathologic fractures, and hypercalcemia are complicated by proteinuria and kidney failure. However, many patients present to nephrologists primarily with symptoms of kidney fail-

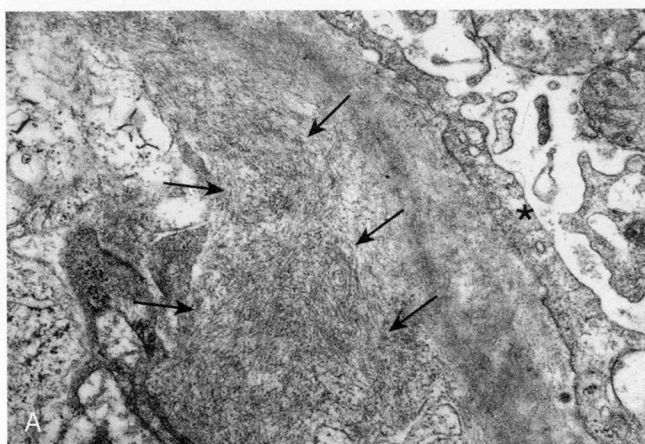
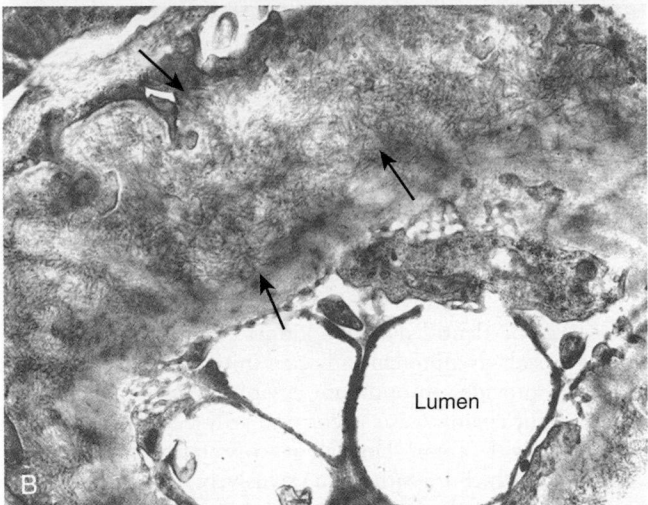

• **Fig. 28.4 Glomeruli.** (A) Electron micrograph of a glomerulus from a patient with AL-type amyloidosis. Note the randomly arranged, relatively straight fibrils with an approximate diameter of 7 to 10 nm (*arrows*). A useful distinction from fibrillary glomerulonephritis is that amyloid fibrils will stain with Congo red or thioflavin T. Note fusion of the foot processes (*asterisk*) of the adjacent epithelial cell. (B) Electron micrograph of a glomerulus from a patient with fibrillary glomerulonephritis. The same random arrangement of nonbranching fibrils (*arrows*) is seen. Careful examination demonstrates that the fibrils are larger (approximately 20 nm in diameter). The overall ultrastructural appearance resembles amyloid, except that the fibrils are approximately twice as thick. (A courtesy Dr. J. Charles Jennette, Department of Pathology, University of North Carolina at Chapel Hill; B courtesy Dr. William Cook, Department of Pathology, University of Alabama at Birmingham.)

ure or undefined proteinuria; further evaluation then confirms a malignant process. Cast nephropathy should be strongly considered in any patient who presents with acute kidney injury and has a monoclonal serum free light chain level >500 mg/L. The diagnosis of cast nephropathy should also be entertained when proteinuria (often more than 3 g/day), particularly without concomitant hypoalbuminemia or significant albuminuria, is found in a patient who is in the fourth decade of life or older. Hypertension is not common with cast nephropathy. Diagnosis of myeloma may be confirmed by finding monoclonal immunoglobulins or light chains in the serum and urine and by bone marrow examination, although typical intraluminal cast formation on kidney biopsy is virtually pathognomonic.

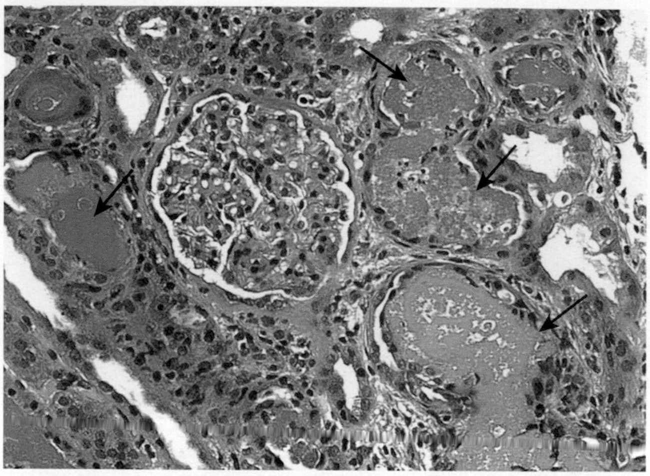

• **Fig. 28.5** Kidney biopsy tissue from a patient with cast nephropathy. The findings include tubules filled with homogenous material (*arrows*) and presence of multinucleated giant cells. Glomeruli are typically normal in appearance (hematoxylin-eosin stain, magnification × 20).

Pathogenesis

Intravenous infusion of nephrotoxic human light chains in rats elevates proximal tubule pressure and simultaneously decreases the single nephron glomerular filtration rate (GFR); intraluminal protein casts can be identified in these kidneys. Myeloma casts contain Tamm-Horsfall glycoprotein and occur initially in the distal nephron, which provides an optimum environment for precipitation with free light chains. Casts occur primarily because light chains coaggregate with Tamm-Horsfall glycoprotein. Tamm-Horsfall glycoprotein, which is synthesized exclusively by cells of the thick ascending limb of the loop of Henle, comprises the major fraction of total urinary protein in healthy individuals and is the predominant constituent of urinary casts. Cast-forming Bence Jones proteins bind to the same site on the peptide backbone of Tamm-Horsfall glycoprotein; binding results in coaggregation of these proteins and subsequent occlusion of the tubule lumen by the precipitated protein complexes. Intranephronal obstruction and kidney failure ensue. Light chains that bind to Tamm-Horsfall glycoprotein are potentially nephrotoxic. The CDR3 domain of the light chain determines binding affinity.

Coaggregation of Tamm-Horsfall glycoprotein with light chains also depends on the ionic environment and the physicochemical properties of the light chain, and not all patients with myeloma develop cast nephropathy, even when the urinary excretion of light chains is high. Increasing concentrations of sodium chloride or calcium, but not magnesium, facilitate coaggregation. The loop diuretic, furosemide, augments coaggregation and accelerates intraluminal obstruction in vivo in the rat. Finally, the lower tubule fluid flow rates of the distal nephron allow more time for light chains to interact with Tamm-Horsfall glycoprotein and subsequently to obstruct the tubular lumen. Conditions that further reduce flow rates, such as volume depletion, can accelerate tubule obstruction or convert nontoxic light chains into cast-forming proteins. Volume depletion and hypercalcemia are recognized factors that promote acute kidney injury (AKI) from cast nephropathy.

Treatment and Prognosis

The principles used to guide therapy in cast nephropathy include rapidly decreasing the concentration of circulating light chains and preventing coaggregation of light chains with Tamm-Horsfall glycoprotein (Box 28.3). Prompt and effective chemotherapy should start upon diagnosis of multiple myeloma. The traditional treatment with alkylating agents and steroids has been replaced by HDT/SCT, particularly in younger patients. A possible advantage with a more aggressive approach is the potential for rapid reductions in the levels of circulating monoclonal light chain. Several randomized trials showed that patients who received HDT/SCT experienced an improvement in overall survival versus patients who received conventional chemotherapy. Chemotherapy is usually initiated before HDT/SCT to reduce the plasma cell clone. Induction therapy with combinations of immunomodulatory drugs (thalidomide and lenalidomide) and proteasome inhibitors (bortezomib and carfilzomib), along with steroids, alkylators, or anthracyclines, followed by autologous hematopoietic cell transplantation (HCT), has improved the median overall survival for patients with multiple myeloma from 36 months to more than 5 years. Treatment with alkylating agents is often avoided before HDT/SCT, because these drugs may impede peripheral stem cell harvest and are associated with myelodysplasia and acute myelogenous leukemia. Almost all patients after autologous SCT ultimately relapse and need further treatment. Monoclonal antibodies, deacetylase inhibitors, kinase inhibitors, and immune checkpoint inhibitors have been tested in clinical trials with promising results; however, nephrotoxicity has been an associated complication.

Patients with advanced kidney failure and refractory myeloma have been treated successfully with bortezomib- and thalidomide-based therapies. These agents have gained wide acceptance and may ultimately obviate the need for HDT/SCT. Nonmyeloablative allogeneic stem-cell transplantation, so-called *mini-allograft therapy*, may also provide beneficial results in myeloma but is not without attendant complications that include graft-versus-host disease.

Studies suggest that interstitial fibrosis can develop rapidly in cast nephropathy, promoting persistent and ultimately irreversible kidney failure. Because clinical evidence suggests that prompt reduction in circulating free light chains accelerates kidney recovery in cast nephropathy, the delay in reduction of free light-chain levels associated with chemotherapy has provoked exploration of extracorporeal removal of circulating free light chains, with mixed results in the era of modern highly effective chemotherapy. Recent randomized trials (MYRE and EuLITE) that examined outcomes of use of high-cutoff hemodialysis (HCHD) treatments to remove circulating light chains have produced mixed results. EuLITE showed no benefit on kidney recovery (with increased adverse effects), while MYRE showed no benefit for kidney recovery at 3 months but did show a benefit at 6 and 12 months. Neither trial showed an improvement in mortality. While it is clear that in cases where HCHD provided a robust free light chain response that the rate of recovery from initially dialysis-dependent cast nephropathy increased, the side effects of the treatment may have mitigated

---

BOX 28.3

Standard Therapy for Cast Nephropathy

Chemotherapy to decrease light-chain production
Increase free water intake to 2 to 3 L/day as tolerated
Treat hypercalcemia aggressively

Avoid exposure to diuretics, radiocontrast agents, and nonsteroidal anti-inflammatory agents.

the potential benefit; accordingly, this approach continues to be examined in the experimental setting. Until additional data are provided, although it seems likely that there may be a subset of patients with AKI from cast nephropathy who will respond favorably to this additional intervention, it is probably not prudent to recommend routinely extracorporeal therapies for treating cast nephropathy, but rather emphasize highly effective chemotherapy. An exception is hyperviscosity syndrome, which remains an indication for extracorporeal removal of the offending monoclonal proteins.

Although the nephrotoxicity of individual monoclonal light chains varies, patients whose serum monoclonal light chain protein exceeds 500 mg/L should be considered at risk of developing cast nephropathy. Along with reducing circulating light chains, prevention of aggregation of light chains with Tamm-Horsfall glycoprotein is a cornerstone of therapy. Volume repletion, normalization of electrolytes, and avoidance of complicating factors such as loop diuretics and nonsteroidal anti-inflammatory agents are helpful in preserving and improving kidney function. Although not all patients with light-chain proteinuria develop AKI following exposure to radiocontrast agents, caution should be used with radiocontrast agent administration in all patients with myeloma. Daily intake up to 3 L of electrolyte-poor fluid should be encouraged. Alkalinization of the urine with oral sodium bicarbonate (or citrate) to keep the urine pH greater than 7 may also be therapeutic but may be mitigated by the requisite sodium loading, which favors coaggregation of these proteins and also should be avoided in patients who have symptomatic extracellular fluid volume overload.

Hypercalcemia occurs during the course of the disease in more than 25% of patients with multiple myeloma. In addition to being directly nephrotoxic, hypercalcemia enhances the nephrotoxicity of light chains. Treatment of volume contraction with the infusion of saline often corrects mild hypercalcemia. Loop diuretics also increase calcium excretion, but diuretics may also facilitate nephrotoxicity from light chains and should be avoided, if possible. Glucocorticoid therapy (such as methylprednisolone) is helpful for acute management of myeloma as well as hypercalcemia. Bisphosphonates, such as pamidronate and zoledronic acid, are used to treat moderate hypercalcemia (serum calcium greater than 3.25 mmol/L, or 13 mg/dL) that is unresponsive to other measures. Bisphosphonates lower serum calcium by interfering with osteoclast-mediated bone resorption. Although hypercalcemia of myeloma responds to bisphosphonates, these agents can be nephrotoxic and should be administered only to euvolemic patients. Kidney function should be monitored closely during therapy. Treatment with pamidronate or zoledronic acid allows outpatient management of mild hypercalcemia. In addition to controlling hypercalcemia, bisphosphonates appear to inhibit growth of plasma cells and are used to treat multiple myeloma, particularly in patients with osseous lesions and bone pain.

If indicated, kidney replacement therapy, with either hemodialysis or peritoneal dialysis, may be used in patients with kidney failure from monoclonal light-chain–related kidney diseases. Recovery of kidney function sufficient to survive without dialysis occurs in as many as 5% of patients with multiple myeloma, although in some patients, this goal requires months to achieve and depends upon the rapidity with which circulating light-chain levels are reduced. Despite the susceptibility to infection in multiple myeloma, the peritonitis rate for peritoneal dialysis, one episode every 14.4 months, is not unacceptably high. Neither peritoneal dialysis nor hemodialysis appears to provide a superior survival advantage in myeloma patients. Kidney transplant also has been performed successfully in selected myeloma patients in remission. Because the light chain is the underlying cause of cast nephropathy, tests that ensure absence of circulating free light chains are useful in the evaluation of candidacy for kidney transplantation.

Other Tubulointerstitial Kidney Lesions Including Proximal Tubulopathy

Proximal tubular injury and tubulointerstitial nephritis can occur. A classic kidney presentation of multiple myeloma is Fanconi syndrome, which is characterized by a proximal renal tubular acidosis (type II) and defective sodium-coupled cotransport processes, producing aminoaciduria, glycosuria, and phosphaturia. Kidney biopsy typically shows crystals of light-chain protein within the epithelium of the proximal tubule. Fanconi syndrome may precede overt multiple myeloma. Plasma cell dyscrasia should, therefore, be considered in the differential diagnosis when this syndrome occurs in adults.

Unlike most endogenous low-molecular-weight proteins, monoclonal light chains have a propensity to produce tubular injury. Although the more common lesion is cast nephropathy, patients occasionally present with kidney failure from an isolated proximal tubulopathy that is distinct from the pathology associated with Fanconi syndrome. Kidney failure from isolated proximal tubular damage generally improves with effective chemotherapy that reduces the circulating monoclonal free light chain. A major mechanism of damage to the proximal epithelium is related to accumulation of toxic light chains in the endolysosome. Light chains appear to catalyze sufficient amounts of hydrogen peroxide to generate intracellular oxidative stress that promotes cytotoxicity as well as the production of inflammatory chemokines such as monocyte chemotactic factor-1 and pro-fibrotic growth factors such as TGF-β. Loss of proximal tubular epithelial cells and generation of a proinflammatory milieu may also promote nephron dropout and the tubulointerstitial scarring and inflammation that are prevalent findings in cast nephropathy.

Waldenström Macroglobulinemia

This disorder constitutes about 5% of monoclonal gammopathies and is characterized by the presence of a monoclonal B-cell malignancy consisting of lymphocytoid plasma cells. The origin of these cells is thought to be a postantigen-stimulated memory B cell that has undergone malignant transformation through somatic hypermutation. This condition clinically behaves more like lymphoma, although the malignant cell secretes IgM (macroglobulin), which usually produces most of the clinical symptoms. Lytic bone lesions are uncommon, but hepatosplenomegaly and lymphadenopathy are frequently identified. IgM is a large molecule that is not excreted and accumulates in the plasma to produce hyperviscosity syndrome, which consists of neurologic symptoms (headaches, stupor, deafness, dizziness), visual impairment (from retinal hemorrhages and edema), bleeding diathesis (related to IgM complexing clotting factors and to platelet dysfunction), kidney failure, and symptoms of hypervolemia. Reduced GFR occurs in about 30% of patients, and hyperviscosity syndrome and precipitation of IgM in the lumen of glomerular capillaries are the most common causes. Approximately 10% to 15% of patients also develop AL-type amyloidosis, but cast nephropathy is rare. Because of the typically advanced age at presentation (sixth to seventh decade) and slowly progressive course, the major therapeutic goal is relief of symptoms. All patients with IgM levels greater than 4 g/dL should have serum viscosity determined. Plasmapheresis is indicated in symptomatic patients and should be continued until symptoms resolve and serum viscosity normalizes. Kidney failure requiring kidney replacement therapy is uncommon. The course of the disease can vary but is often protracted. Factors that portend a worse outcome include age greater than 65 years and organomegaly. Patients lacking these risk factors have a median survival of 10.6 years, whereas patients with either of these risk factors have a median survival of 4.2 years. Symptomatic patients are usually treated with combination chemotherapy that includes an alkylating agent along with rituximab, because these malignant cells express CD20.

Complete bibliography is available at Elsevier eBooks for Practicing Clinicians.

Key Bibliography

Bridoux F, Carron PL, Pegourie B, et al. Effect of high-cutoff hemodialysis vs conventional hemodialysis on hemodialysis independence among patients with myeloma cast nephropathy: a randomized clinical trial. *JAMA*. 2017;318:2099–2110.

Cavo M, Rajkumar SV, Palumbo A, et al. International Myeloma Working Group consensus approach to the treatment of multiple myeloma patients who are candidates for autologous stem cell transplantation. *Blood*. 2011;117:6063–6073.

Drayson M, Begum G, Basu S, et al. Effects of paraprotein heavy and light chain types and free light chain load on survival in myeloma: an analysis of patients receiving conventional-dose chemotherapy in Medical Research Council UK multiple myeloma trials. *Blood*. 2006;108:2013–2019.

Gertz MA, Landau H, Comenzo RL, et al. First-in-human phase I/II study of NEOD001 in patients with light chain amyloidosis and persistent organ dysfunction. *J Clin Oncol*. 2016;34:1097–1103.

Ghobrial IM, Fonseca R, Gertz MA, et al. Prognostic model for disease-specific and overall mortality in newly diagnosed symptomatic patients with Waldenstrom macroglobulinaemia. *Br J Haematol*. 2006;133:158–164.

Hutchison CA, Cockwell P, Moroz V, et al. High cutoff versus high-flux haemodialysis for.

Myeloma cast nephropathy in patients receiving bortezomib-based chemotherapy (EuLITE): a phase 2 randomised controlled trial. *Lancet Haematol*. 2019;6:e217–e228.

Joseph NS, Kaufman JL, Dhodapkar MV, et al. Long-term follow-up results of lenalidomide, bortezomib, and dexamethasone induction therapy and risk-adapted maintenance approach in newly diagnosed multiple myeloma. *J Clin Oncol*. 2020;38:1928–1937.

Katzmann JA, Kyle RA, Benson J, et al. Screening panels for detection of monoclonal gammopathies. *Clin Chem*. 2009;55:1517–1522.

Kyle RA, Gertz MA. Primary systemic amyloidosis: clinical and laboratory features in 474 cases. *Semin Hematol*. 1995;32:45–59.

McTaggart MP, Lindsay J, Kearney EM. Replacing urine protein electrophoresis with serum free light chain analysis as a first-line test for detecting plasma cell disorders offers increased diagnostic accuracy and potential health benefit to patients. *Am J Clin Pathol*. 2013;140:890–897.

Nasr SH, Valeri AM, Cornell LD, et al. Renal monoclonal immunoglobulin deposition disease: a report of 64 patients from a single institution. *Clin J Am Soc Nephrol*. 2012;7:231–239.

Rajkumar SV, Dimopoulos MA, Palumbo A, et al. International Myeloma Working Group updated criteria for the diagnosis of multiple myeloma. *Lancet Oncol*. 2014;15:e538–e548.

Rosenstock JL, Markowitz GS, Valeri AM, et al. Fibrillary and immunotactoid glomerulonephritis: distinct entities with different clinical and pathologic features. *Kidney Int*. 2003;63:1450–1461.

Royal V, Leung N, Troyanov S, et al. Clinicopathologic predictors of renal outcomes in light chain cast nephropathy: A multicenter retrospective study. *Blood*. 2020;135:1833–1846.

Wanchoo R, Abudayyeh A, Doshi M, et al. Renal toxicities of novel agents used for treatment of multiple myeloma. *Clin J Am Soc Nephrol*. 2017;12:176–189.

Yadav P, Sathick IJ, Leung N, et al. Serum free light chain level at diagnosis in myeloma cast nephropathy-a multicentre study. *Blood Cancer J*. 2020;10:28.

Ying WZ, Allen CE, Curtis LM, et al. Mechanism and prevention of acute kidney injury from cast nephropathy in a rodent model. *J Clin Invest*. 2012;122:1777–1785.

Ying WZ, Li X, Rangarajan S, et al. Immunoglobulin light chains generate proinflammatory and profibrotic kidney injury. *J Clin Invest*. 2019;129:2792–2806.

29

Cardiorenal Syndrome

JEFFREY M. TURNER, JEFFREY M. TESTANI

Cardiorenal syndrome (CRS) is a heterogenous disorder that is broadly characterized as interrelated dysfunction of the heart and kidneys. It is predominantly thought of as an entity that occurs in the setting of heart failure, although other cardiac abnormalities such as coronary artery disease, valvular disease, and arrythmias are often present. The specific kidney pathophysiologies that encompass CRS include abnormalities of filtration, sodium and water handling, blood pressure regulation, neurohormonal activation, and responsiveness to diuretics, among others. In this chapter we discuss a pragmatic approach to defining CRS and provide insights into the pathophysiology and therapeutic strategies for this disorder.

The Challenge in Defining Cardiorenal Syndrome

There have been several attempts at defining CRS over the years. These efforts have had limited success and, to date, there is no consensus definition or consensus diagnostic criteria, making synthesis of research and clinical data more challenging. Despite the deployment of several biomarkers in recent years that individually assess heart or kidney function (Table 29.1), the clinical application of these for the diagnosis and treatment of CRS remains somewhat elusive and varies based on clinical preferences. For the purposes of this discussion, we will take a cardio-centric viewpoint, meaning a syndrome in which cardiac dysfunction is primary in the cascade of organ dysfunction, with kidney dysfunction a secondary effect. Previous classification systems have referred to this as *acute and chronic CRS* based on the time frame in which injury occurs. The focus of this chapter will primarily be on the acute phenotype. It is important for the reader to be aware that primary kidney injury leading to acute or chronic cardiac dysfunction is likely an important pathophysiologic entity, although, for the practical purposes of this chapter, kidney-centric CRS is beyond our scope. In addition, much of the recent research efforts that have broadened our understanding of CRS have taken a cardio-centric approach.

Given that the kidneys receive approximately 25% of the blood flow from cardiac output, it seems intuitive that changes in cardiac hemodynamics impact kidney function. What is less obvious is that CRS is not simply due to hemodynamic alterations, but often more importantly, a result of disturbed neurohormonal regulation. In addition, increases in systemic inflammation are increasingly recognized as playing an important role. Notably, CRS is a challenge to define because the mere occurrence of these abnormalities alone is insufficient. After all, even with mild congestive heart failure, NYHA Class I-II patients can have some degree of cardiac-related hemodynamic dysfunction or neurohormonal upregulation that results in abnormal kidney function (mostly in the form of inappropriate sodium avidity); however, it is of limited clinical utility to consider such patients as having CRS. A more applicable characterization of acute CRS is that in which decompensated heart failure directly mediates an acute reduction in kidney function that is accompanied by both a decrease in glomerular filtration rate as well as an increase in tubular sodium avidity. The major clinical implication of these changes is that they complicate strategies that target venous decongestion. This scenario can be seen in patients with acute onset of de novo heart failure as well as in those with an acute decompensation of chronic heart failure; they most commonly occur in such patients with a level of illness severity that requires hospitalization. Common clinical manifestations include shortness of breath at rest or with mild exertion, increased jugular venous distention, tachycardia, crackles on auscultation, and significant lower extremity edema. Box 29.1 highlights the signs and symptoms of heart failure in more detail.

Prognostic Impact of Changes in Kidney Function in Heart Failure

Heart failure impacts approximately 6 million Americans, with over 650,000 new cases diagnosed each year. Up to 50% of patients with heart failure with either preserved ejection fraction or reduced ejection fraction also have chronic kidney disease (CKD), and this negatively impacts prognosis in this population. In a meta-analysis of over 1 million individuals with heart failure, those with CKD (defined as an estimated glomerular filtration rate [eGFR] < 60 mL/min/1.73 m^2) had double the risk of all-cause mortality. It, therefore, is important to appreciate that CKD significantly worsens the prognosis in subjects with heart failure.

In terms of CRS, observational data show that patients with acute decompensated heart failure (ADHF) admitted to the hospital who have an acute change in their kidney function also have a worse prognosis than similar patients with no acute change in kidney function. Cardiorenal syndrome effects about 30%–50% of hospitalized heart failure patients. Earlier studies demonstrated that an acute rise in creatinine was associated with worse outcomes in patients with ADHF, including nearly a two fold increase in mortality. However, newer data have demonstrated that this is an oversimplification of the relationship between kidney function and prognosis in patients hospitalized with ADHF. Recent studies show that, when a rise in creatinine occurs, its impact on mortality is based on the context in which

TABLE 29.1	Heart and Kidney Biomarkers

Blood Biomarkers

Heart
NT-pro-BNP
Troponin I
Troponin C
H-FABP

Kidney
Glomerular Function
Creatinine
Cystatin C
BUN

Tubular Function
NGAL
β2- macroglobulin
Calprotectin

Urine Biomarkers

Glomerular Function
Creatinine
Urea
Albumin

Tubular Function
NGAL
KIM-1
NAG
L-FABP
IGFBP7
TIMP2

NT-pro-BNP, N terminal pro-B-type natriuretic peptide; *H-FABP,* heart-type fatty acid-binding protein; *BUN,* blood urea nitrogen; *NGAL,* neutrophil gelatinase-associated lipocalin; *TNF-α,* tumor necrosis factor α; *KIM-1,* kidney injury molecule 1; *NAG,* N-acetyl-β-D-glucosaminidase; *L-FABP,* liver fatty acid-binding protein; *IGFBP7,* insulin-like growth factor-binding protein 7; *TIMP2,* tissue inhibitor of metalloproteinases 2

BOX 29.1

Clinical Manifestations of Heart Failure

Heart failure is a clinical syndrome in which patients have the following features:
- Symptoms typical of heart failure
  - Breathlessness at rest or on exercise, fatigue, tiredness
- Signs typical of heart failure
  - Tachycardia, tachypnea, pulmonary rales, pleural effusion, raised jugular venous pressure, peripheral edema, hepatomegaly
- Objective evidence of a structural or functional abnormality of the heart at rest
  - Cardiomegaly, third heart sound, cardiac murmurs, abnormality on echocardiogram, raised concentration of natriuretic peptide

Modified from the 2008 European Society of Cardiology Guidelines for the Diagnosis and Treatment of Acute and Chronic Heart Failure.

---

the change in kidney function is occurring. In other words, when the rise in creatinine coincides with worsening markers of venous congestion, there is a higher risk of death. However, this risk is not present, or is blunted, if the rise in creatinine coincides with improving markers of venous congestion. Other data demonstrate that an improvement in eGFR during hospitalization for ADHF can also be associated with negative outcomes if it coincides with worsening venous congestion or incomplete decongestion. This speaks to two important points to be made about CRS: (1) The etiology of the change in kidney function is heterogeneous in this disorder and (2) a mild or moderate rise in creatinine may often be an acceptable outcome, so long as it coincides with a positive therapeutic intervention for the patient.

Pathophysiology of Cardiorenal Syndrome

Changes in hemodynamics and neurohormones are important factors in the pathophysiology of CRS. In addition, emerging data have also implicated the role of inflammation as a key mediator in CRS. A schematic overview of the complex and multifactorial pathways involved in CRS is presented in Fig. 29.1.

It is well recognized that kidney blood flow is reduced in heart failure. Traditional viewpoints have explained this change as secondary to a reduction in cardiac output; however, more contemporary observations have questioned the completeness of this assumption. In multiple studies, cardiac index has not been associated with reductions in kidney function in patients hospitalized with ADHF. In addition, in the ADHERE Registry (Acute Decompensated Heart Failure National Registry), kidney dysfunction was equally prevalent in patients with and without a reduced ejection fraction. Finally, ultrasonographic studies show that blunting of venous blood flow in the kidneys precedes changes in left ventricular filling pressures when heart failure patients are volume expanded. These findings have shifted viewpoints about the pathophysiology of CRS from being solely an entity of perceived hemodynamic changes in the arterial vasculature to the viewpoint that hemodynamic changes in the venous vasculature are equally, if not more, important in the development of CRS.

Along these lines, several studies have concluded that an increase in venous pressure as well as a raised intrabdominal pressure are associated with kidney dysfunction in ADHF. In the ESCAPE trial (Evaluation Study of Congestive Heart Failure and Pulmonary Artery Catheterization Effectiveness), right atrial pressure was the only hemodynamic parameter associated with kidney dysfunction, and this observation has been confirmed in other studies. Increases in central venous pressure, as well as increases in intraabdominal pressures, lead to renal venous hypertension and, subsequently, an imbalance between the kidney arterial perfusion pressure and the kidney venous outflow pressure. In this setting, the net result is a reduction in kidney perfusion, impaired autoregulation, and a deterioration in GFR. Venous congestion also leads to changes outside of the kidney vasculature that similarly result in a decrease in GFR. The primary example of this is an elevation of pressure in the interstitium. Given that the kidney is an encapsulated organ, pressure elevation in the kidney veins can be transmitted to the interstitium and Bowman's capsule. This can lead to extrinsic pressure on tubules, resulting in collapse and a reduction in GFR due to back pressure in Bowman's capsule as well as an increase in sodium avidity.

Maladaptive neurohormonal changes are also important in CRS. Given the varying phenotypes of heart failure (Table 29.2), it is important to note that these changes have mostly been studied in individuals with heart failure with reduced ejection fraction, in whom a reduction in cardiac output triggers hemodynamic changes that are sensed via baroreceptors and mechanoreceptors located in critical areas of the vascular tree that include the carotid

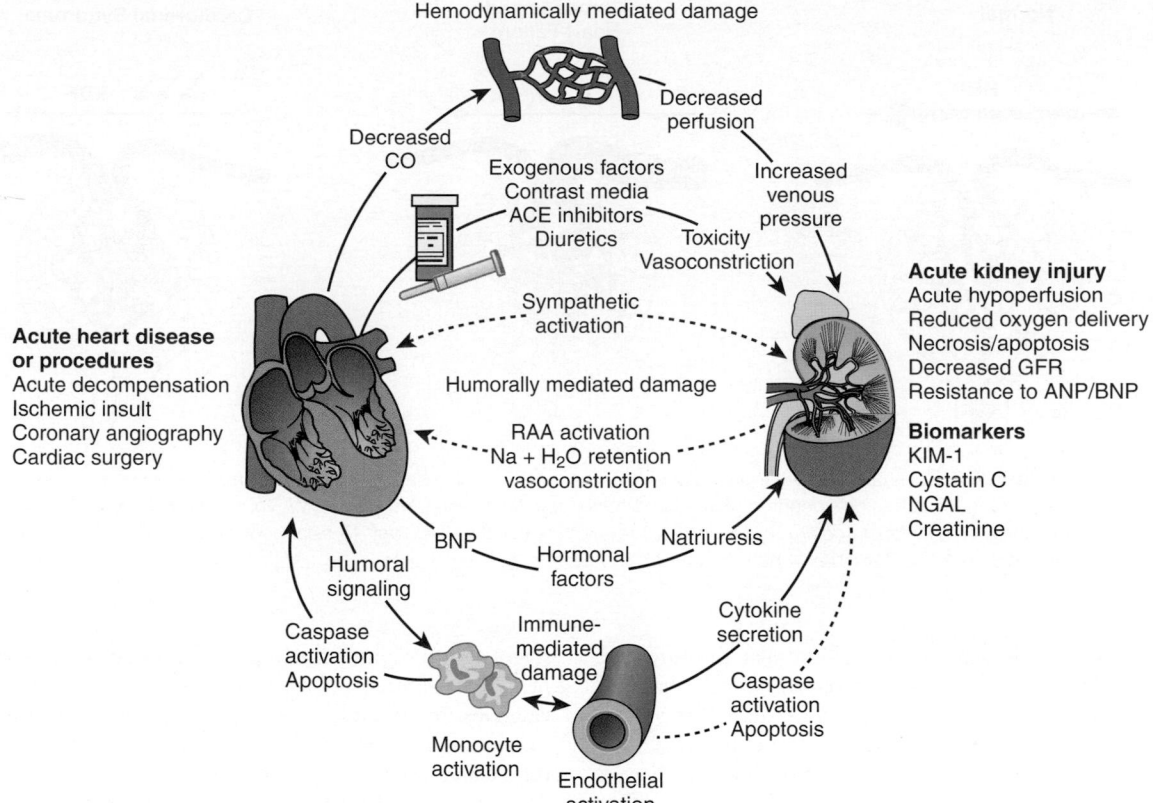

• **Fig. 29.1** Pathophysiologic interactions between the heart and kidney in cardiorenal syndrome. *ACE,* Angiotensin-converting enzyme; *ANP,* atrial natriuretic peptide; *BNP,* B-type natriuretic peptide; *CO,* cardiac output; *GFR,* glomerular filtration rate; *KIM,* kidney injury molecule; *Na,* sodium; *NGAL,* neutrophil gelatinase-associated lipocalin; *RAA,* renin angiotensin aldosterone. (Reproduced from Ronco C, Haapio M, House AA, et al. Cardiorenal syndrome. *J Am Coll Cardiol.* 2008;52:1527–1539, with permission from Elsevier. Original illustration by Rob Flewell.)

TABLE 29.2	Heart Failure Phenotypes: Preserved, Midrange, and Reduced Ejection Fraction		
Type of HF	HFrEF	HFmrEF	HFpEF
Criteria	Symptoms ± signs LV ejection fraction <40%	Symptoms ± signs LV ejection fraction 40%–49% Elevated natriuretic peptides Structural heart disease and/or diastolic dysfunction	Symptoms ± signs LV ejection fraction ≥50% Elevated natriuretic peptides Structural heart disease and/or diastolic dysfunction

HF, Heart failure; *HFmrEF,* heart failure with midrange ejection fraction; *HFpEF,* heart failure with preserved ejection fraction; *HFrEF,* heart failure with reduced ejection fraction; *LV,* left ventricle.
Adapted from the European Society of Cardiology; Heart Failure Association of the ESC (HFA); et al. ESC guidelines for the diagnosis and treatment of acute and chronic heart failure 2016. *Eur Heart J.* 2016;37:2129–2200.

sinus, aortic arch, afferent glomerulus, and the superior and inferior vena cava. Triggers of neurohormonal activation in heart failure with preserved ejection fraction, or whether there is chronic neurohormonal upregulation outside of acute exacerbations, are not as well described. However, it is reasonable to assume that acute exacerbations of heart failure, irrespective of whether there is a reduced or preserved ejection fraction, result in similar neurohormonal changes leading to CRS.

Activation of the sympathetic nervous system, with simultaneous deactivation of the parasympathetic nervous system, leads to increased levels of catecholamines, including norepinephrine and epinephrine. The net effect of this is peripheral vasoconstriction of vascular beds that supply flow to the skin, skeletal muscle, splanchnic organs, and kidneys. As kidney perfusion declines, stimulated renin release within the kidney leads to upregulation of the renin-angiotensin-aldosterone system (RAAS). Elevations in systemic angiotensin II further contribute to systemic arterial vasoconstriction. In addition, angiotensin II specifically constricts the peri-glomerular arterioles. This vasoconstriction effect is predominant in the efferent arteriole as compared to the afferent

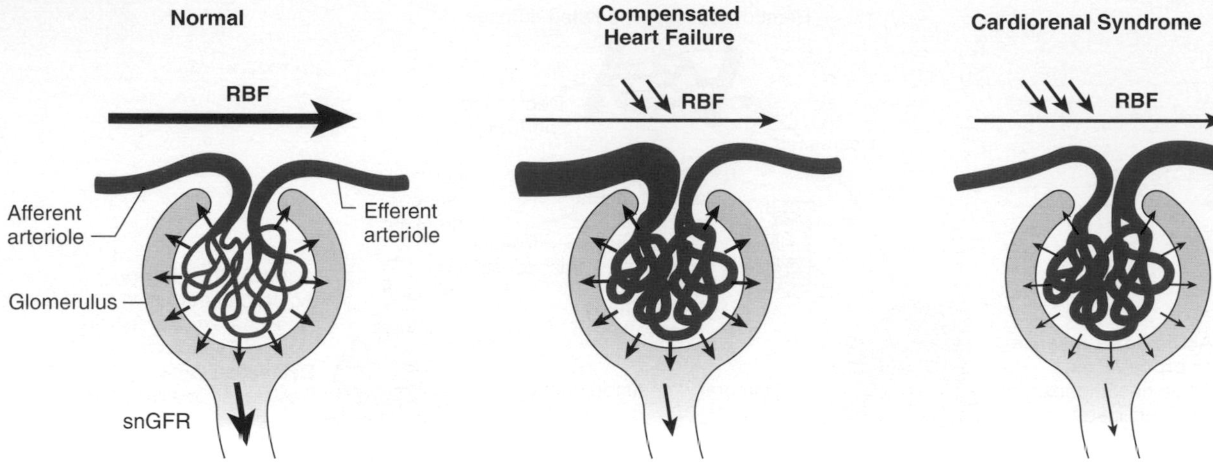

• **Fig. 29.2** Renal autoregulation in various states: normal, compensated heart failure, and cardiorenal syndrome. snGFR: single nephron glomerular filtration rate. (Adapted from Mullens W, Verbrugge FH, Nijst P, Tang WHW. *Renal sodium avidity in heart failure: from pathophysiology to treatment strategies.* Eur Heart J. 2017;38(24):1872–1882.)

arteriole, leading to an increase in intraglomerular pressure and subsequent increase in the filtration fraction. These changes, referred to as *kidney autoregulation* (Fig. 29.2), allow for preservation of GFR in heart failure despite the reduction in kidney blood flow that results from systemic vasoconstriction. However, in more severe degrees of heart failure with CRS, efforts in place to preserve GFR begin to fail. This is likely due to ongoing elevations in systemic vasoconstrictors, notably from the sympathetic nervous system and RAAS, leading to further reductions in kidney blood flow that cannot be compensated for by the previously mentioned kidney autoregulation measures. In addition, in the setting of higher levels of angiotensin II, endothelin, and adenosine, significant vasoconstriction of the afferent arteriole can occur and also contribute to GFR collapse.

Elevated neurohormone levels also lead to significant upregulation of sodium and water retention by the kidney. Angiotensin II directly stimulates sodium reabsorption in the early proximal tubule and mediates the secretion of aldosterone, which enhances sodium reabsorption in cortical collecting tubule. Catecholamines stimulate sodium transport in the proximal tubule and loop of Henle via stimulation of $\alpha 1$-adrenergic receptors, and they also lead to a reduction in postglomerular capillary pressure with increased oncotic pressure, further enhancing proximal tubule sodium reabsorption. Arginine vasopressin (also called *antidiuretic hormone* or *ADH*) release also is increased in heart failure. Elevated levels exacerbate vasoconstriction and lead to free water retention, which can result in hyponatremia in heart failure. Vasopressin also has important synergistic activities on sodium transport in conjunction with neurohormones such as angiotensin II.

Prostaglandins and natriuretic peptides are also increased, and these two classes of molecules work to blunt many of the maladaptive neurohormonal pathways previously listed. There are multiple hormones within the prostaglandin system. The majority of these act as vasodilators within the kidney and their release is stimulated by elevations in angiotensin II, vasopressin, and catecholamines. They act as counterregulatory factors in response to increases in vasoconstrictor peptides. Atrial natriuretic peptide (ANP) and brain natriuretic peptide (BNP) secretions are stimulated by myocardial stretch. Their primary function in the kidney is to increase GFR and inhibit tubular sodium reabsorption. In more severe stages of heart failure, the impact of prostaglandins and natriuretic peptides is blunted and the balanced effect is dominated by that of vasoconstriction and sodium avid pathways. This, in part, is due to enzymes such as neprilysin, which is abundant in the proximal tubule and leads to degradation of natriuretic peptides, rendering them inactive. Therapeutics that inhibit neprilysin have emerged as important new tools for treating heart failure.

Inflammation in the setting of both chronic congestive heart failure and ADHF is increasingly recognized as playing a maladaptive role in disease progression. Inflammatory responses are designed to provide protection and to promote healing in disease states, but, left unchecked, these responses may promote further tissue damage or may prolong injury. Cardiac myocytes, in response to mechanical stretch or ischemia, are capable of producing a broad array of inflammatory cytokines, and elements of the innate immune response may also be upregulated. Furthermore, venous congestion may increase gut absorption of endotoxin, leading to further augmentation of inflammatory responses—whereas venous congestion itself is a stimulus for peripheral synthesis and release of inflammatory mediators. Clinical evidence for this proinflammatory state is derived from observations that patients with severe heart failure experience markedly elevated levels of tumor necrosis factor-α (TNF-α); upregulation of soluble receptors for TNF and a number of interleukins (IL), including IL-1β, IL-18, and IL-6; and upregulation of several cellular adhesion molecules. It is conceivable that these systemic responses to heart failure could contribute to distant organ damage, such as AKI. Virzi and colleagues demonstrated that incubating renal tubular epithelial cells with plasma from patients with acute CRS led to increased expression of proinflammatory cytokines, release of tubular damage markers, and increased apoptosis. The ischemic kidney is capable of producing a postischemic inflammatory state that can induce cardiac apoptosis and, in turn, contribute to ongoing apoptosis and fibrosis in the kidney. The more indolent response to this heightened proinflammatory state almost certainly contributes to CRS. Furthermore, various inflammatory mediators can contribute to vascular endothelial dysfunction and capillary leak, leading to the movement of fluid into the interstitial compartment. Not only does this add to the signs and symptoms of heart failure through worsening pulmonary and peripheral edema, but movement of fluid into the interstitium further contracts the effective circulating volume, and edema within the peritubular interstitium of the kidneys contributes to tubular dysfunction and impaired GFR.

Therapeutic Strategies for Cardiorenal Syndrome

The most evidence-based treatment of CRS is the relief of venous congestion. Numerous observations show a direct correlation between effective measures to reduce volume overload and improved outcomes in patients with CRS. The challenge occurs when first-line therapies, namely, diuretics, either lead to a significant decline in GFR or are ineffective. In these settings, clinicians must decide on adjunctive strategies that have shown mixed results in various clinical trials.

Loop diuretics remain the primary therapy for patients with acute heart failure and venous congestion, including individuals with CRS. Upon admission to the hospital, loop diuretics should be administered by the intravenous route and with a dose uptitration. Doubling the home diuretic dose is typically a reasonable course of action in this setting. Furosemide, torsemide, and bumetanide are the prototypical loop diuretics used in heart failure, and the dose equivalency of these agents is: furosemide 80 mg oral = furosemide 40 mg intravenous = torsemide 20 mg oral = bumetanide 1 mg oral or intravenous. While torsemide and bumetanide both have a high bioavailability rate (> 90%), the bioavailability of furosemide can range from 10%–90% (mean, 50%), which explains the difference in the dose equivalency between oral and intravenous furosemide. The Diuretic Optimization Strategies Evaluation (DOSE) trial found no efficacy difference between bolus versus continuous infusion dosing strategies; therefore, there is not a clear advantage of one treatment course over the other in most patients with CRS. In patients with a GFR less than 30 mL/min/1.73 m² who require high doses of diuretics, bumetanide may be a safer alternative than furosemide as its excretion is minimally impacted by changes in kidney function. Furthermore, reflecting data from animal models, bumetanide is less likely to cause ototoxicity or other side effects.

Patients' responses to the initial diuretic dosing should be closely monitored and titration of the dose should be employed early. Measurement of daily weight and net fluid output are typically used to assess the diuretic response. However, some data suggest that these markers can often be poor surrogates for venous congestion and diuretic effectiveness, and typically they require at least 24 hours to pass before a decision can be made about the need to adjust the dose. This can result in a delay of effective venous decongestion therapy and prolong intensive care unit and overall hospital length of time. Emerging data support the use of cumulative urine sodium output and sodium concentration in the first several hours following a diuretic dose as an effective means to more rapidly determine if a dose titration is warranted, and innovative strategies to more precisely and accurately assess diuretic response are sorely needed.

Poor diuretic effectiveness, or diuretic resistance, is common in CRS. When inadequate diuresis occurs with a loop diuretic, the addition of a thiazide diuretic such as metolazone should be used. Close monitoring of electrolytes is critical when so-called *dual nephron blockade* is employed, especially being diligent about hypokalemia and hypomagnesemia. Traditional dogma has questioned the effective response of thiazides in subjects with GFR below 30 mL/min/1.73 m²; however, newer observations support their use in patients with a severely reduced GFR, especially when co-administered with a loop diuretic. The addition of a mineralocorticoid receptor antagonist can also be employed to increase the natriuretic response in CRS. However, the use of these agents needs to be balanced against the risk for hyperkalemia, especially when co-administered with RAAS blocking agents. Finally, sodium glucose transporter 2 (SGLT2) inhibitors have emerged as important protective therapy in patients with heart failure. Robust data support their use as long-term therapy in patients with stable chronic heart failure with diabetes, and some observations also support their efficacy for enhancing natriuresis in acute CRS. Therefore, they can be considered as additional agents for proximal nephron blockade when severe diuretic resistance is encountered.

Additional therapies that do not specifically inhibit sodium reabsorption in the kidney tubule are also sometimes used for therapy in acute CRS, especially when the previously mentioned therapies fail to achieve adequate natriuresis and/or the GFR significantly declines with those therapies. This includes both pharmacological and non-pharmacological treatments.

In patients with cardiogenic shock, the use of inotropic therapies such as dopamine, milrinone, and dobutamine should be considered. With that said, the routine use of these agents in patients with CRS, especially in the absence of cardiogenic shock, is not recommended. Specific attention has been given to dopamine, as smaller observational studies have shown a kidney-protective effect of low-dose dopamine as it inhibits renal dopaminergic receptors and results in renal vasodilation and increased renal blood flow. However, two larger randomized control trials, the Renal Optimization Strategies Evaluation (ROSE) Trial and the Dopamine in Acute Heart Failure (DAD-HF), did not demonstrate a benefit from dopamine in natriuresis or kidney end points in patients hospitalized with acute heart failure. An important caveat while interpreting ROSE and DAD-HF is that these were not trials of cardio-renal or diuretic-resistant patients. Thus, in some scenarios, low-dose dopamine may be worthwhile to try in patients with acute CRS not responding to first-line efforts for venous decongestion, but it is difficult to predict who will benefit from this therapy and who will not. Neseritide, a recombinant natriuretic peptide, was also investigated in the ROSE trial as well as in the Acute Study of Clinical Effectiveness of Neseritide and Decompensated Heart Failure (ASCEND-HF) trial. Despite having venous and arterial vasodilatory properties as well as purported natriuretic effects, there was no benefit found in cardiorenal end points in ROSE nor in acute heart failure end points in ASCEND-HF. This agent is, therefore, not recommended for use in CRS.

The use of hypertonic saline in combination with high-dose loop diuretics showed promise in several small-scale studies. This strategy is controversial given the traditional viewpoint that sodium excess drives morbidity and mortality in patients with acute heart failure. However, improvements in loop diuretic response and creatinine have consistently been noted in these studies, including a recent retrospective study in a US population. These positive results need further validation in better-designed studies to identify which patients are most likely to benefit from this therapy, but an important takeaway from the currently published data is the lack of reported harmful effects from hypertonic saline administration to patients with CRS. This challenges the previously mentioned assumptions that sodium infusion is an absolute contraindication in the heart failure population. Speculation about mechanisms that involve effects on non-osmotic sodium stores within the soft tissue have been suggested as to how this therapy may be effective, but a firm understanding of the physiologic actions involved with this potential therapy are yet to be elucidated. Currently, some clinicians do use hypertonic saline with high-dose loop diuretics in patients with severe CRS when other reasonable treatment options have been exhausted, but more studies are needed before wider adoption is seen.

There is significant interest in non-pharmacological therapies for cardiorenal syndrome. Most prominent have been investigations of ultrafiltration for acute CRS. While earlier studies showed positive outcomes with ultrafiltration, the Cardiorenal Rescue Study in Acute Decompensated Heart Failure (CARESS-HF) trial failed to demonstrate a benefit of ultrafiltration when compared to aggressively stepped pharmacologic diuretic therapy. Ultrafiltration is often considered a last resort in patients with few options for additional medical therapy; however, prognosis for kidney improvement and overall mortality is quite poor in this population. Peritoneal dialysis is favored by some clinicians for treatment of patients with CRS, especially when preceded with frequent hospitalizations for acute heart failure. Intermittent therapy with overnight icodextrin in conjunction with diuretics is a plausible treatment regimen, and often these patients still have moderate residual kidney function with a GFR higher than what is typical when most other patients are initiated on kidney replacement therapy. The innovative use of intermittent therapy with zero sodium dialysate solutions has also recently been studied and offers promise as a future therapy. Additional mechanical therapies are currently being studied and may offer new treatment options in years to come. This includes a device that intermittently occludes the superior vena cava to reduce cardiac-filling pressures, an infrarenal inferior vena cava catheter that modulates venous flow and renal venous congestion, as well as a biofeedback system designed to modulate infusion of a sodium-containing solution and high-dose loop diuretic based on urine output in order to maximize sodium excretion and diuretic effect. These therapies remain in preliminary phases of investigation.

Summary

Cardiorenal syndrome is a complex disease process that involves simultaneous heart and kidney dysfunction. In patients hospitalized for exacerbations of heart failure, the occurrence of acute CRS complicates therapies aimed at venous decongestion and often requires innovative strategies. Emerging data have added to our understanding of the pathophysiology of this disorder, and no longer is CRS thought to solely be driven by changes in arterial kidney prefusion, but, rather, it is a result of multifactorial insults involving venous congestion with kidney venous hypertension, neurohormonal dysregulation with impairment of autoregulation, and abnormalities of the immune system leading to direct tissue injury. Treatment strategies aimed at reducing venous congestion remain central to obtaining improved outcomes in these patients, and a modest rise in creatinine should not deter these efforts. The use of multiple diuretics with differing sites of action are often warranted and, while more data are needed for adjunctive therapies such as hypertonic saline in combination with high-dose

loop diuretics, the use of inotropic agents, peritoneal dialysis-based therapies, and newer devices, many clinicians are currently employing these as a last resort when other therapies have failed. Additional data and new innovations will hopefully allow for better deployment of treatments in the future.

Bibliography

Ahmad T, Jackson K, Rao VS, et al. Worsening renal function in patients with acute heart failure undergoing aggressive diuresis is not associated with tubular injury. *Circulation.* 2018;137(19):2016–2028.

Bart BA, Goldsmith SR, Lee KL, et al. Ultrafiltration in decompensated heart failure with cardiorenal syndrome. *N Engl J Med.* 2012;367(24):2296–2304.

Chen HH, Anstrom KJ, Givertz MM, et al. Low-dose dopamine or low-dose nesiritide in acute heart failure with renal dysfunction: the ROSE acute heart failure randomized trial. *JAMA.* 2013;310(23):2533–2543.

Di Lullo L, Reeves PB, Bellasi A, Ronco C. Cardiorenal syndrome in acute kidney injury. *Semin Nephrol.* 2019;39(1):31–40.

Felker GM, Ellison DH, Mullens W, Cox ZL, Testani JM. Diuretic therapy for patients with heart failure: JACC State-of-the-art review. *J Am Coll Cardiol.* 2020;75(10):1178–1195.

Felker GM, Lee KL, Bull DA, et al. Diuretic strategies in patients with acute decompensated heart failure. *N Engl J Med.* 2011;364(9):797–805.

Gandhi S, Mosleh W, Myers RB. Hypertonic saline with furosemide for the treatment of acute congestive heart failure: a systematic review and meta-analysis. *Int J Cardiol.* 2014;173(2):139–145. doi:10.1016/j.ijcard.2014.03.020. Epub 2014 Mar 14. PMID: 24679680.

Hanberg JS, Sury K, Wilson FP, et al. Reduced Cardiac Index Is Not the Dominant Driver of Renal Dysfunction in Heart Failure. *J Am Coll Cardiol.* 2016;67(19):2199–2208.

House AA, Wanner C, Sarnak MJ, et al. Heart failure in chronic kidney disease: conclusions from a Kidney Disease: Improving Global Outcomes (KDIGO) Controversies Conference. *Kidney Int.* 2019;95(6):1304–1317. doi:10.1016/j.kint.2019.02.022. Epub 2019 Apr 30. PMID: 31053387.

Mullens W, Abrahams Z, Francis GS, et al. Importance of venous congestion for worsening of renal function in advanced decompensated heart failure. *J Am Coll Cardiol.* 2009;53(7):589–596.

Mullens W, Damman K, Testani JM, et al. Evaluation of kidney function throughout the heart failure trajectory - a position statement from the Heart Failure Association of the European Society of Cardiology. *Eur J Heart Fail.* 2020;22(4):584–603.

Mullens W, Verbrugge FH, Nijst P, Tang WHW. Renal sodium avidity in heart failure: from pathophysiology to treatment strategies. *Eur Heart J.* 2017;38(24):1872–1882.

Rangaswami J, Bhalla V, Blair JEA, et al. Cardiorenal syndrome: classification, pathophysiology, diagnosis, and treatment strategies: a scientific statement from the American Heart Association. *Circulation.* 2019;139(16):e840–e878.

Tang WHW, Kiang A. Acute cardiorenal syndrome in heart failure: from dogmas to advances. *Curr Cardiol Rep.* 2020;22(11):143.

Virzì GM, de Cal M, Day S, et al. Pro-apoptotic effects of plasma from patients with cardiorenal syndrome on human tubular cells. *Am J Nephrol.* 2015;41(6):474–484. doi:10.1159/000438459. Epub 2015 Jul 25. PMID: 26228789.

Zelniker TA, Braunwald E. Clinical benefit of cardiorenal effects of sodium-glucose cotransporter 2 inhibitors: JACC State-of-the-art review. *J Am Coll Cardiol.* 2020;75(4):435–447.

30

Liver Disease, Acute Kidney Dysfunction, and the Hepatorenal Syndrome

ARNALDO LOPEZ-RUIZ, JUAN CARLOS Q. VELEZ, LUIS A. JUNCOS

Systemic homeostasis is normally maintained by a neurohumoral communication-feedback loop between major organs. Any dysregulation of this organ cross talk can contribute to organ dysfunction during times of illness; that is, injury to one organ can have direct or indirect (via medical therapies) deleterious repercussions on the other. There are few circumstances in which this link is as extensive as it is between the kidneys and liver (Table 30.1). These organs can be concurrently affected through two main mechanisms. First, systemic factors, including toxins, genetic ailments, or infections, can concomitantly affect the liver and the kidneys, such that kidney dysfunction is secondary to the systemic disorder and not due to liver disease. Second, the kidney dysfunction may be driven by the presence of liver disease/cirrhosis, reflecting an abnormal neurohumoral feedback loop causing systemic vasodilation with renal vasoconstriction in individuals with advancing cirrhosis. This decrease in effective arterial blood volume is often exacerbated by volume depletion due to gastrointestinal bleeding, therapies that promote gastrointestinal or urinary volume losses (e.g., lactulose and diuretics), and large volume paracentesis (LVP). Moreover, these individuals are often exposed to nephrotoxic antibiotics to treat infections, including spontaneous bacterial peritonitis (SBP).

Along with the heightened risk of common forms of acute kidney injury (AKI), cirrhosis is also linked to progressive kidney dysfunction that culminates in a specific form of prerenal AKI that does not respond to volume expansion, the hepatorenal syndrome (HRS). An association between the presence of ascites and kidney failure was first described in 1863. Later studies found that this form of severe kidney failure was associated with little to no histological abnormalities, suggesting HRS is a functional disorder and may be potentially reversible. Subsequent studies demonstrated that the marked alterations in kidney perfusion and function can be reversed by transplanting the kidneys into non-cirrhotic patients or curing the liver disease via liver transplantation, further supporting the notion that HRS is reversible. Two clinical patterns of HRS have been described: an acute form (type 1 HRS, HRS-1, or AKI-HRS), characterized by rapid decline in kidney function over less than 2 weeks, and a chronic form (type 2 HRS, HRS-2, or CKD-HRS), with a more insidious onset, progressing slowly over weeks to months.

Despite the potential reversibility, HRS is associated with a high mortality rate. Even after resolution of the AKI episode, cirrhotic patients who developed AKI have worse survival compared to those who did not. Among HRS-1 patients requiring hospitalization, mortality approaches 80% in 3 months if untreated, three times higher than seen in individuals with cirrhosis without HRS. While the introduction of vasoconstrictor therapy for HRS treatment and better patient care have improved survival, kidney dysfunction cannot be reversed in many patients, with important prognostic and therapeutic implications. We review the mechanisms that may contribute to AKI in patients with liver disease, and then use these concepts to provide an update to the diagnosis, prevention, and treatment of AKI and HRS.

Pathophysiology of AKI in Liver Disease and HRS

Several mechanisms interact in cirrhosis to increase the risk of AKI (Fig. 30.1). The presence of hepatorenal physiology, defined by the combined effects of cirrhosis-induced circulatory dysfunction and maladaptive kidney perfusion, renders the kidney very susceptible to dysfunction and injury. Moreover, increased exposure to non-hemodynamic factors and other nephrotoxic elements, such as hypovolemia, infections, endogenous toxins, and nephrotoxic medications, not only further increases susceptibility to AKI, but can also directly cause AKI through more common etiologies including perfusion-related AKI and acute tubular injury (ATI). Although perfusion-related AKI and ATI are more common than HRS-1 and differ in their pathogenic mechanisms, AKI in these patients is likely multifactorial, with a considerable overlap in mechanism (Fig. 30.2). Perhaps this explains why fewer than 40% of patients with HRS respond to appropriate vasoconstrictor therapy, and that responsiveness to therapy and recovery of kidney function decreases with the duration of AKI/HRS. Thus, it is imperative that clinicians understand the hemodynamic and non-hemodynamic mechanisms underlying AKI and HRS in each individual patient in order to develop an optimal diagnostic and therapeutic strategy.

Splanchnic Vasodilation and Circulatory Dysfunction

Arterial vasodilatation, the main circulatory derangement leading to hepatorenal physiology, is generated by the following cascade of events. First, damage to the hepatic parenchyma results

TABLE 30.1 Causes of Kidney Disease in Patients with Liver Disease

Diseases Primarily Affecting the Liver

Cirrhosis	AKI-non-HRS	• Hypovolemia-induced AKI • Acute tubular necrosis • Acute interstitial nephritis
	AKI-HRS	• Type 1 HRS
	CKD-HRS	• Type 2 HRS
	Cirrhotic glomerulopathy (e.g., IgA deposition)	
Primary sclerosing cholangitis	Tubulointerstitial nephritis, hyperoxaluria/nephrolithiasis, RTA	
Primary biliary cirrhosis	Tubulointerstitial nephritis, membranous glomerulonephritis, RTA	
Autoimmune hepatitis	Immune-mediated and membranous glomerulonephritis	
NASH	Diabetic nephropathy	

Infectious Diseases

Hepatitis B	Membranous glomerulonephritis, membranoproliferative glomerulonephritis, polyarteritis nodosa
Hepatitis C	Membranoproliferative Glomerulonephritis, cryoglobulinemic glomerulonephritis, membranous glomerulonephritis
Schistosomiasis	Immune-mediated glomerulonephritis, AA amyloidosis
Leishmaniasis	Interstitial nephritis

Systemic Diseases Affecting Both Organs

Hemodynamic shock	Hypovolemic, ischemic, or septic AKI
Amyloidosis	Amyloidosis
Sarcoidosis	Granulomatous tubulointerstitial nephritis, nephrolithiasis, RTA
Sjogren syndrome	Tubulointerstitial nephritis, RTA

Congenital and Hereditary

Polycystic liver disease	Autosomal dominant polycystic kidney disease
Congenital hepatic fibrosis	Autosomal recessive polycystic kidney disease, nephronophthisis
Arteriohepatic dysplasia	Renal dysplasia, tubulointerstitial nephritis,
α1-antitrypsin deficiency	Membranoproliferative glomerulonephritis, anti-GBM disease

Pregnancy-Associated Diseases

Eclampsia	
HELLP syndrome	
Fatty liver of pregnancy	Tubulointerstitial nephritis

Drugs and Toxins (Other Than Alcohol) That Can Cause Combined Liver and Kidney Injury

Acetaminophen toxicity	Antineoplastic agents	Elemental phosphorus
Reye syndrome	Methoxyflurane	Copper
Tetracyclines	Phenytoin	Amatoxins
Allopurinol	Carbon tetrachloride	Arsenic
Methotrexate	Trichloroethylene	Chromium
Rifampin	Chloroform	Barium

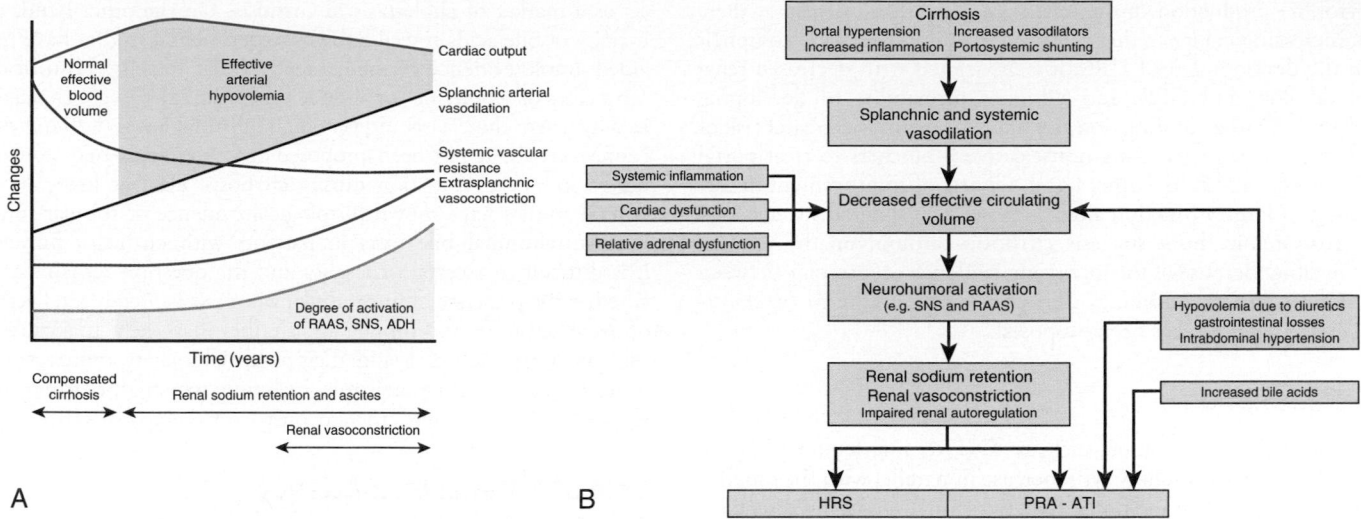

• **Fig. 30.1** (A) Temporal evolution of the hemodynamic, neurohumoral, and renal functional changes occurring in patients with cirrhosis. (B) Summary of the hepatorenal pathophysiologic changes occurring in cirrhosis that predispose to hepatorenal syndrome and acute kidney injury (AKI). (A adapted from Arroyo V, Fernández J. Management of hepatorenal syndrome in patients with cirrhosis. *Nat Rev Nephrol.* 2011;7:517–526.)

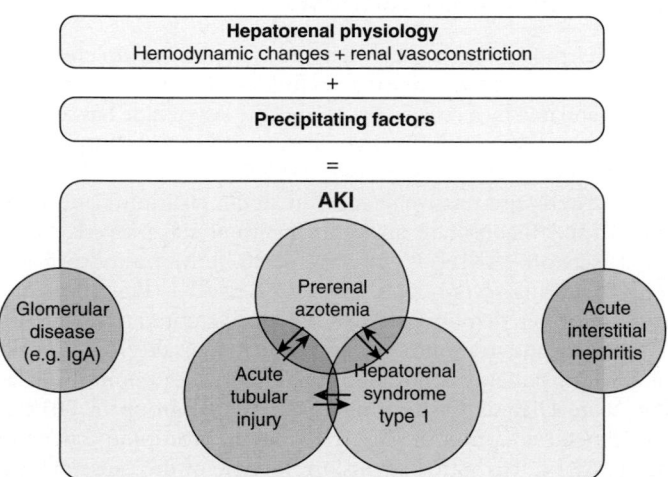

• **Fig. 30.2** Schematic representation of the distinct overlapping pathogenic mechanisms that may be present and contributing to acute kidney injury (AKI) in patients with cirrhosis.

in increased resistance to blood flow through the liver, causing portal hypertension, portosystemic shunting, and increased local production of various vasodilators, particularly nitric oxide (NO). Subsequently, these vasodilators spill over into the splanchnic and systemic circulation, causing arterial vasodilation and decreased effective arterial blood volume. This arterial underfilling triggers activation of the sympathetic nervous system (SNS) and the renin–angiotensin-aldosterone system (RAAS) in an attempt to restore effective circulatory volume and maintain blood pressure. In the pre-ascites phase and in the setting of diuretic-responsive ascites, compensatory increases in heart rate, sodium retention, and cardiac output caused by activation of these systems are sufficient to normalize effective circulating volume and blood pressure. However, elevated levels of angiotensin II, norepinephrine, and other vasoconstrictors, resulting from SNS and RAS activation, provoke vasoconstriction of localized vascular beds, including the

liver, brain, muscle, and the kidney. With worsening severity of underlying liver disease, splanchnic and systemic arterial vasodilation can overwhelm the compensatory capacity, leading to a reduction in blood pressure, potentially compromising tissue and organ perfusion. Indeed, in late-stage cirrhosis (diuretic-resistant ascites and beyond), these compensatory mechanisms fail to maintain an effective circulating volume, and renal vasoconstriction worsens, facilitating the development of HRS.

Kidney Microcirculatory Abnormalities

Activation of the SNS and RAAS is associated with increased angiotensin II, norepinephrine, and other vasoconstrictors (e.g., endothelin, thromboxane, isoprostanes, adenosine), which decrease renal blood flow and shunt perfusion away from the cortex toward the salt-avid juxtamedullary nephrons. Moreover, there is a rightward shift of the autoregulatory curve (indicating lower renal blood flow for any given renal perfusion pressure) and abnormal vascular reactivity; the preglomerular arterioles become less responsive to vasodilators and more responsive to vasoconstrictors. These changes restrict the kidney's capacity to adapt to reductions in perfusion pressure and increase its dependency on renal vasodilators to maintain perfusion. Indeed, there is a compensatory increase in intrarenal vasodilating peptides (e.g., prostaglandin I2 and E2), which may explain the reason why cirrhotics are more susceptible to NSAID-induced AKI.

Cirrhotic Cardiomyopathy

In earlier stages of cirrhosis, the effective circulatory volume and blood pressure are maintained by increased cardiac output. However, as the disease progresses, cardiac output falls due to blunted cardiac responsiveness, impaired diastolic relaxation, and conductance abnormalities. The etiology of cirrhotic cardiomyopathy is unclear but may be related to sympathetic myocardial toxicity (a variant of catecholamine-cardiomyopathy) or increased cytokine production during cirrhosis. Regardless of cause, there is increasing evidence that cirrhotic cardiomyopathy is complicit in the development of HRS; it is associated with decreased renal blood flow and GFR, and a higher probability of developing HRS-1. Cardiac dysfunction might also explain the greater risk of HRS in patients receiving nonselective β-blockers to treat portal hypertension. On the other hand, reports of improvement in cardiac and kidney function after placing a transjugular intrahepatic portosystemic shunt suggests cirrhotic cardiomyopathy may be reversible. Because of the increasing evidence of interplay between the liver, heart, and kidney during cirrhosis, the term *hepatocardiorenal syndrome* has been proposed.

Inflammation

Markers of inflammation such as TNF-α, interleukin-6 (IL-6), and C-reactive protein (CRP) increase in parallel with the progression of liver disease and portal hypertension, even in the absence of clinical evidence of active infection. This inflammation is primarily initiated by translocation of bacteria and/or pathogen-associated molecular patterns from the intestinal lumen and from damage-associated molecular patterns from the injured liver. The subsequent activation of innate host immunity leads to the release of proinflammatory cytokines and oxidative stress, which impair cardiovascular function and exacerbate endothelial dysfunction, thus damaging the function of several organs and directly promoting renal tubular injury. Indeed, elevation of proinflammatory markers can occur with any infection, especially SBP, leading to further deterioration of the circulatory dysfunction and precipitating HRS. This progression is now recognized to be part of a complex syndrome, acute on chronic liver failure (ACLF), characterized by multiorgan failure. Its importance in the pathogenesis of AKI and HRS is further supported by studies showing that gut decontamination with rifaximin improves systemic hemodynamics and kidney function in cirrhotic patients with ascites and that norfloxacin reduces the risk of HRS, independent of SBP prevention.

Intraabdominal Hypertension (IAH)

The main determinant of kidney perfusion is mean arterial pressure (MAP). However, abdominal organ venous outflow pressure (AVOP) can also impact organ perfusion, particularly when MAP is low. AVOP is best represented as the greater of central venous pressure and intraabdominal pressure (IAP). Under normal conditions, IAP ranges from 4–7 mm Hg and has little impact on AVOP; however, if IAP rises, venous pressure in the abdomen increases, resulting in venous congestion and end-organ edema and dysfunction as well as a decrease in abdominal perfusion pressure (the difference between MAP and IAP). Tense ascites increases IAP causing IAH and, thus, may impair kidney perfusion. Accordingly, there are reports of AKI resolution following large volume paracentesis (LVP) to reduce intraabdominal pressure. However, LVP can also worsen circulatory dysfunction and precipitate AKI, especially when intravenous albumin is not given. Thus, when and how to use IAP measurements and reactive LVP remain to be determined.

Kidney Toxicity of Bile Acids

Individuals with cirrhosis have differing degrees of cholestasis and, thus, elevated levels of bilirubin and bile acids. Bilirubin is a powerful antioxidant and considered to be a renoprotective mediator of heme-oxygenase activation. As such, it is often considered to mainly act as a marker of cholestasis in cirrhosis. On the other hand, the toxicity of bile acids is well known. Experimental studies have provided ample evidence of their direct tubular toxicity. Historically, most cases of "cholemic" or "bile acid nephropathy" were characterized by severe cholestasis and very high bilirubin levels (>20 mg/dL). More recently, it has been proposed that bile acids may contribute to kidney dysfunction during cirrhosis, even at lower levels. Several studies have shown histological evidence of tubular injury with intraluminal bile casts in patients with cirrhosis; however, it is difficult to ascertain causality and the question remains as to whether the presence of intratubular bile casts is merely a reflection of decreased GFR and tubular stasis rather than the actual cause of tubular injury. Hence, despite their potential toxicity, more research is needed to determine their role, including why high bilirubin levels predict poor responses to vasoconstrictor therapy in HRS.

Role of Adrenal Insufficiency

Relative adrenal insufficiency (inadequate cortisol production) has been observed in 25%-80% of patients with cirrhosis. Its prevalence is higher in patients with HRS, suggesting a role for adrenal insufficiency in HRS development. Its etiology is not known but may be related to the arterial vasoconstriction affecting the adrenal glands.

Definitions and Diagnosis

AKI in cirrhosis was classically defined as a rise in serum creatinine of 50% to a level ≥1.5 mg/dL, a definition that was arbitrary and never validated by a prospective study. The last decade has seen the development of new AKI criteria that correlate with hospital and out-of-hospital mortality among individuals who develop AKI. These criteria use relative changes in serum creatinine and urine output and incorporate an escalating three-stage severity score [AKI Network (AKIN) Criteria; Table 30.2]. Mortality correlates with increasing severity and progression of AKI (Fig. 30.3), and studies further demonstrate that the AKIN criteria also predict in-hospital and 6-month out-of-hospital mortality in critically ill cirrhotic patients admitted to the intensive care unit. This led the Acute Dialysis Quality Initiative (ADQI) group in 2012 to recommend adoption of the AKIN serum creatinine criteria to define AKI in cirrhotic patients, irrespective of the cause of AKI. HRS-1 was now considered AKI-HRS and HRS-2 was categorized as a form of CKD. In 2015, the International Club of Ascites (ICA) published a new definition for AKI in cirrhosis that aligns with the Kidney Disease Improving Global Outcomes (KDIGO) serum creatinine criteria, a slightly modified version of the AKIN criteria. Their definition of HRS was also modified to incorporate the KDIGO creatinine criteria. While the ICA did not adopt the urine output criteria, worsening oliguria has been reported to be a marker for AKI and associated with adverse outcomes in critically ill cirrhotic patients and should, therefore, be considered as AKI.

One limitation of the above criteria, especially relevant in cirrhotic patients, is the use of serum creatinine as a marker of GFR. Serum creatinine levels, like BUN levels, may be low despite the presence of significant GFR reduction because of the presence of volume overload, poor nutrition, reduced lean body mass, and a low urea generation rate (from the liver failure and low protein intake). Moreover, high bilirubin levels and other substances (to a lesser degree) can interfere with the measurement of serum creatinine. Therefore, there has been increasing efforts at identifying more accurate markers of GFR. Cystatin C is a low-molecular-weight

TABLE 30.2	International Club of Ascites Definitions of Acute Kidney Injury and Hepatorenal Syndrome in Patients with Cirrhosis	
Definition of AKI	sCr increase of ≥0.3 mg/dL (≥26.5 µmol/L) within 48 hr, or sCr increase of ≥50% occurring within 7 days	
Staging of AKI	Stage 1	sCr increase of ≥0.3 mg/dL (26.5 µmol/L), or by 1.5- to 2-fold Stage 1A: sCr increases to a value <1.5 mg/dL Stage 1B: sCr increases to a value ≥1.5 mg/dL
	Stage 2	sCr increase of >2-fold to 3-fold from baseline
	Stage 3	sCr increase of >3-fold from baseline or sCr ≥4.0 mg/dL (353.6 µmol/L) with an acute increase ≥0.3 mg/dL (26.5 µmol/L), or initiation of KRT
Progression of AKI	Progression	Progression of AKI to higher stage and/or need for KRT
	Regression	Regression of AKI to a lower stage
Response to Treatment	No Response	No regression of AKI
	Partial Response	Regression of AKI stage but sCr remains ≥0.3 mg/dL (26.5 µmol/L) above baseline
	Full Response	sCr returns to within 0.3 mg/dL (26.5 µmol/L) of baseline
Diagnostic Criteria for HRS	• Diagnosis of cirrhosis with ascites • Diagnosis of AKI • No response to diuretic withdrawal and plasma volume expansion with albumin • Absence of shock • No current or recent use of nephrotoxic drugs • No macroscopic signs of structural kidney injury	Proteinuria <500 mg/day Hematuria <50 RBCs per HPF Normal kidney ultrasound findings

AKI, Acute kidney injury; *KRT*, kidney replacement therapy.
Preterm includes 29–34 WGA (weeks gestational age).
Modified from Angeli P, Gines P, Wong F, et al. Diagnosis and management of acute kidney injury in patients with cirrhosis: revised consensus recommendations of the International Club of Ascites. *J Hepatol.* 2015;4(62):968–974.

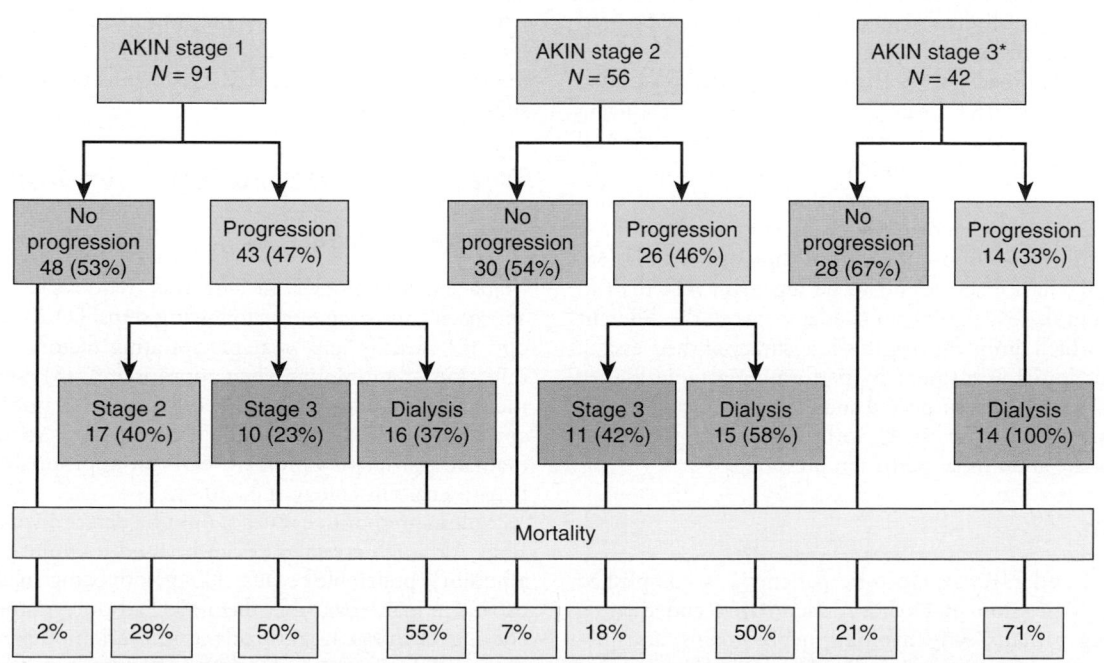

• **Fig. 30.3** Incidence, progression, and prognosis by initial acute kidney injury Network (AKIN) stage. *Three patients were initiated on dialysis on the day of enrollment. Adapted from Belcher JM, Garcia-Tsao G, Sanyal AJ, et al. Association of AKI with mortality and complications in hospitalized patients with cirrhosis. *Hepatology.* 2013;2(57):753–762.

protein that is freely filtered by the glomerulus and subsequently metabolized in the proximal tubules. Its generation and quantification are independent of age, sex, muscle mass, or bilirubin level, which makes it an attractive biomarker to assess kidney function in cirrhosis, but its use requires further validation in this population.

Identifying the cause of AKI in cirrhosis can be challenging. The first step is to identify whether AKI is volume responsive. This is established by the history (e.g., diarrhea, GI bleed, over-diuresis, etc.), physical exam, and other measures of central filling (e.g., point-of-care ultrasound) as well as whether kidney function improves with intravascular volume expansion with 1 to 1.5 g/kg per day of albumin administration in the absence of hypervolemia. Further volume expansion should be guided by the patient's volume status and/or hemodynamic response. We prefer using this tailored approach to volume expansion to ensure the patient has reached optimal intravenous volume expansion. Urinalysis and urine microscopy are mainly helpful to look for alternative causes contributing to AKI. The current ICA criteria call for exclusion of HRS-1 when urine microscopy reveals >50 RBCs per high-power field or proteinuria >500 mg/day. However, care must be taken when applying these criteria because some patients with liver disease may have underlying IgA nephropathy, hepatitis C-associated membranoproliferative glomerulonephritis, or other kidney diseases. Likewise, while the presence of muddy brown casts suggests ATI, whether this is perfusion related cannot be determined by urinalysis. Moreover, care must be taken to avoid confusing muddy brown casts with the bile-stained casts, which can be seen in prerenal AKI and HRS and have a similar appearance. Urinary indices (U_{Na} and FE_{Na}) may help differentiate between inadequate perfusion and ATI; however, more recent studies demonstrate that urinary indices can also be low in patients with ATI and did not differentiate between prerenal and intrinsic causes in cirrhotic patients with AKI. Using more stringent criteria (FE_{Na} <0.1%) or the FE_{Urea} may offer improved diagnostic utility but needs to be further validated and can have significant limitations. Therefore, although urinary indexes are still frequently used in the evaluation of AKI in cirrhosis in clinical practice, they should not be used alone to identify a specific diagnosis.

An attractive approach to differentiating perfusion-related (functional) causes of AKI from ATI could be by measuring biomarkers associated with AKI. Urinary and serum neutrophil gelatinase-associated lipocalin (NGAL), urinary IL-18, kidney injury molecule 1, liver-type fatty acid binding protein, insulin-like growth factor, and tissue inhibitor metalloproteinase have been studied with this purpose. Several of these (NGAL, IL-18, KIM-1, L-FABP) have been found to be higher in ATI than in HRS or PRA, but there is significant overlap between the different causes of AKI, which limits the diagnostic accuracy of these assays. We finalize our initial assessment by performing a rapid kidney ultrasound if obstruction is suspected and measuring bladder pressure in the presence of tense ascites with relative hypotension to ensure appropriate abdominal perfusion pressure.

Prevention

Preventing AKI and HRS in cirrhotic patients is accomplished by inhibiting progression of cirrhosis, identifying and treating decompensating patients early, avoiding nephrotoxins, and preventing events that can exacerbate circulatory dysfunction and precipitate AKI and ACLF.

It is imperative to avoid volume depletion while treating ascites. Thus, a stepwise approach, while monitoring volume loss, is recommended. All patients should follow a low-sodium diet (60–90 mEq/day or 1.5–2 g of salt per day). Spironolactone is added when needed at 50–100 mg/day and increased every 3–5 days as needed up to 400 mg/day. If required, 40–80 mg of furosemide is added, increasing the dose every 2 days up to 160 mg/day. Diuretic dosage should be adjusted to a daily weight loss of ≤500 g/day in patients without peripheral edema and 1 kg/day in patients with peripheral edema. In patients with diuretic resistance, therapeutic paracentesis is indicated but accompanied by an intravenous infusion of albumin (8 g/L of ascites removed) to decrease the incidence of postparacentesis circulatory dysfunction and prevent HRS.

The use of RAAS blockers and nephrotoxic agents, like NSAIDs, aminoglycosides, and radiocontrast media, should be avoided. Beta-blockers, for primary or secondary prophylaxis of variceal bleeding, may reduce MAP and GFR and may increase short-term mortality in patients with cirrhosis. They should be used cautiously in these patients.

Cirrhotic patients with bacterial infections, particularly SBP, bacteremia, and urinary tract infection, are at higher risk of developing HRS. Significant predictive factors for SBP in those who have never developed it include low ascites protein levels (<15 g/L), advanced liver failure (Child-Pugh score ≥9 or MELD score ≥20), increased serum bilirubin (≥3 mg/dL), or impaired kidney function (serum creatinine ≥1.2 mg/dL). Long-term antibiotic therapy with norfloxacin or ciprofloxacin significantly reduces first occurrence of SBP and AKI-HRS in this population. Norfloxacin protects by reducing bacterial translocation and its downstream effects on inflammation, NO generation, and hemodynamics. In confirmed SBP, administration of albumin (1.5 g/kg at diagnosis and 1 g/kg at day 3) in combination with cefotaxime or ceftriaxone may prevent subsequent development of AKI-HRS and improve short-term survival. Patients with severe acute alcoholic hepatitis (Maddrey score >32) may benefit from pentoxifylline due to its inhibitory effect on tumor necrosis factor-α.

Patients with acute gastrointestinal bleeding (esophageal or gastric varices) have a 30%–40% incidence of bacterial infections within 48 hours after admission. Administering prophylactic antibiotics (ceftriaxone or ciprofloxacin) for 7 days to these patients reduces the incidence of AKI-HRS, infections, rebleeding, and, subsequently, mortality.

Treatment of Hepatorenal Syndrome

General Approach

Management of AKI in cirrhosis requires a comprehensive approach consisting of the following steps: (1) Ascertain the etiology, (2) identify and treat precipitating factors (including early initiation of antibiotics when appropriate), (3) assess and correct the patient's volume status, (4) initiate early vasoconstrictor therapy, (5) provide support to the failing systems as needed, and (6) evaluate transplant candidacy early in appropriate patients with hepatorenal physiology (Fig. 30.4).

Volume-responsive states should be determined as early as possible. Although crystalloids can be used for volume resuscitation, albumin is preferable because, along with being an effective plasma expander, it also has other theoretical advantages that may be beneficial in cirrhosis. Its antioxidant, immunomodulator, and detoxification functions may bind and inactivate pathogen-associated molecular patterns (PAMPs), NO, and reactive oxygen species, all of which play a role in the pathogenesis of inflammation and circulatory dysfunction of this disease. Thus, administration of albumin may restore these biological functions in addition to expanding

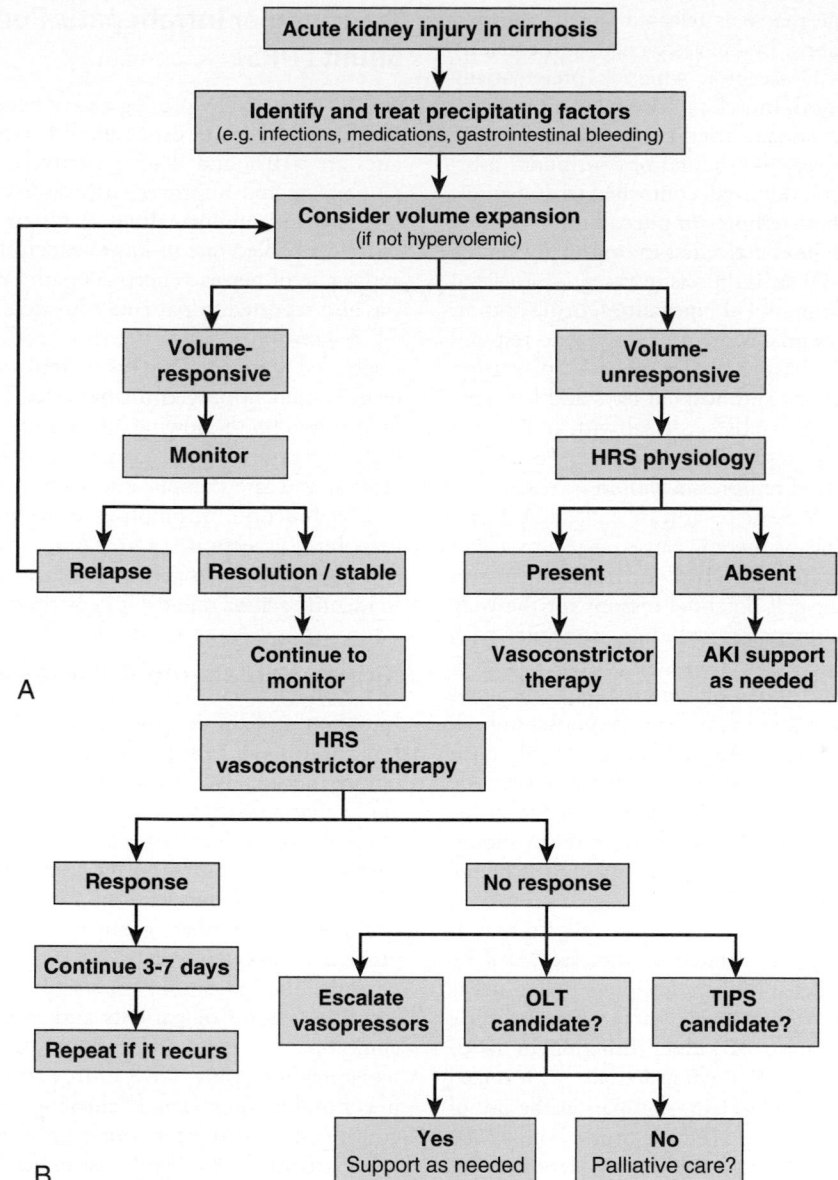

• **Fig. 30.4** (A) Proposed algorithm for the management of acute kidney injury (AKI) in cirrhotic patients based on their volume responsiveness. *Note*: Albumin is the preferred plasma expander (see text). (B) Proposed algorithm for management of vasoconstrictor therapy. Terlipressin is the agent of choice where available. Octreotide and midodrine are usually started where terlipressin is not available. If patients do not respond to octreotide/midodrine, it may be escalated to norepinephrine with a target increase in blood pressure of 15 mm Hg. Albumin should be given to all patients as appropriate.

the plasma volume. Indeed, reversal of hepatic encephalopathy by albumin, but not by colloid, has been reported. Regardless of its mechanism, albumin decreases the incidence of AKI and mortality in SBP (when added to antibiotics) and has been used concurrently in almost all vasoconstrictor trials.

Volume-unresponsive patients with hepatorenal physiology require distinct therapy. The principal treatment strategy in HRS-AKI is to decrease splanchnic vasodilation and increase effective circulating blood volume, to increase cardiac output and MAP. Indeed, studies have shown a strong direct correlation between the magnitude of rise in MAP and the improvement in kidney function during vasoconstrictor therapy, irrespective of the vasoconstrictor used. Because of the profound renal vasoconstriction and impaired microcirculatory function present in AKI-HRS (MAP levels average

70 mm Hg in published studies), targeting a higher MAP than in sepsis may not be unreasonable; achieving MAP of 85–90 mm Hg has been reported to have higher kidney recovery rates, fewer kidney replacement therapy (KRT) requirements, and better short-term and long-term survival. However, optimal targets are not yet known.

Vasoconstrictors

Vasoconstrictor agents in combination with albumin are the cornerstone of HRS therapy. There are three vasoconstrictors currently available for the treatment of HRS: terlipressin, norepinephrine (NE), and the combination of midodrine and octreotide. Of these, the most studied is terlipressin, a vasopressin analogue that is metabolized by exopeptidases to lysine vasopressin. This metabolite has the advantage that it is released slowly, allowing for intermittent bolus injections. Lysine vasopressin subsequently binds to the vasopressin (V1) receptor, which is preferentially expressed in the vascular smooth muscles of the splanchnic circulation, leading to splanchnic vasoconstriction. Terlipressin can be given as a bolus (0.5–1 mg every 4–6 hours) or continuous infusion (2–12 mg/day). Several randomized, controlled trials demonstrated that the combination of terlipressin plus albumin is more effective than albumin alone; its effectiveness in improving kidney function ranged from 25%–70%. Terlipressin was also associated with improvement in neurohumoral abnormalities, urine output, blood pressure, and hyponatremia. Moreover, those who respond to terlipressin and albumin have a better posttransplantation course (e.g., fewer complications and hospital days and less need for dialysis). The median time to HRS reversal with terlipressin is 7 days and all patients who respond do so within 14 days of treatment. Note that the dose of terlipressin should be titrated up if serum creatinine does not decrease by at least 25% after 3 days of treatment. Discontinuation of therapy caused a recurrence of HRS in <20% of patients with AKI-HRS and retreatment was usually effective. There are several potential reasons for the wide variability in efficacy between studies, including stringency with endpoints, timing, and patient selection. For instance, higher serum creatinine, bilirubin, or tubular biomarker levels, HRS precipitated by infections, and lower blood pressure responses were all associated with lower response rates. Adverse effects of terlipressin are diarrhea, abdominal cramps, nausea, and headache. Severe side effects have been described, such as angina, cardiac arrhythmias, intestinal ischemia, and severe hypertension. Terlipressin should be used with utmost caution, if at all, in patients with ischemic heart disease and peripheral vascular disease.

Norepinephrine is a potent α-1 adrenergic agonist that is used as an infusion (0.5–3 µg/hr titrated to increase MAP by ≥10 mm Hg). It is less expensive than terlipressin but needs continuous monitoring in the intensive care unit. An early report found it transiently improved kidney function in 10 of 12 patients. Since then, several small, clinical trials (with mixed population of AKI-HRS and CKD-HRS) comparing the use of terlipressin to continuous infusion of NE have found both agents to be similarly efficacious. While some studies have reported less severe ischemic side effects, others have found similar side effect profiles between the two agents. Because of the small sample sizes and the fact that not all studies have found the vasoconstrictors to be equally efficacious, larger studies are necessary before drawing definitive conclusions.

Midodrine, another α-adrenergic agonist, is metabolized in the liver to the active metabolite desglymidodrine. It is inexpensive, has a favorable side-effect profile, and can be given orally, making it an attractive option for the outpatient management of type-2 HRS patients. When administered as monotherapy to HRS patients, midodrine produced a modest increase in blood pressure but no improvement in kidney function. However, if given with octreotide (a somatostatin analogue) and albumin, it improved kidney function in 40% of patients. It does not appear to be as effective as terlipressin with albumin though, with a head-to-head, randomized, controlled trial finding terlipressin plus albumin significantly more effective at improving kidney function and reducing short-term mortality. Midodrine is started at 5 mg three times daily and increased up to 15 mg three times daily if serum creatinine does not fall by ≥25% on day 3. Octreotide is started at 100 mcg three times daily and can be increased to a maximum of 200 mcg three times daily.

Transjugular Intrahepatic Portosystemic Shunt (TIPS)

A TIPS is created by placing a stent between branches of the portal and hepatic veins. In experienced hands, morbidity and mortality rates are >10% and 2%, respectively. Its insertion reduces portal pressure and improves cirrhosis-associated neurohumoral and hemodynamic abnormalities. A systematic review of nine studies showed a pooled rate of improvement in kidney function of 93% and a rate of hepatic encephalopathy of 46%. Improved survival was also reported in patients who were not transplant candidates. TIPS insertion has also been successful in patients who partially responded to vasoconstrictor therapy; renal blood flow, GFR, and urine output improved further after TIPS. The improvement in kidney function following TIPS is usually delayed by 2–4 weeks. Although generally well tolerated, TIPS is associated with periprocedural and late complications including transient deterioration in liver function, thrombosis or occlusion of the shunt, fistulae, hemolysis, infections, and cardiac decompensation worsening encephalopathy. Altogether, the lack of studies limits our ability to identify a clear role for it in cirrhosis.

Kidney Replacement Therapy (KRT)

Initiation of KRT in patients with HRS remains a contentious topic as it is still commonly viewed only as a bridge to transplantation. Indeed, given the lack of evidence showing a survival benefit, a consensus statement from the ADQI group recommended withholding KRT in HRS-AKI, unless there is an acute reversible component or plan for liver transplantation. However, 28-day mortality in patients with ACLF is better predicted by severity of illness and number of organs failed, rather than the presence of AKI. Consequently, a trial of KRT may be reasonable in select patients. The indications for starting KRT are similar to those in any other group of patients and individualized to the patient's clinical picture. Intermittent hemodialysis and continuous kidney replacement therapy (CKRT) are equally effective in these patients in controlling uremia and achieving target volume balance. However, because of the tenuous hemodynamic status often seen in HRS patients, CKRT may be preferable. A clear indication for CKRT is in patients with fulminant hepatic failure and increased intracranial pressure, as intermittent hemodialysis can worsen intracranial pressure and cause brainstem herniation. Finally, it is important to note that kidney transplant teams often request intraoperative CKRT. Beyond the logistical difficulties, the utility of such a slow therapy is unclear. In most circumstances, any need for intraoperative KRT could have been addressed prior to the surgery. More importantly, the intraoperative electrolyte and volume shifts are such that should they require KRT, intermittent hemodialysis would be better suited to achieve these goals within the time constraints of the surgery.

Peritoneal dialysis (PD) can also be used in cirrhotic patients. It offers several advantages over hemodialysis in that it allows for continuous removal of a fixed amount of ascitic fluid, does not cause acute hemodynamic changes, bleeding and infection rates are low, and it is less expensive. Its main drawback appears to be protein losses, herniation, and fluid leaks. Outcomes of PD patients are similar to those observed in matched PD patients without cirrhosis and perhaps better than those receiving hemodialysis. Patients and families need to be aware of the limited chance of kidney recovery and the high mortality rates associated with HRS, in excess of 90% within 6 months, especially in patients who are not candidates for liver transplantation (LT) or have not responded to vasoconstrictors therapy. The decision to perform KRT must be individualized to avoid futile treatment.

Extracorporeal Liver Support

Extracorporeal liver support systems have been used as a bridge to transplantation or recovery in patients with acute liver failure or ACLF. They remove lipophilic and protein-bound molecules (e.g., bilirubin, bile acids, aromatic amino acids) using either biological (human or animal hepatocytes) or nonbiologic methods. Two nonbiological systems have been tested in humans: the molecular adsorbent recirculating system (MARS) and the fractionated plasma separation and adsorption system (FPSA). Several early studies reported that MARS and FPSA were beneficial in patients with type-1 HRS. However, two randomized control trials showed that, despite some benefit (improved encephalopathy), MARS therapy did not improve survival. A sub-analysis that only included patients with HRS suggested that reversal of HRS tended to be higher in MARS-treated patients. A third trial found that FPSA did not affect overall survival, but a significant improvement was found in patients with MELD scores >30. Thus, while extracorporeal liver support does not appear to improve outcomes in the general HRS/cirrhosis population, it remains to be determined whether it is beneficial in specific patient subtypes.

Liver Transplantation

Orthotopic liver transplantation (OLT) is the definitive treatment for AKI-HRS. It corrects liver dysfunction and portal hypertension. Improvement in blood pressure, RAAS levels, renal vasoconstriction, and sodium excretion all follow. If HRS-AKI was present pre-OLT, its reversal post-OLT is associated with improved 1-year survival (90%) compared to those who do not reverse their AKI (60%). However, normalization of kidney function after OLT occurs in only two-thirds of patients who required pre-OLT KRT. Although several calculators have been developed to predict who will recover kidney function after OLT, this is most accurately predicted by the duration of KRT pre-OLT. In one study of patients on KRT for <30 days, 31–60 days, 61–90 days, and >90 days, the percent of patients who recovered their kidney function was 71%, 56%, 23%, and 11%, respectively. Because of this clear association between the pre-OLT duration of KRT and post-OLT kidney recovery, the United Network for Organ Sharing organization in the United States has recommended that patients with HRS-AKI who have had KRT for more than 8 weeks be considered for a combined liver-kidney transplant (CLKT). European guidelines suggest >30% fibrosis and glomerulosclerosis on biopsy should also receive CLKT (Table 30.3). Other contributing factors to delayed kidney recovery in the post-OLT period include intraoperative hypotension and bleeding (as measured by the number of

TABLE 30.3	Guidelines for Simultaneous Liver-Kidney Transplantation	
Author	**Year**	**Recommendations**
Davies et al.	2007	• Patients with AKI/HRS on dialysis for ≥6 wk • Patients with AKI with kidney biopsy showing fixed kidney damage • Patients with CKD with measured Cl_{Cr} ≤30 mL/min • SLK not recommended in patients with AKI not receiving dialysis
Eason et al.	2008	• Patients with AKI/HRS on dialysis for ≥8 wk • Patients with CKD with GFR ≤30 mL/min • Kidney biopsy showing >30% glomerulosclerosis or 30% fibrosis • Presence of comorbid conditions such as diabetes, hypertension, older age (>65), other preexisting kidney disease; proteinuria, kidney size, and duration of elevated S_{Cr} were also recommended criteria

Nadim et al.	2012	• Candidates with AKI for ≥4 wk with one of the following:
		  • Stage 3 AKI (i.e., 3-fold increase in S_{Cr} from baseline or on KRT)
		  • eGFR ≤35 mL/min/1.73 m² (by the six-variable MDRD Study equation) or
		  • mGFR ≤25 mL/min (by iothalamate clearance)
		• Candidates with CKD with one of the following:
		  • eGFR ≤40 mL/min/1.73 m² (by the six-variable MDRD Study equation) or
		  • mGFR ≤30 mL/min (by iothalamate clearance)
		  • Proteinuria ≥2 g/day
		  • Kidney biopsy showing >30% global glomerulosclerosis or >30% interstitial fibrosis
		  • Metabolic disease

Organ Procurement & Transplantation Network	2017	• AKI for ≥6 consecutive wk with one or both (weekly documentation)
		  • Dialysis
		  • eGFR/CrCl Proteinuria ≤25 mL/min
		• CKD for ≥6 consecutive wk with one or both (weekly documentation)
		  • ESKD
		  • eGFR ≤30 mL/min at the time or after registration on kidney waiting list
		• Metabolic disease
		• Safety net
		  • Patients registered on the kidney waitlist between 60 and 365 days after OLT and are either on dialysis or have an eGFR ≤20 mL/min qualify for increased priority
		  • Documentation required by transplant nephrologist

units of packed red blood cells transfused), need for surgical re-exploration, older donor age, and post-OLT allograft dysfunction. Delaying initiation of calcineurin inhibitor may be beneficial in enhancing kidney recovery following OLT.

Conclusion

AKI is common in patients with hepatic cirrhosis and portends a grim prognosis. HRS is a specific type of AKI that occurs in patients with advanced cirrhosis, ascites, portal hypertension, and hyperdynamic circulation (hepatorenal physiology). The diagnostic criteria for AKI and HRS have recently been modified, but differentiating between HRS and other causes of AKI in cirrhotic patients remains challenging, perhaps because of significant overlap between the entities. Vasoconstrictor therapy is the cornerstone of HRS treatment and can improve outcomes in some patients, but the definitive treatment for severe HRS is liver transplantation.

Complete bibliography is available at Elsevier eBooks for Practicing Clinicians.

Key Bibliography

Allegretti AS, Ortiz G, Wenger J, et al. Prognosis of acute kidney injury and hepatorenal syndrome in patients with cirrhosis: a prospective cohort study. *Int J Nephrol.* 2015;108139:2015.

Angeli P, Gines P, Wong F, et al. Diagnosis and management of acute kidney injury in patients with cirrhosis: revised consensus recommendations of the International Club of Ascites. *J Hepatol.* 2015;4(62):968–974.

Angeli P, Rodriguez E, Piano S, et al. Acute kidney injury and acute-on-chronic liver failure classifications in prognosis assessment of patients with acute decompensation of cirrhosis. *Gut.* 2015;10(64):1616–1622.

Bernardi M, Moreau R, Angeli P, et al. Mechanisms of decompensation and organ failure in cirrhosis: From peripheral arterial vasodilation to systemic inflammation hypothesis. *J Hepatol.* 2015;5(63):1272–1284.

Belcher JM, Sanyal AJ, Peixoto AJ, et al. Kidney biomarkers and differential diagnosis of patients with cirrhosis and acute kidney injury. *Hepatology.* 2014;2(60):622–632.

Cavallin M, Kamath PS, Merli M, et al. Terlipressin plus albumin versus midodrine and octreotide plus albumin in the treatment of hepatorenal syndrome: A randomized trial. *Hepatology.* 2015;2(62):567–574.

Davenport A, Sheikh MF, Lamb E, et al. Acute kidney injury in acute-on-chronic liver failure: where does hepatorenal syndrome fit? *Kidney Int.* 2017;5(92):1058–1070.

European Association for the Study of the Liver. EASL clinical practice guidelines on the management of ascites, spontaneous bacterial peritonitis, and hepatorenal syndrome in cirrhosis. *J Hepatol.* 2010;3(53):397–417.

Garcia-Martinez R, Caraceni P, Bernardi M, et al. Albumin: pathophysiologic basis of its role in the treatment of cirrhosis and its complications. *Hepatology.* 2013;5(58):1836–1846.

Guevara M, Gines P, Bandi JC, et al. Transjugular intrahepatic portosystemic shunt in hepatorenal syndrome: effects on renal function and vasoactive systems. *Hepatology.* 1998;2(28):416–422.

Jalan R, Fernandez J, Wiest R, et al. Bacterial infections in cirrhosis: a position statement based on the EASL Special Conference 2013. *J Hepatol.* 2014;6(60):1310–1324.

Krag A, Bendtsen F, Henriksen JH, et al. Low cardiac output predicts development of hepatorenal syndrome and survival in patients with cirrhosis and ascites. *Gut.* 2010;1(59):105–110.

Martin P, DiMartini A, Feng S, et al. Evaluation for liver transplantation in adults: 2013 practice guideline by the American Association for the Study of Liver Diseases and the American Society of Transplantation. *Hepatology.* 2014;3(59):1144–1165.

Moreau R, Jalan R, Gines P, et al. Acute-on-chronic liver failure is a distinct syndrome that develops in patients with acute decompensation of cirrhosis. *Gastroenterology.* 2013;7(144):1426–1437, 1437.e1421–1429.

Nazar A, Pereira GH, Guevara M, et al. Predictors of response to therapy with terlipressin and albumin in patients with cirrhosis and type 1 hepatorenal syndrome. *Hepatology.* 2010;1(51):219–226.

Sort P, Navasa M, Arroyo V, et al. Effect of intravenous albumin on renal impairment and mortality in patients with cirrhosis and spontaneous bacterial peritonitis. *N Engl J Med.* 1999;6(341):403–409.

Tandon P, James MT, Abraldes JG, et al. Relevance of new definitions to incidence and prognosis of acute kidney injury in hospitalized patients with cirrhosis: a retrospective population-based cohort study. *PLoS One.* 2016;8(11):e0160394.

Thabut D, Massard J, Gangloff A, et al. Model for end-stage liver disease score and systemic inflammatory response are major prognostic factors in patients with cirrhosis and acute functional renal failure. *Hepatology.* 2007;6(46):1872–1882.

Valerio C, Theocharidou E, Davenport A, et al. Human albumin solution for patients with cirrhosis and acute on chronic liver failure: Beyond simple volume expansion. *World J Hepatol.* 2016;7(8):345–354.

Velez JCQ, Therapondos G, Juncos LA. Reappraising the spectrum of AKI and hepatorenal syndrome in patients with cirrhosis. *Nat Rev Nephrol.* 2020;3(16):137–155.

PART 5

Acute Kidney Injury

31

Clinical Approach to the Diagnosis of Acute Kidney Injury

ETIENNE MACEDO, RAVINDRA L. MEHTA

Pathophysiology

The main causes of acute kidney injury (AKI) are associated with decreased kidney perfusion. A decrease in oxygen delivery severe or prolonged enough to impair cellular function can cause tubular or vascular endothelial dysfunction. The mismatch between oxygen delivery and demand is more prominent in certain regions of the kidney because variations in blood flow are characteristic of the kidney circulation. Because the kidneys receive up to 25% of the cardiac output, any decrease in mean arterial pressure may affect kidney perfusion. The most common causes of AKI are severe transitory decline in kidney perfusion, as with hemorrhage, shock, and burns, prolonged moderate decline, as with vomiting, diarrhea, and poor oral intake, impaired cardiac output, decreased vascular resistance, and kidney vasoconstriction.

Acute tubular necrosis (ATN) describes the pathologic result from severe or prolonged hypoperfusion or toxic injury determining lethal injury. However, the most common findings described in AKI—detachment of renal tubular epithelial (RTE) cells from the basement membrane, effacement and loss of the brush border in proximal tubular segments, formation of tubular casts derived from sloughed cells and tubular debris, interstitial edema, and congestion of the peritubular capillaries—are not necessarily present in human biopsy samples. ATN is often focal, with its extent varying according to the severity and duration of the ischemic insult. Sublethal injury that does not incur histologic changes is an important component in AKI, leading to decline in GFR and kidney blood flow that can be rapidly reversed. The extent of the recovery to a sublethal injury is determined by the degree to which cells can restore normal function and promote regeneration. In addition, the degree of glomerular filtration rate (GFR) reduction and these pathologic alterations in AKI are often not correlated, demonstrating the complex interplay of vascular and tubular processes that determine kidney dysfunction in AKI.

The classification of AKI into initiation, extension, maintenance, and recovery phases can be helpful for understanding the interactions of inflammation with tubular and vascular factors in determining the extent of injury. The *initiation* phase occurs when kidney blood flow decreases to a level that results in ATP depletion, or a toxin induces acute cell injury and/or dysfunction. The severity and duration of ischemia or toxic damage define the degree of the endothelial and/or tubular cell dysfunction. During this initiation phase, upregulation of cytokines triggers the inflammatory cascade, further worsening kidney perfusion. In addition, several endothelial mechanisms may affect kidney perfusion, including the regulation of intrinsic vascular constriction and the response to vasoconstrictors or vasodilators. In the *extension* phase, the subsequent necrosis and apoptosis define the extent of injury and fall in GFR. Although the inflammatory cell infiltration can be detected within 24 hours following ischemia and leukocytes may appear within 2 hours, this period is the most favorable phase to allow a therapeutic intervention to contain the amplification of the inflammatory response and prevent further deterioration of kidney function. In the *maintenance* phase, blood flow normalizes, GFR stabilizes, and the process of cell repair, migration, and proliferation initiates. In the following *recovery* phase, cellular differentiation continues and epithelial polarity is reestablished.

It is important to note that the degree of cell injury and dysfunction is heterogeneous in the kidney. While cells in the cortical region can remain viable and able to functionally and structurally recover, cells within the proximal tubule and the thick ascending limb in the outer medulla are more likely to suffer lethal injury. With sublethal injury, disruption of the actin cytoskeleton and loss of polarity lead to tubular back leak and obstruction. In more severe AKI, cell death occurs and can be confirmed by the presence of cellular debris and casts in the urine sediment. Two processes are associated with cell death: *Necrosis* results in a profound inflammatory response as a trigger, while *apoptosis* initiates a regulated program, leading to DNA fragmentation and cytoplasmic condensation without triggering an inflammatory response.

The remarkable efficiency of the reparative process after acute injury is attributable to the capacity of tubular epithelial cells to re-differentiate and restore the functional integrity of the kidney. New techniques of functional genomics and complementary DNA microarray have been able to demonstrate the complex pathways leading to kidney repair. Some of the genes upregulated in the reparative process are involved in cell-cycle regulation, inflammation, cell death regulation, and growth factor or cytokine production. The identification of these genes led to the discovery of early biomarkers of AKI, such as KIM-1, neutrophil gelatinase–associated lipocalin (NGAL), tissue inhibitor of metalloproteinase 2 (TIMP-2), insulin-like growth factor binding protein 7 (IGFBP7), and interleukin 18. In addition to their value for early AKI detection, these new biomarkers may also play a role in the process of injury and/or repair after AKI. The therapeutic application of these and other molecules is currently being extensively investigated and shedding light on future treatment opportunities for this syndrome.

Acute Kidney Injury Definition

Great progress on the definition and classification of AKI took place with the development of the Risk, Injury, Failure, Loss, and End-stage Kidney (RIFLE) classification scheme (Fig. 31.1). Since then, Acute Kidney Injury Network (AKIN) and, more recently,

the Kidney Disease International Global Outcomes (KDIGO) schemes have been widely used in the clinical and research setting. The criteria maintain a 48-hour time interval for absolute changes in creatinine and a 7-day time interval for relative changes in creatinine. The KDIGO group has also proposed a new term, *acute kidney disease* (AKD), to address the problem that changes in

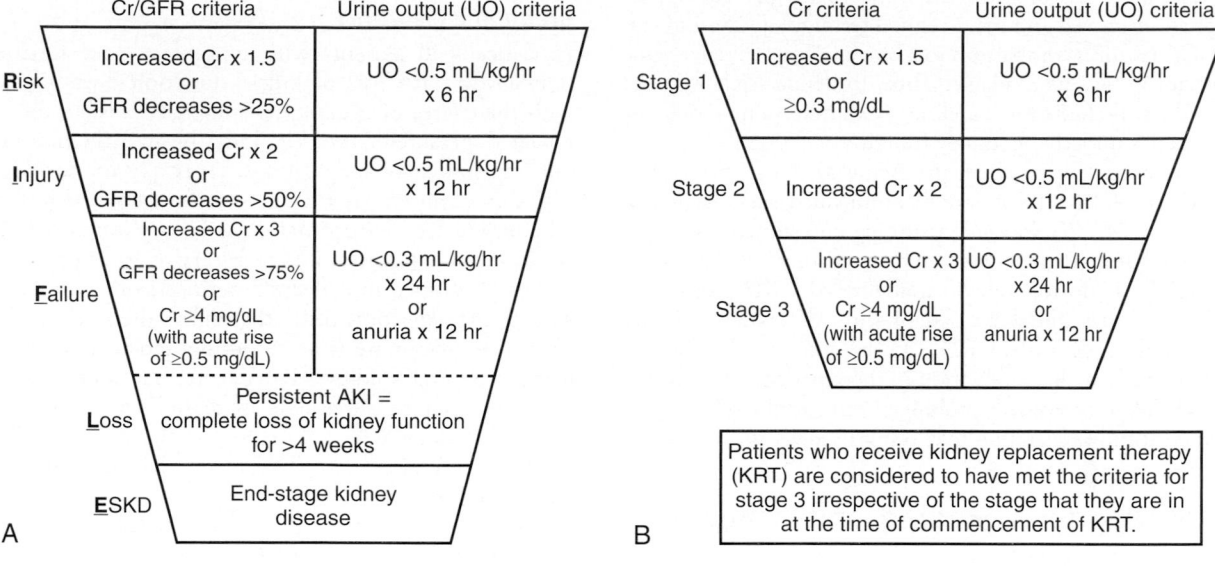

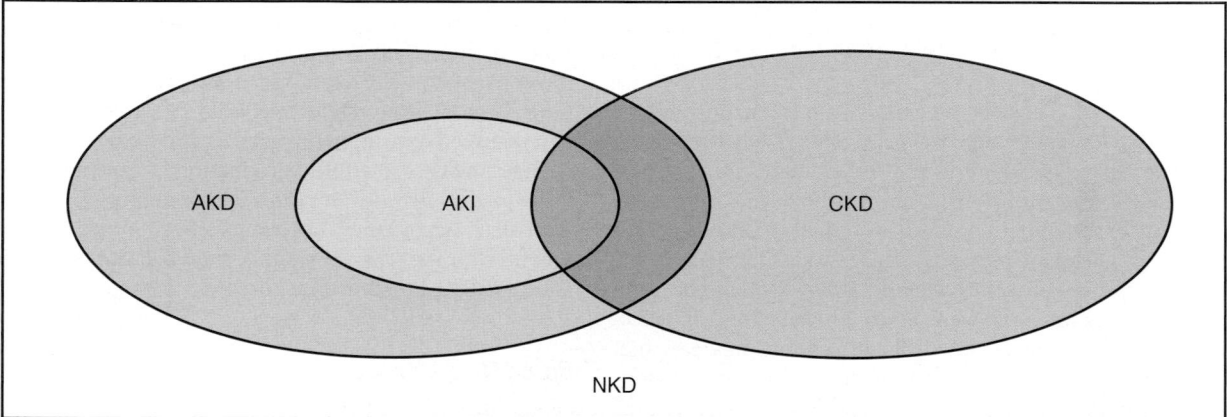

	Functional criteria	Structural criteria
AKI (acute kidney injury)	Increase in SCr by 50% within 7 days, *or* increase in SCr by 0.3 mg/dL within 2 days, *or* oliguria	No criteria
CKD (chronic kidney disease)	GFR <60 for >3 mo	Kidney damage for >3 mo
AKD (acute kidney diseases and disorders)	AKI, or GFR <60 for <3 mo, *or* decrease in GFR by ≥35% *or* increase in SCr by >50% for <3 mo	Kidney damage for <3 mo
NKD (no known kidney disease)	GFR ≥60, stable SCr	No kidney damage

• **Fig. 31.1** Risk, Injury, Failure, Loss, and End-stage Kidney (RIFLE), Acute Kidney Injury Network (AKIN), and Kidney Disease: Improving Global Outcomes (KDIGO) classification systems. (A) Risk, injury, failure, loss, and end-stage kidney. (B) AKIN and KDIGO Classification Systems. The KDIGO definition has modified the serum creatinine criteria for stage 1 (minimum stage for diagnosis) to include an absolute change in serum creatinine of ≥0.3 mg/dL over 48 hours or a relative change of ≥50% over 7 days. (C) Definitions of kidney disease and their overlapping relationship. eGFR does not reflect measured GFR as accurately in AKI as in CKD. *AKD,* Acute kidney disease; *AKI,* acute kidney injury; *CKD,* chronic kidney disease; *Cr,* creatinine; *eGFR,* estimated glomerular filtration rate; *ESKD,* end-stage kidney disease; *GFR,* glomerular filtration rate; *KRT,* kidney replacement therapy; *mGFR,* measured glomerular filtration rate; *NKD,* no known kidney disease; *SCr,* serum creatinine; *UO,* urine output.

creatinine may evolve over periods longer than 7 days and, thus, not meet the AKI definition. AKD can occur with or without other acute or chronic kidney diseases (CKDs) and disorders (see Fig. 31.1C).

Although the use of standardized definitions has greatly improved the current knowledge of AKI, there are still shortcomings with the criteria to define AKI. The definition is still evolving, and the expansion of biomarker use will certainly provide opportunity for an improved and more refined terminology. Serum creatinine (sCr) requires comparison to a baseline or a reference value that may not always be available. Thus, to define AKI, we need two sCr values, including a "baseline" creatinine value representing the patient's underlying kidney function.

In the absence of a baseline, the Acute Dialysis Quality Initiative (ADQI) and KDIGO have recommended *back-calculation of sCr from the MDRD formula*, assuming an estimated GFR of 75mL/min/1.73m². This method can be used when there is no evidence of CKD. Unfortunately, in unidentified CKD, estimating the baseline sCr may mislabel a patient with AKI, when in reality the diagnosis is unidentified CKD. On the other hand, using the minimum sCr during hospitalization in those patients that recover may be helpful. However, in prolonged critical illness or sepsis, decreased creatinine generation may result in lower sCr values.

Tools for Diagnosis, Staging, and Evaluation of Acute Kidney Injury

Standard Lab Tests

Serum Creatinine

Although the use of creatinine to assess kidney function is not ideal, it is widely available, easy to measure, and has been used for more than 80 years. Many factors other than kidney function, such as age, sex, muscle mass, and catabolic rate, influence creatinine concentration. The sCr has a stable concentration, which makes it inadequate to access kidney filtration, a parameter that fluctuates continually. Thus, changes in GFR often correlate poorly with changes in sCr concentration. Three factors influence the sCr concentration: the actual GFR, fluctuations in creatinine production, and fluid balance, affecting the volume of distribution. Furthermore, in patients with normal kidney reserve, sCr may not change, despite acute tubular injury, because of compensatory increases in the function of other nephrons, creating a delay in diagnosis after injury.

In AKI, sCr generation is not equal to filtration and excretion, resulting in retention of creatinine with a rising plasma level. Until the levels of creatinine reach a plateau at a new steady state, usually 24 to 72 hours after a known injury event, sCr can overestimate kidney function. Fluid administration is another common factor delaying AKI diagnosis by sCr, as fluid accumulation increases total body water (TBW), altering the volume of distribution of creatinine and resulting in potential overestimation of kidney function (Fig. 31.2). The masking of AKI severity by volume expansion may be especially problematic in settings where the creatinine is rising relatively slowly because of either lower creatinine generation, as might be expected in the elderly or patients with less muscle mass, or to more modest overall injury. Analysis of the Fluids and Catheters Treatment Trial (FACTT) noted that sCr values corrected for fluid accumulation identified a larger number of patients with AKI who had been misclassified. These patients had outcomes similar to those with AKI.

Standardized creatinine assessments with the isotope dilution mass spectrometry (IDMS) method will improve the comparison across values and will improve agreement between values across centers. However, standardizing the assays has no effect on the individual variation of sCr. Normal sCr is frequently associated with low creatinine clearance (CrCl), especially in critically ill patients.

Creatinine Clearance

In critically ill patients with unstable kidney function in the non-steady state, loss of kidney function does not correspond with the degree of decline in estimated GFR. In those patients, repeated measurement of CrCl may be an early indicator of AKI. For adjustment of medications, especially for toxic, antimicrobial, and chemotherapy drugs, it is fundamental to have a more reliable and accurate estimation of kidney function (Table 31.1). In those circumstances, it is necessary to consider a CrCl, which can be performed in collection periods from 1 to 24 hours. The shorter the collection time, the higher the likelihood for errors caused by inaccurate time recording and incomplete urine collection. Several studies have shown that short duration (1 to 4 hours) CrCl measurements are feasible in the critically ill, and studies have validated the method compared with 24-hour clearance. The use of 4-hour CrCl in the detection of AKI is also a useful method.

Commonly used formulas to estimate GFR are the Cockcroft-Gault and the four-variable Modification of Diet in Renal Disease (MDRD) equations. Particularly in older, underweight, or overweight people, these equations may misrepresent GFR. The CKD Epidemiology Collaboration (EPI) equation performs better in these patients. The Jelliffe equation was developed to estimate GFR in non-steady state conditions; it accounts for the difference between creatinine production and excretion, using the daily changes in sCr. Creatinine production is adjusted for age and for CKD status because creatinine production generally decreases with declining kidney function. The modified Jelliffe equation accounts for the effect of positive fluid balance in variations of sCr and correlates best with measured CrCl.

Blood Urea Nitrogen

Blood urea nitrogen (BUN) is also used to evaluate kidney function, but elevations in BUN level are often, but not always, due to a reduction in GFR. Conditions such as gastrointestinal bleeding, corticosteroid therapy, and high-protein diet enhance urea production and can increase BUN independently of eGFR. In the noncatabolic patient with mildly reduced GFR, daily BUN usually increases less than 10 to 15 mg/dL/day, whereas high catabolic states and high-protein diets are associated with greater urea nitrogen production that can exceed 50 mg/dL.

Blood urea nitrogen concentration is primarily regulated by proximal tubular reabsorption and, thus, highly dependent on urine flow rate. In the presence of decreased effective circulating volume or congestive heart failure, decreased tubular flow increases urea absorption and serum urea concentration. BUN increment will not be proportional to the rise in sCr level and fall in GFR. Normally, the BUN:sCr ratio is about 15:1, with the BUN and sCr increasing by 10 to 15 and 1.0 to 1.5 mg/dL/day, respectively, in the absence of glomerular filtration. Thus, in situations characterized by decreased glomerular perfusion pressure such as heart failure, BUN can increase independently from sCr.

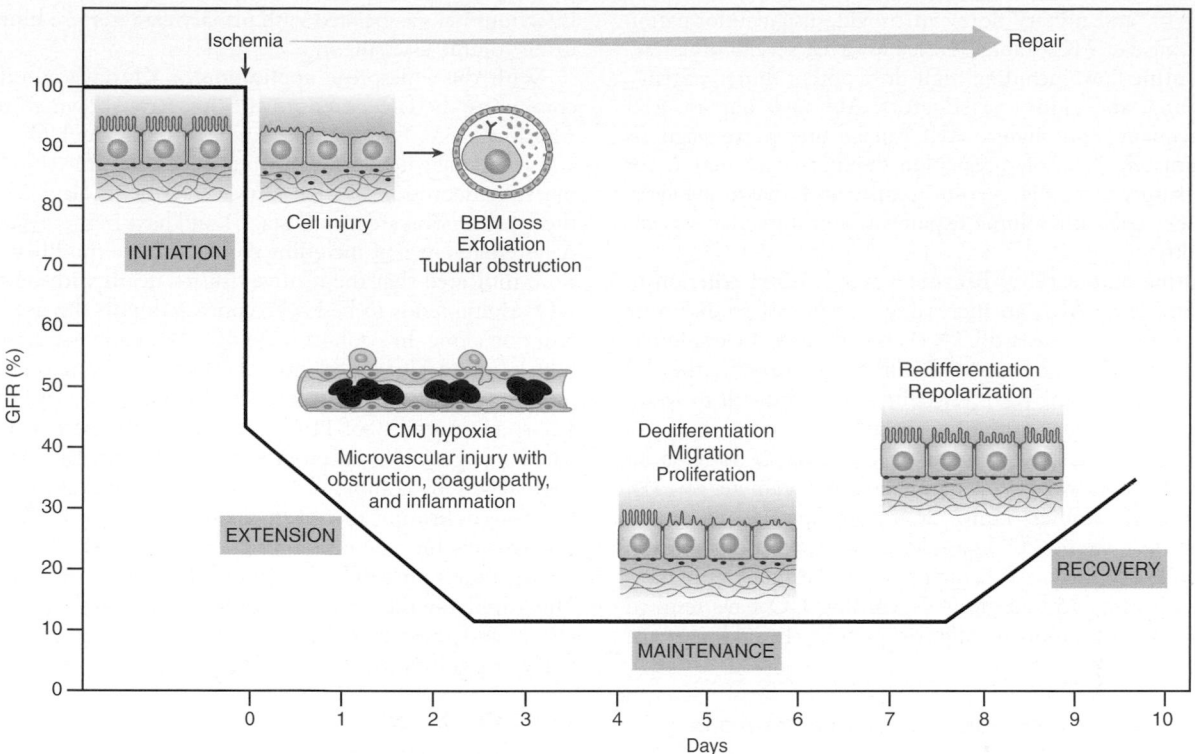

• **Fig. 31.2** Relationship between the clinical phases and the cellular phases of ischemic acute kidney injury (AKI) and the temporal impact on organ function as represented by glomerular filtration rate (GFR). A variety of cellular and vascular events are involved in the development of AKI. The initiation phase occurs when a reduction in kidney blood flow results in cellular injury, particularly the renal tubular epithelial cells, and a decline in GFR. Vascular and inflammatory processes that contribute to further cell injury and further decline in GFR usher in the extension phase. During the maintenance phase, GFR reaches a stable nadir as cellular repair processes are initiated to maintain and reestablish organ integrity. The recovery phase is marked by a return of normal cell and organ function that results in an improvement in GFR. *BBM,* Brush border membrane; *CMJ,* corticomedullary junction. (Data from Basile DP, Anderson MD, Sutton TA. Pathophysiology of acute kidney injury. *Compr Physiol.* 2012;2:1303–1353.)

TABLE 31.1	Clinical Situations Where Assessment of Glomerular Filtration Rate Is Important for Diagnosis and Management of Acute Kidney Injury	
Clinical Decisions	**Change in Level of GFR**	
Diagnosis	Extremes of age (elderly, children)	
	Extremes of body size (obesity, low body mass index <18.5 kg/m²)	
	Severe malnutrition (cirrhosis, end-stage kidney disease, cancer)	
	Grossly abnormal muscle mass (amputation, paralysis, myopathy)	
	High or low intake of creatinine (vegetarian diet, dietary supplements)	
	Pregnancy	
Management	Dose and monitoring for medications cleared by the kidney	
	Determine safety of diagnostic tests or procedures	
	Referral to nephrologists	
	Referral for kidney transplantation	
	Placement of dialysis access	

GFR, Glomerular filtration rate.
Adapted from Stevens LA, Levey AS. Measured GFR as a confirmatory test for estimated GFR. *J Am Soc Nephrol.* 2009;20:2305–2313.

Cystatin C

Cystatin C (CysC) is a low-molecular-weight, 13.36-kDa, non-glycosylated protein, freely filtered by the glomerulus, reabsorbed and metabolized in the proximal tubule, and without tubular or extrarenal secretion. Unlike creatinine, serum CysC levels are not significantly affected by sex, race, or muscle mass. However, concentrations of CysC are affected by age, glucocorticoid excess or supplementation, thyroid disorders, inflammation, cigarette smoking, and some proliferative disorders. As such, CysC is an alternative marker for estimating GFR. In AKI, CysC has potential advantages over sCr as its volume of distribution is one-third of creatinine, thus reaching a new steady state three times faster than creatinine. Despite this potential advantage for earlier recognition of AKI with CysC, there is no clinical evidence of the impact of using this marker on managing AKI. Nevertheless, CysC and sCr have the same limitations associated with positive fluid balance.

Urine Studies

Urine Flow: Oliguria

The normal response of the kidney to decreased effective circulating volume and kidney perfusion is to concentrate the urine and increase sodium reabsorption. As such, AKI associated with ineffective perfusion is often accompanied by urine output less than

0.5 mL/kg/hr, and urinary flow can provide useful information about the cause of AKI (Table 31.2). However, several other factors affect urine flow, including high-dose potent diuretic agents, hypercalcemia, and kidney vasodilators. Although oliguric AKI is more frequent, non-oliguric AKI can be present at diagnosis in approximately 33% of cases. Non-oliguric states may occur following surgery, trauma, nephrotoxins, and rhabdomyolysis, mainly associated with volume expansion and impaired concentrating ability.

Since urine output (UO) became a standardized criterion to diagnose and stage AKI, an increasing number of studies were able to confirm that decreased UO, even without sCr elevation, is a specific marker that correlates with outcomes. However, the UO criterion as stated by the KDIGO definition is difficult to apply. A major barrier is that an accurate hourly UO measurement is difficult to obtain, and assessment of UO over 6- to 12-hour blocks has also been validated as an adequate parameter for AKI in epidemiologic studies. However, for prospective diagnostic and intervention studies, UO should be measured hourly. Thus, non-availability of automatic urine meters and difficulties in measuring, monitoring, and accurately recording UO have resulted in a lack of identification of oliguric periods. In addition, the infectious risks associated with urinary catheter use limit accurate urine volume assessment.

With the widespread application of KDIGO criteria, studies combining the UO criterion with sCr have shown an increase in AKI incidence. For example, studies adding the UO criterion to sCr reveal that up to 80% of intensive care unit (ICU) patients meet the definition of AKI. However, patients classified solely by the UO criterion are mostly stage 1 and have higher recovery rates. A systematic review, including studies using a modified UO criterion, indicated that the relative risk for death with both sCr and UO criteria tends to be lower, compared with the use of the sCr criterion alone. In a cohort of 23,866 AKI patients, those reaching both sCr and UO criteria for AKI had worse outcomes. Patients reaching AKI stage 3 by sCr in the absence of any UO criteria had a hospital mortality of 11.6%, but mortality increased to 38.6% when a stage 1 UO criterion was also present. Patients who met AKI stage 3 by combined criteria had the highest mortality rate, 51.1%, confirming that even small increments in sCr (stage 1) dramatically increase mortality in oliguric patients and emphasizing the importance of both UO and sCr in the assessment of AKI. Thus, applying the AKI classification system without the UO criterion underestimates the incidence and severity of AKI and is likely to significantly delay AKI recognition.

Urine Microscopy

In AKI, urine microscopy traditionally has been used as a tool to discriminate between functional and intrinsic kidney disorders. Cast scoring indices have been developed to standardize the sediment analysis and showed good performance to detect ATN. Lack of RTE cells or granular casts in patients with an initial diagnosis of decreased kidney perfusion is associated with functional AKI, fewer histologic changes, and higher probability of AKI reversal, whereas higher scores are associated with dose-dependent increased risk of delayed recovery and further worsening of kidney function. In a study evaluating urine microscopy and urine NGAL levels in 363 emergency room (ER) patients, of whom 76 (21%) had AKI, the presence of RTE cell, RTE cell cast, or granular cast had high specificity (93.0% to 98.6%) to discriminate AKI versus non-AKI patients. The presence of these elements as a group showed a higher sensitivity (6% to 22%) and good specificity (91%), determining a low negative but high positive predictive value (81.6%). In the same study, urine NGAL at ER admission had a sensitivity of 64.5% and specificity of 64.5% to predict AKI development.

When ATN is present, brownish-pigmented cellular casts and many RTE cells are observed in more than 75% of patients. Sufficient red blood cells to cause microscopic hematuria, especially if dysmorphic, are traditionally thought to result from glomerulonephritis or structural kidney disorders (stones, tumor, infection, or trauma). Red blood cell casts suggest the presence of glomerular or kidney vascular inflammatory disease and, rarely, if ever, occur with ATN. Red blood cell casts, however, can occasionally be seen in acute interstitial nephritis (AIN). The presence of large numbers of polymorphonuclear leukocytes, singly or in clumps, suggests acute pyelonephritis or papillary necrosis.

In AIN, white blood cell casts or eosinophilic casts on Hansel stain of the urine sediment may be diagnostically helpful. Eosinophiluria may be also present in some forms of glomerulonephritis and in atheroembolic kidney disease. However, eosinophiluria is neither sensitive nor specific as a biomarker of AIN. It is possible that novel cytokine biomarkers will be able to differentiate AIN from ATN. In one single-center study, urine TNF-α and

TABLE 31.2	Fractional Excretion of Sodium and Urea in Clinical Studies		
Performance Measure	FE_{Na} (<1% or >3%)		FE_{Urea} (<35%)
Sensitivity			
For perfusion-related azotemia	78%–96%		48%–92%
For perfusion-related azotemia on diuretic	29%–63%		79%–100%
For intrinsic causes	56%–75%		68%–75%
Specificity			
For perfusion-related azotemia	67%–96%		75%–100%
For perfusion-related azotemia on diuretic	81%–82%		33%–91%
For intrinsic causes	78%–100%		48%–98%
Positive Predictive Value			
For perfusion-related azotemia	86%–98%		79%–100%
For perfusion-related azotemia on diuretic	86%–89%		71%–98%
For intrinsic causes	64%–100%		43%–94%
Negative Predictive Value			
For perfusion-related azotemia	60%–86%		43%–83%
For perfusion-related azotemia on diuretic	18%–49%		44%–83%
For intrinsic causes	82%–86%		79%–86%

Although cutoff values differ among studies, in a patient with acute kidney injury, an FE_{Na} lower than 1% suggests a perfusion-related cause, whereas a value higher than 3% suggests an intrinsic cause. Similarly, an FE_{Urea} less than 35% suggests a functional cause of altered kidney function, whereas a value higher than 50% suggests an intrinsic one. The FE_{Na} can be falsely high in patients taking a diuretic; it can be falsely low in a number of intrinsic kidney conditions, such as contrast-induced nephropathy, rhabdomyolysis, and acute glomerulonephritis.

FE_{Na}, Fractional excretion of sodium; FE_{Urea}, fractional excretion of urea.

interleukin-9 were higher in AIN participants than in ATN controls and helped discriminate AIN from ATN (area under curve 0.83 [0.73–0.92]).

The combination of brownish-pigmented granular casts and positive occult blood tests on urine in the absence of hematuria indicates either hemoglobinuria or myoglobinuria. The finding of large numbers of "football-shaped" uric acid crystals in fresh, warm urine may suggest a diagnosis of acute uric acid nephropathy when AKI is present, whereas the finding of large numbers of "back-of-envelope-shaped" oxalic acid crystals suggests ethylene glycol toxicity. Other agents (e.g., indinavir, atazanavir, sulfadiazine, acyclovir, and methotrexate) can also induce AKI with characteristic crystal appearance on urinalysis.

Urinary Chemical Indices

The rationale behind the use of urinary chemical indices is that, following an insult, the proportion of viable cells that maintain enough function to appropriately absorb Na^+ and other electrolytes is a reflection of intact cellular structure and likelihood for recovery. The fractional excretion of sodium estimates the percent of filtered sodium that is excreted in the urine: FE_{Na} = [Urine Na^+/Plasma Na^+]/[Urine creatinine/Plasma creatinine] × 100. It was initially thought to be useful in differentiating between reversible perfusion-related AKI and ATN. However, the relevance of using spot urine chemistries as a diagnostic tool has been questioned, as their values are widely variable, influenced by medications (diuretics, aminoglycosides, contrast), and affected by concomitant diseases (cirrhosis, sepsis). Studies demonstrate conflicting results of these parameters for establishing the underlying pathophysiology of AKI and correlating with its duration (transient vs. persistent). In experimental studies of sepsis, decreasing urine Na^+ and FE_{Na} have been demonstrated in the context of increasing kidney blood flow. In this context, it is inappropriate to consider low urine Na^+ and FE_{Na} as diagnostic of kidney hypoperfusion, and their use to guide fluid therapy is not recommended. Thus, although urinary electrolytes can be a supportive tool in the diagnosis of AKI characterized by oliguria, low effective circulating volume, and avid sodium reabsorption (urine Na^+ <10 mEq/L, and FENa <1%), they should not be used in isolation to determine the AKI etiology.

Although these caveats have reduced routine use of urinary biochemistry, nearly all studies of spot chemistries were performed at a single time point, often relatively late in the course of AKI. The lack of serial data is of fundamental importance because AKI is a dynamic process. For example, in early phases of AKI, kidney tubular function may be intact, while in later phases, cell injury may result in the loss of tubular cell polarity and dysfunction. The ensuing urine chemistries, therefore, are dependent on the AKI phase in which they were obtained. As shown in Table 31.2, the sensitivity, specificity, and predictive value of these tests is variable and influenced by the volume status and prior use of diuretics. The combination of sequential evaluation of these urinary indices, along with the urinalysis and urine sediment assessment, may be more relevant in the differential diagnosis of AKI to determine if structural changes are occurring. Predicting the response to diuretic therapy may be an additional use of urinary biochemistry, as some studies suggested that oliguric patients with AKI have lower values for FE_{Na} and higher values for urine-to-plasma osmolality.

The fractional excretion of uric acid and urea nitrogen have been proposed as an alternative marker to evaluate the degree of tubular injury. Because intact nephrons reabsorb urea nitrogen from the urine, functional changes without nephron damage should inherently have a low FE_{urea}, with a threshold value of less than 35%. With tubular damage, high FE_{urea} (>50%) is expected to parallel changes in FE_{Na}, with the possible advantage of being less affected by diuretic use. However, given the multitude of factors associated with urea production, the FE_{urea} also suffers from poor sensitivity and specificity in AKI evaluation.

Uric acid is another marker that is absorbed by the proximal tubule with the advantage that is not affected by loop or thiazide diuretics. $FE_{Uric\ acid}$ below 12% have been associated with a higher likelihood of rapid recovery, whereas levels above 20% are suggestive of ATN. Over the next few years, we expect that novel urinary and serum biomarkers that detect tubular injury will become a more accurate tool to determine the extent of injury and likelihood for rapid recovery.

Clearance Measurements

As GFR cannot be measured directly, the urinary clearance of a filtration marker is used as a surrogate. Inulin is the ideal marker to assess eGFR, being freely filtered and not absorbed or secreted by the tubule. Thus, inulin clearance is the gold standard for GFR measurement. However, it is expensive and requires continuous infusion with multiple blood sample collections. Clearance of other filtration markers, such as iothalamate, iohexol, and ethylenediaminetetraacetic acid (EDTA), are more accurate than creatinine clearance and are more frequently used in research protocols.

Iothalamate urinary clearance tends to overestimate GFR because of its tubular secretion. Iohexol is inexpensive and widely available but associated with rare adverse reactions. The main limitation is the expense of the high-performance liquid chromatography or mass spectroscopy assay. 51Cr-EDTA clearance underestimates GFR compared with inulin clearance by 5% to 15%, suggesting tubular reabsorption. Diethylenetriamine pentaacetic acid (DTPA), an analog of EDTA that is available for use in the United States, has a shorter half-life (5 hours) that minimizes radiation exposure.

The development of less expensive and simpler assays may increase their utility in patients who need a more accurate estimation of kidney function. Visible fluorescent injectate (VFI) consists of a large 150-kD rhodamine derivative and small 5-kD fluorescein carboxymethylated dextrans and is a promising exogenous biomarker to assess GFR. Recent studies have shown that after a single intravenous injection of VFI, plasma volume and measured GFR can be determined on the basis of the pharmacokinetics of the rhodamine derivative and the fluorescein carboxymethylated dextrans, respectively. Further studies are needed to validate the assessment in patients with CKD and in those with very large body weights. The advantage is that the fluorescent dyes in VFI will allow for a rapid and frequent read-out, enabling more accurate assessment of kidney function and better assessment of response to therapies during the development phase of AKI.

New Biomarkers

The discovery of early biomarkers of tubular injury allowed acute kidney injury to join other ischemic events, such as acute chest pain syndromes and stroke, to consider interventions based on "windows of opportunity." Earlier detection of tubular injury before the established diagnosis of AKI provides a window to perform supportive and therapeutic interventions. Several promising candidates for early biomarkers for AKI diagnosis have emerged, demonstrating reasonable performance for detecting AKI up to 48 hours before a significant sCr change.

Although the studies with these new biomarkers started more than a decade ago, their clinical use is still limited. Initial studies in a homogenous population showed high diagnostic and prognostic ability, but in heterogeneous populations, in which the time of kidney injury was poorly defined, their performance to improve clinical evaluation and AKI management was questioned. Other factors have prevented the widespread clinical use of biomarkers for AKI. The influence of inflammatory states such as sepsis, underlying kidney function, and sex imposes a challenge in determining meaningful thresholds for clinical practice. Furthermore, the pattern of elevation, in situations other than following cardiopulmonary bypass or exposure to iodinated contrast, is not completely understood.

Recent studies using biomarkers to select patients at increased risk for AKI to implement a care bundle to prevent AKI showed a reduction in the frequency and severity of AKI in different populations, including the postoperative period of cardiac and abdominal surgery. These findings may dispel the myth that AKI is inevitable and demonstrate that implementation of care bundles in high-risk patients can improve outcomes.

Kidney Function Reserve

Studies evaluating eGFR have shown that, rather than being a fixed quantity, in reality GFR is variable and responsive to periods of variable demand. Thus, while in captive animals provided with steady nutrition GFR appears invariable, the same animals in the wild vary their GFR in response to variable protein intake. This led to the development of the concept of kidney functional reserve (KFR). The *KFR* refers to the number of nephrons initially inactive that are available for increased filtration in higher demand states. It can be measured by the increment in GFR in response to either a protein meal, amino acid infusion (especially glycine and arginine), or dopamine infusion. Studies have demonstrated that as GFR decreases in the course of CKD, so does the magnitude of reserve. AKI studies demonstrate increased susceptibility to acute ischemia in patients with lower KFR.

Loss of KFR as a new, early, subclinical measure of kidney injury has been investigated. Clearly, patients with decreased KFR would more readily experience an increase in serum filtration markers such as creatinine, compared with patients with a larger reserve. Moreover, KFR has been shown to be activated in critical care situations, when 24-hour creatinine clearances may be as high as 170 mL/min for many days in patients on ventilators and on vasopressors ("augmented kidney clearance").

Recently, a reduced KFR in the preoperative period was the more sensitive predictor of post-AKI injury. In a 3-month follow-up of postsurgery patients stratified by postoperative AKI and cell-cycle arrest (CCA) biomarkers with apparently normal kidney GFR, AKI patients displayed a significant decrease in KFR with a high oral protein load from 14.4 (interquartile range [IQR] 9.5–24.3) to 9.1 (IQR 7.1 to 12.5) mL/min/1.73 m²; $P < 0.001$. Patients without AKI but with positive postoperative CCA biomarkers also experienced a similar decrease of KFR from 26.7 (IQR 22.9–31.5) to 19.7 (IQR 15.8–22.8) mL/min/1.73 m²; $P < 0.001$. In contrast, patients with neither clinical AKI nor positive biomarkers had no such decrease of KFR. Finally, of the three patients who developed new CKD, two sustained AKI and one had positive CCA biomarkers but without AKI. AKI or elevated postoperative CCA biomarkers were associated with decreased KFR at 3 months despite normalization of serum creatinine. Larger prospective studies to validate the use of KFR to assess kidney recovery in combination with biochemical biomarkers may be warranted.

Imaging

Ultrasonographic evaluation of the kidney can also assist in the diagnosis of AKI. Ultrasound is an excellent modality for structural imaging of kidney parenchyma, size, scarring, calcification, and kidney cysts. Small kidney size strongly supports a diagnosis of CKD, helping to differentiate acute from chronic kidney injury. Cortical echogenicity can be assessed, with a hyperechoic cortex (normal cortex is hypoechoic to liver) present in most causes of CKD. In ATN, ultrasound usually shows enlarged kidneys with normal cortical echogenicity and a normal or hypoechoic medulla, primarily due to interstitial edema. Obstructed kidneys are typically normal in size with a dilated pelvicalyceal system. The urine-filled structures appear as anechoic areas with posterior acoustic enhancement. The ureter and kidney collecting system can be dilated without being obstructed, most commonly after previous obstruction with residual changes, normal pregnancy, or as an anatomic variant (enlarged extrarenal pelvis). False negatives can occur in the hyperacute setting if the kidney collecting system has not had time to dilate or if associated with retroperitoneal fibrosis or ureteral encasement.

Doppler ultrasonography is an emerging tool to characterize the likelihood of early AKI recovery because the renal arteries can be evaluated for the resistive index (RI). RI is defined as the systolic velocity minus diastolic velocity divided by systolic velocity ([Vs – Vd]/Vs). Alterations in RI (normal range ≤0.70) have been correlated with the severity of AKI. However, these techniques are operator dependent and have not been widely used.

Direct measurement of GFR with magnetic resonance imaging can be performed shortly after injection of gadolinium-DTPA and gadolinium-DOTA. These are widely available, and immunoassay techniques are easily performed. However, the potential risk of systemic nephrogenic fibrosis in subjects with very low GFR will limit use of these agents. Safer contrast agents may facilitate GFR measurement with MRI, but the logistics of transporting critically ill patients are difficult.

Diffusion-weighted MRI (DW-MRI) without contrast media is a promising tool for detecting microstructural and functional changes of kidney parenchyma before morphologic differences become evident. Novel analysis utilizing an intravoxel incoherent motion (IVIM) model allows measuring the perfusion fraction (f), the pseudodiffusion coefficient (D*), and the diffusion coefficient (D). These analyses evaluate medullary fractional anisotropy diffusion and perfusion pressure to help determine degree of fibrosis and tissue infiltration. Application of these techniques in AKI may assist in assessing the likelihood and timing of complete or partial recovery.

Other techniques to evaluate kidney perfusion are currently under investigation. Evaluating renal artery blood flow may identify perfusion alterations in diseases that change microcirculation. Some pathophysiologic processes may be associated with increased global kidney blood flow despite loss of kidney function. Therefore, correlations between kidney blood flow and GFR are not linear, and techniques evaluating the microcirculatory parameters and regional tissue oxygenation measurement may be more valuable in understanding loss of function in AKI.

Kidney Biopsy

A kidney biopsy is usually considered when the cause of AKI is not obvious, with a prolonged course (>2 to 3 weeks), or when AKI is accompanied by heavy proteinuria and/or persistent hematuria.

In clinical practice, most nephrologists choose to perform a biopsy when they are not confident of the cause of the AKI, or when kidney injury has an obscure etiology. Unfortunately, the lack of effective therapeutic options coupled with the risks of kidney biopsy decreases the likelihood that the clinician will recommend the procedure. The most common minor complications include hematuria, arteriovenous fistulae formation, which is seen in approximately 15% of cases, and perinephric hematomas that occur in 20%–86% of cases, depending on the timing and modality of the postbiopsy imaging. The interventional radiology guidelines consider kidney biopsy in the highest risk category for postprocedure bleeding. Major complications occur in approximately 2%–8% of procedures and include need for a blood transfusion, need for intervention to stop bleeding, and urinary tract obstruction. Major risk factors for bleeding include use of larger biopsy needles, lower prebiopsy hemoglobin, and higher baseline serum creatinine. AKI imposes a twofold to sevenfold increased risk of major bleeding complications over kidney biopsies performed for other indications, because of more frequent concomitant uremia, anemia, lower degree of kidney function at the time of biopsy, and greater likelihood of patient receiving antiplatelet agents due to the relatively urgent nature of the biopsies. The transjugular approach has also enhanced our ability to obtain tissue, particularly in patients who are at high risk for bleeding and cannot be placed in the prone position. The complication rates appear similar to ultrasound-guided percutaneous biopsies.

Nevertheless, a kidney biopsy should be considered when the underlying clinical AKI diagnosis is not consistent with ATN. Patients with an undefined cause of AKI may benefit from identifying a treatable form of AKI with biopsy, such as AIN. In addition, significant discordance between prebiopsy and postbiopsy diagnoses in the setting of AKI exists. In the elderly, the clinical diagnosis was incorrect in 34% of cases biopsied, many of them involving potentially treatable diseases. Among elderly patients with rapidly progressive kidney injury, 71% and 17% were noted to have crescentic glomerulonephritis and AIN, respectively. Prebiopsy and histopathologic diagnoses differed in 15% of patients, and both groups benefited from therapeutic intervention.

These data emphasize the value of the kidney biopsy in the management of AKI of uncertain origin, regardless of the age of the patient. Accurate diagnosis is important to direct appropriate treatment, especially in vasculitis and crescentic GN where delay in diagnosis may affect outcome.

Differential Diagnosis and Evaluation

Widespread use of KDIGO classification for AKI has improved our knowledge of AKI epidemiology and risk factors for nonrecovery. Nevertheless, the current definition does not consider whether AKI refers only to ATN and other parenchymal diseases or includes reversible functional changes. Using elevations of sCr or reduction in UO as criteria, it is not known whether the kidney dysfunction in AKI is reversible, likely including cases of intravascular volume depletion, relative hypotension, compromised cardiac output, and hepatorenal syndrome (Fig. 31.3). Thus, the definition does not differentiate conditions that vary considerably in pathophysiology and includes ATN as well as conditions that are likely to reverse with improved kidney perfusion.

However, there is no agreement on the degree or timing of recovery to establish nonreversibility. In most cases, the response to fluid expansion or hemodynamic support on kidney function is retrospective and frequently evaluated by trial and error. The return of kidney function to the previous baseline within 24 to 72 hours is considered a perfusion-related or reversible condition. Diagnostic

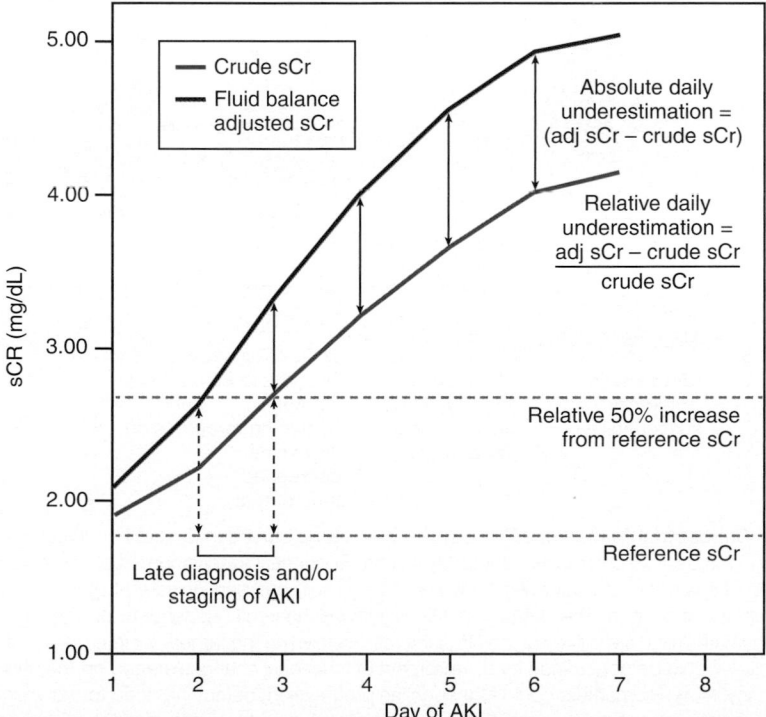

• **Fig. 31.3** Difference between mean crude and adjusted serum creatinine during the follow-up period (late recognition of severity group). *AKI,* Acute kidney injury; *sCr,* serum creatinine. (Data from Macedo E, Bouchard J, Soroko SH, et al. Fluid accumulation, recognition and staging of acute kidney injury in critically-ill patients. *Crit Care.* 2010;14:R82.)

strategies are based on demonstrating a fluid-responsive change in kidney function; however, unnecessary fluid administration and fluid overload are potential complications of this approach. With the availability of new biomarkers of kidney injury, refined paradigms for defining reversible states are emerging (Fig. 31.4). The diagnosis of reversible functional changes requires a consideration of several factors, including preexisting kidney disease, time frame for kidney function changes, and the response to interventions. There are some promising new biomarkers that may be helpful in distinguishing between reversible and established AKI. During the reversible state, persistent vasoconstriction associated with metabolic changes and inflammation promotes the release of cell functional markers that can be detected in the blood and urine. Urinary NGAL levels were evaluated in ER patients, with very little overlap in values in patients with reversible and established AKI. Conversely, sCr values overlapped significantly. However, currently there are no specific markers identifying reversible conditions. Some studies have shown a correlation between urinary biomarker concentration and functional severity. While it is accepted that urinary biomarker concentrations increase with functional reversible injuries, the concentrations differ from patients with established structural damage. It is likely that the clinical application of biomarkers of tubular injury may help to improve the definition and classification of AKI with a more precise delineation of the pathophysiology, site, mechanisms, and severity of injury. In addition, the ability to recognize the various pathophysiologic processes mediating AKI will likely be critical in developing targeted therapies and designing pharmacologic trials.

In the clinical setting, known scenarios are more often associated with reversible AKI. Volume depletion, recent diuretic use, and the presence of decreased kidney blood flow from severe bilateral renal artery stenosis are all contributing factors for perfusion-related AKI. Renin-angiotensin blockade with a resultant decrease in both kidney perfusion pressure and efferent arteriolar vasodilation can precipitously decrease GFR without the presence of kidney injury. About one-third of patients with severe congestive heart failure experience an abrupt rise in sCr concentration following renin-angiotensin blockade. In this setting, the increase in sCr following renin-angiotensin blockade tends to be mild and readily reversible on drug discontinuation. In addition, studies have shown that an eGFR decline of 20% in the setting of initiating renin-angiotensin blockade is not associated with increased risk of mortality in a long term follow up of 1–2 years. Once reversible and obstructive AKI have been excluded, a variety of kidney disorders can lead to a prolonged or sustained AKI. In hospitalized adults, many of these cases are the result of ATN. Three major categories of insults are associated with ATN: prolonged or severe kidney ischemia, nephrotoxins, and pigmenturia (myoglobinuria and hemoglobinuria). ATN is often the result of multiple insults. The most common predisposing factor in the development of ATN is kidney ischemia from a functional or structural reduction in kidney perfusion. Sepsis, and particularly septic shock, has assumed an ever-increasing role as a major predisposing factor in the occurrence of ATN. Nephrotoxins are involved in about 20% of all cases of ATN. Nephrotoxins commonly encountered include aminoglycosides, radiographic contrast materials, NSAIDs, and

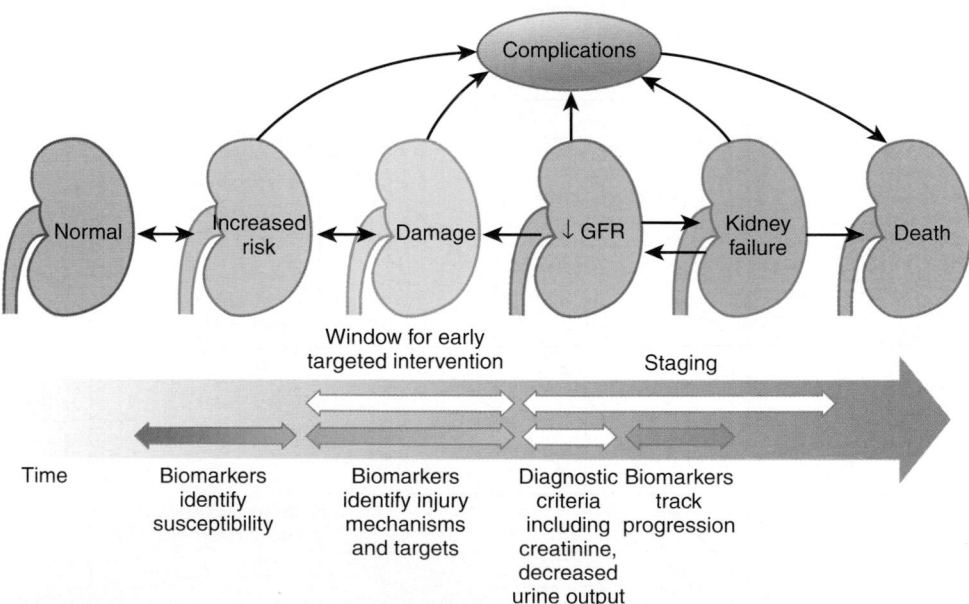

• **Fig. 31.4 Conceptual framework for acute kidney injury.** Surveillance could be initiated for high-risk individuals on the basis of clinical and biomarker criteria. Sequential assessment of biomarkers may permit identification of a window of opportunity in which kidney injury has been initiated but has not progressed to kidney functional change. The duration of this window is inherently dependent on the type and site of injury and the nature and specificity of the biomarkers to determine the targets for intervention. Progression of kidney injury would be determined by development of functional changes staged on the basis of the severity of kidney injury. Biomarkers could further define progression, determine need for additional interventions, and predict prognosis. By combining biomarkers—for example, urine flow (functional change) and neutrophil gelatinase–associated lipocalin (structural damage)—clinicians will have better tools to characterize patients with respect to reversibility and more clearly identify phases of the disease. *GFR,* Glomerular filtration rate. (Modified from Mehta RL. Timed and targeted therapy for acute kidney injury: a glimpse of the future. *Kidney Int.* 2010;77:947–949.)

antineoplastic agents. A high proportion of patients with HIV infection develop drug-induced nephrotoxicity.

Diagnostic Approach

Currently, clinicians classify patients with AKI as perfusion-related (prerenal), intrinsic (intrarenal), or obstructive (postrenal) based on the clinical presentation. However, this approach may be somewhat limiting because there is usually no histopathology to confirm the diagnosis. A revised framework for approaching patients with AKI based on reversibility is noted in Table 31.3. The first step is to establish a patient's prior level of kidney function to determine whether there is de novo AKI or AKI superimposed on CKD. In several instances, information on prior kidney function is not available. Nevertheless, a detailed history including comorbidities, medication use, and prior lab tests should be obtained. Urinary abnormalities such as proteinuria can help identify prior damage. It is preferable to consider sCr values from greater than 3 months earlier to determine whether a patient has CKD. However, baseline sCr is either not available or unknown in many instances. Using a surrogate such as sCr at the time of hospitalization for baseline sCr has a marked effect on the incidence and severity of AKI. Current recommendations are to assess baseline kidney function with an estimating equation. Nevertheless, assuming a normal eGFR in patients with long-standing diabetes or multiple risk factors for CKD are likely to overestimate kidney function and erroneously classify a CKD patient as AKI. Misclassification in AKI diagnosis and severity can ultimately lead to different therapeutic approaches and influence prognosis.

Accurate identification of AKI risk factors for patients is fundamental to achieve early diagnosis and accurate assessment of AKI severity. This is essential to developing approaches for earlier intervention, correcting reversible factors, and mitigating the downstream effects of AKI (Table 31.4). Advanced age, which is often associated with some degree of preexisting kidney disease, is another common risk factor associated with AKI. Administration of potentially nephrotoxic drugs increases the risk of AKI, as seen with the concurrent use of furosemide and intravenous contrast agents. Congestive heart failure, nephrotic syndrome,

TABLE 31.4	Nonmodifiable and Modifiable Risk Factors for Acute Kidney Injury	
Nonmodifiable	**Modifiable**
Chronic kidney disease	Hypertension
Diabetes mellitus	Hypoalbuminemia
Older age	Anemia
Chronic liver disease	Sepsis
Congestive heart failure	Nephrotoxic drugs
Renal artery stenosis	Mechanical ventilation
Peripheral vascular disease	Hypercholesterolemia
AIDS	Rhabdomyolysis
Prior kidney surgery	Hyponatremia

and liver disease are common predisposing conditions associated with AKI due to tenuous effective circulating volume. As shown in Table 31.4, modifiable risk factors can be targets for prevention and intervention.

Knowledge of underlying CKD status and potential risk factors should prompt a search for specific insults for AKI. While AKI associated with one specific cause is common outside the ICU, most patients have several etiologic factors contributing to AKI development. The most common are failure of kidney autoregulation, direct nephrotoxicity, ischemia/reperfusion, and inflammatory states. With multiple factors directly influencing kidney function, the nature and timing of the inciting event are often unknown. If a specific etiology can be identified, such as exposure to contrast agents or nephrotoxic antibiotics, the course can be somewhat predictable. However, clinicians should be vigilant in their search for additional reversible factors that may influence the course, such as volume depletion.

Diagnostic strategies using the established parameters of urinalysis, urine microscopy, urine chemistries, and imaging should be combined with newer biomarkers to better differentiate patients with functional reversible changes from those with structural kidney injury. For example, our current concepts of perfusion-related AKI represent conditions wherein tubular function is intact and restoration of perfusion reverses the kidney dysfunction. Alternatively, structural injury leads to a more protracted course and highlights conditions where biomarkers such as NGAL and KIM1 are elevated. In the reversible conditions, markers would more likely be below thresholds associated with injury, although there may be some overlap. As we begin to use AKI biomarkers, specific combinations will provide better fingerprints to enable clinicians to more optimally assess AKI patients. Once the diagnosis and severity stage have been established, directed interventions can be further designed based on the AKI stage.

Finally, although several individual risk factors are associated with AKI occurrence, the development of risk-stratification scores could better predict AKI in specific patient populations (e.g., after cardiac surgery, contrast exposure, hospital acquired, general surgery, and high-risk surgery). Access to large data sets in electronic health records has contributed to machine learning approaches for identifying phenotypes of patients at risk for AKI. In a large US Veterans Affairs (VA) longitudinal data set of more than 700,000 patients across diverse clinical settings, a model predicted 55.8% of all inpatient episodes of AKI and 90.2% of all dialysis-requiring AKI episodes within 90 days of the initial onset. However, the algorithm generated two false positives for every true alert. In a

TABLE 31.3	Clinical Approach to Acute Kidney Injury

1. Reversible AKI

- Decreased effective kidney perfusion
- Extrarenal obstruction to urine flow

2. Self-Limited AKI

- Acute tubular necrosis
- Acute interstitial nephritis
- Intrarenal obstruction, drugs, uric acid
- Acute glomerulonephritis

3. Irreversible AKI

- Cortical necrosis
- Large vessel occlusion
- Certain nephrotoxins: methoxyflurane
- Microvascular occlusions

AKI, Acute kidney injury.

separate study, a predictive model for AKI development with internal and external validation from three hospital systems and almost 500,000 patients showed an area under the curve as high as 0.92 for AKI and as high as 0.97 for dialysis. However, in both these studies the overall low prevalence of events reduced the positive predictive value, making it difficult for clinical application. Few models have examined the clinical risk factors for AKI among the ICU population, but risk profiling can be used to establish appropriate criteria for surveillance for AKI in hospitalized patients. The use of models to predict the AKI risk can help clinicians identify patients at high risk of developing AKI, perform clinical decisions based on this risk, and provide better patient counseling. A combination of risk assessment, active surveillance, early recognition, rapid response, and targeted intervention can be standardized to optimally manage these patients and improve outcomes.

Thus, as AKI is a common condition that is prevalent in outpatient and inpatient settings, a practical clinical approach to diagnosis is required. Our understanding of the pathophysiology, mechanisms, and pathways has been enhanced in recent years from experimental models and epidemiologic studies. With the availability of new biomarkers, we are now better positioned to approach patients for earlier recognition, active surveillance, and targeted interventions. Strategies for management should focus on identifying reversibility and intervening early to prevent further progression. Several tools are now available to clinicians to manage patients with AKI.

Complete bibliography is available at Elsevier eBooks for Practicing Clinicians.

Key Bibliography

Basile DP, Anderson MD, Sutton TA. Pathophysiology of acute kidney injury. *Compr Physiol.* 2012;2:1303–1353. doi:10.1002/cphy.c110041.

Bouchard J, Macedo E, Soroko S, et al. Comparison of methods for estimating glomerular filtration rate in critically ill patients with acute kidney injury. *Nephrol Dial Transplant.* 2010;25:102–107.

Bragadottir G, Redfors B, Ricksten SE. Assessing glomerular filtration rate (GFR) in critically ill patients with acute kidney injury—true GFR versus urinary creatinine clearance and estimating equations. *Crit Care.* 2013;17:R108.

Gotfried J, Wiesen J, Raina R, Nally JV. Finding the cause of acute kidney injury: which index of fractional excretion is better? *Cleve Clin J Med.* 2012;79:121–126. doi:10.3949/ccjm.79a.11030.

Haase M, Bellomo R, Matalanis G, Calzavacca P, Dragun D, Haase-Fielitz A. A comparison of the RIFLE and Acute Kidney Injury Network classifications for cardiac surgery-associated acute kidney injury: a prospective cohort study. *J Thorac Cardiovasc Surg.* 2009;138:1370–1376. doi:10.1016/j.jtcvs.2009.07.007.

Haase M, Devarajan P, Haase-Fielitz A, et al. The outcome of neutrophil gelatinase-associated lipocalin-positive subclinical acute kidney injury: a multicenter pooled analysis of prospective studies. *J Am Coll Cardiol.* 2011;57:1752–1761.

Hoste EA, Damen J, Vanholder RC, et al. Assessment of renal function in recently admitted critically ill patients with normal serum creatinine. *Nephrol Dial Transplant.* 2005;20:747–753. doi:10.1093/ndt/gfh707.

Hsu RK, McCulloch CE, Dudley RA, Lo LJ, Hsu CY. Temporal changes in incidence of dialysis-requiring AKI. *J Am Soc Nephrol.* 2013;24:37–42.

Kellum JA, Sileanu FE, Murugan R, Lucko N, Shaw AD, Clermont G. Classifying AKI by urine output versus serum creatinine level. *J Am Soc Nephrol.* 2015;26:2231–2238.

Macedo E, Bouchard J, Soroko SH, et al. Fluid accumulation, recognition and staging of acute kidney injury in critically-ill patients. *Crit Care.* 2010;14:R82.

Macedo E, Mehta RL. Measuring renal function in critically ill patients: tools and strategies for assessing glomerular filtration rate. *Curr Opin Crit Care.* 2013;19:560–566.

Mehta RL. Timed and targeted therapy for acute kidney injury: a glimpse of the future. *Kidney Int.* 2010;77:947–949. doi:10.1038/ki.2010.79.

Perazella MA, Coca SG, Hall IE, Iyanam U, Koraishy M, Parikh CR. Urine microscopy is associated with severity and worsening of acute kidney injury in hospitalized patients. *Clin J Am Soc Nephrol.* 2010;5:402–408.

Pickering JW, Frampton CM, Walker RJ, Shaw GM, Endre ZH. Four hour creatinine clearance is better than plasma creatinine for monitoring renal function in critically ill patients. *Crit Care.* 2012;16:R107.

Prowle JR, Kirwan CJ, Bellomo R. Fluid management for the prevention and attenuation of acute kidney injury. *Nat Rev Nephrol.* 2014;10:37–47.

Schneider AG, Goodwin MD, Bellomo R. Measurement of kidney perfusion in critically ill patients. *Crit Care.* 2013;17:220. doi:10.1186/cc12529.

Siew ED, Matheny ME, Ikizler TA, et al. Commonly used surrogates for baseline renal function affect the classification and prognosis of acute kidney injury. *Kidney Int.* 2010;77:536–542.

Siew ED, Ware LB, Gebretsadik T, et al. Urine neutrophil gelatinase-associated lipocalin moderately predicts acute kidney injury in critically ill adults. *J Am Soc Nephrol.* 2009;20:1823–1832.

Stevens LA, Levey AS. Measured GFR as a confirmatory test for estimated GFR. *J Am Soc Nephrol.* 2009;20:2305–2313.

Tangri N, Stevens LA, Schmid CH, et al. Changes in dietary protein intake has no effect on serum cystatin C levels independent of the glomerular filtration rate. *Kidney Int.* 2011;79:471–477.

32

Acute Tubular Injury and Acute Tubular Necrosis

SAMANTHA GUNNING, JAY L. KOYNER

Acute tubular injury (ATI) characterizes damage to renal tubular epithelial cells and is the leading cause of acute kidney injury (AKI) in hospitalized patients. ATI is defined by a sudden decline in kidney function from ischemic or toxic insults and can occur at any epithelial segment along the nephron but is typically most profound in the proximal tubule. Packed with mitochondria and dependent on oxidative phosphorylation, the proximal tubule is particularly vulnerable to injury and ultimately cell death. The term *ATI* has largely replaced the term *acute tubular necrosis* (ATN) as we understand more about pathways of damage to and regeneration of the renal tubular epithelium. Damage can result in necrosis but is often limited to highly susceptible areas such as the outer medullary region largely due to its relative lack of oxygen supply. Damage can also result in cellular repair and apoptosis more broadly within the proximal tubule. This chapter will focus on the major ischemic and nephrotoxic mechanisms of acute tubular injury.

Ischemic Acute Tubular Injury

The renal tubular epithelium becomes susceptible to ischemic injury in pathologic states when autoregulation of blood flow and perfusion pressure to the renal microvasculature is disturbed. Pathologic microvascular ischemia manifests on a continuum between functional changes in glomerular filtration, often referred to as *prerenal injury*, to direct tubular cell injury, often referred to as *intrarenal injury*. The process is often patchy and does not occur in an all-or-none fashion due to normal variations in regional blood flow and differences in energy and oxygen consumption along the nephron. Modern classifications of tubular injury have attempted to move away from the pre-, intra-, and postrenal definitions, instead opting to classify cases based on changes in functional and damage biomarkers of kidney injury.

The point at which microvascular ischemia causes direct cellular injury rather than just functional change in glomerular filtration (as measured by serum creatinine or cystatin C) is incompletely understood. Generally, the more severe the perfusion defect, the greater the injury is at the cellular level. A number of comorbidities, including sepsis, chronic kidney disease (CKD), hypertension, and atherosclerosis, as well as a kidney's reserve capacity to hyper-filter, will lower the threshold at which cellular injury begins to occur. There are numerous causes of renal microvascular ischemia that fall into two general categories. The first is hypotension-induced ischemia, resulting from decreased systemic arterial pressure and subsequent end-organ hypoperfusion. The second is localized obstruction or constriction within the renal vasculature that results in ischemia in downstream tissues. From the second category, this chapter will cover cholesterol atheroembolic kidney disease and kidney infarction.

Hypotension-Induced Ischemia

Causes

Renal microvascular ischemia often results from systemic disorders that cause decreased arterial pressure and subsequent end-organ hypoperfusion. These include septic shock, cardiogenic shock, hypovolemic shock, autonomic dysfunction, and iatrogenic sources.

Septic shock creates a particularly pathologic environment for the kidney. Historically, well-recognized organ dysfunction from hypoperfusion and tissue hypoxia plays an important role. More recently, the role of inflammatory cytokines has been recognized as a critical additional mechanism of injury. The inflammatory milieu is thought to create variation in renal macro- and microcirculation, diffusion limitation, disruption of the endothelial barrier and glycocalyx, and mitochondrial dysfunction, all of which contribute to and perpetuate ATI. While large animal models suggest all of this can occur in the absence of hypotension, clinical correlation in humans is under-investigation. Human sepsis seems to be associated with ischemic and inflammatory injury to the tubular epithelium.

Acute decompensated heart failure creates two cardinal issues that lead to renal microvascular ischemia and tubular injury: significant compromise to renal blood flow and venous congestion. In cardiogenic shock, there is underfilling of the systemic arterial vascular bed, including the kidneys, which leads to pathologic compensatory increases in sympathetic nervous system and renin-angiotensin-aldosterone system activity. This leads to maladaptive renal microvascular vasoconstriction. In states of overt volume overload in the setting of decreased forward flow rather than frank cardiogenic shock, it is venous congestion and related increases in intraabdominal pressure that drive hydraulic alterations in microvascular blood flow that result in ischemic injury.

Hypovolemic shock commonly occurs secondary to significant volume loss in the setting of diuresis, hemorrhage, vomiting, or diarrhea. Markedly reduced oncotic pressure from low albumin states such as cirrhosis, nephrotic syndrome, and protein-losing enteropathies can also result in severe intravascular volume depletion, despite an excess of total body fluid. Signs and symptoms of organ dysfunction do not typically manifest clinically until approximately 20% to 25% of effective arterial blood volume has been removed. Hypotension related to autonomic dysfunction is most commonly seen in the setting of diabetes mellitus; however, it is also associated with liver disease, Guillain-Barré syndrome, cerebral vascular accidents, dementia, and other processes.

Iatrogenic causes of hypotension include medications, such as excessive exposure to antihypertensive agents, antiarrhythmics, narcotics, and sedatives. Medications that interfere with the autoregulation of renal blood flow can also contribute to or exacerbate tubular injury from other primary causes. Nonsteroidal antiinflammatory drugs (NSAIDs) can reduce blood flow through relative constriction of the afferent arteriole and can impair medullary blood flow in prostaglandin-dependent patients. Angiotensin-converting enzyme (ACE) inhibitors and angiotensin receptor blockers (ARBs) can reduce GFR by altering intrarenal hemodynamics through efferent arteriolar dilation, and could thereby perpetuate ischemia from other causes. This potential mechanism is not fully understood and there is no consensus that discontinuation of ACE inhibitors and ARBs improves outcomes in acute tubular injury, although there is mounting evidence that restarting ACE inhibitors and ARBs following an episode of AKI may improve short- and long-term outcomes.

Diagnosis

Along with history and clinical suspicion, urinalysis and urine microscopy remain the mainstay of diagnosis of ischemic acute tubular injury. Laboratory studies in ATI reflect dysfunction of the proximal tubule and include a blood urea nitrogen-to-creatinine ratio of less than 20, fractional excretion of sodium greater than 2%, and fractional excretion of urea more than 50%. However, the fractional excretion of sodium (FENa) may be found to be less than 1% in several circumstances where there is a mix of functional change in glomerular filtration and tubular cell injury (e.g., presence of diuretics, exposure to radio-contrast or calcineurin inhibitors). As such, the clinical utility of the FENa in the differential diagnosis of AKI remains unclear. Other common features on urinalysis include isosthenuria with a specific gravity of 1.010 and urine osmolality less than 350 mOsm/kg. This latter biomeasure reflects impairment in distal tubule and collecting duct ability to effectively concentrate or dilute urine.

Manual urine microscopy provides crucial diagnostic and prognostic information. The classic finding of dense granular or "muddy brown" casts (Fig. 32.1) is specific for the diagnosis of ATI. Fine granular casts, renal tubular epithelial cell casts, and renal tubular epithelial cells are also commonly found in ATI. While several urine sediment scoring systems have been published, there has been limited external validation of these scores. A urine sediment scoring system developed by Patel and colleagues from prospective clinical work had positive predictive value of 100% and negative predictive value of 91% for the diagnosis of ATI. Perazella and colleagues showed scores had prognostic significance by associating higher urine sediment severity scores with dose-dependent, increased relative risk for worsening acute kidney injury (higher AKI stage, dialysis requirement, or death).

Owing to the imprecision of many of the aforementioned ATI diagnostic tools, innovation in the detection and management of ATI is a large focus in current clinical research. Tissue inhibitor of metalloproteinases (TIMP2) and insulin-like growth-factor binding protein 7 (IGFBP7) are two biomarkers that have been combined in use commercially (NephroCheck, Biomerieux, France) in both

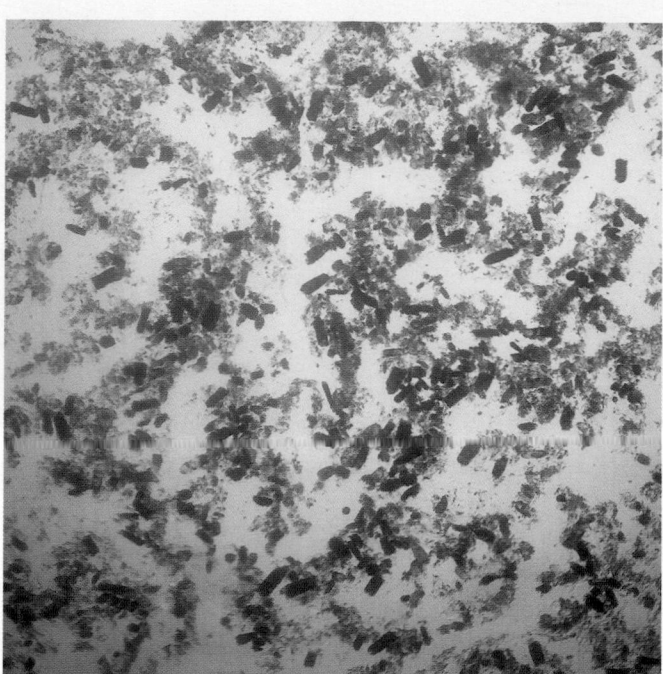

• **Fig. 32.1** Low-power view of the urine sediment demonstrates a low-power field (×40) of ATI with a large number of muddy brown casts. (Courtesy Randy Luciano, MD, Yale University.)

the United States and Europe for detection and risk stratification of severe AKI. Prediction of moderate to severe post-CABG AKI (KDIGO stage 2 or higher) with this test has been extremely good with an area under the curve (AUC) of 0.80 to 0.90. In high-risk groups (postcardiac surgery, intensive care unit), detection of ATI using these biomarkers combined with deploying AKI care bundles has been shown in several investigations to improve patient outcomes (less severe AKI, shorter ICU stays, decreased cost of care). Internationally, other biomarkers have been approved for clinical use and several others remain under investigation, including neutrophil gelatinase-associated lipocalin (NGAL), kidney injury molecule-1 (KIM-1), and proenkelphalin (Penkid). Several of these markers have been shown to correlate with adverse patient outcomes (dialysis requirement, prolonged length of stay, inpatient mortality) even in the absence of changes in serum creatinine or urine output, leading to the concept of "subclinical ATI." While the data supporting this concept are emerging, they have yet to be validated with prospective trials and human biopsy samples. In general, adoption of biomarkers has been somewhat slow, perhaps related to a sense that there is no targeted "therapeutic" for ATI. However, the positive findings from deployment of AKI care bundles (kidney-focused care aimed to optimize kidney perfusion, prevent volume overload, and avoid additional kidney stressors) as well as recent inclusion of biomarkers in perioperative cardiac surgery guidelines are expected to spur increased adoption in the near future.

Cholesterol Atheroembolic Disease

Clinical Presentation

Cholesterol atheroembolic kidney disease describes the result of disruption of atheromatous plaques within walls of arterial beds, which release cholesterol crystals that flow downstream and lodge in various blood vessels and organs including the kidney. This phenomenon leads to ischemic kidney injury due to vessel obstruction from cholesterol crystals and the subsequently provoked inflammatory response. Plaque disruption is generally iatrogenic from vessel cannulation for cardiac catheterization (aortic plaques) and various vascular procedures (including both open and closed vascular surgery). The incidence of this syndrome appears to have decreased substantially over time. Retrospective analyses and case series from the 1970s and 1980s report incidence rates as high as 25%-30%, but more recent retrospective and prospective analyses from the 1990s and early 2000s show incidence rates consistently less than 2%. Study heterogeneity complicates assessment, but it is felt that widespread statin use and less invasive modes of vessel cannulation and manipulation (radial artery approaches, advances in technology, and surgical technique including distal clot-catching devices) have had a significant effect in disease reduction.

The disease can present in one of three ways. The first is an acute process with fulminant AKI occurring within one week of the triggering event. This scenario is often the result of a large burden of cholesterol emboli with multi-organ involvement. Severity can range from catastrophic tissue necrosis characterized by severe (stage 3) AKI, GI bleeding, necrotic skin ulcerations, spinal cord infarction, and rapid death, to less severe presentations with abdominal pain, livedo reticularis, and acalculous cholecystitis. A second presentation is a subacute decline in kidney function, with AKI appearing several weeks after the initial insult. Kidney dysfunction occurs in a stepwise fashion, representing ongoing cholesterol crystal embolization. The third presentation is with a chronic or delayed course, in which significant kidney impairment may not be noted until up to 6 months after the trigger. These cases are likely under-recognized and typically attributed to other causes of CKD, such as hypertensive nephrosclerosis. Kidney biopsy, however, demonstrates the classic needle-shaped clefts within the intrarenal vasculature.

Diagnosis

Laboratory test findings are often non-specific and can include anemia, leukocytosis, thrombocytopenia, and elevated inflammatory markers such as ESR and CRP. Eosinophilia and hypocomplementemia are more specific laboratory findings that have been described, but the negative predictive value of these markers is quite low. Urinalysis typically reveals a bland sediment with minimal proteinuria. Kidney biopsy is regarded as the definitive method for diagnosis. However, the benefit of biopsy may be limited as there are no definitive therapeutic options, with anticoagulation, steroids, or other specific treatments not having shown consistent benefit in improving patient outcomes (see therapy section below).

Pathology

After entering the renal artery, cholesterol crystals typically settle within the arcuate and interlobular arterioles of the kidney, but they can reach the afferent arteriole and glomerular capillary as well. An inflammatory reaction ensues that is characterized initially by granulocyte infiltration and then mononuclear cell infiltration and giant cell formation. Endothelial proliferation occurs, which leads to intimal thickening and concentric fibrosis. Ultimately this process results in arteriole obstruction and ischemic infarction of downstream tissues, including the glomeruli, tubules, and interstitium. Histologically, cholesterol crystal emboli are identified in the lumen of arcuate and interlobular arteries as biconvex, needle-shaped, and empty clefts, referred to as *ghost cells* because they dissolve during specimen processing. The tissue damage caused by these crystal emboli is patchy. Glomerular and interstitial changes are mainly ischemic, with a varying extent of glomerular obsolescence and interstitial fibrosis. In the early phases, areas of acute tubular necrosis can be identified.

Therapy and Outcomes

Primary prevention remains the most effective target at this time, with data extrapolated from the cardiac disease prevention literature as there are no formal clinical trials specifically looking at atheroembolic kidney disease. This includes aggressive management of underlying predisposing conditions (e.g., hypertension, hyperlipidemia, and tobacco use) and careful consideration of the risks and benefits of initiation or continuation of anticoagulant or antithrombotic therapy (as these may increase risk for plaque disruption) and of proceeding with intervention at all. Once atheroembolic disease develops, there are no rigorously studied therapies that have shown consistent improvement in kidney outcomes. Steroids have been used in severe cases with acute multi-organ involvement with limited success but are not currently thought to be beneficial more generally. Other experimental therapies such as low-density lipoprotein (LDL) apheresis have been used but have not been evaluated in controlled settings.

Few outcome studies have been done in patients with atheroembolic kidney disease. The data available suggest kidney prognosis is poor with as many as 40%–60% of patients requiring dialysis at the time of initial presentation, and 25% of patients remaining dialysis-dependent in the two studies with more long-term follow-up. Statin use has been associated with improved outcomes in retrospective analyses. Preexisting CKD, longstanding hypertension, and presence of eosinophilia have all been identified as poor prognostic markers.

Kidney Infarction

Kidney infarction is an uncommon condition resulting from sudden disruption of blood flow in the main renal artery or in one of its segmental branches. A large autopsy series of over 14,000 people from the 1940s estimated prevalence of this condition at 0.014%. Recent estimation of incidence based on emergency department series of 250,000 patients over 4 years was 0.007%. However, it is felt that this may be an underestimate as the clinical diagnosis could be missed, given presenting symptoms mimic other much more common conditions. A small but more recent case series coming from a specialized hypertension ward in France has reported an incidence of 0.07%.

Clinical Presentation and Diagnosis

The presentation is generally symptomatic, given acute onset and lack of collateral blood supply. Typically, patients present with abdominal and/or unilateral flank pain. Other common symptoms include nausea, vomiting, and fever. Infarcted tissues release renin, so an abrupt rise in blood pressure often accompanies these symptoms. Oliguric acute kidney injury is rare unless both kidneys or a single functioning kidney is involved. Laboratory findings include microscopic hematuria, leukocytosis, elevated lactate dehydrogenase (LDH), and elevated C-reactive protein (CRP). Imaging is required to make the diagnosis, given the non-specific nature of these other symptoms and signs. Computed tomography (CT) imaging with intravenous contrast will often make the diagnosis with the finding of a wedge-shaped lesion demarcating the area of hypoperfusion. Other diagnostic imaging tools include nuclear scan with dimercaptosuccinic acid and renal artery angiogram, with both studies showing perfusion defects.

Causes and Treatment

Etiologies can be divided into four broad categories—cardioembolic, renal artery injury, thrombophilic, and idiopathic—each with a number of different causes (Table 32.1). The relative frequency of each diagnosis has been described in three recent case series. Two of these series were derived from general internal medicine and nephrology wards and found that cardioembolic diagnoses were most common (30%-55%). The third was from a specialty hypertension ward at a tertiary care center and found that renal artery injury diagnoses were most common (80%). However, larger investigations of a more general hospital-based population are lacking. It is not known if the long-term kidney outcomes based on etiology differ, although making the correct diagnosis likely has treatment and outcome implications.

Long-term anticoagulation is important for the prevention of recurrent loss of blood supply in the cardioembolic and thrombophilic diagnoses. Surgical or percutaneous revascularization should be explored in cases of renal artery injury. Data are extremely sparse regarding outcomes associated with different treatment strategies. The largest series with 438 patients and a 20-month median follow-up only found 5% mortality and 2% progression to ESRD with anticoagulation prescribed for 80% of patients. A small series of 42 participants compared patients with and without revascularization and found higher mortality (17% versus 7%) in patients without revascularization, but higher eGFR decline (19.5 mL/min versus 6 mL/min) in patients with revascularization.

Acute Tubular Injury by Endogenous Nephrotoxins

Accumulation of naturally occurring substances in specific clinical scenarios can have nephrotoxic effects and lead to acute tubular injury. Most notably, these include rhabdomyolysis, hemoglobinuria, and tumor lysis. Unlike cases of iatrogenic nephrotoxins, these exposures may not be readily apparent based on a patient's medical records. As such, a high degree of clinical suspicion and knowledge of the specific clinical scenarios associated with these toxic substances are important. Preventing ongoing exposure of the kidney to these toxic agents can be difficult, so management of these conditions often involves manipulating the biochemical environment to limit the kidney's interaction with the toxic substance to limit injury.

TABLE 32.1	Causes of Kidney Infarction		
Cardioembolic	**Renal Artery Injury**	**Thrombophilic**	**Idiopathic**
-Atrial Fibrillation	-Atherosclerosis	-Hypercoagulable	
-Valve Replacement	-Fibromuscular	Disorder	
-Endocarditis	Dysplasia	-JAK2 Mutation	
-LV or Aortic	-Dissecting or	-Malignancy	
Thrombus	Aneurysmal		
-Patent Foramen	Arterial Disease		
Ovale	-Trauma		
	-Ehlers-Danlos		
	-Arteritis		

Rhabdomyolysis

The term *rhabdomyolysis* refers to the clinical scenario of breakdown of striated skeletal muscle resulting in the release of cellular contents into the circulation. It is diagnosed by acute neuromuscular weakness or dark urine in addition to elevation of serum creatine kinase (CK) to levels greater than 2000 U/L. Bywaters and Beall are credited with the initial description of kidney failure from rhabdomyolysis in four cases involving crush injuries during the bombing of London in World War II. The outcomes of rhabdomyolysis vary widely from being benign and asymptomatic to life-threatening electrolyte abnormalities, AKI, including the need for kidney replacement therapy (KRT), and death. Among hospitalized patients with rhabdomyolysis, 13% to 50% develop creatinine and urine output based AKI, 4% to 13% require KRT, and 1.7% to 46% die during hospitalization. In-hospital mortality rates are significantly higher in rhabdomyolysis patients who develop AKI compared to those without AKI (22% to 62% vs. 7% to 18%).

Causes and Pathophysiology

Etiologies of rhabdomyolysis are listed in Box 32.1. Overexertion may cause necrosis in otherwise normal muscles because of a mismatch in energy supply and demand. This is most commonly seen in poorly conditioned persons who partake in extreme exercise activities, although there have been case reports of well-trained marathon runners developing rhabdomyolysis and AKI. The most frequent etiology in a series of 475 hospitalized patients in the United States was from medications and toxin ingestions. Alcohol and cocaine were the two most abused substances associated with rhabdomyolysis. A number of medications also cause muscle injury; the most frequently implicated agents are antipsychotics, statins, and selective serotonin release inhibitors. Incidence of statin-induced rhabdomyolysis has recently been estimated at 1 case per 100,000 patients based on a review of over 400,000 health claims.

The mechanism by which rhabdomyolysis causes AKI is not certain but several processes have been implicated. These include renal vasoconstriction and ischemic tubular injury, cast formation, and myoglobin-induced direct tubular toxicity. Renal vasoconstriction results from muscle necrosis via activation of the renin-angiotensin system due to volume depletion from third spacing as well as endotoxin and cytokine release. Acellular, red-brown-pigmented casts result from the precipitation of myoglobin with Tamm-Horsfall proteins when the tubular concentration of myoglobin is increased and the urinary space is acidic. These casts cause kidney injury by tubular obstruction, which eventually leads to a reduction in GFR. Finally, while the exact mechanisms are not known, myoglobin is felt to be a direct tubular toxin through some combination of lipid peroxidation, inflammation, and oxidative injury.

Diagnosis

Rhabdomyolysis is classically characterized by the triad of muscle pain, weakness, and dark urine. Cases may be either asymptomatic or patients may be incapacitated. Clinical suspicion or known history of immobilization, trauma, or ingestion can be important to identify. Diagnosis is made by serum chemistries with elevated levels of CK, myoglobin, and other muscle enzymes. While an elevated CK suggests the presence of rhabdomyolysis, the degree of its elevation alone is a weak predictor of the development of AKI and the need for KRT. The risk of AKI is typically not significant until the CK levels are greater than 15,000 to 20,000 U/L. Other

BOX 32.1

Causes of Rhabdomyolysis

1. Physical injury
   a. Trauma
   b. Crush injury
   c. Compartment syndrome
   d. Immobilization
2. Muscle fiber exhaustion
   a. Excessive exercise
   b. Seizures
   c. Heat stroke
   d. Neuroleptic malignant syndrome
   e. Malignant hyperthermia
3. Medications, illicit drugs, and dietary supplements
   a. Statins
   b. Fibrates
   c. Zidovudine
   d. Phenytoin
   e. Selective serotonin reuptake inhibitors
   f. Isoniazid
   g. Colchicine
   h. Antipsychotics
   i. Antimalarials
   j. Trimethoprim-sulfamethoxazole in HIV infection
   k. Cocaine
   l. Amphetamines
   m. Heroin
   n. Methadone
   o. Phencyclidine
   p. Creatine
   q. Ephedra
4. Toxins
   a. Alcohol
   b. Toluene
   c. Carbon monoxide
   d. Hydrocarbons
   e. Quail poisoning
   f. Mushroom poisoning
5. Electrolyte disturbances
   a. Hypokalemia
   b. Hypophosphatemia
   c. Excessive fluid shifts
6. Inflammatory states
   a. Dermatomyositis and polymyositis
   b. Vasculitis
   c. Systemic inflammatory response
   d. Viral infections (e.g., influenza, parainfluenza, coxsackie, HIV, EBV, CMV, herpes)
   e. Bacterial infection (e.g., Legionnaire disease, tularemia, toxic shock syndrome, streptococci, staphylococci, *Clostridium*, *Salmonella*)
   f. Protozoal infections (e.g., *Plasmodium falciparum* malaria)
7. Deficiencies in metabolic enzymes
   a. Muscle phosphorylase deficiency (McArdle disease)
   b. Carnitine palmitoyl transferase deficiency
   c. Phosphofructokinase deficiency in muscle (Tarui disease)

CMV, Cytomegalovirus; *EBV*, Epstein-Barr virus; *HIV*, human immunodeficiency virus.

---

biochemical laboratory abnormalities may include hyperkalemia, hyperphosphatemia, hyperuricemia, elevated LDH, and hypocalcemia. These labs result from their release from necrotic muscle and accumulation due to reduced kidney clearance. Hypocalcemia occurs due to the complexing of calcium with phosphorus in necrotic tissue beds.

The presence of myoglobin in the urine may make it appear reddish-brown in color. Urine dipstick shows significant heme protein positivity with few or no red blood cells on urine sediment evaluation. This apparent discrepancy occurs because the peroxidase agent in the dipstick test reacts with heme found in both hemoglobin and myoglobin and is, therefore, unable to differentiate between the two. An additional characteristic feature of rhabdomyolysis is a fractional excretion of sodium <1% early in the disease course, although this is not universal. Approximately 50% of cases will have some level of proteinuria detected on urinalysis (>1+). Under the microscope, red-brown-pigmented, granular casts will be seen.

Risk Factors and Prognosis

The McMahon Rhabdomyolysis Risk Score (Table 32.2) has been developed and retrospectively validated on a separate cohort as a risk prediction score for the composite outcome of need for KRT and in-hospital mortality. Important clinical variables that predict these outcomes include age, female sex, initial serum creatinine, and serum concentrations of CK (>40,000), phosphorus (>5.4),

TABLE 32.2 Rhabdomyolysis Risk Score

Variable	Score
Age, in years	
>50 to ≤70	1.5
>70 to ≤80	2.5
>80	3
Female sex	1
Initial creatinine	
1.4 to 2.2 mg/dL (124-195 µmol/L)	1.5
>2.2 mg/dL (>195 µmol/L)	3
Initial calcium <7.5 mg/dL (<1.88 mmol/L)	2
Initial CPK >40,000 U/L	2
Origin not seizures, syncope, exercise, statins, or myositis	3
Initial phosphate, mg/dL	
4.0 to 5.4 mg/dL (1.0-1.4 mmol/L)	1.5
>5.4 (>1.4 mmol/L)	3
Initial bicarbonate <19 mEq/L (19 mmol/L)	2

Interpretation:
Score <5: 2.3% risk of death or requiring KRT
Score >10: 61.2% risk of death or requiring KRT

KRT, Kidney replacement therapy.

calcium (<7.5), and bicarbonate (<19). Scores below 5 have a negative predictive value of 97% for the composite outcome of KRT and in-hospital mortality. Every 1-point increase in the score is associated with almost 1.5 times the increase in odds of the composite outcome. The score was validated in a retrospective study of patients with rhabdomyolysis in the intensive care unit (ICU) setting and found that a score of 6 on admission was 83% sensitive and 55% specific for the prediction of need for KRT.

Treatment

Overall, rhabdomyolysis care is primarily supportive with efforts to prevent continued muscle damage, avoid kidney injury when possible, and correct electrolyte disturbances. Aggressive resuscitation with isotonic intravenous fluids is a critical preventive measure, as patients with rhabdomyolysis are usually significantly volume depleted from fluid sequestration into injured muscles. Although there have been no randomized controlled trials to determine the ideal composition and dose of resuscitative fluid in this setting, it is generally agreed that isotonic solutions such as 0.9% normal saline at a rate to maintain urine output above 200 mL/hr is advisable. Theoretical benefits of urinary alkalinization have been proposed to reduce precipitation of myoglobin in the renal tubule; however, the potential adverse outcomes of worsened hypocalcemia and calcium-phosphate deposition in the kidney limit the advisable use of alkaline fluids. Growing evidence indicates that use of balanced solutions is associated with lower risk of AKI. However, lactated Ringer, which contains potassium, is often avoided in this scenario because of the hyperkalemia that is associated with rhabdomyolysis. In the setting of adequate intravascular volume, diuretics (mannitol, loop diuretics) have been used in concert with intravenous fluids in an effort to maintain intravascular volume, promote high urinary flow, and prevent myoglobin precipitation, but there is no clear evidence that these prevent AKI.

Heme Pigment Nephropathy

Free circulating hemoglobin occurs in the setting of intravascular hemolysis. There are several different etiologies of hemolysis that have been associated with free circulating hemoglobin (see Box 32.2).

BOX 32.2

Causes of Hemolysis

Within the Red Cell

1. Membrane defects (hereditary)
2. Enzyme defects (G6PD, pyruvate kinase)
3. Hemoglobin defects (sickle cell anemia, thalassemias)

Outside the Red Cell

1. Autoimmune
   a. Autoimmune hemolytic anemia
   b. Transfusion reactions
2. Nonimmune
   a. Hypersplenism
   b. Fragmentation syndromes (heart valves, mechanical circulatory devices)
   c. Infections (malaria, Bartonella)
   d. Drugs
   e. Liver disease
   f. Paroxysmal nocturnal hemoglobinuria

Mechanical trauma to erythrocytes liberates hemoglobin into plasma, which is bound by haptoglobin. This haptoglobin-hemoglobin complex is then taken up by reticuloendothelial cells and is degraded. When plasma haptoglobin is fully saturated, free plasma hemoglobin dissociates to dimeric hemoglobin, which can undergo appreciable glomerular filtration. Filtered hemoglobin is endocytosed by proximal tubular cells or contributes to intratubular heme pigment cast formation.

Pathophysiology

Within the nephron, excess heme pigments cause renal vasoconstriction, tubular obstruction, increased oxidative stress, and inflammation. Impaired renal blood flow occurs because of a decrease in the vasodilator nitric oxide, which is avidly scavenged by heme proteins, and an increase in vasoconstrictors such as endothelin and isoprostanes. The consequent decrease in renal perfusion results in further ischemic injury to renal tubular cells. Tubular obstruction occurs in an acidic urinary space, which denatures heme proteins to a conformation that promotes binding with Tamm-Horsfall protein, leading to tubular cast formation. Increased oxidative stress can occur by way of tubular obstruction due to prolonged exposure of tubular epithelial cells to heme proteins. Longer duration of exposure to heme proteins is associated with increased uptake into tubular cells and direct cell injury by free radical formation and lipid peroxidation. Finally, there is an increasing body of evidence that heme can trigger the nucleotide-binding domain-like receptor protein 3 (NLRP3) inflammasome-signaling cascade and lead to release of proinflammatory cytokines such as IL-1β and IL-18.

Prognosis and Management

Treatment is supportive and similar to management of rhabdomyolysis. Early aggressive fluid administration helps to limit cast formation and excessive heme protein concentrations within the tubule. Animal studies have shown benefit to urinary alkalinization by reducing hemoglobin binding with Tamm-Horsfall protein and inhibiting the reduction-oxidation cycling of hemoglobin that leads to lipid peroxidation. However, there is no clear clinical evidence suggesting superiority of isotonic bicarbonate-containing fluid administration over other fluids. Small, non-randomized case series have shown antioxidant agents, including pentoxifylline, vitamin E, and vitamin C, to be of benefit, but these therapies have not been rigorously studied. Several preclinical studies have investigated the use of inflammasome inhibitors such as glyburide and other novel sulfonylurea-containing compounds (MCC950) in AKI, but their therapeutic efficacy has not yet been tested in models of pigment nephropathy.

Two recent kidney biopsy cohorts from India and the United States have been able to describe outcomes related to AKI in the setting of hemolysis. In the Indian cohort of 3300 cases of AKI, 2.9% had evidence of hemolysis and, of those, 20% (20 patients) had biopsy-proven heme pigment nephropathy. The most common sources of hemolysis were medications (rifampin) and disseminated intravascular coagulation (DIC). All except one patient (95%) required HD, three patients (15%) died during their hospitalization, but only three patients (15%) had CKD at mean follow-up of 14 months. In the United States cohort of all native kidney biopsies from a centralized pathology lab, 0.78% had heme pigment nephropathy. The most common sources of hemolysis were autoimmune hemolytic anemia and medications (rifampin, trimethoprim-sulfamethoxazole). Clinical information was available for 23 patients, of whom 57% required HD, 14%

died during their hospitalization, and 78% experienced normalization of serum creatinine at median 13-month follow-up.

Acute Nephropathy Associated with Tumor Lysis Syndrome

Pathophysiology

Tumor lysis syndrome (TLS) is a constellation of specific metabolic derangements that arise when tumor cells die and intracellular contents are released into the systemic circulation. Characteristic findings include hyperkalemia, hyperphosphatemia, hypocalcemia, and hyperuricemia, which range from mild to severe and life threatening. Diagnosis, both laboratory and clinical, is made by the Cairo-Bishop scoring system (Table 32.3). TLS typically occurs after the administration of chemotherapeutic agents for the treatment of lymphomas and leukemias, but does occur with other malignancies, and it can rarely occur spontaneously in rapidly dividing solid tumors that outgrow their blood supply. Acute crystalline nephropathy is a common occurrence and is a direct consequence of uric acid and calcium-phosphate precipitation within the renal tubules.

Management

Intravenous saline is employed to maintain high urine flow rates with the aim of preventing crystal formation and volume depletion. Urinary alkalinization is no longer recommended due to risk for calcium-phosphate and xanthine crystal precipitation within tubules. Allopurinol and febuxostat (xanthine oxidase inhibitors) can be used to preemptively prevent hyperuricemia, but rasburicase, a recombinant urate oxidase enzyme, is often required to rapidly and effectively correct hyperuricemia with TLS. These medications should be considered as prophylaxis in high-risk patients planned for chemotherapy.

Other Endogenous Toxins

Other endogenous substances can accumulate within the renal tubules and cause tubular injury. Similar to the previous causes, this occurs when pathologic states lead to elevated plasma levels of substances that are relatively benign under normal conditions. In myeloma, free monoclonal light chains are filtered by the glomerulus before inducing direct proximal tubule cellular injury (see Chapter 27).

Plasma levels of oxalate can be elevated as a result of either endogenous production or exogenous ingestion. In primary hyperoxaluria, oxalate overproduction occurs as a result of an inborn error in the metabolism of glyoxylate. This leads to urine oxalate concentrations at supersaturated levels. Calcium oxalate precipitation occurs and results in crystal aggregation, tubular injury, and nephrocalcinosis. Hyperoxaluria can also occur following gastric bypass surgery (Roux-en-Y bypass, gastric sleeve, and gastric banding) and with other causes of malabsorption (pancreatitis, Crohn disease). This occurrence is a result of increased gut absorption of oxalate from dietary sources. Exogenous etiologies include ingestion of ethylene glycol (antifreeze), large doses of orlistat, excessive vitamin C intake, and overconsumption of high-oxalate food (kale, spinach, and teas).

SARS-CoV-2-Related Acute Tubular Injury

A third novel coronavirus leading to severe respiratory infection (coronavirus disease 2019, COVID-19) was first identified in Wuhan, China, in December 2019 and, as of the summer of 2020, was responsible for over half a million deaths. Based on available data, AKI is a fairly common complication of COVID-19 infection in hospitalized patients. AKI incidence rates vary by setting and patient population with rates as low as 3%–5% in those with mild disease to 75% of those requiring ICU admission and advanced forms of life support. While there are only limited case series with biopsy information of those with AKI in the setting of COVID-19, the most prominent pathologic feature seems to be ATI, although glomerular and other injury patterns have been reported.

While it appears that the majority of cases follow a pattern consistent with other forms of critical illness, some cases may be related to direct invasion of the virus into tubular cells. In the setting of COVID-19 and critical illness, AKI and tubular injury are often multifactorial with relative or absolute hypotension, organ cross-damage from acute lung injury/acute respiratory distress syndrome (ARDS), mechanical ventilation, and nephrotoxin exposure all being frequently implicated. Nephrotoxin exposure aside, many of these processes do not correlate with direct tubular injury (e.g., the decreased cardiac output and renal perfusion associated with positive pressure ventilation) but rather prime the kidney for impending injury from a "second hit." As for nephrotoxins, while many of them are known to cause tubular injury, they are beyond the scope of this chapter and will be discussed in Chapter 34. Separate from critical illness-associated forms of AKI, tubular obstruction by endogenous nephrotoxins has been reported. These include the aforementioned rhabdomyolysis, hyperoxaluria from vitamin C administration, and hyperuricemia from a theorized catabolic state without creatine kinase (CK) elevation.

Direct viral tubular toxicity is also possible, although available data are far from conclusive. Viral RNA has been demonstrated in urine samples, but the virus is not consistently evident in tissue samples from the largest biopsy/autopsy series as yet. The

TABLE 32.3	Cairo-Bishop Definitions
Laboratory Tumor Lysis Syndrome (LTLS)*	**Clinical Tumor Lysis Syndrome (CTLS)****
Serum uric acid ≥476 μmol/L or 25% increase from baseline	Creatinine ≥1.5 times greater than the institutional ULN if below the age/gender-defined ULN, for patients >12 years of age
Serum potassium ≥6 mmol/L or 25% increase from baseline	Cardiac arrhythmia/sudden death not directly or probably attributable to a therapeutic agent
Serum phosphorus ≥2.1 mmol/L in children, ≥1.45 mmol/L in adults, or 25% increase from baseline	Seizure not directly or probably attributable to a therapeutic agent
Serum calcium ≤1.75 mmol/L or 25% decrease from baseline	

*The Cairo-Bishop definition of LTLS requires that two or more metabolic abnormalities are present within the 3 days preceding or 7 days following the initiation of chemotherapy. The required 25% change in metabolite serum concentration assumes the patient has received adequate hydration and a hypouricemic agent.

**The Cairo-Bishop definition of CTLS requires one or more clinical manifestations along with criteria for LTLS.

angiotensin-converting enzyme 2 (ACE2) receptor on tubular epithelial cells does seem to serve as a binding domain for the virus to gain access to tubular cells. The growing recognition of other pathologic features on tissue specimens (podocytopathy, thrombotic microangiopathy, other glomerulopathy) points to the role of cytokine-mediated effects and an adaptive immune response that will be discussed in other chapters. Future investigations into COVID-associated AKI are needed to examine the specific incidence and impact of tubular injury.

Complete bibliography is available at Elsevier eBooks for Practicing Clinicians.

Key Bibliography

Abuelo JG. Normotensive ischemic acute renal failure. *N Engl J Med*. 2007;357:797–805.

Antopolsky M, Simanovsky N, Stalnikowicz R, et al. Renal infarction in the ED: 10-year experience and review of the literature. *Am J Emerg Med*. 2012;30:1055–1060.

Cavanaugh C, Parazella MA. Urine sediment examination in the diagnosis and management of kidney disease: core curriculum 2019. *Am J Kid Dis*. 2019;73(2):258–272.

Dvanajscak Z, Walker PD, Cossey LN, et al. Hemolysis associated hemoglobin cast nephropathy results from a range of clinicopathologic disorders. *Kidney Int*. 2019;96:1400–1407.

Giuliani KTK, Kassianos AJ, Healy H, et al. Pigment nephropathy: novel insights into inflammasome mediated pathogenesis. *Int J Mol Sci*. 2019;20(8):1997–2014.

Gómez H, Kellum JA. Sepsis-induced acute kidney injury. *Curr Opin Crit Care*. 2016;22:546–553.

Hirsch J, Ng JH, Ross DW, et al. Acute kidney injury in hospitalized patients with COVID-19. *Kidney Int*. 2020;98(1):209–218.

Howard SC, Jones DP. Pui C-H. The tumor lysis syndrome. *N Engl J Med*. 2011;364:1844–1854.

Huerta-Alardín AL, Varon J, Marik PE. Bench-to-bedside review: rhabdomyolysis - an overview for clinicians. *Crit Care*. 2005;9(2):158–169.

Koyner JL, Shaw AD, Chawla LS, et al. Tissue inhibitor metalloproteinase-2 (TIMP-2)IGF binding protein-7 (IGFBP7) levels are associated with adverse long-term outcomes in patients with AKI. *J Am Soc Nephrol*. 2015;26:1747–1754.

McMahon GM, Zeng X, Waikar SS. A risk prediction score for kidney failure or mortality in rhabdomyolysis. *JAMA Intern Med*. 2013;173(19):1821–1828.

Melli G, Chaudhry V, Cornblath DR. Rhabdomyolysis: an evaluation of 475 hospitalized patients. *Medicine (Baltimore)*. 2005;84(6):377–385.

Parikh CR, Mansour SG. Perspective on clinical application of biomarkers in AKI. *J Am Soc Nephrol*. 2017;28(6):1677–1685.

Rangaswami J, Bhalla V, Blair JEA, et al. Cardiorenal syndrome. Classification, pathophysiology, diagnosis, and treatment strategies: a scientific statement from the American Heart Association. *Circulation*. 2019;139(16):e840–e878.

Silverberg D, Menses T, Rimon U, et al. Acute renal artery occlusion: presentation, treatment, and outcome. *J Vasc Surg*. 2016;64(4):1036–1042.

Simpson JP, Taylor A, Sudhan N, et al. Rhabdomyolysis and acute kidney injury: creatine kinase as a prognostic marker and validation of the mcmahon score in a 10-year cohort: a retrospective observational evaluation. *Eur J of Anaesthesiol*. 2016;33(12):906–912.

Sun J, Zhu A, Li H, et al. Isolation of infectious SARS-CoV-2 from urine of a COVID-19 patient. *Emerg Microbes Infect*. 2020;9(1):991–993.

Sury K. Update on the prevention and treatment of tumor lysis syndrome. *J Onco-Nephrol*. 2019;3:19–30.

Toriu N, Sumida K, Mizuno H, et al. Long-term outcomes of biopsy proven cholesterol crystal embolism. *J Interven Exp Nephrol*. 2019;23:1181–1187.

Zhou F, Yu T, Du R, et al. Clinical course and risk factors for mortality of adult inpatients with COVID-19 in Wuhan, China: a retrospective cohort study. *Lancet*. 2020;395:1054–1062.

33

Acute Interstitial Nephritis

URSULA C. BREWSTER, RANDY L. LUCIANO

In 1898, W. T. Councilman defined acute interstitial nephritis (AIN) as "an acute inflammation of the kidney characterized by cellular and fluid exudation in the interstitial tissue, accompanied by, but not dependent on, degeneration of the epithelium; the exudation is not purulent in character, and the lesions may be both diffuse and focal." This was seen on postmortem examination of patients with scarlet fever and, less commonly, other systemic infectious diseases that had no evidence for direct bacterial invasion of the kidney parenchyma.

More than a century later, definitive diagnosis of AIN requires the pathologic findings of interstitial edema and infiltration with acute inflammatory cells, including polymorphonucleocytes (PMNs), eosinophils, and lymphocytes. In the years since Councilman's description, the causes of AIN have changed dramatically, with pharmacologic agents now being the most common etiology (more than 75%). In this chapter we will focus primarily on acute tubulointerstitial inflammation, while briefly covering direct parenchymal invasion by infectious agents.

The incidence of AIN varies greatly, depending on the clinical scenario. An incidence of 0.7% is seen in asymptomatic patients with proteinuria or hematuria, whereas hospitalized patients with acute kidney injury (AKI) of unknown etiology experience an incidence of 10% to 15%. Although AIN can occur in all age groups, it is more common in the elderly. In one report, biopsy-proven AIN was seen in 3.0% of the elderly compared with 1.9% of younger subjects. This may reflect greater exposure of elderly patients to drugs and other inciting factors.

Clinical Presentation

The presenting symptoms of AIN include an acute or subacute decline in kidney function, often in patients exposed to multiple drugs. Although the "classic" presentation of skin rash, arthralgia, and eosinophilia is occasionally seen, this triad occurs in only 5% to 10% of unselected patients. This presentation more commonly occurs in association with certain drugs, such as penicillin derivatives, compared with nonsteroidal antiinflammatory drugs (NSAIDs). Fever, the most common clinical sign, is present in up to 50% of patients with drug-induced AIN but only in 30% of unselected patients. Skin rash is reported in one-third of patients and is usually maculopapular or morbilliform, typically involving the trunk. More often, a rash is seen when AIN is related to a drug hypersensitivity reaction. No clinical symptoms or signs are sensitive or specific enough to establish a definitive diagnosis. Nonoliguric AKI usually accompanies AIN, but oliguric AKI with a rapid rise in creatinine also occurs. Increasingly, AIN develops in patients with underlying chronic kidney disease (CKD) and multiple comorbidities, which make a diagnosis challenging. AIN should, therefore, be considered in any patient with acute or subacute decline in kidney function with no clear inciting factor.

Laboratory Findings

Common laboratory findings in AIN are summarized in Table 33.1. The most frequent abnormality is a slow and steady decline in the glomerular filtration rate (GFR). When dealing with drug-induced AIN, the GFR typically falls 7 to 10 days after starting the medication. Rapid and fulminant presentation of AIN occurs less often, unless there has been previous drug exposure. However, drugs such as the NSAIDs and proton pump inhibitors (PPIs) may not develop AIN for many weeks or months after initial exposure. The time course for AIN related to systemic disease, metabolic disturbances, or infection is more varied and prolonged. Other major laboratory findings include eosinophilia, eosinophiluria, and urinary sediment abnormalities. Eosinophilia is common in β-lactam antibiotic–associated AIN, reported in up to 80% of cases, where only one-third of other drug-induced AIN cases develop eosinophilia. Hyperkalemia, with or without hyperchloremic metabolic acidosis, is occasionally seen. Other tubulopathies may rarely occur. Anemia is also commonly described in AIN. This finding is rather nonspecific, especially in the setting of systemic inflammation, AKI, or underlying CKD. Anemia with AIN is most likely the result of decreased erythropoietin production from the medullary interstitium and underlying erythropoietin hyporesponsiveness in the setting of inflammation or infection.

Urinalysis and the examination of the urine sediment are often the most useful laboratory tests. Low-grade proteinuria (1–2+) and positive leukocyte esterase are noted on urine dipsticks in most patients. Leukocyte esterase has been noted to be positive in approximately 80% of patients with AIN, but ranges from 20%–80% in published studies. Quantitative proteinuria measurements are usually less than 1 g/day, with the majority being non-albumin proteinuria. (Albuminuria would be more indicative of glomerular disease.) Macroscopic hematuria is rare, whereas microscopic hematuria is present less than 50% of the time. Leukocytes are present on urine microscopy in virtually all cases of methicillin-induced AIN but may be absent in as many as 50% of patients with AIN due to other drugs. The absence of leukocyturia, therefore, should not rule out this diagnosis. Classically, urine microscopy will show hematuria, leukocyturia, leukocyte casts, and renal tubular epithelial (RTE) cells (Fig. 33.1). However, urinary leukocyte casts are an insensitive test for diagnosing AIN. Red blood cell casts and mixed red blood cell and white blood cell casts have also been reported. Cellular casts are seen in most cases

TABLE 33.1	Laboratory Findings in Acute Interstitial Nephritis	
Eosinophilia	Inconsistent Finding Seen More Commonly in Drug-Induced AIN	
Eosinophiluria (>1% and >5%)	Sensitivity 19.8%–30.8%, specificity 68.2%–91.2%, PPV 15.6%–30%, NPV 83.7%–85.6%, positive LR 0.97–2.3, negative LR 0.9–1.01	
Urinary sediment	Hematuria, leukocyturia, leukocyte casts, RTE cells, and RTE casts	
Protein excretion	Less than 1 g/24 hours	
Fractional excretion of sodium (FeNa)	Greater than 1%	
Proximal tubular defect	Glycosuria, phosphaturia, bicarbonaturia, aminoaciduria	
Distal tubular defect	Hyperkalemia, distal RTA, sodium wasting	
Medullary defect	Nephrogenic diabetes insipidus, anemia	

AIN, Acute interstitial nephritis; *LR*, likelihood ratio; *NPV*, negative predictive value; *PPV*, positive predictive value; *RTA*, renal tubular acidosis; *RTE*, renal tubular epithelial.

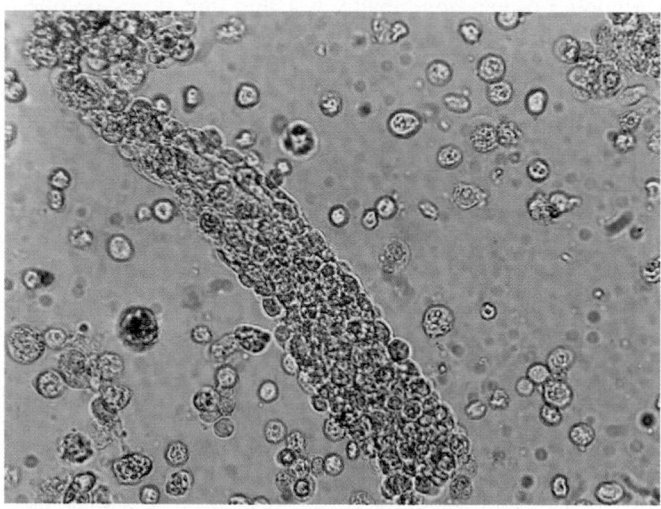

• **Fig. 33.1** Urine microscopy showing a white blood cell cast and surrounding white blood cells (× 60).

of methicillin-associated AIN, and in up to 50% of patients with AIN from other exposures. However, up to 20% of AIN cases can have a bland urinary sediment.

Eosinophiluria, once thought to be a hallmark of this disease, is neither sensitive nor specific and should not be used to make a diagnosis. When using a cutoff of greater than 1% urinary eosinophils, the sensitivity and specificity are 30.8% and 68.2%, respectively. A 5% urinary eosinophil cutoff increases specificity to 91.2% but decreases sensitivity to 19.8%. Various techniques used to stain urine for eosinophils and enhance detection (Wright stain and Hansel stain) have proven unreliable and cumbersome. In addition, other disease states, such as cystitis, pyelonephritis, atheroembolic kidney disease, and rapidly progressive glomerulonephritis may present with eosinophiluria, highlighting the poor specificity of this test.

Recent studies have looked at the role of urinary biomarkers, including soluble C5b-9, tumor necrosis factor-α (TNF-α), and interleukin-9 (IL-9) in the diagnosis of AIN. Urinary TNF-α and IL-9 were highly sensitive and specific in differentiating biopsy-proven AIN from other kidney lesions (in particular, acute

tubular injury/necrosis) diagnosed on kidney biopsy. While these biomarkers are not currently clinically available, they raise the possibility of future noninvasive methods of diagnosing AIN.

Imaging

Kidney ultrasound in the setting of AIN typically shows normal to enlarged kidneys with normal echogenicity. However, these findings are also nonspecific and may be seen with other forms of kidney disease. Although a gallium-67 scan was initially reported as highly sensitive in AIN, this has not been supported over time, and its only role may be to differentiate AIN from acute tubular necrosis (ATN) in those patients who cannot undergo a kidney biopsy. Positron emission tomography has shown diagnostic promise in several AIN cases but needs further evaluation before widespread use.

Pathology

Although suspicion of AIN is based on clinical clues, definitive diagnosis often requires a kidney biopsy. Major pathologic findings include interstitial edema, inflammation, and tubulitis without glomerular or vascular involvement (Fig. 33.2). Interstitial infiltration may be diffuse but is often patchy in nature and consists of lymphocytes, mononuclear cells, eosinophils, neutrophils, and plasma cells. T lymphocytes are primarily composed of CD4 and CD8 cells. The number of eosinophils is highly variable and is more prominent in drug-induced AIN. Granulomas are uncommon but occasionally seen, especially with sarcoidosis and drug-induced AIN. Tubulitis, characterized by the invasion of inflammatory cells through the tubular basement membrane, results in tubular injury and is often seen in association with severe inflammation. The severity of interstitial inflammation, however, does not always correlate with clinical outcome. Poor prognosis is more directly related to the degree of interstitial fibrosis and tubular atrophy. Immunofluorescence and electron microscopic studies are usually unrevealing. NSAID-related AIN is sometimes associated with glomerular features of minimal change disease or membranous nephropathy. In contrast to isolated AIN, full-blown nephrotic syndrome accompanies AKI in NSAID-related cases.

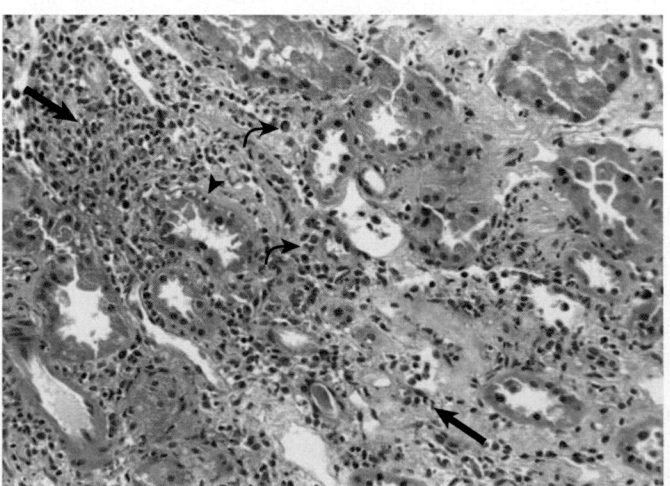

• **Fig. 33.2** Kidney biopsy showing acute interstitial nephritis. A diffuse interstitial infiltrate is present (*arrows*) along with severe tubular injury and tubulitis (*arrowhead*), where lymphocytes have crossed the tubular basement membrane. Also present are eosinophils (*curved arrows*) (hematoxylin and eosin ×40).

Pathogenesis

The clinical and histopathologic findings summarized earlier strongly point to an immune-mediated mechanism initiating and sustaining tubulointerstitial damage. The immunologic basis of injury is supported by the low frequency of AIN in persons exposed to a drug, lack of dose dependency, presence of systemic symptoms in some patients, and recurrence of AIN upon re-exposure. The antigens initiating the immune-mediated injury could be of endogenous origin (Tamm-Horsfall protein, megalin, and tubular base membrane components) or exogenous, such as drugs and chemicals. Exogenous antigens may be trapped directly or may circulate as immune complexes that are deposited in the kidney interstitium. They may bind to a tubular antigen acting as a hapten or mimic a normal tubular or interstitial antigen, thereby triggering an immune reaction. In animal models, both cell-mediated and humoral immunity is involved. The injury is initiated by the presentation of endogenous or exogenous antigens to antigen-presenting lymphocytes, resulting in the activation of T cells. These cells induce differentiation and proliferation of other T cells responsible for delayed hypersensitivity and cytotoxicity. The resultant inflammatory infiltrates within the interstitium produce a variety of fibrinogenic cytokines and chemokines, such as transforming growth factor-β (TGF-β), platelet-derived growth factor-BB (PDGF-BB), epidermal growth factor (EGF), and fibroblast growth factor-2 (FGF-2). The fibroblasts invading the interstitium are the product of epithelial-to-mesenchymal transition. Ultimately, this inflammatory process results in the accumulation of extracellular matrix, interstitial fibrosis, and tubular loss.

NSAID-induced interstitial nephritis appears to have a different mechanism of action. NSAIDs inhibit cyclooxygenase-1 and cyclooxygenase-2, enzymes that catalyze the conversion of arachidonic acid into prostaglandin H2. When this reaction is inhibited, arachidonic acid can then be converted preferentially to leukotrienes through the action of lipoxygenase. This results in an imbalance of inflammatory mediators with an abundance of the proinflammatory leukotrienes and a paucity of prostaglandins, which serve to regulate the inflammatory cascade.

Causes of Acute Interstitial Nephritis

There are multiple causes of AIN, but pharmacologic agents are the most common (Table 33.2). Diagnosis of AIN should trigger a review of the medication list to identify culpable agents and limit further drug exposure. In addition to various drugs, certain infectious agents may induce AIN. Although less common in the antibiotic era, infectious agents must be considered when the clinical scenario is consistent. Finally, systemic diseases, primarily rheumatologic, are associated with the pathologic findings of AIN. These diseases are usually evident from the clinical presentation (Table 33.3).

Drug-Associated Interstitial Nephritis

Antibiotics

β-Lactam Antibiotics

Methicillin and other β-lactam antibiotics are common agents associated with AIN. Methicillin is immunogenic and leads to a hypersensitivity syndrome more often than other drugs, including those in the β-lactam class. The time course is variable, but AIN usually develops 10 to 14 days following drug exposure, unless previous sensitization has occurred. Patients with β-lactam–induced

TABLE 33.2 Common Drugs Associated With Acute Interstitial Nephritis

Drug Class	Examples
Antibiotics	β-lactams, sulfonamides, fluoroquinolones, rifampin, vancomycin, erythromycin, ethambutol, chloramphenicol
Antivirals	Acyclovir, atazanavir, abacavir, indinavir
Analgesics	NSAIDs, selective COX-2 inhibitors
GI medications	PPIs, H2-receptor blockers, 5-aminosalicylates
Anticonvulsants	Phenytoin, carbamazepine, phenobarbital
Diuretics	Hydrochlorothiazide, furosemide, triamterene, chlorthalidone
Anticancer agents	Tyrosine kinase inhibitors, immune-checkpoint inhibitors, B-RAF inhibitors
Others	Allopurinol, Chinese herbs

COX-2, Cyclooxygenase-2; *GI,* gastrointestinal; *NSAIDs,* nonsteroidal antiinflammatory drugs; *PPIs,* proton pump inhibitors.

TABLE 33.3 Common Diseases Associated With Acute Interstitial Nephritis

Bacterial infection	*Legionella, Staphylococcus, Streptococcus, Yersinia*
Viral infection	Hantavirus, CMV, EBV, HIV, herpes simplex, Hep C, SARS-CoV-2 (?)
Autoimmune	Systemic lupus erythematosus, Sjögren syndrome, sarcoidosis, Crohn disease, IgG4 disease
Neoplastic diseases	Lymphoproliferative disorders, plasma cell dyscrasias

CMV, Cytomegalovirus; *EBV,* Epstein-Barr virus; *Hep C,* hepatitis C virus; *HIV,* human immunodeficiency virus.

AIN frequently manifest systemic symptoms of fever, rash, arthralgias, and eosinophilia, along with AKI. These symptoms may be fleeting or nonexistent, making them unreliable clinical tools for diagnosing AIN. Urinalysis and urine microscopy demonstrate low-grade proteinuria, hematuria, and leukocyturia in approximately 75% of cases (see Fig. 33.1). Given its association with AIN, methicillin is rarely used because of the availability of other, less-inciting β-lactam agents. Cephalosporins may cause a similar clinical presentation of AIN; however, this is less common than with traditional penicillins. On withdrawal of the drug, kidney function usually recovers, although CKD may persist in some.

Non β-Lactam Antibiotics

Rifampin-induced AIN can be severe and appears to occur more frequently with intermittent dosing as compared with continuous dosing regimens. AIN develops in a dose-dependent fashion in most but not all patients, and, at times, circulating antibodies to rifampin may be detected. Systemic manifestations include fever, chills, abdominal pain, and myalgia. Laboratory abnormalities include elevated liver transaminases, hemolytic anemia, and thrombocytopenia. Kidney histopathology demonstrates interstitial inflammation with infiltration of mononuclear cells and occasional eosinophils. Tubular epithelial cell injury and tubular necrosis related to vasomotor injury may also occur. Patients with a history of a severe reaction should not be reexposed to the agent, because of the potential risk of hemodynamic collapse.

Sulfonamides are widely used antibiotics associated with kidney injury. When these drugs were introduced in the first half of the 20th century, the most common kidney injury was tubular obstruction from crystalline deposition of insoluble drug and/or metabolite. Currently, AIN is the most common cause of kidney injury reported with these agents. Patients exposed to these drugs often present with an acute hypersensitivity syndrome characterized by fever, rash, and eosinophilia. Patients with human immunodeficiency virus (HIV) infection, kidney transplant recipients, or those with underlying CKD appear to be more susceptible to an allergic reaction, but the increased use of agents such as trimethoprim-sulfamethoxazole in these populations may account for this observation. Patients who are slow acetylators of sulfonamides may be at higher risk because of drug accumulation, even with routine dosing schedules.

Fluoroquinolones, particularly ciprofloxacin, may cause kidney injury by several mechanisms; however, AIN is the most common kidney complication. AIN often presents with a slowly progressive decline in kidney function, despite the absence of a hypersensitivity syndrome. Ciprofloxacin, based on its widespread use, is the most common agent in this class to cause AIN.

Azithromycin, erythromycin, ethambutol, gentamicin, nitrofurantoin, tetracycline, vancomycin, and multiple antiviral agents have all been associated with AIN. No drug is beyond suspicion, and every agent must be considered in the evaluation.

Nonsteroidal Antiinflammatory Agents

Nonsteroidal antiinflammatory agents are widely used by patients, including those with chronic illness and chronic pain. Both NSAIDs and the selective cyclooxygenase-2 (COX-2) inhibitors are associated with AIN. Given the high frequency of NSAID use, AIN remains a relatively rare event, supporting an idiosyncratic drug reaction. NSAIDs cause several kidney syndromes (see Chapter 34), marked by hemodynamic AKI, electrolyte/acid-base disturbances, and nephrotic syndrome. AIN associated with NSAIDs presents more insidiously than that seen with antibiotics. It often occurs months after starting therapy, with an average onset time of 6 to 18 months. Classically, patients do not develop a hypersensitivity syndrome, and fever, eosinophilia, and rash are rare. An interstitial infiltrate, which is less intense and has fewer eosinophils than that seen with other culprit agents, and tubulitis are noted on kidney histopathology. Despite multiple classes of NSAIDs with a variety of chemical structures, the pattern of kidney injury is remarkably similar across all agents, arguing against a single epitope-induced immune response.

Gastrointestinal Agents

PPIs have emerged as the most frequent cause of AIN worldwide. In many countries, these agents are available over the counter, further increasing their use. Since omeprazole became available in the early 1990s, the number of prescriptions for PPIs has continued to increase. The mean time to AIN diagnosis from drug initiation is approximately 11 weeks, although it can occur after months of therapy. Only 10% of patients with PPI-induced AIN will present with the classic hypersensitivity syndrome of fever, rash, and eosinophilia, and, therefore, symptoms are either absent or very mild and nonspecific. Early recognition and treatment of AIN are associated with a relatively good prognosis, and AIN induced by PPIs rarely requires kidney replacement therapy, although CKD may occur in a percentage of these patients. CKD

itself has been implicated as a complication of PPI use, with studies showing a 29% to 50% higher risk of CKD in patients exposed to PPIs.

5-Aminosalicylates are the mainstay of therapy for patients with inflammatory bowel disease. Most patients require long-term treatment and many years of drug exposure. Kidney impairment is rare with these drugs, occurring in 1 in 200 to 500 patients on therapy. A hypersensitivity reaction can occur and cause AIN. In the absence of early recognition, CKD from chronic interstitial fibrosis may develop. This reaction usually occurs within the first year of therapy, but it can develop at any time in a dose-independent fashion.

Diuretics

Diuretic-induced AKI is almost always related to kidney hypoperfusion from decreased intravascular volume. There are, however, multiple case reports of diuretic-induced AIN from furosemide, hydrochlorothiazide, chlorthalidone, and triamterene. AIN is relatively rare, despite widespread use of these drugs. In published reports, most patients experience systemic symptoms, including fever, rash, and eosinophilia, suggesting a hypersensitivity syndrome. Drug discontinuation generally leads to kidney recovery.

Oncologic Agents

Many classic chemotherapeutic agents can cause AKI from acute tubular injury, but in recent years, AIN has also emerged with the increased utilization of immunotherapy. Cancer cells resist the immune system by downregulating surface antigens that would be otherwise detected as foreign by T-cells. They also deactivate T-cells by expressing antigens that bind inhibitory T-cell receptors. Immunotherapy drugs such as pembrolizumab, ipilimumab, and nivolumab, known as *immune-checkpoint inhibitors*, are designed to boost the host's immune T-cells to recognize tumor cells and destroy them. This boosting of immunity, which causes a form of autoimmunity, has been shown to cause AIN and AKI in a small percentage of patients (2%-5%). AIN induced by these drugs has been successfully treated with oral prednisone and cessation of the medication, but decisions on restarting therapy can be complicated if it is the best agent to treat the malignancy. AIN can certainly recur upon reexposure to the drug (23%-40% of patients), so a collaborative plan between the nephrologist and oncologist is required.

Infections

Invasive Infections

In the preantibiotic era, streptococcal and diphtheria infections caused inflammatory reactions in the kidney in the absence of direct tissue invasion. However, infection-related AIN diminished in frequency after antibiotics became readily available. Now, when AKI develops in the setting of an infection treated with antibiotics, the drug is assumed to be the culprit. If AKI persists despite antibiotic withdrawal, an acute postinfectious glomerulonephritis or AIN should be considered.

Tubulointerstitial injury can occur either from direct invasion by an organism, as in pyelonephritis, or indirectly by an immune-mediated mechanism. Unlike AIN, pyelonephritis is usually confined to one pyramid in the kidney. In the setting of urinary obstruction, it becomes more diffuse, resulting in AKI. Although clinical history usually differentiates the two conditions readily, CT imaging showing a wedge-shaped area of inflammation supports a diagnosis of pyelonephritis rather than AIN.

A number of infectious agents have been linked with invasive AIN. These include Epstein-Barr virus (EBV), legionella, mycoplasma, cytomegalovirus (CMV), adenovirus, rickettsial Rocky Mountain spotted fever, babesiosis, and fungal infections. Leptospirosis is a classic example of invasive AIN. The spirochete enters the bloodstream through the skin or mucosa before transiently invading glomerular capillaries and migrating into the tubulointerstitium. Once in this compartment, the organism induces inflammation and direct tubular injury that, over time, manifests as large, edematous kidneys. In addition, ischemic ATN may co-exist with AIN in patients who develop septic shock from overwhelming leptospiral infection. Eradication of infection is associated with recovery of kidney function.

Hantavirus is an RNA virus associated with interstitial edema with infiltration of polymorphonuclear leukocytes, eosinophils, and monocytes. Interstitial hemorrhage accompanies kidney inflammation and is associated with gross or microscopic hematuria. Candidemia has been associated with an interstitial inflammatory reaction initially limited to the kidney cortex. With time, large fungus balls can form, obstruct the collecting system, and cause AKI as a result of obstructive uropathy.

Infection with severe acute respiratory syndrome corona virus 2 (SARS-CoV-2), also known as *COVID-19,* is a described cause of AKI. While critically ill COVID-19 patients develop AKI, often requiring kidney replacement therapy, most do not undergo kidney biopsy. The AKI in some of these cases is characterized by tubular proteinuria (albuminuria/proteinuria ratio of 0.23 ± 20), indicating predominant tubulointerstitial injury. While unknown, it is possible that the virus or medications employed to treat this infection may cause AIN.

Noninvasive Infections

Even without direct invasion of the kidney, infectious agents have been associated with AIN. Historically, streptococcal infections were commonly associated with AIN. The clinical syndrome associated with AIN develops early in the course of infection (9 to 12 days). Given the rapidity with which streptococcal infections are treated currently, infection-related AIN has disappeared as a clinical entity.

Systemic Diseases

The classic lesions of acute tubulointerstitial inflammation may also complicate a variety of systemic diseases. Whereas rheumatologic processes primarily cause immune-mediated glomerular disease, they can also induce AIN. Metabolic diseases and malignancy are also associated with interstitial inflammation and AKI.

Tubulointerstitial Nephritis and Uveitis

Tubulointerstitial nephritis and uveitis (TINU) is a rare condition of unclear etiology that presents most frequently in adolescent girls but may appear in adulthood. Weight loss, fever, anemia, and hyperglobulinemia occur before ocular and kidney manifestations. Fanconi syndrome with glucosuria, proteinuria, and aminoaciduria is the initial kidney manifestation, followed by a tubulointerstitial infiltrate, sometimes with granulomas. Certain infections such as toxoplasmosis, Epstein-Barr infection, and giardiasis have been associated with TINU. However, there is no clearly elucidated immune or genetic cause. Steroids are the mainstay of therapy for both the ocular and kidney manifestations of the disease. Fortunately, the prognosis is good in treated patients.

Immunologic Diseases

The vast majority of rheumatologic conditions complicated by AKI have underlying glomerular disease, from antiglomerular basement membrane (GBM) antibody disease (i.e., Goodpasture disease), immune deposition diseases (lupus or IgA nephropathy among others), or antineutrophil cytoplasmic antibody (ANCA)–related pauci-immune vasculitides. However, there are some rheumatologic ailments, such as Sjögren and sarcoidosis, that may present with tubulointerstitial inflammation in the absence of glomerular involvement. In the right clinical scenario, these causes of AIN should remain high on the differential diagnosis of kidney injury.

Immune-related injury in a transplanted kidney (cellular rejection) manifests primarily as tubulointerstitial inflammation with or without vascular involvement. The workup and classification of this interstitial disease can be found in Chapter 60.

Malignancy

Patients with underlying cancer are at high risk for AKI because of the malignancy itself or therapies used in its management. Primary lymphoma of the kidney is a rare cause of AKI, whereas non-Hodgkin lymphoma and acute lymphoblastic leukemias commonly invade the kidney parenchyma. Although it is seen on rare occasions in Hodgkin lymphoma, infiltrates are usually bilateral and diffuse, and kidneys may appear enlarged on imaging. Multiple myeloma and the plasma cell dyscrasias cause kidney injury when filtered light chains coalesce and obstruct tubular lumens. These obstructive "casts" are accompanied by varying degrees of tubular injury, necrosis, and an interstitial inflammatory reaction on kidney biopsy that resembles classic interstitial nephritis.

Treatment

Treatment of AIN depends on the process that is driving the inflammatory reaction. When the inflammation is associated with an underlying disease such as a malignancy, therapy is directed at the identified cause. In rheumatologic disease, treatment of the inflammatory condition often improves kidney function as well. In the setting of infection-related interstitial nephritis, eradication of the infection is often associated with kidney recovery.

Treatment of drug-induced AIN is more complicated and controversial. The most important intervention is early recognition of disease and its causative agent and drug discontinuation. This can be a complicated endeavor in patients taking multiple essential medications, making it challenging to identify the culprit drug. Careful scrutiny of the medication record for exposure dates and history of previous drug treatment may point to the offending agent. When a drug is suspected, it should be immediately discontinued and replaced, if necessary, with an agent from a different class. A drug-free trial should be undertaken to determine if kidney function recovers without further intervention. If no improvement is noted after a period of observation (3 to 5 days), or if kidney function is declining rapidly, a trial of corticosteroids is reasonable. Prognosis appears to depend on the timing of diagnosis and drug withdrawal. In general, earlier is better, with data supporting a 1- to 2-week time frame. Despite this, a substantial proportion of patients (up to 35%) may develop CKD.

The data published on use of corticosteroids for AIN remain incomplete. Assuming the offending drug is withdrawn, steroids improved the rate of kidney recovery in several small studies (fewer than 20 patients). A review of seven nonrandomized, retrospective studies, including up to 100 patients, showed no benefit of steroids in recovery of kidney function or prevention of CKD. However, many of the retrospective studies were biased against steroids, as more severely affected patients were treated, confounding the results.

Early steroid therapy, initiated 1 to 2 weeks after diagnosis, is more likely to improve kidney function compared with courses started later. In addition, it is reasonable to offer steroids to those with severe AIN, where kidney replacement therapy is or will likely be required in the absence of rapid kidney recovery. Steroid therapy is recommended for 4 to 6 weeks with a slow taper. If there is no substantial improvement in kidney function after 3 to 4 weeks, response is unlikely and steroids should be discontinued.

There are limited data available on other forms of immunosuppression. In a small case series of eight patients, mycophenolate mofetil (MMF) improved or stabilized kidney function in patients with steroid-dependent or steroid-resistant AIN. As a result, MMF may offer an alternative therapy to corticosteroids, but more data are required before this agent can be recommended.

Complete bibliography is available at Elsevier eBooks for Practicing Clinicians.

Key Bibliography

Brewster UC, Perazella MA. Proton pump inhibitors and the kidney: critical review. *Clin Nephrol*. 2007;68:65–72.

Caravaca-Fontán F, Fernández-Juárez G, Praga M. Acute kidney injury in interstitial nephritis. *Curr Opin Crit Care*. 2019;25(6):558–564.

Clarkson MR, Giblin L, O'Connell FP, et al. Acute interstitial nephritis: clinical features and response to corticosteroid therapy. *Nephrol Dial Transplant*. 2004;19:2778–2783.

Cortazar FB, Kibbelaar ZA, Glezerman IG, et al. Clinical features and outcomes of immune checkpoint inhibitor-associated AKI: a multicenter study. *J Am Soc Nephrol*. 2020;31(2):435–446.

Fogazzi GB, Ferrari B, Garigali G, Simonini P, Consonni D. Urinary sediment findings in acute interstitial nephritis. *Am J Kidney Dis*. 2012;60:330–332.

Fernandez-Juarez G, Perez JV, Caravaca-Fontán F, et al. Duration of treatment with corticosteroids and recovery of kidney function in acute interstitial nephritis. *Clin J Am Soc Nephrol*. 2018;13(12):1851–1858.

González E, Gutiérrez E, Galeano C, et al. Early steroid treatment improves the recovery of renal function in patients with drug-induced acute interstitial nephritis. *Kidney Int*. 2008;73:940–946.

Moledina DG, Parikh CR. Differentiating Acute interstitial nephritis from acute tubular injury: A challenge for clinicians. *Nephron*. 2019;143(3):211–216.

Moledina DG, Perazella MA. Drug-induced acute interstitial nephritis. *Clin J Am Soc Nephrol*. 2017;12(12):2046–2049.

Moledina DG, Wilson FP, Pober JA, et al. Urine TNF-alpha and IL-9 for clinical diagnosis of acute interstitial nephritis. *JCI Insight*. 2019;4(10):e127456.

Muriithi AK, Nasr SH, Leung N. Utility of urine eosinophils in the diagnosis of acute interstitial nephritis. *Clin J Am Soc Nephrol*. 2013;8:1857–1862.

Oliva-Damaso N, Oliva-Damaso E, Payan J. Acute and chronic tubulointerstitial nephritis of rheumatic causes. *Rheum Dis Clin North Am*. 2018;44(4):619–633.

Perazella MA. Clinical approach to diagnosing acute and chronic tubulointerstitial disease. *Adv Chronic Kidney Dis*. 2017;24(2):57–63.

Perazella MA, Bomback AS. Urinary eosinophils in AIN: farewell to an old biomarker? *Clin J Am Soc Nephrol*. 2013;8:1841–1843.

Perazella MA, Markowitz GS. Drug-induced acute interstitial nephritis. *Nat Rev Nephrol*. 2010;6:461–470.

Praga M, González E. Acute interstitial nephritis. *Kidney Int*. 2010;77:956–961.

Preddie DC, Markowitz GS, Radhakrishnan J, et al. Mycophenolate mofetil for the treatment of interstitial nephritis. *Clin J Am Soc Nephrol*. 2006;1:718–722.

Raghavan R, Eknoyan G. Acute interstitial nephritis—a reappraisal and update. *Clin Nephrol*. 2014;82:149–162.

Rubin S, Orieux A, Prevel R, et al. Characterization of acute kidney injury in critically ill patients with severe coronavirus disease 2019. *Clin Kidney J*. 2020;13(3):354–361.

Spanou Z, Keller M, Britschgi M, et al. Involvement of drug-specific T cells in acute drug-induced interstitial nephritis. *J Am Soc Nephrol*. 2006;17:2919–2927.

PART 6

Drugs and the Kidney

34

Kidney Disease Caused by Therapeutic Agents

MARK A. PERAZELLA, ANUSHREE C. SHIRALI

Medications are an essential intervention to provide appropriate patient care, and new agents are being introduced into clinical practice at a rapid pace. Although most drugs are well tolerated, kidney injury remains an unfortunate and relatively frequent adverse consequence. Some kidney toxicity is idiosyncratic, while some individuals possess risk factors that predispose them to these syndromes. Not unexpectedly, the general population is regularly exposed to various diagnostic and therapeutic agents with nephrotoxic potential. Although most are prescribed, many other preparations are purchased over the counter. Drugs fall into the categories of diagnostic agents, therapeutic medications, alternative or complementary substances, and drugs of abuse, resulting in a variety of kidney syndromes (Table 34.1).

Kidney Susceptibility to Nephrotoxic Agents

In addition to clearance of endogenous waste products, excretion of sodium and water, electrolyte and acid-base balance, and endocrine activity, the kidney is responsible for the metabolism and excretion of exogenously administered drugs, making it susceptible to various types of injury. There are several factors that increase the kidney's susceptibility to these potential toxins, which can be classified into three simple categories: drug-related factors, kidney-related factors, and host-related factors. Furthermore, these often occur in combination to promote nephrotoxicity, and explain much of the variability and heterogeneity of drug-related kidney disease noted among patients.

Drug-related factors are the critical first step to the development of nephrotoxicity. Innate drug toxicity is important because the drug or its toxic metabolite may cause kidney injury by impairing kidney hemodynamics, direct cellular injury, osmotic injury, or intratubular crystal deposition, to name a few mechanisms. Large doses, extended drug exposure, and nephrotoxic drug combinations further enhance nephrotoxicity.

The kidney's handling of drugs also determines why certain agents cause nephrotoxicity. As kidney blood flow approximates 25% of cardiac output, the kidney is significantly exposed to nephrotoxic drugs. Kidney injury is increased in the loop of Henle where high metabolic rates coexist with a relatively hypoxic environment. Increased drug/metabolite concentrations in the kidney medulla also contribute to direct toxicity. Kidney drug metabolism from cytochrome P450 (CYP450) and other enzymes increases local toxic metabolite and reactive oxygen species (ROS) formation, which promote injury via nucleic acid oxidation/alkylation, DNA-strand breaks, lipid peroxidation, and protein damage.

The kidney pathway of excretion for many therapeutic agents involves proximal tubular cells. Extensive drug trafficking through the cell via luminal and basolateral transporters can lead to cellular injury. Some drugs are endocytosed at the luminal membrane of cells, whereas other drugs are transported into the cell via basolateral ion transporters. Such drug transport can be associated with increased cellular concentrations that injure mitochondria, phospholipid membranes, lysosomes, and other organelles.

Nonmodifiable factors such as older age and female sex increase nephrotoxic risk through reduced total body water leading to more frequent misdosing of drugs. Unrecognized reduced glomerular filtration rate (GFR) and hypoalbuminemia, which result in increased toxic drug concentration, also enhance risk. Pharmacogenetic differences likely explain much of the variable response of patients to drugs. Liver and kidney CYP450 enzyme gene polymorphisms are associated with reduced metabolism and end-organ toxicity. Polymorphisms of genes encoding proteins involved in the metabolism and kidney elimination of drugs are correlated with nephrotoxic risk. In addition, a highly variable host immune response to drugs may play a role; one patient reacts with a heightened allergic response, whereas another has a limited reaction with no kidney lesion. Thus, innate host response genes tend to determine the drug reaction.

Kidney susceptibility to drug injury is also enhanced by true or effective volume depletion, including nausea/vomiting, diarrhea, and diuretic therapy on the one hand, and heart failure, liver disease with ascites, and sepsis on the other. This physiology enhances the nephrotoxicity of drugs that are excreted primarily by the kidney, drugs reabsorbed/secreted by the proximal tubule, and drugs that are insoluble in the urine. Nephrotoxic risk is also increased in patients with acute kidney injury (AKI) or chronic kidney disease (CKD) because of a lower number of functioning nephrons, reduced drug clearance, and a robust kidney oxidative response to drugs and metabolites. Finally, electrolyte and acid-base disturbances present in some patients also contribute to host susceptibility to drug injury.

Kidney Injury Associated With Medications

Therapeutic agents associated with kidney injury can be classified based on the category of the agent or the clinical kidney syndrome. Recognizing that all drugs cannot be covered in this chap-

TABLE 34.1	Drug-Induced Clinical Kidney Syndromes
Kidney Syndrome	**Causative Agents**
Acute Kidney Injury	
Prerenal	Cyclosporine, tacrolimus, radiocontrast, AmB, ACE inhibitors, ARBs, NSAIDs, interleukin-2, exenatide
Intrarenal	
Vascular disease	Gemcitabine, anti-VEGF drugs, propylthiouracil, interferon
ATN	AGs, AmB, cisplatin, tenofovir, ifosfamide, pemetrexed, polymyxins, vancomycin, pentostat, zoledronate, warfarin
AIN	Immune checkpoint inhibitors, penicillins, cephalosporins, sulfonamides, rifampin, NSAIDs, interferon, ciprofloxacin, many others
Crystalline nephropathy	Methotrexate, acyclovir, sulfonamides, indinavir, atazanavir, darunavir, ciprofloxacin, sodium phosphate
Osmotic nephropathy	IVIG, HES, dextran, mannitol
Postrenal	Methysergide, drug-induced stones, alpha-agonists
Proteinuria	Gold, NSAIDs, anti-VEGF drugs, penicillamine, interferon, pamidronate
Tubulopathies	AGs, tenofovir, cisplatin, ifosfamide, AmB, pemetrexed, cetuximab
Nephrolithiasis	Sulfadiazine, atazanavir, indinavir, darunavir, topiramate, zonisamide
CKD	Li+, analgesic abuse, cyclosporine, tacrolimus, cisplatin, nitrosourea

ACE, Angiotensin-converting enzyme; *AmB,* Amphotericin B; *AIN,* acute interstitial nephritis; *AGs,* aminoglycosides; *ARBs,* angiotensin receptor blockers; *ATN,* acute tubular necrosis; *CKD,* chronic kidney disease; *HES,* hydroxyethyl starch; *IVIG,* intravenous immune globulin; *Li+,* lithium; *NSAIDs,* nonsteroidal antiinflammatory drugs; *VEGF,* vascular endothelial growth factor.

ter, we describe drug-induced nephrotoxicity by drug category and highlight the clinical kidney syndrome and the segment of nephron injury by the drug within each category. Drug-induced acute interstitial nephritis (AIN) (see Chapter 33) and CKD (see Chapter 35) are discussed elsewhere in the *Primer*.

Diagnostic Agents

Radiocontrast Agents

Contrast-associated AKI (CA-AKI) is a relatively common cause of hospital-acquired AKI. It is defined by an absolute or percentage rise in serum creatinine from the baseline within 48 to 72 hours of exposure. In general, serum creatinine begins to rise within the first 24 hours of administration, peaks between 2 and 5 days, and returns to baseline by 7 to 14 days. The incidence of CA-AKI depends on the definition used and the population studied, ranging from 5% to 40%, and the course varies depending on the overall patient risk profile. The increased number of imaging studies and percutaneous procedures with radiocontrast throughout the past decade and the ever-enlarging population of patients with underlying CKD have resulted in a rise in the incidence. Patients with CKD stage 4 or greater have the highest risk of CA-AKI.

Radiocontrast media may injure the kidney via several mechanisms. First, vasoactive substances such as adenosine and endothelin mediate vasoconstriction of the afferent arterioles, thereby reducing kidney blood flow and promoting kidney medullary ischemia. Second, kidney epithelial cell necrosis also occurs with isoosmolar radiocontrast agents because their high viscosity causes sluggish blood flow through the peritubular capillaries and promotes hypoxic kidney injury. Lastly, radiocontrast causes direct renal tubular toxicity through hyperosmolar injury, which results in vacuolization of proximal tubular cells, and oxidative stress from free oxygen radicals with associated tubular cell apoptosis and necrosis.

The level of kidney function at the time of exposure is one of the most important determinants of the risk for CA-AKI. In addition, patient-specific risk factors include older age, volume depletion, congestive heart failure, diabetic kidney disease, both hypertension and hypotension, and anemia. Intraaortic balloon pumps are associated with increased AKI risk primarily because they are a surrogate for severe cardiac disease, tenuous cardiac output, and kidney hypoperfusion. Emergent procedures increase risk because of reduced use of contrast prophylaxis and increased severity of patient illness. The type, volume, and route of contrast administration also affect CA-AKI risk. With regard to radiocontrast type, osmolality and viscosity are the two most important characteristics. The osmolality of a solution varies significantly from high-osmolar contrast media (HOCM) to low-osmolar media (LOCM) to isoosmolar media (IOCM). Viscosity, another contrast property, varies from one product to the next, does not correlate with osmolality, and may be associated with CA-AKI. For example, IOCM solutions are about twice as viscous as LOCM products despite having a lower osmolality.

The incidence of CA-AKI is higher with HOCM than with LOCM, and the relative risk is doubled in CKD patients. As a result, LOCM and IOCM agents have replaced HOCM. A meta-analysis of 16 randomized, controlled trials suggested a benefit of using IOCM instead of LOCM, with the relative risk reduction of CA-AKI greatest in CKD patients. The maximum increase in serum creatinine was less in CKD patients given IOCM compared with LOCM. However, a randomized trial comparing IOCM with LOCM noted no significant difference in CA-AKI incidence. Thus, the benefits of low osmolality may be counterbalanced by the detrimental properties of high viscosity, making these agents equal in their risk for CA-AKI. A larger volume of contrast increases CA-AKI, with a recommended upper limit of 150 mL for patients with a serum creatinine 1.5 to 3.4 mg/dL and maximum dose of 100 mL recommended for patients with a creatinine greater than 3.4 mg/dL. The smallest contrast volume required to perform the procedure should be used. Risk of CA-AKI is highest with intraarterial injection, with the intravenous (IV) route presenting a much lower risk. Coronary angiography has an even higher CA-AKI risk than other arterial studies, likely due to the underlying comorbidities of the patient. CKD outpatients have a low CA-AKI risk with nonemergent computed tomography (CT) scans. In fact, an eGFR greater than 30 mL/min per 1.73 m^2 is not considered a substantial risk for CA-AKI in patients dosed by the IV route.

Measures to reduce kidney injury should be undertaken in patients at higher risk for CA-AKI. In addition to limiting the contrast load and using either IOCM or nonionic LOCM, the most important intervention is IV fluid administration. Studies have uniformly demonstrated the benefit of prophylactic isotonic fluids administered both before and after radiocontrast administration.

Because urinary alkalinization is hypothesized to reduce kidney oxidative stress, IV sodium bicarbonate has been studied and initially showed promise. The PRESERVE study, a randomized, controlled trial of IV sodium bicarbonate versus isotonic saline prophylaxis in 4993 relatively high-risk patients exposed to intraarterial contrast, showed no difference in outcomes between the two forms of volume repletion (sodium bicarbonate, 4.4% vs. isotonic saline, 4.7%). Thus, isotonic saline is preferable for radiocontrast prophylaxis due to its low cost and avoidance of the need for pharmacy compounding. For outpatient studies, oral fluids with salt tablets before exposure may provide adequate volume expansion to prevent CA-AKI in CKD, but this approach has not been extensively examined.

N-acetylcysteine (NAC) is an antioxidant that has been used for CA-AKI prevention. However, the Acetylcysteine for Contrast-Induced Nephropathy Trial showed no benefit with NAC in 2308 patients randomized to NAC vs. placebo (the proportion developing CA-AKI was 12.7 among both NAC and placebo recipients). The PRESERVE trial also showed no benefit with NAC prophylaxis (NAC, 4.6% vs. placebo, 4.5%), confirming NAC offers no protection against CA-AKI. In regard to other medications, it is reasonable to avoid nonsteroidal antiinflammatory drugs (NSAIDs) and other potential nephrotoxins before radiocontrast exposure. Regarding renin-angiotensin-aldosterone system (RAAS) blockers, some studies note increased CA-AKI risk, whereas others show nephroprotection. An individualized approach is required for the RAAS blockers prior to contrast exposure.

Based on its size, lack of protein binding, and small volume of distribution, radiocontrast is efficiently removed with hemodialysis (HD). In fact, approximately 80% is removed over 4 hours with a high-flux dialyzer. HD following radiocontrast exposure to prevent CA-AKI, especially in patients with advanced CKD, has been examined in several studies. Although all HD studies have been negative, one small study demonstrated that prophylactic HD in CKD stage 5 patients reduced the need for an acute and chronic dialysis requirement after discharge. Hemofiltration performed 4 to 6 hours before and 18 to 24 hours after contrast reduced the incidence of CA-AKI, in-hospital events, need for acute dialysis, and both in-hospital and 1-year mortality. In contrast, the hemofiltration postprocedure alone offered no benefit beyond standard prophylaxis. A systematic review of 11 studies with 1010 patients concluded that one or more sessions of HD, hemofiltration, or hemodiafiltration performed after contrast administration did not reduce the incidence of CA-AKI or the need for acute or chronic dialysis. Examination of HD and hemofiltration/hemodiafiltration separately shows that HD is associated with increased CA-AKI risk, whereas hemofiltration/hemodiafiltration did not affect the occurrence of CA-AKI but did reduce the receipt of acute dialysis. Therefore, HD and hemodiafiltration are not recommended as a prophylactic measure for CA-AKI.

Gadolinium-Based Contrast Agents

Gadolinium-based contrast agents (GBCAs) were considered a safe and effective diagnostic agent, revolutionizing the world of imaging. However, over time, it became clear that GBCAs were not risk free. Rare reports of AKI surfaced, primarily in patients with underlying kidney disease who received large doses via direct arterial injection. However, GBCA-induced AKI is rare and typically of minor severity, likely caused by the small volume of contrast required for imaging.

GBCAs began to be used widely for imaging patients with kidney disease in the early to mid-1990s as an alternative to radiocontrast.

However, nephrogenic systemic fibrosis (NSF), a severe and largely irreversible sclerosing condition of skin, joints, eyes, and internal organs, was first noted as a complication of GBCAs in 2006. Two factors were required for the development of NSF: GBCA exposure and underlying kidney disease. Certain linear GBCAs (gadodiamide, gadoversetamide, gadopentetate), which were considered unstable, were the primary agents associated with NSF. Other factors that likely further increased the risk for NSF included infection, inflammation, vascular disease, hypercoagulability, hypercalcemia, hyperphosphatemia, erythropoiesis-stimulating agent (ESA), and iron therapy.

The GBCAs were recently categorized into three groups (group I: gadodiamide, gadoversetamide, gadopentetate dimeglumine; group II: gadoterate meglumine, gadobutrol, gadoteridol, gadobenate dimeglumine; and group III: gadoxetate disodium) by the American College of Radiology. Group I GBCAs have the highest risk and have been essentially eliminated from clinical use in the United States. The group II GBCAs, which have been shown to be a safer GBCA option, are now employed. In a 2019 systematic review and meta-analysis of 4931 group II GBCA administrations in patients with CKD stage 4 or 5 (eGFR <30 mL/min/1.73 m^2), the risk of NSF was 0% (0 cases in 4931 subjects). Importantly, 732 CKD stage 5 and 1849 CKD stage 5D patients were included in this study. While these data are reassuring, it is premature to assume no risk.

The best approach to preventing NSF is as follows. High-risk patients should be considered for imaging options such as non-GBCA MR imaging, CT scan, ultrasonography, and other techniques that will provide equivalent diagnostic results. When a GBCA is necessary to make the diagnosis, a group II GBCA with the lowest dose required to obtain a diagnostic image should be used. It is also helpful to extend the time between GBCA studies. In AKI and ESKD patients on hemodialysis, schedule dialysis to follow the GBCA exposure.

Therapeutic Agents

Analgesics

NSAIDs, including selective cyclooxygenase-2 (COX-2) inhibitors, are widely used to treat pain, fever, and inflammation, and are available by prescription or over the counter. Annually, more than 50 million patients in the United States ingest these drugs on an intermittent basis, whereas 15 to 25 million people use NSAIDs daily.

NSAIDs and selective COX-2 inhibitors are associated with various clinical kidney syndromes (Box 34.1). It has been estimated that 1% to 5% of patients who ingest NSAIDs develop some form of nephrotoxicity, perhaps representing as many as 500,000 persons in the United States alone. These adverse effects are caused primarily by prostaglandin (PG) inhibition; however, other effects are idiosyncratic. PGs are produced by COX enzyme metabolism and are secreted locally in the kidney to modulate the effects of various systemic and local substances. For example, PGs enhance afferent arteriolar vasodilatation in the presence of vasoconstrictors such as angiotensin-II, norepinephrine, vasopressin, and endothelin, thereby providing critical counterbalance to the vasoconstriction that predominates in hypovolemic states. Patients with decreased true or effective circulating volume are at highest risk to develop renal vasoconstriction and reduced GFR. Because CKD is a PG-dependent state, these patients are also at higher risk for NSAID-induced kidney injury. In fact, exposure to NSAIDs doubles the risk of hospitalization for AKI in patients with CKD. Similar rates of AKI with NSAID exposure are noted in the elderly, those with cardiac disease, and patients receiving angiotensin-converting enzyme (ACE) inhibitors. As noted in a nested case-control study, the adjusted relative risks of AKI were 4.1 and 3.2 in current NSAID users versus nonusers in the general population, respectively. Patients with hypertension, heart failure, and diuretic therapy had an adjusted relative risk of 11.6 with addition of NSAIDs.

In addition to increasing arteriolar blood flow, PGs also enhance kidney sodium, potassium, and water excretion. PGs modulate kidney potassium excretion through stimulation of the RAAS. Inhibition of PGs can result in hyperkalemia when coexistent conditions such as AKI, CKD, diabetes mellitus, and therapy with certain medications (RAAS blockers, potassium-sparing diuretics) are also present. The classic syndrome of hyporeninemic hypoaldosteronism with hyperkalemic metabolic acidosis (type IV renal tubular acidosis) can be observed with NSAID therapy. Inhibition of PGs is associated with decreased kidney sodium excretion, and all NSAIDs cause some degree of sodium retention. This is especially common in patients with hypertension, heart disease, and other salt-retentive disease states (e.g., cirrhosis, nephrotic syndrome, AKI, and CKD) who are at highest risk for developing edema, hypertension, or heart failure. Hypertension is a particularly important complication, as small changes in blood pressure are associated with increased cardiovascular events. Hyponatremia from impaired water excretion also complicates therapy as PGs act to antagonize water reabsorption in the distal nephron, an effect that is lost with NSAIDs. Reduced GFR also contributes to water retention and hyponatremia.

Idiosyncratic effects of selective and nonselective NSAIDs include proteinuric glomerular diseases. Minimal change disease (MCD) is most common, whereas membranous nephropathy is a relatively rare complication of these drugs. Nephrotic-range proteinuria or full-blown nephrotic syndrome is the typical clinical presentation, sometimes accompanied by AKI. NSAID-induced AIN can occur alone or along with these glomerular diseases.

Chemotherapeutic Agents

Chemotherapeutic agents are critical to halting or slowing tumor growth, but adverse kidney effects often complicate treatment. They are most commonly associated with AKI, but also cause electrolyte and acid-base disturbances, proteinuria, and hypertension.

Antiangiogenesis Drugs

Antiangiogenesis drugs target vascular endothelial growth factor (VEGF) or its tyrosine kinase receptor (VEGF-R). VEGF signaling is critical to tumor angiogenesis, and disruption of the signaling pathways provides novel treatment options for aggressive malignancies. However, VEGF function is also essential to renal microvasculature, peritubular, and glomerular integrity. Podocytes provide local VEGF to glomerular endothelial cells, preserving the integrity of the fenestrated endothelium. Loss of VEGF promotes endothelial dysfunction and injury. A reduction in podocyte-synthesized VEGF by pharmacologic VEGF inhibition or genetic ablation decreases local inhibitory complement factor H and other complement regulators in the glomerulus, increasing susceptibility to complement activation and development of thrombotic microangiopathy (TMA). In animals, pharmacologic reduction in VEGF production or effect causes proteinuria, hypertension, and TMA by damaging the renal microvasculature, in particular, the glomerular endothelium. A similar clinical syndrome marked by proteinuria (rarely nephrotic) and hypertension occurs in patients treated with antiangiogenesis agents such as bevacizumab and the tyrosine kinase inhibitors. TMA is the most common pathologic lesion noted in patients taking these medications who undergo kidney biopsy for AKI (Fig. 34.1). Importantly, nearly 50% of the reported cases of anti-VEGF therapy-related TMA is kidney limited with no systemic findings.

Interferon

Interferon (α, β, γ) is described as causing glomerular injury and proteinuria. Early reported cases showed minimal change lesions, but more recent reports describe collapsing and noncollapsing focal segmental glomerulosclerosis (FSGS) on biopsy. Patients tend to present with nephrotic-range proteinuria and/or AKI within weeks of commencing interferon therapy. The time to clinical presentation is shorter for interferon-α as compared to other subtypes. Although proteinuria declines with cessation of interferon therapy, complete reversal is uncommon. The mechanism underlying interferon-associated glomerular injury is not entirely clear, but it may include

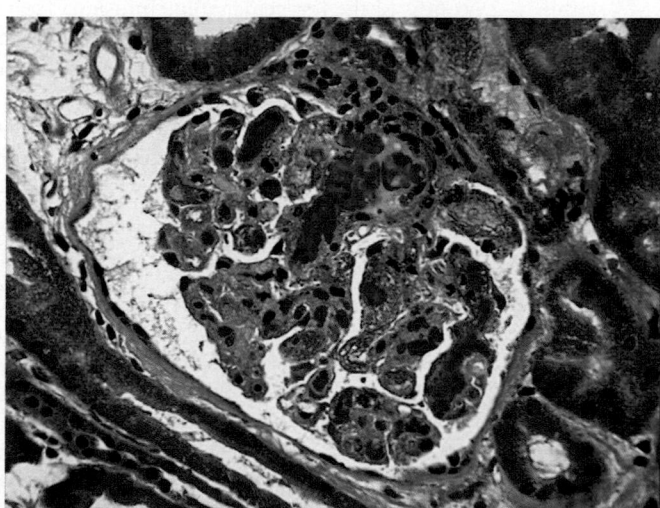

• **Fig. 34.1** Thrombotic microangiopathy as manifested by mesangiolysis, endothelial denudation, red blood cell congestion, and basement membrane duplication in the glomerulus on light microscopy. (Courtesy Michael Kashgarian, Yale University.)

direct binding to podocyte receptors and alteration of normal cellular proliferation. Other postulated effects include macrophage activation and skewing of the cytokine profile toward IL-6 and IL-13, which are purported permeability factors in MCD and FSGS.

Bisphosphonates

The bisphosphonates are effective treatments for malignancy-related bone disorders such as multiple myeloma, hypercalcemia of malignancy, and osteolytic metastases. They are also commonly used in Paget disease and osteoporosis. One of their major adverse effects is nephrotoxicity, seen primarily with pamidronate and zoledronate. Nephrotoxicity is more common with high-dose IV formulations than the oral or low-dose IV preparations used in osteoporosis treatment. Depending on the particular bisphosphonate, glomerular and/or tubular injury may result. Pamidronate-induced kidney injury is dose related, where high dosage and long duration increase risk. Nephrotoxic manifestations include nephrotic-range proteinuria or nephrotic syndrome associated with collapsing FSGS or MCD, consistent with a toxic podocytopathy. Acute tubular necrosis (ATN) may also accompany collapsing FSGS. Nephrotoxicity is sometimes reversible, but progressive CKD and end-stage kidney disease (ESKD) requiring chronic dialysis may develop. IV zoledronate is more commonly associated with AKI from ATN, although rare cases of FSGS are described. Current evidence suggests that ibandronate has the least nephrotoxicity. Because bisphosphonates undergo kidney excretion, prevention of nephrotoxicity hinges on dose reduction in patients with reduced GFR, with clinical guidelines recommending discontinuation of therapy when estimated GFR falls to less than 30 mL/min.

Gemcitabine

Gemcitabine is an effective antineoplastic agent that is associated with AKI from TMA. This lesion is a rare complication with an incidence of 0.015%–0.31%. However, development of TMA with this drug is associated with a high mortality rate (40%–90%). TMA develops when the median cumulative gemcitabine dose exceeds 20,000 mg/m², but may occur at lower doses when combined with mitomycin. In general, most patients develop TMA within 1–2 months of the last gemcitabine infusion. Treatment includes drug discontinuation and supportive care. Plasma exchange is not beneficial, but case reports/series suggest that complement inhibition may be useful for gemcitabine-associated TMA. Correction of hematologic abnormalities and kidney function improvement were observed with eculizumab in some patients who failed drug withdrawal and plasmapheresis.

Platinum Compounds

Platinum-based agents are potent antineoplastic drugs that have a high incidence of nephrotoxicity, particularly in patients with CKD. Nonoliguric AKI from toxic ATN is the most common pattern of kidney injury. Cisplatin has the most nephrotoxic potential, although second- and third-generation drugs such as carboplatin and oxaliplatin are also nephrotoxic at high doses. Cisplatin's mechanism of nephrotoxicity is related to its drug characteristics and kidney handling. Chloride at the *cis*-position of the molecule promotes kidney injury, whereas its uptake into proximal tubular cells via OCT-2 also contributes to damage. Other mechanisms of injury are activation of intracellular injury pathways, inflammation, oxidative stress, and vascular injury. The end result is renal tubular

cell apoptosis or necrosis, manifesting as clinical AKI and/or a tubulopathy. Platinum drugs are also associated with Fanconi syndrome from proximal tubular injury, and sodium-wasting syndrome and hypomagnesemia from cellular injury in the loop of Henle.

In high-risk patients, carboplatin and oxaliplatin are used based on their less nephrotoxic profile. Neither of these molecules is transported by OCT-2, thereby reducing proximal tubular intracellular concentrations. In addition, the chloride at the *cis*-position in cisplatin is replaced by carboxylate and cyclobutane in carboplatin and oxaliplatin, respectively, which may further reduce toxicity. Antioxidants such as sodium thiosulfate and amifostine have been proposed as prophylactic measures against platinum nephrotoxicity, but concerns of decreased anticancer activity and adverse effects limit their utility. Prevention of platinum nephrotoxicity focuses on volume expansion with IV saline administration and avoidance of other nephrotoxins.

Ifosfamide

Ifosfamide is an alkylating agent derived from the parent molecule cyclophosphamide. In contrast to cyclophosphamide, ifosfamide causes renal tubular injury primarily through its nephrotoxic metabolite, chloroacetaldehyde. In addition, ifosfamide enters tubular cells via OCT-2, whereas cyclophosphamide does not. Nephrotoxic manifestations include tubulopathies such as isolated proximal tubular injury, Fanconi syndrome, nephrogenic diabetes insipidus (DI), and AKI from ATN, which is often reversible but can be permanent. Tubular cell injury and necrosis with swollen, dysmorphic mitochondria are noted on kidney histopathology. Risk factors for kidney injury include previous cisplatin exposure, cumulative dose greater than 90 g/m², and underlying CKD.

Preventive measures are limited. IV saline and dose reduction are used. Because this agent is transported into cells via OCT-2, competitive inhibition of this pathway with cimetidine is being evaluated. Treatment is supportive, addressing electrolyte disorders and monitoring for CKD and dialysis-requiring ESKD. Other long-term complications include permanent proximal tubulopathy and isolated phosphaturia.

Pemetrexed

Pemetrexed is a methotrexate derivative that inhibits enzymes involved in purine and pyrimidine metabolism, impairing RNA and DNA synthesis in tumors. It is excreted unchanged by the kidneys, although pemetrexed enters the proximal tubular cell via luminal and basolateral pathways. Luminal drug uptake may occur via the folate receptor-α transport pathway, whereas basolateral entry is by the reduced folate carrier. Intracellular pemetrexed is polyglutamylated, which traps the drug within the cell. The higher intracellular drug concentration more fully impairs RNA and DNA synthesis and causes cell injury. Reversible AKI occurs with high-dose therapy, with kidney lesions consisting of ATN and AIN. Tubular dysfunction consisting of nephrogenic DI and distal renal tubular acidosis occurs. Most patients present with AKI and minimal proteinuria, which stabilizes with drug discontinuation but can lead to CKD from chronic tubulointerstitial nephritis.

Epidermal Growth Factor Receptor Antagonists

Monoclonal antibodies that antagonize epithelial growth factor receptor (EGFR) signaling, including cetuximab and panitumumab, offer promising biologic therapy for colorectal and head and neck tumors. Given the role of EGFR signaling in magnesium homeostasis, these antibodies induce kidney magnesium wasting. The EGFR signaling cascade is necessary for activation of transient receptor potential M6 (TRPM6), the epithelial channel in the distal nephron that facilitates magnesium reabsorption. Monoclonal antibodies against EGFR, which have a much higher affinity for EGFR than epidermal growth factor (EGF), potently inhibit placement of TRPM6 in the luminal membrane and prevent luminal magnesium reabsorption. The incidence of hypomagnesemia approaches 43% with cetuximab in clinical trials, whereas nearly all patients develop some reduction in serum magnesium level. Thus, serum magnesium monitoring should be a standard of care with anti-EGFR therapy. Panitumumab causes hypomagnesemia less commonly. The likelihood of hypomagnesemia increases with duration of therapy and may persist for several weeks after drug discontinuation before resolving. Treatment requires IV magnesium repletion, particularly in cancer patients who tend to have diarrhea, vomiting, and decreased oral intake. Because secondary hypokalemia and hypocalcemia occur with hypomagnesemia, serum potassium and calcium concentrations should be monitored and repletion undertaken when these electrolyte disorders are present.

Immune Checkpoint Inhibitors

Immune checkpoint inhibitors (CPIs) are monoclonal antibodies that prevent the function of immune "checkpoints" that suppress adaptive immune responses. T cells possess surface receptors such as programmed death-1 protein (PD-1) and cytotoxic T lymphocyte-associated antigen-4 (CTLA-4), which bind to their cognate ligands on antigen-presenting cells and inhibit T cell activation. This normally suppresses the development of autoimmunity, though various tumors overexpress ligands that bind these inhibitory T cell receptors. This leads to a decrease of infiltrating activated T cells within the tumor microenvironment and inhibits antitumor T cell responses, resulting in enhanced tumor survival. To combat this, monoclonal antibodies that block ligand binding to PD-1 and CTLA-4 receptors were designed to facilitate T cell rescue and restore antitumor immunity. Ipilimumab (anti-CTLA-4) and the anti-PD-1 drugs nivolumab and pembrolizumab are such examples. However, one concern of blocking immune checkpoints is the potential for pathologic autoimmunity and end-organ injury.

In fact, this concern has been realized in the kidney. The reported incidence of AKI associated with the CPIs varies from 2% to 5%, highest with combination therapy. In addition to other end-organ autoimmune effects, biopsy-proven AIN, some with granulomatous changes, has been observed with these drugs (see Table 34.1). Glomerular lesions such as minimal change disease, focal segmental glomerulosclerosis, and IgA nephropathy have been less frequently described with currently available CPIs. A multi-center cohort study of 138 patients treated with CPIs that developed AKI noted AIN in 93% of 60 biopsied patients. There is no consistent clinical manifestation of drug nephrotoxicity except AKI, though rare presentations of rash and eosinophilia may occur. Urinalysis and urine microscopy have inconsistently shown findings of pyuria, hematuria, and low-grade proteinuria to support a diagnosis of AIN, and kidney biopsy remains necessary for definitive diagnosis. A small number of cases have required dialysis. Most cases respond to drug discontinuation and steroid therapy, with courses as long as 8 to 12 weeks due to the drugs' long half-life and frequent relapse of AIN. However, CKD is seen in a small number of patients. Rechallenge with a CPI following

an episode of AKI is associated with recurrence in approximately one-quarter of patients. Thus, patients should be monitored closely when rechallenged with a CPI.

Several mechanisms of CPI-induced AIN have been postulated. First, inhibition of the CTLA-4 and PD-1 pathways can lead to autoimmunity. As shown in murine models, checkpoint receptor signaling promotes tolerogenic dendritic cells while blunting self-reactive T cells. With genetic deletion of murine PD-1, glomerulonephritis develops, supporting a role for checkpoint signaling in minimizing T cell–mediated kidney inflammation. Alternatively, because patients treated with CPIs are often also on other drugs associated with AIN, disruption of checkpoint signaling that may be critical to maintaining peripheral self-tolerance to these other drug antigens may permit reactivation of exhausted drug-specific T cells previously primed by nephritogenic drugs. Suddenly, because of loss of tolerance, T cells are activated against the other drug. Ultimately, CPI therapy may promote a permissive environment for effector T cells to migrate into the kidney and cause an inflammatory response leading to AIN.

CAR-T Cell Therapy

The newest form of immunotherapy to reach clinical practice is chimeric antigen receptor (CAR)-T cells, which are patient-derived cytotoxic T cells that have been engineered ex vivo with tumor antigen-specific receptors to allow targeted killing of cancer cells. At present, CAR-T cells with antigen specificity for B cell leukemias and lymphomas are approved for clinical use, but trials are underway for other hematologic malignancies and potentially for treatment of solid tumors. The receptors on CAR-T cells are synthetic antibody molecules with an extracellular domain that recognizes peptides unique to tumor cells and intracellular signaling and costimulatory domains that allow expansion of these T cells, particularly in the presence of cytokines such as interleukin (IL)-2. Once CAR-T cells are infused back into the lymphodepleted patient, they have the potential of recognizing antigen on tumor cells to facilitate tumor cell lysis and cytokine production. These events are critical to tumor killing but have the risk of systemic adverse effects, including nephrotoxicity. In particular, *cytokine release syndrome* (CRS) refers to the clinical syndrome of high fever, myalgias, and vasodilatory shock that accompanies the release of inflammatory mediators such as IL–6, IL-10, and interferon-gamma (IFN-γ) upon CAR-T infusion and tumor cell death. Similar to cytokine storm with IL-2 therapy for renal cell carcinoma that historically resulted in volume depletion and hypotension due to severe third spacing, there has been concern that CRS may result in AKI in the prerenal-to-ATN spectrum. Additionally, tumor lysis with standard chemotherapy can cause AKI via a variety of mechanisms, highlighting another potential way in which CAR-T therapy may result in nephrotoxicity. Early data suggest a high prevalence of AKI, from 3%–21.7%, depending on tumor type and grade of AKI. There are no biopsy data from these studies; but, on clinical criteria, decreased kidney perfusion and ATN appear to be the most common reasons for AKI. Electrolyte abnormalities have also been mentioned, including hyponatremia, hypokalemia, and hypophosphatemia, suggesting that TLS seen with standard chemotherapy may not be the dominant mechanism of kidney injury with CAR-T therapy. Importantly, in these studies, most patients with AKI due to CAR-T therapy quickly recovered kidney function. As CAR-T therapy increases in use, particularly in patients with more comorbidities and underlying CKD, we may see greater and sustained nephrotoxicity.

BRAF Inhibitors

Targeting mutations in cancer cells is an effective strategy to combat various malignancies. Melanoma frequently has a BRAF V600 mutation that can be targeted by the selective BRAF inhibitors vemurafenib and dabrafenib. Patient survival has increased with this class of anticancer drugs. However, nephrotoxicity has also been observed in treated patients. A decline in GFR at 1 and 3 months of therapy in 15/16 patients (five with proteinuria) was noted and was complicated by persistent kidney injury after 8 months of follow-up (no kidney histology). Another series of eight patients treated with vemurafenib developed AKI, with acute tubular injury seen on kidney biopsy in one patient. AKI in another four patients treated with vemurafenib was described. All had skin rash and two had eosinophilia suggestive of AIN, but no kidney tissue was obtained. Three of four patients recovered kidney function following drug discontinuation.

A retrospective study of 74 patients exposed to vemurafenib over 3 years described AKI, primarily Kidney Disease: Improving Global Outcomes (KDIGO) stage 1 (80%), in 44 patients. AKI developed within 3 months of drug exposure and 80% recovered kidney function within 3 months of drug discontinuation. Kidney biopsy revealed tubulointerstitial injury in two patients. Examination of the FDA Adverse Events Reporting System over 3 years for BRAF inhibitor nephrotoxicity revealed evidence for nephrotoxicity. The major adverse effect following treatment with vemurafenib was AKI ($n = 132$), with a small number of cases of hyponatremia and hypokalemia. For dabrafenib, 13 cases of AKI, six cases of hyponatremia, and two cases of hypokalemia were noted over slightly more than a year of reporting. Unfortunately, data on proteinuria and histology were not available from these patients.

The mechanism of kidney injury with BRAF inhibitors is unknown; they may interfere with the downstream mitogen-activated protein kinase (MAPK) pathway, increasing kidney susceptibility to ischemic tubular injury.

Antimicrobial Agents

Several widely prescribed antimicrobial medications can result in kidney injury, especially in hospitalized patients. Antimicrobial agents are administered to the most severely ill patients who have coexistent processes that can independently affect kidney function and potentiate nephrotoxicity.

Antibiotics

Aminoglycosides

AGs are frequently associated with kidney injury in hospitalized patients. The reported incidence ranges between 7% and 36% of patients receiving these drugs, increases with the duration of drug administration, and may approach 50% with more than 2 weeks of therapy. AGs are freely filtered by the glomerulus and then reabsorbed by proximal tubular cells. Ultimately, kidney excretion is the major route of elimination. Their cationic and amphophilic properties enhance binding to the luminal membrane of proximal tubular cells, likely via the megalin-cubilin receptor, and lead to accumulation of drug within cortical tubular cells. Nephrotoxicity tracks with charge; the more cationic, the more likely the drug interacts with luminal membranes where they undergo endocytosis and accumulate within intracellular lysosomes. Myeloid (or myelin) bodies (Fig. 34.2) visualized on electron microscopy

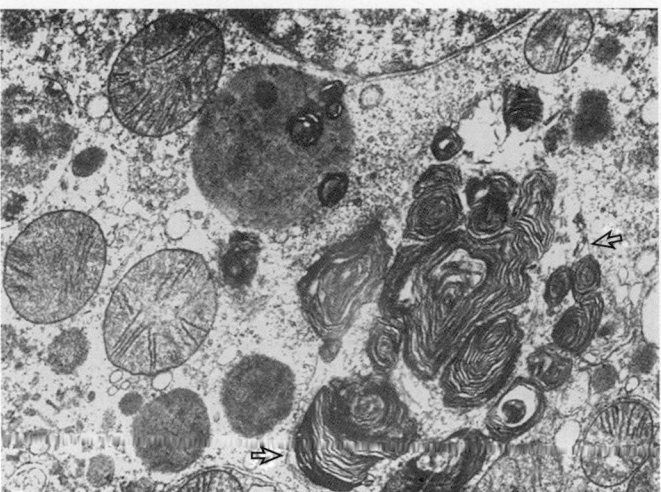

• **Fig. 34.2** Aminoglycoside-induced tubular cell injury manifested by myeloid (myelin) bodies *(arrows)* as seen on electron microscopy. These bodies represent changes in tubular lysosomes caused by the accumulation of polar lipids. (Courtesy Gilbert W. Moeckel, Yale University.)

often develop. These structures are membrane fragments and damaged organelles that result from inhibition of lysosomal enzymes. Nephrotoxicity occurs from mechanisms such as disruption of subcellular organelle activity, induction of oxidative stress, and enhanced mitochondrial dysfunction.

AG nephrotoxicity presents clinically as a rising serum creatinine after approximately 5 to 7 days of therapy, but may occur earlier in the presence of risk factors. AKI is often preceded by a concentrating defect. Low-grade proteinuria and urine sediment containing renal tubular epithelial (RTE) cells or granular casts are seen days before clinical AKI, supporting ongoing subclinical kidney injury. Tubular dysfunction is manifested by an elevated fractional excretion of sodium (>1% to 2%), and urinary potassium, calcium, and magnesium wasting. Gentamicin has been described as causing a proximal tubulopathy or full-blown Fanconi syndrome in some patients, whereas a Bartter-like syndrome has also been noted. The latter lesion is speculated to occur from the activation of the calcium-sensing receptor by cationic gentamicin, thereby inhibiting the $NKCC^-$ transporter in the loop of Henle. AKI progressively worsens, but the course may be limited in severity with early drug discontinuation. Nevertheless, a time lag may occur before kidney function improves.

Several risk factors for AG nephrotoxicity have been identified (Box 34.2). This allows, when alternative antibiotics are unavailable, more intensive monitoring and modification of risk factors, such as volume depletion and electrolyte abnormalities. All members of the AG family can cause nephrotoxicity, but tobramycin exhibits less nephrotoxicity than gentamicin in animal models.

Tailoring AG doses to maintain drug levels within the therapeutic range minimizes nephrotoxicity while maintaining bactericidal drug concentrations. When calculating doses, it should be recognized that changes in the serum creatinine often underestimate the true GFR reduction in elderly, cirrhotic, and malnourished patients. In addition to appropriate dose reduction, single daily-dose regimens may reduce AG nephrotoxicity because tubular absorption is saturable, although the data are mixed. Monitoring of peak and trough drug levels, along with serum creatinine concentration, every 2 to 3 days is prudent, but daily monitoring may be required in patients with serious infections and unstable

BOX 34.2

Risk Factors for Aminoglycoside Nephrotoxicity

- Prolonged course of treatment (>10 days)
- Volume depletion
- Sepsis
- Preexisting kidney disease
- Hypokalemia
- Advanced age
- Combination therapy with certain cephalosporins, particularly cephalothin
- Concomitant exposure to other nephrotoxins (e.g., radiocontrast, amphotericin B, cisplatin)
- Exposure to gentamicin > amikacin > tobramycin

kidney function. Urine microscopic findings may identify kidney injury before changes in serum creatinine.

Vancomycin

Vancomycin is a widely prescribed and typically well-tolerated drug. Although AKI rarely occurs as a complication, two lesions have been classically described. One is an idiosyncratic reaction resulting in AIN, and the other is direct tubular toxicity that occurs with excessive serum concentrations. Kidney biopsies in patients with AKI associated with toxic vancomycin concentrations have demonstrated primarily toxic ATN rather than classic AIN. However, another form of kidney injury, coined *vancomycin cast nephropathy* was described in a series of patients with excessive serum vancomycin levels. The casts contained vancomycin and uromodulin and generated a cellular reaction akin to light chain cast nephropathy. Although an animal model confirmed the findings, confirmation by another group in humans is required before this lesion is accepted. High dose and longer drug exposure are likely risk factors for AKI. More recently, numerous epidemiologic studies have noted a higher incidence of AKI associated with the combination of vancomycin plus piperacillin-tazobactam as compared with vancomycin alone or combined with other antibiotics. This finding remains even after controlling for several potentially confounding variables and risk factors of AKI. Unfortunately, kidney biopsy was not obtained in these patients to help understand the potential mechanism of increased nephrotoxicity. As of now, it is unclear if this is another form of toxic ATN, AIN, or cast nephropathy.

Polymyxins

The polymyxins are a group of antibiotics generally reserved for resistant organisms, primarily because of their high nephrotoxic potential. Colistin and polymyxin B are the two agents that are employed as antimicrobials. Both have a narrow therapeutic window with nephrotoxicity related to their D-amino content and fatty acid component. This increases tubular cell membrane permeability and the influx of cations, resulting in tubular cell injury. Patients with underlying risk often develop AKI within 5–7 days. The risk for AKI is dose dependent and increases with a longer duration of therapy. Drug discontinuation is required in 21%, and up to 28% require dialysis.

Sulfonamides

Sulfa-based antibiotics are effective antimicrobial agents that can cause three distinct kidney lesions: AIN, crystalline nephropathy, and vasculitis. AIN is most common, whereas crystal-induced AKI occurs primarily with high-dose sulfadiazine (and with other sulfonamides to a lesser degree). Vasculitis is probably the least common sulfonamide-related kidney lesion, typically a hypersensitivity reaction that rarely is associated with development of polyarteritis nodosa. The incidence of AKI ranges from 0.4% to 29%. Crystal-induced kidney injury occurs when insoluble sulfa drug precipitates within the tubular lumen of the distal nephron. Because sulfa drugs are weak acids, this is more likely to happen in an acidic urine (pH <6.0), when urine flow rates are low, with hypoalbuminemia, and with excessive dose for the level of GFR.

Although patients are generally asymptomatic, vague abdominal or flank pain along with an increasing serum creatinine and oliguria occur within 7 days of starting therapy. Urine microscopy reveals strongly birefringent sulfonamide crystals (e.g., shocks of wheat and shells), sometimes admixed with white blood cells, RTE cells, and granular casts. Rarely, small radiolucent calculi may also lodge in the kidney parenchyma and/or calyces and appear as layered clusters of echogenic material on kidney ultrasonography. Treatment includes IV fluids, urinary alkalinization, and sulfonamide dose reduction or discontinuation.

Ciprofloxacin

The quinolone antibiotic ciprofloxacin is widely used to treat numerous bacterial infections. As noted with other antibiotics, ciprofloxacin causes AKI in patients primarily through the development of AIN. Experimental studies have demonstrated crystalluria following the administration of ciprofloxacin. Less commonly, this drug can be associated with crystal-induced AKI in humans. Ciprofloxacin is insoluble at neutral or alkaline pH (pH >7.3), and it crystallizes in alkaline urine. Intrarenal crystallization may result from excessive drug doses in patients with advanced age, underlying CKD, volume depletion, and/or alkaline urine. Patients are generally asymptomatic, and the first sign of kidney injury is a rise in serum creatinine after 2 to 14 days of treatment. Urine microscopy shows ciprofloxacin crystals, which appear as strongly birefringent needles, sheaves, stars, fans, butterflies, and other unusual shapes, along with other cellular elements and casts. Kidney biopsy reveals crystals within the tubules. To avoid this complication, ciprofloxacin should be dosed appropriately for the level of kidney function. To prevent AKI and crystalluria, patients receiving ciprofloxacin should be aggressively volume repleted, and alkalinization of the urine should be avoided. Treatment of kidney injury is drug discontinuation or dose reduction, and volume repletion with isotonic IV fluids.

Antiviral Drugs

Acyclovir

Acyclovir is an effective antiviral agent that is widely used to treat herpes virus infections. Although generally safe, it can cause AKI from intratubular crystal deposition when administered intravenously, particularly at high doses. Acyclovir is excreted in the urine through both glomerular filtration and tubular secretion. Acyclovir is relatively insoluble in the urine, which accounts for its intratubular precipitation at high concentration or with low urine flow rates, resulting in intrarenal urinary obstruction. Isolated crystalluria and asymptomatic AKI are most common, but nausea/vomiting and flank/abdominal pain may occur. Crystalline nephropathy typically develops within 24 to 48 hours of acyclovir administration, with an incidence of 12% to 48% when acyclovir is administered as a rapid IV bolus. In contrast, low-dose IV and oral acyclovir therapy rarely cause AKI unless there is severe volume depletion or underlying kidney disease. Urine microscopy usually shows both hematuria and pyuria, along with birefringent, needle-shaped crystals. Prevention hinges on avoiding rapid bolus infusion of acyclovir and by maintaining adequate intravascular volume and urine flow rates during drug exposure. Dose reduction is critical in patients with underlying kidney disease. HD removes significant amounts of acyclovir and is sometimes indicated with severe AKI and concomitant neurotoxicity. Fortunately, most patients recover kidney function with acyclovir discontinuation and volume resuscitation.

Indinavir, Atazanavir, and Darunavir

Indinavir, atazanavir, and darunavir are protease inhibitors used in the treatment of human immunodeficiency virus (HIV) infection. Indinavir revolutionized HIV care, but its use was complicated by a number of toxicities including crystal-induced AKI and nephrolithiasis. Atazanavir has gained widespread use, and it is also associated with crystal-related kidney injury and nephrolithiasis. More recently, darunavir has been added to the armamentarium and has been rarely associated with crystalluria, nephrolithiasis, and crystalline nephropathy.

The kidney clears approximately 20% of indinavir, and intratubular crystal precipitation occurs at urine pH above 5.5 (Fig. 34.3). Intrarenal tubular obstruction and obstructing calculi can also lead to AKI. Complications include kidney colic, dysuria, back/flank pain, or gross hematuria, with an 8% incidence of urologic symptoms. Urine microscopy shows crystals of varying shapes, including plate-like rectangles, fan-shaped crystals, and starburst forms. Although most cases of indinavir-associated AKI are mild and reversible, more severe AKI from obstructing calculi and CKD occurs. Prevention of intrarenal crystal deposition requires intake of 2 to 3 L of fluid per day. Patients with liver disease should receive a dose reduction. Discontinuation of indinavir generally reverses nephrotoxicity; however, chronic tubulointerstitial fibrosis has been noted.

Atazanavir has chemical characteristics and pharmacokinetics similar to indinavir, likely explaining its nephrotoxicity. Crystalline nephropathy, nephrolithiasis, and AIN have been described. Thirty cases of atazanavir-associated nephrolithiasis have been reported to the FDA, whereas another study estimated a 0.97% prevalence of atazanavir stones among those taking the drug. Analysis of kidney stones shows 60% atazanavir metabolite and 40% calcium apatite. Atazanavir-associated crystalline nephropathy has also been described, where rod-like atazanavir crystals were noted on urine

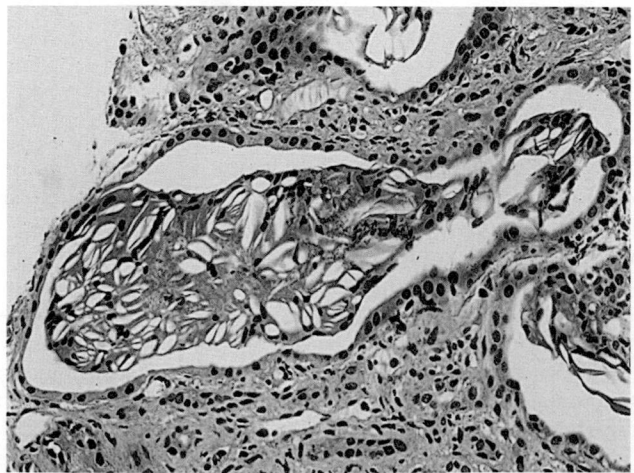

• **Fig. 34.3** Indinavir crystal deposition within renal tubular lumens causes acute and chronic kidney injury, an entity coined *crystalline nephropathy*, as seen on light microscopy. (Courtesy Glen S. Markowitz, Columbia University.)

microscopy and within tubular lumens on kidney biopsy. Prevention is best achieved by avoiding intravascular volume depletion. Treatment hinges on volume resuscitation and stone removal when indicated. Drug discontinuation is sometimes necessary.

Darunavir combined with ritonavir has been associated with increased urinary darunavir levels, with levels 13 times higher in the urine than the plasma. Four of 51 patients treated with darunavir/ritonavir had urinary crystals, which contained darunavir (7.8%). The incidence of nephrolithiasis was lower with darunavir/ritonavir than atazanavir/ritonavir, which resulted in the recommendation of its use in patients at risk for CKD. Finally, intratubular crystals and crystals within tubular cell cytoplasm were observed on light microscopy and within lysosomes on electron microscopy in a patient with darunavir-associated AKI.

Tenofovir Disoproxil Fumarate

Tenofovir disoproxil fumarate (TDF) is an agent used to treat various viral infections, including HIV and hepatitis B virus, and as prophylaxis following exposure. TDF is a prodrug that is metabolized to the active drug, tenofovir diphosphate, which accumulates within renal tubular cells. Animal models note that tenofovir diphosphate causes proximal tubular dilatation, abnormalities in mitochondrial ultrastructure, depleted mitochondrial DNA (mtDNA), and depressed respiratory chain enzyme expression. Clinically, patients present with AKI or a proximal tubulopathy and, less commonly, with nephrogenic DI. AKI may require temporary dialysis, although a degree of kidney recovery often results in CKD. Kidney histology from patients with clinical nephrotoxicity demonstrates proximal tubular injury and varying degrees of chronic tubulointerstitial scarring. On light microscopy, prominent eosinophilic inclusions within proximal tubular cell cytoplasm represent giant, abnormal mitochondria. On electron microscopy, injured mitochondria vary from small and rounded to swollen with irregular contours.

Host factors that potentiate TDF nephrotoxicity include the HIV-infected host's mtDNA depletion, reduced GFR, and genetic defects in drug excretion pathways. TDF is eliminated by a combination of glomerular filtration and proximal tubular secretion, which, in part, explains its compartmental toxicity. It is transported from the basolateral circulation into proximal tubular cells via organic ion transporter-1 (OAT-1), and it is subsequently translocated into the urine through luminal efflux transporters such as multidrug resistance proteins (MRP-2/-4). Reduced GFR enhances the amount of drug that is secreted, increasing traffic through proximal tubular cells. Impaired MRP-driven efflux activity can reduce drug secretion and increase intracellular concentrations. A single nucleotide polymorphism (SNP) in the MRP-2 efflux transporter gene (ABCC2) has been documented in HIV-infected patients with tenofovir-induced nephrotoxicity.

Prevention of and monitoring for tenofovir-related kidney injury are important. Genetic risk factor testing (SNP in ABCC2 gene) to identify high-risk patients and targeted interventions such as probenecid to reduce OAT-1–mediated drug transport into tubular cells may reduce toxicity. Avoidance of tenofovir in patients with advanced CKD, or at least appropriate dose reduction, further reduces nephrotoxicity.

Tenofovir alafenamide fumarate (TAF) is a prodrug that is structurally similar to TDF but contains different lipophilic groups that confer increased stability of the prodrug in plasma. This characteristic allows TAF to enter target cells in prodrug form, prior to conversion into metabolically active tenofovir diphosphate. As a result, the concentration of metabolically active tenofovir diphosphate increases within target cells, while plasma concentrations remain low. Reduced plasma levels result in less tubular exposure to tenofovir diphosphate. In addition, TAF does not interact with OAT-1 transporters, further reducing intracellular accumulation of TAF and potential cytotoxicity. In addition, metabolism of TAF into tenofovir diphosphate is primarily by intracellular lysosomal serine protease cathepsin A.

Phase 1, 2, and 3 trials have shown that TAF has an equivalent or enhanced antiviral potency, similar safety profile, and an early signal for better kidney tolerance than TDF. A multi-center, open-labeled, randomized trial that evaluated the efficacy of virologic suppression in patients with normal baseline kidney function who were switched from a TDF-based to a TAF-based regimen favored TAF. However, a case report described a high-risk HIV-infected patient treated with TAF who developed dialysis-requiring AKI that resolved following TAF cessation, suggesting that TAF is not entirely without risk, at least in those with concomitant risk factors for kidney injury.

Antifungal Agents

Amphotericin B

Amphotericin B is a polyene antibiotic used in treatment of many serious fungal infections, but it is also associated with nephrotoxicity. The degree of kidney injury is roughly proportional to the total cumulative dose. Because this drug is highly bound to cell membranes, it damages membrane integrity and increases permeability. Membrane injury is thought to underlie development of the characteristic clinical syndromes of potassium and magnesium wasting, inability to maximally concentrate urine, and distal tubule acidification defects. These abnormalities, along with urine microscopy findings with RTE cells/casts and granular casts, usually precede the development of clinically apparent AKI. Amphotericin B also produces acute afferent arteriolar vasoconstriction, causing a hemodynamic reduction in the GFR. Tubuloglomerular feedback triggered by increased sodium permeability has been suggested as playing a role in vasoconstriction.

Reduced kidney function is frequently nonoliguric and progressive, but slowly abates after drug discontinuation. However, high doses and repetitive drug exposure can cause CKD. Volume depletion potentiates nephrotoxicity, whereas sodium loading and volume expansion can ameliorate kidney injury, perhaps by blunting tubuloglomerular feedback. Risk factors for kidney injury include a high cumulative dose, prolonged duration of therapy, intensive care unit admission when therapy is initiated, and cyclosporine therapy. Several formulations of amphotericin B in lipid vehicles, including liposomes, have been developed for clinical use and result in fewer constitutional symptoms while retaining antifungal activity. Studies have shown that these formulations are less nephrotoxic, but they can still cause AKI in high-risk patients.

Miscellaneous

Anticoagulant-Related Nephropathy

A little-known complication of warfarin and other anticoagulants is AKI from severe glomerular bleeding and obstructing red blood cell (RBC) casts. This entity was initially termed *warfarin nephropathy* but can occur with any form of excessive anticoagulation in at-risk patients. It has been described in patients with and without CKD who are overanticoagulated with warfarin or other oral anticoagulants. The mechanism appears to be related to glomerular hemorrhage with subsequent obstruction of tubules by RBC casts. Tubular obstruction and/or heme-related tubular injury from lysosomal overload and oxidative damage are thought to play a role. Hemoglobin may enter cells

via megalin-cubilin receptor-mediated endocytosis, with free hemoglobin promoting lipid peroxidation and heme/iron-generating ROS, mitochondrial damage, and apoptosis. Treatment consists of reversal of anticoagulation initially, followed by more judicious anticoagulation in those who truly require it. Unfortunately, many patients are left with CKD, sometimes requiring chronic dialysis.

Osmotic Agents

Osmotic nephropathy refers to kidney injury seen when certain macromolecules enter proximal tubular cells through the luminal membrane. First described in animal studies, sucrose infusion was associated with tubular cell swelling and kidney dysfunction. Similar histopathology and kidney injury have been described with mannitol, dextran, and, more recently, with IV immune globulin (IVIG) and hydroxyethyl starch (HES). Tubular injury begins with drug entry into the tubular cell, followed by accumulation within lysosomes causing tubular epithelia to swell and form vacuoles. This process ultimately disrupts cellular integrity and, if tubular swelling is severe, obstructs tubular lumens and impedes urine flow, causing AKI. Kidney biopsy shows characteristic histopathologic lesions such as swollen, edematous tubules filled with cytoplasmic vacuoles, which represent swollen lysosomes on electron microscopy (Fig. 34.4). With severe injury, tubules may appear degraded, similar to ischemic or toxic ATN.

Osmotic nephropathy is most commonly associated with IVIG stabilized with sucrose and HES. IVIG-related osmotic nephropathy occurs in patients with underlying kidney disease and advanced age. Nonsucrose formulations of IVIG have not been linked to AKI and, thus, are preferred for high-risk patients. HES is a potent volume expander with an amylopectin chain with hydroxyethyl substitutions of varying degrees. Systemic degradation of HES allows glomerular filtration of the smaller HES molecules that enter proximal tubular cells. Similar to sucrose, HES-induced kidney injury has histopathologic features typical of osmotic nephropathy, including tubular cell swelling and vacuolization. Clinically, HES is associated with AKI, sometimes requiring dialysis, especially in patients with sepsis and underlying kidney disease. Prevention is based on avoiding these agents in

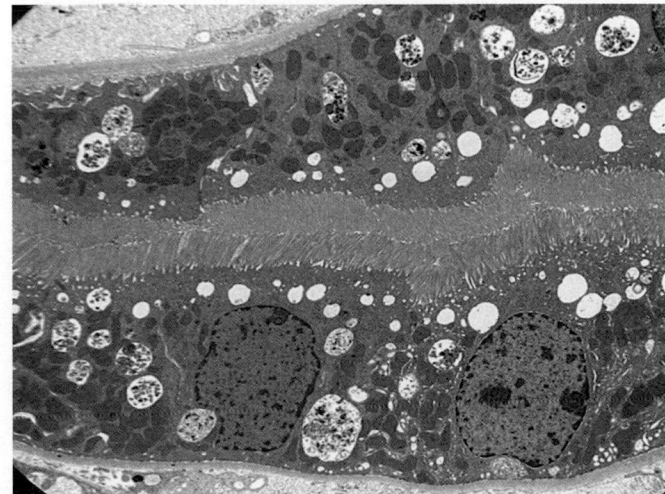

• **Fig. 34.4** Uptake of osmotic substances such as sucrose, hydroxyethyl starch, dextran, and radiocontrast causes acute and chronic tubular injury, an entity known as *osmotic nephropathy*. Electron microscopy demonstrates characteristic cytoplasmic vacuoles. (Courtesy Gilbert W. Moeckel, Yale University.)

high-risk patients, whereas therapy for osmotic nephropathy is supportive with avoidance of further exposure.

The SGLT2 inhibitors are important therapies to prevent progression of CKD. Multiple randomized, controlled trials confirm this beneficial effect without evidence to support increased AKI. However, the FDA Adverse Events Reporting System describes AKI as a relatively frequent event. In addition, there are published case reports of AKI from these drugs. It is likely that the rise in serum creatinine reflects the hemodynamic effects of tubuloglomerular feedback and/or RAS blockade or volume depletion from concurrent diuretic effects. Osmotic nephropathy, observed on light microscopy (dilated proximal tubular cells with numerous vacuoles) and electron microscopy (large lysosomal vacuoles with amorphous debris), has been described in a few cases of severe AKI (one requiring dialysis). Importantly, no other cause for osmotic nephropathy was noted. Induction of severe glucosuria with reabsorption of glucose in the S3 segment by SGLT2 is speculated as the cause of the lysosomal accumulation with vacuolization and cell swelling. As such, patients who develop AKI in the setting of SGLT2 therapy who do not recover after 5-7 days should undergo kidney biopsy to definitively establish the cause of AKI.

Lithium

Lithium (Li$^+$) is one of the most effective medications for the treatment of bipolar disorders, making it a cornerstone of therapy despite its various toxicities. Li$^+$ adversely affects several organ systems, including the kidney, which excretes this cation. Although several kidney syndromes occur, the most common complication is nephrogenic DI. This condition develops in as many as 20% to 30% of patients and is a result of kidney resistance to the actions of antidiuretic hormone (ADH). ADH resistance reduces water permeability in the distal nephron through inhibition of the generation or action of cyclic adenosine monophosphate (cyclic-AMP). This decreases expression and attenuates luminal targeting of aquaporin-2 water channels in tubular epithelial cells. Although polyuria generally improves with Li$^+$ withdrawal, amiloride therapy can further reduce urine volume by antagonizing epithelial sodium channels, which may be useful in patients who must continue on Li$^+$.

Acute Li$^+$ intoxication can occur with intentional overdose or in patients on stable dose who suffer an acute decline in GFR. It is manifested by symptoms ranging from nausea and tremor to seizures and coma. In addition, AKI can occur. The severity of intoxication generally correlates with serum Li$^+$ concentrations. Along with gastric lavage and polyethylene glycol, IV saline is used to reverse volume depletion and induce diuresis, thereby facilitating Li$^+$ excretion. In patients with AKI or CKD, significant neurologic symptoms, and Li$^+$ levels greater than 4.0 mEq/L, HD should be pursued. HD efficiently clears Li$^+$, where a 4-hour treatment can reduce plasma levels by about 1 mEq/L.

Long-term Li$^+$ therapy can cause chronic tubulointerstitial nephritis, characterized by tubular atrophy and interstitial fibrosis, with cortical and medullary tubular microcysts. Rarely, patients develop high-grade proteinuria and FSGS. Although kidney function may improve after drug cessation, irreversible CKD and ESKD may be observed.

Proton Pump Inhibitors

Proton pump inhibitors (PPIs) are a class of drugs that are widely used worldwide, and have emerged as one of the most common

causes of AIN. Recently, PPI exposure has been associated with increased risk for CKD. If this is a true PPI complication, CKD may be due to unrecognized and untreated AIN. However, this area remains unclear and needs further study. Chapter 33 describes the nephrotoxic effects of PPIs in more detail.

Complete bibliography is available at Elsevier eBooks for Practicing Clinicians.

Key Bibliography

Baker M, Perazella MA. NSAIDs in CKD: are they safe? *Am J Kidney Dis.* 2020;76(4):P546–P557. doi:10.1053/j.ajkd.2020.03.023.

Calza L, Sachs M, Colangeli V, et al. Prevalence of chronic kidney disease among HIV-1-infected patients receiving a combination antiretroviral therapy. *Clin Exp Nephrol.* 2019;23(11).1272–1279.

Cortazar FB, Kibbelaar ZA, Glezerman IG, et al. Clinical features and outcomes of immune checkpoint inhibitor-associated AKI: a multicenter study. *J Am Soc Nephrol.* 2020;31(2):435–446.

Davenport MS, Perazella MA, Yee J, et al. Use of intravenous iodinated contrast media in patients with kidney disease: consensus statements from the American College of Radiology and the National Kidney Foundation. *Radiology.* 2020;294(3):660–668.

Davis J, Desmond M, Berk M. Lithium and nephrotoxicity: a literature review of approaches to clinical management and risk stratification. *BMC Nephrol.* 2018;19(1):305–311.

Ermina V, Jefferson A, Kowalewska J, et al. VEGF inhibition and renal thrombotic microangiopathy. *N Engl J Med.* 2008;358:1129–1136.

Gupta S, Seethapathy H, Strohbehn IA, et al. Acute kidney injury and electrolyte abnormalities after chimeric antigen receptor T-cell (CAR-T) therapy for diffuse large B-cell lymphoma. *Am J Kidney Dis.* 2020;76(1):63–71.

Izzedine H, Harris M, Perazella MA. The nephrotoxic effects of HAART. *Nat Rev Nephrol.* 2009;5:563–573.

Perazella MA. Drug-induced acute kidney injury: diverse mechanisms of tubular injury. *Curr Opin Crit Care.* 2019;25(6):550–557.

Perazella MA. Pharmacology behind common drug nephrotoxicities. *Clin J Am Soc Nephrol.* 2018;13(12):1897–1908.

Perazella MA. Advanced kidney disease, gadolinium and nephrogenic systemic fibrosis: the perfect storm. *Curr Opin Nephrol Hypertens.* 2009;18:519–525.

Perazella MA, Moeckel GW. Nephrotoxicity from chemotherapeutic agents: clinical manifestations, pathobiology and prevention/therapy. *Semin Nephrol.* 2010;30:570–581.

Perazella MA, Shirali AC. Immune checkpoint inhibitor nephrotoxicity: what do we know and what should we do? *Kidney Int.* 2020;97(1):62–74.

Rosner MH, Perazella MA. Acute kidney injury in patients with cancer. *N Engl J Med.* 2017;376(18):1770–1781.

Seethapathy H, Zhao S, Chute DF, et al. The incidence, causes, and risk factors of acute kidney injury in patients receiving immune checkpoint inhibitors. *Clin J Am Soc Nephrol.* 2019;14(12):1692–1700.

Sury K, Perazella MA. The changing face of human immunodeficiency virus-mediated kidney disease. *Adv Chronic Kidney Dis.* 2019;26(3):185–197.

Shirali AC, Perazella MA, Gettinger S. Association of acute interstitial nephritis with programmed cell death 1 inhibitor therapy in lung cancer patients. *Am J Kidney Dis.* 2016;68:287–291.

Weisbord SD, Gallagher M, Jneid H, et al. PRESERVE trial group. outcomes after angiography with sodium bicarbonate and acetylcysteine. *N Engl J Med.* 2018;378(7):603–614.

Woolen SA, Shankar PR, Gagnier JJ, et al. Risk of nephrogenic systemic fibrosis in patients with stage 4 and 5 chronic kidney disease receiving a group II gadolinium-based contrast agent: a systematic review and meta-analysis. *JAMA Int Med.* 2019:E1–E8.

35

Principles of Drug Therapy in Patients With Decreased Kidney Function

THOMAS D. NOLIN

Decreased kidney function may be observed in many settings, including patients with chronic kidney disease (CKD), the elderly with age-related decline in glomerular filtration rate (GFR), and patients with acute kidney injury (AKI). In adults, these conditions are associated with high medication use, making these patients particularly vulnerable to the accumulation of a drug or its active or toxic metabolites. Clinicians must have a thorough understanding of the impact of decreased kidney function on drug disposition and the appropriate methods by which to individualize drug therapy as they strive to optimize the outcomes of their patients.

Individualization of therapy for those agents that are predominantly (>70%) eliminated unchanged by the kidney can be accomplished with a proportional dose reduction or dosing-interval prolongation based on the fractional reduction in GFR or its more commonly evaluated clinical counterparts, creatinine clearance (CL_{CR}) and estimated GFR (eGFR). However, decreased kidney function is associated with progressive alterations in the bioavailability, plasma protein binding, distribution volume, and nonrenal clearance (CL_{NR}; i.e., metabolism and transport) of many drugs. Thus, a more complex adjustment scheme may be required for medications that are extensively metabolized by the liver or for which changes in protein binding and/or distribution volume have been noted. Patients with decreased kidney function may also respond to a given dose or serum concentration of a drug (e.g., phenytoin) differently from those with normal kidney function because of the physiologic and biochemical changes associated with progressive CKD.

Using a sound understanding of basic pharmacokinetic principles, the pharmacokinetic characteristics of a drug, and the pathophysiologic alterations associated with decreased kidney function, clinicians can design individualized therapeutic regimens. This chapter describes the influence of decreased kidney function resulting from CKD and, when information is available, from AKI on drug absorption, distribution, metabolism, transport, and excretion. A practical approach to drug-dosage individualization for patients with decreased kidney function and those receiving continuous kidney replacement therapy (CKRT), peritoneal dialysis, or hemodialysis is provided.

Drug Absorption

There is little quantitative information about the influence of decreased kidney function in CKD patients on drug absorption.

Several variables, including changes in gastrointestinal transit time and gastric pH, edema of the gastrointestinal tract, vomiting and diarrhea, and concomitant administration of phosphate binders, have been associated with alterations in the absorption of some drugs, such as digoxin and many of the fluoroquinolone antibiotics. The fraction of a drug that reaches the systemic circulation after oral versus intravenous administration (termed *absolute bioavailability*) is rarely altered in CKD patients. However, alterations in the peak concentration (C_{max}) and in the time to which the peak concentration is attained (t_{max}) have been noted for a few drugs, suggesting that the rate, but not the extent of absorption, is altered. Although the bioavailability of some drugs, such as furosemide or pindolol, is reported as being reduced, there are no consistent findings in patients with CKD to indicate that absorption is actually impaired. However, an increase in bioavailability resulting from a decrease in metabolism during the drug's first pass through the gastrointestinal tract and liver has been noted for some β-blockers and dihydrocodeine.

Drug Distribution

The volume of distribution of many drugs is significantly altered in patients with advanced CKD (Table 35.1), and changes in patients with oliguric AKI are also reported. These changes are predominantly the result of altered plasma protein or tissue binding or of volume expansion secondary to reduced kidney sodium and water excretion. The plasma protein binding of acidic drugs, such as warfarin and phenytoin, typically is decreased in patients with CKD because of decreased concentrations of albumin. Changes in the conformation of albumin-binding sites and accumulation of endogenous inhibitors of binding may also contribute to decreased protein binding. In addition, the high concentrations of some drug metabolites that accumulate in CKD patients may interfere with the protein binding of the parent compound. Regardless of the mechanism, decreased protein binding increases the free or unbound fraction of the drug. On the other hand, the plasma concentration of the principal binding protein for several basic drug compounds, α_1-acid glycoprotein, is increased in kidney transplant patients and in hemodialysis patients. For this reason, the unbound fraction of some basic drugs (e.g., quinidine) may be decreased, and, as a result, the volume of distribution in these patients is decreased.

TABLE 35.1	Volume of Distribution of Selected Drugs in Patients With Chronic Kidney Disease Stage 5		
Drug	Normal (L/kg)	CKD Stage 5 (L/kg)	Change From Normal (%)
Amikacin	0.20	0.29	45
Azlocillin	0.21	0.28	33
Cefazolin	0.13	0.17	31
Cefoxitin	0.16	0.26	63
Cefuroxime	0.20	0.26	30
Clofibrate	0.14	0.24	71
Dicloxacillin	0.08	0.18	125
Digoxin	7.3	4.0	−45
Erythromycin	0.57	1.09	91
Gentamicin	0.20	0.32	60
Isoniazid	0.6	0.8	33
Minoxidil	2.6	4.9	88
Phenytoin	0.64	1.4	119
Trimethoprim	1.36	1.83	35
Vancomycin	0.64	0.85	33

The net effect of changes in protein binding is usually an alteration in the relationship between unbound and total drug concentrations, an effect frequently encountered with phenytoin. The increase in the unbound fraction often more than doubles, to values as high as 20% to 25% from the normal of 10%, which may result in increased hepatic clearance and decreased total concentrations of phenytoin. Although the unbound concentration therapeutic range is unchanged (1 to 2 μg/mL), the therapeutic range for total phenytoin concentration is reduced to 5 to 10 μg/mL (normal, 10 to 20 μg/mL) as GFR fails to account for the doubling of the unbound fraction. Therefore, the maintenance of therapeutic unbound concentrations of 1 to 2 μg/mL provides the best target for individualizing phenytoin therapy in patients with decreased kidney function.

Altered tissue binding may also affect the apparent volume of distribution of a drug. For example, the distribution volume of digoxin is reported as being reduced by 30% to 50% in patients with severe CKD. This may be the result of competitive inhibition by endogenous or exogenous digoxin-like immunoreactive substances that bind to and inhibit membrane adenosine triphosphatase (ATPase). The absolute amount of digoxin bound to the tissue digoxin receptor is reduced, and the resultant serum digoxin concentration observed after administration of any dose is greater than expected.

Therefore, in CKD patients, a normal total drug concentration may be associated with either serious adverse effects secondary to elevated unbound drug concentrations or subtherapeutic responses because of an increased plasma-to-tissue drug concentration ratio. Monitoring of unbound drug concentrations is suggested for drugs that have a narrow therapeutic range, those that are highly protein bound (>80%), and those with marked variability in the bound fraction (e.g., phenytoin, disopyramide).

Drug Metabolism and Transport

CL_{NR} of drugs includes all routes of drug elimination excluding kidney excretion. Several metabolic enzymes and active transporters collectively constitute the primary pathways of CL_{NR}. Alterations in the function of and interactions between them can significantly affect the pharmacokinetic disposition and corresponding patient exposure to drugs that are substrates of nonrenal pathways. The effect of CKD on the expression or function of many of these pathways has been characterized in experimental models of kidney disease. For example, in rat models of end-stage kidney disease, hepatic expression of several cytochrome P450 (CYP) enzymes, including CYP3A1 and CYP3A2 (equivalent to human CYP3A4), is decreased by as much as 85%. CYP2C11 and CYP3A2 activity is also significantly decreased, but CYP1A1 activity is unchanged. CYP functional expression is also decreased in the intestine; CYP1A1 and CYP3A2 are decreased up to 40% and 70%, respectively.

Several hepatic reductase enzymes are also affected by kidney disease. Gene and protein expression of carbonyl reductase-1, aldo-keto reductase-3, and 11β-hydroxysteroid dehydrogenase-1 is decreased by as much as 93% and 76%, respectively, in CKD rats. Hepatic expression of the conjugative enzymes N-acetyltransferases (NAT) is also decreased, while uridine diphosphate-glucuronosyltransferases (UGT) are unchanged. Similarly, functional expression of several intestinal and hepatic transporters is altered in experimental models of kidney disease. The expression and corresponding activities of the efflux transporters P-glycoprotein (P-gp) and multidrug resistance-associated protein 2 (MRP2) are decreased by as much as 65% in the intestine, but the uptake transporter organic anion-transporting polypeptide (OATP) is not affected. Conversely, in the liver, protein expression of P-gp, MRP2, and OATP is increased, unchanged, and decreased, respectively.

In humans with kidney disease, the activities of CYPs and reductases appear to be minimally affected. CYP2D6-mediated clearance of drugs is generally decreased in parallel with kidney function. It was previously reported that CYP3A4 activity was decreased, but recent data indicate minimal impact of decreased kidney function on the pharmacokinetics of CYP3A4 drug substrates, but that OATP uptake activity is decreased. Thus, perceived changes in CYP3A4 activity were likely due to altered transporter activity, not an alteration in CYP activity. The reduction of CL_{NR} of several drugs that exhibit overlapping CYP and transporter substrate specificity in patients with CKD stages 4 or 5 supports this premise (Table 35.2). To date, prediction of the effect of decreased kidney function on the metabolism and/or transport of a particular drug is difficult, and a general quantitative strategy to adjust dosage regimens for drugs that undergo extensive CL_{NR} has not yet been proposed. However, some qualitative insight may be gained if one knows which enzymes or transporters are involved in the clearance of the drug of interest and how those proteins are affected by a decrease in kidney function.

The effect of CKD on the CL_{NR} of a particular drug is difficult to predict, even for drugs within the same pharmacologic class. The reductions in CL_{NR} for CKD patients have frequently been noted to be proportional to the reductions in GFR. In the small number of studies that have evaluated CL_{NR} in critically ill patients with AKI, residual CL_{NR} was higher than in CKD patients with similar levels of CL_{CR}, whether measured or estimated by the Cockcroft-Gault equation. Because an AKI patient may have a higher CL_{NR} than a CKD patient, the resultant plasma concentrations will be

TABLE 35.2   Major Pathways of Nonrenal Drug Clearance and Selected Substrates

CL_{NR} Pathway	Selected Substrates
Oxidative Enzymes	
CYP	
1A2	Polycyclic aromatic hydrocarbons, caffeine, imipramine, theophylline
2A6	Coumarin
2B6	Nicotine, bupropion
2C8	Retinoids, paclitaxel, repaglinide
2C9	Celecoxib, diclofenac, flurbiprofen, indomethacin, ibuprofen, losartan, phenytoin, tolbutamide, S-warfarin
2C19	Diazepam, S-mephenytoin, omeprazole
2D6	Codeine, debrisoquine, desipramine, dextromethorphan, fluoxetine, paroxetine, duloxetine, nortriptyline, haloperidol, metoprolol, propranolol
2E1	Ethanol, acetaminophen, chlorzoxazone, nitrosamines
3A4/5	Alprazolam, midazolam, cyclosporine, tacrolimus, nifedipine, felodipine, diltiazem, verapamil, fluconazole, ketoconazole, itraconazole, erythromycin, lovastatin, simvastatin, cisapride, terfenadine
Reductase Enzymes	
11β-HSD	Bupropion, daunorubicin, prednisone, warfarin
CBR	Bupropion, daunorubicin, haloperidol, warfarin
AKR	Bupropion, daunorubicin, haloperidol, ketoprofen, nabumetone, naloxone, naltrexone, warfarin
Conjugative Enzymes	
UGT	Acetaminophen, morphine, lorazepam, oxazepam, naproxen, ketoprofen, irinotecan, bilirubin
NAT	Dapsone, hydralazine, isoniazid, procainamide
Transporters	
OATP	
1A2	Bile salts, statins, fexofenadine, methotrexate, digoxin, levofloxacin
1B1	Bile salts, statins, fexofenadine repaglinide, valsartan, olmesartan, irinotecan, bosentan
1B3	Bile salts, statins, fexofenadine, telmisartan, valsartan, olmesartan, digoxin
2B1	Statins, fexofenadine, glyburide
P-gp	Digoxin, fexofenadine, loperamide, irinotecan, doxorubicin, vinblastine, paclitaxel, erythromycin
MRP	
2	Methotrexate, etoposide, mitoxantrone, valsartan, olmesartan
3	Methotrexate, fexofenadine

AKR, Aldo-keto reductase; *CYP*, cytochrome P450 isozyme; *CBR*, carbonyl reductase; *11β-HSD*, 11β-hydroxysteroid dehydrogenase; *MRP*, multidrug resistance-associated protein; *NAT*, N-acetyltransferase; *OATP*, organic anion-transporting polypeptide; *P-gp*, P-glycoprotein; *UGT*, uridine 5′-diphosphate glucuronosyltransferase.

lower than expected and possibly subtherapeutic if classic CKD-derived dosage guidelines are followed.

Kidney Excretion of Drugs

Kidney clearance (CL_K) is the net result of glomerular filtration of unbound drug plus tubular secretion, minus tubular reabsorption. An acute or chronic reduction in GFR results in a decrease in CL_K. The degree of change in total body drug clearance is dependent on the fraction of the dose that is eliminated unchanged in individuals with normal kidney function, the intrarenal drug transport pathways, and the degree of functional impairment of each of these pathways. The primary kidney transport systems of clinical importance with respect to drug excretion include the OAT, organic cationic (OCT), P-gp, breast cancer resistance protein, and multidrug resistance-associated protein transporters. Diuretics, β-lactam antibiotics, nonsteroidal antiinflammatory drugs, and glucuronide drug metabolites are eliminated by the family of OAT transporters. The OCT transporters contribute to the secretion and excretion of cimetidine, famotidine, and quinidine. The P-gp transport system in the kidney is involved in the secretion of cationic and hydrophobic drugs (e.g., digoxin, *Vinca* alkaloids). The net clearance of drugs that undergo tubular secretion by the kidney (typically evidenced by $CL_K > 300$ mL/min) may be decreased from impairment in one or more of these kidney transporters.

Despite the different mechanisms involved in the elimination of drugs by the kidney and the availability of several methods for determining kidney function (see Chapter 3), the clinical estimation of CL_{CR} remains the most commonly used index for guiding drug-dosage regimen design. The importance of an alteration in kidney function on drug elimination usually depends primarily on two variables: (1) the fraction of drug normally eliminated by the kidney unchanged and (2) the degree of GFR loss. There are a few drugs for which a metabolite is the primary active entity; in that situation, a key variable is the degree of CL_K of the metabolite.

Estimation of Kidney Function for Drug-Dosing Purposes

The estimation of kidney function by various estimating equations for drug-dosing purposes is a critically important issue. In contrast to measured approaches, estimation of CL_{CR} or GFR requires only routinely collected laboratory and demographic data. The Cockcroft-Gault equation for CL_{CR} and the Chronic Kidney Disease Epidemiology Collaboration (CKD-EPI) equations for eGFR correlate well with CL_{CR} and GFR measurements in individuals with stable kidney function and average body composition (see Chapter 3). The traditional approach of estimating CL_{CR} and using it as a continuous variable of kidney function for drug-dosing adjustment is now being supplemented and, in some institutions, replaced by eGFR. Caution is warranted, however, since the use of eGFR as a guide for drug-dosage adjustment has not been systematically validated. Currently, there are limited prospective pharmacokinetic data and corresponding dosing recommendations based on GFR-estimating equations. In addition, eGFR equations continue to evolve. For example, the inclusion of race in eGFR-estimating equations, including the CKD-EPI equation, and its implications for the diagnosis and management of patients with kidney diseases is being scrutinized. The removal of race from the equation is being implemented at some medical centers currently, and the implications to drug dosing are unclear. Because nearly all of the primary published literature to date have used CL_{CR} to derive the relationship between kidney function and kidney and/or total body clearance of a drug, CL_{CR} is still the standard metric for drug-dosing purposes. Nevertheless, widespread availability of automatically reported eGFR affords clinicians a tool that, if validated for drug dosing, could easily be incorporated into clinical practice. Furthermore, use of eGFR for management of kidney disease and drug dosing, and harmonization of practice in this regard between physicians, pharmacists, laboratories, and other clinicians, would be ideal and warrants further evaluation.

Several issues should be considered by clinicians when assessing CL_{CR} and eGFR data for drug dosing. First, the automatically reported eGFR value provides an estimate that is normalized for body surface area (BSA) in units of mL/min/1.73 m^2. When used for drug dosing, the eGFR value should be individualized (i.e., not normalized for BSA) and converted to units of mL/min, particularly in patients whose BSA is considerably larger or smaller than 1.73 m^2. The individualized value should be compared with CL_{CR} estimates (mL/min). Second, when presented with various kidney function estimates that potentially translate into different drug-dosing regimens, clinicians should choose the regimen that optimizes the risk-benefit ratio, given the patient-specific clinical

scenario. For drugs with a narrow therapeutic range, typically more conservative kidney function estimates and corresponding doses should be used, particularly if therapeutic drug monitoring is not readily available. Because CL_{CR} estimates are more conservative and indicate the need for dose adjustment more often than eGFR, they may be preferred when dosing narrow therapeutic window drugs, especially in high-risk subgroups, such as the elderly. The use of eGFR and a more aggressive dosing strategy may be acceptable for drugs with a wide therapeutic range and a broader margin of safety. Third, when estimating equations are not expected to provide accurate measures of kidney function (i.e., because of altered creatinine generation or unstable serum creatinine concentrations) and therapeutic drug monitoring is not available, it may be reasonable to obtain an accurately timed urine collection to calculate CL_{CR}, particularly for drugs with narrow therapeutic window and high toxicity. Use of cystatin C-based estimated GFR may be a more accurate alternative for dosing drugs that are predominantly cleared by glomerular filtration (e.g., vancomycin). Fourth, the limitations and the study population of the original trials from which the eGFR equations were developed, and subsequent populations in which they have been validated, must be considered before applying them to a specific patient. All of these methods are poor predictors of kidney function in individuals with liver disease, and their use is not recommended for such patients. Finally, although several methods for CL_{CR} estimation in patients with unstable kidney function (e.g., AKI) have been proposed, the accuracy of these methods has not been rigorously assessed, and at the present time their, use cannot be recommended.

Strategies for Drug Therapy Individualization

Design of the optimal dosage regimen for a patient with decreased kidney function depends on the availability of an accurate characterization of the relationship between the drug's pharmacokinetic parameters and the individual's kidney function. An industry guidance report issued by the US Food and Drug Administration (FDA) in May 1998 provided guidelines regarding when a study should be considered, provided recommendations for study design, data analysis, and assessment of the impact of the study results on drug dosing, and recommended use of dose-adjustment categories derived from CL_{CR}. Currently, the FDA is considering including dosing tables based on eGFR and CL_{CR} in a revised version of the 1998 FDA guideline. Drug-dosing recommendations based on eGFR in addition to CL_{CR} increasingly are being included in new FDA-approved drug-dosing labels. However, for drugs already approved by the FDA with existing dose-adjustment recommendations based on CL_{CR}, it is unlikely drug manufacturers will provide additional eGFR-based dosing recommendations.

Most dosage-adjustment reference sources for clinical use have proposed the use of a fixed dose or interval for patients with a broad range of kidney function. Indeed, "normal" kidney function has often been ascribed to anyone who has a CL_{CR} greater than 50 mL/min, even though many individuals (e.g., hyperfiltering early diabetics) have values in the range of 120 to 180 mL/min. The "moderate kidney function impairment" category in many guides encompasses a 5-fold range of CL_{CR}, from 10 to 49 mL/min, whereas severe kidney function impairment or end-stage kidney disease is defined as a CL_{CR} of less than 10 to 15 mL/min. Each of these categories encompasses a broad range of kidney function, and the calculated drug regimen may not be optimal for all patients within that range.

If specific literature recommendations or data on the relationship of the pharmacokinetic parameters of a drug to CL_{CR} are not available, then these parameters can be estimated for a particular patient with the method of Rowland and Tozer, provided that the fraction of the drug that is eliminated unchanged by the kidney (f_e) in normal subjects is known. This approach assumes that (1) the change in drug clearance is proportional to the change in CL_{CR}, (2) kidney disease does not alter the drug's CL_{NR}, (3) any metabolites produced are inactive and nontoxic, (4) the drug obeys first-order (linear) kinetic principles, and (5) it is adequately described by a one-compartment model. If these assumptions are true, then the kinetic parameter or dosage-adjustment factor (Q) can be calculated as follows:

$$Q = 1 - \left[f_e \left(1 - KF \right) \right]$$

where KF is the ratio of the patient's CL_{CR} to the assumed normal value of 120 mL/min. As an example, the Q factor for a patient who has a CL_{CR} of 10 mL/min and a drug that is 85% eliminated unchanged by the kidney would be:

$$Q = 1 - \left[0.85 \left(1 - 10 / 120 \right) \right]$$
$$Q = 1 - \left[0.85 \left(0.92 \right) \right]$$
$$Q = 1 - 0.78$$
$$Q = 0.22$$

The estimated clearance rate of the drug in this patient (CL_{PT}) would then be calculated as:

$$CL_{PT} = CL_n \times Q$$

where CL_n is the respective value in patients with normal kidney function derived from the literature.

For antihypertensive agents, cephalosporins, and many other drugs for which there are no target values for peak or trough concentrations, attainment of an average steady-state concentration similar to that in normal subjects is appropriate. The principal means to achieve this goal is to decrease the dose or prolong the dosing interval. If the dose is decreased and the dosing interval is unchanged, then the desired average steady-state concentration will be near normal; however, the peak will be lower and the trough higher. Alternatively, if the dosing interval is increased and the dose remains unchanged, then the peak, trough, and average concentrations will be similar to those in the patients with normal kidney function. This interval adjustment method is often preferred because it is likely to yield significant cost savings due to less-frequent drug administration. If a loading dose is not administered, then it will take approximately five half-lives for the desired steady-state plasma concentrations to be achieved in any patient; this may require days rather than hours, because of the prolonged half-life of many drugs in patients with decreased kidney function. Therefore, to achieve the desired concentration rapidly, a loading dose (D_L) should be administered for most patients with decreased kidney function. D_L can be calculated as follows:

$$D_L = \left(C_{peak} \right) \times \left(V_D \right) \times \left(\text{Body weight in kilograms} \right)$$

The loading dose is usually the same for patients with decreased kidney function as it is for those with normal kidney function. However, if the V_D in patients with decreased kidney function is significantly different from the V_D in patients with normal kidney function (see Table 35.1), then the modified value should be used to calculate the D_L.

The adjusted dosing interval (τ_{PT}) or maintenance dose (D_{PT}) for the patient with decreased kidney function can then be calculated from the normal dosing interval (τ_n) and normal dose (D_n), respectively:

$$\tau_{PT} = \tau_n / Q$$
$$D_{PT} = D_n \times Q$$

If these approaches yield a time interval or a dose that is impractical, then a new dose can be calculated with a fixed, prespecified dose interval (τ_{FPDI}) such as 24 or 48 hours, as follows:

$$D_{PT} = \left[D_n \times Q \times \tau_{FPDI} \right] / \tau_n$$

Patients Receiving Continuous Kidney Replacement Therapy

CKRT is used primarily in critically ill patients with AKI. Drug therapy individualization for the patient receiving CKRT must take into account the fact that patients with AKI may have a higher residual CL_{NR} of a drug than CKD patients with similar levels of kidney function. In addition to patient-specific differences, there are marked differences in the efficiency of drug removal among different CKRT modalities. The primary variables that influence drug clearance during CKRT are the ultrafiltration rate (UFR), the blood flow rate (BFR), and the dialysate flow rate (DFR), as well as the type of hemofilter used. For example, clearance during continuous venovenous hemofiltration (CVVH) is directly proportional to the UFR as a result of convective transport of drug molecules. Drug clearance in this situation is a function of the membrane permeability of the drug, which is called the *sieving coefficient* (SC), and the UFR. The SC can be approximated by the fraction of drug that is unbound to plasma proteins (f_u), so the clearance can be calculated as follows:

$$CL_{CVVH} = UFR \times SC$$

or:

$$CL_{CVVH} = UFR \times f_u$$

Clearance during continuous venovenous hemodialysis (CVVHD) also depends on the DFR and the SC of the drug. If UFR is negligible, then CL_{CVVHD} can be estimated to be maximally equal to the product of DFR and f_u or SC. Clearance of a drug by continuous venovenous hemodiafiltration (CVVHDF) is generally greater than by CVVHD, because the drug is removed by diffusion as well as by convection/ultrafiltration. CL_{CVVHDF} in many clinical settings can be mathematically approximated as:

$$CL_{CVVHDF} = \left(UFR + DFR \right) \times SC$$

provided the DFR is less than 33 mL/min and BFR is at least 75 mL/min. Changes in BFR typically have only a minor effect on drug clearance by any mode of CKRT, because BFR is usually much larger than the DFR and is, therefore, not the limiting factor for drug removal.

Individualization of therapy for CKRT is based on the patient's residual kidney function and the drug clearance by the mode of CKRT used. The patient's residual drug clearance can be predicted, as described earlier in this chapter. CKRT clearance can also be approximated from published literature reports, although operating conditions are often not disclosed, and it may, thus, be hard to directly apply the findings to a given patient situation. The clearances of several frequently used drugs by CVVH and CVVHDF are summarized in Tables 35.3 and 35.4, respectively. Whenever feasible, plasma drug concentration monitoring for drugs that require achievement of target concentrations to avoid toxicity or maximize efficacy (e.g., aminoglycosides, vancomycin) is highly recommended.

Patients Receiving Chronic Hemodialysis

Drug therapy in patients undergoing hemodialysis should be guided by careful evaluation of the patient's residual kidney function, in addition to the added clearance associated with the patient's dialysis prescription. Dosing recommendations are available for many agents, especially those with a wide therapeutic index. However, for those drugs with a narrow therapeutic index, individualization of the drug therapy regimen based on prospective serum concentration monitoring is highly recommended. Although many new hemodialyzers have been introduced in the past 30 years, and the average delivered dose of hemodialysis has increased, the effect of hemodialysis on the disposition of a drug is rarely reevaluated following its initial introduction to the market. As a result, most of the published dosing guidelines underestimate the impact of hemodialysis on drug disposition,

and clinicians should cautiously consider the prescription of doses that are larger than those conventionally recommended for their critically ill patients. The effect of hemodialysis on a patient's drug therapy depends on the molecular weight, protein binding, and distribution volume of the drug; the composition of the dialyzer membrane and its surface area; BFR and DFR; and whether the dialyzer is reused. Drugs that are small molecules but highly protein bound (>80%) are usually not well dialyzed, because the two principal binding proteins (α_1-acid glycoprotein and albumin) are high-molecular-weight entities. Finally, drugs with a large volume of distribution (i.e., >1 L/kg) are poorly removed by hemodialysis, assuming distribution to extravascular tissues is complete.

Conventional or low-flux dialyzers are relatively impermeable to drugs with a molecular weight greater than 1000 Da. High-flux hemodialyzers allow the passage of most drugs with a molecular weight of 10,000 Da or less.

The determination of drug concentrations at the start and end of dialysis, with subsequent calculation of the half-life during dialysis, has historically been used as an index of drug removal by dialysis. A more accurate means of assessing the effect of hemodialysis is to calculate the dialyzer clearance of the drug. Because drug concentrations are generally measured in plasma, the plasma clearance of the drug by hemodialysis (CL_{pD}) can be calculated as follows:

$$CL_{pD} = Q_p \left(\left[A_p - V_p \right] / A_p \right)$$

TABLE 35.3	Drug Clearance and Dosing Recommendations for Patients Receiving Continuous Venovenous Hemofiltration			
Drug	**Hemofilter**	**CL_T (mL/min, Mean or Range)**	**CL_{CVVH} (mL/min, Mean or Range)**	**Dosage Recommendation**
Acyclovir	PS	0.39	NR	5 mg/kg q12h
Amikacin	PS	10.5	10–16	IND[a]
Amrinone	PS	40.8	2.4–14.4	None provided
Atracurium	PA	502.5	8.25	None provided
Ceftazidime	AN69, PMMA, PS	NR	7.5–15.6	500 mg q12h
Ceftriaxone	AN69, PMMA, PS	NR	NR	300 mg q12h
	PA	39.3	17	1000 mg q24h
Cefuroxime	PS	32	11	0.75–1.0 g q24h
Ciprofloxacin	AN69	84.4	12.4	400 mg q24h
Fluconazole	AN69	25.3	17.5	400–800 mg q24h
Gentamicin	PS	11.6	3.47	IND[a]
Imipenem	PS	108.3	13.3	500 mg q6–8h
Levofloxacin	AN69	42.3	11.5	250 mg q24h
Meropenem	PA	76	16–50	0.5–1.0 g q12h
Phenytoin	PS	NR	1.02	IND[a]
Piperacillin	NR	42	NR	4 g q12h
Ticarcillin	PS	29.7	12.3	2 g q8–12h
Tobramycin	PS	11.7	3.5	IND[a]
Vancomycin	PA, PMMA, PS	14–29	12–24	750–1250 mg q24h

[a]Serum concentrations may vary markedly depending on the patient's condition; therefore, dose individualization is recommended.

AN69, Acrylonitrile; CL_{CVVH}, CVVH clearance; CL_T, total body clearance; *IND*, individualize; *NR*, not reported; *PA*, polyamide filter; *PMMA*, polymethylmethacrylate filter; *PS*, polysulfone filter.

Adapted from Matzke GR, Clermont G. Clinical pharmacology and therapeutics. In: Murray P, Brady HR, Hall JB, eds. *Intensive Care Nephrology*. London: Taylor and Francis; 2006.

TABLE 35.4	Drug Clearance and Dosing Recommendations for Patients Receiving Continuous Venovenous Hemodiafiltration			
Drug	Hemofilter	CL_T (mL/min, Mean or Range)	CL_{CVVHDF} (mL/min, Mean or Range)	Dosage Recommendation
Acyclovir	AN69	1.2	NR	5 mg/kg q12h
Ceftazidime	AN69, PMMA, PS	25–31	13–28	0.5–1 g q24h
Ceftriaxone	AN69	—	11.7–13.2	250 mg q12h
	PMMA, PS	—	19.8–30.5	300 mg q12h
Cefuroxime	AN69	22	14–16.2	750 mg q12h
Ciprofloxacin	AN69	264	16–37	300 mg q12h
Fluconazole	AN69	21–38	25–30	400–800 mg q12h
Ganciclovir	AN69	32	13	2.5 mg/kg q24h
Gentamicin	AN69	20	5.2	IND[a]
Imipenem	AN69, PS	134	16–30	500 mg q6–8h
Levofloxacin	AN69	51	22	250 mg q24h
Meropenem	PAN	55–140	20–39	1000 mg q8–12h
Mezlocillin	AN69, PS	31–253	11–45	2–4 g q24h
Sulbactam	AN69, PS	32–54	10–23	0.5 g q24h
Piperacillin	AN69	47	22	PIP: 4 g q12h
				PIP/TAZO: 3.375 g q8–12h
Teicoplanin	AN69	9.2	3.6	LD: 800 mg
				MD: 400 mg q24h × 2, then q48–72h
Vancomycin	AN69	17–39	10–17	7.5 mg/kg q12h
	PMMA	—	15–27.0	1.0–1.5 g q24h
	PS	36	11–22	0.85–1.35 g q24h

[a]Serum concentrations may vary markedly depending on the patient's condition, therefore dose individualization is recommended.

AN69, Acrylonitrile; *CL_CVVHDF*, CVVHDF clearance; *CL_T*, total body clearance; *IND*, individualize; *LD*, loading dose; *MD*, maintenance dose; *NR*, not reported; *PA*, polyamide filter; *PAN*, polyacrylonitrile filter; *PMMA*, polymethylmethacrylate filter; *PS*, polysulfone filter; *TAZO*, tazobactam.

Adapted from Matzke GR, Clermont G. Clinical pharmacology and therapeutics. In: Murray P, Brady HR, Hall JB, eds. *Intensive Care Nephrology*. London: Taylor and Francis; 2006.

where p represents plasma, A_p is arterial plasma concentration, V_p is venous plasma concentration, and Q_p is the plasma flow rate calculated as:

$$Q_P = BFR \times (1 - Hematocrit)$$

This clearance calculation accurately reflects dialysis drug clearance only if the drug does not penetrate or bind to formed blood elements.

For patients receiving hemodialysis, the usual objective is to restore the amount of drug in the body at the end of dialysis to the value that would have been present if the patient had not been dialyzed. The postdialysis supplementary dose (D_{postHD}) is calculated as follows:

$$D_{postHD} = \left[V_D \times C \right] \left(e^{-k \cdot t} - e^{-k_{HD} \cdot t} \right)$$

where ($V_D \times C$) is the amount of drug in the body at the start of dialysis, $e^{-k \cdot t}$ is the fraction of drug remaining as a result of the patient's residual endogenous total body clearance during the

dialysis procedure, $e^{-k_{HD} \cdot t}$ is the fraction of drug remaining as a result of elimination by the dialyzer, and k_{HD} is:

$$k_{HD} = CL_{pD} / V_D$$

Alternative dosing strategies for some drugs, such as gentamicin and vancomycin, which include drug administration before or during the dialysis procedure, have been proposed. These approaches may save time in the ambulatory dialysis setting but increase drug cost because more drugs will have to be given to compensate for the increased dialysis removal. Values for CL_{pD} of some commonly used drugs are listed in Table 35.5. This information only serves as initial dosing guidance; measurement of predialysis serum concentrations is recommended to guide subsequent drug dosing.

The impact of hemodialysis on drug therapy must not be viewed as a "generic procedure" that will result in removal of a fixed percentage of the drug from the body with each dialysis session; neither should simple "yes/no" answers on the dialyzability of drug compounds be considered sufficient information for

TABLE 35.5	Drug Disposition During Dialysis Depends on Dialyzer Characteristics			
	HEMODIALYSIS CLEARANCE (mL/min)		**HALF-LIFE DURING DIALYSIS (h)**	
Drug	Conventional	High-Flux	Conventional	High-Flux
Ceftazidime	55–60	155 (PA)	3.3	1.2 (PA)
Cefuroxime	NR	103 (PS)	3.8	1.6 (PS)
Foscarnet	183	253 (PS)	NR	NR
Gentamicin	58.2	116 (PS)	3.0	4.3 (PS)
Tobramycin	45	119 (PS)	4.0	NR
Ranitidine	43.1	67.2 (PS)	5.1	2.9 (PS)
Vancomycin	9–21	31–60 (PAN)	35–38	12.0 (PAN)
	—	40–150 (PS)	—	4.5–11.8 (PS)
	—	72–116 (PMMA)	—	NR

NR, Not reported; *PA,* polyamide filter; *PAN,* polyacrylonitrile filter; *PMMA,* polymethylmethacrylate; *PS,* polysulfone filter.

therapeutic decisions. Compounds considered nondialyzable with low-flux hemodialyzers may, in fact, be significantly removed by high-flux hemodialyzers.

Patients Receiving Chronic Peritoneal Dialysis

Peritoneal dialysis has the potential to affect drug disposition, but drug therapy individualization is often less complicated in these patients because of the relative inefficiency of the procedure per unit time. Variables that influence drug removal in peritoneal dialysis include drug-specific characteristics such as molecular weight, solubility, degree of ionization, protein binding, and volume of distribution. Patient-specific factors include peritoneal membrane characteristics such as splanchnic blood flow, surface area, and permeability. The contribution of peritoneal dialysis to total body clearance is often low and, for most drugs, markedly less than the contribution of hemodialysis per unit time. Antiinfective agents are the most commonly studied drugs because of their primary role in the treatment of peritonitis, and the dosing recommendations for peritonitis, which are regularly updated, should be consulted as necessary. Most other drugs can generally be dosed according to the patient's residual kidney function because clearance by peritoneal dialysis is small.

If there is a significant relationship between the desired peak (C_{peak}) or trough (C_{trough}) concentration of a drug for a given patient with decreased kidney function and the potential clinical response (e.g., aminoglycosides) or toxicity (e.g., quinidine, phenobarbital, phenytoin), then attainment of the target plasma concentration value is critical. In these situations, the adjusted dosage interval (τ_{PT}) and maintenance dose (D_{PT}) for the patient with decreased kidney function can be calculated as follows:

$$\tau_{PT} = \left([1/k_{PT}] \times \ln \left[C_{peak} / C_{trough} \right] \right) + t_{inf}$$

$$D_{PT} = \left[k_{PT} \times V_D \times C_{peak} \right] \times \left[1 - e^{-(k_{PT})(\tau_{PT})} / 1 - e^{-(k_{PT})(t_{inf})} \right]$$

where t_{inf} is the infusion duration, V_D is the volume of distribution of the drug that can be obtained from literature values such as those in Table 35.1, k_{PT} is the elimination rate constant of the drug for that patient estimated as:

$$k_{PT} = k_n \times Q$$

k_n is the respective value in patients with normal kidney function derived from the literature and Q is the dosage adjustment factor. This estimation method assumes that the drug is administered by intermittent intravenous infusion and its disposition is adequately characterized by a one-compartment linear model.

Clinical Decision Support Tools

The availability of health information technology, namely, clinical decision support tools, has increased substantially in recent years, and use of these tools may facilitate kidney drug dosing by providing consistent, accurate dosing recommendations in real time. Clinical decision support systems (CDSS) are commonplace in institutional health information computer systems and their computerized provider order entry (CPOE) systems and have been shown to improve medication use in CKD and AKI patient populations. In addition, CDSS make individual assessments and comparisons of kidney function estimates feasible. For example, CDSS can easily accommodate new equations (e.g., CKD-EPI) as they become available and facilitate conversion of eGFR values to individualized values by modifying units of mL/min/1.73 m^2 to units of mL/min.

Numerous other resources are available for kidney drug-dosing information, including online resources, as well as smart phone applications such as Epocrates, Lexicomp, and Micromedex. The American Hospital Formulary Service *Drug Information* text, the *British National Formulary,* Aronoff's *Drug Prescribing in Renal Failure,* and Martindale's *Complete Drug Reference* are excellent resources for drug-dosage recommendations for patients with decreased kidney function and are all accessible electronically and/or online.

Conclusions

The adverse outcomes associated with inappropriate drug use and dosing are largely preventable if the principles illustrated in this chapter are used by the clinician in concert with reliable population pharmacokinetic estimates to design rational initial drug-dosage regimens for patients with decreased kidney function and those needing dialysis. Subsequent individualization of therapy should be undertaken whenever clinical therapeutic monitoring tools, such as plasma drug concentrations, are available. These key recommendations for practice are highlighted in Table 35.6.

TABLE 35.6	Key Recommendations for Clinicians

1. Diligent medication therapy management is essential, including medication reconciliation and frequent assessment for potential medication-related problems.
2. Over-the-counter and herbal products as well as prescription medications should be assessed to ensure they are indicated.
3. The least nephrotoxic agent should be used whenever possible.
4. If a drug interaction is suspected and the clinical implication is significant, alternative medications should be used.
5. Although the Cockcroft-Gault equation for estimating CL_{CR} remains the most commonly used kidney function index for drug-dosage adjustment, eGFR is widely available in units of mL/min/1.73 m² and should be converted to mL/min when considering use of CL_{CR}-based dosing recommendations.
6. The dosage of drugs that are more than 30% eliminated unchanged by the kidney should be verified to ensure that appropriate initial dosage adjustments are implemented in CKD.
7. Maintenance dosage regimens should be adjusted based on patient response and serum drug concentration determinations when indicated and available.

CKD, Chronic kidney disease; *CKD-EPI,* Chronic Kidney Disease Epidemiology Collaboration; *eGFR,* estimated glomerular filtration rate.

Bibliography

Alshogran OY, Nolin TD. Implications of kidney disease on metabolic reduction. *Curr Drug Metab.* 2016;17:663–672.

Aronoff GR, Bennetl WM, Berns JS, et al. *Drug Prescribing in Renal Failure: Dosing Guidelines for Adults and Children.* 5th ed. Philadelphia: American College of Physicians-American Society of Internal Medicine; 2007.

Goldstein SL. Automated/integrated real-time clinical decision support in acute kidney injury. *Curr Opin Crit Care.* 2015;21:485–489.

Heintz BH, Matzke GR, Dager WE. Antimicrobial dosing concepts and recommendations for critically ill adult patients receiving continuous renal replacement therapy or intermittent hemodialysis. *Pharmacotherapy.* 2009;29:562–577.

Hudson JQ, Nolin TD. Pragmatic use of kidney function estimates for drug dosing: the tide is turning. *Adv Chronic Kidney Dis.* 2018;25:14–20.

Lea-Henry TN, Carland JE, Stocker SL, Sevastos J, Roberts DM. Clinical pharmacokinetics in kidney disease: fundamental principles. *Clin J Am Soc Nephrol.* 2018;13:1085–1095.

Li PK, Szeto CC, Piraino B, et al. ISPD peritonitis recommendations: 2016 update on prevention and treatment. *Perit Dial Int.* 2016;36:481–508.

Matzke GR, Aronoff GR, Atkinson Jr AJ, et al. Drug dosing consideration in patients with acute and chronic kidney disease—a clinical update from Kidney Disease: Improving Global Outcomes (KDIGO). *Kidney Int.* 2011;80:1122–1137.

Matzke GR, Clermont G. Clinical pharmacology and therapeutics. In: Murray PT, Brady HR, Hall JB, eds. *Intensive Care in Nephrology.* Boca Raton, FL: Taylor and Francis; 2006:245–265.

Naud J, Nolin TD, Leblond FA, Pichette V. Current understanding of drug disposition in kidney disease. *J Clin Pharmacol.* 2012;52:10S–22S.

Nigam SK, Wu W, Bush KT, et al. Handling of drugs, metabolites, and uremic toxins by kidney proximal tubule drug transporters. *Clin J Am Soc Nephrol.* 2015;10:2039–2049.

Nolin TD. A synopsis of clinical pharmacokinetic alterations in advanced CKD. *Semin Dial.* 2015;28:325–329.

Nolin TD, Aronoff GR, Fissell WH, et al. Pharmacokinetic assessment in patients receiving continuous KRT: perspectives from the kidney health initiative. *Clin J Am Soc Nephrol.* 2015;10:159–164.

Roberts DM, Sevastos J, Carland JE, Stocker SL, Lea-Henry TN. Clinical pharmacokinetics in kidney disease: Application to rational design of dosing regimens. *Clin J Am Soc Nephrol.* 2018;13:1254–1263.

Tan ML, Zhao P, Zhang L, et al. Use of physiologically based pharmacokinetic modeling to evaluate the effect of chronic kidney disease on the disposition of hepatic CYP2C8 and OATP1B drug substrates. *Clin Pharmacol Ther.* 2019;105:719–729.

Verbeeck RK, Musuamba FT. Pharmacokinetics and dosage adjustment in patients with renal dysfunction. *Eur J Clin Pharmacol.* 2009;65:757–773.

Vidal L, Shavit M, Fraser A, et al. Systematic comparison of four sources of drug information regarding adjustment of dose for renal function. *BMJ.* 2005;331:263–266.

Whittaker CF, Miklich MA, Patel RS, Fink JC. Medication safety principles and practice in CKD. *Clin J Am Soc Nephrol.* 2018;13:1738–1746.

Yoshida K, Sun B, Zhang L, et al. Systematic and quantitative assessment of the effect of chronic kidney disease on CYP2D6 and CYP3A4/5. *Clin Pharmacol Ther.* 2016;100:75–87.

PART 7

Hereditary Kidney Disease

36

APOL1-Mediated Kidney Disease

ETTY KRUZEL-DAVILA, LIJUN MA, BARRY I. FREEDMAN[a]

Ancestry and Chronic Kidney Disease

Racial disparities in the incidence rates of chronic kidney disease (CKD) are widely appreciated. Compared to Americans of European descent, Americans of African descent face approximately a 4-fold higher risk for developing end-stage kidney disease (ESKD) with an estimated lifetime risk for ESKD approaching 8% (versus 2%–3% in European Americans). Although lower socioeconomic status and poorer access to healthcare contribute to this disparity, epidemiologic studies demonstrating familial aggregation of disparate causes of ESKD in families of African descent suggested an inherited basis.

Genetic association between two coding "kidney-risk variants" (KRVs) in the apolipoprotein L1 gene (*APOL1*) on chromosome 22q12 with nondiabetic ESKD ultimately proved this concept. The ancestral allele, designated G0, does not increase the risk of nephropathy. The derived KRVs include G1 (encoding S342G and I384M substitutions) and G2 (encoding N388 and Y389 amino acid deletions). The two variants constituting G1 are in near perfect linkage disequilibrium; however, G342 is causative because it confers the same risk as possessing both variants. It is rare for the G1 and G2 KRVs to occur on a single chromosome. Allele frequencies of *APOL1* KRVs are extremely high; approximately 38% of Americans of African descent possess one KRV and 13% have two KRVs comprising *APOL1* high-risk genotypes with increased risk for CKD (e.g., G1G1, G2G2, or G1G2). Based on these frequencies, it is estimated that more than 70 million people worldwide, including approximately 6 million Americans of African descent, have *APOL1* high-risk genotypes.

APOL1 KRVs are among the most powerful common variants causing complex disease. G1 and G2 arose in sub-Saharan Africa less than 10,000 years ago, and a selective sweep likely led to today's high frequencies. Their current frequencies stem from an evolutionary advantage that confers protection from *Trypanosoma brucei rhodesiense*, a parasite causing African sleeping sickness. Enhanced survival was seen in those with one or two KRVs, at the expense of increased risk for CKD later in life among those with two KRVs.

Clinical Implications of *APOL1*

In Americans of African descent, *APOL1* underlies approximately 70% of cases of idiopathic focal segmental glomerulosclerosis (FSGS) and HIV-associated nephropathy (HIVAN); the popula-

tion-attributable risk approximates 70%. In essence, the risk for nondiabetic ESKD in Americans of African vs European descent would approach unity if G1 and G2 KRVs did not occur.

The most common reported cause of nondiabetic ESKD in Americans of African descent is "hypertension-attributed" nephropathy. This term is applied to nondiabetic patients with CKD, low-level (or absent) proteinuria, and hypertension. However, discovery of *APOL1* made it clear that many such patients had secondary hypertension related to CKD and not hypertensive nephropathy. In most cases, *APOL1*-associated solidified glomerulosclerosis is present. Significant proteinuria does not develop due to the lack of patent capillaries (reduced perfusion) in solidified glomerular tufts. Compared to arteriolar nephrosclerosis, solidified glomeruli lack collagen deposition in the urinary space, ischemic collapse of capillaries, or thickening of Bowman's capsule. *APOL1*-associated nephropathy reveals that the primary glomerular disease "solidified glomerulosclerosis" typically presents without heavy proteinuria and forces us to reconsider the interpretation of likely sites of kidney injury based on the urinalysis.

Results from the National Institutes of Health (NIH)-sponsored "African American Study of Kidney Disease and Hypertension" (AASK) trial revealed that aggressively lowering blood pressure with high-dose angiotensin-converting enzyme (ACE) inhibitors in nondiabetic Americans of African descent felt to have essential hypertension as the cause of kidney disease does not slow progression of nephropathy. AASK recruitment criteria include hypertensive and nondiabetic Americans of African descent between the ages of 18–70 years, with an estimated glomerular filtration rate (eGFR) of 20–65 mL/min/1.73 m², proteinuria <2.5 g/day, and no other known cause of CKD. After almost 10 years of follow-up, nearly 70% of AASK participants developed ESKD, doubling of serum creatinine concentration, or death. Antihypertensive medication class and blood pressure target failed to predict the risk of CKD progression. *APOL1* genotypes were the strongest predictor of kidney outcomes, an effect independent from the blood pressure treatment arm. The AASK and "Systolic Blood Pressure Intervention Trial" (SPRINT) provide evidence that intensive blood pressure control in patients felt to have "hypertension-attributed" CKD does not delay progression of CKD. Results support that mild-moderate hypertension is an infrequent initiator of CKD.

The odds ratio for *APOL1* association with "hypertension-attributed" ESKD, FSGS, HIVAN, progressive lupus nephritis, and collapsing glomerulopathy (on backgrounds of other glomerular diseases, interferon, and HIV or SARS-CoV-2 infection) approach those reported in Mendelian disorders; they range from 7 to 89. Accelerated failure of transplanted kidneys from African-ancestry donors with *APOL1* high-risk genotypes also occurs.

[a]*Disclosure*: Wake Forest University Health Sciences and Dr. Freedman have rights to an issued U.S. patent related to *APOL1* genetic testing. Dr. Freedman is a consultant for AstraZeneca and RenalytixAI.

These disorders share common molecular mechanisms leading to progressive nephropathy and are considered the spectrum of *APOL1*-associated nephropathy.

Second Hits and Modifying Factors

Although the odds ratios in *APOL1*-associated nephropathy are among the highest reported in common nonmonogenic disease, only a minority of individuals with the high-risk genotype develop kidney disease. The lifetime risk for FSGS in individuals with *APOL1* high-risk genotypes is 4%, whereas the risk is 50% in untreated individuals with HIV infection and the high-risk genotypes. Overall, approximately 15%-20% of individuals with *APOL1* high-risk genotypes develop nephropathy.

Autopsy and biopsy studies demonstrate that *APOL1* high-risk genotypes associate with exaggerated age-related nephron loss, solidified glomerulosclerosis, thyroidization-type tubular atrophy, and "disappearing glomeruli," often with enlargement of remaining glomeruli. Findings suggest that subclinical kidney disease may often be present, manifested as systemic hypertension prior to recognition of reduced eGFR or proteinuria. A likely paradigm explaining the variable lifetime risk for CKD is that a clinically silent pathology exists that can evolve to progressive CKD with exposure to a second hit.

Environmental factors and genetic background likely alter the risk for developing CKD. Environmental modifiers that transform *APOL1* genetic risk into CKD include robust induction of *APOL1* by administration of exogenous interferon, increased susceptibility to collapsing glomerulopathy in patients with HIV or SARS-CoV-2 infection, and systemic lupus erythematosus.

Second hits appear to increase the transcription of *APOL1* mRNA and produce higher levels of toxic APOL1 KRV protein in kidney cells. The most powerful environmental influence on *APOL1*-asssociated nephropathy is untreated HIV infection, with an odds ratio of 29 to 89 for developing HIVAN in individuals with *APOL1* high-risk genotypes (odds ratio 2–5 reported in Africans with only one G1 allele). Interestingly, the frequency of HIVAN has decreased after the introduction of highly active antiretroviral treatment. Therefore, we consider antiretroviral treatment reno-protective in individuals who harbor *APOL1* high-risk genotypes.

In contrast to infection with HIV and SARS-CoV-2 infection, JC polyomaviruria (signifying active kidney and/or urinary tract viral replication) associates with a paradoxically lower risk of *APOL1* and non-*APOL1* etiologies of CKD. This protective association may reflect reduced immune system activation, where kidneys fail to restrict replication of the nonpathogenic JC polyomavirus. Individuals who lack JC polyomaviruria likely cleared their childhood infections; thus, they may have a more robust immune system. Immune activation appears to promote development of *APOL1*-associated (and other) kidney diseases. Additional protective environmental and inherited risk factors accounting for low rates of progressive kidney disease in individuals with *APOL1* high-risk genotypes remain to be discovered. These factors could have therapeutic implications (Fig. 36.1).

It is debated whether *APOL1* initiates CKD or is a risk factor for its progression. We believe APOL1 KRV proteins promote more rapid progression of nephropathy to ESKD. We base this on the observations that a minority of individuals with *APOL1* high-risk genotypes develop CKD, and it is more strongly associated with advanced CKD and ESKD than mildly reduced eGFR or low-level proteinuria. An early study in patients with lupus

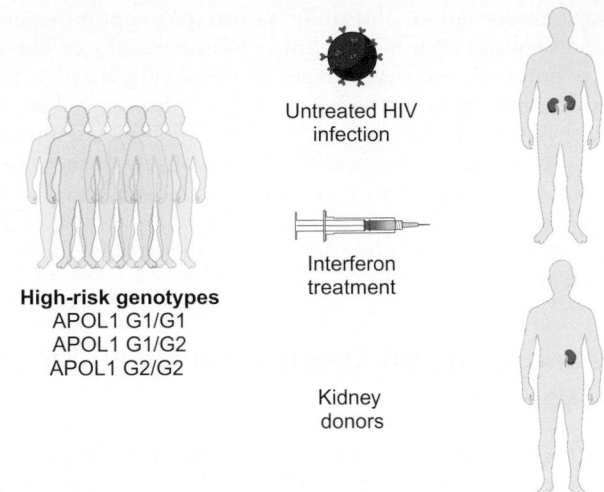

• **Fig. 36.1** Identifying individuals with *APOL1* high-risk genotypes at increased risk for chronic kidney disease (CKD). A minority of individuals harboring *APOL1* high-risk genotypes (*left*) develop CKD (*right*). Risk factors associated with development of CKD include untreated HIV infection and administration of interferon. Reducing or treating these factors may reduce risk for development and progression of CKD.

nephritis failed to detect *APOL1* association, but most of the cases had mild CKD with preserved eGFR. However, robust association exists between *APOL1* and lupus nephritis in patients with ESKD. Thus, available evidence more strongly supports *APOL1* as a progression factor for CKD.

APOL1 and Kidney Transplantation: Insights into Disease Pathogenesis

Kidney transplantation provides important insights related to the biologic effects of kidney-produced APOL1 protein versus circulating (predominantly liver-synthesized) APOL1. The risk of shortened kidney allograft survival and more rapid decline in kidney function was associated with two *APOL1* KRVs in donor kidneys, not recipient *APOL1* genotypes. Hence, *APOL1* KRV-induced allograft injury is mediated by endogenous (not circulating) APOL1. Similar to the observation that only a minority of individuals with *APOL1* high-risk genotypes develop CKD, most *APOL1* two-KRV donor kidneys do not fail early after engraftment; many function beyond 5 years. As in native CKD, this suggests other genetic and/or environmental second-hits influence allograft survival.

Similar results were seen in living kidney donors of African descent, individuals felt to be healthy (without kidney disease) at the time of donor nephrectomy. Doshi et al. reported that living kidney donors of African descent with high-risk *APOL1* genotypes had significantly faster rates of decline in eGFR compared to those with low-risk genotypes. In addition, significantly more living donors with high-risk genotypes developed an eGFR <60 mL/min/1.73 m^2 after 12-year median follow-up (67% high-risk vs. 36% low-risk, p = 0.01) and 11% of 19 *APOL1* high-risk live donors developed ESKD (versus none of 117 low-risk donors).

The NIH "APOL1 Long-term Kidney Transplant Outcomes" (APOLLO) Network is prospectively assessing effects of donor and recipient *APOL1* genotypes in deceased donor and live donor kidney transplantation. This study is expected to optimize guidelines and policies regarding allocation of deceased donor kidneys from donors with recent African ancestry (individuals with similar genetic makeup to those who now reside in Africa), as well as maximize the safety of live kidney donation. APOLLO results may lead to reductions in the discard of good-quality kidneys from deceased donors with recent African ancestry who have *APOL1* low-risk genotypes. If true, this could increase the number of kidneys transplanted, reduce healthcare costs, and improve outcomes for all patients with ESKD.

Trypanosoma Sub-Species and *APOL1* Kidney Risk Variants

APOL1 is a member of a series of clustered paralogous innate immunity genes (*APOL1–6*). *APOL1* is the only member of this gene family that encodes a signal peptide; this enables APOL1 protein secretion from liver cells into the circulation. The circulating protein functions as a trypanolytic factor and renders humans innately resistant to some members of the *Trypanosoma* family of parasites.

Circulating APOL1 protein is comprised of several domains essential for trypanolytic function. These include an N-terminal domain, which forms a colicin-like domain with the potential to perforate membranes, a BH3-only subdomain (located within the N-terminal domain) that may affect apoptosis and autophagy, a membrane-addressing domain with a putative pH-dependent apparatus enabling APOL1 activation in acidic pH, and a C-terminal domain (including a coiled coil domain) with a leucine zipper motif important for interactions with other proteins and possibly lipids. The C-terminus domain contains the G1 and G2 KRVs.

African trypanosomiasis is a parasitic disease caused by trypanosomes that infect humans and animals residing in sub-Saharan Africa. In humans, the parasite causes sleeping sickness, which is fatal if untreated. APOL1 is the innate immune protein that protects humans against *Trypanosoma brucei* (*T. brucei*). The absence of *APOL1* in chimpanzees renders them susceptible to *T. brucei* infection. APOL1 circulates in serum complexes identified as trypanosome lytic factors (TLFs), TLF1 and TLF2. Once TLF1 and/or TLF2 are taken up by trypanosomes, APOL1 is released from the carrier complex and inserts into the parasite's endosomal membranes at an acidic pH. Death of the parasite results from APOL1 ion channel activity causing transmembrane ionic flux, osmotic swelling of the lysosome, and mitochondrial membrane permeabilization. *T. br. Rhodesiense* evolved resistance to APOL1 via a virulence factor designated serum-resistant activity (SRA). SRA binds the C-terminus of APOL1 in an acidic endolysosome organelle, thereby overriding the APOL1-mediated lysis. The KRVs, which are located at the interaction site of APOL1 with SRA, restore trypanolytic activity by reducing SRA binding affinity to APOL1.

Mode of Inheritance

A recessive mode of inheritance is widely reported with *APOL1* association with nondiabetic CKD. Recessive inheritance is not typically associated with gain-of-function mutations, as some have proposed for *APOL1*. Several hypotheses attempt to explain this paradoxical observation, including KRV association with a threshold inflection point needed to mediate injury, enhanced multimerization of the KRV compared to the G0 variant leading to cell death, a protective role of G0, and a loss of inhibition model.

With regard to the last hypothesis, disruption of the putative autoinhibitory domain in the SRA-binding region of the KRV may cause loss of function of the inhibitory domain, leading to overall gain of function of APOL1 protein. Alternatively, an as-yet-unidentified interacting human protein/lipid that attenuates toxicity by binding the C-terminal domain and has a reduced affinity to the KRV, similar to the APOL1 and SRA interaction system in trypanosomes, may play a role.

Given preserved toxicity of the KRVs in various model organisms (such as yeast, flies, and mice that do not normally express *APOL1*), the intrinsic autoinhibitory loss of function of the C-terminal hypothesis may explain why different mutations in the C-terminus lead to the same gain of function, which is actually a loss-of-inhibition effect. These hypotheses are not mutually exclusive.

Mechanism of Kidney Injury

While a causative role of *APOL1* KRVs was identified in mice with inducible podocyte-specific expression of *APOL1* G0, G1, or G2, the mechanism(s) mediating human kidney injury by KRVs and their relationship to pathways involved in trypanolysis are less clear. *In vitro* and *in vivo* models suggest a gain-of-function injury, but several aspects require clarification. Pathways including disrupted autophagic flux, impaired acidification of the endolysosomal organelles, and endosomal trafficking pathways, increased potassium efflux with activation of stress protein kinases, endoplasmic reticulum stress, pyroptotic cell death, and interaction with soluble urokinase-type plasminogen activator receptor have been implicated in the cellular injury induced by *APOL1* KRVs.

Two independent reports detected *APOL1* KRV reductions in mitochondrial function. *APOL1* KRVs can induce cell death by opening the inner mitochondrial membrane permeability transition pore and/or inducing mitochondrial fission, resulting in depletion of the mitochondrial membrane potential. Given the plethora of potentially involved pathways and cross talk between them, it has been a challenge to identify the initial injurious event. However, mounting evidence supports a key role for mitochondrial dysfunction in the earliest stages of *APOL1* nephropathy.

Genetic Testing and Involvement of Communities of African Descent

Given the magnitude of the *APOL1* effect on nephropathy, allowing for the fact that approximately one in five with high-risk genotypes ultimately develop kidney disease, there has been ongoing discussion on the appropriate use of *APOL1* genotyping in clinical practice. Testing is widely available, simple, and relatively inexpensive. With this capability, we must address ethical concerns, and it is critical that communities of African descent be engaged in this process.

APOL1 genotyping may be useful in the setting of kidney transplantation. Recruitment of live kidney donors in APOLLO requires discussion of *APOL1* genetic testing in candidates with recent African ancestry prior to donor nephrectomy. Many US transplant programs now discuss *APOL1* with live donor candidates of African descent. In addition, many programs genotype candidates as part of the donor evaluation. APOLLO will determine whether rapidly performing *APOL1* genotyping in deceased organ donors (and replacing the race-based component of the Kidney Donor Risk Index with *APOL1* genotype) more accurately defines the quality of donor kidneys. If APOLLO confirms results from retrospective studies, *APOL1* genotyping may be useful in the evaluation of deceased and living kidney donors who possess recent African ancestry.

Genotyping may also prove useful for determining subsequent risk for nephropathy in Americans of African descent with systemic lupus erythematosus, HIV infection, and sickle cell disease. Patients who display suboptimal adherence to therapy might benefit from knowledge of whether or not they face heightened risk for ESKD. *APOL1* genotyping could also prove useful for family planning, particularly in those with multiple family members with ESKD.

It is clear that genetic testing will have its greatest impact when treatment trials for *APOL1*-associated nephropathy are underway, especially if safe and proven therapies become available. At present, genotyping can provide information as to the cause of nephropathy and prognosis for kidney outcomes in individuals who wish to know their genotype. This knowledge may allow them to participate in future clinical trials, perhaps involving *APOL1* antisense oligonucleotide therapy, small molecule inhibitors, or other novel approaches. If a therapy proves effective, we predict a major shift in practice. At that time, many individuals at risk for nephropathy or with early kidney disease will likely request genetic testing.

From the research standpoint, genotyping provides the ability to tell which patients with CKD have a disease in the *APOL1* spectrum. Most Americans of African descent presumed to have diabetic kidney disease (DKD) do not undergo kidney biopsy. It may be difficult to differentiate between patients with diabetes mellitus and coincident proteinuric FSGS from those with DKD. Type 2 diabetes and FSGS are both more common in Americans of African than European descent. If a treatment for *APOL1* nephropathy becomes available, it will be critical to genotype Americans of African descent with presumed DKD, especially those with atypical courses who lack retinopathy or heavy proteinuria. Those with high-risk genotypes can be offered kidney biopsies to determine the cause of nephropathy and guide whether therapy directed against *APOL1* KRVs or treatment of diabetes have the highest likelihood of success.

Studies are addressing views of communities of African descent on *APOL1* testing and participation in clinical research that include genetic testing. Recent NIH studies include community advisory councils comprised of individuals with recent African ancestry and firsthand knowledge of kidney disease, kidney transplantation, and kidney donation in the development and performance of clinical trials. As with any controversial scientific topic, there will never be uniform agreement among all parties, but it is clear that communities of African descent wants a voice in deliberations on how to proceed.

The majority of the Americans of African descent in these reports favored making *APOL1* testing broadly available to those who want it and returning test results to patients along with appropriate information and counseling. It is striking that these opinions held even in the absence of treatments or lifestyle changes that would alter risk for CKD. Physicians, researchers, and community members agree that testing should never be mandated, information regarding *APOL1* and the implications of being tested discussed *prior* to ordering the test, and patients should be asked whether they want to learn their result. In the same way that determining someone has an *APOL1* high-risk genotype does not mean they will develop nephropathy, possession of a low-risk genotype only means the individual will not develop *APOL1*-associated nephropathy. They should still maintain a healthy diet, participate in an exercise program, avoid smoking, and control other risk factors such as hyperlipidemia, hypertension, and hyperglycemia to minimize the risk for developing another kidney disease. Finally, we must ensure adherence to the Genetic Information Nondiscrimination Act (GINA), preventing discrimination due to genetic risk for a disease. Decisions on health insurance and employment should not be influenced by genetic test results.

Conclusions

Although the precise mechanisms mediating *APOL1*-associated kidney injury are not fully clear, the *APOL1* discovery provides an exciting opportunity for precision medicine in the treatment of CKD. Personalized interventions may soon improve the allocation of deceased donor kidneys and better predict risk for CKD after live kidney donation. In addition, identification of genetic and environmental "second hits" for *APOL1* nephropathy may lead to preventive strategies. In the near future, platforms for high-throughput screening may discover drugs that attenuate the deleterious effects of APOL1 protein. The clinical utility of *APOL1* antisense oligonucleotide therapy to reduce *APOL1* mRNA expression and small molecule inhibitors may soon undergo testing. As such, the *APOL1* discovery could yield clinical screening capabilities and therapies to mitigate risk for ESKD in populations with African ancestry.

Bibliography

Beckerman P, et al. Transgenic expression of human APOL1 risk variants in podocytes induces kidney disease in mice. *Nat Med.* 2017;23:429–438.

Doshi MD, et al. APOL1 genotype and renal function of black living donors. *J Am Soc Nephrol.* 2018;29:1309–1316.

Freedman BI, Cohen AH. Hypertension-attributed nephropathy: what's in a name? *Nat Rev Nephrol.* 2016;12:27–36.

Freedman BI, Locke JE, Reeves-Daniel AM, Julian BA. Apolipoprotein L1 gene effects on kidney transplantation. *Semin Nephrol.* 2017;37:530–537.

Freedman BI, Skorecki K. Gene-gene and gene-environment interactions in apolipoprotein L1 gene-associated nephropathy. *Clin J Am Soc Nephrol.* 2014;9(11):2006–2013.

Freedman BI, Spray BJ, Tuttle AB, Buckalew VM Jr. The familial risk of end-stage renal disease in African Americans. *Am J Kidney Dis.* 1993;21:387–393.

Freedman BI, et al. End-stage renal disease in African Americans with lupus nephritis is associated with APOL1. *Arthritis Rheumatol.* 2014;66:390–396.

Freedman BI, et al. APOL1 Long-term Kidney Transplantation Outcomes Network (APOLLO): design and rationale. *Kidney Int Rep.* 2020;5:278–288.

Genovese G, et al. Association of trypanolytic ApoL1 variants with kidney disease in African Americans. *Science.* 2010;329:841–845.

Granado D, et al. Intracellular APOL1 risk variants cause cytotoxicity accompanied by energy depletion. *J Am Soc Nephrol.* 2017;28(11):3227–3238.

Kopp JB, et al. APOL1 genetic variants in focal segmental glomerulosclerosis and HIV-associated nephropathy. *J Am Soc Nephrol.* 2011;22:2129–2137.

Kruzel-Davila E, Wasser WG, Skorecki K. APOL1 nephropathy: A population genetics and evolutionary medicine detective story. *Semin Nephrol.* 2017;37:490–507.

Kruzel-Davila E, et al. JC Viruria is associated with reduced risk of diabetic kidney disease. *J Clin Endocrinol Metab.* 2019;104:2286–2294.

Larsen CP, et al. Histopathologic findings associated with APOL1 risk variants in chronic kidney disease. *Mod Pathol*. 2015;28:95–102.

Lipkowitz MS, et al. Apolipoprotein L1 gene variants associate with hypertension-attributed nephropathy and the rate of kidney function decline in African Americans. *Kidney Int*. 2013;83:114–120.

Ma L, et al. APOL1 kidney-risk variants induce mitochondrial fission. *Kidney Int Rep*. 2020. https://doi.org/10.1016/j.ekir.2020.03.020.

Ma L, et al. APOL1 renal-risk variants induce mitochondrial dysfunction. *J Am Soc Nephrol*. 2017;28:1093–1105.

Shah SS, et al. APOL1 kidney risk variants induce cell death via mitochondrial translocation and opening of the mitochondrial permeability transition pore. *J Am Soc Nephrol*. 2019;30:2355–2368.

Tzur S, et al. Missense mutations in the APOL1 gene are highly associated with end stage kidney disease risk previously attributed to the MYH9 gene. *Hum Genet*. 2010;128:345–350.

Umeukeje EM, et al. You are just now telling us about this? African American perspectives of testing for genetic susceptibility to kidney disease. *J Am Soc Nephrol*. 2019;30:526–530.

37

Genetically Based Kidney Transport Disorders

STEVEN J. SCHEINMAN

The coming of age of clinical chemistry in the latter half of the 20th century, bringing with it the routine measurement of electrolytes and minerals in patient samples, produced descriptions of distinct inherited syndromes of abnormal tubular transport in the kidney. Clinical investigation led to speculation, often ingenious and sometimes controversial, regarding the underlying causes of these syndromes. More recently, the tools of molecular biology made possible the cloning of mutated genes found in patients with monogenic disorders of kidney tubular transport. These diseases represent experiments of nature, and for anyone interested in pathophysiology, and specifically for kidney physiologists, the insights they have revealed are exciting. Some provide gratifying confirmation of our existing knowledge of transport mechanisms along the nephron. Examples include mutations in diuretic-sensitive transporters in the Bartter and Gitelman syndromes. In other cases, positional cloning led to the discovery of previously unknown proteins, often surprising ones that appear to play important roles in epithelial transport. For example, the chloride transporter CLC-5 (gene name *CLCN5*), the tight junction claudin 16 (paracellin 1), and the phosphaturic hormone fibroblast growth factor 23 (FGF23) were discovered through positional cloning in the study of Dent disease, inherited hypomagnesemic hypercalciuria, and autosomal dominant hypophosphatemic rickets (ADHR), respectively.

Table 37.1 summarizes genetic diseases of kidney tubular transport for which the molecular basis is known. The diseases listed are explained by abnormalities in the corresponding gene product. They are all inherited in Mendelian fashion, either autosomal or X-linked, with the single exception of a syndrome of hypomagnesemia with maternal inheritance that results from mutation in a mitochondrial tRNA rather than in the nuclear genome.

Disorders of Proximal Tubular Transport Function

Selective Proximal Transport Defects

Sodium resorption in the proximal tubule occurs through secondary active transport processes in which the entry of sodium is coupled either to the entry of substrates (e.g., glucose, amino acids, or phosphate) or to the exit of protons. Autosomal recessive conditions of impaired transepithelial transport of glucose and dibasic amino acids have been shown to be caused by mutations in sodium-dependent transporters that are expressed in both kidney and intestine, resulting in urinary losses and intestinal malabsorption of these solutes. Other disorders with kidney-selective transport defects result from mutations in transporters expressed specifically in kidney.

Impaired Proximal Phosphate Reabsorption

Hypophosphatemic rickets can be inherited in X-linked, autosomal dominant, and autosomal recessive patterns. All three modes are associated with kidney phosphate wasting, with a reduced maximal transport capacity for phosphate. In all three, serum levels of the phosphate-regulating hormone (phosphatonin) FGF23 are elevated, and serum levels of 1,25-dihydroxyvitamin D are not elevated despite the stimulus of hypophosphatemia.

X-linked (dominant) hypophosphatemic rickets (XLHR) is the most common form of hereditary rickets. Mutations in XLHR involve a phosphate-regulating gene with homologies to a neutral endopeptidase on the X chromosome (*PHEX*) that is expressed in bone and is indirectly involved in the degradation and processing of FGF23. Elevations in FGF23 are sufficient to explain the kidney phosphate wasting, but other factors independent of FGF23 appear to contribute as well to the bone demineralization and rickets. Recent studies demonstrate the effectiveness of a monoclonal anti-FGF23 antibody, burosumab, to correct hypophosphatemia and improve bone mineralization in children with XLHR, further validating a central role for FGF23 in this disease.

The rare ADHR is associated with mutations in the gene encoding FGF23 that protects the phosphatonin from proteolytic cleavage. FGF23 disrupts kidney phosphate reabsorption by inhibiting expression of two genes encoding sodium-dependent phosphate transporters in proximal tubule, *SLC34A1* (encoding the Na-dependent phosphate transporter Npt2a) and *SLC34A3* (encoding Npt2c). FGF23 inhibits the 1-hydroxylation of 25-hydroxyvitamin D, likely explaining why hypophosphatemia in these three conditions is not associated with either elevated levels of 1,25-dihydroxyvitamin D or hypercalciuria. A single kindred has been reported with autosomal dominant hypophosphatemia and rickets with mutation in *SGK3*, encoding a proximal tubular protein kinase SGKL.

Autosomal recessive inheritance of hypophosphatemic rickets has been reported in association with mutations in one of three genes. In ARHR type 1, the mutated gene is *DMP1*, encoding the dentin matrix protein 1 (DMP-1), a bone matrix protein that appears to play a role with PHEX in regulating bone mineralization

TABLE 37.1 Molecular Bases of Genetic Disorders of Renal Transport

Inherited Disorder	Defective Gene Product
Proximal Tubule	
Glucose-galactose malabsorption syndrome	Sodium-glucose transporter 1
Dibasic aminoaciduria	Basolateral dibasic amino acid transporter (lysinuric protein intolerance)
XLHR	PHEX
ADHR	FGF23 (excess)
	SGKL
Autosomal recessive hypophosphatemic rickets	DMP1
	ENPP1
	FAM20C
HHRH	Sodium-phosphate cotransporter NPT2c
Familial hyperostosis-hyperphosphatemia	FGF23 (deficiency)
	GalNac transferase 3
	Klotho (FGF23 co-receptor)
Fanconi syndrome	
Autosomal dominant	Glycine amidinotransferase
	Peroxisomal enoyl-CoA Hydratase-L-3-hydroxyacyl-CoA dehydrogenase (L-PBE)
	Nuclear hormone receptor HNF4A
Autosomal recessive	Sodium-phosphate cotransporter NPT2a
	NADH:ubiquinone oxidoreductase complex assembly factor 6
Hereditary fructose intolerance	Aldolase B
Fanconi-Bickel syndrome	Facilitated GLUT2
Oculocerebrorenal syndrome of Lowe	Inositol polyphosphate-5-phosphatase (OCRL1)
Dent disease (X-linked nephrolithiasis)	Chloride transporter (ClC-5)
	Inositol polyphosphate-5-phosphatase (OCRL1)
Cystinuria	Apical cystine-dibasic amino acid transporter rBAT
	Light subunit of rBAT
Autosomal recessive proximal RTA	Basolateral sodium-bicarbonate cotransporter NBC1
TAL of Loop of Henle	
Bartter syndrome	
Type I	Bumetanide-sensitive Na-K-2Cl cotransporter NKCC2
Type II	Apical potassium channel ROMK
Type III	Basolateral chloride channel ClC-Kb
Type IV, with sensorineural deafness	Barttin (ClC-Kb–associated protein)
Familial hypocalcemia with Bartter features	CaSR (activation)
Type V, transient antenatal with polyhydramnios	Melanoma antigen, Family D2 (MAGED2)
Familial hypomagnesemia with hypercalciuria and nephrocalcinosis	
Without ocular abnormalities	Claudin-16 (paracellin-1)
With ocular abnormalities	Claudin-19
Familial hypocalciuric hypercalcemia[a]	CaSR (inactivation)
Neonatal severe hyperparathyroidism[b]	CaSR (inactivation)
Autosomal dominant hypercalciuric hypocalcemia	CaSR (activation) (type 1)
	$G\alpha_{11}$ G-protein (type 2)
Familial juvenile hyperuricemic nephropathy	Uromodulin (Tamm-Horsfall protein)
Distal Convoluted Tubule	
Gitelman syndrome	Thiazide-sensitive NaCl cotransporter NCC
Pseudohypoparathyroidism type Ia[c]	Guanine nucleotide-binding protein (Gs)
Familial hypomagnesemia with secondary hypocalcemia	TRPM6 cation channel[d]
Isolated recessive renal hypomagnesemia	EGF
Autosomal dominant hypomagnesemia with hypocalciuria	γ subunit of Na/K-ATPase
	HNF1B transcription factor
	PCBD1 dimerization cofactor
SeSAME/EAST syndromes	Kir4.1 potassium channel
Dominant hypomagnesemia with ataxia	Kv1.1 potassium channel
Familial tubulopathy with hypomagnesemia	Mitochondrial tRNAisoleucine
Dominant or recessive hypomagnesemia	CNNM2 (cyclin M2)
De novo severe infantile hypomagnesemia with seizures and intellectual disability	α1 subunit of Na/K-ATPase

TABLE 37.1	Molecular Bases of Genetic Disorders of Renal Transport—cont'd	

Inherited Disorder	Defective Gene Product
Collecting Duct	
Liddle syndrome	α, β, γ subunits of epithelial Na channel ENaC
Pseudohypoaldosteronism	
Type 1	
Autosomal recessive	α, β, γ subunits of ENaC
Autosomal dominant (Geller syndrome)	Mineralocorticoid (type I) receptor
Type 2 (Gordon syndrome)	WNK1, WNK4 kinases
	Cullin-3 scaffold protein
	Kelch3 adaptor protein
Glucocorticoid-remediable aldosteronism	11β-hydroxylase and aldosterone synthase (chimeric gene)[e]
Syndrome of AME	11β-hydroxysteroid dehydrogenase type II
Distal RTA	
Autosomal dominant	Basolateral anion exchanger (AE1) (band 3 protein)
Autosomal recessive, with hemolytic anemia	Basolateral anion exchanger (AE1) (band 3 protein)
Autosomal recessive (with hearing deficit)	β1 subunit of proton ATPase
	Forkhead transcription factor FOXI1
Autosomal recessive (hearing deficit variable)	α4 isoform of α subunit of proton ATPase
Carbonic anhydrase II deficiency[f]	Carbonic anhydrase type II
Nephrogenic diabetes insipidus	
X-linked	AVP 2 (V2) receptor
Autosomal	AQP-2 water channel

[a]Results from heterozygous mutation.
[b]Results from homozygous mutation.
[c]Gene also expressed in proximal tubule where functional abnormalities are clinically apparent.
[d]Gene also expressed in intestine.
[e]Gene expressed in adrenal gland.
[f]Clinical phenotype can be of proximal RTA, distal RTA, or combined.

ADHR, Autosomal dominant hypophosphatemic rickets; *AME*, apparent mineralocorticoid excess; *AQP-2*, aquaporin 2; *AVP*, arginine vasopressin; *CaSR*, calcium-sensing receptor; *DMP1*, dentin matrix protein 1; *EAST*, epilepsy, ataxia, sensorineural deafness, and tubulopathy; *EGF*, epidermal growth factor; *ENPP1*, ectonucleotide pyrophosphatase/phosphodiesterase 1; *FGF23*, fibroblast growth factor 23; *GLUT2*, glucose transporter; *GRA*, glucocorticoid-remediable aldosteronism; *HHRH*, hereditary hypophosphatemic rickets with hypercalciuria; *NCCT*, sodium chloride cotransporter; *NKCC2*, Na⁺-K⁺-2Cl⁻ cotransporter; *PHEX*, phosphate-regulating gene with homologies to endopeptidases on the X chromosome; *RTA*, renal tubular acidosis; *SeSAME*, seizures, sensorineural deafness, ataxia, mental retardation, and electrolyte imbalance; *TAL*, thick ascending limb; *XLHR*, X-linked hypophosphatemic rickets.

and FGF23 production. ARHR2 is associated with mutations in *ENPP1*, encoding ectonucleotide pyrophosphatase/phosphodiesterase 1. Patients with either subtype resemble those with autosomal dominant (i.e., FGF23 mutations) and X-linked (PHEX mutations) hypophosphatemic rickets. ARHR3 is associated with mutations in *FAM20C*, encoding a protein kinase that phosphorylates FGF23; this subtype may also manifest features of osteosclerosis.

Hereditary hypophosphatemic rickets with hypercalciuria (HHRH), an autosomal recessive disorder, is different from XLHR, ADRH, and ARHR, all of which are associated with reduced urinary calcium excretion. In contrast, hypophosphatemia in HHRH is associated with appropriate elevations of 1,25-dihydroxyvitamin D levels, and FGF23 levels are normal or reduced. This profile in HHRH is consistent with a primary defect in phosphate transport and, indeed, the disease is associated with mutations in *SLC34A3*, encoding the proximal tubule phosphate transporter Npt2c. Expression of this transporter, as well as that of *SLC34A1* encoding the more abundant transporter Npt2a, responds to physiologic stimuli such as parathyroid hormone (PTH) and dietary phosphate. Knockout of the mouse homologue of *SLC34A1* reproduces the features of human HHRH except for rickets, mouse knockout of *SLC34A3* manifests hypercalcemia and hypercalciuria, but not hypophosphatemia, nephrocalcinosis, or rickets, and a double knockout of both genes produces mice with the full phenotype of hypophosphatemia, hypercalciuria,

nephrocalcinosis, and rickets. In one human kindred, apparent autosomal dominant inheritance of HHRH was associated with compound heterozygosity for *SLC34A3* and *SLC34A1*.

Excessive Proximal Phosphate Reabsorption

Inherited hyperphosphatemia in the familial hyperostosis-hyperphosphatemia syndrome represents a mirror image of ADHR and XLHR, with excessive kidney phosphate reabsorption, persistent hyperphosphatemia, inappropriately normal levels of 1,25-dihydroxyvitamin D, and low levels of FGF23. This can result from mutations in one of three genes identified to date. These genes encode FGF23 itself, a Golgi-associated biosynthetic enzyme, *N*-acetylglucosaminyl (GalNac) transferase 3 that is involved in glycosylation of FGF23 and is necessary for its secretion, and Klotho, a transmembrane protein that complexes with the FGF23 receptor and regulates its affinity for FGF23. Together, these discoveries augment our understanding of the role of bone in the complex regulation of mineral metabolism.

Impaired Proximal Bicarbonate Transport

Selective proximal renal tubular acidosis (RTA) is inherited in an autosomal recessive manner and is associated with mutations that inactivate the basolateral sodium bicarbonate cotransporter NBC1, encoded by the gene *SLC4A4*. These patients typically exhibit short stature and often suffer blindness from ocular abnormalities, including band keratopathy, cataracts, and glaucoma; these ocular manifestations probably are a consequence of impaired bicarbonate transport in the eye. Mutations in the *SLC4A4* gene result in impaired transporter function or aberrant trafficking of the protein to the basolateral surface. This gene belongs to the same group as the gene encoding the anion exchanger AE1 (now designated *SLC4A1*), which is mutated in distal RTA. Proximal RTA can also be inherited in an autosomal dominant fashion, though the responsible gene(s) have not yet been identified.

Inherited Fanconi Syndrome: Hereditary Fructose Intolerance, Lowe Syndrome, and Dent Disease

The Fanconi syndrome represents a generalized impairment in reabsorptive function of the proximal tubule and comprises proximal RTA with aminoaciduria, glycosuria, hypouricemia, and hypophosphatemia. Some or all of these abnormalities are present in individual patients with Fanconi syndrome. Generalized Fanconi syndrome is genetically heterogeneous. It has been reported with autosomal dominant inheritance in association with mutations in genes encoding glycine amidinotransferase, the enzyme L-PBE, and the nuclear hormone receptor HNF4A (associated with MODY), and with recessive inheritance in the cases of genes encoding the sodium-phosphate transporter NaPi-IIa and the NADH:ubiquinone oxidoreductase complex assembly factor 6. Inherited causes of partial or complete Fanconi syndrome also include hereditary fructose intolerance, Lowe syndrome, and Dent disease.

Hereditary fructose intolerance is caused by mutations that result in deficiency of the aldolase B isoenzyme, which cleaves fructose-1-phosphate. Symptoms are precipitated by intake of sweets. Massive accumulation of fructose-1-phosphate occurs, leading to sequestration of inorganic phosphate and deficiency of adenosine triphosphate (ATP). Acute consequences can include hypoglycemic shock, severe abdominal symptoms, and impaired function of the Krebs cycle that produces metabolic acidosis; this is exacerbated by impaired kidney bicarbonate reabsorption. ATP deficiency leads to impaired proximal tubular function in general, including the full expression of the Fanconi syndrome with consequent rickets and stunted growth. ATP breakdown can be so dramatic as to produce hyperuricemia, as well as hypermagnesemia from the dissolution of the magnesium-ATP complex. Avoiding dietary sources of fructose can minimize acute symptoms and chronic consequences such as liver disease.

Characteristic features of the oculocerebrorenal syndrome of Lowe include congenital cataracts, mental retardation, muscular hypotonia, and the Fanconi syndrome. In contrast, Dent disease is confined to the kidney. In both syndromes, low-molecular-weight (LMW) proteinuria is a prominent feature along with other evidence of proximal tubulopathy such as glycosuria, aminoaciduria, and phosphaturia. One important and puzzling difference is that proximal RTA with growth retardation can be severe in patients with Lowe syndrome, but it is not a part of Dent disease. Some patients with Lowe syndrome or Dent disease may have rickets, which is thought to be a consequence of hypophosphatemia and, in Lowe syndrome, of acidosis as well. Hypercalciuria is a characteristic feature of Dent disease and is associated with nephrocalcinosis in most and kidney stones in many patients with Dent

disease; nephrocalcinosis and nephrolithiasis are less common in Lowe syndrome. Kidney failure is common in both of these conditions, typically occurring in young adulthood in Dent disease and even earlier in patients with Lowe syndrome.

Dent disease is caused in most cases by mutations that inactivate the chloride transporter CLC-5. This transport protein is expressed in the proximal tubule, the medullary thick ascending limb (MTAL) of the loop of Henle, and the α-intercalated cells of the collecting tubule. In the cells of the proximal tubule, CLC-5 co-localizes with the H$^+$-ATPase in subapical endosomes. These endosomes are important in the processing of proteins that are filtered at the glomerulus and taken up by the proximal tubule through adsorptive endocytosis. The activity of the H$^+$-ATPase acidifies the endosomal space, releasing the proteins from membrane-binding sites and making them available for proteolytic degradation. CLC-5 mediates electrogenic exchange of chloride for protons in these endosomes, facilitating endosomal acidification. Mutations that inactivate CLC-5 in patients with Dent disease interfere with the mechanism for reabsorption of LMW proteins and explain the consistent finding of LMW proteinuria. Glycosuria, aminoaciduria, and phosphaturia occur commonly but less consistently and may reflect altered membrane protein recycling, as CLC-5 interacts directly with several trafficking proteins. Hypercalciuria appears largely to reflect a dysregulation of kidney 1-hydroxylation of 25(OH)-vitamin D.

Lowe syndrome is associated with mutations in *OCRL1*, which encodes a phosphatidylinositol-4,5-bisphosphate-5-phosphatase. In tubular epithelial cells, this phosphatase is localized to the *trans*-Golgi network, which plays an important role in directing proteins to the appropriate membrane. The CLC-5 protein and the OCRL1 phosphatase interact with the actin cytoskeleton and are involved in assembly of the endosomal apparatus. Similarities in the kidney features of these two syndromes may be the result of defective membrane trafficking. A subset of patients with mutations in *OCRL1* have no cataracts or cerebral dysfunction and no RTA ("Dent 2" disease). Such mutations occur predominantly in the 5' end of the gene and are critical to expression of the gene in the kidney, but apparently not to expression of transcripts in eye or brain.

Disorders of Transport in the Medullary Thick Ascending Limb of Henle

Bartter Syndrome

Solute transport in the MTAL involves the coordinated functions of a set of transport proteins depicted in Fig. 37.1. These proteins are the loop diuretic-sensitive Na$^+$-K$^+$-2Cl$^-$ cotransporter (NKCC2) and the renal outer medullary potassium channel (ROMK) on the apical surface of cells of the MTAL, and the chloride channel ClC-Kb on the basolateral surface. Optimal function of the ClC-Kb chloride channel requires interaction with a subunit called *barttin*. Mutations in any of the genes encoding these four proteins lead to the phenotype of Bartter syndrome. In addition, activation of the epithelial CaSR inhibits activity of the ROMK potassium channel. Mutations producing constitutive activation of the CaSR cause familial hypocalcemic hypercalciuria. Some patients with hypocalcemic hypercalciuria have the phenotype of Bartter syndrome, and mutations in the CaSR may be considered a fifth molecular cause of this syndrome. However, defects in these five genes still do not account for all patients with Bartter syndrome.

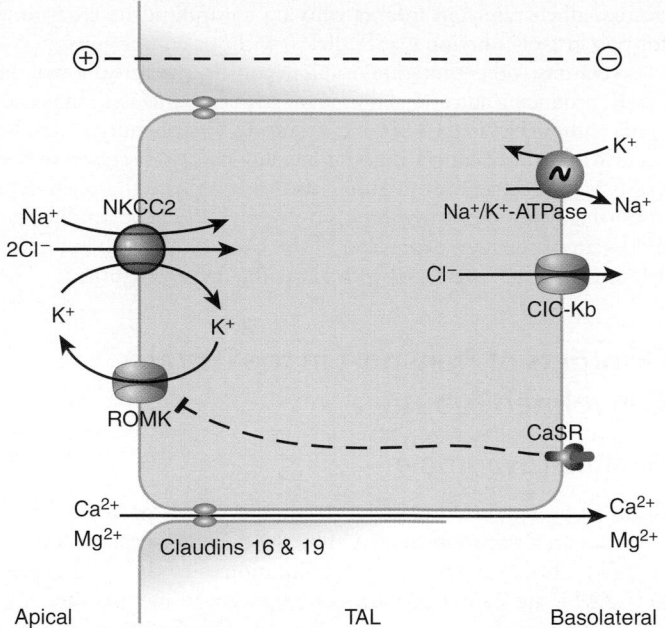

• **Fig. 37.1** Transport mechanisms in the thick ascending limb of the loop of Henle. Reabsorption of sodium chloride occurs through the electroneutral activity of the loop diuretic-sensitive Na⁺-K⁺-2Cl⁻ cotransporter (NKCC2). Activity of the basolateral sodium-potassium adenosine triphosphatase (Na⁺,K⁺-ATPase) provides the driving force for this transport and also generates a high intracellular concentration of potassium, which exits through the ATP-regulated apical potassium channel, ROMK. This ensures an adequate supply of potassium for the activity of the NKCC2 and also produces a lumen-positive electrical potential, which itself is the driving force for paracellular reabsorption of calcium, magnesium, and sodium ions through the tight junctions, involving the protein paracellin 1. Chloride transported into the cell by NKCC2 exits the basolateral side of the cell through the voltage-gated chloride channel, ClC-Kb. Activation of the extracellular calcium-sensing receptor, CaSR, inhibits solute transport in the TAL by inhibiting activity of the ROMK and possibly by other mechanisms. Mutations that inactivate the CaSR are associated with enhanced calcium transport and hypocalciuria in familial benign hypercalcemia, and mutations that activate the CaSR occur in patients with familial hypercalciuria with hypocalcemia. *ROMK,* Renal outer medullary potassium channel; *TAL,* thick ascending limb.

The ClC-Kb basolateral chloride channel provides the route for chloride exit to the interstitium. Flow of potassium through the ROMK channel ensures that potassium concentrations in the tubular lumen do not limit the activity of the NKCC2 while maintaining a positive electrical potential in the lumen of this nephron segment. This positive charge is the driving force for paracellular reabsorption of calcium and magnesium.

Bartter syndrome manifests in infancy or childhood with polyuria and failure to thrive, often occurring after a pregnancy with polyhydramnios. It is characterized by hypokalemic metabolic alkalosis, typically with hypercalciuria, and these patients resemble patients chronically taking loop diuretics that inhibit activity of NKCC2 pharmacologically. Defective function of NKCC2, ROMK, ClC-Kb, or barttin leads to impaired salt reabsorption in the MTAL, resulting in volume contraction and activation of the renin-angiotensin-aldosterone axis, which subsequently stimulates distal tubular secretion of potassium and protons, resulting in hypokalemic metabolic alkalosis. Despite impaired reabsorption of magnesium, serum magnesium levels are usually normal or only mildly reduced in patients with Bartter syndrome. Severity, age at

onset of symptoms, and particular clinical features vary with the gene abnormality. For example, nephrocalcinosis as a consequence of hypercalciuria is most common in individuals with mutations in genes encoding NKCC2 and ROMK. Barttin is expressed in the inner ear, and patients with mutations in its gene have sensorineural deafness. As Barttin is also expressed beyond the TAL in the DCT, patients with type IV Bartter syndrome often have more severe salt wasting and typically lack hypercalciuria; they often develop progressive GFR loss. Cases of severe but transient antenatal Bartter syndrome have been reported with mutations in *MAGED2* on the X chromosome, which regulates expression of NKCC2 in the MTAL, and of the thiazide-sensitive sodium-chloride cotransporter NCC in DCT.

Bartter syndrome is discussed further in Chapter 10.

Inherited Hypomagnesemic Hypercalciuria

Reabsorption of calcium and magnesium in the MTAL occurs through the paracellular route, driven by the positive electrical potential in the tubular lumen. The tight junctions between the epithelial cells determine the selective movement of cations (i.e., calcium, magnesium, and sodium). Disturbance of this selective paracellular barrier would be expected to produce parallel disorders in the reabsorption of calcium and magnesium.

Familial hypomagnesemia with substantial kidney magnesium losses, hypercalciuria, and nephrocalcinosis (FHHNC) is inherited in an autosomal recessive fashion. These patients develop kidney failure and kidney stones. Investigation of families first led to identification by positional cloning of the gene encoding a tight junction protein designated claudin 16 (also called *paracellin 1*). This was the first instance of a disease shown to result from mutations that alter a tight junction protein. Another member of this family, claudin 19, is mutated in other pedigrees in whom FHHNC is associated with ocular abnormalities (e.g., macular colobomas, myopia, horizontal nystagmus) with severe visual impairment. Both claudin 16 and claudin 19 are expressed in the thick ascending limb (TAL; Fig. 37.2), but claudin 19 also is expressed in the retina. These two proteins interact in the tight junction to regulate cation permeability. It is unclear why a defect in tight junctions is associated with hyperuricemia, a consistent finding in this disease.

Familial Hypocalciuric Hypercalcemia

The extracellular CaSR is expressed in many tissues in which ambient calcium concentrations trigger cellular responses. In the parathyroid gland, activation of the CaSR suppresses synthesis and release of PTH. In the kidney, the CaSR is expressed on the basolateral surface of cells of the TAL (cortical more than medullary), on the luminal surface of the cells of the papillary collecting duct, and in other portions of the nephron. Activation of the CaSR in the TAL probably mediates the known effects of hypercalcemia to inhibit the transport of calcium, magnesium, and sodium in this nephron segment. For example, CaSR activation inhibits activity of the ROMK potassium channel (see Fig. 37.1). This can be expected to reduce the positive electrical potential in the lumen and thereby suppress the driving force for reabsorption of calcium and magnesium. The CaSR also interacts with claudins to reduce the permeability of the tight junction to calcium and magnesium. In the papillary collecting duct, activation of the apical CaSR may explain how hypercalciuria impairs the hydroosmotic response to vasopressin, resulting in nephrogenic diabetes insipidus. Notably,

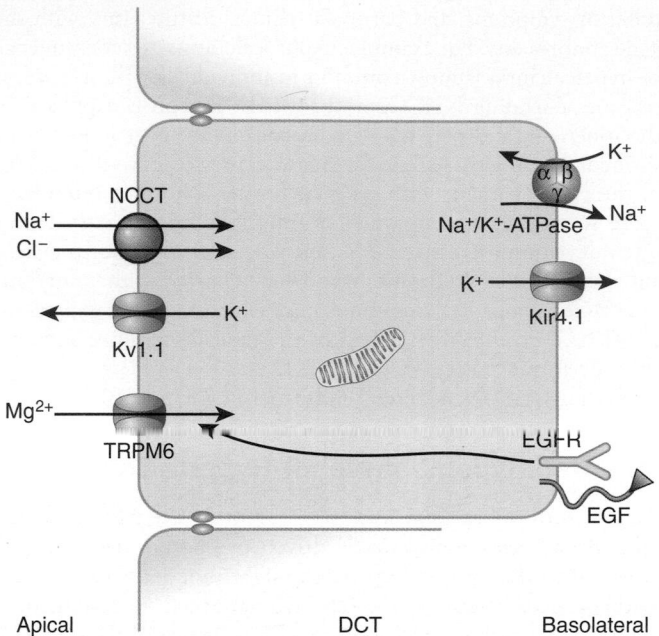

• **Fig. 37.2** Transport mechanisms in the distal convoluted tubule. The basolateral sodium-potassium adenosine triphosphatase (Na+/K+-ATPase), composed of α, β, and γ subunits, establishes the low-intracellular-sodium concentration that provides the driving force for coupled sodium and chloride entry across the apical NCC transporter. It also maintains the high intracellular potassium concentration that drives potassium exit across the apical Kv1.1 potassium channel, which establishes a positive lumen-to-cytosol electrical gradient that drives magnesium entry across the apical TRPM6 cation channel. The basolateral Kir4.1 potassium channel allows potassium exit that may serve to assure an adequate potassium supply for the Na+/K+-ATPase. The EGF receptor stimulates trafficking of TRPM6 to the apical membrane and stimulates activity of that transporter. Genes encoding these proteins are responsible for inherited electrolyte disturbances discussed in the text. *DCT,* Distal convoluted tubule; *EGF,* epidermal growth factor; *EGFR,* epidermal growth factor receptor; *NCC,* sodium chloride cotransporter.

the presence of a large volume of dilute urine produced in this situation is potentially protective against the development of nephrocalcinosis or nephrolithiasis in the setting of hypercalciuria due to hypercalcemia and an increased filtered load.

In familial hypocalciuric hypercalcemia (FHH), loss-of-function mutations of the *CASR* gene increase the set point for calcium sensing, resulting in hypercalcemia with relative elevation of PTH levels. Urinary calcium excretion is low because of enhanced calcium reabsorption in the TAL and PTH-stimulated calcium transport in the distal convoluted tubule (DCT). FHH occurs in patients heterozygous for such mutations. It is benign, as tissues are resistant to the high serum calcium levels, although cases of pancreatitis have been reported, and chondrocalcinosis may occur in older patients. Rare cases of FHH have been reported in association with two other genes involved in signal transduction from the CaSR: *GNA11*, encoding $G\alpha_{11}$ (FHH type 2), and *AP2S1*, encoding AP2σ (FHH type 3). A family history helps to differentiate FHH from primary hyperparathyroidism, which is important because parathyroidectomy should not be performed in FHH.

Infants of consanguineous parents with FHH can be homozygous for these mutations, resulting in a syndrome of severe hypercalcemia with marked hyperparathyroidism, fractures, and failure to thrive, known as *neonatal severe hyperparathyroidism.* This also

occurs, albeit rarely, in infants who are compound heterozygotes for two loss-of-function CaSR alleles, without consanguinity.

In contrast, other mutations result in constitutive activation of the CaSR, producing autosomal dominant hypocalcemia with hypercalciuria without elevated PTH concentrations. This phenotype can also occur with gain-of-function mutations in $G\alpha_{11}$. As discussed earlier, CaSR gain-of-function mutations also can produce the phenotype of Bartter syndrome. Polymorphism in the *CASR* gene producing a mild gain-of-function expression of the CaSR without frank hypocalcemia has been associated with idiopathic hypercalciuria.

Disorders of Transport in the Distal Convoluted Tubule

Gitelman Syndrome

Reabsorption of sodium chloride in the DCT occurs through electroneutral transport mediated by the thiazide-sensitive sodium chloride cotransporter (NCC). Mutations in the NCC gene (*SLC12A3*) are associated with Gitelman syndrome, another condition of hypokalemic metabolic alkalosis. The phenotype of type 3 Bartter syndrome (CLC-Kb mutation) can overlap with Gitelman, particularly regarding the presence of hypomagnesemia. Gitelman syndrome once was viewed as a variant of Bartter syndrome; however, an essential distinction between these two conditions is the presence of *hypo*calciuria in Gitelman syndrome, in contrast to the *hyper*calciuria that occurs in Bartter syndrome or in patients taking loop diuretics. Hypocalciuria in Gitelman syndrome resembles the reduction in calcium excretion that occurs in patients taking thiazide diuretics. These findings are satisfying in that they connect the clinical physiology with molecular physiology. However, our understanding of kidney transport does not allow us to explain the fact that significant hypomagnesemia with kidney magnesium wasting is typical of Gitelman syndrome, whereas in Bartter syndrome it is much less common and, when it does occur, milder.

Impaired Distal Magnesium Reabsorption

Our understanding of the mechanisms involved in distal tubular magnesium transport has been substantially enriched by the identification in recent years of genes responsible for several distinct syndromes of hypomagnesemia. The TRPM6 apical magnesium channel is critical to magnesium transport in the gut as well as in the distal tubule, and mutations in the gene encoding this channel cause a hypomagnesemic syndrome sufficiently severe as to impair PTH release and function, with secondary hypocalcemia. Potassium channels expressed on the apical (Kv1.1) and basolateral (Kir4.1) membranes are also expressed in the brain, and mutations result in hypomagnesemia as well as neurologic dysfunction including ataxia. Hypomagnesemia also results from inherited defects in distal tubule basolateral membrane proteins epidermal growth factor (EGF), the γ subunit of the Na+/K+ ATPase, and a protein of unknown function, CNNM2.

Familial Hypomagnesemia with Secondary Hypocalcemia

Patients with this syndrome experience severe hypomagnesemia, often with neonatal seizures and tetany. If not recognized and treated early, the hypomagnesemia can be fatal. Serum magnesium levels fall low enough to impair PTH release or responsiveness, and this is presumed to be the mechanism of the hypocalcemia that commonly accompanies hypomagnesemia in these patients. The primary defect appears to be in intestinal magnesium absorption, although kidney magnesium conservation also is deficient. These patients have mutations in a gene (TRPM6) encoding the TRPM6 protein. TRPM6 is a member of the long transient receptor potential channel family and is expressed in both the intestine and the DCT. Under experimental conditions, TRPM6 forms functional heteromers with its close homologue TRPM7, which, like TRPM6, has an α-kinase domain. Activity of the cation channel formed by these heteromers involves a protein, RACK1, that regulates the α-kinase. To date, mutations have not been described in TRPM7 or RACK1.

Isolated Recessive Renal Hypomagnesemia

This has been described in a single consanguineous Dutch pedigree, in which two sisters presented with hypomagnesemia with kidney magnesium wasting, otherwise normal serum and urinary electrolyte metabolism, and associated mental retardation. This disease is linked to the locus encompassing the gene encoding the epidermal growth factor (EGF), and both patients had homozygous mutation in this gene. This mutation leads to abnormal basolateral sorting of autocrine pro-EGF. EGF receptors are expressed on DCT cells and elsewhere in the tubular epithelium and vasculature, and activation of EGF receptors stimulates activity of TRPM6 magnesium channels, whereas blockade of EGF receptors with the monoclonal antibody cetuximab prevents this stimulation. This observation is consistent with the clinical experience of hypomagnesemia seen with cetuximab use as therapy for colon cancer.

Autosomal-Dominant Hypomagnesemia with Hypocalciuria

A syndrome of inherited hypomagnesemia with seizures, tetany, chondrocalcinosis, kidney magnesium wasting, and hypercalciuria has been described in association with mutation in the FXYD2 gene encoding the γ subunit of the basolateral Na⁺/K⁺-ATPase. The mechanism of a dominant-negative effect of heterozygous mutations in this gene is not fully understood. It has been speculated that the mutant subunit results in destabilization of the enzyme complex, leading to a reduced membrane potential in the DCT cells, and a reduced drive for magnesium entry across the apical TRPM6 channel. There is also evidence that the γ subunit can mediate basolateral extrusion of magnesium.

The HNF1B transcription factor is involved in tubular embryonic development and tissue-specific gene expression. HNF1B interacts with FXYD2 and with a dimerization cofactor PCBD1 that is expressed in the distal collecting duct. Mutations in the genes encoding both NHF1B and PCBD1 are associated with hypomagnesemia and kidney magnesium wasting.

SeSAME/EAST Syndromes

The KCNJ10 gene encoding the Kir4.1 potassium channel is expressed in the brain and distal tubule, and mutations produce an autosomal recessive syndrome that has been labeled "SeSAME syndrome" (for seizures, sensorineural deafness, ataxia, mental retardation, and electrolyte imbalance) and "EAST syndrome" (epilepsy, ataxia, sensorineural deafness, and tubulopathy). In the DCT, the Kir4.1 channel allows potassium recycling from cytosol back to the interstitium. This maintains a negative intracellular potential and also assures adequate extracellular potassium for optimal functioning of the Na⁺/K⁺-ATPase, which, in turn, provides the driving force for apical sodium and chloride influx through NCC. Loss of function of Kir4.1, therefore, results in abnormal electrolyte handling resembling that of NCC inactivation in Gitelman syndrome, with salt wasting, secondary activation of the renin-angiotensin-aldosterone axis, hypokalemic metabolic alkalosis, and hypocalciuria, in addition to hypomagnesemia. The neurologic findings separate SeSAME/EAST syndromes from Gitelman syndrome, and the metabolic abnormalities distinguish this from other neurodevelopmental diseases.

Isolated Hypomagnesemia with KCNA1 Mutation

The Kv1.1 apical potassium channel is important in establishing the negative potential across the DCT luminal membrane that provides the driving force for magnesium transport through TRPM6. Mutation is associated with autosomal dominant inheritance of isolated hypomagnesemia, without other electrolyte disturbances. The Kv1.1 channel is also expressed in the cerebellum, and mutations in KCNA1 are also associated with the rare episodic ataxia type 1, which, however, is not associated with hypomagnesemia. This paradox may relate to tissue-specific splice variants of the gene or differential interactions with tissue-specific Kv1 units.

Hypomagnesemia with Mitochondrial Inheritance

A single but very instructive family has been reported with maternal rather than Mendelian inheritance of symptomatic hypomagnesemia with hypocalciuria and hypokalemia, associated with mutation in a mitochondrial gene encoding a tRNA for isoleucine. The DCT has the highest energy consumption of any nephron segment and is, therefore, presumably more susceptible to impairment in energy supply for ATP-dependent sodium transport. Electrolyte abnormalities cluster in this family with hypertension and hypercholesterolemia, suggesting a possible role for mitochondria in the metabolic syndrome.

CNNM2 Mutations in Dominant Hypomagnesemia

CNNM2 encodes a protein, cyclin M2, that is expressed in the brain and other organs and on the basolateral surface of TAL and DCT in the kidney. It was identified through studies of families with either dominant or recessive inheritance of symptomatic hypomagnesemia with kidney magnesium wasting. Clinical manifestations include seizures and muscle weakness, but other electrolytes are normal. Its expression in cultured DCT cells is increased in magnesium deprivation, and functional studies of the mutant protein demonstrate reduction in magnesium-sensitive currents. Cyclin M2 may represent the postulated basolateral transporter mediating magnesium efflux or a magnesium sensor.

De Novo Mutation in ATP1A1 Causing Dominant Hypomagnesemia With Refractory Seizures and Intellectual Disability

A syndrome of severe hypomagnesemia with generalized seizures and significant intellectual disability has been described in several unrelated infants presenting as early as 6 days after birth. Heterozygous mutations in the ubiquitously expressed α1 subunit of Na$^+$/K$^+$-ATPase were identified in the children but not parents, indicating that they were *de novo*. *In vitro* expression of these variants confirmed that they were functionally significant. Hypomagnesemia was accompanied by massive kidney magnesium wasting and was only partially corrected by aggressive supplementation.

Disorders of Transport in the Collecting Tubule

Liddle Syndrome

Sodium reabsorption by the principal cells of the cortical collecting duct is physiologically regulated by aldosterone. As in other cells, low intracellular sodium concentrations are maintained by the basolateral Na$^+$/K$^+$-ATPase, and this drives sodium entry through amiloride-sensitive epithelial sodium channels (ENaC) on the apical surface. Mutations that render the ENaC persistently open produce a syndrome of excessive sodium reabsorption and low-renin hypertension (i.e., Liddle syndrome). This autosomal dominant condition often manifests in children with severe hypertension and hypokalemic alkalosis. It resembles primary hyperaldosteronism, but serum aldosterone levels are quite low, and, for this reason, the disease also has been called *pseudohyperaldosteronism*. In their original description of the syndrome, Liddle and colleagues demonstrated that aldosterone excess was not responsible for this disease, and that, although spironolactone had no effect on the hypertension, patients did respond well to triamterene or dietary sodium restriction. They proposed that the primary abnormality was excessive kidney salt conservation and potassium secretion independent of mineralocorticoid. This hypothesis proved to be correct, and it is explained by persistent sodium channel activity. Kidney transplantation in Liddle's original proband led to resolution of the hypertension, consistent with correction of the defect intrinsic to the kidneys.

In Liddle syndrome, gain-of-function mutations in the ENaC produce channels that are resistant to downregulation by physiologic stimuli such as volume expansion. Three homologous subunits, designated αENaC, βENaC, and γENaC, form the ENaC. Missense or truncating mutations in patients with Liddle syndrome alter the carboxyl-terminal cytoplasmic tail of the β or γ subunit in a domain that is important for interactions with the cytoskeletal protein that regulates activity of the ENaC. In contrast, reported mutation in αENaC produces gain of function, increasing intrinsic channel activity. In addition to the severe phenotype of Liddle syndrome resulting from these mutations, it has been speculated that polymorphisms in the ENaC sequence that have less dramatic effects on sodium channel function may contribute to the much more common low-renin variant of essential hypertension.

Pseudohypoaldosteronism Types 1 and 2

Pseudohypoaldosteronism types 1 and 2 are referred to as *pseudohypoaldosteronism,* because they feature hyperkalemia and metabolic acidosis without aldosterone deficiency. Type 1 disease is associated with salt wasting and results from mutations that inactivate either the mineralocorticoid receptor (autosomal dominant; Geller syndrome) or the ENaC (autosomal recessive). The autosomal-recessive form is milder and resolves with time, but the autosomal dominant form is more severe and persistent. Type 2 disease differs from hypoaldosteronism in that it is a hypertensive condition. Type 2 pseudohypoaldosteronism is also known as *Gordon syndrome* or *familial hyperkalemic hypertension*. It is a mirror image of Gitelman syndrome, with hyperkalemia, metabolic acidosis, and hypercalciuria, although serum magnesium levels are normal.

The first insights into the genes responsible for Gordon syndrome emerged from the discovery that it is associated with mutations in two kinases known as *WNK1* and *WNK4* (with no lysine [K]). Both are expressed in the DCT and collecting duct. WNK4 downregulates the activity of both the NCC and the ENaC. Inactivating mutations in *WNK4* result in increased activity of both pathways for sodium reabsorption. WNK4 also regulates the ROMK potassium channel, but mutations that relieve WNK4's inhibition of sodium transport enhance its inhibition of ROMK, contributing to the hyperkalemia in Gordon syndrome. WNK1 is a negative regulator of WNK4, and gain-of-function *WNK1* mutations indirectly increase NCC activity. Coordinated regulation of distal ion transport by these WNK kinases may explain how the kidney balances the two effects of aldosterone on sodium reabsorption and potassium secretion, and polymorphisms in this pathway may be relevant to the mechanisms of essential hypertension.

More recently, it has been appreciated that the majority of families with Gordon syndrome have mutations not in these WNK proteins but in two genes encoding proteins involved in the degradation of WNK kinases: *CUL3* encoding the Cullin-3 scaffold protein in an ubiquitin-E3 ligase, and *KLHL3* encoding the adaptor protein Kelch3.

Other Disorders Resembling Primary Hyperaldosteronism

Two other hereditary conditions produce hypertension in children with clinical features resembling primary hyperaldosteronism. The syndrome of apparent mineralocorticoid excess (AME) is an autosomal recessive disease in which the kidney isoform of the 11β-hydroxysteroid dehydrogenase enzyme is inactivated by mutation. In a sense, this is a genetic analogue of the ingestion of black licorice, which contains glycyrrhizic acid that inhibits this enzyme. Inactivation of the enzyme results in failure to convert cortisol to cortisone locally in the collecting duct, allowing cortisol to activate mineralocorticoid receptors and produce a syndrome resembling primary hyperaldosteronism but, like Liddle syndrome, with low circulating levels of aldosterone. AME presents in infancy with low birth weight, failure to thrive, severe hypertension, hypokalemia, metabolic alkalosis, hypercalciuria, and nephrocalcinosis, progressing to kidney failure. As in Liddle syndrome, kidney transplantation has resulted in resolution of hypertension in patients with AME syndrome.

The autosomal dominant condition known as *glucocorticoid-remediable aldosteronism* (GRA) is caused by a chromosomal rearrangement that produces a chimeric gene in which the regulatory region of the gene encoding the steroid 11β-hydroxylase (which is part of the cortisol biosynthetic pathway and is normally regulated by adrenocorticotropic hormone [ACTH]) is fused to distal sequences of the aldosterone synthase gene. This results in production of aldosterone that responds to ACTH rather than normal regulatory stimuli. Patients with GRA may have variable elevations in plasma aldosterone levels and are often normokalemic. Aldosterone levels are suppressed by glucocorticoid therapy.

Elevated urinary levels of 18-oxacortisol and 18-hydroxycortisol are characteristic of GRA.

Hereditary Renal Tubular Acidosis

Secretion of acid by the α-intercalated cells of the collecting duct is accomplished by the apical H^+-ATPase. Cytosolic carbonic anhydrase catalyzes the formation of bicarbonate from hydroxyl ions, and the bicarbonate then exits the cell in exchange for chloride through the basolateral anion exchanger, AE1 (encoded by the gene *SLC4A1*). Mutations affecting each of these proteins have been documented in patients with hereditary forms of RTA. Autosomal recessive distal RTA is associated with mutations in the β_1 subunit of the H^+-ATPase or in the forkhead transcription factor, FOXI1. This form of RTA is often severe, manifesting in young children, and typically is accompanied by hearing loss, consistent with the fact that these genes are expressed in the cochlea, endolymphatic sac of the inner ear, and kidney. Other patients with autosomal-recessive distal RTA have mutations in the gene encoding a noncatalytic α_4 isoform of the α accessory subunit of the ATPase, and these patients have less severe or no hearing deficit. Autosomal dominant RTA, a milder disease that often is undetected until adulthood, is associated with mutations in the AE1, which is also the band 3 erythrocyte membrane protein. In patients of Asian ancestry, mutations in the AE1 occur with recessive inheritance of distal RTA and hemolytic anemia.

Other genetic loci appear to be responsible for additional familial cases of distal RTA. Familial deficiency of carbonic anhydrase II is also characterized by cerebral calcification and osteopetrosis, and the latter condition reflects the important role of carbonic anhydrase in osteoclast function. The acidification defect in carbonic anhydrase II deficiency affects bicarbonate reabsorption in the proximal tubule and the collecting duct.

Nephrogenic Diabetes Insipidus

Reabsorption of water across the cells of the collecting duct occurs only when arginine vasopressin (AVP) is present. AVP activates V2 receptors on the principal cells and cells of the inner medullary collecting duct, initiating a cascade that results in fusion of vesicles containing aquaporin 2 (AQP-2) water channels into the apical membranes of these cells (Chapter 8). A gene on the X chromosome encodes the V2 receptor, and inactivating mutations in the V2 receptor gene cause the most common form, accounting for 90% of cases, of inherited nephrogenic diabetes insipidus. This results in vasopressin-resistant polyuria that typically is more severe in male patients and is associated with impaired responses to the effects of AVP that are mediated by extrarenal V2 receptors, specifically, vasodilatation and endothelial release of factor VIIIc and von Willebrand factor. Less commonly, families have been described with autosomal recessive inheritance of nephrogenic diabetes insipidus, and these patients have mutations in the gene encoding AQP-2 that result in either impaired trafficking of water channels to the luminal membrane or defective pore function. Rare autosomal dominant occurrence of nephrogenic diabetes insipidus with a mutation in AQP-2 has also been reported. Patients with defective aquaporin channels can be distinguished by intact extrarenal responses to exogenous AVP.

Complete bibliography is available at Elsevier eBooks for Practicing Clinicians.

Key Bibliography

Bichet DG. Pathophysiology, diagnosis and treatment of familial nephrogenic diabetes insipidus. *Eur J Endocrinol.* 2020;183:R29–R40.

Bockenhauer D, Bichet DG. Pathophysiology, diagnosis and management of nephrogenic diabetes insipidus. *Nat Rev Nephrol.* 2015;11:576–588.

Bockenhauer D, Feather S, Stanescu HC, et al. Epilepsy, ataxia, sensorineural deafness, tubulopathy, and KCNJ10 mutations. *N Engl J Med.* 2009;360:1960–1970.

Downie ML, Lopez Garcia SC, Kleta R, Bockenhauer D. Inherited tubulopathies of the kidney: insights from genetics. *Clin J Am Soc Nephrol.* 2020 online ahead of print.

Goldsweig BK, Carpenter TO. Hypophosphatemic rickets: lessons from disrupted FGF23 control of phosphorus homeostasis. *Curr Osteoporos Rep.* 2015;13:88–97.

Hannan FM, Babinsky VN, Thakker RV. Disorders of the calcium-sensing receptor and partner proteins: insights into the molecular basis of calcium homeostasis. *J Mol Endocrinol.* 2016;57:127–142.

Hou J, Rajagopal M, Yu AS. Claudins and the kidney. *Annu Rev Physiol.* 2013;75:479–501.

Jonsson KB, Zahradnik R, Larsson T, et al. Fibroblast growth factor 23 in oncogenic osteomalacia and X-linked hypophosphatemia. *N Engl J Med.* 2003;348:1656–1663.

Kahle KT, Ring AM, Lifton RP. Molecular physiology of the WNK kinases. *Annu Rev Physiol.* 2007;70:329–355.

Kleta R, Bockenhauer D. Bartter syndromes and other salt-losing tubulopathies. *Nephron Physiol.* 2006;104:73–80.

Konrad M, Schlingmann KP. Inherited disorders of renal hypomagnesaemia. *Nephrol Dial Transplant.* 2014;29:iv63–iv71.

O'Shaughnessy KM. Gordon syndrome: a continuing story. *Pediatr Nephrol.* 2015;30:1903–1908.

Scheinman SJ. Dent's disease. In: Lifton R, Somlo S, Giebisch G, Seldin D, eds. *Genetic Diseases of the Kidney.* San Diego, CA: Elsevier; 2009.

Scheinman SJ, Guay-Woodford LM, Thakker RV, et al. Genetic disorders of renal electrolyte transport. *N Engl J Med.* 1999;340:1177–1187.

Simon DB, Lu Y, Choate KA, et al. Paracellin-1, a renal tight junction protein required for paracellular Mg resorption. *Science.* 1999;285:103–106.

Viering DHHM, de Baaij JHF, Walsh SB, Kleta R, Bockenhauer D. Genetic causes of hypomagnesemia: a clinical overview. *Pediatr Nephrol.* 2017;32:1123–1135.

Wagner CA, Imenez Silva PH, Bourgeois S. Molecular pathophysiology of acid-base disorders. *Sem Nephrol.* 2019;39:340–352.

Wilson FH, Hariri A, Farhi A, et al. A cluster of metabolic defects caused by mutation in a mitochondrial tRNA. *Science.* 2004;306:1190–1194.

38

Sickle Cell Nephropathy

KABIR O. OLANIRAN, VIMAL K. DEREBAIL

Sickle cell anemia is the most common monogenic disorder in the world and is caused by the homozygous inheritance of the sickle β-globin gene (HbSS), produced by a single-point mutation in chromosome 11. The resultant β chain of the hemoglobin molecule possesses a substitution of valine for glutamic acid at position 6, leading to an unstable form of hemoglobin (hemoglobin S). Under conditions of low-oxygen tension, acidity, extreme temperatures, and other stressors, the altered hemoglobin undergoes polymerization, leading to the "sickling" of red blood cells (Fig. 38.1). These red cells are rigid, leading to both microvascular obstruction and the activation of inflammation and coagulation. Sickle cell disease (SCD) is also seen in the double heterozygous inheritance of hemoglobin mutations, HbS gene, and another mutation, such as in hemoglobin SC disease and sickle β-thalassemia.

The prevalence of sickle cell trait (SCT; HbAS) in the United States is between 6% and 9% among Blacks, with sickle cell anemia occurring in approximately 1 of 500 Black live births. Globally, the prevalence of the hemoglobin S mutation varies greatly and is often highest where malaria is endemic due to the protection it affords against malarial disease. The highest prevalence is seen in sub-Saharan Africa, the Middle East, parts of the Mediterranean, and India. In 2010, an estimated 312,000 neonates were born worldwide with sickle cell anemia.

Although SCD affects multiple systems throughout the body and is characterized by acute pain crises and progressive multiorgan damage, the kidney is a particularly susceptible organ. The renal medulla, with its lower oxygen tension, high osmolarity, lower pH, and relatively sluggish blood flow, is an ideal environment for "sickling" and microvascular obstruction. As a result, kidney manifestations are common in SCD (Table 38.1).

Pathophysiology

Although the classic understanding of SCD is based on microvascular obstruction, its pathophysiology is better understood in the context of recurrent vasoocclusion with ischemia-reperfusion injury and hemolytic anemia. In addition to triggering hemoglobin polymerization, inflammation and other stressors also initiate erythrocyte adhesion to endothelium and leukocytes, beginning the process of microvascular obstruction. These processes are dynamic, resulting in ischemia followed by the restoration of blood flow and the subsequent reperfusion injury, with resultant oxidative stress and inflammatory cytokine production. Intravascular hemolysis is another contributor to disease burden, with the

release of free hemoglobin into the plasma, generating reactive oxygen species and depleting nitric oxide. These processes produce endothelial dysfunction and activate the coagulation system.

Disease severity in SCD appears to be modulated by the relative concentration of sickle hemoglobin (HbS). The presence of fetal hemoglobin (HbF), which can be increased with hydroxyurea therapy, reduces the relative content of hemoglobin S; accordingly, haplotypes of the mutation that correlate with lower HbF production, most notably the Central African Republic haplotype, typically have the most severe disease manifestations. Similarly, coinheritance of α-thalassemia mutations reduces intracellular HbS concentration and leads to reduced hemolysis and fewer complications.

Within the kidney, these pathologic mechanisms lead to changes in kidney hemodynamics, tubulointerstitial damage, and, in some patients, glomerular disease.

Kidney Hemodynamics

Much like the systemic circulation in sickle cell disease, the kidney exhibits contrasting macrovascular hyperperfusion and microvascular hypoperfusion. Systemically, plasma volume and cardiac output are both increased in young SCD patients, and systemic blood pressure and vascular resistance are low. This results in increased systemic and regional large-vessel blood flow, contrasted by microcirculatory defects that cause underperfusion in small vascular beds. The kidney reflects this same incongruity in perfusion with overall increased renal blood flow but hypoperfusion of the microcirculation of the renal medulla.

Glomerular hyperfiltration is extraordinarily common among patients with SCD and can be detected before 13 months of age. Glomerulomegaly is evident even in patients without clinical kidney disease and may contribute to hyperfiltration. Glomerular hyperfiltration is likely driven by vasodilatation of the afferent arteriole, which may occur as a compensatory response to chronic tissue hypoxia in the renal medulla. The exact mechanisms behind this response are not fully known but may be mediated by up-regulation of the prostaglandin and nitric oxide systems. Indomethacin and other prostaglandin inhibitors, administered at doses that would not affect the GFR in normal individuals, can reduce GFR to more normal values in patients with SCD. Hemolysis and production of free heme may also play a role in the process. Sickle cell animal models have demonstrated that hemolysis induces up-regulation of heme-oxygenase-1 (HO-1) with subsequent production of carbon monoxide (CO), a local vasodilator.

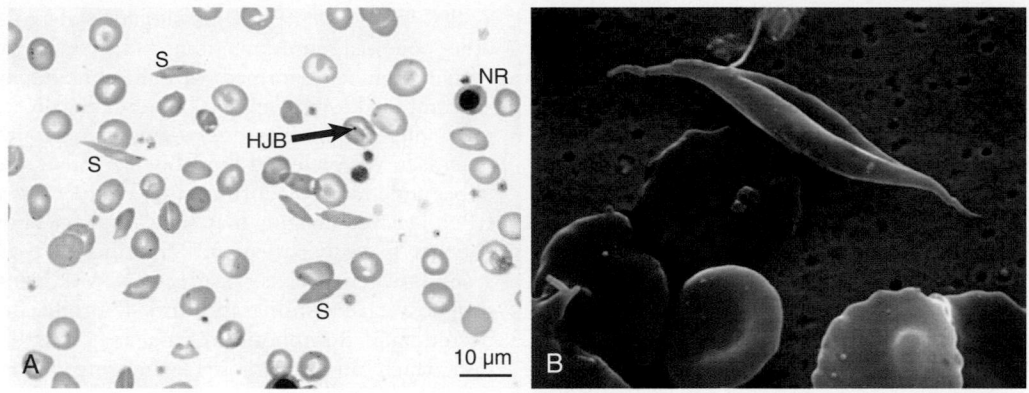

• **Fig. 38.1** (A) Peripheral blood smear of a patient with sickle cell anemia. This blood film shows irreversibly sickled cells (S), a nucleated red blood cell (NR), and a Howell-Jolly body (HJB); these last two features are mainly associated with hyposplenism (stained with May-Grunwald-Giemsa). (B) Scanning electron microscopic image of sickled and other red blood cells, false-colored red. Photographed with Philips 501 SEM. (A from Rees DC, Williams TN, Gladwin MT. Sickle cell disease. *Lancet*. 2010;376:2018–2031; B from EM Unit, UCL Medical School, Royal Free Campus, Wellcome Images.)

TABLE 38.1	Kidney Pathology in Sickle Cell Disease
Kidney Abnormality	**Clinical Consequence**
Glomerulus	
Hyperfiltration	Increased GFR (early), albuminuria/proteinuria, sickle glomerulopathy, CKD (late)
Proximal Tubule	
Enhanced proximal tubule activity	Increased creatinine secretion, increased phosphate resorption (hyperphosphatemia)
Depressed renin	Hyporeninemic hypoaldosteronism (hyperkalemia)
Distal Tubule/Cortical Collection Duct	
Impaired hydrogen ion secretion	Metabolic acidosis (type 4 RTA)
Impaired potassium secretion	Hyperkalemia
Impaired urinary concentration	Hyposthenuria
Interstitium	
Chronic "sickling" in vasa recta	Hematuria, renal papillary necrosis (due to ischemia), renal medullary carcinoma, CKD

CKD, Chronic kidney disease; *GFR*, glomerular filtration rate; *RTA*, renal tubular acidosis.

Tubulointerstitial Disease

Impaired Urinary Concentration

The most commonly reported kidney manifestation in patients with SCD is the loss of maximal urinary concentrating ability. Typically, the generation of concentrated urine requires an intact collecting duct and a medullary concentration gradient. The juxtamedullary nephrons, which extend deepest into the medulla and are most capable of producing a high concentration gradient, are also those most likely to be affected by sickling in the medullary vasa recta. Microangiographic studies demonstrate the obliteration of the vasa recta in these patients, with subsequent fibrosis and shortening of the renal papilla. The functional result of these anatomic changes ultimately manifests as an inability to achieve a urinary osmolarity above 400 mOsm/kg. Early in life, this defect is partially reversible following blood transfusions that rapidly increase normal hemoglobin A (HbA) and reduce sickling in the vasa recta. However, impaired urinary concentration becomes fixed later in life (as early as age 15) and no longer improves with transfusion. As a result, depending on water and solute intake, patients with SCD may have obligatory water losses of up to 2.0 L/day, predisposing them to higher serum osmolality and thereby potentially exacerbating sickle crises. The ability to produce a maximally dilute urine and to excrete free water remains intact.

Hematuria

Hematuria can be one of the most dramatic kidney presentations in patients with SCD and may range from microscopic hematuria to gross hematuria. Gross hematuria may occur in patients of any age, including young children. Although the etiology of hematuria remains unclear, vasoocclusion occurring in the acidic, hyperosmolar, low-oxygen-tension environment of the medulla is thought to play a central role. Studies of kidneys removed from sickle cell patients with severe hematuria demonstrate severe stasis of peritubular capillaries, particularly those in the medulla, as well as erythrocytes extravasated into the collecting tubules. In addition to the aforementioned vascular occlusion–mediated ischemia and oxidative/reperfusion injury, sickling in these vessels may also lead to vessel wall injury and necrosis, which could cause the structural changes leading to hematuria.

Typically, hematuria is unilateral and occurs nearly four times more often from the left kidney. The longer course and higher venous pressures of the left renal vein as it traverses between the aorta and superior mesenteric artery likely lead to this phenomenon.

Although bleeding is typically benign and self-limited, massive hemorrhage can occur and can be potentially life threatening.

Treatment consists of conservative management, including bed rest and the maintenance of high urine output to prevent clots. Alkalinization of the urine may help by raising medullary pH, thereby reducing sickling; however, no studies have shown a proven benefit of this intervention. Intravenous fluids may be used to ensure high urine flow but must be used with caution in patients at risk for congestive heart failure or acute chest syndrome. Diuretics can increase urine flow rates, but care must be taken to avoid volume depletion.

For patients with massive and persistent hematuria despite conservative therapy, antifibrinolytic agents, such as ε-aminocaproic acid (EACA) or tranexamic acid, may be beneficial. Reports have demonstrated improvement with EACA, although no standard dose regimen or length of therapy has been defined. However, these agents are prothrombotic and must be used with caution in SCD patients who are already at risk for thrombotic events. Currently, EACA use is recommended only for a limited period and at the lowest dose necessary to achieve inhibition of urinary fibrinolytic activity. In addition to EACA, intravenous vasopressin to limit hematuria has been successful in case reports.

In patients who are refractory to medical therapy, invasive intervention may be necessary. Mechanical tamponade or percutaneous embolization, if bleeding can be localized by imaging, may be attempted. Rarely, unilateral nephrectomy of the affected kidney is required. In all patients with hematuria, and particularly in those with persistent or massive hematuria, alternative causes should be considered, including acquired or hereditary bleeding disorders or kidney abnormalities such as nephrolithiasis, polycystic kidney disease, or renal medullary carcinoma (RMC; see next sections).

Renal Papillary Necrosis

Renal papillary necrosis (RPN) is common in SCD, occurring in more than 60% of patients in some series. Although often accompanied by hematuria, a similar proportion of patients may be asymptomatic. With severe sickling in the vasa recta, the renal papillae that depend on these vessels can undergo focal, repetitive infarcts leading to necrosis (Fig. 38.2). If hematuria is present,

as described earlier, patients should undergo an evaluation for other potential causes, including kidney masses or nephrolithiasis. Imaging can be performed with ultrasonography, although a helical computed tomography (CT) scan may detect RPN earlier. CT urography with intravenous contrast timed for the excretory phase is, in fact, the preferred modality. Persistent streaking contrast at upper and lower pole fornices may be the most specific feature for RPN. Delayed imaging may show evidence of prior RPN in SCD patients. In many patients, RPN ultimately results in calcification around the renal pelvis. Treatment, as with hematuria, is generally supportive, using similar measures. If significant sloughing occurs, necrotic and thrombotic material may lead to ureteral obstruction, which can be diagnosed by imaging and relieved by stenting.

Renal Medullary Carcinoma

RMC is extremely rare and seen almost exclusively in patients with SCT, although there are a few reports in patients with SCD (<10% of cases). The vast majority of cases have been reported in patients younger than 40 years of age, with a median age at presentation of 21–24 years. Men appear to be affected more than twice as often as women. In contradistinction to hematuria and papillary necrosis, RMC has a predilection for the right kidney (>70% of cases). The typical presentation is gross hematuria, often painless but sometimes accompanied by flank or lumbar pain or abdominal masses. Some patients may not present with a clinically evident mass but may have suspected kidney abscesses or urinary tract infection. Constitutional symptoms of weight loss, fevers, and fatigue may be present. Repetitive ischemic injuries to the tubules are postulated to drive the development of this lesion. Loss of SMARCB1, a component of chromatin remodeling and a tumor suppressor gene, has been identified as a feature of RMC. Disease is often metastatic at diagnosis with regional lymph nodes, liver, and lungs as the most common sites, followed by bone and adrenal glands. Median survival is only 6 to 12 months, and mortality approaches nearly 95% even with treatment. For these reasons, presentation of gross hematuria in patients with SCT or

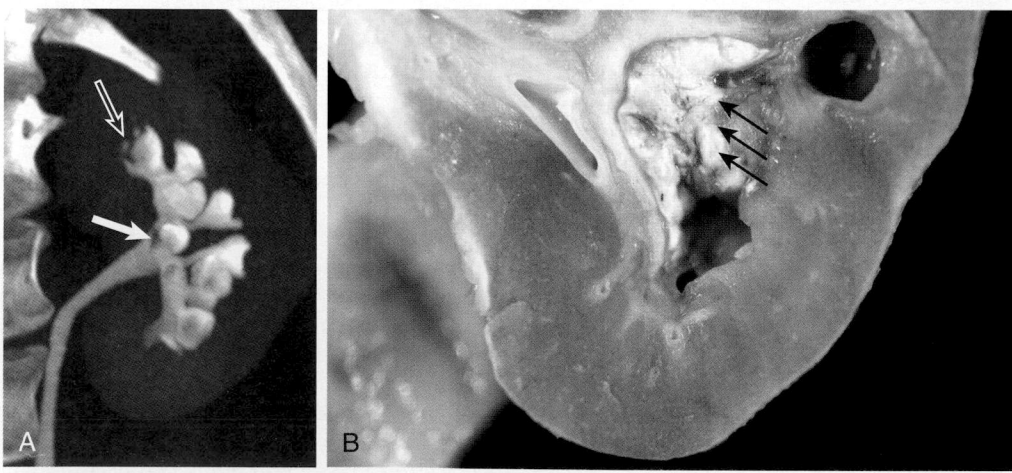

• **Fig. 38.2** (A) Maximum-intensity projection (MIP) images from computed tomography urography in a 23-year-old woman with sickle cell trait presenting with intermittent gross hematuria for 5 days. Pooling of contrast material within multiple papillae bilaterally *(open arrow)* is consistent with papillary necrosis. Filling defect within left renal pelvis *(solid arrow)* was shown to represent blood clot at ureteroscopy. (B) Gross photomicrograph of a bivalved kidney demonstrating necrosis of a renal papilla *(arrows)*. Over time, this area will form a scar with cystic dilation of the calices. (A from Chow LC, Kwan SW, Olcott EW, et al. Split-Bolus MDCT urography with synchronous nephrographic and excretory phase enhancement. *Am J Roentgenol.* 2007;189:314–322. B courtesy Vincent Moylan Jr, MS, PA.)

SCD should prompt consideration of imaging via ultrasonography or preferably CT scan to allow early diagnosis.

Acidification, Potassium Excretion, and Other Tubular Abnormalities

Metabolic acidosis may be found in up to 40% of patients even in the absence of overt kidney failure. Although some patients may manifest an incomplete distal renal tubular acidosis (dRTA), as in prior reports, recent data suggest that the acidosis is more commonly driven, in part, by impaired urinary acidification and impaired ammonium (NH_4^+) excretion. Hyperkalemia may accompany acidosis; however, this is rare without significant potassium ingestion or medications that interfere with potassium handling. The inability of the damaged distal nephron to excrete ammonium and titratable acids as well as an inability to respond to aldosterone, lead to these findings. If necessary, treatment with potassium restriction, sodium bicarbonate, and loop diuretics can be effective.

The aforementioned abnormalities generally indicate impaired distal tubule secretory function. In contrast, the proximal tubule demonstrates enhanced activity. Sodium reabsorption is increased, leading to less urinary excretion as well as a relative resistance to loop diuretics. Accompanying this increase in sodium reabsorption is an enhancement of proximal phosphate reabsorption that may cause hyperphosphatemia in settings of increased phosphorus loads (hemolysis, rhabdomyolysis). In addition, uric acid secretion is increased, perhaps as an adaptive mechanism to the increased uric acid load from chronic hemolysis. Finally, secretion of creatinine in the proximal tubule is also heightened, diminishing the usefulness of creatinine clearance and creatinine-based equations to estimate GFR.

Sickle Cell Glomerulopathy

The presence of glomerular involvement has long been noted in SCD, with levels of proteinuria ranging from low-level albuminuria to overt nephrotic syndrome. Initial reports of glomerular lesions were those of immune complex deposition and pathology consistent with membranoproliferative glomerulonephritis. However, more recent studies have demonstrated glomerulomegaly often with features of focal segmental glomerulosclerosis (FSGS) in the majority of patients with sickle cell nephropathy (Fig. 38.3). In children,

mesangial hypercellularity may be a more common feature and perhaps a precursor to later sclerosis. As in other forms of FSGS, immunofluorescence of biopsy samples may demonstrate minimal staining with immunoglobulin M (IgM), C1q, and C3, but electron microscopy usually fails to identify any electron-dense deposits. Collapsing lesions have also been reported, presumably due to vascular occlusion and ischemia; however, the role of concurrent APOL1 inheritance remains to be defined in these cases. Hemosiderin deposition is often prominent in the tubular epithelium, but also may be present focally in glomerular epithelial cells (Fig. 38.4). Sickled erythrocytes are often noted in medullary vasculature and less commonly in glomeruli. The clinical sequelae of these composite lesions are thought to begin with albuminuria and evolve into overt proteinuria, loss of kidney function, and development of advanced CKD.

Albuminuria and Proteinuria

Albuminuria and overt proteinuria clearly increase as patients with SCD age, with more than 60% of adults over the age of 35 exhibiting low-level albuminuria. However, children below the age of 10 rarely demonstrate these findings. Recent evidence suggests that albuminuria and proteinuria in children is preceded by persistent glomerular hyperfiltration occurring between the ages of 4 and 10 years, defined by GFR estimated with cystatin above 180 mL/min. Over 20% of adults with low-level albuminuria will progress to overt proteinuria and progressive GFR decline. The presence of albuminuria, especially mild or low-grade albuminuria, may wax and wane, but one prospective study found that a baseline urine albumin-to-creatinine ratio ≥100mg/g was associated with persistent albuminuria over time. The nephrotic syndrome itself is fairly rare, but it portends a poor kidney prognosis. An uncommon but well-recognized cause of acute onset of the nephrotic syndrome is parvovirus B19 infection, which often leads to the collapsing variant of FSGS. Abnormalities in albumin excretion are more frequent in sickle cell anemia (HbSS disease) and in sickle-β^0-thalassemia than in other sickle hemoglobinopathies (HbSC disease, HbS-β^+-thalassemia). The presence of APOL1 and MYH9 has also been associated with proteinuria in sickle cell nephropathy. In contrast, the presence of alpha thalassemia appears to be protective. The severity of SCD in some series also seems to correlate with the development of albuminuria.

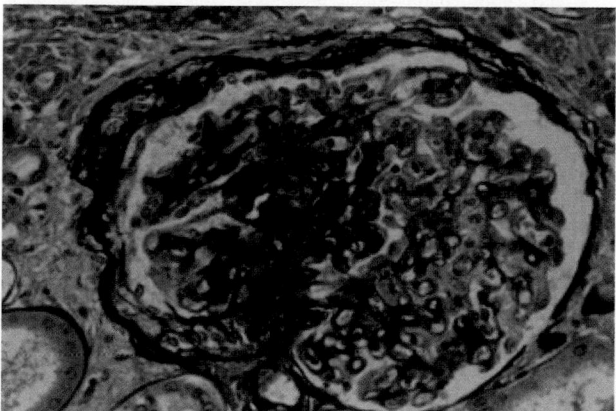

• **Fig. 38.3** Individuals with sickle cell disease and proteinuria may exhibit glomerulomegaly and focal segmental glomerulosclerosis (FSGS), most often the perihilar variant. (Jones' silver methenamine stain with hematoxylin–eosin counterstain, ×300). (From Falk RJ, Scheinman J, Phillips G, et al. Prevalence and pathologic features of sickle cell nephropathy and response to inhibition of angiotensinconverting enzyme. *N Engl J Med*. 1992;326:910.)

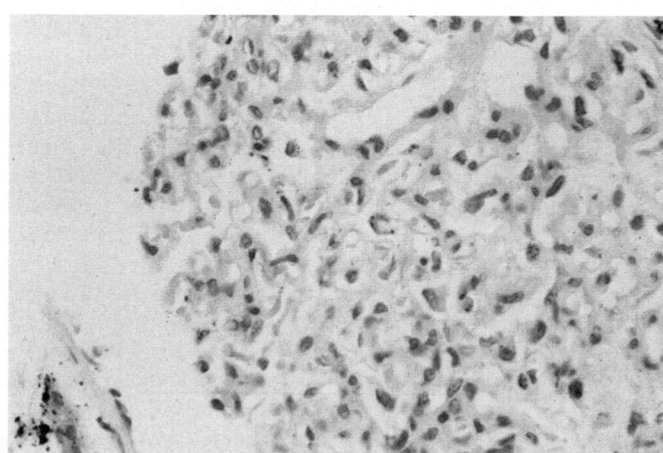

• **Fig. 38.4** Sickle cell nephropathy with iron deposits in glomerular visceral epithelial cells and tubular epithelial cells (*bottom left*) (Prussian blue iron stain). (From Lusco MA, Fogo AB, Najafian B, et al. AJKD atlas of renal pathology: sickle cell nephropathy. *Am J Kidney Dis*. 2016;68:e1.)

The underlying pathophysiology of albuminuria is multifactorial and probably related to a variety of pathologic developments in SCD. Persistence of glomerular hyperfiltration, as in other diseases with this feature, results in albuminuria and eventual GFR decline. As repetitive sickling occurs and interstitial fibrosis leads to the dropout of affected nephrons, hyperfiltration is further accentuated in the remaining glomeruli. In addition, evidence suggests that endothelial dysfunction from both direct injury related to sickling and the release of free heme during hemolysis contributes to the glomerulopathy. Subsequently, markers of hemolysis, such as reticulocyte hemoglobin and lactate dehydrogenase (LDH), may correlate with albuminuria, as do mediators of endothelial dysfunction including soluble fms-like tyrosine kinase-1 (sFLT-1). Endothelin-1 (ET-1) also appears to mediate glomerular injury via reactive oxygen species.

Treatment

The role of kidney biopsy in SCD to guide treatment has not been established. In general, kidney biopsy should be considered, when safe, in adult SCD patients with persistent proteinuria in excess of 1 g/24 hours, and performed in all SCD patients with persistent nephrotic-range proteinuria. While the assumption that all proteinuria in SCD patients is due to underlying SCD may be largely true, severe pathologies, such as collapsing FSGS, may go undiagnosed, and concurrent diseases not uncommon among Blacks, such as lupus nephritis or primary FSGS, could also be missed. Furthermore, due to limitations of serum creatinine in SCD (discussed later), interstitial fibrosis may not correlate with estimated GFR, and kidney biopsies may provide prognostic information and bolster the need for disease-modifying therapies in SCD.

Therapies for reducing albuminuria and proteinuria due to sickle cell nephropathy have been advocated in the hope of delaying the progression of CKD, although little prospective data exist to determine whether any therapy is truly effective. As with many diseases in which proteinuria is a feature, inhibition of the renin-angiotensin system forms the mainstay of therapy. Several studies have demonstrated a short-term reduction in both proteinuria and hyperfiltration with the use of angiotensin-converting enzyme (ACE) inhibitors and angiotensin receptor blockers (ARBs). These effects seem to be independent of any blood pressure lowering and are likely related to the reduction of glomerular capillary hypertension. Current guidelines suggest screening for proteinuria beginning at age 10, and then annually if negative. If detected, ACE inhibitors or ARBs should be initiated. With the institution and dose titration of these agents, both kidney function and serum potassium must be monitored closely, as SCD patients are prone to the metabolic effects of reduced GFR and impaired potassium secretion. Animal studies suggest that ARBs carry less potential harm compared to ACE inhibitors because ARBs only block the fibrotic effects of angiotensin and not the urine concentrating effects. These effects have yet to be examined in depth in humans.

Hydroxyurea, or hydroxycarbamide, is now recommended for all SCD patients with symptomatic disease regardless of severity. Its role in the management of albuminuria and CKD is less well defined. The mechanism of action is not completely understood but is, in part, due to the ability of hydroxyurea to induce HbF production and thereby reduce the overall concentration of hemoglobin S. Hydroxyurea may also affect the synthesis of nitric oxide and has other beneficial effects. The addition of hydroxyurea to ACE inhibitors may provide further reduction in proteinuria. Other data have been conflicting regarding hydroxyurea use in the prevention of hyperfiltration in children with

SCD. However, recent cross-sectional data and interventional studies in adults with SCD have demonstrated hydroxyurea may be associated with a reduction in albuminuria. At present, albuminuria alone in SCD is not a clear indication for hydroxyurea, but its use should be considered, particularly in the setting of any other identifiable sickle cell disease symptoms.

In recent years, several new therapeutic agents for the prevention of frequent pain crises have been approved by the FDA including L-glutamine, voxelotor, and crizanlizumab. However, their effect on albuminuria and proteinuria in SCD remains to be seen, although it remains plausible that improvement of underlying disease would potentially benefit the associated kidney disease. Table 38.2 contains a summary for management of proteinuria in patients with SCD.

Management of Chronic Kidney Disease in Sickle Cell Disease

Identification of reduced GFR in the setting of SCD may be difficult. Traditional methods using serum creatinine to estimate GFR are hampered in SCD because of enhanced secretion of creatinine. Typical estimating equations when compared with radionucleotide measures of GFR demonstrated significant bias. The CKD-EPI

TABLE 38.2	Approach to Proteinuria in Sickle Cell Disease

- Important components of the history unique to sickle cell disease include hydration practices, frequency of pain episodes managed at home, frequency of admissions/emergency room visits for pain episodes, prior history of severe complications (acute chest syndrome, priapism, lower extremity ulcers not caused by hydroxyurea, strokes, and renal papillary necrosis), and a history of sickle cell retinopathy.
- Screening for proteinuria/albuminuria by quantitative measurement at least yearly and correlate levels with hemolysis labs.
- Confirmation of significantly elevated spot proteinuria/albuminuria by 24-hour urine studies at least once due to tubular hypersecretion of creatinine.
- In patients with proteinuria sustained >500 mg/24 hours, assess HIV, RPR, hepatitis B, hepatitis C, complement, antinuclear antibodies, and urine sediment. Serum protein electrophoresis and free light chains should also be evaluated in older patients. Parvovirus should be evaluated in nephrotic-range proteinuria. Where available, consider genetic testing for APOL1 for prognostication.
- We recommend considering a kidney biopsy under the following circumstances, if safe:
  - Stable baseline serum creatinine with new onset urine protein equivalent ≥1 g/24 hr that is sustained over 4 weeks and cannot be explained by acute pain episodes, NSAID use, medications, or any other known kidney insult.
  - Progressively rising serum creatinine from baseline with new-onset sustained urine protein equivalent to ≥0.5 g/24 hours with no known cause described above.
  - New-onset urine protein equivalent to ≥3 g/24 hours, regardless of kidney function, if safe.
- Avoid NSAID use once proteinuria is detected.
- Consider ACE inhibitors or ARBs if there are no contraindications. Target blood pressure in those with concurrent hypertension is <130/80 mmHg.
- Discuss the initiation of additional sickle cell disease-modifying therapies with the patient's hematologist.

Adapted from Ataga KI, Derebail VK, Archer DR. The glomerulopathy of sickle cell disease. Am J Hematol. 2014 Sep; 89(9):907–914.

equation seems to afford the best creatinine-based assessment of eGFR, although it still can overestimate GFR. Elevated creatinine may, therefore, be a late indicator of CKD in patients with SCD. Use of serum cystatin C (without creatinine) for estimating eGFR may perform better than serum creatinine-based equations; however, this measure is not as widely available.

Nevertheless, changes in creatinine and estimated GFR over time may be used to determine progression. Therefore, an early baseline serum creatinine should be established in SCD. Retrospective studies have identified several risk factors for faster GFR decline in SCD including severe phenotypes (HbSS and S-beta thalassemia zero), male sex, more than one admission per year for pain crisis, lower hemoglobin, and concurrent comorbid conditions (hypertension, diabetes mellitus, and cardiovascular disease). One prospective study found that persistent albuminuria is also associated with more rapid GFR decline.

The management of SCD patients who have CKD is similar to patients with CKD due to other causes, with a few exceptions. The first relates to the management of anemia. With chronic ischemic kidney insults and ongoing hemolysis, SCD patients typically have a greater stimulus for erythropoietin and exhibit higher endogenous erythropoietin levels. However, with progressive kidney disease, the ability to produce adequate endogenous erythropoietin is lost, typically occurring when GFR falls below 60 mL/min in SCD. As with other forms of CKD, erythropoiesis-stimulating agents (ESAs) are used to maintain hemoglobin levels and reduce transfusion needs, but SCD patients usually require much larger ESA doses, and the target hemoglobin is different from what is typical in other CKD or ESKD populations. In general, a maximum achieved hemoglobin level of 10 mg/dL is recommended to avoid precipitation of vasoocclusive crises. Iron stores should be maintained to maximize erythropoiesis in those not receiving chronic transfusions, although care must be taken to avoid iron overload in this susceptible population.

Finally, even though patients with SCD are at greater risk for advanced CKD, hypertension is an uncommon feature in this population. Despite a prevalence of hypertension of 28% in the general Black population, only about 2% to 6% of Blacks with SCD exhibit hypertension. Various explanations for this finding have been posited, including relative volume depletion and reduced systemic vascular resistance. However, pediatric data suggest the SCD patient may manifest primarily masked hypertension that requires ambulatory readings to detect, and hypertension may simply be underdiagnosed. If hypertension is detected in patients with SCD, therapy should be initiated as in any patient with CKD or at risk for CKD. Most would consider a goal blood pressure of 130/80 mm Hg. Some suggest avoidance of diuretics unless overt hypervolemia is present given the predisposition of individuals with SCD to volume depletion, which can induce a pain crisis and microvascular thrombosis.

End-Stage Kidney Disease in Sickle Cell Disease

Once patients with SCD reach ESKD, either peritoneal dialysis or hemodialysis presents viable dialysis options. Early referral to a nephrologist is particularly important for this population of patients. In the United States, patients with kidney failure due to SCD have a 26% mortality rate in their first year of dialysis. European data suggest mortality may not be as pronounced but is still 2-fold higher than the non-SCD population. Overall,

cardiovascular mortality, infections, and thromboembolic events may be more likely in SCD patients receiving dialysis as compared to non-SCD dialysis patients. There is no strong clinical evidence regarding the preferred dialysis modality in SCD. Peritoneal dialysis (PD) may confer benefits with gentler ultrafiltration and, therefore, lower risk for rapid hemoconcentration precipitating pain crisis or hospitalizations. The potential mortality benefit of PD versus hemodialysis (HD) in SCD has not yet been demonstrated. SCD patients receiving HD should be educated to minimize interdialytic weight gains and carefully monitored to avoid high ultrafiltration rates. Additionally, high dialysate sodium and cooler dialysate temperatures could promote red blood cell sickling and should be avoided. The target hemoglobin in SCD dialysis patients may be even lower and should be guided by the baseline hemoglobin prior to initiating dialysis and evaluation for symptoms of anemia. The primary hematologist should be consulted in setting hemoglobin targets especially in the first several months after dialysis initiation.

Although SCD patients are less likely to be listed for kidney transplantation and less likely to receive a transplant, this kidney replacement modality appears to offer survival benefit similar to other causes of kidney failure. In the more recent era of kidney transplantation, the 6-year survival of SCD patients receiving kidney transplantation has approached 70% (compared with ~55% in earlier reports). Overall mortality for SCD kidney transplant recipients is now comparable to that of patients with diabetes. Furthermore, the likelihood of graft failure does not seem to be greater in SCD recipients. After transplantation, SCD patients must be monitored for allograft thrombosis, an increase in vasoocclusive crises, and a recurrence of sickle glomerulopathy, which has been reported as early as 3 years after transplantation. Hydroxyurea and exchange transfusion have been used in the posttransplant period, and simultaneous bone marrow transplantation could be curative of the disease as a whole.

Sickle Cell Trait

Patients with a single hemoglobin S mutation are deemed to have SCT, HbAS. Although generally viewed as a benign condition, SCT does have manifestations more akin to an intermediate phenotype. Kidney manifestations are by far the most commonly reported comorbidities in SCT and are similar to those seen in SCD.

Impaired urinary concentration is common, albeit not as severe as that seen in SCD. Again, the severity of the concentrating defect seems to be modulated by the coinheritance of α-thalassemia. Hematuria and RPN also occur in this population. As noted earlier, RMC, rarely described in SCD, has been nearly exclusively reported in patients with SCT.

With its numerous reported kidney abnormalities, speculation as to whether SCT contributes to the development of CKD has been longstanding. An early study demonstrated accelerated progression to kidney failure among those with concurrent SCT and adult polycystic kidney disease, and high prevalence of SCT has been reported in Black kidney failure patients. Although there were early conflicting reports, multiple recent, population-based studies have shown SCT to be associated with faster eGFR decline, albuminuria, incident and prevalent CKD, and kidney failure. These studies have provided more definitive evidence that SCT may be a risk factor for CKD.

Complete bibliography is available at Elsevier eBooks for Practicing Clinicians.

Key Bibliography

Alvarez O, Miller ST, Wang WC, et al. Effect of hydroxyurea treatment on renal function parameters: results from the multi-center placebo-controlled BABY HUG clinical trial for infants with sickle cell anemia. *Pediatr Blood Cancer*. 2012;59:668–674.

Alvarez O, Rodriguez MM, Jordan L, et al. Renal medullary carcinoma and sickle cell trait: a systematic review. *Pediatr Blood Cancer*. 2015;62:1694–1699.

Asnani MR, Lynch O, Reid ME. Determining glomerular filtration rate in homozygous sickle cell disease: utility of serum creatinine based estimating equations. *PLoS ONE*. 2013;8:e69922.

Ataga KI, Derebail VK, Archer DR. The glomerulopathy of sickle cell disease. *Am J Hematol*. 2014;89:907–914.

Aygun B, Mortier NA, Smeltzer MP, et al. Hydroxyurea treatment decreases glomerular hyperfiltration in children with sickle cell anemia. *Am J Hematol*. 2013;88:116–119.

Bartolucci P, Habibi A, Stehlé T, et al. Six months of hydroxyurea reduces albuminuria in patients with sickle cell disease. *J Am Soc Nephrol*. 2016;27:1847–1853.

Boyle SM, Jacobs B, Sayani FA, et al. Management of the dialysis patient with sickle cell disease. *Semin Dial*. 2016;29:62–70.

Cazenave M, Audard V, Bertocchio JP, et al. Tubular acidification defect in adults with sickle cell disease. *Clin J Am Soc Nephrol*. 2020;15:16–24.

Guasch A, Navarrete J, Nass K, et al. Glomerular involvement in adults with sickle cell hemoglobinopathies: prevalence and clinical correlates of progressive renal failure. *J Am Soc Nephrol*. 2016;17:2228–2235.

Heimlich JB, Speed JS, O'Connor PM, et al. Endothelin-1 contributes to the progression of renal injury in sickle cell disease via reactive oxygen species. *Br J Pharmacol*. 2016;173(2):386–395.

Huang E, Parke C, Mehrnia A, et al. Improved survival among sickle cell kidney transplant recipients in the recent era. *Nephrol Dial Transplant*. 2013;28:1039–1046.

Key NS, Connes P, Derebail VK. Negative health implications of sickle cell trait in high income countries: from the football field to the laboratory. *Br J Haematol*. 2015;170:5–14.

Kato GJ, Piel FB, Reid CD, et al. Sickle cell disease. *Nat Rev Dis Primers*. 2018;4:18010 Mar 15.

McClellan AC, Luthi JC, Lynch JR, et al. High one year mortality in adults with sickle cell disease and end-stage renal disease. *Br J Haematol*. 2012;159:360–367.

Nath KA, Hebbel RP. Sickle cell disease: renal manifestations and mechanisms. *Nat Rev Nephrol*. 2015;11:161–171.

Naik RP, Derebail VK, Grams ME, et al. Association of sickle cell trait with chronic kidney disease and albuminuria in African Americans. *JAMA*. 2014;312:2115–2125.

Nielsen L, Canouï Poitrine F, Jais JP, et al. Morbidity and mortality of sickle cell disease patients starting intermittent haemodialysis: a comparative cohort study with non-sickle dialysis patients. *Br J Haematol*. 2016;174:148–152.

Niss O, Lane A, Asnani M, et al. Progression of albuminuria in patients with sickle cell anemia: a multicenter, longitudinal study. *Blood Adv*. 2020;4(7):1501–1511 April 14.

Olaniran K, Allegretti A, Zhao S, et al. Kidney Function Decline among Black Patients with Sickle Cell Trait and Sickle Cell Disease: An Observational Cohort Study. *J Am Soc Nephrol*. 2020;31(2):393–404 Feb.

U.S. Department of Health and Human Services, National Institutes of Health, National Heart, Lung, and Blood Institute. 2014. Evidence-based management of sickle cell disease: expert panel report. Retrieved from https://www.nhlbi.nih.gov/sites/www.nhlbi.nih.gov/files/sickle-cell-disease-report.pdf.

39

Polycystic and Other Cystic Kidney Diseases

ARLENE B. CHAPMAN, FREDERIC F. RAHBARI-OSKOUI, JARED COOK, DANA V. RIZK

Autosomal Dominant Polycystic Kidney Disease

Autosomal dominant polycystic kidney disease (ADPKD) is the most common inherited kidney disorder, occurring in 1 of 400 to 1000 live births. It is the most common of all hereditary cystic disorders (Table 39.1). ADPKD affects all ethnic groups equally, and it has been reported worldwide. It accounts for approximately 5% of the end-stage kidney disease (ESKD) population in the United States and 10% of those under 60 years of age. ADPKD is a systemic disorder that affects almost every organ, resulting in significant extrarenal manifestations; however, its hallmark is the gradual and massive cystic enlargement of the kidneys, ultimately resulting in kidney failure.

Pathogenesis

At least three genes have been implicated in the pathogenesis of ADPKD. Approximately 80% of patients with ADPKD have mutations in the *PKD1* gene, close to 15% of ADPKD patients have mutations in the *PKD2* gene, and approximately 5% of patients are found to have mutations in other genes including the *GANAB* gene. Although mutations in *PKD1* and *PKD2* lead to the same phenotype, patients with *PKD2* mutations have milder disease with fewer kidney cysts, later onset of hypertension, later onset of kidney failure (median age of onset of 74 vs. 54 years, respectively), and an approximately 10-year longer life expectancy. Given the milder phenotype associated with *PKD2*, when surveillance autopsies are performed, the relative frequency of *PKD2* increases, accounting for up to 27% of all ADPKD cases. *GANAB* mutation cases are still relatively rarely reported; however, they appear to have a milder phenotype than *PKD1,* with hepatic cystic disease predominating.

PKD1 is located on the short arm of chromosome 16 (16p13.3) and codes for polycystin-1 (PC1), an integral membrane protein made up of 4304 amino acids. PC1 has a large extracellular N-terminal, 11 transmembrane regions, and a short intracellular C-terminal. PC1 is located in the primary cilium, focal adhesions, tight junctions, desmosomes, and adherens junctions. PC1 plays an important role in cell-cell interactions and cell-matrix interactions. *PKD2* is located on the long arm of chromosome 4 (4q12.2) and encodes for polycystin-2 (PC2), a 968 amino acid protein with a short cytoplasmic N-terminal, six transmembrane regions, and a short cytoplasmic C-terminal. It localizes to the endoplasmic reticulum, plasma membrane, primary cilium, centrosome, and mitotic spindles in dividing cells. PC2 belongs to the family of voltage-activated calcium channels (e.g., transient receptor potential polycystin-2 [TRPP-2]) and is involved in intracellular calcium regulation through several pathways. PC1 and PC2 are co-localized in the primary cilium of renal epithelial cells, which function as a mechanosensor. Primary cilia create transmembrane calcium currents in the presence of stretch or luminal flow. PC1 and PC2 contribute to ciliary function, and the physical interaction between PC1 and PC2 is required for a membrane calcium channel to operate properly. Normal polycystin function increases intracellular calcium, which initiates a signaling cascade leading to vesicle fusion and a change in gene transcription. The magnitude of these changes contributing to the PKD epithelial phenotype has recently been challenged because the reservoir of calcium released from primary ciliary stimulation is relatively low.

Polycystins affect cell proliferation, differentiation, and fluid secretion through G-coupled protein receptors and JAK-STAT-mediated signaling pathways. The interaction of PC1 ligand on the basolateral surface with adenylate cyclase and the G protein–coupled response of adenylate cyclase to binding of vasopressin to the vasopressin V_2 receptor produces similar results. Both result in increased intracellular concentrations of cyclic adenosine monophosphate (cAMP) and, ultimately, in chloride secretion across the luminal membrane. This chloride-rich fluid secretion is a critical component of cystogenesis, enabling expansion of cysts even after they detach from their parent nephron. The accumulation of cyst fluid, rich in chloride and sodium, relies on the active luminal excretion of chloride primarily through the cystic fibrosis transmembrane conductor regulator (CFTR) (Fig. 39.1).

ADPKD cystic disease is focal, with less than 5% of all nephrons becoming cystic. It is thought that each kidney cyst is derived from a single, clonal, hyperproliferative epithelial cell that has genetically transformed through somatic mutations. The clonal cystic epithelia proliferate because of an additional somatic mutation in the *PKD1* or *PKD2* gene, indicating that a "second hit" is involved in cyst growth and development. Epithelial cell proliferation, fluid secretion, and alterations in extracellular matrix ultimately result in focal out-pouching from the parent nephron. Most cysts detach from the parent nephron when cyst size exceeds 2 cm and continue to secrete fluid autonomously, resulting in cyst and kidney enlargement, and, ultimately, progressive loss of kidney function.

TABLE 39.1	Genes and Proteins of Inherited Cystic Disorders of the Kidney				
Disease	Frequency	Chromosome	Gene Locus	Protein	Function
ADPKD	1:1000	16p13.3	PKD1	Polycystin 1, which co-localizes with polycystin 2 in the primary cilium	Regulates intracellular cAMP, mTOR, planar polarity
	1:15,000	4q21.2	PKD2	Polycystin 2, which colocalizes with polycystin 1 in the primary cilium and ER	Regulates intracellular Ca levels through ER Ca release, activates Ca channels
ARPKD	1:20,000	6q24.2	PKHD	Fibrocystin or polyductin, located throughout the primary cilium	Serves as receptor to maintain intracellular cAMP levels
VHL	1:36,000	3p25	VHL	VHL, located at the base of the primary cilium	Inhibits HIF-1α and cell turnover, maintains planar polarity, allows ciliogenesis
TSC	1:6000	9q34.3	TSC1	Hamartin	Interacts with tuberin to suppress mTOR activity
		16p13.3	TSC2	Tuberin	Interacts with hamartin to suppress mTOR activity

ADPKD, Autosomal dominant polycystic kidney disease; *ARPKD*, autosomal recessive polycystic kidney disease; *cAMP*, cyclic adenosine monophosphate; *ER*, endoplasmic reticulum; *HIF*, hypoxia-inducible factor; *mTOR*, mammalian target of rapamycin; *PKHD*, polycystic kidney and hepatic disease; *TSC*, tuberous sclerosis complex; *VHL*, von Hippel-Lindau.

Diagnosis

Kidney imaging by ultrasound remains the primary method for diagnosing ADPKD. The characteristic findings include enlarged kidneys and the presence of multiple cysts throughout the kidney parenchyma (Fig. 39.2). Unified diagnostic ultrasonographic criteria for at-risk individuals independent of genotype were developed by Pei and colleagues in 2009. In individuals at risk for inheriting ADPKD (an affected parent) aged 15 to 39, the presence of at least three (unilateral or bilateral) kidney cysts is sufficient to establish a diagnosis of ADPKD. In those individuals 40 to 59 years of age, two cysts in each kidney are required, and in those older than 60, in whom acquired cystic disease is common, four or more cysts in each kidney are required for diagnosis. For patients with no family history, the diagnostic criteria are more stringent with at least 20 cysts bilaterally by the age of 30 and a phenotype consistent with ADPKD required (see later).

When disease status must be determined with certainty, such as when an at-risk family member is being evaluated as a potential kidney donor or for family-planning purposes, then initial computed tomography (CT) or magnetic resonance imaging (MRI) should be pursued if ultrasound imaging is negative. Genetic testing should also be considered in individuals under the age of 40 if imaging is negative, given that PKD2 disease appears later than PKD1 disease. If the mutation in the family is known and is a PKD1 mutation, then negative screening over the age of 30 is sufficient. Mutation screening with direct sequencing of the *PKD1* or *PKD2* genes is commercially available. Both the high cost of the test and its ability to detect mutations in up to 86% of PKD1 individuals restrict its use. However, after a genetic diagnosis is confirmed in a patient, which often requires a diagnosis in other affected members, other at-risk family members can be screened at a reduced cost by performing targeted exon-specific sequencing of the identified mutation. Current mutation detection rates are up to 86% and 95% for *PKD1* and *PKD2* genes, respectively.

Kidney Manifestations and Complications

Kidney enlargement is a universal feature of ADPKD, and individuals with multiple cysts in small kidneys, particularly in the setting of reduced glomerular filtration rate (GFR), should be screened for other cystic diseases. Kidney function among ADPKD patients remains normal for decades despite significant cyst expansion and kidney enlargement. After kidney function becomes impaired, progression is typically universal and rapid, with an average decline in GFR of 4.0 to 5.0 mL/min/year. More recent data from contemporary clinical trials show the rate of kidney function decline is slower (perhaps due to clinical trial involvement or due to improved patient care). There are a number of clinical and genetic predictors for risk of progression to ESKD in ADPKD, such as male sex, *PKD1* genotype, early-age onset of hypertension, early-onset hematuria, and the presence of detectable proteinuria.

Total kidney volume (TKV) incorporates all of the aforementioned clinical and genetic risk factors and is the strongest predictor of future GFR loss. In the Consortium for Radiologic Imaging in the Study of Polycystic Kidney Disease (CRISP), a large multicenter study of 241 ADPKD patients with intact kidney function, patients were followed prospectively with serial MRIs and demonstrated a 5.2%/year increase in TKV. Cysts accounted for the increase in TKV seen and increased at a continuous rate, resulting in an overall increase of approximately 55% over 8 years. *PKD2* patients had smaller TKV at baseline (694 ± 221 vs. 986 ± 204 mL) and lower age-adjusted cyst number per kidney when compared with *PKD1* patients but demonstrated similar rates of growth (4.9 ± 2.3% vs. 5.2 ± 1.6%/year), indicating that the age of cyst formation and cyst number, rather than the rate of cyst expansion, differ between the two genotypes. More recently, data from the CRISP study showed that height-adjusted total kidney volume (HtTKV) of greater than 600 mL/m accurately predicts progression to CKD stage 3 within 8 years. For each 100 mL/m change in HtTKV, there was a 48% relative risk of reaching CKD stage 3. Therefore, TKV is a good predictive biomarker for the development of future GFR loss, with potential application for risk stratification in clinical practice.

Patients can now be grouped into risk classes (1A to 1E) based on age, sex, ethnicity, and measured HtTKV. Patients in class 1A and 1B are at a low risk for loss of kidney function, and patients in class 1C to 1E are at a high risk for progression of kidney disease and would benefit from aggressive monitoring with regard

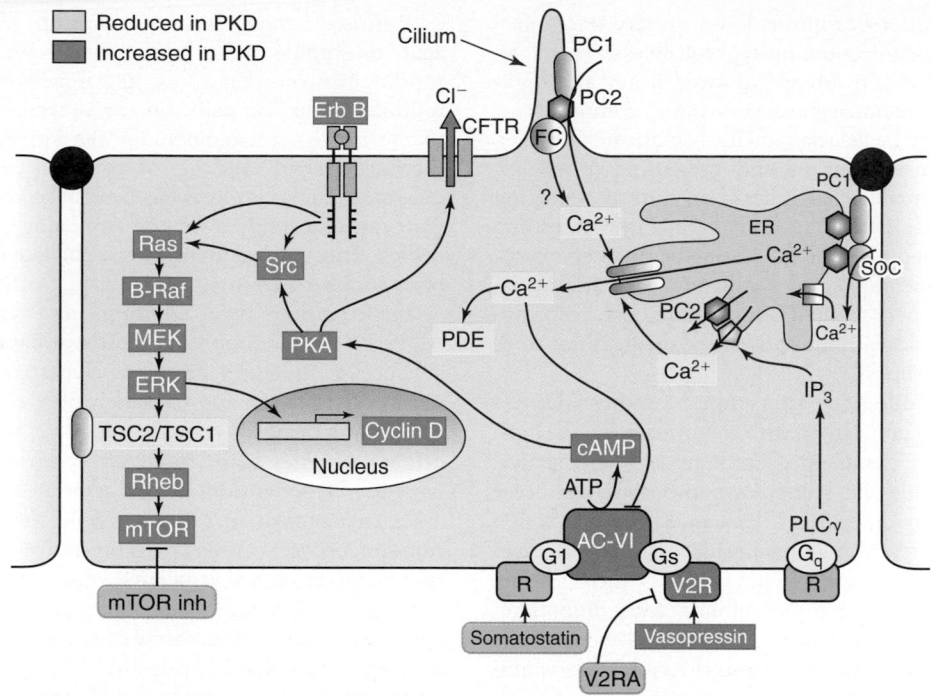

• Fig. 39.1 Renal tubular epithelial cell showing location and interactions of polycystin 1 and polycystin 2. *(Top)* The luminal surface with a single cilium. *(Both sides and bottom)* The basolateral surfaces. Mutations in PC1 *(gold ovals)* or PC2 *(blue hexagons)* result in changes in the intracellular calcium level or increases in the level of cAMP. A change in the balance of these two critical intracellular components leads to alterations in the Ras pathway, the mTOR pathway, cell turnover, apoptosis, and fluid secretion through the CFTR channel. Mutations in PC1 and PC2 colocalize to the primary cilium and the basolateral membranes. PC2 resides alone in the ER. G-coupled receptor activation increases the concentration of cAMP. Interference with G-coupled receptor processes can return the increased cAMP level seen in ADPKD to normal. Blockade of the vasopressin 2 (V_2) receptor by a V_2 receptor antagonist is one example. PC1 interacts with the tuberous sclerosis complex proteins (TSC2 and TSC1) regulating the mTOR pathway. Therapies aimed at reducing G-coupled receptor, FGF receptor, CFTR channel, mTOR, and cyclin activity or increasing ER release of calcium may normalize epithelial cell function in ADPKD. *AC-VI,* Adenylate cyclase; *ADPKD,* autosomal dominant polycystic kidney disease; *B-Raf,* proto-oncogene serine/threonine-protein kinase; *cAMP,* cyclic adenosine monophosphate; *CFTR,* cystic fibrosis transmembrane conductance regulator; *EGF,* epithelial growth factor; *ER,* endoplasmic reticulum; *Erb,* epidermal growth factor (erythroblastic leukemia, viral); *ERK,* extracellular signal-regulated kinase; *Inh,* inhibitor; IP_3, inositol triphosphate; *MEK,* mitogen signal-regulated kinase; *mTOR,* mammalian target of rapamycin; *PC1,* polycystin 1; *PC2,* polycystin 2; *PDE,* phosphodiesterase; *PKA,* phosphokinase A; *PKD,* polycystic kidney disease; *R,* receptor; *Ras,* renin-angiotensin system; *Rheb,* Ras homolog enriched in brain; *SOC,* store-operated channels; *Src,* nonreceptor (cytoplasmic) protein tyrosine kinase; *V2R,* vasopressin V_2 receptor; *V2RA,* vasopressin V_2 receptor antagonist.

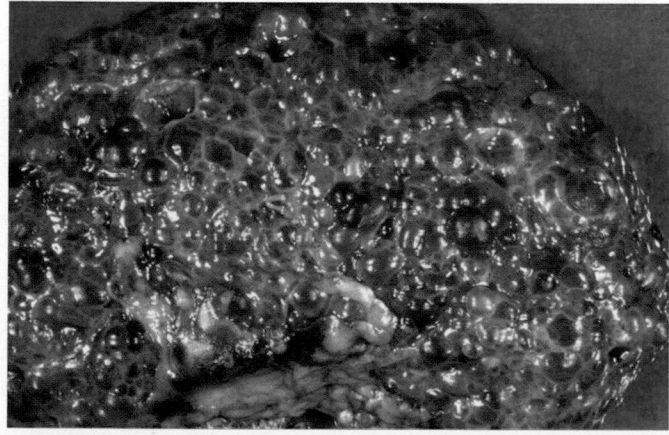

• Fig. 39.2 Gross pathology of autosomal dominant polycystic kidney disease.

to blood pressure and diet and potentially from participating in clinical trials, as well as approved disease-modifying therapies. TKV can be measured by ultrasound; however, ultrasound measurements are less precise and TKV measurements are inaccurate when used over short periods of time. US measurements use the ellipsoid formula, where maximum length, width, and depth are determined. This approach typically overestimates the TKV by close to 11%. Because of its lack of precision, ultrasound cannot be used to measure short-term disease progression, but single measurements can be used for risk stratification. Similar to MRI, ultrasound-measured HtTKV of greater than 650 mL/m or simply a kidney length over 16.5 cm predicts the development of CKD stage 3 within 8 years.

Hematuria, whether gross or microscopic, occurs in about 35% to 50% of patients and often precedes loss of kidney function. It is associated with increased TKV and with worse kidney outcomes. Hematuria can be precipitated by an acute event such as trauma, heavy exertion, cyst rupture, lower urinary tract infection, pyelonephritis, cyst infection, or nephrolithiasis. Therefore, ADPKD patients are typically advised to avoid heavy and high-impact exercise. Cyst hemorrhage occurs more commonly as kidneys enlarge and may be associated with hematuria and fever. However, localized pain is often the only presenting complaint. The diagnosis of a cyst hemorrhage is based on clinical evaluation and can be difficult to differentiate from kidney cyst infection. CT scan occasionally can be helpful in locating hemorrhagic cysts. The management for uncomplicated cyst hemorrhage and hematuria is supportive and includes fluid resuscitation, rest, pain control, and, often, withholding antihypertensive medications until the acute episode has resolved.

Lower urinary tract infections are common among ADPKD patients, as in the general population, with coliforms being the most common pathogens. The treatment is the same as in the general population. Pyelonephritis and kidney cyst infections can occur and may be challenging to differentiate. Patients with cyst infection commonly present with fever, abdominal pain, and, often, elevated C-reactive protein. Typically, blood cultures identify the offending pathogen more frequently than urine cultures. Most important, treatment of cyst infections requires a prolonged, 4-week course of antibiotics that adequately penetrate into the cyst, such as quinolones, vancomycin, chloramphenicol, or trimethoprim-sulfamethoxazole. Recent reports have suggested that positron emission tomography with fluorodeoxyglucose (FDG-PET) may be a promising diagnostic tool for detecting infected cysts in challenging cases.

The incidence of nephrolithiasis is about 5 to 10 times higher among patients with ADPKD compared with the general population. About 25% of those afflicted with kidney stones are symptomatic. Increased urinary stasis and metabolic disturbances, including hypocitraturia, low urinary pH, and abnormal renal transport of ammonium, account for the high incidence of nephrolithiasis. The most common stone type in ADPKD is uric acid, responsible for approximately 50% of all stones, followed by calcium oxalate. Nephrolithiasis should be suspected in any ADPKD patient with acute flank pain. Diagnosis by imaging is difficult, given the radiolucent nature of the stones and the presence of calcified cyst walls. Noncontrast CT remains the imaging modality of choice for detecting nephrolithiasis. The management of nephrolithiasis in ADPKD is similar to that in non-ADPKD patients. Noninvasive or minimally invasive interventions such as extracorporeal shock-wave lithotripsy and percutaneous nephrolithotomy have been performed on ADPKD patients; however, long-term studies regarding safety in this patient population are lacking.

Patients with ADPKD commonly complain of increased thirst, polyuria, nocturia, and urinary frequency. A decrease in urinary concentrating ability is one of the earliest manifestations of ADPKD. It is initially mild and worsens with increasing age and declining kidney function. The urinary concentrating defect is closely related to the severity of anatomic deformities induced by the cysts, independent of age and GFR. Approximately 60% of affected children demonstrated a decreased response to desmopressin, possibly because of disruption of tubular architecture and alterations in principal cell function.

Proteinuria is typically mild in ADPKD with an average of 260 mg of protein excretion per day, and only 18% of ADPKD adults have detectable proteinuria on point-of-care urinalysis or dipstick (greater than 300 mg/day of protein excretion). Although the level of proteinuria is low-grade in ADPKD, the presence of proteinuria and albuminuria is associated with increased TKV and more rapid decline in kidney function.

Pain is the most common symptom in ADPKD and can be acute or chronic. Acute pain episodes are usually related to cyst rupture or hemorrhage, cyst or parenchymal infection, or nephrolithiasis. Chronic pain, on the other hand, is typically related to the massive enlargement of the kidneys and liver and their increased weight. The site of pain can be in the lower back as increased lumbar lordosis has been observed in ADPKD patients. Pain can also result from the stretching of the renal capsule or pedicle. Pain management can be challenging and should include both nonpharmacologic as well as pharmacologic interventions.

Hypertension is a common and early manifestation of ADPKD, affecting more than 60% of patients before any detectable decline in kidney function. Hypertension precedes the diagnosis of ADPKD in approximately 30% of cases, with the average age of onset being 29 years. Studies show that hypertension occurs earlier and tends to be more severe among *PKD1* versus *PKD2* patients. Hypertension is also associated with a greater rate of TKV enlargement (6.2%/year vs. 4.5%/year), suggesting a relationship between cyst expansion and elevations in blood pressure. Hypertension is associated with worse kidney outcomes and increased cardiovascular morbidity and mortality. ADPKD kidneys have an attenuated vasculature with angiographic evidence of intrarenal arteriolar tapering. MRI-based measurements demonstrate a reduction of renal blood flow that correlates inversely with TKV and occurs before loss of kidney function. These findings suggest that renal ischemia induced by cyst expansion plays a role in the development of hypertension, with intrarenal activation of the renin-angiotensin-aldosterone system (RAAS). Data from the HALT-PKD trial showed that in young patients (15 to 49 years) with preserved kidney function, treatment with inhibitors of the RAAS with a goal blood pressure of <110/75 mmHg resulted in a 14.2% slower increase in TKV over 5 years, reduced urinary albumin excretion, and a greater decline in left ventricular mass index. The overall rate of decline in estimated GFR (eGFR) in the strict and the standard blood pressure group was similar overall but slower in the lower blood pressure group during the chronic phase of the 5-year study. The overall lack of difference in eGFR decline was due to the more rapid decline in eGFR in the strict blood pressure group during the first 4 months of the trial. Importantly, when ADPKD patients with mild disease severity or class 1A and 1B patients (those unlikely to progress) were excluded from the analysis, then significant benefits in change in TKV and slope of eGFR were found in the low BP control group.

Kidney transplantation remains a viable option for patients approaching ESKD. ADPKD transplant recipients tend to survive longer than those transplanted for other kidney pathologies. Native polycystic kidneys do not have to be removed before transplantation unless chronic infections are present or their large size interferes with nutritional intake or quality of life. Overall, post-transplant complications specific to ADPKD tend to be related to intraabdominal complications, such as perforated diverticuli.

Extrarenal Manifestations

Polycystic Liver Disease

Liver cysts are the most common extrarenal manifestation in ADPKD. Liver cysts occur in more than 80% of patients by the age of 30 (Fig. 39.3), with women more often affected and with a greater liver cyst burden. Previous estrogen or progesterone exposure, through birth control pills, hormone replacement therapy, or pregnancy, is associated with significant polycystic liver disease.

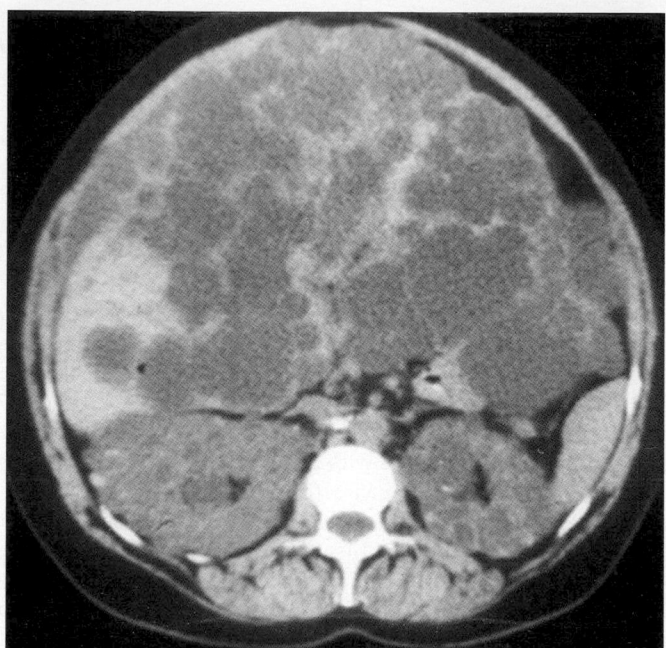

• Fig. 39.3 Computed tomography scan with evidence of kidney and liver cysts in autosomal dominant polycystic kidney disease.

Liver function is preserved even in the presence of massive liver cystic disease, and standard biochemical tests are normal except for mild elevation in the serum concentration of alkaline phosphatase. Isolated autosomal dominant polycystic liver disease (ADPLD) without kidney cysts exists. ADPLD can be a distinct disease genetically unrelated to ADPKD and instead linked to mutations in two genes: *PRKCSH* (protein kinase C substrate 80K-H) located on chromosome 19 and *SEC63* located on chromosome 6.

Liver enlargement results in symptoms of shortness of breath, pain, early satiety, gastroesophageal reflux, decreased mobility, ankle swelling, and, rarely, inferior vena cava compression. Symptoms occur because of compression of surrounding organs by the enlarged liver. This severe form of polycystic liver disease is uncommon, occurring in fewer than 20% of all cases. It predominantly affects women and may require surgical cyst deroofing, fenestration, partial liver resection, or, in extreme cases, liver transplantation. Recently, the use of somatostatin analogues in the treatment of polycystic liver disease was inconclusive (see below). Mammalian target of rapamycin (mTOR) inhibitors have also generated a lot of interest: an observational study in ADPKD kidney transplant recipients showed that those who were treated with sirolimus had a reduction in polycystic liver volumes by 12% compared with an increase of 14% among patients not receiving sirolimus.

Cardiovascular Manifestations

Intracranial aneurysms (ICAs) are the most feared complication of ADPKD. The prevalence of ICA in patients with ADPKD is 7% to 12%, compared with 2% to 3% in the general population. The prevalence increases to 22% to 27% in patients with a family history of hemorrhagic stroke or ruptured ICA. Recent meta-analyses demonstrated that hypertension and smoking exposures are two modifiable risk factors associated with ICA in ADPKD. The aneurysms occur most often in the anterior cerebral circulation, and multiple ICAs are common in ADPKD patients, similar to what is observed among non-ADPKD familial ICAs. Average age of ICA rupture in patients with ADPKD is approximately 40 years. Risk of mortality or permanent morbidity after ICA rupture has not changed over the last 50 years and is more than 50%, with ruptured ICA contributing to 4% to 7% of deaths among ADPKD patients. Screening is indicated in asymptomatic patients with a positive family history for ICA or with a previous history of intracranial hemorrhage, those with high-risk occupations, or before major elective surgery that would affect intracranial hemodynamics. Persons without a family history of ICAs and without these additional concerns do not warrant routine screening. There are suggestions that ADPKD individuals pursuing kidney transplant should consider pretransplant screening. Time-of-flight, three-dimensional magnetic resonance angiography (MRA) without gadolinium is the imaging modality of choice. Although rupture of an ICA is associated with significant morbidity and mortality, only 50% of ADPKD individuals with ICAs have a rupture during their lifetime. Postoperative complications related to surgical clipping are common, and recovery from elective surgery can be prolonged. For larger aneurysms (greater than 10 mm), the risk of rupture is significantly increased, and the anticipated complications from rupture outweigh the benefits of no intervention; elective surgical intervention is recommended in these cases. For asymptomatic unruptured ICAs between 5 and 10 mm, the management is less straightforward and should be individualized in consultation with the treating neurosurgeon and neuroradiologist. Monitoring the rate of growth of these ICAs with periodic imaging is warranted. For those with an ICA smaller than 5 mm, longitudinal studies have not demonstrated significant growth of the ICA, and the risk of rupture is relatively small. Stability of asymptomatic small aneurysms (<7 mm) should be assessed within 6 months to 1 year. Patients with a negative initial MRA and a positive family history of ICA or subarachnoid hemorrhage are at low risk for demonstrating new ICA on future imaging studies. Risk factors for aneurysmal growth include smoking and hypertension, and counseling about smoking cessation as well as blood pressure control is warranted as part of conservative management of ICA. The current indications for surgical repair of these smaller ICAs are unclear. With the development of less invasive therapies (i.e., interventional, nonsurgical coiling or stenting), alternative treatment of small, asymptomatic ICAs may be used more frequently.

Left ventricular hypertrophy (LVH) with echocardiographic imaging is common in ADPKD patients, and it has been reported in as many as 48% of hypertensive individuals. More recent data derived from the HALT-PKD study using cardiac MRI in a contemporary cohort of hypertensive ADPKD patients younger than 50 years of age showed a much lower incidence of LVH (less than 4%). However, more than 50% of patients in this cohort were previously receiving long-term RAAS blockers. Other studies have shown that young, normotensive ADPKD patients have increased left ventricular mass index (LVMI) and diastolic dysfunction.

Other cardiovascular manifestations of ADPKD include coronary aneurysms, valvular heart disease including mitral valve prolapse and mitral regurgitation (26% of ADPKD individuals, compared with 3% of the general population), and aortic insufficiency (11%).

Effects on Fertility and Pregnancy

Overall, fertility rates in ADPKD men and women not yet on dialysis are similar to those in the general population despite a higher incidence of ectopic pregnancies, congenital absence of the seminiferous tubules, seminal vesical cysts, and immotile spermatozoa. Affected women with a normal GFR and normal blood pressure experience pregnancy outcomes similar to those of the general population. Pregnancy-induced hypertension, worsening hypertension, and preeclampsia occur with increased frequency in women with ADPKD, and they have a higher rate of premature delivery. Patients with a reduced GFR before pregnancy are at high risk for midgestation fetal loss and progressive loss of kidney function.

Autosomal Dominant Polycystic Kidney Disease in Children

ADPKD children with cysts are usually asymptomatic, with only about 1% to 2% of patients presenting with symptoms before the age of 15 years. TKV, when regressed against age increases exponentially in children with ADPKD, and the annual growth rate in children has been reported to be 7.4% (greater than high risk individuals in the CRISP consortium). Glomerular hyperfiltration is seen early in the course of ADPKD, and children with glomerular hypertension had a faster decline in kidney function and higher rate of kidney growth.

Other kidney manifestations in children include urinary concentrating defects, present in about 60% of affected individuals. Proteinuria is usually low-grade and relatively uncommon; however, it is more common in ADPKD children than in adults. Thirty percent of children have albuminuria, and 23% have overt proteinuria, as compared with 25% and 17% of adults, respectively. Similar to the adult population, proteinuria in children with ADPKD correlates with diastolic hypertension and more severe cystic kidney disease.

Studies in children with ADPKD show that hypertension is the earliest and most prevalent systemic feature, occurring in up to 44% of cases, and children with hypertension have increased TKV and more pronounced increase in TKV compared with normotensive ADPKD children. Moreover, ADPKD children demonstrate abnormal circadian blood pressure patterns with increased nocturnal blood pressure. Other cardiovascular abnormalities found in affected children include mitral valve prolapse, increased LVMI, and hyperlipidemia, defined as a fasting cholesterol or triglyceride level above the 95th percentile for age and sex. Although rare among children, cases of ruptured ICA have been reported. Extrarenal manifestations in children include liver cysts, which are typically benign. Rare cases of congenital hepatic fibrosis have been described in children with ADPKD. Importantly, inguinal hernias are a common manifestation, and children with ADPKD should be screened for this. At-risk offspring should have regular blood pressure measurements and urinalyses, but current guidelines indicate no role for systematic screening of asymptomatic, at-risk children, given that there are no currently approved pharmacologic therapies for this disorder. Once clinical trials in adolescents with tolvaptan are completed, these recommendations may change.

Therapy

Randomized, controlled clinical trials evaluating angiotensin-converting enzyme (ACE) inhibitors, rigorous blood pressure control, and dietary protein restriction have failed to demonstrate kidney protection in ADPKD when studied late in the course of disease. Lifestyle and dietary changes are recommended for all patients with ADPKD. There is a positive correlation between urinary sodium excretion and rate of HtTKV increase in ADPKD participants in the CRISP study. Based on these findings, dietary salt (<2 g/day) restriction is recommended. Vasopressin stimulates the production of intracellular cAMP, which associates with epithelial proliferation and cyst development and growth in ADPKD and can be inhibited by increased fluid intake. Water intake greater than 3 L/day can suppress vasopressin secretion in individuals with a usual solute load, and ADPKD patients with preserved kidney function are asked to increase fluid intake to at least this amount. Caution should be exercised in patients with more advanced stages of CKD because increasing water intake to extremely high levels can result in a dilutional hyponatremia. Long-term effects of increased water intake on kidney function are under investigation in the ongoing prevent kidney failure (PREVENT-ADPKD) trial, which will be completed in 2021. Other dietary modifications, such as limiting caffeine intake due to its theoretical positive effects on cAMP production, have been suggested based on animal studies but not formally established in prospective, randomized clinical trials in patients with ADPKD.

Due to the early intrarenal activation of the renin-angiotensin-aldosterone system, ACE inhibitors or angiotensin receptor blockers are recommended as first-line treatment for hypertension in ADPKD. In the HALT-PKD trial-Study A, strict blood pressure control to less than 110/75 mmHg with renin-angiotensin blockade was associated with slower increase in HtTKV over time, reduced urinary albumin excretion, and a greater reduction of left ventricular mass index. The impact of this was greatest in those with the largest cyst burden (Mayo class 1C, 1D, and 1E). Longer-term follow-up data on the effect of intensive blood pressure control during participation in the HALT A trial on kidney function will be available in 2022. The goal blood pressure for all patients with ADPKD is below 130/80 mm Hg, with a lower target of less than 110/75 mmHg in young adult patients (age <50) with preserved kidney function.

Pravastatin showed beneficial effects on HtTKV, LVMI, and urinary albumin excretion in a randomized, double-blind, placebo-controlled trial conducted on 56 children, even without dyslipidemia; however, statins are not currently approved for this indication.

Therapy aimed at reducing intracellular cAMP accumulation by blocking the vasopressin V_2 receptor has successfully slowed disease progression in four distinct genetic murine forms of cystic disease: the *PKD2* WS25 mouse, the Han:SPRD rat, the pcy mouse (a mouse model for familial juvenile nephronophthisis), and the polycystic kidney (pck) rat (a murine model for autosomal recessive polycystic kidney disease). Phase II studies of vasopressin V_2 receptor antagonists in ADPKD subjects demonstrated effective inhibition of the V_2 receptor, resulting in decreased water reabsorption and urinary osmolality over 24 hours. This medication was well tolerated, with patients maintaining serum sodium concentrations and tolerating mild increases in the frequency of nocturia. The Tolvaptan Efficacy and Safety Management of Autosomal Dominant Polycystic Kidney Disease and Its Outcomes (TEMPO) 3:4 trial is a phase 3, randomized, double-blind, placebo-controlled trial. Among 1445 participants over 3 years of follow-up, the tolvaptan-treated group had a slower rate of kidney volume growth (2.8% vs. 5.5%/year). The slope of kidney function decline, measured as the reciprocal of the serum creatinine, also favored tolvaptan therapy. Tolvaptan also showed a beneficial effect on kidney pain and frequency of urinary tract infections. The Replicating Evidence of Preserved Renal Function: An Investigation of Tolvaptan Safety and Efficacy in ADPKD (REPRISE trial) was subsequently conducted in 1370 patients aged 18–65 with eGFRs between 25 and 65 mL/min/1.72 m^2 and showed similar protective effects; at 12 months, the change from baseline eGFR was lower among those assigned tolvaptan compared with placebo (−2.34 versus −3.61 mL/min/1.73 m²).

It is worth mentioning that, aside from expected side effects related to aquaresis in the tolvaptan group, 5.6% of treated participants had liver enzyme elevations. These abnormalities were reversed when the drug was discontinued. Tolvaptan is the only disease-modifying agent that is approved for use in ADPKD patients in the US, Japan, Europe, and Canada. In the United States, the Food and Drug Administration approved Tolvaptan use in April 2018 for ADPKD patients at increased risk for progression to ESRD.

Risk stratification or prognostic biomarkers for disease progression are available in ADPKD. It is critical to be familiar with the prognostic tools that have recently been developed to define rapid progression. The Mayo prognostic classification divides typical ADPKD patients (Class I) into five subcategories, ranging from IA to IE, representing increasing order of severity. The classification is based on a calculation of the HtTKV captured by MRI or CT scan and adjusted to the patient's age. Class IA patients have extremely slow progression (HtTKV growth rate of <1.5%/year and predicted annual eGFR loss <0.23 mL/min/1.72 m²), with a predicted age of ESRD of 77 years and a majority never reaching ESRD. In contrast, Class IE patients have a very aggressive course of disease (HtTKV growth rate of >6.5%/year and a predicted annual eGFR loss of 4.78 mL/min/m²), with a predicted age of onset of ESRD of 42 years of age (Fig. 39.4). In patients for whom longitudinal follow-up data are available, the rate of decline of kidney function can also suggest rapid progression if eGFR is less than 65 mL/min prior to the age of 55 or if the annual rate of GFR decline is greater than 2.5 mL/min/1.73 m².

The PROPKD score (ranging from 0–9) is another validated prognostication tool for ADPKD that combines clinical parameters (sex, presence of hypertension before 35 years of age, occurrence of the first urologic event before 35 years of age) with genetic information (PKD1 versus PKD2 mutation, and truncating versus nontruncating PKD1 mutation). The PROPKD score categorizes patients into low risk (0 to 3 points), intermediate risk (4 to 6 points), and high risk (7 to 9 points) for progression to ESKD, with corresponding median ages for ESKD onset of 70.6, 56.9, and 49 years. This scoring system is limited in that individuals less than 35 years of age cannot be fully scored and genetic testing is required. It is currently unknown if the PROPKD score functions independently of HtTKV in prognostication as age of onset of complications are tightly linked to cyst burden or HtTKV.

We propose the following practical criteria to justify the use of tolvaptan:

(1) Mayo classes 1C, 1D, or 1E
(2) Age ≤ 55 years and an eGFR <65 mL/min/1.73 m²
(3) Kidney length (by ultrasound, MRI, or CT) >16.5 cm in a patient aged <50 years
(4) PROPKD score >6
(5) A documented annual decline rate of greater than 2.5 mL/min/1.73 m²/year over a 6-month period without any other causes for kidney injury.

Tolvaptan is contraindicated in patients with known hypersensitivity to the drug, baseline abnormal liver function tests (three times upper limit of the normal on alanine aminotransferase [ALT], aspartate aminotransferase [AST]) and concomitant use of strong inhibitors of the CYP3A, dysnatremias (particularly hypernatremia), inability to sense or respond to thirst, hypovolemia, or uncorrected urinary outflow obstruction. The starting dose of tolvaptan should be 30 mg in the morning and 15 mg 8 hours later. Dose titration can be done every 1 to 4 weeks, as tolerated, to a maximum of 90 mg in the morning and 30 mg in the afternoon to achieve an optimal urinary dilution (urine osmolality < 150 mmol/L).

It is important to note that tolvaptan was approved by the US Food and Drug Administration under the restricted drug dispensing program called the *Risk Evaluation and Mitigation Strategy* (REMS) program. The REMS program requires that patients

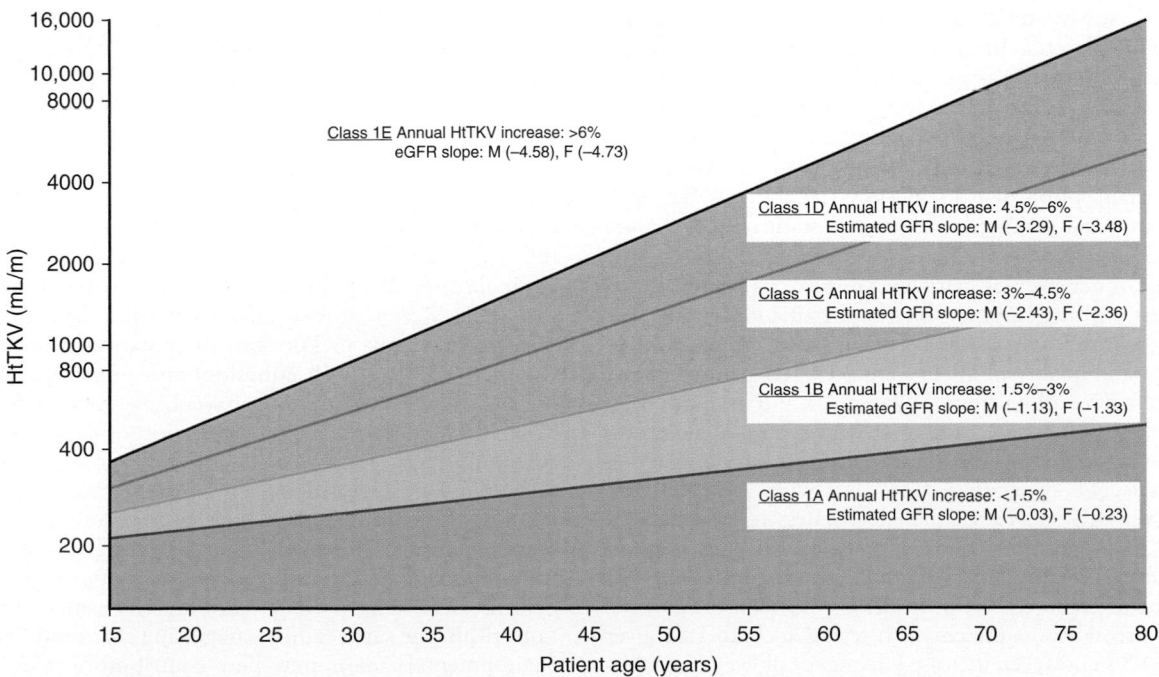

• **Fig. 39.4 Mayo prognostic classification for typical ADPKD.** HtTKV, Height-adjusted total kidney volume; GFR, glomerular filtration rate; M, males; F, females. (From Irazabal. *J Am Soc Nephrol* 2015; 26:160–172.)

consent to have their liver enzymes ([ALT], [AST], and bilirubin) measured before initiating treatment, at 2 and 4 weeks after initiation of therapy, then monthly for 18 months (20 liver function tests during the first 18 months), and then quarterly while on the medication. In case of symptomatic liver injury or elevation of ALT, AST, or bilirubin to greater than 2 times the upper limit of normal, the treatment should be discontinued and liver tests repeated within 72 hours. If laboratory abnormalities stabilize or resolve, tolvaptan may be reinitiated and continued as long as ALT and AST levels remain <3 times the ULN. However, it should not be restarted if ALT or AST increased to greater than 3 times the upper limit of normal with tolvaptan identified as the causative agent. Importantly, alternate vasopressin V2 receptor antagonists have been developed that are predicted in silico not to impact liver function. Clinical trials are underway to explore this alternative avenue as frequent blood monitoring is a significant patient burden.

Longer-term data on the effectiveness of tolvaptan are currently missing, but hypothetical extrapolations of the data from the TEMPO and REPRISE trials suggest a prolongation of the kidney lifespan by 6–9 years among patients who start tolvaptan with an eGFR <60 mL/min/1.73 m^2 and even longer among those who start tolvaptan earlier. The decision to initiate tolvaptan therapy should be individually made after careful assessment of risks (liver toxicity, polyuria, polydipsia), benefits, and affordability.

Somatostatin is an inhibitor of intracellular cAMP accumulation through inhibition of the G-coupled protein receptor and adenylate cyclase pathway. Somatostatin analogues, octreotide and lanreotide, have been studied in ADPKD and, despite their effectiveness in reducing the annual rate of increase in HtTKV, they failed to show any beneficial effect in slowing the rate of decline in eGFR, significant loss of kidney function (>30%), or reaching ESKD.

Polycystic liver disease has also been investigated with regard to somatostatin analogues. In a small, single-center, double-blind, placebo-controlled trial of a long-acting somatostatin (octreotide), the investigators showed that over a 12-month period, liver volumes decreased by 4.95% ± 6.77% in the active drug group compared with placebo. In another randomized, double-blind, placebo-controlled trial, lanreotide 120 mg given monthly for 6 months demonstrated a 2.9% decrease in the liver volume as compared with 1.6% increase with placebo. Importantly, somatostatin analogues were well tolerated and patients experienced an improved perception of pain and physical activity. The most common symptoms reported with somatostatin analogues are abdominal cramps and diarrhea.

Treatment of massive polycystic liver disease has demonstrated partial success utilizing surgical resection (hepatic lobectomy, surgical cyst deroofing), which has been shown to improve symptomatic relief and quality of life in some ADPKD patients. Most of these results have arisen from single centers and have not been easily reproduced elsewhere. Additionally, a recent single-center report of 4-year follow-up on the use of octreotide long-acting release in selected symptomatic patients with ADPKD and polycystic liver disease showed the effectiveness of treatment in arresting PLD progression, alleviating symptoms, and improving health-related quality of life. Interestingly, discontinuation of treatment led to organ regrowth. In the DIPAK consortium, the impact of octreotide was present with regard to both total liver volume and TKV; however, increased frequency of liver cyst infections occurred, most likely secondary to retrograde biliary flow due to changes in biliary peristalsis.

Recent evidence indicates that normal PC1 interacts with the tuberous sclerosis complex (TSC1/TSC2), and this interaction plays a role in the inhibition of mTOR activity. In support of these findings, the inhibitor of mTOR, sirolimus, has been shown to decrease kidney cyst burden in the Han:SPRD rat. ADPKD patients who received sirolimus following kidney transplantation demonstrated a significant decline in the size of their native kidneys over time. However, two recent trials involving the mTOR inhibitors failed to show the anticipated benefit on kidney disease progression. In an 18-month, open-label, randomized, controlled trial, 100 patients with early polycystic kidney disease were assigned to receive sirolimus versus standard of care. At the conclusion of this study, the investigators found that sirolimus therapy had no effect on rate of TKV growth or GFR. However, the sirolimus dose used in this study was low, raising the possibility that the drug dose chosen limited its efficacy.

In another 2-year, double-blind trial, 433 patients with ADPKD were randomly assigned to receive everolimus versus placebo. At the conclusion of this trial, everolimus significantly slowed the increase in TKV but not the progression of GFR loss. In fact, the everolimus group experienced a greater decline in the eGFR. In addition, at the end of the 2-year study, proteinuria had significantly increased in the everolimus-treated group when compared with the placebo group. Finally, everolimus use was associated with a high rate of serious adverse events (37.4% of patients who received at least one dose of the drug) and an extremely high rate of study withdrawal (greater than 35%). Short trial duration, inadequate dosing, and lack of availability of risk stratification using HtTKV classes 1C-1E may have limited a true assessment of the mTOR inhibitors.

Autosomal Recessive Polycystic Kidney Disease

Autosomal recessive polycystic kidney disease (ARPKD) occurs in 1 in 20,000 live births. Its etiology is linked to mutations in the polycystic kidney and hepatic disease (PKHD1) gene located on the short arm of chromosome 6 (6p21.1). The gene encodes for a protein product called *fibrocystin* (also known as *polyductin*), an integral membrane protein of 4074 amino acids with a large extracellular N-terminal and a short cytoplasmic tail. Fibrocystin is expressed primarily in the renal collecting ducts and ascending loop of Henle as well as biliary epithelial and pancreatic epithelial cells. The function of fibrocystin remains to be fully elucidated but, similar to other proteins involved in kidney cystic diseases, it has been localized to the basal body and primary cilia. Recent studies have shown that epithelial cells with PKHD1 knockout or knockdown mutations exhibit decreased cell matrix and cell-cell adhesion with greater cell deformability and motility. Mutations have been identified in 42% to 87% of cases. Homozygous mutations that predict immediate stop codons or truncated proteins lead to the most severe phenotype and are associated with increased perinatal mortality. Most patients are compound heterozygotes having two missense mutations. Mutations tend to be unique to each pedigree. Importantly, there is significant variability in the severity of kidney disease among patients carrying the same PKHD1 mutation within the same family, suggesting that modifier genes and environmental factors may play contributory roles. The use of PKHD1 sequencing data for clinical decision making or prenatal counseling is currently limited.

ARPKD is characterized by fibrocystic kidney and liver involvement of variable severity. The kidney cystic disease is a result of fusiform dilatation of renal collecting tubules. Up to 90% of collecting tubules are involved and, unlike ADPKD cysts, are diffuse, and continue to retain their connection to the parent nephron. Most ARPKD patients have severely enlarged kidneys perinatally with poor cortico-medullary differentiation that can be detected in utero on routine prenatal ultrasound. Affected fetuses can present with oligohydramnios secondary to poor kidney function and reduced urinary output, the Potter phenotype with pulmonary hypoplasia, and deformed facies, spine, and limbs. In this setting, hypoxia due to pulmonary hypoplasia is the leading cause of death, with approximately a 30% perinatal mortality. Not surprisingly, kidney survival correlates with age at diagnosis, with those diagnosed before the age of 1 having significantly higher risk of progression to ESKD. Cyst distribution also carries prognostic information. High-resolution ultrasonography is more sensitive in detecting kidney pathology limited to the medulla, and cystic anomalies limited to the medulla are associated with a milder kidney disease. On the other hand, corticomedullary anomalies that present perinatally are associated with a faster decline in kidney function. Hypertension is diagnosed in up to 80% of children with ARPKD and is usually associated with reduced GFR. Studies in animal models of ARPKD suggest intrarenal renin and ACE upregulation. The treatment of hypertension includes salt restriction and blockade of the renin-angiotensin-aldosterone system, but often requires multiple agents to achieve control. Hyponatremia has been reported in about 26% of neonates diagnosed with ARPKD.

The liver disease in ARPKD consists of dilation of intrahepatic and extrahepatic bile ducts, which predisposes them to recurrent ascending cholangitis. Patients can also have biliary dysgenesis and periportal fibrosis, known as *congenital hepatic fibrosis*, which leads to portal hypertension with subsequent splenomegaly and esophageal varices. When cystic dilation of the intrahepatic bile ducts is seen in the context of portal hypertension and congenital hepatic fibrosis, it is referred to as *Caroli syndrome*. Liver involvement rarely leads to hepatocellular damage with synthetic dysfunction, and, although liver involvement is histologically universal, clinical manifestations of portal hypertension are variable, making early diagnosis difficult. A retrospective study of a large NIH cohort found that platelet count and ultrasound (US) elastography were the best predictors of portal hypertension and hepatic fibrosis, respectively. Acoustic radiation force impulse (ARFI) US elastography of the left hepatic lobe has a high sensitivity and specificity for detecting liver disease in ARPKD and may be useful as a screening tool and clinical trial endpoint. Current therapy includes portosystemic shunts for esophageal varices. Children with advanced liver disease may be eligible for liver or combined kidney-liver transplantation. Tesevatinib, a multikinase inhibitor, has been shown to reduce kidney and liver disease in mouse models of ARPKD, and a phase 1 trial of tesevatinib in human subjects has recently been completed.

Growth retardation is common among ARPKD children and cannot be solely attributed to chronic kidney disease or lung disease. A recent study of 22 children with ARPKD compared to two matched control groups of children with other causes of congenital CKD found no difference in annual change in height or growth hormone use, suggesting no disease-specific mechanism for growth retardation in ARPKD. However, the small sample size may not have been sufficiently powered to find a difference, and further study is needed. Treatment with growth hormone can be helpful, as in other etiologies of CKD.

Tuberous Sclerosis Complex

TSC is an autosomal dominant disease estimated to occur in 1 in 6000 births. TSC results from mutations in either the *TSC1* gene, located on chromosome 9, or the *TSC2* gene, located on chromosome 16. *TSC2* is 50 base pairs away from *PKD1,* lying in a head-to-head orientation. Deletions in both genes result in the contiguous gene syndrome characterized by severe early onset of a polycystic phenotype with cutaneous and neurologic manifestations of TSC. *TSC1* and *TSC2* are tumor suppressor genes, and, consistent with the two-hit hypothesis, a mutation in both alleles of either gene is required for disease manifestation. About 70% to 80% of patients have no family history of the disorder. Most of the spontaneous cases involve *TSC2* mutations and are associated with a more severe phenotype. In familial cases, mutations in *TSC1* are twice as likely to be the culprit. The gene products of *TSC1* and *TSC2*, hamartin and tuberin, are co-expressed in cells of many organs including the kidney, brain, lung, and pancreas. Both proteins are bound to form a heterodimer with an inhibitory effect on the mammalian target of rapamycin (mTOR) complex 1. Under normal circumstances, protein kinase (Akt)-mediated inactivation of tuberin results in degradation of the tuberin-hamartin complex, allowing mTOR signaling. The mTOR pathway plays a key role in cell growth and proliferation as well as angiogenesis. In TSC cases, allelic mutations in either *TSC1* or *TSC2* followed by a second somatic mutation in the normal allele result in disruption of the tuberin-hamartin complex, with unabated mTOR activation. This results in the growth of nonmalignant tumors (known as *hamartomas*) throughout the body. Although benign, these tumors lead to organ dysfunction characteristic of this disease.

In 1998, the National Institutes of Health sponsored a TSC consensus conference that led to the establishment of diagnostic criteria for TSC. In 2011, an international TSC consensus conference was organized with a mission to update the diagnostic criteria and provide surveillance and treatment guidelines for the disease. Currently, genetic testing alone can establish the diagnosis of TSC if a pathogenic mutation that disrupts the synthesis or function of the protein product is identified. In affected individuals, it is estimated that about 10% to 25% of genetic screening is negative, but this does not rule out the diagnosis. Clinical diagnostic criteria were also updated and include 11 major criteria (≥3 hypomelanotic macules at least 5 mm in size, ≥3 angiofibromas or fibrous cephalic plaque, ≥2 ungual fibromas, shagreen patch, multiple retinal hamartomas, cortical dysplasias, subependymal nodules, subependymal giant cell astrocytoma, cardiac rhabdomyoma, lymphangioleiomyomatosis, and angiomyolipomas) and six minor criteria ("confetti" skin lesions, >3 dental enamel pits, ≥2 intraoral fibromas, retinal achromic patch, multiple kidney cysts, non-kidney hamartomas). The clinical diagnosis of TSC requires the presence of two major criteria, or one major and two minor (Table 39.2).

Most features of the disease become evident after 3 years of age. Approximately 85% of TSC patients experience central nervous system (CNS) complications that include epilepsy and cognitive impairment, and are referred to as *TSC-associated neuropsychiatric disorders* or *TAND*. It is recommended that all TSC patients undergo baseline brain MRI as well as electroencephalogram. Kidney manifestations are the second most common finding. Fifty percent of patients have cystic kidney disease, and 80% have angiomyolipomas (AMLs) identified by non-contrast abdominal MRI. MRI is recommended for screening as well as for follow-up every 1 to 3 years. Secondary hypertension is common, and

TABLE 39.2	Diagnostic Criteria for Tuberous Sclerosis Complex	
Major features	**Minor features**	
1. Hypomelanotic macules (≥3, at least 5 mm in diameter)	1. "Confetti" skin lesions	
2. Angiofibromas (≥3) or fibrous cephalic plaque	2. Dental enamel pits (>3)	
3. Ungual fibromas (≥2)	3. Intraoral fibromas (≥2)	
4. Shagreen patch	4. Retinal achromic patch	
5. Multiple retinal hamartomas	5. Multiple renal cysts	
6. Cortical dysplasias	6. Non-renal hamartomas	
7. Subependymal nodules		
8. Subependymal giant cell astrocytoma		
9. Cardiac rhabdomyoma		
10. Lymphangioleiomyomatosis (LAM)		
11. Angiomyolipomas (≥2)		

Definite diagnosis: Two major features or one major feature with ≥2 minor features

Possible diagnosis: Either one major feature or ≥2 minor features

routine blood pressure checks should be performed. The abundant abnormal vascular structures in AML are prone to aneurysmal formation, and the risk of bleeding increases substantially after lesions enlarge beyond 4 cm or aneurysms enlarge beyond 5 mm in diameter. Currently, the standard of care to control active bleeding is arterial embolization. Postembolectomy syndrome is common within 48 hours of the procedure and manifests as nausea, pain, fever, and hemodynamic instability, and should be treated with corticosteroids. For AML larger than 3 cm, the first-line treatment is an mTOR inhibitor. Recently published results from the EXIST-1 and EXIST-2 (Everolimus for angiomyolipoma associated with tuberous sclerosis complex or sporadic lymphangioleiomyomatosis) trials showed that everolimus treatment was safe and effective in reducing the volume of AML and helped to preserve eGFR in most patients, supporting its use for asymptomatic growing AML.

Angiomyolipomas are also thought to underlie the pathogenesis of lymphangioleiomyomatosis (LAM), a devastating pulmonary complication that occurs almost exclusively among women, leading to cystic and interstitial lung disease, pneumothoraces, and chylous pleural effusions. Screening with high-resolution CT scans is recommended every 5 to 10 years for asymptomatic at-risk patients, but the frequency of imaging studies should increase once symptoms arise. In cases of moderate to severe lung disease, mTOR inhibitors can be used. The combination of simvastatin with everolimus has been shown to kill LAM cells in preclinical studies and is currently being investigated in clinical trials.

Currently, everolimus is being investigated in clinical trials for many other manifestations of TSC including dermatitis, cognitive and attention deficit disorders, seizures, and glioblastomas. Recent results of the EXIST-3 trial have shown that everolimus decreases seizure frequency in patients with treatment-refractory seizures, and phase 3 trials are ongoing. Preliminary data did not, however, show improvement in neuropsychological deficits with the use of everolimus.

Von Hippel-Lindau Disease

Von Hippel-Lindau (VHL) is a rare autosomal dominant disease with an incidence of 1 in 36,000 live births, characterized by benign and malignant tumors in multiple organs. The term "VHL disease" was coined in 1936 to honor Drs. Eugen von Hippel and Arvid Lindau who had respectively described retinal angiomas and spinal hemangioblastomas (HBs) in a small group of VHL patients. Characteristic tumors in VHL include retinal and CNS HB, clear cell renal carcinomas (RCCs), pheochromocytomas (PCCs), pancreatic islet tumors, and endolymphatic sac tumors (ELSTs). Other common benign findings include kidney and pancreatic cysts. The clinical diagnosis of VHL requires the presence of one of the abovementioned tumors in the setting of a positive family history of VHL or two tumors (excluding epididymal and kidney cysts) in the absence of a family history.

Approximately 20% of VHL cases arise from de novo mutations. VHL disease is further categorized as type 1 (absence of PCC), type 2A (presence of PCC but without RCC), type 2B (presence of PCC and RCC), and type 2C (only PCC). The VHL gene has been mapped to chromosome 3p25 and encodes two protein isoforms: $pVHL_{30}$, a 30-kD protein of 213 amino acids, and $pVHL_{19}$, a smaller 19-kD protein lacking 53 amino acids from $pVHL_{30}$. Both isoforms are believed to have similar function. VHL is a tumor suppressor gene and, in accordance with the two-hit hypothesis, a biallelic mutation is required for tumors to develop. Under normoxic conditions, the α-subunits of the hypoxia-inducible factor (HIF) are hydroxylated, and pVHL binds and promotes their degradation. In conditions of hypoxia, or in the absence of functional pVHL, the HIF α-subunits are stabilized, escape degradation, and translocate to the nucleus. There they form heterodimers with HIF β-subunits, leading to the activation of a cascade of hypoxia-inducible genes, including vascular endothelial growth factor (VEGF), erythropoietin (EPO), tumor growth factor alpha (TGFα), and platelet-derived growth factor (PDGFβ). It is the biochemical consequence of this activation that leads to tumor formation. Another role of pVHL is its effect on microtubule orientation and stability. Cyst formation in VHL disease can be explained by the pVHL effect on HIF and microtubules, both of which are essential to the integrity of the primary cilia. pVHL has also been shown to be integral in mediating the differentiation of nephron progenitor cells through alterations in cell metabolism.

Disease-causing mutations can be detected in almost all patients with classic clinical features of VHL (95% to 100% detection rate), and those that carry mutations have a very high penetrance (>90%). Genetic testing is recommended in at-risk relatives with a family history of VHL or those with suspected disease. Genotype-phenotype correlations have been established but, so far, do not affect our clinical management practice. Surprisingly, VHL mutations are also detected in a substantial number of individuals who have sporadic cases of VHL-associated tumors, including retinal HBs (30% to 50%), CNS hemangioblastomas (CNS HB) (4% to 40%), and ELST (20%). These observations led to the guideline recommendations by the American College of Medical Genetics and Genomics and the National Society of Genetic Counselors that patients with isolated retinal or CNS HB, PCC, or ELST, as well as clear cell RCC diagnosed before the age of 50, bilateral or multifocal tumors, or with a family history of clear cell RCC, be screened for VHL mutations.

VHL disease is clinically characterized by the development of benign and malignant tumors in many organs. CNS HBs occur in 60% to 80% of VHL patients and most commonly occur in the cerebellum, spinal cord, and brainstem. Although benign in nature, CNS HBs enlarge over time and cause symptoms related to increased intracranial pressure and mass effect. Their biologic behavior is unpredictable with intermittent phases of growth and quiescence. These tumors tend to be multiple and recurrent, which make routine radiologic screening mandatory. MRI of the brain and cervical spine is recommended every 1 to 2 years starting at age 16. When symptomatic, CNS HBs are best treated by surgical removal. Retinal angiomas are identical histopathologically to CNS HBs and are the most common presenting feature of VHL disease. They tend to be bilateral and can lead to vision loss in 35% to 55% of cases. Annual eye examinations with indirect ophthalmoscopy are recommended from birth. Most lesions respond well to laser photocoagulation. VEGF inhibitors such as ranibizumab and tyrosine kinase inhibitors such as sunitinib have been studied with some improvement in those with severe exudative lesions.

RCCs are the most common malignant tumors in VHL and are an important cause of death. The lifetime risk of RCC varies based on the VHL mutation but can be as high as 70%. Most RCCs are of the clear cell variety and tend to be multifocal and bilateral. The mean age at presentation is 40 years. The best management strategy remains close surveillance for RCCs with serial imaging using abdominal MRI with and without contrast every 2 years starting at age 16. When RCCs reach 3 cm in size, the risk of metastasis increases, and kidney-sparing surgery or ablation is recommended. PCCs are seen in 7% to 20% of patients, with the risk varying based on the underlying mutation. They tend to be bilateral, occur at a young age (mean age 28 years), and can be extraadrenal. Screening is recommended annually starting at age 5. Asymptomatic VHL patients scheduled for elective surgery should be screened for PCC to prevent hemodynamic and cardiac complications associated with anesthesia and surgery. ELSTs arise from the membranous labyrinth of the inner ear and, when bilateral, are pathognomonic of VHL. They can lead to tinnitus, vertigo, and hearing loss. Pancreatic cysts are common but rarely lead to organ dysfunction. Pancreatic tumors occur in 5% to 10% of cases, are typically multiple, and are usually non-secretory islet cell tumors. Surgery may be indicated when these tumors reach a size greater than 3 cm to avoid obstructive pancreatitis.

Tyrosine kinase inhibitors have been investigated in several pilot and retrospective studies and show promise in treating RCCs, pancreatic lesions, PCCs, and retinal CNS HBs, though further study is warranted.

Acquired Cystic Kidney Disease

Acquired cystic kidney disease (ACKD) refers to the sporadic, non-inherited development of kidney cysts in patients with chronic kidney disease or ESKD. Its distinction from inherited cystic kidney disorder (particularly ADPKD) is important, and helpful hints include the lack of family history and extrarenal manifestations (particularly liver cysts, which are very common in ADPKD) and the ability to distinguish normal parenchyma between cysts with preservation of the corticomedullary junction. Kidneys are usually small or normal in size, and the cysts tend to be of different morphology and size, although classically they are less than 3 cm.

The prevalence of ACKD is around 7% in the predialysis population. It increases with time on dialysis and has been reported to go from 10% to 20% after 1 to 3 years of dialysis to more than 90% after 5 to 10 years of dialysis. Men and African-Americans are at higher risk for developing ACKD.

Most patients with ACKD are asymptomatic, but cysts can rupture causing hematuria or retroperitoneal hemorrhage with flank pain. This latter complication occurs mostly in patients on hemodialysis, likely related to the concomitant use of anticoagulation. RCCs remain the most feared complication, affecting about 3% to 6% of patients with ACKD, which is approximately a 100-fold increase in incidence compared with the general population. The tumors tend to occur at a younger age than the general population and are more frequently multifocal and bilateral when compared with sporadic RCCs. Papillary cell carcinomas are the most common histologic variant of RCCs in ACKD, as opposed to clear cell carcinomas in sporadic cases. Risk factors for developing RCCs include male sex, older age, ACKD and ESKD due to tuberous sclerosis, FSGS, or obstruction.

More recently, two tumor types exclusive to ACKD patients have been described. Together they represent 60% of ACKD-associated RCCs. The first tumor is acquired cystic disease-associated RCC characterized by a well-circumscribed tumor that arises within cysts. A dense, fibrous capsule separates the tumor from surrounding kidney tissue. The hallmark of this tumor is the presence of oxalate crystals seen under the polarizing microscope. Acquired cystic disease-associated RCC typically has an indolent course. The second type of tumor is the clear cell papillary RCC seen among ESKD patients with or without ACKD. Characteristically, tumor cells reveal signs of inverted polarity with their nuclei positioned away from the basement membrane. These two types of tumors are distinguished by morphology, cytogenetics, and immunohistochemistry. To date, there are no clear recommendations regarding the screening of ESKD patients for ACKD and RCC. A decision analysis model showed that screening provides significant benefits only for patients with a life expectancy of at least 25 years. Due to the poor life expectancy of patients with ESKD, it is not beneficial or cost effective to screen the entire ESKD population. It may, however, be beneficial to screen high-risk individuals (i.e., the young, men, African-Americans, patients on dialysis for more than 3 years). Ultrasound is a good screening modality; however, CT or MRI is more sensitive and recommended for patients who have signs or symptoms suggestive of carcinoma (e.g., hematuria, unexplained anemia, back pain, weight loss). Cysts that appear solid or moderately complex on ultrasound should be further investigated with a contrasted CT or MRI. Screening guidelines for kidney transplant candidates or recipients are equally controversial. A recent meta-analysis of greater than 100,000 kidney transplant recipients showed an absolute risk of about 1% for developing RCC 10 years after transplant. Risk factors for RCC in that study included older age, male sex, and duration of dialysis. Another study that included 516 kidney transplant recipients determined a prevalence of RCC of about 5%, and almost all cases were diagnosed in the setting of ACKD of the native kidneys. Risk factors for RCCs in that study included older age, male sex, history of heart disease, larger kidneys, and the presence of kidney calcifications. The prevalence of ACKD after transplant was lower than among ESKD patients, suggesting that better kidney function and/or immunosuppressive therapies may have a protective influence on cyst formation. A study comparing RCC diagnosed in ESKD patients on dialysis versus those transplanted suggested that tumors diagnosed after transplant have more benign features and are associated with superior clinical survival rates. It remains to be determined whether this advantage is related to more aggressive surveillance practices in transplant recipients or to an altered biology of these tumors. When detected, treatment of RCC depends on staging and tumor size. Tumors <4 cm are often treated with partial nephrectomy, especially in the predialysis CKD population, while radical nephrectomy is preferred in the ESRD population and in those with local metastasis. Metastatic RCC can be treated with tyrosine kinase inhibitors, checkpoint inhibitors, bevacizumab, and mTOR inhibitors.

Complete bibliography is available at Elsevier eBooks for Practicing Clinicians

Key Bibliography

Bae KT, Zhu F, Chapman AB, et al. Magnetic resonance imaging evaluation of hepatic cysts in early autosomal-dominant polycystic kidney disease: the Consortium for Radiologic Imaging Studies of Polycystic Kidney Disease cohort. *Clin J Am Soc Nephrol.* 2006;1(1):64–69.

Bernts LHP, Neijenhuis MK, Edwards ME, et al. Symptom relief and quality of life after combined partial hepatectomy and cyst fenestration in highly symptomatic polycystic liver disease. *Surgery.* 2020;168(1):25–32.

Binderup ML, Budtz-Jørgensen E, Bisgaard ML. Risk of new tumors in von Hippel-Lindau patients depends on age and genotype. *Genet Med.* 2016;18:89–97.

Bissler J, Kingswood J, Radzikowska E, et al. Everolimus for angiomyolipoma associated with tuberous sclerosis complex or sporadic lymphangioleiomyomatosis (EXIST-2): a multicenter, randomized, double-blind, placebo-controlled trial. *Lancet.* 2013;381:817–824.

Bonsib S. Renal cystic diseases and renal neoplasms: a mini-review. *CJASN.* 2009;4:1998–2007.

Cadnapaphornchai MA, George DM, McFann K, et al. Effect of pravastatin on total kidney volume, left ventricular mass index, and microalbuminuria in pediatric autosomal dominant polycystic kidney disease. *Clin J Am Soc Nephrol.* 2014;9(5):889–896.

Caroli A, Perico N, Perna A, et al. Effect of long acting somatostatin analogue on kidney and cyst growth in autosomal dominant polycystic kidney disease (ALADIN): a randomised, placebo-controlled, multicentre trial. *Lancet.* 2013;382(9903):1485–1495.

Chapman AB, Bost JE, Torres VE, et al. Kidney volume and functional outcomes in autosomal dominant polycystic kidney disease. *Clin J Am Soc Nephrol.* 2012;7(3):479–486.

Chapman AB, Devuyst O, Eckardt KU, et al. Autosomal-dominant polycystic kidney disease (ADPKD): executive summary from a kidney disease: Improving Global Outcomes (KDIGO) controversies conference. *Kidney Int.* 2015;88(1):17–27.

Chapman AB, Rubinstein D, Hughes R, et al. Intracranial aneurysms in autosomal dominant polycystic kidney disease. *N Engl J Med.* 1992;327(13):916–920.

Chebib FT, Perrone RD, Chapman AB, et al. A practical guide for treatment of rapidly progressive ADPKD with tolvaptan. *J Am Soc Nephrol.* 2018;29(10):2458. Epub 2018 Sep 18.

Cornec-Le Gall E, Audrézet MP, Rousseau A, et al. The PROPKD Score: A new algorithm to predict renal survival in autosomal dominant polycystic kidney disease. *J Am Soc Nephrol.* 2016;27(3):942–951. Mar Epub 2015 Jul 6.

Grantham JJ, Torres VE, Chapman AB, et al. Volume progression in polycystic kidney disease. *N Engl J Med.* 2006;354(20):2122–2130.

Hartung EA, Guay-Woodford LM. Autosomal recessive polycystic kidney disease: a hepatorenal fibrocystic disorder with pleiotropic effects. *Pediatrics.* 2014;134(3):e833–e845.

Hogan MC, Masyuk T, Bergstralh E, et al. Efficacy of 4 years of octreotide long-acting release therapy in patients with severe polycystic liver disease. *Mayo Clin Proc.* 2015;90(8):1030–1037.

Irazabal MV, Rangel LJ, Bergstralh EJ, et al. Imaging classification of autosomal dominant polycystic kidney disease: a simple model for selecting patients for clinical trials. *J Am Soc Nephrol.* 2015;26(1):160–172.

Krueger D, Northtrup H. International Tuberous Sclerosis Complex Consensus Group. Tuberous sclerosis complex surveillance and management: recommendations of the 2012 International Tuberous Sclerosis Complex Consensus Conference. *Pediatr Neurol.* 2013; 49:255–265.

Meijer E, Visser FW, van Aerts RMM, et al. DIPAK-1 Investigators. Effect of lanreotide on kidney function in patients with autosomal dominant polycystic kidney disease: The DIPAK 1 randomized clinical trial. *JAMA.* 2018;320(19):2010–2019 Nov 20.

Wong ATY, Mannix C, Grantham JJ, et al. Randomised controlled trial to determine the efficacy and safety of prescribed water intake to prevent kidney failure due to autosomal dominant polycystic kidney disease (PREVENT-ADPKD). *BMJ Open.* 2018;8(1):e018794. doi:10.1136/bmjopen-2017-018794. Jan 21 PMID: 29358433.

Torres VE, Chapman AB, Devuyst O, et al. REPRISE Trial Investigators. Tolvaptan in later-stage autosomal dominant polycystic kidney disease. *N Engl J Med.* 2017;377(20):1930. Epub 2017 Nov 4.

40

Nephronophthisis and Medullary Cystic Kidney Disease

DANIELA A. BRAUN, FRIEDHELM HILDEBRANDT

Nephronophthisis (NPHP) and medullary cystic kidney disease (MCKD) represent a set of rare genetic kidney diseases with a similar kidney histopathology, which includes interstitial fibrosis with tubular atrophy, changes in the tubular basement membrane (TBM), and cyst formation. These two diseases can be distinguished clinically by their inheritance pattern and often by their age of onset. NPHP has an autosomal recessive inheritance pattern and results in kidney failure within the first three decades of life. MCKD has an autosomal dominant inheritance pattern and usually results in kidney failure between the fourth and seventh decades of life. While NPHP is frequently accompanied by defects in various other organ systems, gout is the only extrarenal manifestation described in MCKD thus far (Table 40.1). Clinical presentation, family history, and findings on kidney biopsy can suggest a diagnosis of NPHP or MCKD. However, the only definitive diagnostic modality is genetic testing. NPHP is genetically heterogenous with 20 different gene loci known to date. For MCKD, two gene loci are known, and researchers have finally succeeded in identifying the two underlying genes. As the term *MCKD* may be misleading in some cases, a Kidney Disease: Improving Global Outcomes (KDIGO) consensus report in 2015 suggested a new terminology for this syndrome, namely, *autosomal dominant tubulointerstitial kidney disease (ADTKD)* and proposed a gene-based subclassification. As a new development, recent genetic studies have shown that gene mutations thus far predominantly implicated in pediatric kidney disease appear to be more relevant in the adult-onset chronic kidney disease (CKD) than was previously assumed.

Epidemiology

NPHP is recognized as a rare cause of ESKD worldwide, but it is one of the most common genetic causes of ESKD in the pediatric population. Historically, the incidence of NPHP alone has been quoted as between 1 in 50,000 and 1 in 1 million live births. The 2007 annual report of the United States Renal Data System (USRDS) indicated that the overall incidence and prevalence of ESKD related to NPHP or MCKD were both about 0.1% in the United States. For the period 2012–16, USRDS data reported a combined incidence of 1.5% for MCKD and NPHP in pediatric patients with ESKD.

The incidence and prevalence of these diseases reported in databases may be an underestimate because patients often come to clinical attention only after kidney failure when the identification of the underlying diagnosis may no longer be possible. In addition, urinalysis in these disorders is typically bland without significant proteinuria or hematuria, limiting opportunities for screening and making aggressive diagnostic procedures such as biopsy less likely to be pursued. Although a presumptive diagnosis of NPHP or MCKD can be made based on clinical features and kidney histopathology, the only way to definitively diagnose these disorders is through genetic testing. Unfortunately, despite recent advances in next-generation sequencing and drastic cost reduction, access to molecular diagnostics in clinical settings is still limited.

Pathology

The similar appearance of the kidney histology between NPHP and MCKD led to the historic association of these two disorders. The classic triad of kidney pathology findings that are shared by all genetic types of NPHP except NPHP type 2 (NPHP2) includes interstitial fibrosis with tubular atrophy, TBM disruption, and corticomedullary cysts. Periglomerular fibrosis and sclerosis have also been noted. Cysts range in size from 1 to 15 mm, are typically located at the corticomedullary junction, and usually arise from the distal convoluted tubule or medullary collecting duct. Kidney size is normal or reduced in these types of NPHP, and cysts may not be apparent by imaging early in the course of the disease. Although NPHP frequently presents with extrarenal involvement, cysts have not been observed in other organs in contrast to autosomal dominant and autosomal recessive polycystic kidney disease (ADPKD/ARPKD).

NPHP2, or infantile NPHP, is caused by mutations in the *inversin (INVS)* gene, and its kidney pathology and clinical course are distinct from those of other types of NPHP. NPHP2 results in kidney failure in the first decade of life, often within the first 2 years, and is characterized by the cystic enlargement of the kidneys bilaterally. Kidney pathology is characterized by more remarkable cyst formation, which appears more prominently in the cortex, but it can also be present in the medulla. Cysts seem to arise from the proximal and distal tubules, and cystic enlargement of the glomerulus has occasionally been noted. Tubulointerstitial nephritis is another prominent finding in NPHP2, which it shares with the other forms of NPHP. Compared to other types of NPHP, TBM disruption is less commonly observed in the setting of NPHP2.

The gross appearance of the kidney in MCKD is normal to slightly reduced in size, similar to NPHP. Histologically, the kidney pathology of MCKD is virtually indistinguishable from

TABLE 40.1	Genetic Causes of Nephronophthisis and Medullary Cystic Kidney Disease				
Disease	Gene	Protein	Mode of Inheritance	Chromosomal Localization	Extrarenal Manifestations
NPHP1	NPHP1	Nephrocystin 1	AR	2q13	Retinitis pigmentosa, oculomotor apraxia, cerebellar vermis hypoplasia (rare)
NPHP2	INVS	Inversin	AR	9q31.1	Retinitis pigmentosa, *situs inversus*, liver fibrosis, pulmonary hypoplasia
NPHP3	NPHP3	Nephrocystin 3	AR	3q22.1	Retinitis pigmentosa, liver fibrosis, Meckel-Gruber syndrome
NPHP4	NPHP4	Nephroretinin	AR	1q36.22	Retinitis pigmentosa, oculomotor apraxia
NPHP5	IQCB1	Nephrocystin 5	AR	3q13.33	Retinitis pigmentosa (all described cases)
NPHP6	CEP290	Nephrocystin 6	AR	12q21.32	Retinitis pigmentosa, cerebellar vermis hypoplasia, liver fibrosis, Meckel-Gruber syndrome
NPHP7	GLIS2	GLIS 2	AR	16p13.3	Not reported
NPHP8	RPGRIP1L	Nephrocystin 8	AR	16q12.2	Retinitis pigmentosa, cerebellar vermis hypoplasia, liver fibrosis, Meckel-Gruber syndrome
NPHP9	NEK8	NEK8	AR	17q11.2	Liver fibrosis, congenital heart defects, Meckel-Gruber syndrome
NPHP10	SDCCAG8	SDCCAG8	AR	1q43–q44	Retinitis pigmentosa, Bardet-Biedl syndrome
NPHP11	TMEM67	Meckelin	AR	8q22.1	Retinitis pigmentosa, cerebellar vermis hypoplasia, liver fibrosis, polydactyly, Meckel-Gruber syndrome
NPHP12	TTC21B	TTC21B	AR	2q24.3	Cerebellar vermis hypoplasia, skeletal involvement
NPHP13	WDR19	WDR19/IFT144	AR	4p14	Retinitis pigmentosa, skeletal involvement, liver fibrosis
NPHP14	ZNF423	ZNF423	AR	16q12.1	Retinitis pigmentosa, cerebellar vermis hypoplasia
NPHP15	CEP164	CEP164	AR	11q23.3	Retinitis pigmentosa, cerebellar vermis hypoplasia
NPHP16	ANKS6	ANKS6	AR	9q22.33	Liver fibrosis, congenital heart disease
NPHP17	IFT172	IFT172	AR	2p23.3	Retinitis pigmentosa, skeletal involvement, liver fibrosis
NPHP18	CEP83	CEP83/CCDC41	AR	12q22	Retinitis pigmentosa, brain involvement
NPHP19	DCDC2	DCDC2	AR	6p22.3	Liver fibrosis
NPHP20	MAPKBP1	MAPKBP1	AR	15q15.1	None reported
MCKD1 (ADTKD-*MUC1*)	MUC1	Mucin 1	AD	1q22	Hyperuricemia, gout
MCKD2 (ADTKD-*UMOD*)	UMOD	Uromodulin	AD	16p12.3	Hyperuricemia, gout

AD, Autosomal dominant; *ADTKD*, autosomal dominant tubulointerstitial kidney-disease; *AR*, autosomal recessive; *MCKD*, medullary cystic kidney disease; *NPHP*, nephronophthisis.

NPHP, which has led to the historic nomenclature of these diseases as the *NPHP-MCKD disease complex*.

Pathogenesis

The molecular causes of NPHP are very heterogeneous. In addition to 20 genes that cause NPHP types 1 to 20 if mutated (see Table 40.1), NPHP-like kidney involvement has been described for many of the ~90 monogenic diseases that are collectively termed *ciliopathies*. This term was chosen because encoded proteins localize to the primary cilium, a cellular organelle that arises from the apical surface of virtually every cell of the human body. Consequently, the genes have a broad tissue expression pattern. NPHP is inherited in an autosomal recessive manner, is fully penetrant, and typically manifests in childhood or adolescence. Disease manifestation in heterozygous carriers has never been shown. The most common form of NPHP is type 1, which accounts for approximately 25% of all cases. Nearly 85% of mutations in *NPHP1* consist of large deletions, which typically include the whole gene. The remaining genetic causes of NPHP each account for only a small fraction of diagnosed cases.

The first monogenic causes of NPHP were identified with the help of positional cloning and linkage analysis. More recently, advances in next-generation sequencing have facilitated gene discovery and resulted in a rapid increase in the number of newly identified human disease genes. The study of NPHP genes and their related gene products, the nephrocystins, has provided important insight into pathogenic mechanisms underlying NPHP. Interestingly, all nephrocystin proteins share a common subcellular localization to the cilia-basal body-centrosome complex, suggesting that primary cilia play an essential role in the pathogenesis of cystic kidney diseases, a conclusion supported by experimental data from mouse studies. Many nephrocystin proteins show molecular interactions with other nephrocystins, indicating that these proteins and other ciliary proteins may be part of a common functional network. Molecular research has shown that primary cilia represent signaling hubs that convert extracellular stimuli into intracellular signals. It appears that numerous different signaling pathways, including the developmental pathways Sonic Hedgehog and Wnt signaling, require primary cilia for proper function. By regulating these pathways, nephrocystin proteins seem to control kidney fibrosis and the maintenance of proper kidney architecture. More recently, it was shown that centrosomal proteins, which give rise to NPHP and other ciliopathies if their genes are mutated, play a critical role in the regulation of cell cycle progression, mitotic spindle orientation, and DNA damage response signaling. The fact that all these signaling pathways or selective signal pathways may be defective depending on the severity of the mutation could explain the broad phenotypic spectrum and the multitude of extrarenal symptoms that can be present in patients with NPHP. Despite intense research, the exact pathogenic mechanism by which mutations in NPHP genes result in kidney disease is still unknown; however, it seems plausible that dysregulation in several pathways results in a common kidney histopathology of interstitial fibrosis, tubular atrophy, and degenerative cysts.

Two gene loci have been identified for MCKD: *MCKD1* on 1q21 and *MCKD2* on 16p12. Fifteen years after the initial description of the *MCKD1* locus and after numerous failed attempts, researchers finally identified single nucleotide insertions in very long and highly GC-rich tandem repeat areas (VNTRs) of the gene *MUC1*, encoding Mucin 1, as the molecular cause of MCKD type 1. The mutation causes a shift of the reading frame, resulting in a truncated protein (MUC1-fs) that lacks several characteristic domains of the wild-type protein, including the transmembrane domain, resulting in subcellular mislocalization of Mucin 1. The mutated protein is expressed in tubular epithelial and collecting duct cells of affected patients, and detection of MUC1-fs in kidney biopsies can be used for molecular diagnostics. As seen in neurodegenerative diseases, such as Alzheimer, MUC1-fs appears to act as a toxic protein, which accumulates intracellularly and causes cell injury by endoplasmic reticulum stress, an evolving target for therapy.

Mutations in the gene *UMOD*, encoding uromodulin, the Tamm-Horsfall protein, have been shown to cause MCKD2, familial juvenile hyperuricemic nephropathy (FJHN), and glomerulocystic kidney disease (GCKD). Uromodulin is expressed in the thick ascending limb of the loop of Henle and is the most abundant protein found in the urine. The excretion of uromodulin is reduced in these patients, and pathologic intracellular accumulation of uromodulin occurs in the tubular epithelial cells of the thick ascending limb. The exact molecular pathogenesis of MCKD2 remains unknown.

According to the new KDIGO classification, MCKD1 has been renamed ADTKD-*MUC1* and MCKD2 has been renamed ADTKD-*UMOD*. Additionally, the group of ADTKD includes ADTKD-*REN*, caused by mutations in the *REN* gene that encodes renin, a condition previously termed *FJHN type 2*, and ADTKD-*HNF1B*, describing patients with *HNF1B* mutations who present predominantly with kidney phenotypes. Typically, *HNF1B* mutations give rise to various extrarenal manifestations, mostly diabetes mellitus, resulting in two syndromic diseases known as *maturity-onset diabetes mellitus of the young type 5 (MODY5)* and *kidney cyst and diabetes syndrome*. The ADTKD classification furthermore includes ADTKD-NOS (not otherwise specified) for patients with a typical clinical phenotype who cannot be attributed to a specific gene mutation. All types of ADTKD are inherited in an autosomal-dominant manner.

Clinical Features and Diagnosis

The age of onset of clinically apparent kidney disease and the pattern of inheritance in familial cases are different in NPHP and MCKD (see Table 40.1). Although biopsy findings in conjunction with the appropriate clinical presentation and patient history can suggest a diagnosis of NPHP or MCKD, the only definitive diagnostic modality is genetic testing. With recent technical advances and cost reduction in next-generation sequencing, molecular genetic testing has become more feasible. However, the accessibility of clinical genetic testing in certified diagnostic laboratories for patients with chronic kidney diseases is still limited, and many patients thus remain without a definitive molecular diagnosis. A list of research and clinical laboratories offering genetic testing is available at http://www.genetests.org. Considering the broad phenotypic and genetic heterogeneity of NPHP, the method of choice for genetic testing should be whole-exome sequencing rather than targeted sequencing of a limited number of candidate genes. For technical reasons, genetic testing for *MUC1* mutations is still challenging and availability is extremely limited. Therefore, family history, clinical features, and staining of MUC1-fs protein in kidney biopsies oftentimes have to suffice for diagnostics in clinical practice.

Nephronophthisis

Kidney function decline begins early in NPHP, typically progressing to kidney failure within the first three decades of life. The earliest clinical manifestation of NPHP is a urinary concentrating defect that results in the clinical symptoms of polyuria, secondary enuresis, and nocturnal polydipsia. These findings may precede the onset of glomerular filtration rate (GFR) loss. A family history of affected siblings with an autosomal recessive inheritance pattern is strongly suggestive of the diagnosis, but given the rarity of the disease, sporadic cases are more common.

Historically, the age of onset has been considered an important clinical distinction among the various types of NPHP, leading to categorization of the disease as infantile (only NPHP2), juvenile (NPHP1 and NPHP4), or adolescent (NPHP3). However, with the exception of NPHP2, which leads to ESKD in the first decade of life, it is not clear whether there is truly a predictable difference in the age of onset for the other types of NPHP.

The extrarenal manifestations of NPHP (see Table 40.1) include retinitis pigmentosa, which has been present in all cases of NPHP5 identified thus far but can also be present in other types of NPHP. Many cases of NPHP6 are initially identified as Joubert syndrome, a brain developmental defect, which has the characteristic features of cerebellar vermis hypoplasia, ataxia, and other impairment of motor coordination. Beyond NPHP6, Joubert syndrome has been described in other types of NPHP. Oculomotor apraxia type Cogan is typically associated with mutation in the genes *NPHP1* and *NPHP4*. Laterality defects, such as *situs inversus* or congenital heart defects, are frequently observed in patients with NPHP2. Liver involvement is most frequent in patients with mutations in the genes *NPHP3*, *TMEM67* (NPHP11), *ANKS6* (NPHP16), and *DCDC2* (NPHP19). NPHP-like kidney involvement has also been described as part of several clinical syndromes, including the COACH (Cerebellar vermis hypoplasia, Oligophrenia, Ataxia, Coloboma, and Hepatic fibrosis), Arima, Jeune, Sensenbrenner, and Bardet-Biedl syndromes.

Physical findings of NPHP include growth retardation and anemia. Interestingly, compared to other causes of chronic kidney disease, both symptoms have been noted as being more pronounced when adjusted to the GFR level. Conversely, elevated blood pressure is typically less prevalent than would be expected for the given GFR.

The laboratory evaluation of NPHP patients includes a urinalysis of the first morning void, which usually is normal except for a low specific gravity, reflecting a urinary concentrating defect. The absence of proteinuria or hematuria helps to distinguish NPHP from other heritable kidney diseases such as focal segmental glomerulosclerosis and Alport syndrome, respectively. Other laboratory abnormalities are commensurate with the degree of GFR loss.

The most relevant diagnostic test is an ultrasound examination of the kidneys, which demonstrates normal to slightly reduced kidney size, increased echotexture, and a loss of corticomedullary differentiation. Cysts are typically located at the corticomedullary junction, but cysts are not always visible on imaging and are not a prerequisite for the diagnosis of NPHP. The imaging findings for patients with NPHP2 are substantially different from those of other types of NPHP: kidney size is often increased, and cysts are a prominent finding.

In summary, the diagnosis of NPHP should be entertained when an individual presents in the first three decades of life with reduced kidney function, a bland urine sediment, and normal to small kidneys on ultrasound with increased echotexture and loss of corticomedullary differentiation. The most common extrarenal manifestation associated with NPHP is retinitis pigmentosa, which often leads to blindness in the first decade of life and occurs in about 10% of patients. The occurrence of similarly affected siblings strongly suggests NPHP. The parents of affected children are not affected because NPHP is inherited as an autosomal-recessive disease. The recessive inheritance pattern differentiates NPHP from MCKD, which is transmitted as an autosomal-dominant disease (i.e., one parent of the affected individual should also be affected).

While generally considered a disease of children, a recent study detected deletions of the *NPHP1* gene in a small fraction of patients with adult-onset CKD (>30 years). This finding is in line with other studies that detected mutations in genes typically associated with pediatric kidney disease in adults with CKD of unknown origin, thus suggesting that monogenic diseases may be more relevant in the setting of adult-onset CKD than was previously assumed.

Medullary Cystic Kidney Disease

MCKD usually presents in the fourth to seventh decades of life. Two exceptions to this pattern are FJHN and GCKD, which are allelic (i.e., caused by mutations in the same gene) to MCKD2 but manifest within the first three decades of life. MCKD, FJHN, and GCKD are all inherited in an autosomal dominant pattern. The only extrarenal manifestation associated with these diseases, aside from those attributable to reduced kidney function, is hyperuricemia with gouty arthritis.

There are no other distinctive findings on physical examination associated with MCKD. Laboratory findings are notable for a urinary concentration defect with reduced fractional excretion of uric acid, but the urinalysis is otherwise unremarkable. Ultrasound examination demonstrates normal to slightly reduced kidney size, increased echogenicity, loss of corticomedullary differentiation, and medullary cysts. However, especially in early stages of the disease, the changes may be too subtle for detection with ultrasound or computed tomography studies.

Treatment

Despite significant advances in understanding the molecular mechanisms of NPHP, no curative or targeted treatment is available at this point, and no systematic clinical trials have been undertaken to examine different treatment regimens for NPHP or MCKD in people. Accordingly, treatment of NPHP and MCKD centers on the sequelae of chronic kidney disease, including anemia, acidosis, electrolyte imbalance, mineral and bone disorder, and growth retardation. Kidney failure typically develops within the first three decades of life in patients with NPHP and between ages 40 and 70 years in patients with MCKD. Patients with NPHP and MCKD have successfully undergone kidney transplantation without evidence of recurrent disease in the transplant.

Bibliography

Braun DA, Schueler M, Halbritter J, et al. Whole exome sequencing identifies causative mutations in the majority of consanguineous or familial cases with childhood onset increased renal echogenicity. *Kidney Int*. 2016;89:468–475.

Chaki M, Airik R, Ghosh AK, et al. Exome capture reveals ZNF423 and CEP164 mutations, linking renal ciliopathies to DNA damage response signaling. *Cell*. 2012;150:533–548.

Connaughton DM, Kennedy C, Shril S, et al. Monogenic causes of chronic kidney disease in adults. *Kidney Int*. 2019;95:914–928.

Dahan K, Devuyst O, Smaers M, et al. A cluster of mutations in UMOD gene causes familial hyperuricemic nephropathy with abnormal expression of uromodulin. *J Am Soc Nephrol*. 2003;14:2883–2893.

Eckardt KU, Alper SL, Antignac C, et al. Autosomal dominant tubulointerstitial kidney disease: diagnosis, classification, and management—A KDIGO consensus report. *Kidney Int*. 2015;88:676–683.

Halbritter J, Porath JD, Diaz KA, et al. Identification of 99 novel mutations in a worldwide cohort of 1,056 patients with a nephronophthisis-related ciliopathy. *Hum Genet*. 2013;132:865–884.

Hart TC, Gorry MC, Hart PS, et al. Mutations of the UMOD gene are responsible for medullary cystic disease 2 and familial hyperuricemic nephropathy. *J Med Genet*. 2002;39:882–892.

Hildebrandt F. Nephronophthisis-medullary cystic kidney disease. In: Avner ED, Harmon WE, Niaudet P, eds. *Pediatric Nephrology*. 5th ed. Philadelphia: Lippincott, Williams and Wilkins; 2004:665–673.

Hildebrandt F, Benzing T, Ciliopathies Katsanis N. *N Engl J Med*. 2011;364:1533–1543.

Hildebrandt F, Otto E. Cilia and centrosomes: a unifying pathogenetic concept for cystic kidney disease? *Nat Rev Genet*. 2005;6:928–940.

Kirby A, Gnirke A, Jaffe DB, et al. Mutations causing medullary cystic kidney disease type 1 lie in a large VNTR in MUC1 missed by massively parallel sequencing. *Nat Genet*. 2013;45:299–303.

Knaup KX, Hackenbeck T, Popp B, et al. Biallelic Expression of Mucin-1 in Autosomal Dominant Tubulointerstitial Kidney Disease: Implications for Nongenetic Disease Recognition. *J Am Soc Nephrol*. 2018;29:2298–2309.

Rampoldi L, Caridi G, Santon D, et al. Allelism of MCKD, FJHN and GCKD caused by impairment of uromodulin export dynamics. *Hum Mol Genet*. 2003;12:3369–3384.

Sang L, Miller JJ, Corbit KC, et al. Mapping the NPHP-JBTS-MKS protein network reveals ciliopathy disease genes and pathways. *Cell*. 2011;145:513–528.

Simons M, Gloy J, Ganner A, et al. Inversin, the gene product mutated in nephronophthisis type II, functions as a molecular switch between Wnt signaling pathways. *Nat Genet*. 2005;37:537–543.

Snoek R, van Setten J, Keating BJ, et al. NPHP1 (Nephrocystin-1) Gene Deletions Cause Adult-Onset ESRD. *J Am Soc Nephrol*. 2018;29:1772–1779.

United States Renal Data System. United States Renal Data System. *USRDS Annual Data Report: Epidemiology of Kidney Disease in the United States*. Bethesda, MD: National Institutes of Health, National Institute of Diabetes and Digestive and Kidney Diseases; 2018.

Vivante A, Hildebrandt F. Exploring the genetic basis of early-onset chronic kidney disease. *Nat Rev Nephrol*. 2016;12:133–146.

Wolf MT. Nephronophthisis and related syndromes. *Curr Opin Pediatr*. 2015;27:201–211.

41

Alport Syndrome and Related Disorders

MARTIN C. GREGORY

Alport syndrome is a disease of type IV collagen that always affects the kidneys, usually the ears, and often the eyes. Cecil Alport described the association of hereditary hematuric nephritis with hearing loss in a family whose affected male members died in adolescence. Genetic advances have broadened the scope of the condition to include optical defects, late-onset kidney failure, and normal hearing in some families. Approximately 85% of kindreds have X-linked disease, resulting from a mutation of *COL4A5*, the gene located at Xq22 that codes for the α5 chain of type IV collagen, α5(IV). Autosomal inheritance occurs in perhaps 15% of cases from mutations in COL4A3 or COL4A4.

Phenotypic Variability in X-Linked Alport Syndrome

Kidney failure tends to occur at a broadly similar age in all male members of a family, but this age varies widely among families, with kidney failure in males occurring in childhood or adolescence in some families and in adulthood in others. Forms with early onset of kidney failure in affected males have been called *juvenile*, while those with kidney failure in middle age are *adult type*. Some authors use the term *hypomorphic* to describe mutations that cause very mild or delayed kidney manifestations. Extrarenal manifestations tend to be more prominent in juvenile kindreds. Because boys in juvenile kindreds do not commonly survive to reproduce, these kindreds tend to be small and frequently arise from new mutations, whereas adult-type kindreds are typically much larger without new mutations (Table 41.1).

Biochemistry

The open mesh of interlocking type IV collagen molecules that form the framework of the glomerular basement membrane (GBM) is composed of heterotrimers of α chains. In fetal life, these heterotrimers consist of two α1(IV) chains and one α2(IV) chain, but early in postnatal development, production switches to α3(IV), α4(IV), and α5(IV) chains. The primary chemical defect in Alport syndrome involves the α5(IV) chain or, less commonly, the α3(IV) chain, but faulty assembly of the α3,4,5-heterotrimer produces similar pathology in glomerular, aural, and ocular basement membranes, regardless of which α chain is defective. As an illustration of failure of normal heterotrimer formation, most patients whose genetic defect is in the gene coding for the α3(IV) chain lack demonstrable α5(IV) chains in GBMs.

Genetics

In most kindreds, inheritance of Alport syndrome is X-linked. Causative mutations of COL4A5, the gene coding for α5(IV), are located at Xq22 and appear consistently in many kindreds. These mutations include deletions, point mutations, and splicing errors. There is some correlation between the mutation type and the clinical phenotype: deletions and some splicing errors cause severe kidney disease and early hearing loss. Missense mutations may cause juvenile disease with hearing loss or adult disease with or without hearing loss. Deletions involving the 5′ end of the *COL4A5* gene and the 5′ end of the adjacent *COL4A6* gene occur consistently in families with Alport syndrome and esophageal and genital leiomyomatosis.

Homozygotes or mixed heterozygotes for mutations of the *COL4A3* or *COL4A4* genes (chromosome 2) develop autosomal recessive Alport syndrome. Heterozygotes for these mutations account for many cases of benign familial hematuria or familial thin basement membrane disease (TBMD). Cases of digenic inheritance with one mutation in COL4A3 and one in COL4A4 have also been described. As mentioned above for COL4A5 mutations, COL4A3 and COL4A4 mutations are variably pathogenic so that phenotypic variability occurs and some heterozygotes can develop GFR loss or even kidney failure. The frequency of autosomal dominant Alport syndrome is debated: several reports suggest that it may be more common than previously thought.

Patients with autosomal dominant hematuria and kidney failure with thrombocytopenia, giant platelets (Epstein syndrome), and leukocyte inclusions (Fechtner syndrome) have mutations in the *MYH9* gene on chromosome 22 (see below). These patients should no longer be considered to have Alport syndrome but rather have MYH9-related disorders.

Immunochemistry

Male patients with X-linked Alport syndrome and patients with autosomal recessive Alport syndrome frequently lack the α3, α4, and α5 chains of type IV collagen in the GBM, and hemizygous males with X-linked Alport syndrome often lack α5(IV) chains in the epidermal basement membrane (EBM). Monoclonal antibodies specific to the α2 and α5 chains of type IV collagen are commercially available and can be used to assist in the diagnosis of Alport syndrome. The GBM and EBM of normal individuals, as well as those of all Alport patients, react with the α2 antibody, but most male and female patients with autosomal recessive Alport

TABLE 41.1	Alport Syndrome Types With Chromosomal and Gene Locations and Relative Frequencies		
Type	Chromosome	Gene	Relative Frequency[a]
X-linked	X	*COL4A5*	85%
Juvenile type			90% of families, 50% of patients
Adult type			8% of families, 25% of patients
Adult type with "normal" hearing			2% of families, 25% of patients
Autosomal recessive	2	*COL4A3, COL4A4*	15%
Autosomal dominant	2	*COL4A3, COL4A4*	Debated, but likely less than 1%

[a]Relative frequencies of the X-linked, autosomal recessive, and autosomal dominant forms are fairly well accepted. The frequencies of "juvenile" (mean age of end-stage kidney disease [ESKD] in males <30 years), "adult" (mean age of ESKD in males >30 years), and adult type with near-normal hearing are rough estimates from the numbers of patients and families known to the University of Utah Alport Study. In the United States, C1564S is a common mutation causing adult-type Alport syndrome, and L1649R is a common mutation causing adult-type Alport syndrome with near-normal hearing.

syndrome and most male patients hemizygous for a COL4A5 mutation show no staining of the GBM with the α5 antibody. Males with X-linked disease commonly show no staining of EBM with antibody to α5, whereas females heterozygous for a COL4A5 mutation show interrupted staining of the GBM and EBM, consistent with mosaicism.

After kidney transplants, fewer than 5% of male patients with Alport syndrome develop anti-GBM glomerulonephritis, presumably because they are exposed for the first time to normal collagen chains including a 26-kDa monomer of the α3(IV) chain to which tolerance has never been acquired. Recurrences of anti-GBM glomerulonephritis are usual but not inevitable after repeat transplantation. The serum antibodies to GBM developing after transplantation are heterogeneous; all stain normal GBM, and some stain EBM.

Pathology

In young children, light microscopy of the kidneys may be normal or near normal. Glomeruli with persistent fetal morphology may be seen. As disease progresses, interstitial and tubular foam cells, which arise for reasons that are unclear, may become prominent (Fig. 41.1), although they are nonspecific and can also be found in many other conditions. Eventually, progressive glomerulosclerosis and interstitial scarring develop. The histology may eventually be that of secondary focal segmental glomerular sclerosis (FSGS), or FSGS may develop without ultrastructural changes of Alport syndrome. Genome-wide searches have shown that an appreciable proportion of adult patients with FSGS have mutations in the COL4A genes despite not presenting with Alport syndrome features. The results of routine immunofluorescence examination for immunoglobulins and complement are negative, and lack of staining for the α5(IV) chain may be informative (see "Immunochemistry").

The GBM is up to three times its normal thickness, split into several irregular layers, and frequently interspersed with electron-dense granules about 40 nm in diameter (Fig. 41.2). In florid cases of juvenile types of Alport syndrome, the basement membrane lamellae may branch and rejoin in a complex basket-weave pattern. Early in the development of the lesion, thinning of the GBM may predominate or be the only abnormality visible. The abnormalities in boys, adolescent males, and females heterozygous for adult-type Alport syndrome may be unimpressive or indistinguishable from those of TBMD disease (see below).

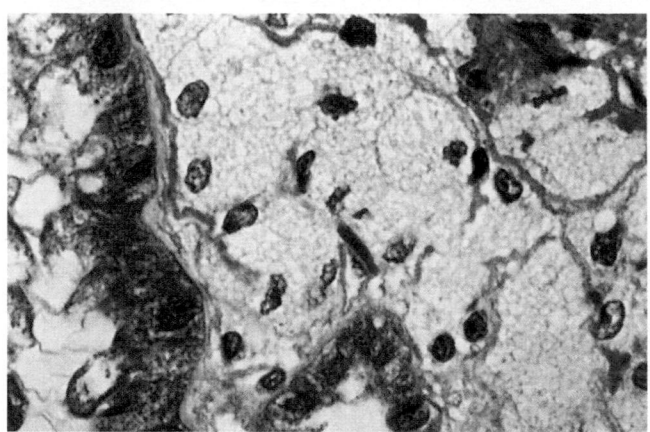

• **Fig. 41.1** High-power photomicrograph shows foam-filled tubular and interstitial cells in a kidney biopsy specimen from a patient with Alport syndrome. Relatively normal proximal tubular cytoplasm stains red in the tubules on the left and at the bottom. The remaining cells appear "foamy" because of the spaces left where lipids have been eluted during processing.

Clinical Features

Kidney Features

Uninterrupted microscopic hematuria occurs from birth in affected males. Hematuria may become visible after exercise or during fever; this is more common in juvenile kindreds. Microscopic hematuria has a penetrance of approximately 90% in heterozygous females in adult-type kindreds. In juvenile kindreds, the penetrance of hematuria in females has been studied less extensively but appears to be common. Urinary erythrocytes are dysmorphic, and red-cell casts usually can be found in affected males. The degree of proteinuria varies, but it occasionally reaches nephrotic levels.

Hemizygous males inevitably progress to end-stage kidney disease (ESKD). This occurs at widely different ages, but, within each family, the age of ESKD is fairly constant. Heterozygous females are usually much less severely affected. About one-fourth of them develop ESKD, usually after the age of 50 years, but ESKD can occur earlier. In families with autosomal inheritance, females are affected as severely and as early as males, and kidney failure often occurs before the age of 20 in those who are homozygous for autosomal recessive Alport syndrome. Microscopic hematuria is a consistent feature.

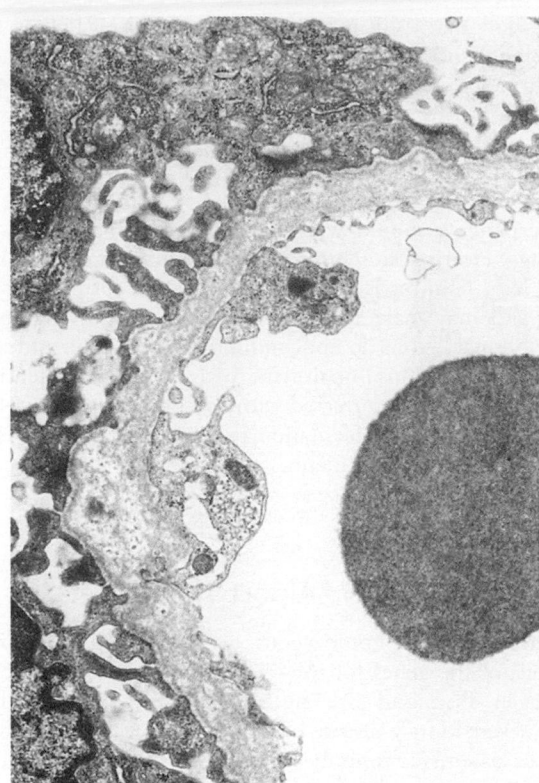

• **Fig. 41.2** High-resolution electron micrograph shows a glomerular basement membrane from a patient with Alport syndrome that varies in thickness. It is split into several layers, which in some areas are separated by lucencies containing small, dense granules. (Courtesy Dr. Theodore J. Pysher.)

Extrarenal Features

Hearing Loss

Bilateral, high-frequency cochlear hearing loss occurs in many kindreds, but X-linked disease progressing to ESKD can occur in families without overt hearing loss. It is easy to miss the diagnosis of Alport syndrome if hearing loss is expected as a constant feature (see Table 41.1). In families with juvenile-type disease, hearing loss is almost universal in male hemizygotes and common in severely affected female heterozygotes.

Patterns of hearing loss vary. Often, the most severe loss is at 2 kHz to 6 kHz, but it may occur at a higher frequency if there has been superimposed noise damage. In adult-type Alport syndrome with hearing loss, there is typically no perceptible deficit until 20 years of age, but loss progresses to 60 to 70 dB at 6 to 8 kHz after 40 years of age. It is important to realize that about half of those with adult-type Alport syndrome will have no overt hearing loss; failure to recognize this is a common reason for overlooking the diagnosis in adults. Hearing loss occurs earlier in juvenile kindreds. The rate at which hearing is lost is not well established in juvenile kindreds, but many adolescents require hearing aids.

Ocular Defects

Ocular defects are common in juvenile kindreds. Three changes that are present in a minority of kindreds but that are almost diagnostic are anterior lenticonus, posterior polymorphous corneal dystrophy, and retinal flecks. Anterior lenticonus is a forward protrusion of the anterior surface of the ocular lens. It results from

a weakness of the type IV collagen forming the anterior lens capsule. The resulting irregularity of the surface of the lens causes an uncorrectable refractive error. The retina cannot be clearly seen by ophthalmoscopy, and with a strong positive lens in the ophthalmoscope the lenticonus often can be seen through a dilated pupil as an "oil drop" or circular smudge on the center of the lens (Fig. 41.3). Retinal flecks are small, yellow or white dots scattered around the macula or in the periphery of the retina (Fig. 41.4). If sparse, they may be difficult to distinguish from small, hard

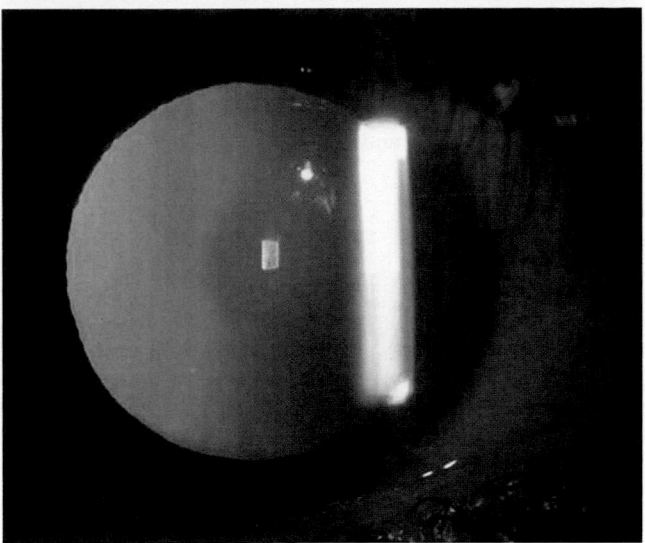

• **Fig. 41.3** Retroilluminated lens photography shows the "oil-drop" appearance of anterior lenticonus, a pathognomonic feature of Alport syndrome. The bulging area of the lens is the dark circular area just to the left of the vertical reflected light artifact from the slit-lamp examination. This is similar to the view obtained through a direct ophthalmoscope with a strong positive lens.

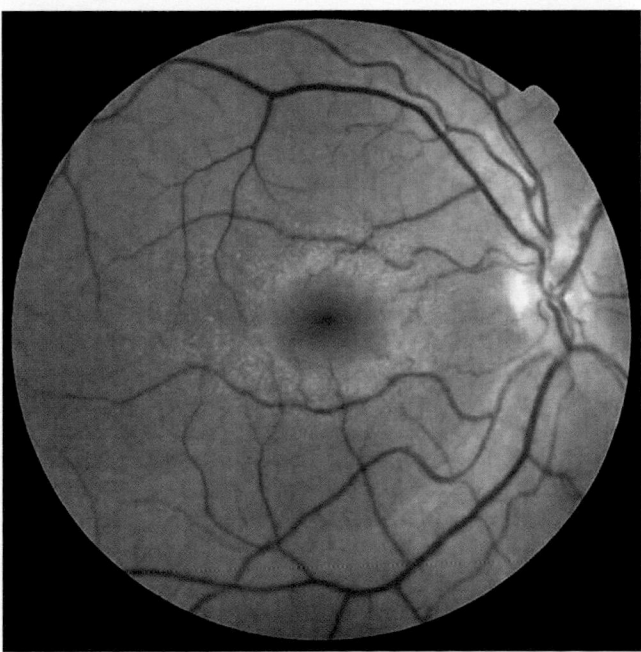

• **Fig. 41.4** Retinal photograph of right fundus from a 14-year-old boy with Alport syndrome shows perimacular dots and flecks that spare the foveola and are more discrete at the outer margin of the ring. Alport retinopathy varies from occasional dots and flecks in the temporal macula to this appearance. (Courtesy Drs. Judith Savige and Deb Colville.)

exudates. Macular holes occur rarely but can severely affect sight. Ocular manifestations are often subtle, and consultation with an ophthalmologist familiar with Alport syndrome is invaluable.

Optical coherence tomography is a simple, inexpensive test that shows thinning of the temporal retina in patients with Alport syndrome. This test appears to have high sensitivity and specificity, but more study is needed.

Leiomyomatosis

Young members of several families with X-linked Alport syndrome develop striking leiomyomas of the esophagus and female genitalia. Patients frequently have multiple large tumors, which may bleed or cause obstruction, and their resection can be difficult. All described families have had a deletion at the 5′ ends of the contiguous *COL4A5* and *COL4A6* genes.

Diagnosis

No single clinical feature is pathognomonic of Alport syndrome. The diagnosis is based on finding hematuria in many family members, a history of kidney failure in related males, and a kidney biopsy showing characteristic ultrastructural changes in the proband or a relative. Immunofluorescence examination of the biopsy specimen should include staining with antibodies specific to GBM or to α5(IV); the lack of staining in most male patients with Alport syndrome helps to differentiate Alport syndrome from familial TBMD, in which staining is normal. If the skin of affected family members is known to lack immunofluorescent staining with antibodies to α5(IV), an α5(IV) immunofluorescence examination of a skin biopsy from a suspected case in the family may be diagnostic.

Molecular diagnosis is almost 100% sensitive and specific but only after a mutation has been found in the family. Sequencing the *COL4A3*, *COL4A4*, and *COL4A5* genes is at least 80% sensitive for mutations, and is now readily available.

The key to diagnosis is clinical suspicion of Alport syndrome in any patient with otherwise unexplained hematuria, glomerulopathy, or kidney failure. In many cases, the familial nature of the condition is not immediately apparent. Inquiry into the family history must be detailed and complete. The patient is usually a boy or young man, and, given the X-linked transmission, he may have one or more male relatives with kidney failure in his mother's family. Urine samples from both of the patient's parents, particularly his mother, should be checked for hematuria.

Although it is a helpful clue, it is crucial to remember that hearing loss is neither a sensitive nor a specific marker of Alport syndrome; it is neither necessary nor sufficient for the diagnosis. Many adults with kidney failure from Alport syndrome do not have conspicuous hearing loss, particularly those with the *COL4A5* L1649R mutation. In addition, many patients with hearing loss and kidney disease do not have Alport syndrome but instead have other kidney disorders, most often glomerulonephritis, with a more common cause for hearing loss, such as noise exposure, aminoglycoside therapy, or unrelated inherited hearing loss.

Treatment

There is no specific treatment for Alport syndrome, but clinical trials are currently under way. General measures to retard the progression of kidney failure, such as treatment of hypertension, specifically with angiotensin-converting enzyme (ACE) inhibitors, are warranted. Animal studies and observational data from Europe show that ACE inhibition delays onset of kidney failure and prolongs survival, although controlled trials are still lacking. Unconfirmed reports claim benefit from cyclosporine in reducing proteinuria and retarding progression of kidney disease; however, other investigators have found little benefit with risk of cyclosporine nephrotoxicity. Bardoxolone methyl has shown benefit in trials but is not currently FDA approved.

Male patients should wear hearing protection in noisy surroundings. Hearing aids improve but do not completely restore hearing loss. Tinnitus is usually resistant to all forms of therapy; hearing aids may make it less disruptive by amplifying ambient sounds. Retinal lesions do not commonly affect vision and require no therapy. The serious impairment to vision caused by lenticonus or cataract cannot be corrected with spectacles or contact lenses. Lens removal with reimplantation of an intraocular lens is standard and satisfactory treatment.

Related Disorders

Autosomal Recessive Alport Syndrome

Children may have homozygous or compound heterozygous mutations of the genes for the α3(IV) or α4(IV) chains of type IV collagen. Boys and girls are equally affected, and both may develop severe kidney disease before the age of 20 years. The heterozygous parents commonly have TBMD (discussed later), but not all have persistent hematuria.

Autosomal Dominant Alport Syndrome

Several recent studies show that families with autosomal dominant Alport syndrome as a consequence of heterozygous mutations of the genes for the α3(IV) or α4(IV) chains of type IV collagen appear to be more common than previously reported.

Alport Syndrome with Thrombocytopathy: Epstein Syndrome and Fechtner Syndrome

The Epstein and Fechtner syndromes are uncommon autosomal dominant syndromes of hematuria and progressive kidney failure associated with moderate thrombocytopenia and severe hearing loss in males and females. Platelets (about 7 μm in diameter) are much larger than normal (1 to 1.5 μm), and there is a mild or moderate bleeding tendency. In families with Fechtner syndrome, an additional feature is inclusion bodies (Fechtner bodies) in leukocytes. These syndromes are caused by a mutation in the nonmuscle myosin heavy chain 9 gene *(MYH9)* on chromosome 22q12.3–13.1.

Familial Thin Basement Membrane Disease

TBMD, or benign familial hematuria, is an autosomal dominant basement membrane glomerulopathy. Many cases result from heterozygous mutations of the *COL4A3* or *COL4A4* genes at chromosome 2q35 to 2q37; those patients who carry homozygous or compound heterozygous mutations in trans in these same genes develop autosomal recessive Alport syndrome. Ultrastructurally, the GBM is uniformly thinned to about one-half its normal thickness. There is no disruption or lamellation of the GBM, nor are any other abnormalities of the glomeruli, tubules, vessels, or interstitium visible by light, immunofluorescence, or electron microscopy. Kidney failure seldom occurs. Longevity is unaffected by this condition, with survivors into the ninth decade documented. Minor degrees of lamellation of the GBM and hearing loss have been described in some families, but these families might have had unrecognized Alport syndrome.

After a precise molecular diagnosis is established, the patient and family can be spared further invasive tests, and an appropriate prognosis can be provided to them and to health insurers. However, the distinction between Alport syndrome and benign familial hematuria is not always easy to make.

Familial Focal Segmental Glomerulosclerosis

COL4A3, COL4A4, and *COL4A5* mutations are emerging as the most common cause of familial FSGS presenting in adults.

Approach to the Patient with 'Hereditary Nephritis'

Although Alport syndrome is less common than polycystic kidney disease, it is probably more common than generally appreciated. Important conditions comprising the differential diagnoses of hematuria in young persons include IgA nephropathy or other glomerulonephritides, kidney stones, and medullary sponge kidney. The differential diagnosis of familial kidney disease with hematuria includes TBMD, familial IgA nephropathy, Fabry disease, and polycystic kidney disease. Familial kidney diseases without hematuria that may be confused with Alport syndrome include polycystic kidney disease, medullary cystic disease, and rare forms of inherited glomerular and tubulointerstitial kidney disease.

If a patient with unexplained hematuria or kidney failure has a family history of hematuria or kidney failure, the family history should be extended, concentrating particularly on the mother's male relatives. Identifying hearing loss strengthens, and finding a specific ocular lesion greatly strengthens, suspicion for Alport syndrome. Kidney biopsy may be indicated for one family member, but the easy availability of genetic testing has greatly reduced the need for biopsy. After the diagnosis of a heritable basement membrane disease is established in a family, it is difficult to justify biopsies in other members unless there are features that suggest another diagnosis. The extent of investigation is guided by clinical judgment and relates inversely to the strength of the family history. For example, a young man on the line of descent of a known Alport family whose urine contains dysmorphic erythrocytes needs minimal investigation. He may need no further workup other than an assessment of the glomerular filtration rate and urine protein quantification, unless there are additional clinical features suggesting a systemic disease. A patient with hematuria and an uncertain family history may merit the standard nephrologic and/or urologic workup for hematuria. If suspicion of Alport syndrome is moderate or strong, and the test is available, a skin biopsy with staining for the α5(IV) chain may be considered, particularly if a known affected family member is available as a positive control.

Genetic testing generally will start with next-generation sequencing of the *COL4A3, COL4A4,* and *COL4A5* genes. After a mutation is defined in a family, targeted mutation analysis is an inexpensive way to determine whether other family members

carry the mutant gene and may be spared the need for a kidney biopsy. Sequencing of the three genes is still reasonable for family members and may be no more expensive.

Patients with any hereditary nephropathy should be informed about the nature of the disease and perhaps be given a copy of the genetic analysis or kidney biopsy report to avoid unnecessary further investigation. Similar recommendations apply to family members who are potential gene carriers. Those with Alport syndrome should be followed regularly for elevation of blood pressure and changes in kidney function. The frequency of follow-up depends on the anticipated age of onset of kidney function deterioration in the family. Those with familial TBMD should be checked about every 2 years, because some may ultimately turn out to have Alport syndrome.

Bibliography

Barker DF, Hostikka SL, Zhou J, et al. Identification of mutations in the *COL4A5* collagen gene in Alport's syndrome. *Science.* 1990;248:1224–1227.

Bekheirnia MR, Reed B, Gregory MC, et al. Genotype-phenotype correlation in X-linked Alport syndrome. *J Am Soc Nephrol.* 2010;21:876–883.

Gleeson MJ. Alport's syndrome: audiological manifestations and implications. *J Laryngol Otol.* 1984;98:449–465.

Govan JA. Ocular manifestations of Alport's syndrome: a hereditary disorder of basement membranes? *Br J Ophthalmol.* 1983;67:493–503.

Gregory MC. Alport's syndrome and thin basement membrane nephropathy: unraveling the tangled strands of type IV collagen. *Kidney Int.* 2004;65:1109–1110.

Gregory MC, Shamshirsam A, Kamgar M, et al. Alport's syndrome, Fabry's disease, and nail-patella syndrome. In: Schrier RW, ed. *Diseases of the Kidney.* 8th ed. Boston, MA: Little Brown; 2007:540–569.

Groopman EE, Marasa M, Cameron-Christie S, et al. Diagnostic utility of exome sequencing for kidney disease. *New Eng J Med.* 2019;380:142–151.

Gross O, Licht C, Anders HJ, et al. Early angiotensin-converting enzyme inhibition in Alport syndrome delays renal failure and improves life expectancy. *Kidney Int.* 2012;81:494–501.

Heath KE, Campos-Barros A, Toren A, et al. Nonmuscle myosin heavy chain IIA mutations define a spectrum of autosomal dominant macrothrombocytopenias: May-Hegglin anomaly and Fechtner, Sebastian, Epstein, and Alport-like syndromes. *Am J Hum Genet.* 2001;69:1033–1045.

Jais JP, Knebelmann B, Giatras I, et al. X-linked Alport syndrome: natural history in 195 families and genotype-phenotype correlations in males. *J Am Soc Nephrol.* 2000;11:649–657.

Jais JP, Knebelmann B, Giatras I, et al. X-linked Alport syndrome: natural history and genotype-phenotype correlations in girls and women belonging to 195 families. A "European Community Alport Syndrome Concerted Action" study. *J Am Soc Nephrol.* 2003;14:2603–2610.

Kashtan CE, Ding J, Gregory M, et al. Clinical practice recommendations for the treatment of Alport syndrome: a statement of the Alport Syndrome Research Collaborative. *Pediatr Nephrol.* 2013;28:5–11.

Kashtan CE, Kleppel MM, Gubler M-C. Immunohistologic findings in Alport syndrome. In: Tryggvason K, ed. *Molecular Pathology and Genetics of Alport's Syndrome.* Basel: Karger; 1996:142–153.

Lemmink HH, Nielsson WN, Mochizuki T, et al. Benign familial hematuria due to mutation of the type 4 collagen gene. *J Clin Invest.* 1996;98:1114–1118.

Tiebosch TA, Frederik PM, van Breda Vriesman PJ, et al. Thin basement membrane nephropathy in adults with persistent hematuria. *N Engl J Med.* 1989;320:14–18.

42

Fabry Disease

GERE SUNDER-PLASSMANN, MANUELA FÖDINGER, RENATE KAIN

Fabry disease (OMIM 301500) is an X-linked lysosomal storage disorder that results from absent or deficient activity of the enzyme α-galactosidase A (αGAL; EC 3.2.1.22). This enzyme is encoded by the *GLA* gene on Xq22 (Fig. 42.1), with more than 1000 different variants so far described. Importantly, many of these genetic variants are seemingly benign, and carriers are not candidates for specific enzyme replacement or chaperone therapy (Table 42.1). Chaperone therapy is now available in the US, and novel experimental therapies, including second-generation enzymes, substrate synthesis inhibitors, and gene therapy, are in development.

A recent newborn-screening study reported the incidence of variants, including benign variants, in *GLA* to be 1 in 3859 births in Austria. The enzyme defect leads to progressive accumulation of glycosphingolipids, predominantly globotriaosylceramide (Gb3), in all organs (Fig. 42.2).

Early manifestations during childhood include pain, anhidrosis, and gastrointestinal symptoms, among others (Box 42.1). Later, chronic kidney disease (CKD) (Fig. 42.3) leading to kidney failure, hypertrophic cardiomyopathy (Fig. 42.4), and cerebral events (Fig. 42.5) are the clinically most important organ manifestations resulting in a reduced life span of hemizygous men and heterozygous women. Most male patients develop the classic phenotype with involvement of all organ systems, whereas alterations in X-inactivation lead to highly variable disease expression in women. Furthermore, kidney or heart variant phenotypes with later onset of disease, probably linked to some residual enzyme activity, have also been described. Importantly, because of the nonspecific nature of complaints, there is often a delay of more than 10 to 20 years from the earliest symptoms of disease until the correct diagnosis is established. Therefore, it is prudent to include Fabry disease in the differential diagnosis if two or more of the clinical problems indicated in Box 42.2 are present in young adults.

Beyond screening individuals with a family history of Fabry disease (Fig. 42.6), many cases are identified by means of kidney biopsy on patients referred to nephrologists for proteinuria or other signs of kidney damage. Other cases are found among high-risk populations, such as patients with kidney failure, left ventricular hypertrophy, or stroke. Reduced or absent activity of αGAL in leukocytes confirms the diagnosis in male patients. In women, genetic testing is mandatory because αGAL activity may be normal in a significant proportion. Urinary excretion of Gb3 is increased in many instances, and lyso-Gb3 in the plasma is used as a marker for diagnosis and treatment monitoring. Proteomics, the large-scale study of the entire complement of proteins, is another valuable research tool directed at finding biomarkers for diagnosis, disease progression, and responsiveness to therapy in the urine or serum of patients with Fabry disease.

Kidney Manifestations of Fabry Disease

Kidney disease is a major complication of Fabry disease related to glycosphingolipid accumulation throughout the nephron, with interstitial fibrosis and focal segmental glomerulosclerosis observed early in the course of disease. Kidney failure occurs in almost all affected men around the fourth or fifth decade of life but can also be seen in adolescents. The course of the disease is less severe in women, who may also eventually progress to kidney failure.

In affected individuals, the urine sediment may show red and white blood cells, hyaline or granular casts, and lipid particles with Maltese cross appearance upon polarization. Early in the course, dysfunction of the proximal and distal tubules includes reduced net acid excretion or a urinary concentrating defect with polyuria, nocturia, and polydipsia. Albuminuria or overt proteinuria sometimes develops during childhood but is present by the age of 35 years in approximately 50% of men and 20% of women. Kidney imaging may show cortical or parapelvic cysts, the cause of which is unknown. Increased blood pressure above 130/80 mm Hg was present in 57% of men and 47% of women in a large analysis of 391 patients presenting with various stages of CKD. A retrospective analysis of 168 women and 279 men with Fabry disease from 27 sites in five countries showed a more rapid decline of estimated glomerular filtration rate (eGFR) of –6.8 mL/min/1.73 m²/year in men with an eGFR less than 60 mL/min/1.73 m² versus –3.0 mL/min/1.73 m² in men with eGFR greater than 60 mL/min/1.73 m². The corresponding progression rates for women were –2.1 mL/min/1.73 m²/year and –0.9 mL/min/1.73 m²/year, respectively. Similar to other nephropathies, proteinuria and hypertension are also associated with more rapid decline in kidney function. End-stage kidney disease (ESKD) developed in 49 men and eight women described in this report. The prevalence of Fabry disease among patients undergoing dialysis enrolled in large US and European registries was 0.017% and 0.019%, respectively, but most of the case-finding studies during the last decade have shown a prevalence of 0.2% to 0.5% among men with ESKD. In patients with an established diagnosis of Fabry disease, a routine kidney biopsy is not mandatory. Annual monitoring should include measurements of serum creatinine and urinary albumin- or protein-to-creatinine ratio.

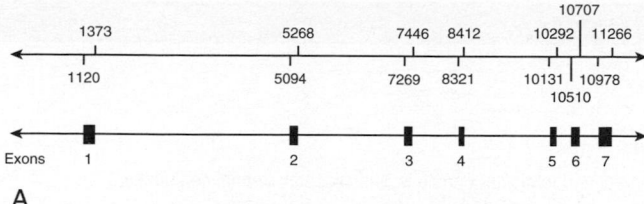

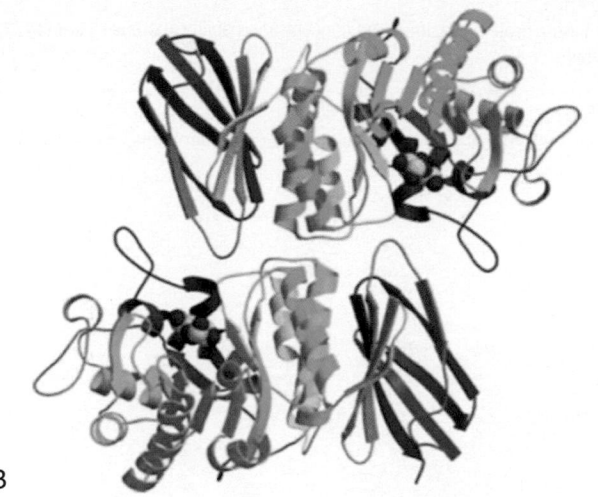

• **Fig. 42.1** (A) Organization of the *GLA* gene on Xq22.1. The whole gene spans 12.4 kb of genomic DNA and contains seven exons. *Black boxes* in the lower scheme indicate seven coding regions (exons) of the *GLA* gene. The upper scheme shows the exon position numbering according to the GenBank database entry X14448.1. (B) The structure of α-galactosidase A (αGAL). The structure of the human αGAL dimer is shown in ribbon representation. The ribbon is colored from blue to red as the polypeptide goes from *N*- to *C*-terminus. The active site is identified by the catalytic product galactose, shown in sphere Corey-Pauling Koltun format. Each monomer in the homodimer contains two domains, a (β/α)8 barrel containing the active site *(blue to yellow)* plus a *C* terminal antiparallel β domain *(yellow to red)*. (A from Anita Jallitsch-Halper, doctoral thesis, Medical University of Vienna, 2012; B from Garman SC. Structure-function relationships in alpha-galactosidase A. *Acta Paediatr Suppl.* 2007;96:6.)

Pathology of Kidney Disease in Fabry Disease

Gross Pathology

There are few gross descriptions of the kidneys in Fabry disease, although enlargement caused by both storage and cysts is described.

Light Microscopy

Histologic changes show characteristically vacuolated "foamy" podocytes. However, other cell types, including endothelial cells, vascular myocytes, and tubular epithelial cells, may be similarly affected by accumulation of glycosphingolipid. In conventional light microscopy on formalin-fixed and paraffin-embedded material, these inclusions appear empty, as their content is removed during processing. Fixation with osmium and embedding in epoxy resins retains the stored material that can easily be visualized by either electron microscopy or light microscopy on 1-μm-thin

TABLE 42.1	Benign and Likely Benign Genetic Missense Variants of *GLA*	
cDNA	**Protein**	
c.159C>A	p.N53K	
c.196G>C	p.E66Q	
c.52C>T	p.R118C	
c.76A>G	p.S126G	
c.427G>A	p.A143T*	
c.454T>C	p.Y152H	
c.685T>G	p.F229V	
c.870G>C	p.M290I	
c.870G>A	p.M290I	
c.937G>T	p.D313Y	
c.989A>G	p.Q330R	
c.1067G>A	p.R356Q	
c.1102G>A	p.A368T	

*May be pathogenic in some patients.
Adapted from Doheny D, Srinivasan R, Pagant S, et al. Fabry disease: prevalence of affected males and heterozygotes with pathogenic *GLA* mutations identified by screening renal, cardiac and stroke clinics, 1995–2017. *J Med Genet.* 2018;55:261–268.

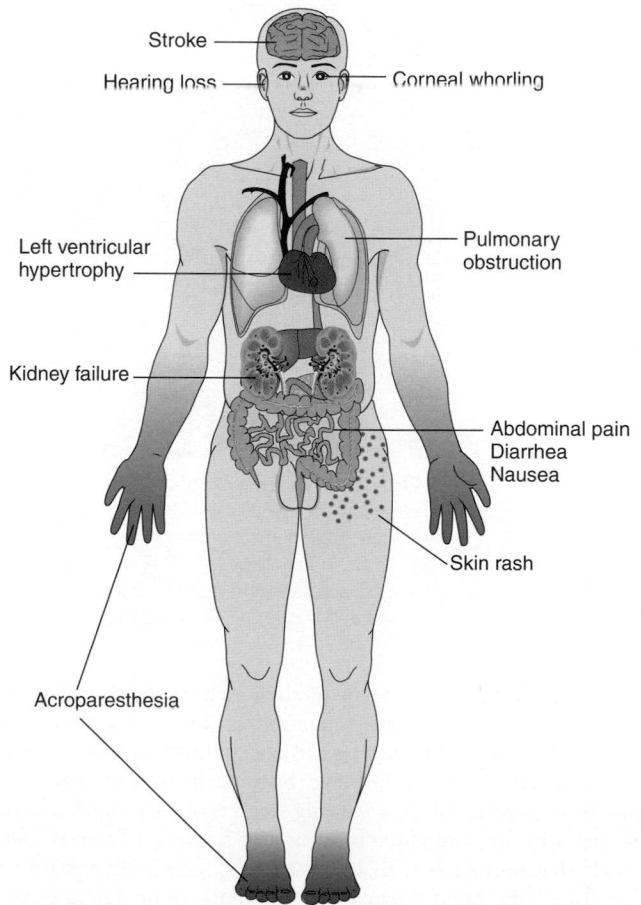

• **Fig. 42.2** Organ manifestations in patients with Fabry disease.

Early Signs and Symptoms of Fabry Disease

Nervous System

Acroparesthesias, nerve deafness, heat intolerance, tinnitus

Gastrointestinal Tract

Nausea, vomiting, diarrhea, postprandial bloating and pain, early satiety, difficulty gaining weight

Skin

Angiokeratoma, hypohidrosis

Eyes

Corneal and lenticular opacities, vasculopathy (retina, conjunctiva)

Kidneys

Albuminuria, proteinuria, impaired concentrating ability, increased urinary Gb3 excretion

Heart

Impaired heart rate variability, arrhythmias, ECG abnormalities (shortened PR interval), mild valvular insufficiency

ECG, Elecvtrocardiogram; *Gb3,* globotriaosylceramide.
Adapted from Germain DP. Fabry disease. *Orphanet J Rare Dis.* 2010;5:30.

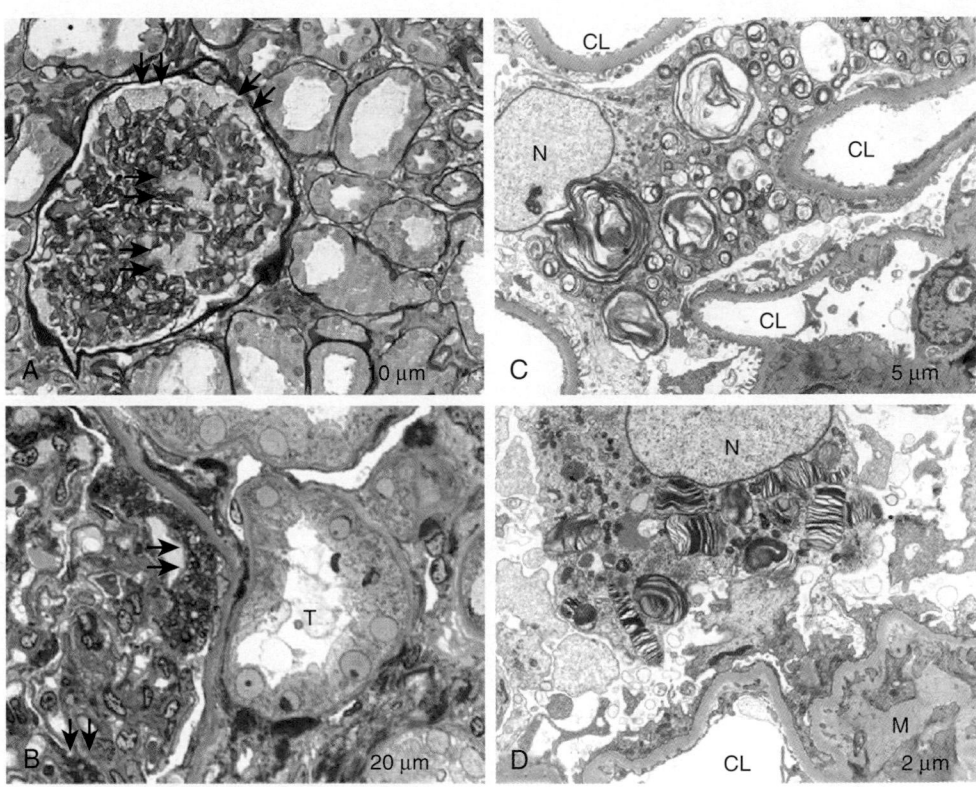

• **Fig. 42.3** Histopathology and electron microscopy of kidney manifestations in Fabry disease. (A) Light microscopy of formalin-fixed and paraffin-embedded material shows "foamy" podocytes *(double arrows)* resulting from numerous empty cytoplasmic vacuoles (periodic acid–Schiff). (B) Cytoplasmic inclusions are osmiophilic *(double arrows)* in a toluidine blue on Epon-embedded thin section. Electron microscopy showing lamellated membrane inclusion bodies with either "myelin-like" (C) or "zebroid" (D) appearance in secondary lysosomes. *CL,* Capillary lumen; *M,* mesangium; *N,* nucleus of podocytes; *T,* proximal tubule.

sections with toluidine blue or methylene blue staining. The lipid content of the inclusions is sudanophilic and stains with oil red O on frozen section. It may be further characterized by immunohistochemistry or lectin binding. Specific histologic changes are usually accompanied by a varying degree of mesangial sclerosis, tubular atrophy, interstitial fibrosis, and sclerosis of arterial blood vessels that correlates with the stage of CKD. Kidney biopsy is, therefore, considered a valuable instrument in the baseline assessment of Fabry nephropathy, and a validated scoring sheet has been developed to record progression on serial biopsies by light microscopy (see Fig. 42.3).

Electron Microscopy

Electron microscopy shows podocytes with lamellated membrane inclusion bodies in secondary lysosomes. These consist of concentric "myelin-like" rings or have a striped "zebroid" appearance (see Fig. 42.3).

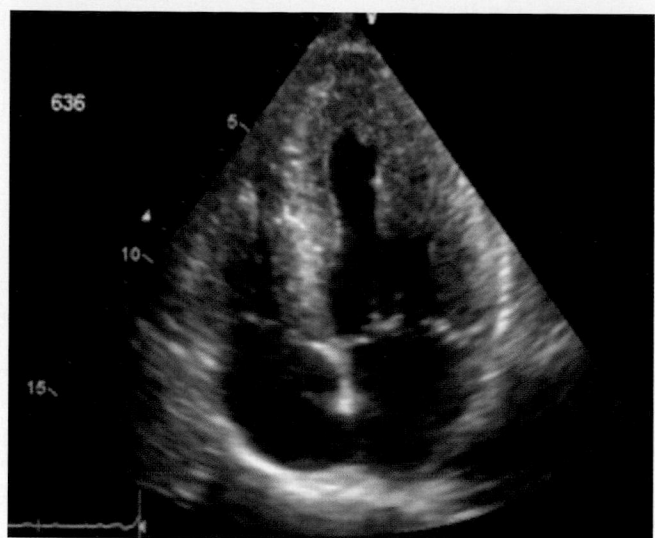

• **Fig. 42.4** Cardiac sonography of a 53-year-old man with Fabry disease showing cardiac hypertrophy. (Courtesy Gerald Mundigler, MD, Medical University of Vienna.)

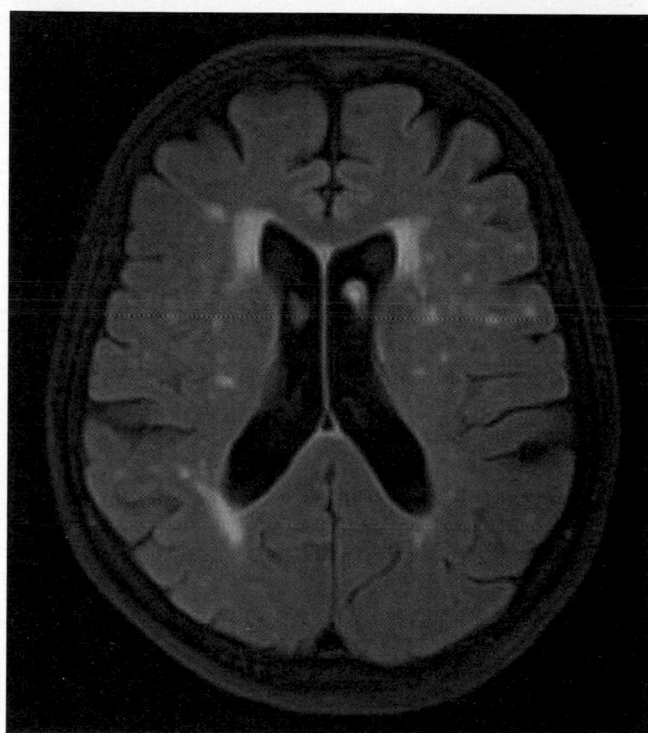

• **Fig. 42.5** Magnetic resonance imaging of the brain of a 63-year-old woman with Fabry disease showing typical white matter lesions on a T2-weighted image. (Courtesy Paulus Rommer, MD, Medical University of Vienna.)

BOX 42.2

Signs and Symptoms Suggestive of Fabry Disease[a]

1. Acroparesthesia or neuropathic pain in hands or feet beginning in later childhood, precipitated by illness, fever, exercise, emotional stress, or exposure to heat
2. Persistent proteinuria of unknown cause
3. Hypertrophic cardiomyopathy, especially with prominent diastolic dysfunction[b]
4. Progressive CKD
5. Cryptogenic stroke or transient ischemic attack
6. Family history of ESKD, stroke, or hypertrophic cardiomyopathy showing an X-linked pattern of transmission that primarily, but not solely, affects men
7. Vague, persistent, or recurrent abdominal pain associated with nausea, diarrhea, and tenesmus

CKD, Chronic kidney disease; *ESKD*, end-stage kidney disease.
[a]Any combination of two or more of these problems is highly suggestive of Fabry disease in either sex.
[b]This may be the only clinical manifestation of Fabry disease in patients of either sex with variants of classical Fabry disease.
Adapted from Clarke JT. Narrative review: Fabry disease. *Ann Intern Med.* 2007;146:425–433.

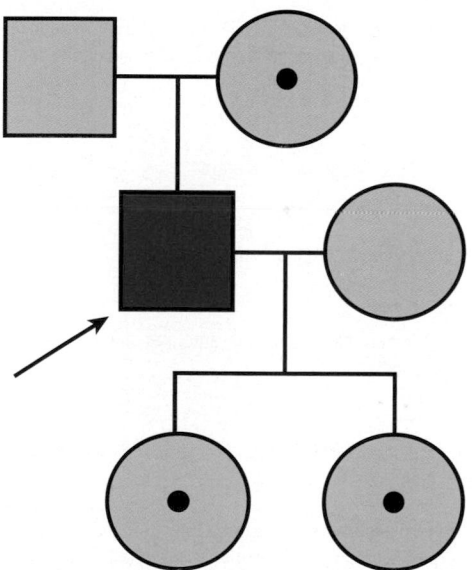

• **Fig. 42.6** Pedigree of a family with Fabry disease. The index case *(arrow)* was diagnosed by a nationwide case-finding study among Austrian patients undergoing dialysis. His mother and the two daughters *(dots)* carry the same mutation and were asymptomatic at the time of screening. (From Kotanko P, et al. Results of a nationwide screening for Anderson-Fabry disease among dialysis patients. *J Am Soc Nephrol.* 2004;15:1323–1329.)

Differential Diagnosis

Similar histologic features as seen in Fabry disease have been reported in small series of patients receiving chloroquine for auto-immune diseases. Despite the very similar appearance of zebroid or lamellar inclusion bodies in kidney biopsies by transmission electron microscopy (TEM), curvilinear bodies (twisted microtu-bular structures) seem to be a unique distinguishing feature of chloroquine-induced nephropathy for which the pathogenetic

mechanisms remain inconclusive. αGLA deficiency should be ruled out genetically and biochemically in those patients, even if systemic iatrogenic phospholipidosis is suspected.

Treatment Issues in Fabry Disease

Fabry disease can affect every organ system. Therefore, various symptoms may require specific therapy (Box 42.3). The most debilitating early symptom, often starting in childhood, is chronic

Concomitant Therapy in Patients with Fabry Disease

Acroparesthesia

Painful crisis: avoiding quick temperature changes, nonsteroidal antiinflammatory drugs
Chronic pain: anticonvulsants

Hypohidrosis

Appropriate temperature and environment

Angiokeratoma

Cosmetic removal with argon laser therapy

Proteinuria

ACE inhibitors or ARBs

Kidney Failure

Dialysis, transplantation, conservative kidney care

Gastrointestinal Symptoms

Pain relief, H2-blockers, motility agents, pancreatic enzyme supplementation

Hypertension

Regular monitoring and rigorous surveillance following general guidelines (avoid beta-blockers because they can cause sinus bradycardia)

Hyperlipidemia

Regular routine surveillance, statin therapy

Edema

Diuretics, compression stockings, lymph drainage

Stroke Prevention

Management of hypertension, diabetes, smoking, and dyslipidemia; antiplatelet agents

Depression

Selective serotonin reuptake inhibitors, serotonin norepinephrine reuptake inhibitors

ACE, Angiotensin-converting enzyme; *ARB*, angiotensin receptor blocker.
Adapted from Whybra-Trümpler C. Symptomatic and ancillary therapy. In: Elstein D, Altarescu G, Beck M, eds. *Fabry Disease*. Dordrecht, Heidelberg, London, New York: Springer; 2010: 481–487.

pain; this is typically triggered by vigorous exercise and temperature changes. Pain (and depression) management agents include gabapentin, carbamazepine, phenytoin, amitriptyline, and other antidepressants.

Renin-Angiotensin-Aldosterone System Blockade

The role of renin-angiotensin-aldosterone system (RAAS) blockade remains an unresolved issue in Fabry disease. One uncontrolled study of 11 patients suggested reduction of proteinuria and stabilization of kidney function with angiotensin-converting enzyme (ACE) inhibitors or angiotensin receptor blockers (ARB); however, in the Fabry Outcome Survey (FOS), 208 subjects had a nonstatistically significant reduction in eGFR with ACE inhibitor or ARB use. Furthermore, recombinant αGAL may interact with endogenous ACE and inhibit its activity, resulting in lower blood pressure during enzyme infusion.

Kidney Replacement Therapy

European and US studies have shown that patients with Fabry disease receiving dialysis have a poorer 3-year survival rate as compared with nondiabetic controls. The 5-year survival after kidney transplantation is also lower than that of controls. However, Fabry nephropathy does not recur in the allograft, and transplanted Fabry patients appear to have better overall outcomes than those maintained on dialysis. Therefore, kidney transplantation should be recommended as a first-choice therapy for patients with kidney failure from Fabry disease.

Specific Therapies

Currently available therapies for Fabry disease include intravenous enzyme replacement and oral pharmacologic chaperone therapy (Table 42.2). However, disease progression cannot be halted in a significant proportion of treated patients. Thus, novel therapeutic strategies are needed to further improve outcomes in patients with this disease. Current drug developments include novel enzyme preparations with longer half-life and better tissue penetration, substrate synthesis inhibition, and gene therapy (Fig. 42.7).

Enzyme Replacement Therapy

Specific enzyme replacement therapy with intravenous recombinant human αGAL has been available for treatment of Fabry disease since 2001. It can be considered for every adult male patient, for symptomatic boys, and for symptomatic women.

Two preparations are currently available, with other products in clinical development (see Table 42.2). The first, agalsidase alfa (Takeda Pharmaceutical Company limited, Tokyo, Japan), is produced in human skin fibroblasts with gene activation technology. It is approved at a dose of 0.2 mg/kg every-other week (infusion time: 40 minutes) in the European Union and many other countries, but not in the United States. The other product, agalsidase beta (Fabrazyme, Sanofi Genzyme, Cambridge, Massachusetts), is produced in Chinese hamster ovary cells and is registered for use at 1.0 mg/kg every-other week (infusion time: several hours). Fabrazyme is the only currently available enzyme replacement in the United States.

Side effects of enzyme replacement therapy include fever, rigors, and chills, typically mild to moderate in nature. These occur in more than half of the patients during the first months of treatment. Infusion-related reactions may be due to IgG or IgE antibodies that have been detected in several patients. In case of reactions, the infusion rate should be decreased or stopped, and the administration of antihistamines and/or corticosteroids should be considered. The infusion can be continued in the case of mild reactions. Some patients need premedication with antihistamines, paracetamol/acetaminophen, or corticosteroids. In patients receiving maintenance dialysis therapy, the infusion can be administered during the dialysis treatment.

The clinical effect of both products was examined in two small pivotal trials, a few controlled studies, and numerous uncontrolled studies and registry reports. In a double-blind, placebo-controlled

	TABLE 42.2 Specific Therapy of Fabry Disease			
	Enzyme Replacement Therapy (ERT)		Chaperone Therapy
	RECOMBINANT A-GALACTOSIDASE A		SMALL MOLECULE
	Agalsidase Alfa	Agalsidase Beta	Migalastat
Licensed for specific variants of *GLA*	No	No	Yes
Licensed in the US	No	Yes	Yes
CKD stage	1 to 5D*	1 to 5D*	1 to 3
Route of administration	Intravenous	Intravenous	Oral
Dosing	0.2 mg/kg	1.0 mg/kg	123 mg capsules
Frequency	Every other week	Every other week	Every other day
Duration of infusion	40 min	15 mg/hr	—
Frequent side-effects	Infusion reactions, anti-drug antibodies	Infusion reactions, anti-drug antibodies	Headache, nasopharyngitis
Treatment during pregnancy	Yes	Yes	No
Registration trials	1 published study Placebo controlled 26 male participants	1 published study Placebo controlled 58 participants (2 females)	2 published studies 1 placebo controlled 1 comparison with ERT 124 participants (75 females)

*Can be administered during dialysis.

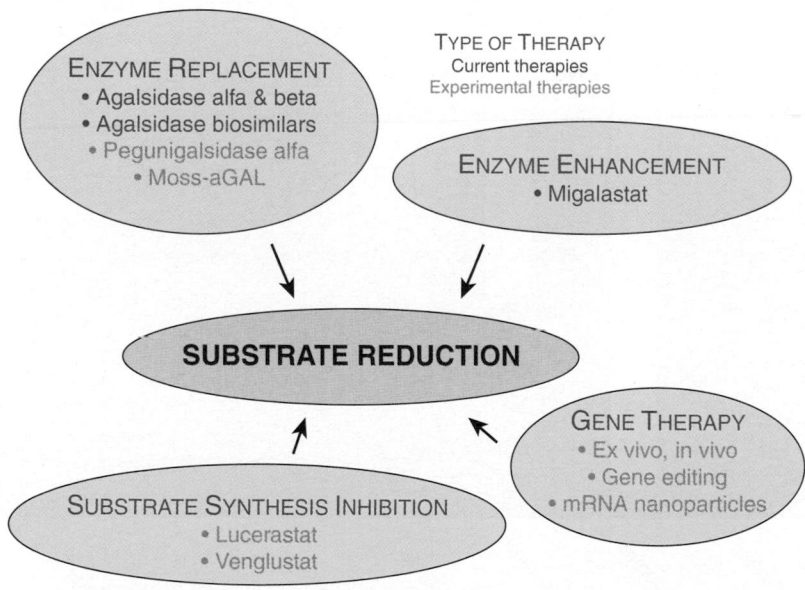

• **Fig. 42.7** Established and experimental therapies for Fabry disease.

trial, Schiffmann et al. randomized 26 men to receive agalsidase alpha at a dosage of 0.2 mg/kg (*n* = 14) or placebo (*n* = 12) every-other week for a total of 12 doses. Neuropathic pain, the primary endpoint, improved during therapy with agalsidase alpha as assessed by a pain questionnaire. Similarly, pain-related quality of life improved during active treatment. Secondary endpoints included kidney function, with no significant difference in the change of measured GFR or kidney tissue Gb3 content.

In the other pivotal trial, Eng et al. examined the effect of agalsidase beta in 58 adults (56 men, two women) with Fabry disease by examining the percentage of patients in whom kidney microvascular endothelial Gb3 deposits were cleared. After 20 weeks of treatment (11 infusions), 20 of the 29 participants (69%) in the agalsidase beta group had no microvascular endothelial Gb3 deposits, as compared with 0 of 29 participants in the placebo group. Among secondary endpoints, there was no difference in pain between active treatment and placebo.

A subsequent randomized, controlled study by Banikazemi et al. failed to show an effect of agalsidase beta on the primary composite endpoint (time to first clinical kidney, heart, or cerebrovascular event or death) in 82 individuals (10 women and 72 men) with advanced Fabry disease and a mean serum creatinine of 1.6 mg/dL; there were only 27 outcomes in this trial, potentially limiting power. A per-protocol analysis, adjusted for baseline proteinuria, however, suggested a beneficial effect of agalsidase beta as compared with placebo.

Uncontrolled studies suggest stabilization or even improvement of kidney and heart disease manifestations during enzyme replacement therapy in many patients. Quality of life, gastrointestinal symptoms, hypohidrosis, pulmonary obstruction, and other clinical symptoms also showed improvement. Kidney function, proteinuria, and blood pressure are important predictors of the kidney response to enzyme replacement therapy. In a recent analysis of 213 patients treated with agalsidase beta for at least 2 years enrolled in the Fabry Registry, a higher urinary protein level, worse initial kidney function, and delayed initiation of enzyme replacement therapy after the onset of symptoms were strong predictors of kidney disease progression in men. A history of cardiac or cerebral events was also associated with a steeper slope of eGFR decline. A total of 75% of the male patients had an eGFR slope of −2.8 mL/min/1.73 m² to −15.5 mL/min/1.73 m² during enzyme therapy. In a report from the FOS, kidney function was assessed in 208 patients treated with agalsidase alpha for at least 5 years. The mean annual change in eGFR was −2.2 mL/min/1.73 m² in men and −0.7 mL/min/1.73 m² in women. Patients with protein excretion greater than 1 g/day had worse kidney function at baseline and follow-up compared with patients with protein excretion of 500 to 1000 mg/day or less than 500 mg/day. Kidney function was worse in patients with baseline hypertension, and there was a more rapid annual decline compared with normotensive patients. Taken together, these data suggest that agalsidase alpha or agalsidase beta cannot halt kidney disease progression in many patients. However, a comparison of treated and untreated patients suggests a somewhat attenuated slope of eGFR decline in treated patients (Fig. 42.8). The largest head-to-head comparison of both enzymes, a retrospective comparison of patients treated in one Canadian and several European centers reported by Arends and colleagues, showed no clear advantage of one drug, but clinically relevant disease progression in a significant proportion of patients.

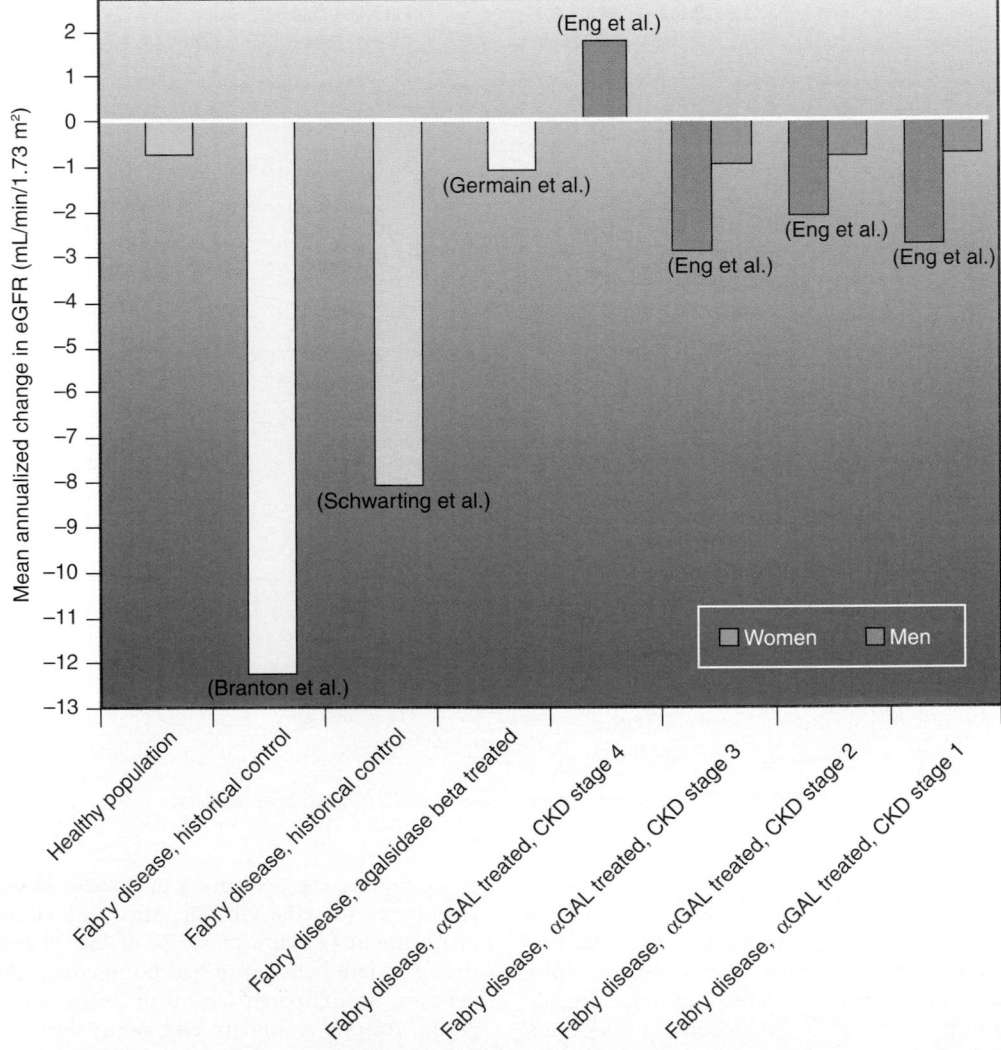

• **Fig. 42.8** Comparison of the annual decline of estimated glomerular filtration rate (*eGFR*) in patients without and with enzyme replacement therapy. *CKD*, Chronic kidney disease. (Adapted from Mehta A, Beck M, Elliott P, et al. Enzyme replacement therapy with agalsidase alfa in patients with Fabry's disease: an analysis of registry data. *Lancet.* 2009;374:1986.)

Potential reasons for disease progression during enzyme replacement therapy include low physical stability of recombinant αGAL, a short circulating half-life, and variable uptake into different tissues. Importantly, antibodies to recombinant human αGAL can be detected in about 40% of treated men and are associated with greater left ventricular mass and substantially lower GFR, among other disease manifestations, as compared with antibody-negative patients.

Pharmacologic Chaperones

A pharmacologic chaperone (or pharmacoperone) acts as a "protein chaperone" and is a small molecule that causes mutant proteins to fold and route correctly within the cell. Missense mutations in Fabry disease may cause misfolding of αGAL, leading to retention in the endoplasmic reticulum and subsequent degradation. A potent αGAL inhibitor, the iminosugar 1-deoxygalactonojirimycin (migalastat hydrochloride; Amicus Therapeutics, Cranbury, New Jersey), is an analogue of the terminal galactose of Gb3. It binds to the active site of αGAL, thereby improving stability and trafficking to the lysosomes (Fig. 42.9). It reduces Gb3 storage in vitro and in vivo and stabilizes wild-type and mutant forms of αGAL. Furthermore, co-administration improves the pharmacologic properties of recombinant human αGAL. It prevents denaturation and activity loss in vitro and results in substantially higher cellular αGAL and greater Gb3 reduction compared to recombinant human αGAL alone in vivo. Migalastat hydrochloride increases enzyme activity and reduces Gb3 in the tissue of patients with specific mutations in *GLA*. An in vitro assay can be used to identify subjects with mutations that are likely to respond to chaperone treatment.

A double-blind, placebo-controlled phase 3 study examined the safety and efficacy of migalastat hydrochloride (150 mg orally every-other day for 6 months) in 67 patients with Fabry disease. Kidney biopsy samples were available for 64 patients and showed a ≥50% reduction in the number of Gb3 inclusions per kidney interstitial capillary in 41% of patients who received migalastat hydrochloride and 28% of patients who received placebo ($P = .3$). Of note, among 45 patients with responsive mutations, therapy with migalastat hydrochloride was associated with a greater reduction in the mean number of Gb3 inclusions per kidney interstitial capillary compared with placebo (-0.25 ± 0.10 vs. 0.07 ± 0.13; $P = .008$). Among other secondary endpoints, therapy with migalastat hydrochloride reduced plasma levels of lyso-Gb3 and gastrointestinal symptoms but showed no effect on urinary Gb3, kidney function, or left ventricular mass. In patients who received migalastat hydrochloride for ≥18 months, kidney function remained stable and left ventricular mass index significantly decreased.

In 2016 and 2018, respectively, the European Medical Agency and the FDA approved migalastat hydrochloride for the treatment of Fabry disease in patients with suitable mutations based on this trial and another phase III study that also showed stable kidney function and an improvement of left ventricular mass. Other studies showed substantial Gb3 clearance from podocytes and improvement of gastrointestinal symptoms. Taken together, these data suggest an important clinical potential for this newer therapeutic tool, alone or in combination with enzyme replacement therapy.

Complete bibliography is available at Elsevier eBooks for Practicing Clinicians.

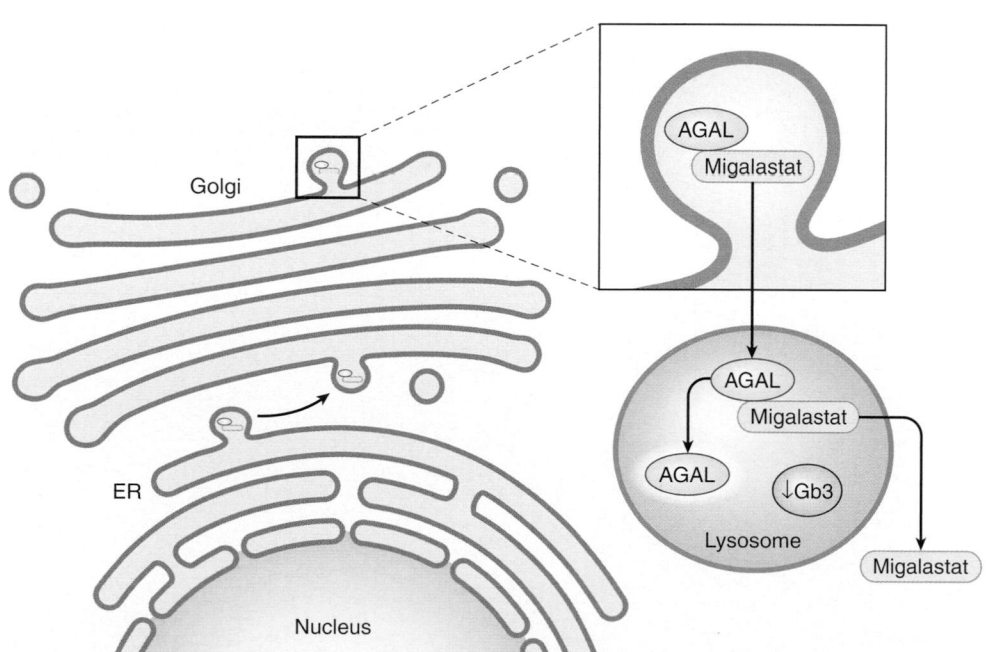

• **Fig. 42.9** Mechanism of action of migalastat hydrochloride. Binding of migalastat to catalytically active but unstable α-galactosidase (*AGAL*) allows for proper folding and trafficking of the enzyme from the endoplasmic reticulum (*ER*) through the Golgi apparatus to the lysosome. In the lysosome, dissociation of migalastat restores enzyme activity and allows degradation of globotriaosylceramide (*Gb3*). (From Gaggl M, Sunder-Plassmann G. Fabry disease – a pharmacological chaperone on the horizon. *Nat Rev Nephrol.* 2016;12:653.)

Key Bibliography

Banikazemi M, Bultas J, Waldek S, et al. Agalsidase-beta therapy for advanced Fabry disease: a randomized trial. *Ann Intern Med.* 2007;146:77–86.

Benjamin ER, Khanna R, Schilling A, et al. Co-administration with the pharmacological chaperone AT1001 increases recombinant human alpha-galactosidase A tissue uptake and improves substrate reduction in Fabry mice. *Mol Ther.* 2012;20:717–726.

Branton MH, Schiffmann R, Sabnis SG, et al. Natural history of Fabry renal disease: influence of alpha-galactosidase A activity and genetic mutations on clinical course. *Medicine (Baltimore).* 2002;81:122–138.

Clarke JT. Narrative review: Fabry disease. *Ann Intern Med.* 2007;146: 425–433.

Domm JM, Wootton SK, Medin JA, West ML. Gene therapy for Fabry disease: Progress, challenges, and outlooks on gene-editing. *Mol Genet Metab.* 2021;134(1-2):117–131.

Eng CM, Guffon N, Wilcox WR, et al. Safety and efficacy of recombinant human alpha-galactosidase A replacement therapy in Fabry's disease. *N Engl J Med.* 2001;345:9–16.

Fogo AB, Bostad L, Svarstad E, et al. Scoring system for renal pathology in Fabry disease: report of the International Study Group of Fabry Nephropathy (ISGFN). *Nephrol Dial Transplant.* 2010;25:2168–2177.

Gaggl M, Sunder-Plassmann G. Fabry disease—a pharmacological chaperone on the horizon. *Nat Rev Nephrol.* 2016;12:653–654.

Gal A. Molecular genetics of Fabry disease and genotype-phenotype correlation. In: Elstein D, Altarescu G, Beck M, eds. *Fabry Disease.* Dordrecht: Springer; pp. 3–19.

Germain DP, Hughes DA, Nicholls K, et al. Treatment of Fabry's disease with the pharmacologic chaperone migalastat. *N Engl J Med.* 2016;375:545–555.

Hughes DA, Nicholls K, Shankar SP, et al. Oral pharmacological chaperone migalastat compared with enzyme replacement therapy in Fabry disease: 18-month results from the randomised phase III ATTRACT study. *J Med Genet.* 2017;54:288–296.

Khan A, Barber DL, Huang J, et al. Lentivirus-mediated gene therapy for Fabry disease. *Nat Commun.* 2021;12(1):1178.

Lenders M, Stypmann J, Duning T, et al. Serum-mediated inhibition of enzyme replacement therapy in Fabry disease. *J Am Soc Nephrol.* 2016;27:256–264.

Linhart A, Kampmann C, Zamorano JL, et al. Cardiac manifestations of Anderson-Fabry disease: results from the international Fabry outcome survey. *Eur Heart J.* 2007;28:1228–1235.

Mechtler TP, Stary S, Metz TF, et al. Neonatal screening for lysosomal storage disorders: feasibility and incidence from a nationwide study in Austria. *Lancet.* 2012;379:335–341.

Müller-Höcker J, Schmid H, Weiss M, Dendorfer U, Braun GS. Chloroquine-induced phospholipidosis of the kidney mimicking Fabry's disease: case report and review of the literature. *Hum Pathol.* 2003;34:285–289.

Schiffmann R, Kopp JB, Austin HA 3rd, et al. Enzyme replacement therapy in Fabry disease: a randomized controlled trial. *JAMA.* 2001;285:2743–2749.

Schiffmann R, Warnock DG, Banikazemi M, et al. Fabry disease: progression of nephropathy, and prevalence of cardiac and cerebrovascular events before enzyme replacement therapy. *Nephrol Dial Transplant.* 2009;24:2102–2111.

Warnock DG, Bichet DG, Holida M, et al. Oral migalastat HCl leads to greater systemic exposure and tissue levels of active alpha-galactosidase A in Fabry patients when co-administered with infused agalsidase. *PLoS One.* 2015;10:e0134341.

West M, Nicholls K, Mehta A, et al. Agalsidase alfa and kidney dysfunction in Fabry disease. *J Am Soc Nephrol.* 2009;20:1132–1139.

PART 8

Tubulointerstitial Diseases

43

Chronic Tubulointerstitial Disease

MARK A. PERAZELLA, CYNTHIA C. NAST

Primary interstitial kidney disease comprises a diverse group of disorders that elicit interstitial inflammation associated with tubular damage. Traditionally, interstitial nephritis has been classified morphologically and clinically into acute and chronic forms. Acute interstitial nephritis (AIN) generally induces rapid deterioration in kidney function with a marked interstitial inflammatory response characterized by mononuclear cell infiltration with or without eosinophils, interstitial edema, and varying degrees of tubular cell injury. This process typically spares both glomerular and vascular structures, and is discussed more fully in Chapter 33. By contrast, chronic interstitial nephritis (CIN) follows a more indolent course and is characterized by interstitial fibrosis, tubular atrophy, and most often an interstitial mononuclear cell infiltrate. Over time, glomerular and vascular structures are involved, with progressive parenchymal fibrosis and sclerosis. Overlap can occur between these two clinical conditions; AIN sometimes presents as a more insidious disease with progression to chronic kidney disease (CKD). Similarly, some forms of CIN are associated with acute tubular cell injury.

Histopathology

The histopathology of CIN is remarkably consistent despite the varied causes (Box 43.1). CIN is characterized by the development of tubular atrophy with interstitial fibrosis typically with associated predominantly mononuclear cell inflammation with or without inflammation in atrophied tubules (Fig. 43.1). Certain forms of CIN may have minimal inflammation (e.g., lead, lithium) or have interstitial granulomas (e.g., sarcoidosis). Glomerular and vascular structures may be relatively preserved early in the course of disease but ultimately become involved in progressive sclerosis and fibrosis. Ongoing development of tubulointerstitial fibrosis is observed in all forms of progressive kidney disease, including primary tubulointerstitial, glomerular, and vascular disorders, as a final common pathway to kidney failure.

Mononuclear cell infiltrates generally accompany CIN, suggesting a pathogenic immune-mediated mechanism for disease progression. One hypothesis concerning immune recognition of the interstitium suggests that portions of infectious particles or drug molecules cross-react with or alter endogenous kidney antigens. An immune response directed against these inciting agents would, therefore, also target the interstitium (molecular mimicry). Intriguing results of a study examining kidney biopsy samples obtained over 8 years at a single center suggest a prominent role of Epstein-Barr virus (EBV) in cases of CIN previously deemed idiopathic. Investigators detected EBV DNA and its receptor, CD21, primarily in proximal tubular cells of all 17 patients with

primary idiopathic interstitial nephritis but not in 10 control kidney biopsy specimens. Such observations imply a more prominent role than previously appreciated for occult viral infections in eliciting chronic deleterious immune responses that target the tubulointerstitium.

Mechanisms of Tubulointerstitial Fibrosis

Irrespective of initiating events, tubulointerstitial fibrosis is the final common pathway leading to CKD. Tubulointerstitial fibrosis involves the loss of renal tubules and the accumulation of fibroblasts and matrix proteins, such as collagen, fibronectin, and laminin. Although cells infiltrating the interstitium were thought to play a major role in tubulointerstitial fibrosis, fibroblasts have been identified as the principal effector mediating tubulointerstitial fibrosis. Observations from the experimental literature suggest that renal tubular epithelial-mesenchymal transition (EMT) may play a role in the initiation and progression of tubulointerstitial fibrosis. As the renal epithelium develops from the metanephric mesenchyme via a process of mesenchymal-epithelial transition, observations suggest a unique paradigm of tubulointerstitial response to injury whereby dedifferentiation pathways are activated within the epithelium, resulting in a transition to cells of more mesenchymal characteristics. Dysregulation of such processes in vivo could induce more fibrogenic responses (Fig. 43.2). Renal EMT in this setting could thus facilitate accumulation of fibroblasts and myofibroblasts that are characteristic of CIN and other kidney diseases associated with tubulointerstitial fibrosis.

The ability of renal tubular epithelial cells to transform in vitro to fibroblasts and myofibroblasts is well documented. Although the processes relevant for primary CIN in humans have not been elucidated, experimental models of injury and many in vitro studies have implicated a major role for transforming growth factor-β and other fibrogenic mediators, such as fibroblast growth factor-2, advanced glycation end products, and angiotensin II. These factors regulate the renal fibrogenic responses and renal tubular EMT (see Fig. 43.2). Chronic ischemia also contributes to the development of tubulointerstitial nephritis. Induction of angiotensin-II and suppression of nitric oxide underlie chronic vasoconstriction, which contributes to tissue ischemia and hypoxia and stimulates EMT. Loss of peritubular capillaries, or rarefaction in areas of tubulointerstitial fibrosis, may develop due to downregulation of VEGF, which contributes to further ischemia. Reduction of interstitial capillary blood flow, leading to starvation of tubules, may underlie tubular atrophy and loss. Numerous human kidney biopsy studies have demonstrated the colocalization of epithelial and mesenchymal markers in tubular cells in areas of injury,

BOX 43.1

Chronic Interstitial Nephritis

Drugs/Toxins

Analgesics
Heavy metals (lead, cadmium, mercury)
Lithium
Chinese herbs (aristolochic acid)
Calcineurin inhibitors (cyclosporine, tacrolimus)
Cisplatin
Nitrosoureas
Herbicides (glyphosate, paraquat, others)

Hereditary Disorders

Polycystic kidney disease
Medullary cystic disease–juvenile nephronophthisis
Hereditary nephritis
Karyomegalic interstitial nephritis

Metabolic Disturbances

Hypercalcemia/nephrocalcinosis
Hypokalemia
Hyperuricemia
Hyperoxaluria
Cystinosis

Immune-Mediated Disorders

Kidney allograft rejection
Systemic lupus erythematosus
Sarcoidosis
Granulomatosis with polyangiitis (Wegener granulomatosis)
Vasculitis
Sjögren syndrome
Tubulointerstitial nephritis and uveitis (TINU) syndrome
IgG4 disease
Anti-low-density lipoprotein receptor-related protein 2 (LRP2) nephropathy

Hematologic Disturbances

Multiple myeloma
Light chain disease
Dysproteinemias
Lymphoproliferative disease
Sickle cell disease

Infections

Kidney
Systemic

Obstruction/Mechanical Disorders

Tumors
Stones
Vesicoureteral reflux

Miscellaneous Disorders

Balkan nephropathy (aristolochic acid)
Chronic kidney disease of unknown origin (Mesoamerican nephropathy, Sri Lankan agricultural nephropathy, chronic interstitial nephritis in agricultural communities)
Radiation nephritis
Aging
Hypertension
Kidney ischemia

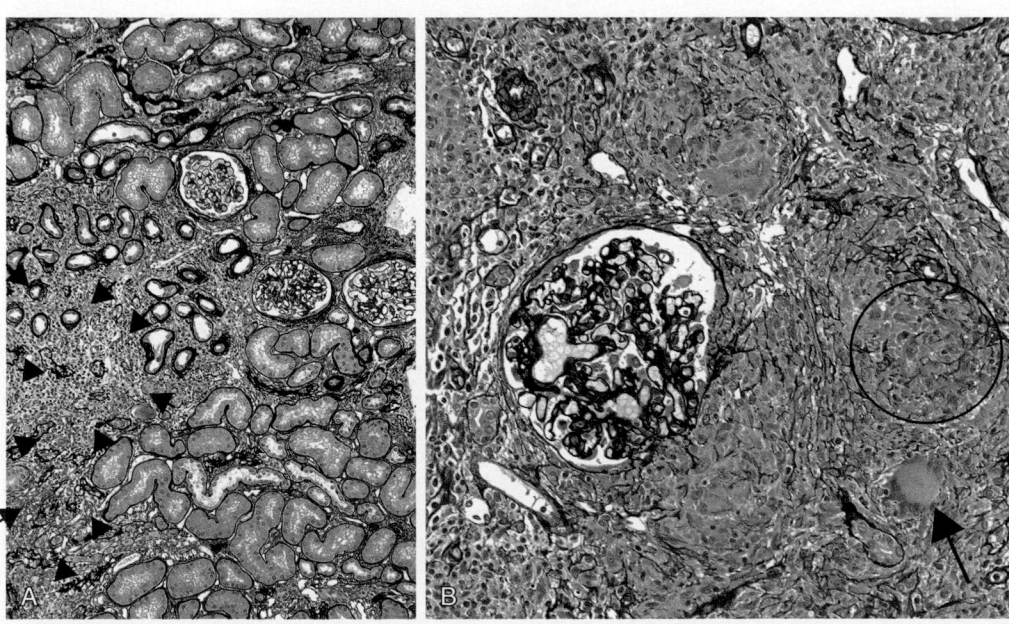

• **Fig. 43.1** Chronic interstitial nephritis. (A) There is renal cortical focal tubular atrophy and interstitial fibrosis with an associated heavy lymphocytic infiltrate (*arrowheads*). Note there is no inflammation in the preserved tubulointerstitium, and the glomeruli and artery do not show sclerosis. (Jones methenamine silver). (B) There is tubular atrophy and the interstitium contains several non-necrotizing granulomas (*black circle*) with giant cells (*arrow*) and adjacent lymphocytes. The glomerulus is spared (Jones methenamine silver).

[AU2]

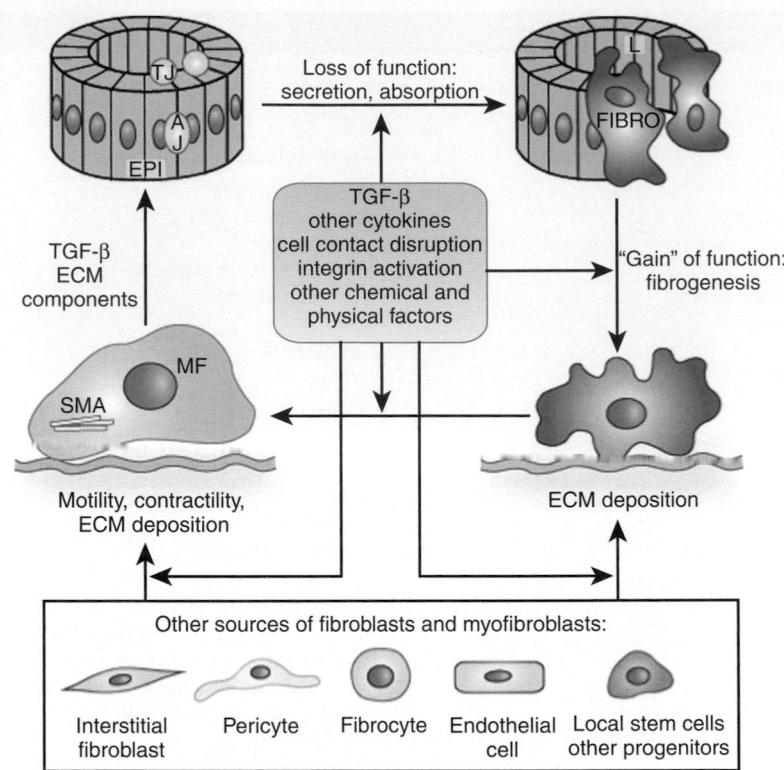

• **Fig. 43.2** The development and progression of kidney fibrosis. Fibroblasts and myofibroblasts (MF) originate from other cell types (as noted in the *bottom box*) and play a significant role in the process of kidney fibrosis. The paradigm of tubular epithelial-mesenchymal transition suggests an additional pathway to kidney fibrosis, in that tubular epithelium undergoes profound phenotypic changes after exposure to fibrogenic stimuli *(center box)*. This results in loss of epithelial characteristics and gain of mesenchymal characteristics. The transitioning cells might remain in the tubular wall or migrate into the interstitium. Epithelial-derived fibroblasts contribute to the deposition of extracellular matrix (ECM), and a subpopulation may begin expressing α-smooth muscle actin (SMA), a hallmark of the MF phenotype. Activated fibroblasts and MF secrete elevated amounts of transforming growth factor-β (TGF-β), whereas the enhanced contractility of MFs contributes to activation of latent TGF-β through an integrin-mediated mechanochemical pathway. Increasing TGF-β levels along with ECM accumulation might facilitate transformation of previously intact tubules, thereby creating a positive feedback loop of epithelial injury. *AJ*, Adherens junction; *EPI*, epithelium; *FIBRO*, fibroblasts; *L*, lumen; *TJ*, tight junction. (From Macmillan Publishers Ltd: Quaggin SE, Kapus A. Scar wars: mapping the fate of epithelial-mesenchymal-myofibroblast transition. *Kidney Int.* 2011;80:41-50.)

supporting the notion that renal tubular EMT is associated with progressive tubulointerstitial fibrosis in a variety of kidney diseases. However, recent fate-mapping studies, which allow the tagging and tracking of renal epithelial cells in vivo in experimental models of disease, have generated apparently conflicting observations regarding the role of EMT in progressive kidney injury. Future studies will likely better characterize pathways that both initiate and propagate renal fibrogenic processes.

Clinical Features

As shown in Box 43.1, CIN occurs in a variety of clinical settings, most commonly following exposure to drugs or toxins, or in settings of genetic disorders, metabolic disorders, immune-mediated diseases, hematologic disturbances, infections, or obstruction. It may also be idiopathic. Because CIN tends to occur as a slowly progressive disease, most patients diagnosed with CIN present with systemic complaints of the primary underlying disease, if one exists, or with symptoms of advanced CKD. Laboratory findings in these patients often include low-grade (tubular) proteinuria, microscopic

hematuria, and sterile pyuria. As listed in Table 43.1, other frequently reported urinary abnormalities, such as glucosuria, phosphaturia, and sodium wasting, reflect tubular defects. Serologic studies in CIN, such as anti-DNA antibodies, antinuclear antibodies, and complement levels, are typically normal, except when CIN occurs in the setting of a systemic autoimmune disorder.

Affected patients may also have elevated urinary excretion of low-molecular-weight (LMW) proteins that are commonly associated with tubular injury (e.g., lysozyme, β_2-microglobulin, and retinol-binding protein), and increased enzymuria with *N*-acetyl-β-D-glucosaminidase, alanine aminopeptidase, and intestinal alkaline phosphatase. However, routine assessment of urinary LMW proteins and enzymes is not typically conducted because they are neither diagnostic nor prognostic. Hypertension is another common clinical feature of CIN, although in many forms of CIN it is not apparent until the patient approaches ESKD. With progressive CIN, kidney ultrasonography in patients without significant structural abnormalities (e.g., cystic kidney disease) typically reveals shrunken, echogenic kidneys. Irregular renal contours and renal calcifications are seen in some forms of CIN.

TABLE 43.1	Laboratory Findings in Interstitial Nephritis
Parameter	**Finding**
Urinary sediment	Erythrocytes, leukocytes (eosinophils), leukocyte casts
Fractional excretion of sodium	Usually >1%
Proximal tubular defects	Glucosuria, bicarbonaturia, phosphaturia, aminoaciduria, proximal RTA
Distal tubular defects	Hyperkalemia, sodium wasting, distal RTA
Medullary defects	Sodium wasting, urine-concentrating defects

RTA, Renal tubular acidosis.

Clinical Course and Therapy

Because of the slowly progressive loss of kidney function observed in most cases of CIN, general therapeutic considerations include treating an underlying systemic disorder (sarcoidosis, Sjögren syndrome), avoiding the drug or toxin exposure (analgesics, lead), or eliminating the condition that has induced the chronic interstitial lesion (obstruction). Tubulointerstitial fibrosis, along with the resultant impairment in kidney function, is not currently amenable to therapeutic intervention. Although definitive diagnosis of CIN requires kidney biopsy, it is probably of limited usefulness in those with advanced CKD. Therapy is, therefore, largely supportive, with kidney replacement therapy initiated in kidney failure patients if desired and/or available. More specific therapies for interstitial lesions associated with lead exposure or immune-related injury are discussed in the following section.

Distinct Causes of Chronic Tubulointerstitial Nephritis

Many causes of CIN listed in Box 43.1 are more fully described in other chapters of this text. This section focuses on the common causes of primary CIN. It is also noted that progression to kidney failure and end-stage kidney disease (ESKD) has been reported with all forms of AIN, which likely follow a path to CIN over time if resolution of the injury does not occur.

Analgesic Nephropathy

In the last three decades of the 20th century, analgesic nephropathy was considered the most common form of drug-induced CIN, particularly in the United States, Europe, and Australia. The condition is associated with chronic excessive consumption of combined analgesic preparations over many years. Affected patients typically have regularly ingested combination analgesic products (e.g., aspirin, phenacetin, and paracetamol) that also contain codeine or caffeine. However, over the last several decades, recognition of the association of analgesic nephropathy with chronic use of over-the-counter combination analgesic products resulted in a marked reduction in availability of these products to the public, as well as a marked reduction in the incidence of this disease. Phenacetin-containing combination products were particularly noted for their association with analgesic nephropathy, although the disorder continues to be reported even after these products were removed from the market. The subsequent removal of other combination analgesic products resulted in a further decrease in the incidence of analgesic nephropathy worldwide. Since 2002, the United States Renal Data System (USRDS) Annual Data Report reported approximately 180 cases of ESKD due to analgesic nephropathy each year in the United States. The prevalence of analgesic nephropathy in a Swiss autopsy study was 0.2% in 2000.

The nephrotoxicity of combination analgesics appears to be dose-dependent, with medullary lesions most prominent early in the disease course. Early medullary capillary and tubular changes then extend to interstitial injury and fibrosis, as well as renal papillary necrosis (RPN) with calcification. RPN is characteristic, but not diagnostic, of analgesic nephropathy, as it occurs in other kidney disorders such as diabetes mellitus, sickle cell disease, renal tuberculosis, and urinary tract obstruction. It has also been reported with use of single reagent analgesic preparations, such as nonsteroidal antiinflammatory drugs or aspirin. The mechanism of nephrotoxicity is not completely understood. Ingested compounds and their metabolites are concentrated along the medullary osmotic gradient, likely achieving chronic high levels within the medulla to induce the early renal medullary lesions. In addition to high local metabolite concentrations, the relatively vulnerable vascular supply in the medulla could play a major role in initiating and propagating kidney injury.

The clinical manifestations are nonspecific and insidious. Patients typically present with sterile pyuria, mild proteinuria, and slowly progressive glomerular filtration rate (GFR) decline. As kidney disease progresses, anemia and hypertension develop. The disease has been reported more commonly in women than in men, with 50% to 80% of cases reported in women across several studies. The age range extends from 30 to 70 years of age, previously with a peak incidence in the early 50s. More recently, an Australian study found ESKD due to analgesic nephropathy is markedly decreasing among those below 75 years old. Daily use of analgesics to treat a chronic pain condition is common among those who develop analgesic nephropathy, and estimates suggest that nephropathy develops after a cumulative ingestion of 2 to 3 kg of analgesic preparations.

Diagnosis of analgesic nephropathy relies on clinical history, urinary findings, and kidney imaging studies, but can be difficult because early signs and symptoms are generally nonspecific. Computerized tomography (CT) scanning without intravenous contrast findings of bilateral reduction in kidney volume, cortical scarring with irregular kidney contours, and evidence of papillary damage and calcification suggest analgesic nephropathy. While these typical CT features are not generally noted in other forms of CIN, studies assessing their sensitivity and specificity for analgesic nephropathy have yielded inconsistent findings.

The clinical course of analgesic nephropathy is variable and depends largely on the extent of irreversible kidney scarring that has occurred at the time of diagnosis. Removal of the offending agent before irreversible kidney fibrosis has occurred is essential for preserving kidney function. Several reports of analgesic nephropathy have described stabilization or mild improvement in kidney function with cessation of analgesic use.

Chronic Lead Nephropathy

Exposure to high levels of lead over years to decades is associated with a progressive CIN, referred to as *chronic lead nephropathy*. Most such exposures are occupational and seen in the manufacturing or use of lead-containing paints, ammunition, radiators, batteries, wires, ceramic glazes, solder, and metal cans. Environmental lead exposure can occur with use of lead pipes and solder joints in drinking water lines, consuming crops grown in lead-contaminated soil, or ingesting lead-based paint scraps or "moonshine" generated in lead-lined car radiators. Lead exposure sufficient to induce lead nephropathy in developed countries was considered rare because recognition of its toxicity has resulted in routine removal of lead from most sources. However, this paradigm changed with the recognition of lead (and other heavy metals) intoxication from drinking water from the Flint River in Michigan. Lead toxicity occurred when the town of Flint switched its water supply from Lake Huron to the Flint River in 2014. While acute lead toxicity was observed, only time will tell if chronic lead nephropathy will also develop. Since the recognition of this disaster, other drinking water supplies around the United States have been noted to have excessive levels of heavy metals and other pollutants.

There are eosinophilic intranuclear inclusions in the proximal tubular cells composed of a lead-protein complex in the early stage of lead-induced kidney damage, suggesting proximal reabsorption with subsequent intracellular lead accumulation. Early clinical manifestations reflect proximal tubular dysfunction with hyperuricemia, aminoaciduria, and glucosuria (see Table 43.1). Because the kidney disease is slowly progressive, affected patients typically present with CKD, hypertension, hyperuricemia, and gout; therefore, chronic urate nephropathy and hypertensive nephrosclerosis are in the differential diagnosis. Patients presenting with hypertension, hyperuricemia, and CKD should be evaluated for lead exposure before assuming these other diagnoses.

The diagnosis of chronic lead intoxication is generally established with a lead mobilization test, performed by measuring urinary lead excretion after administering ethylenediaminetetraacetic acid (EDTA). X-ray fluorescence can also be used to determine bone lead levels. The diagnosis of lead nephropathy, however, is frequently made on the basis of a history of lead exposure in the setting of hyperuricemia, hypertension, and slowly progressive kidney disease consistent with CIN. In late-stage kidney disease, the histology is non-specific as the nuclear inclusions are absent and the tubulointerstitium lacks significant inflammation. Treatment of lead intoxication consists of chelation therapy with EDTA or oral succimer. In view of the side effects associated with EDTA administration, chelation therapy should be carefully considered, particularly if there is significant preexisting irreversible kidney fibrosis.

Recent population-based studies have observed a trend of increased blood lead levels in the general population with a related inverse trend in creatinine clearance. It is unclear, however, whether these population-based observations reflect an increase in chronic lead nephropathy or an increase in kidney disease that induces lead retention. These studies suggest that chronic low-level lead exposure in developing countries, and an insufficient occupational limit on blood lead levels, may confer additional risk for CKD progression. In addition, some studies have suggested that chelation therapy may slow progression of CKD in these patients.

Aristolochic Acid Nephropathy and Balkan Nephropathy

Rapidly progressive fibrosing interstitial nephritis has been described in clusters of patients in weight-loss programs who ingested Chinese herbal preparations tainted with a plant nephrotoxin derived from *Aristolochia fangchi* (aristolochic acid). Kidney lesions are characterized by predominantly cortical interstitial fibrosis and tubular atrophy with minimal inflammation, which also may involve the medullary rays and outer medulla. Several hundred cases have been reported in the literature thus far, although some cases were observed in patients who ingested herb preparations not containing aristolochic acid. Other reports from Asia suggest that herbal therapy–induced kidney damage is not uncommon. Kidney disease in affected individuals is typically progressive and irreversible despite withdrawal of toxin exposure, with many patients requiring dialysis or transplantation within 1 year of presentation.

The putative nephrotoxin, aristolochic acid, induces tubulointerstitial fibrosis in animal models of disease following chronic daily exposure. Women may be at higher risk for aristolochic acid nephropathy, and the observation that some patients exposed to toxic herbs do not develop kidney disease further suggests variability in patient susceptibility to kidney injury. In addition, variability in herbal products could significantly alter toxin concentration in batched preparations. Studies in animal models indicate that both toxin exposure and concurrent renal vasoconstriction may be required to precipitate the characteristic progressive kidney disease. A frequent association of upper urinary tract urothelial cell atypia and carcinoma has also been reported in experimental animals and in many affected patients. The mechanism of aristolochic acid–induced nephrotoxicity (AAN) has not been delineated. Identification of aristolactam-DNA adducts, as well as tumor suppressor *p53* gene mutations, in genitourinary tumors has implicated these factors in malignant urothelial transformation. Because many affected patients have undergone kidney transplantation with immunosuppressive therapy, routine surveillance of urinary cytology is generally recommended in view of this association with urothelial malignancy.

Balkan nephropathy (BN) is a form of CIN observed in farmers that is endemic to the areas of Bulgaria, Romania, Serbia, Croatia, Bosnia, and Herzegovina, most commonly along the confluence of the Danube River. Several recent studies suggest that BN is induced by chronic exposure to aristolochic acid in susceptible individuals. Because *Aristolochia* plants grow abundantly in agricultural areas, harvesting of crops, such as wheat, from contaminated fields could introduce aristolochic acid into the local food supply and expose the population to the nephrotoxin. BN and AAN are both linked to aristolochic acid exposure, have similar kidney pathology, and are associated with urothelial, and less often renal cell, carcinomas. A wide range of tumor incidence, from 2% to 47%, has been reported in these patients. Kidney and urothelial cancer tissue isolated from BN patients also identified DNA adducts from aristolochic acid and *p53* gene mutations—features that characterize aristolochic acid–induced tumors in experimental models and patients with AAN. Interestingly, with the advent of more modern wheat harvesting techniques that prevent contamination with *Aristolochia*, the incidence of BN is declining.

BN is a slowly progressive kidney disease that is typically observed after the fourth decade of life and rarely affects patients younger than 20 years of age. Patients generally present with normal blood pressure and either normal or slightly reduced kidney size on ultrasonography. Hematuria and tubular dysfunction may be present. There currently is no specific treatment or preventive strategy for the disorder, although corticosteroids may slow progression of CKD.

Sarcoidosis

The most common kidney manifestation of sarcoidosis is mediated through disordered calcium metabolism resulting in hypercalcemia and hypercalciuria, occasionally inducing nephrolithiasis (10%) and nephrocalcinosis (<5%). Although interstitial inflammation, often with non-necrotizing granuloma formation, is relatively common in sarcoidosis (15% to 30%) and the most frequent finding on kidney biopsy, autopsy series indicate that it is unusual for the interstitial abnormalities to result in clinically significant kidney dysfunction (see Fig. 43.1B). Moreover, it is unusual to observe interstitial disease in the absence of extrarenal involvement in sarcoidosis. Although most patients with impaired kidney function respond well to corticosteroid therapy, recovery of kidney function is frequently incomplete because of chronic interstitial inflammation and fibrosis. Presentation with hypercalcemia has been associated with a more sustained response to corticosteroid therapy 1 year following therapy. Relapse of kidney functional impairment during steroid taper has been reported, but progression to ESKD is rare.

Sjögren Syndrome

Sjögren syndrome, a disorder characterized by lymphocyte and plasma cell infiltration in salivary, parotid, and lacrimal glands, results in progressive organ dysfunction and sicca syndrome. Involvement of other organs, including the kidney, is frequently reported. Circulating autoantibodies (anti-Ro/SSA and anti-La/SSB antibodies) are associated with Sjögren syndrome. Kidney involvement occurs in up to 67% of affected patients. The kidney lesion consists predominantly of tubulointerstitial lymphocytic inflammation with tubular injury and without associated immune complex deposits. Cortical granuloma formation has rarely been reported and may suggest the diagnosis of sarcoidosis or tubulointerstitial nephritis and uveitis (TINU) syndrome. These other conditions, however, are not associated with sicca syndrome. With disease chronicity in Sjögren syndrome, tubular atrophy and interstitial fibrosis are more extensive, and patients may exhibit biochemical disorders from tubular dysfunction. Response to immunosuppression is variable, with patients often not improving or slowly worsening, with rare development of ESKD.

Tubulointerstitial Nephritis and Uveitis Syndrome

TINU syndrome is a relatively rare autoimmune process that results in eye and kidney disease. Both AIN and CIN are observed with this syndrome, which can occur at any age but is more common in adolescents. Eye symptoms may precede, coincide, or, more often, occur up to 14 months after tubulointerstitial nephritis is noted. Fever, weight loss, fatigue, abdominal and/or flank pain, arthralgias, and polyuria may also be seen. TINU should be considered in any patient presenting with unexplained tubulointerstitial disease, which often manifests with acute or CKD, minimal proteinuria, and sterile pyuria. Typical kidney biopsy findings with chronic TINU are tubulointerstitial fibrosis with a lymphocyte predominant infiltrate. Occasionally there may be non-necrotizing granulomas, and sarcoidosis needs to be excluded. Treatment includes prednisone 1 mg/kg/day for 3 to 6 months (depending on kidney response) with a slow taper.

IgG4-Related Tubulointerstitial Nephritis

Immunoglobulin (Ig)G4-related interstitial nephritis is often part of a systemic disease process with multiorgan involvement, now known as *IgG4-related disease* (IgG4D). This disease is characterized by an elevated serum IgG4 level (positive in 60% of patients) and dense infiltration of IgG4-positive plasma cells within the involved organ. Predominantly affecting middle-aged to elderly men, other organ involvement often causes aortitis/periaortitis, cholangitis, sialadenitis, pancreatitis, and hypophysitis. Other features include elevated serum IgG and IgE levels, eosinophilia, and hypocomplementemia, although these features are not consistently present in all patients.

Kidney involvement in IgG4D includes acute and chronic interstitial disease, membranous nephropathy, nodular masses within the kidneys, and obstructive uropathy from retroperitoneal fibrosis. CIN in IgG4D is characterized histopathologically by a lymphoplasmacytic infiltrate with a predominance of IgG4-positive plasma cells and T-lymphocytes, a specific swirling or storiform pattern of interstitial fibrosis, which may encase small collections of leukocytes ("birds' eye" pattern), and, less often, obliterative phlebitis (Fig. 43.3). Before the development of

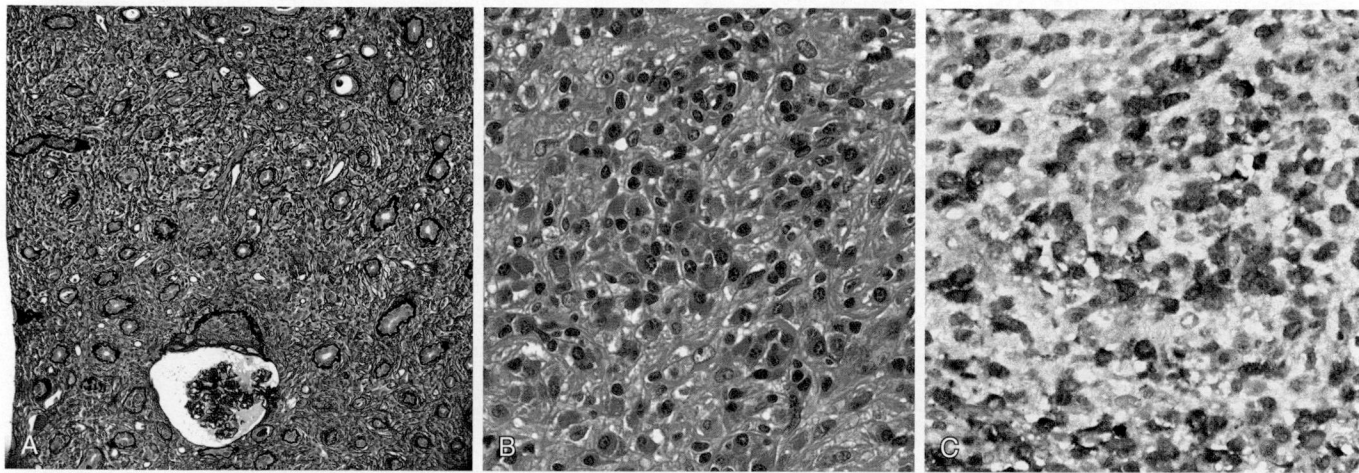

• **Fig. 43.3** Immunoglobulin G4 disease. (A) There is tubular atrophy and the interstitium contains a dense inflammatory infiltrate with a storiform and "birds-eye" pattern of fibrosis (Jones methenamine silver). (B) There is a dense interstitial inflammatory infiltrate composed of plasma cells and lymphocytes in a fibrotic background (hematoxylin-eosin). (C) Immunohistochemistry for immunoglobulin (Ig)G4 shows a large number of positive staining cells.

extensive fibrosis, IgG4D is generally glucocorticoid responsive. However, relapse often occurs with steroid taper, and rituximab has been successfully used to treat steroid-dependent or steroid-resistant disease.

Chronic Kidney Disease of Unknown Origin (CKDu)

An epidemic of CKD in Central America was identified in the late 1990s, predominantly in male agricultural workers between the ages of 20 and 50 years, and is termed *Mesoamerican nephropathy*. Another chronic interstitial disease, initially described in agricultural workers in 1994, is Sri Lankan agricultural nephropathy (SAN). Subsequently, similar cases were found in several other countries around the world in Asia, the Middle East, Europe, and North America, earning the name *Chronic Interstitial Nephritis in Agricultural Communities (CINAC)*. The term employed to encompass many of these entities is *CKD of unknown origin (CKDu)*.

The clinical features of these diseases are similar and include working or living in an agricultural area, especially in the sugarcane or paddy fields in the initial descriptions, tubular proteinuria, a progressive decline in kidney function, and often hyperuricemia and/or hypokalemia. There is an absence of traditional CKD risk factors such as diabetes, primary glomerular disease, and hypertension, although there may be mildly elevated blood pressure. Some, but not all, affected individuals have a history of manual labor under extremely hot conditions. Histopathologically these diseases also are similar, characterized primarily by tubulointerstitial fibrosis with variable associated inflammation and dysmorphic proximal tubular cell lysosomes. There may be glomerulomegaly, ischemic-type glomerular changes, and global and secondary focal segmental glomerulosclerosis (Fig. 43.4).

The cause of the disease is unknown; however, the two leading hypotheses are severe heat exposure with recurrent volume depletion and environmental agrochemical toxin exposure causing proximal tubular injury. Environmental exposure to low levels of heavy metals, silica, and infection with leptospirosis or hantavirus also have been suggested to play a role in the pathogenesis of the disease. It is possible some of these factors occur together, and additional use of nonsteroidal antiinflammatory agents and excessive hyperuricosuria are considered other potential exacerbating factors.

There may be slow or more rapid progression of CKD, which can occur in as little as 3 years after diagnosis, minimal proteinuria with bland sediment, and small echogenic kidneys on ultrasound. Treatment is supportive for CKD, and it is unknown if removal from agricultural work and its environment would slow disease progression.

Chronic Pyelonephritis

Chronic pyelonephritis was considered a leading cause of inflamed tubulointerstitial scarring in the past. However, it is now recognized that this is relatively uncommon and typically occurs following episodes of recurrent urinary tract infections, reflux nephropathy, or urinary obstruction. The morphologic features include mononuclear inflammation, often with plasma cells, in the fibrotic interstitium and atrophied tubules of the cortex and medulla. The plasma cells may stain for IgG4 and requires differentiation from IgG4D. Thyroidization of tubules has been reported as a hallmark lesion but is not specific for any single cause of CIN.

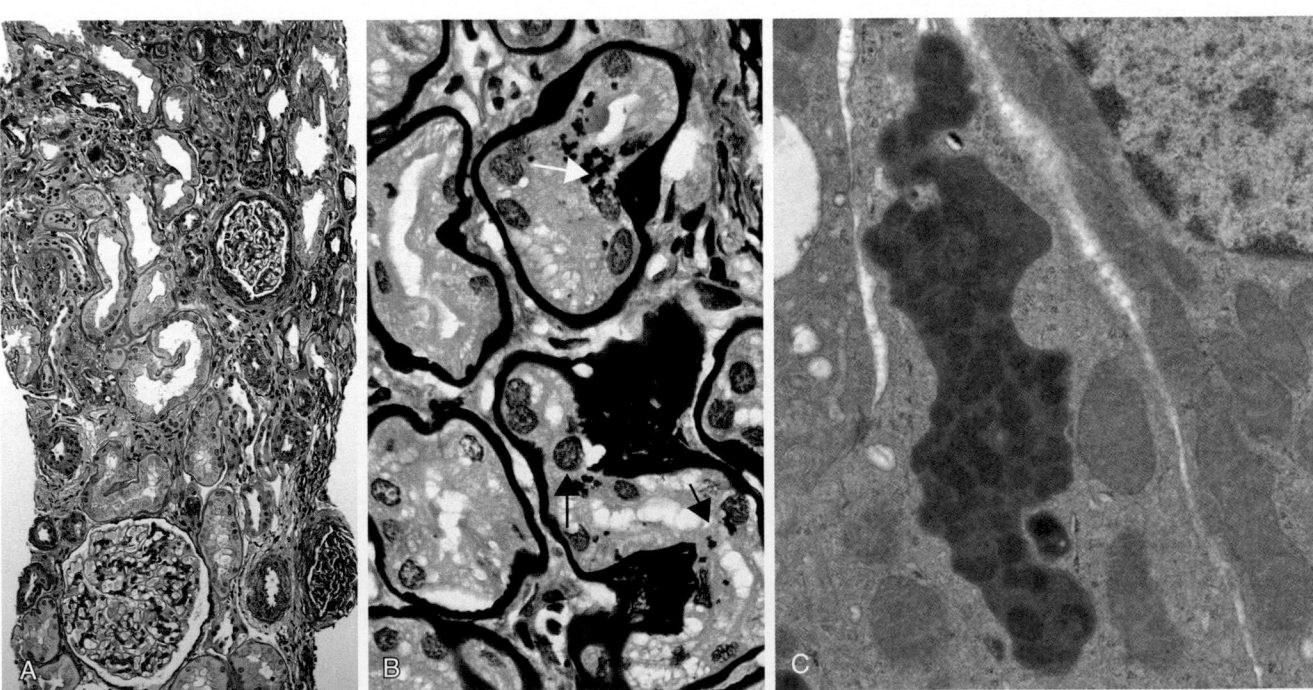

• **Fig. 43.4** Mesoamerican nephropathy (CKDu). (A) There is focal tubular atrophy with interstitial fibrosis and a mild lymphocytic infiltrate. One glomerulus is enlarged and the other two have mild ischemic-type capillary wall corrugation (periodic acid-Schiff). (B) Proximal tubular cells containing large, irregular, silver-positive granules (*arrow*) (Jones methenamine silver). (C) Electron micrograph of a proximal tubular cell with a large, dysmorphic lysosome containing dispersed electron dense aggregates, corresponding to the silver-positive granules seen on light microscopy (×8000).

Other forms of infection-related CIN include xanthogranulomatous pyelonephritis, malakoplakia, and megalocytic interstitial nephritis. These are associated with macrophage dysfunction, typically in the setting of gram-negative infections, resulting in kidney infiltration with abnormal macrophages forming foam cells, von Hansemann histocytes with cytoplasmic calcifications, or with PAS-positive granular cytoplasm, respectively. When bilateral, kidney failure results often with enlarged kidneys and may simulate an infiltrative process such as lymphoma or amyloidosis. Therapy involves treating any active infection and underlying reflux or obstruction. Nephrectomy may be required if the kidney is irreversibly scarred.

Complete bibliography is available at Elsevier eBooks for Practicing Clinicians.

Key Bibliography

Abed L, Merouani A, Haddad E, Benoit G, Oligny LL, Sartelet H. Presence of autoantibodies against tubular and uveal cells in a patient with tubulointerstitial nephritis and uveitis (TINU) syndrome. *Nephrol Dial Transplant.* 2008;23:1452–1455.

Anumudu S, Eknoyan G. Pyelonephritis: a historical reappraisal. *J Am Soc Nephrol.* 2019;30:914–917.

Bhandari S, Kalowski S, Collett P, et al. Karyomegalic nephropathy: an uncommon cause of progressive renal failure. *Nephrol Dial Transplant.* 2002;17:1914–1920.

Bruggeman LA. Common mechanisms of viral injury to the kidney. *Adv Chronic Kidney Dis.* 2019;26:164–170.

Correia FASC, Marchini GS, Torricelli FC, et al. Renal manifestations of sarcoidosis: from accurate diagnosis to specific treatment. *Int Braz J Urol.* 2020;46:15–25.

Clive DM, Vanguri VK. The syndrome of tubulointerstitial nephritis with uveitis (TINU). *Am J Kidney Dis.* 2018;72:118–128.

Correa-Rotter R, García-Trabanino R. Mesoamerican nephropathy. *Semin Nephrol.* 2019;39(3):263–271.

Cortazar FB, Stone JH. IgG4-related disease and the kidney. *Nat Rev Nephrol.* 2015;11(10):599–609.

Esparza AR, McKay DB, Cronan JJ, Chazan JA. Renal parenchymal malakoplakia. Histologic spectrum and its relationship to megalocytic interstitial nephritis and xanthogranulomatous pyelonephritis. *Am J Surg Pathol.* 1989;13:225–236.

Gifford FJ, Gifford RM, Eddleston M, Dhaun N. Endemic nephropathy around the world. *Kidney Int Rep.* 2017;2:282–292.

Goules A, Geetha D, Arend LJ, Baer AN. Renal involvement in primary Sjögren's syndrome: natural history and treatment outcome. *Clin Exp Rheumatol.* 2019;118(3):123–132 37 Suppl.

Herrera Valdés R, Almaguer López M, Orantes Navarro CM, et al. Chronic interstitial nephritis of nontraditional causes in Salvadoran agricultural communities. *Clin Nephrol.* 2020;93:60–67.

Jayasumana C, Gunatilake S, Siribaddana S. Simultaneous exposure to multiple heavy metals and glyphosate may contribute to Sri Lankan agricultural nephropathy. *BMC Nephrol.* 2015;16:103–110.

Jelakovic B, Dika Z, Arlt VM. et al. Balkan endemic nephropathy and the causative role of aristolochic acid. *Semin Nephrol.* 2019;39:284–296.

Jelaković B, Karanović S, Vuković-Lela I, et al. Aristolactam-DNA adducts are a biomarker of environmental exposure to aristolochic acid. *Kidney Int.* 2012;81:559–567.

Kritz W, Kaissling B, Le Hir M. Epithelial-mesenchymal transition (EMT) is kidney fibrosis: fact or fantasy? *J Clin Invest.* 2011;121:468–474.

Markowitz GS, Perazella MA. Drug-induced acute interstitial nephritis. *Nat Rev Nephrol.* 2010;6:461–470.

Raissian Y, Nasr SH, Larsen CP. et al. Diagnosis of IgG4-related tubulointerstitial nephritis. *J Am Soc Nephrol.* 2011;22(7):1343–1352.

Verveat BA, Nast CC, Jayasumana C. et al. Chronic interstitial nephritis in agricultural communities (CINAC): a toxic lysosomal tubulopathy. *Kidney Int.* 2020;97:350–369.

Wallace ZS, Naden RP, Chari S, et al. The 2019 American College of Rheumatology/European League Against Rheumatism classification criteria for IgG4-related disease. *Ann Rheum Dis.* 2020;79:77–87.

44

Obstructive Uropathy

RICHARD W. SUTHERLAND

Obstruction of the urinary tract can occur anywhere between the collecting duct and the urethral meatus. Microcrystals in the collecting duct, urinary calculi, tumors, and luminal strictures all may block the normal flow of urine. Regardless of the cause, the ultimate effect is the same: an increase in the hydrostatic pressure of the collecting system, which is transmitted into Bowman space. This reduces the glomerular filtration rate (GFR) and initiates a cascade of events that, if not reversed, will result in kidney scarring and loss of overall kidney function. The extent of kidney injury and the damage to the physical structures of the collecting system vary depending on the duration and completeness of the obstruction. The reduction of kidney function is determined by two components: loss of GFR and the loss of tubular function. Although both are critical, GFR is the dominant contributor. Even in an unobstructed kidney, tubular function collapses when glomerular filtration is disrupted as the glomerular filtrate is necessary to provide the substrate (i.e., Na^+ ions) for tubular function. In cases of prolonged obstruction to the kidney, both glomerular and tubular functions are compromised.

Unilateral Ureteral Obstruction

Historically, unilateral and bilateral ureteral obstructions (BUOs) are discussed separately because of distinct changes in kidney physiology. In the first hours after obstruction, differences between the two types of obstructions occur in glomerular blood flow and ureteral pressure profiles. In unilateral ureteral obstruction (UUO), a triphasic event of vascular blood flow and ureteral pressure is seen. Only two phases are seen in BUO. In UUO (Fig. 44.1), there is an initial elevation in the luminal hydrostatic pressure. GFR is maintained by a simultaneous increase in the glomerular capillary pressure induced by afferent arteriolar dilation. Prostaglandin E_2 (PGE_2) and nitrous oxide (NO) are considered the initial mediators. Studies using inhibitors of PGE_2 and NO attenuate this increase in renal blood flow and GFR. The exact triggering mechanisms for the production of PGE_2 and NO are less well understood but may be due to the decreased presentation of Na^+ and Cl^- to the macula densa. The changes in GFR and luminal pressure define the first phase.

The second phase of UUO begins with the decrease of glomerular blood flow. Between 12 and 24 hours after the initial obstruction, afferent arteriolar vasodilation transitions to vasoconstriction. Activation of the renin-angiotensin system occurs during the first phase and becomes the dominant process affecting GFR, whereupon efferent and partial afferent arteriole vasoconstriction overwhelms PGE_2- and NO-mediated vasodilation. Experimental data show that the administration of angiotensin-converting enzyme (ACE) inhibitors blunts the vasoconstriction and GFR

reduction. Thromboxane A2 and endothelin reduce glomerular blood flow during UUO. This second phase of UUO is defined by a persistent elevation of hydrostatic pressure from the obstructed lumen, even with the reduction of GFR.

The third and last phase of UUO is marked by decreased luminal hydrostatic pressure and renal blood flow. Glomerular capillary blood flow and luminal pressure remain below baseline until the obstruction is relieved. It is during this last phase that the majority of permanent damage is done to the kidney. The return to baseline function is dependent on the overall duration and severity of the initial obstruction. A partial obstruction may be present for 14 days or more with complete return of function. A total obstruction will leave permanent fibrosis within a week.

Bilateral Ureteral Obstruction

The primary difference between UUO and BUO is persistent vasoconstriction of the efferent artery, which maintains GFR in BUO. Luminal pressure remains elevated for longer than 24 hours in BUO, whereas it begins to decrease by 6 hours with UUO. To account for the persistent afferent arteriolar dilation and efferent arteriolar vasoconstriction, it is likely that additional vasoactive substances accumulate or are produced in BUO but not in UUO. One substance, atrial natriuretic peptide (ANP), is produced as volume overload occurs and an increase in diuresis is required. Vasodilators PGE_2 and NO are likely present because blockade of their production magnifies the already blunted increase in GFR seen in BUO. This suggests that although ANP produces afferent arteriolar dilation, PGE_2 and NO enhance this process.

Tubular Dysfunction

Loss of tubular function during obstruction occurs primarily from a decrease in GFR rather than direct hydrostatic pressure injury to the tubular cells. Sodium and potassium homeostasis, water handling, and urinary acidification are altered. The decline in GFR initiates a series of compensatory yet maladaptive events that are mediated by vasoactive substances, cytokines, and ischemia. These maladaptive events alter the amount of filtrate, the composition of the filtrate, tubular transport proteins, and tubular blood flow (Table 44.1).

Sodium Reabsorption

Obstruction of the kidney impairs Na^+ reabsorption throughout the nephron. The luminal Na^+/H^+ exchanger (NHE3), the luminal $Na^+/K^+/2Cl^-$ cotransporter (NKCC2), and the basolateral

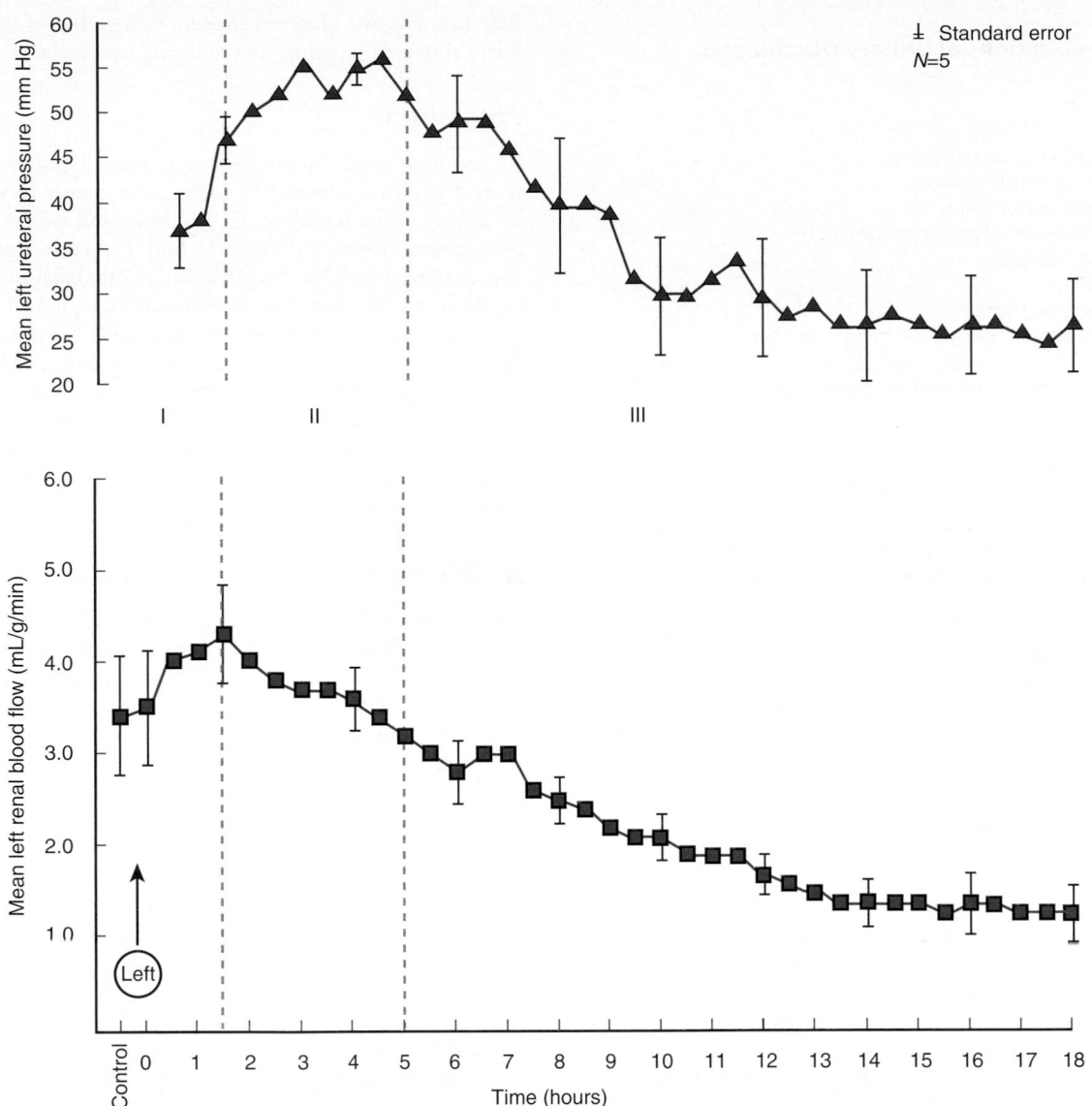

• **Fig. 44.1** Renal resistance in ureteral occlusion. Triphasic relationship of left ureteral luminal pressure and left renal blood flow after occlusion of the left ureter. (From Moody TE, Vaughn ED Jr, Gillenwater JY. Relationship between renal blood flow and ureteral pressure during 18 hours of total unilateral urethral occlusion: implications for changing sites of increased renal resistance. *Invest Urol.* 1975;13:246–251.)

Na$^+$/K$^+$-ATPase pump are all downregulated in obstructed kidneys. Cell suspension studies of distinct nephron segments support this conclusion. In the proximal tubule, reduction of NHE3 activity is seen. In the medullary portion of the collecting system, NHE3 expression is suppressed and energy consumption is reduced. In the loop of Henle, decreased activity of the NKCC2 cotransporter is noted in cells studied from the thick ascending limb. Na$^+$ reabsorption also requires luminal transport into the cell. This process is affected by furosemide, supporting disruption of the NKCC2 transporter. Many of these transport processes are energy dependent and require ATP. Although a reduction in the amount of available ATP has been hypothesized because of ischemia, it is the downregulation of the receptors and enzymes that appears to be the rate-limiting step in Na$^+$ transport.

The actual triggers for the loss of receptor and enzyme activity are still an area of active research. Possible signals include decreased filtrate substrates, natriuretic substances, and direct tubular hydrostatic pressure. Decreased GFR reduces Na$^+$ ion presentation to the loop of Henle, which could downregulate its receptor and transport proteins. Additionally, loss of luminal Na$^+$ reduces the electrochemical gradient, whereas blockade of Na$^+$ movement into obstructed medullary thick ascending limb cells results in a loss of ouabain-sensitive ATPase. Taken together, decreased Na$^+$ presentation to cells could downregulate Na$^+$/K$^+$-ATPase at the translational or posttranslational level.

PGE$_2$ levels change as a result of obstruction and eventually begin to affect Na$^+$ reabsorption. PGE$_2$ is released during obstruction from increased COX-2 production. COX-2 inhibition reduces the loss of NKCC2 and Na$^+$/K$^+$-ATPase activity, implying an effect of PGE$_2$ to impair Na$^+$ reabsorption.

Na$^+$ reabsorption in BUO differs from UUO because of the presence of volume expansion. The addition of ANP and the loss of aldosterone reduce tubular reabsorption of Na$^+$. Much of the impaired Na$^+$ handling in UUO is amplified by the effect of ANP, which blocks release of renin and reduces the ultimate creation of

TABLE 44.1 Complications of Urinary Obstruction

1. **Natriuresis**
   Decreased NHE3, NKCC2, and Na$^+$/K$^+$ ATPase activity
2. **Impaired urinary concentration**
   Disruption of osmotic gradient
   Damaged urea recycling
   Loss of aquaporin receptors (nephrogenic DI)
3. **Metabolic acidosis**
   Distal RTA
4. **Kidney scarring/fibrosis**
   Increased extracellular matrix MP/TIMP imbalance
   Increased fibroblast/myofibroblast activity
   Growth factors/cytokines/enzymes/protein shifts: TGF-β, SMADs, PAI-1
5. **Apoptosis**
   Extrinsic pathway: TNF-α, TRADD
   Intrinsic pathway: Oxidative stress, mitochondrial breakdown

MP, Metalloproteinases; *NHE3,* Na$^+$/H$^+$ exchanger; *NKCC2,* Na$^+$/K$^+$/2Cl$^-$ cotransporter; *RTA,* renal tubular acidosis; *TIMP,* tissue inhibitors of metalloproteinases; *TRADD,* tumor necrosis factor receptor type 1–associated death domain.

angiotensin II. ANP also directly reduces Na$^+$ reabsorption in the collecting duct and blocks angiotensin II's effect on Na$^+$ reabsorption, the net effects being diuresis and natriuresis.

Urinary Concentration

Obstruction disrupts normal urinary concentration. With a reduced GFR, less Na$^+$ is available to create the osmolar gradient in the medullary interstitium. As with the defects in Na$^+$ reabsorption, there is loss of the luminal and basolateral membrane proteins, NKCC2 and Na$^+$/K$^+$-ATPase. This prevents Na$^+$ transport from the tubular lumen into the medullary interstitium, which is critical to the countercurrent multiplier that creates the gradient for water reabsorption. Without the ability to reabsorb Na$^+$ in the ascending limb and dilute the filtrate as it enters the distal convoluted tubule, the solutes required to maintain the gradient are excreted. In the collecting duct of an obstructed kidney, action of antidiuretic hormone (ADH) to increase water permeability is blunted because of decreased AQP-2 in the luminal membrane. Several studies have shown this to be a post-cAMP defect. Reduced transcription of AQP-2 mRNA and a decrease in the phosphorylation necessary to incorporate AQP-2 vesicles into the luminal membrane explain this effect. Finally, a decrease in basolateral membrane AQP-3 and AQP-4 is also noted. After obstruction is relieved, overall urinary concentration returns, paralleling the return of the AQP-2 channel to the luminal membrane.

Urea recycling is another process used by the nephron to increase the gradient for urinary concentration. Urea within the filtrate passively exits the collecting duct at its inner medullary segment and enters the interstitium. The vasa recta and the thin portion of the loop of Henle reabsorb it. A maximum medullary interstitial osmotic gradient is created with the recycling of urea. Urea permeability in the collecting duct tubules is controlled by urea transporters UT-A1 and UT-A3. ADH enhances the permeability of urea, allowing it to flow into the interstitium. Urea reabsorption by the vasa recta is stimulated by UT-B receptors under ADH control. In the obstructed kidney, expression of urea transporters UT-A1, UT-A3, and UT-B is reduced. Urea transporter

defects reduce the maximal concentrating effect of the gradient by disrupting urea recycling and allowing urea to be excreted.

Potassium

K$^+$ handling in the nephron is not affected directly by obstruction. The initial disturbance in K$^+$ homeostasis is best explained by defects in Na$^+$ handling, H$^+$ handling, and reduced GFR. With obstruction, there is a decrease in both Na$^+$ reabsorption (reduced Na$^+$ channels) and Na$^+$ presentation to the distal tubule (reduced GFR). In the low-flow state of obstruction, high urinary potassium concentrations in the collecting duct blunt the gradient between the lumen and the tubular cells, resulting in a reduction in K$^+$ movement into the lumen, impaired K$^+$ excretion, and ultimately hyperkalemia. Additionally, pseudohypoaldosteronism (PHA) can be seen when obstruction damages the distal tubules and blunts their ability to respond to aldosterone, resulting in hyperkalemia, hyponatremia, and metabolic acidosis.

Acidification

Urinary obstruction produces a metabolic acidosis best understood as a form of distal (type 1) renal tubular acidosis (RTA) with hyperkalemia, or "voltage-dependent" RTA. It is characterized by a failure of distal H$^+$ and K$^+$ secretion. The Na$^+$ channel defects play a central role in this acidosis. Loss of Na$^+$ reabsorption from the distal tubule results in impaired urinary acidification in the obstructed kidney. Na$^+$/K$^+$-ATPase dysfunction on the basolateral surface of the cell ultimately disrupts Na$^+$ removal from the lumen of the collecting duct. This decrease in cation reabsorption reduces the passive H$^+$ excretion into the collecting duct lumen down the electrochemical gradient, and a "voltage-dependent acidosis" occurs. Simultaneous hyperkalemia occurs from failure of Na$^+$/K$^+$-ATPase and Na$^+$ reabsorption. Decreased expression of the H$^+$-ATPase in the collecting duct adds to the metabolic acidosis. However, a defect of the H$^+$-ATPase transporter cannot account completely for the acidosis seen in hyperkalemic distal RTA due to urinary obstruction. Urinary acidification occurs in the early phases of obstruction, suggesting an intact proton pump. A similarity is noted between voltage-dependent RTA and type 4 RTA. In neither of these two processes is H$^+$ secretion felt to be the primary defect.

Fibrosis

Persistent obstruction produces tubulointerstitial fibrosis. The activated pathways producing fibrosis do not differ significantly from fibrosis noted with other kidney disease processes. An imbalance in normal kidney homeostasis results in excess accumulation of extracellular matrix (ECM) with the subsequent development of tubulointerstitial fibrosis and, in later stages, glomerular and vascular sclerosis.

Maintenance of the ECM has classically been described as a balance of metalloproteinases (MMPs) and tissue inhibitors of metalloproteinases (TIMPs). The upregulation of fibroblast-produced TIMPs, which decrease the activity of the MMPs, results in a deposition of collagen I and III. Work in the last decade has shown this simple explanation is incomplete. TIMP 3 may prevent fibrosis, whereas TIMP 2 may promote fibrosis through activation of MMP 2. Different classes of presenting fibroblasts produce different cytokines and growth factors.

At the cellular level, there is an increase in the number of fibroblasts and myofibroblasts. Infiltrating macrophages and fibroblasts responding to injury release cytokines, including TGF-β, plasminogen activator inhibitor-1 (PAI-1), BMP-7, interleukin (IL)-2, and IL-6. Through the process of epithelial-mesenchymal transition (EMT) and endothelial-mesenchymal transition (EndMT), additional fibroblasts are produced as epithelial tubular cells and endothelial cells transform into mesenchymal cells. The end result is an increased number of fibroblasts are necessary for the pathologic collagen deposition.

The presence of angiotensin II, triggered by obstruction, stimulates the expression of TGF-β, a key facilitator of fibrosis. TGF-β fibrosis occurs through SMAD and non-SMAD pathways. SMAD3 is the best described promoter of fibrosis. SMAD3 is counterbalanced by SMAD2, which is regulated by bone morphogenetic protein-7 (BMP-7), an ECM fibrotic protector.

PAI-1 appears to be an additional pathway for the creation of fibrosis. While direct inhibition of urokinase (uPA) and tissue plasminogen activator (tPA) may be one mechanism that promotes fibrosis, an independent action of PAI-1 affecting the ECM fibrosis is suspected. Additional growth factors, cytokines, and vasoactive compounds promote cell growth and fibrosis, such as TNF-α, NF-κB, platelet-derived growth factor (PDGF), vascular cell adhesion molecule-1 (VCAM-1), and basic fibroblast growth factor (bFGF).

Several therapeutic strategies to reduce fibrosis within the ECM are available not only in obstructive uropathy but also in other diseases, such as diabetes mellitus. These include manipulation of PAI-1 and TXA2 and ACE inhibition. In obstructive uropathy, these continue to be hypothetical and not applicable to clinical medicine. Many of the possible treatments that would block these fibrotic pathways also disrupt the pathways that are needed for normal wound healing, thereby exacerbating the fibrosis. This has been seen when ACE inhibitors and TGF-β blockade have been used in an attempt to inhibit fibrosis. The most important therapeutic treatment is to relieve the obstruction.

Apoptosis

Apoptosis, or programmed cell death, is a normal physiologic remodeling mechanism that occurs within the kidney and throughout other organ systems of the body. During obstruction, apoptosis is increased through external and internal cellular signals. Extrinsic activation with obstruction occurs from an increase in the tissue levels of TNF-α, which binds to its receptor, TNFR1. This complex then combines with the cell death domain (TRADD) to activate apoptotic pathways, resulting in cell death. Intrinsic activation occurs from oxidative stress, which causes intracellular release of a number of substances from damaged organelles. Mitochondrial release of cytochrome-c is a known trigger for apoptosis in many organ systems, including the kidney. Stress to the endoplasmic reticulum upregulates the apoptotic c-JUN NH2 terminal kinase, resulting in increased inflammation and subsequent fibrosis. The external and internal pathways converge on a common pathway to continue apoptosis through effector caspases, which cleave the nucleus to create apoptotic bodies. There are 12 different apoptotic caspases, with 3, 8, and 12 identified within the obstructed kidney tissue. Attempts at manipulating the apoptotic pathways to ameliorate fibrosis continue to be exploratory.

Postobstructive Diuresis

Postobstructive diuresis is a normal physiologic event in patients with prolonged BUO. The rate of diuresis is based on the severity of volume overload, urea accumulation, and electrolyte disturbances developing during obstruction. There is no rate of urine output that defines postobstructive diuresis. However, rates of 250 mL/h are common, and 750 mL/h can be seen.

Several factors facilitate the physiologic diuresis. Before release of the obstruction, there is downregulation of Na+ transporters, and this inability to reabsorb Na+ diminishes the osmotic gradient necessary for urinary concentration. In the distal tubule, reduced aquaporin activity promotes aquaresis. ANP is released because of activation of the cardiac atrial stretch receptors from increased preload, further increasing urine output.

Initial treatment of the postobstructive diuresis is free access to fluids. In the postsurgical patient who is unable to drink, approximately 75% of the urine volume is replaced with 0.45% (1/2 normal) saline. Intravenous fluids are adjusted based on volume status, subsequent urine osmolality, serum osmolality, and serum electrolyte measurements every 12 hours, depending on the rate of the diuresis and illness of the patient. The aggressive resuscitation to "chase" the volume of fluid excreted, rather than kidney pathology, results in "iatrogenic" diuresis after relief of obstruction.

Pathologic postobstructive diuresis does occur. Ongoing excretion of dilute urine can result in severe volume depletion. Initial treatment is the same as in physiologic postobstructive diuresis, with resuscitation with water and electrolytes and frequent measurement of serum chemistries. In severe cases, laboratory testing every 4 to 6 hours may be required until a stable balance has been created with oral and intravenous fluid and electrolyte therapy. In infancy and the pediatric population, persistent polyuria can create a state of chronic hyperosmolality. The hyperosmolality results in the intracellular and extracellular loss of volume and a metabolic acidosis with failure to thrive and poor growth.

Specific Causes of Obstructions

Causes of urinary obstruction are listed in Box 44.1.

Nephrolithiasis

Nephrolithiasis produces an intrinsic obstruction, anywhere from the ureteropelvic junction (UPJ) to the urethral meatus. Renal pelvic stones cause obstruction at the UPJ, with ureteral stones commonly producing an obstruction at two locations: (1) the ureter where it crosses the iliac vessels and (2) the ureterovesicular junction (UVJ). A ureteral stricture can produce a narrowing and resulting obstruction from a stone. Bladder stones can block the urethra at the bladder neck. Rarely, urethral stones, generally with prior urethral stricture disease or surgical reconstruction, occlude the urethra or urethral meatus.

Treatment of obstructing stones depends on the location and severity of illness. Stones in the calyces from infundibular stenosis produce pain and infection. The location of the infundibulum deep within the kidney parenchyma makes open surgical management difficult. Endoscopic laser incision of the stenosis may relieve the obstruction. Extended narrowing tends to restricture, making laser ablation of the entire calyx a consideration with partial loss of function.

Once within the renal pelvis, a small calcification can form a nidus to create a larger obstructing stone. Renal pelvis stones are excellent candidates for extracorporeal shock wave lithotripsy (ESWL). The retroperitoneal location of the kidney, away from other vital structures and bowel gas, allows for shock waves to penetrate the kidney and fragment the stone. Larger stones require prolonged and repetitive shock-wave treatment, which

BOX 44.1

Causes of Urinary Obstruction

Intrinsic Obstructions

Nephron
1. Uric acid and drug crystals/stones
2. Sloughed papillae
3. Gross hematuria with clot

Renal Pelvis
1. Malignancy, primary/metastatic
2. Renal cyst
3. Ureteropelvic junction (UPJ) stenosis

Ureteral
1. Ureteral stricture
2. Ureteral stone
3. Aperistaltic ureter (i.e., megaureter or prune belly syndrome)
4. Ureterocele
5. Ectopic ureter

Bladder
1. Neurogenic (i.e., spina bifida, diabetes)
2. Malignancy, transitional cell carcinoma
3. Fibrosis (i.e., radiation, chronic inflammation)

Urethra
1. Posterior urethral valves
2. Benign prostatic hyperplasia
3. Malignancy
4. Stricture
5. Prostatic abscess
6. Phimosis

Extrinsic Compressions

Renal Pelvis
1. Peripelvic cyst
2. Cancer, primary kidney or metastatic
3. Trauma

Ureter
1. UPJ crossing vessel
2. Retrocaval ureter
3. Tumor (pelvic malignancy)
4. Retroperitoneal fibrosis
5. Pregnancy
6. Endometriosis
7. Ovarian vein thrombosis

Bladder
1. Bladder neck contraction (previous surgery, malignancy)

PCN because of the ability to use larger and more powerful instruments with better visualization.

While ESWL works well for kidney stones, it has a significantly lower success rate for mid-ureteral stones. ESWL requires focalization of a pressure wave through tissue to fragment the stone. Gas within adjacent bowel impedes shock-wave migration to the stones. Ureteroscopy becomes the treatment of choice for the majority of mid- and lower ureteral stones. Retrograde access is again the preferred choice, but antegrade access through the renal pelvis and down the ureter can be performed.

Strictures

Strictures found within the urinary tract suggest a previous event, such as trauma, infection, or systemic disease. They occur from the UPJ to the urethral meatus. Balloon dilation with a simultaneous full-thickness ureteral wall incision of the stricture is a good option. In short, isolated strictures, a long-term success rate of 85% to 90% is expected. Postprocedure, temporary stenting facilitates drainage and minimizes extravasation of acidic urine, which can impair healing and result in restenosis. Extensive stricture disease of the ureter or urethra from tuberculosis, infection, or malignancy may require open surgical resection of the diseased portion with reanastomosis.

Malignancy

There are numerous malignancies that can obstruct the urinary tract extrinsically, but few obstruct the system intrinsically. The most common internal malignancy is transitional cell carcinoma (TCC), which is derived from epithelial cells of the urinary mucosa. It is a friable, frondular tumor with a solid stalk found primarily in older patients with a history of tobacco use. Treatment of obstruction is dependent on tumor location; those that fill the renal pelvis can be treated initially with a ureteral stent. TCC can also produce obstruction at the UVJ. Initial treatment includes an attempt at local cystoscopic excision or unroofing the orifice. When unresectable by cystoscopy, a temporizing stent or nephrostomy tube can be placed until surgical reconstruction with ureteral reimplantation or a possible cystectomy can be completed.

Extrinsic compression of the ureter from malignancies occurs more frequently. The most common are primary pelvic tumors in women. Retroperitoneal adenopathy along the aorta or vena cava adjacent to the ureter can also produce obstruction. Tumors can directly invade into the ureteral wall and occlude the lumen. Initial treatment with a stent is suggested. Large pelvic masses may obliterate the normal anatomy of the bladder and ureteral orifices. This can make ureteral stent placement impossible. In this situation, an initial PCN tube can be placed with subsequent antegrade internalization of the stent.

Benign Prostatic Hyperplasia/Prostate Cancer

An enlarged prostate creates urinary obstruction through bladder decompensation and failure rather than a fixed urethral obstruction. The relatively slow and gradual prostatic enlargement can come from benign or malignant causes. Enlargement of prostate tissue produces a partial obstruction that increases the patient's voiding pressure. The chronic increase in voiding pressure produces a hydrostatic stress to the smooth muscles of the bladder, resulting in bladder muscle hypertrophy. A subsequent increase in fibroblast and smooth muscle results in bladder wall trabeculations

may damage the surrounding parenchyma. Percutaneous nephrolithotripsy (PCNL) or ureteroscopy may be a better option in these cases.

Ureteroscopy is a very effective technique (greater than 85% success) in selected cases. It treats the stone and allows for direct visualization of the ureter and renal pelvis. This ensures there is no structural pathology that may have predisposed the patient to produce the original stone. Abnormal anatomy can make ureteroscopy difficult, requiring direct access through a percutaneous nephrostomy (PCN) tube. With PCN access to the kidney, PCNL can be performed with either laser or ultrasonic probes. Treatment of larger (>2 cm) and harder stones may benefit from and eventual bladder wall deterioration. The loss of muscle tone culminates in bladder dysfunction with the ultimate cause of the uropathy being urinary retention. It is this bladder deterioration that produces the functional obstruction and uropathy.

Initial treatment of symptomatic benign prostatic hyperplasia (BPH) uses α-blockers (tamsulosin, terazosin) to reduce prostatic smooth muscle tone. This increases the size of the urethral lumen and allows voiding pressures to decrease. Phosphodiesterase (PD-5) inhibitors are another class of medications that affect smooth muscle and are associated with subjective improvement in voiding symptoms. Combining the PD-5 inhibitor with an α-blocker synergistically improves symptoms better than either medication alone. If medical therapy proves inadequate, transurethral resection of the prostate, open surgical excision, and clean intermittent catheterization (CIC) may be used.

Neurogenic Bladder

Patients with neurogenic bladder must be monitored closely for new-onset obstructive uropathy. This was a leading cause of morbidity and uropathy in the adult neurogenic bladder population before the acceptance of CIC in the 1970s. Spinal cord trauma and myelomeningocele are the most common causes of neurogenic bladder in the adult and pediatric population, respectively. The normal voiding reflex in the adult relaxes the urinary sphincter during bladder contraction. Loss of this coordinated reflex in patients with neurogenic bladders results in bladder contraction against a closed sphincter, known as *detrusor sphincter dyssynergia (DSD)*. High-pressure voiding puts the patient at risk of bladder deterioration and upper urinary tract damage similar to BPH (Figs. 44.2 and 44.3). Chronic elevated bladder pressure is a more significant risk factor. The bladder fills to a maximum safe volume, but the patient does not sense the continued urine production. As the volume increases further, the constant resting pressure of the bladder rises. A resting pressure above 40 cm H_2O prevents flow into the bladder by overwhelming the maximum ureteral pressure of ureteral peristalsis. This results in upper tract dilation and subsequent uropathy. Patients with a small, low-volume bladder and tight urethral sphincter are at increased risk of GFR loss.

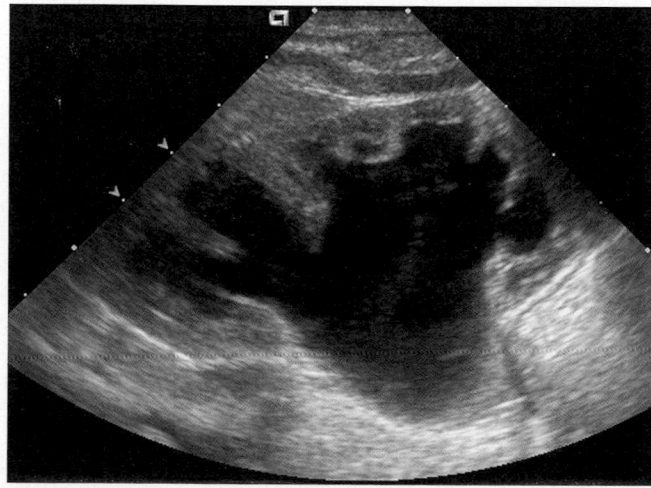

• **Fig. 44.2** Society of Fetal Urology grade IV hydronephrosis, which can be seen with or without vesicoureteral reflux, in a patient with a neurogenic bladder and a resting bladder pressure greater than 40 cm H_2O.

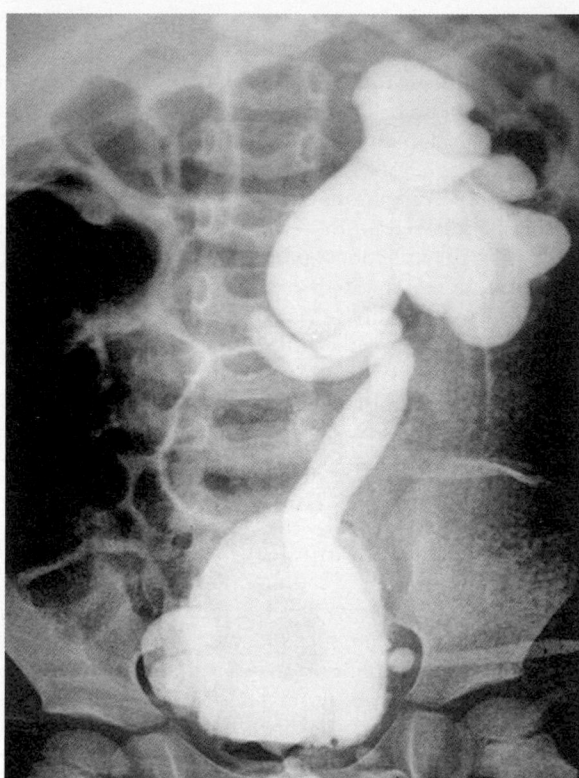

• **Fig. 44.3** Voiding cystourethrogram in a patient with a neurogenic bladder. High resting pressures and dysfunctional voiding result in bladder trabeculations and cellules, with the development of secondary grade 5 reflux.

Treatment involves lowering the resting pressure within the bladder. This can be achieved with anticholinergic medication, CIC, urethral dilation, or surgical reconstruction. Urinary diversions, such as ileal conduits or cutaneous ureterostomies, are other options. Many patients prefer a continent reconstruction with intermittent catheterization through the urethra or cutaneous stoma, such as a Mitrofanoff or Indiana pouch. Upper urinary tract deterioration with hydroureteronephrosis is generally seen before the irreversible uropathy. A screening kidney ultrasound should be considered annually in a high-risk asymptomatic patient to monitor for silent development of hydronephrosis.

Congenital Defects in the Adult Population

Congenital defects of the collecting system can present in adults. Defects of the UPJ and UVJ, ectopic ureters, ureteroceles, and even posterior urethral valves can present after childhood. Management depends on the specific signs and symptoms. Patients presenting with pain, infection, or reduced kidney function should be surgically repaired. Intervention can be endoscopic, laparoscopic, or open surgical correction. Asymptomatic abnormalities identified incidentally do not always require treatment. In the adult, there are several anatomic defects that can obstruct the urinary system. UPJ obstruction is identified when stones or infection occur as a result of urinary stasis. Chronic intermittent flank pain previously believed to be of gastrointestinal origin is another common presentation. Treatment of stones and infection will improve the symptoms, but recurrent stone formation or infection is common. Balloon dilation with simultaneous incision of the stricture with the specifically designed Acucise balloon has a success rate approaching 85% in the appropriately selected patient with a UPJ lesion. Long segments of dysplasia at the UPJ have a high failure rate with the Acucise balloon technique. Open surgery or laparoscopic/robotic pyeloplasty is an excellent option for reconstruction, approaching a 95% to 97% success rate. In asymptomatic patients with hydronephrosis from a UPJ narrowing, intervention should be reserved for those with decreased kidney function. Determination of a functional problem may require a furosemide nuclear scan to reveal if kidney dysfunction is caused by obstruction. In a cooperative adult, it is possible to recreate pain during the high urinary flow of the furosemide phase of the study. In the rare equivocal patient with intermittent pain, an indwelling double-J stent can be placed to bypass a possible obstruction to observe if the pain is relieved.

Congenital Defects in the Pediatric Population

Congenital obstruction in the pediatric patient occurs throughout the urinary tract. The most common locations are the UPJ, the UVJ, and the posterior urethral valves. Prenatal obstruction from a congenital defect can produce dramatic damage to the urinary tract and kidney function. Fortunately, the majority of children will have a continuation of normal development with growth of the ureter and its lumen after birth, resulting in an unaffected urinary system. The goal of managing prenatal congenital defects is to identify the 10% to 30% that will develop progressive disease if left untreated.

Up to 80% of significant partial UPJ obstructions will resolve without loss of kidney function. Dramatic hydronephrosis with parenchymal thinning can be monitored if kidney function is comparable to the unaffected contralateral kidney. Megaureters (Fig. 44.4), associated with UVJ obstruction, correct themselves without intervention in 70% of cases. Hydronephrosis does not necessarily mean obstruction.

In the young child with symptomatic UPJ obstruction, pyeloplasty continues to be the best surgical option. A success rate of 95% to 97% should be expected. Laparoscopic pyeloplasty is an excellent technique, except in children less than 1 year old, where a slightly higher failure rate is seen. Acucise balloon dilation is rarely indicated in the young child.

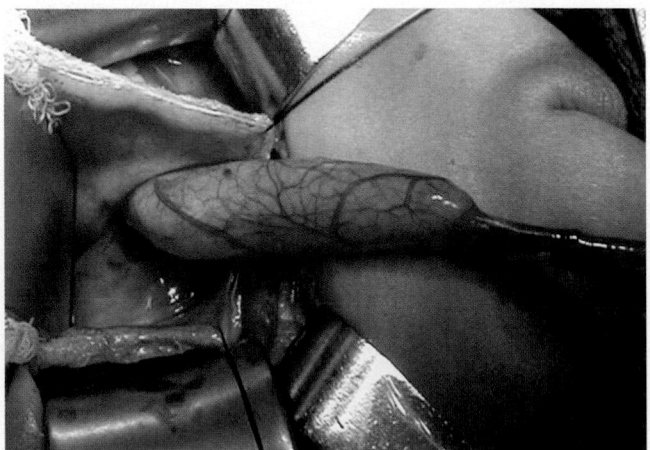

• **Fig. 44.4** Intraoperative megaureter reconstruction. The patient's bladder is open. Initial dissection shows the dilated ureter pulled up into the opened bladder. The distal ureteral narrowing is to the right with proximal healthy, but dilated, vascularized ureter to the left.

Pregnancy

Hydronephrosis is commonly seen in pregnancy but is rarely pathologic. Hydronephrosis occurs in 40% to 100% of pregnant women depending on the amount of dilation considered abnormal. Postpartum dilation may be seen for up to 6 weeks and is not considered pathologic. Two mechanisms contribute to the hydroureteronephrosis of pregnancy: ureteral compression and hormonal relaxation. By the 20th week, the gravid uterus achieves adequate size to reach the pelvic rim and extrinsically compress the ureter, producing a partial mechanical obstruction. The right kidney is more likely to be dilated because of the position of the uterus. A total of 10% to 15% of women will have hydronephrosis during the first trimester. Hormones present during pregnancy, including estrogen and progesterone that relax the smooth muscle of the ureters, also contribute to hydroureteronephrosis. Identification of hydronephrosis frequently occurs during routine prenatal ultrasound. Follow-up for even moderate hydroureteronephrosis is not needed unless the individual becomes symptomatic.

Treatment of true obstruction from severe extrinsic compression or nephrolithiasis can be performed cystoscopically with ureteral stent placement. Early stent encrustation will require frequent stent exchange to prevent stent obstruction. PCN can be performed if stent placement is not possible or if the stent is not tolerated.

Obstruction With Infection

An obstructed urinary system with an active infection is a medical emergency. Active infection requires close management with early surgical intervention for any systemic progression of illness. Decompression must be accomplished to prevent significant morbidity and mortality. Regardless of the cause of the obstruction, the urgency and means of decompression are dependent on illness severity in the affected patient. Infection is a relative contraindication for many reconstructive surgeries because of the inflammatory process hindering wound healing and promoting fibrosis, scarring, and recurrent obstruction.

Treatment can be as simple as a Foley catheter in an adult man with a urethral stricture to an open pyelostomy or PCN tube in an infant with a ruptured UPJ. Ureteral obstruction from a stone or a tumor is common and is best treated early with cystoscopic stent placement. Definitive reconstruction can be done after the infection and its inflammation resolves. Voiding complaints due to stents irritating the bladder are common. Anticholinergic medications are indicated for symptomatic patients with bladder hypercontractility.

A PCN tube is particularly beneficial in the ill patient. The tube can frequently be placed with mild sedation rather than the riskier general anesthesia required for stents. An advantage of a PCN tube is the ability to monitor drainage and to ensure adequate decompression, whereas internalized stents can obstruct asymptomatically. Irrigation of the PCN tube is simple compared to a possible stent exchange. Open surgical drainage is rarely performed and is reserved for the patient with abnormal anatomy where stenting or PCN is not possible. Patients with severe contractures or ectopic kidneys are in this category. Newborn boys with small urethras will not always accept a cystoscope. If the newborn kidney is not significantly hydronephrotic, PCN placement is difficult, and an open decompression procedure may be required. Dilated distal ureters, when present, can be brought to the skin as a cutaneous ureterostomy. A pyelostomy can be performed to protect the ureter for future reconstruction.

Bibliography

Batlle DC, Arrunda J, Kurtzman NA. Hyperkalemic distal renal tubular acidosis associated with obstructive uropathy. *N Engl J Med.* 1981;304:373–380.

Canbay A, Friedman S, Gores GJ. Apoptosis: The nexus of liver injury and fibrosis. *Hepatology.* 2004;39:273–278.

Edgtton KL, Gow RM, Kelly DJ, et al. Plasmin is not protective in experimental renal interstitial fibrosis. *Kidney Int.* 2004;66:68–76.

Flevaris P, Vaughan D. The role of plasminogen activator inhibitor type-1 in fibrosis. *Semin Thromb Hemost.* 2016;43(2):169–177.

Gu C, Zhang J, Noble NA, et al. An additive effect of anti-PAI-1 antibody to ACE inhibitor on the slowing the progression of diabetic kidney disease. *Am J Physiol Renal Physiol.* 2016;311:F852–F863.

Halachmi S, Pillar G. Congenital urological anomalies diagnosed in adulthood—management considerations. *J Pediatr Urol.* 2008;4: 2–7.

Hijmans RS, Rasmussen DG, Yazdani S, et al. Urinary collagen degradation products as early markers of progressive renal fibrosis. *J Transl Med.* 2017;15:63.

Jensen AM, Bae EH, Fenton RA, et al. Angiotensin II regulates V2 receptor and pAQP2 during ureteral obstruction. *Am J Physiol Renal Physiol.* 2009;296:F127–F134.

Jensen AM, Li C, Praetorius HA, et al. Angiotensin II mediates downregulation of aquaporin water channels and key renal sodium transporters in response to urinary tract obstruction. *Am J Physiol Renal Physiol.* 2006;291:F1021–F1032.

Kouba E, Wallen EM, Pruthi RS. Management of ureteral obstruction due to advanced malignancy: Optimizing therapeutic and palliative outcomes. *J Urol.* 2008;180:444–450.

Li C, Klein JD, Wang W, et al. Altered expression of urea transporters in response to ureteral obstruction. *Am J Physiol Renal Physiol.* 2004;286:F1154 -F1162.

McVary KT, Roehrborn CG, Avins AL, et al. Update on AUA guideline on the management of benign prostatic hyperplasia. *J Urol.* 2011;185:1793–1803.

Meng XM, Chung AC, Lan HY. Role of the TGF-B/BMP-7/Smad pathways in renal diseases. *Clin Sci.* 2013;124:243–254.

Mirone V, Imbimbo C, Longo N, et al. The detrusor muscle: An innocent victim of bladder outlet obstruction. *Eur Urol.* 2007;51:57–66.

Misseri R, Meldrum DR, Dinarello CA, et al. TNF-alpha mediates obstruction-induced renal tubular cell apoptosis and proapoptotic signaling. *Am J Physiol Renal Physiol.* 2005;288:F406–F411.

Sands JM. Critical role of urea in the urine-concentrating mechanism. *J Am Soc Nephrol.* 2007;18:670–671.

Sands JM, Layton HE. The physiology of urinary concentration: an update. *Semin Nephrol.* 2009;29:178–195.

Stødkilde L, Nørregaard R, Fenton RA, et al. Bilateral ureteral obstruction induces early downregulation and redistribution of AQP2 and phosphorylated AQP2. *Am J Physiol Renal Physiol.* 2011;301:F226–F235.

Wang Z, Famulski K, Lee J, et al. TIMP2 and TIMP3 have divergent roles in early renal tubulointerstitial injury. *Kidney Int.* 2014;85:82–93.

Wang G, Ring T, Li C, et al. Unilateral ureteral obstruction alters expression of acid-base transporters in rat kidney. *J Urol.* 2009;182:2964–2973.

Wolf G. Renal injury due to renin-angiotensin-aldosterone system activation of the transforming growth factor-beta pathway. *Kidney Int.* 2006;70:1914–1919.

Yao L, Wright MF, Farmer BC, et al. Fibroblast-specific plasminogen activator inhibitor-1 depletion ameliorates renal interstitial fibrosis after unilateral ureteral obstruction. *Nephrol Dial Transplant.* 2019;34:2042–2205.

45

Nephrolithiasis

ANJA PFAU, FELIX KNAUF

Epidemiology

The prevalence of nephrolithiasis in the US population rose from 3.8% in the late 1970s to 8.8% in the late 2000s, and it is estimated that more than 5 billion US dollars are spent on stone disease annually. Nephrolithiasis appears to be more common in non-Hispanic white populations than in black populations, and it is positively correlated with male sex, age, and obesity. School-aged children and adolescents are incrementally affected, and the prevalence increases with age in women at a greater rate than in men.

The risk of the first recurrent stone after the incident stone in untreated patients remains controversial. Early studies reported frequencies of stone recurrences ranging from 30%-50% at 5 years, yet the rate of stone recurrence might be underestimated when focusing on symptomatic stones requiring intervention. In a recent, multicenter, prospective cohort study, the risk to develop a recurrent stone by 5 years after a first episode was found to be 19% for symptomatic stones resulting in clinical care, but 67% when considering symptomatic, self-reported, and asymptomatic, radiographically detected stones. When assessing the risk for recurrence in an individual patient, the Recurrence of Kidney Stone (ROKS) nomogram might serve as a helpful tool in daily practice. Based on several clinical features (age, sex, family history, etc.), it estimates the risk of recurrence of symptomatic and asymptomatic nephrolithiasis 2, 5, and 10 years after the first event. Thus, patients can be identified who will most benefit from a complete metabolic workup and further dietary and medical interventions.

Nephrolithiasis as a Systemic Disease

During the last two decades, large epidemiologic studies have led to a shift in the perception of nephrolithiasis; it is no longer considered an isolated condition, but has been recognized as part of metabolic disorders such as metabolic syndrome and cardiovascular disease. Waist circumference, obesity, and weight gain have been shown to be independent risk factors for the development of kidney stones. This risk tends to be higher for women than for men. In parallel, nephrolithiasis and diabetes are reciprocally correlated; the diagnosis of nephrolithiasis increases the risk of future diabetes mellitus and, in turn, diabetes may favor formation of kidney stones, mainly uric acid and calcium oxalate stones. In addition, stone formers have a higher risk for developing incident hypertension, atherosclerosis, and coronary artery disease even after adjustment for typical cardiovascular risk factors. A history of nephrolithiasis predisposes to metabolic and hypertensive complications during pregnancy, such as preeclampsia. All these epidemiologic findings emphasize

the potential role of stone formation as part of a systemic metabolic disease and suggest that nephrolithiasis and cardiovascular disease share common risk factors or pathophysiologic pathways.

Furthermore, recurrent kidney stone formers are at a higher risk to develop chronic kidney disease (CKD) and end-stage kidney disease (ESKD). A large, retrospective survey of almost 7000 stone formers and 25,000 controls calculated the attributable risk of ESKD from symptomatic stone disease at 5.1% within the study population. As putative mechanisms, inflammation and ischemia caused by obstruction and increased intratubular pressure, chronic pyelonephritis, or papillary necrosis in the presence of large staghorn calculi are being discussed. Additionally, stone formers who develop ESKD are more likely to suffer from urologic comorbidities such as a solitary kidney or ileal conduit than nonstone formers with ESKD. Moreover, an elegant study has recently demonstrated that not only kidney stones but also higher urinary oxalate excretion in general are associated with progression of CKD.

Acute Renal Colic

With the passage of a stone from the kidney pelvis into the ureter resulting in partial or complete obstruction, there is sudden onset of unilateral flank pain of sufficient severity that the individual usually seeks medical attention. Despite the use of the misnomer "colic," the pain does not completely remit but rather waxes and wanes. Nausea and vomiting may accompany the pain. The pattern of pain depends on the location of the stone: if it is in the upper ureter, pain may radiate anteriorly to the abdomen; if it is in the lower ureter, pain may radiate to the ipsilateral testicle in men or labium in women; if it is lodged at the ureterovesical junction (UVJ), the primary symptoms may be urinary frequency and urgency. A less common acute presentation is gross hematuria without pain.

The symptoms from a ureteral stone may mimic those of several other acute conditions. A stone lodged in the right ureteropelvic junction can mimic acute cholecystitis. A stone lodged in the lower right ureter as it crosses the pelvic brim can mimic acute appendicitis. A stone lodged at the UVJ on either side can mimic acute cystitis. A stone lodged in the lower left ureter as it crosses the pelvic brim can mimic diverticulitis. An obstructing stone with proximal infection can mimic acute pyelonephritis. Note that infection in the setting of obstruction is a medical emergency ("pus under pressure") that requires emergent drainage by placement of a ureteral stent or a percutaneous nephrostomy tube. However, because nephrolithiasis is common, the simple presence of a stone in the kidney does not confirm the diagnosis of renal colic in a patient presenting with acute abdominal pain.

Other conditions to consider in the differential diagnosis of suspected renal colic include muscular or skeletal pain, herpes zoster, duodenal ulcer, abdominal aortic aneurysm, gynecologic causes, ureteral obstruction resulting from other intraluminal factors (e.g., blood clot, sloughed papilla), and ureteral stricture. Extraluminal factors causing compression tend not to result in a presentation with symptoms of renal colic.

The physical examination alone rarely allows for diagnosis, but clues guide the evaluation. The patient typically is in obvious pain and is unable to achieve a comfortable position. There may be ipsilateral costovertebral angle tenderness or, in cases of obstruction with infection, symptoms and signs of sepsis.

Although blood tests are typically normal, there may be a leukocytosis resulting from stress or infection. The GFR is typically normal, but it may be reduced in the setting of volume depletion, bilateral ureteral obstruction, or unilateral obstruction, particularly in a patient with a solitary functioning kidney. The urinalysis classically shows red blood cells and white blood cells, and occasionally crystals. If ureteral obstruction by the stone is complete, there may be no red blood cells because urine will not be flowing through that ureter into the bladder.

Because of the often nonspecific physical examination and laboratory findings, imaging studies play a crucial role in making the diagnosis. A recent study suggested that a kidney ultrasound can be used as the first imaging study in the emergency department (Fig. 45.1A). However, it should be noted that ultrasonography can image only the kidney and proximal ureter and might miss more distal or smaller stones (<5 mm). The imaging modality that provides the most detailed information is a noncontrast helical (spiral) computed tomography (CT), because it can detect stones as small as 1 mm. Even pure uric acid stones, traditionally considered "radiolucent," are identified. Typically, the study shows a ureteral stone or evidence of recent passage, such as perinephric stranding or hydronephrosis. Of note, many centers have implemented low-dose CT techniques (Fig. 45.1B), which still provide excellent sensitivity to detect stones, while reducing radiation exposure (<3 vs. 14 mSv with standard CT). A plain abdominal radiograph of the kidney, ureter, and bladder (KUB) might be helpful to monitor the progress of a known kidney stone, but due to its low sensitivity, its utility is limited, especially in acute settings. MRI allows imaging without radiation, and its sensitivity to detect stones is higher than that of ultrasonography, but less than that of CT scan. Its widespread use is prevented by high costs and the time-consuming imaging process. Yet, MRI might be useful as an additional diagnostic tool in pregnant patients if ultrasonography is inconclusive.

Renal colic is one of the most excruciating types of pain, and pain control is essential. Narcotics and parenteral nonsteroidal antiinflammatory drugs are effective, with the latter preferable because they cause fewer side effects. The majority of stones pass spontaneously, especially those smaller than 5 mm. As shown by a recent meta-analysis, administration of alpha blockers (e.g., tamsulosin 0.4 mg once daily) can effectively facilitate passage of stones 5-10 mm in diameter.

Types of Stones

Almost 90% of stones in first-time stone formers contain calcium, most commonly as calcium oxalate. Other types of stones, such as pure uric acid, cystine, and struvite, are much less common. However, these types of stones also deserve careful attention because recurrences are common.

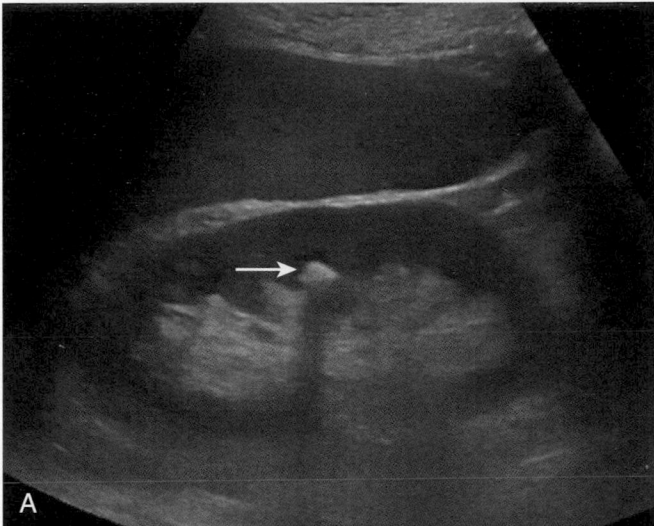

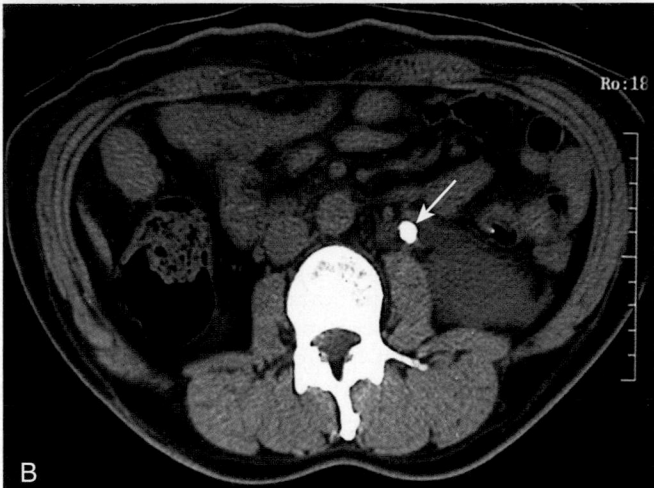

• **Fig. 45.1** (A) A kidney stone (*arrow*) revealed by ultrasound. Note echo shadow. (B) Non-contrast-enhanced CT scan shows a radiopaque obstructing stone (*arrow*) in the left ureter. (A courtesy Professor Thomas Fischer, Charité, Berlin.)

Pathogenesis

General Pathophysiology

The urinary concentrations of calcium, oxalate, and other solutes that influence stone formation are high enough that they should result in crystal formation in the urine of most individuals, but this is clearly not the case. This condition is termed *supersaturation*. Substances in the urine that prevent crystal formation are called *inhibitors*. The most clinically important inhibitor is citrate, which works by chelating calcium cations in the urine and decreasing the free calcium available to bind with oxalate or phosphate anions. If the supersaturation is sufficiently high or there are insufficient inhibitors, precipitation occurs with resulting crystalluria.

Calcium-based stones have a multifactorial etiology. Traditionally, stone formation was believed to occur from (1) crystal formation in the kidney tubule, followed by (2) attachment of the crystal to the tubular epithelium, usually at the tip of the papilla, and (3) growth of the attached crystal by deposition of additional crystalline material. However, it now appears that the initial event occurs when calcium phosphate deposits in the medullary interstitium. The calcium phosphate material may then erode through the papillary epithelium, upon which calcium oxalate is subsequently deposited.

The remainder of this chapter summarizes the role of urinary composition, nutrition and lifestyle, and other predisposing factors in regard to formation of calcium oxalate stones, except where noted.

Urinary Risk Factors

Urinary variables that increase the risk of calcium oxalate stone formation are higher concentrations of calcium and oxalate, whereas a higher concentration of citrate and a higher total urine volume decrease the risk, as illustrated in Fig. 45.2. Although higher urinary uric acid concentration had been postulated to increase the risk of calcium oxalate stone formation, larger studies were unable to confirm this finding.

The traditional approach to urinary abnormalities is based on 24-hour urinary excretion. The reference ranges for urinary factors vary by laboratory; this is because there are no universally accepted normal ranges. Commonly used definitions of "abnormal values" are presented in Table 45.1. Further treatment is directed at correcting the abnormalities identified in the 24-hour urine collections.

Although this approach has been used for decades, it has several limitations. Stone formation is a disease of concentration. Therefore, it is not just the absolute amount of substances that determines the likelihood of stone formation. The traditional definitions of "abnormal" excretion must be applied cautiously for several reasons. First, there are insufficient data supporting the cutoff points used regarding the risk of actual stone formation. For example, the traditional definition of hypercalciuria is 50 mg/day greater in men than in women, but there is no justification with respect to stone formation for having a higher upper limit of normal in men, particularly because the mean 24-hour urine volume is lower in men than in women. Similarly, another common definition of hypercalciuria is urinary calcium excretion in excess of 4 mg/kg of body weight per day. However, by this definition, an individual who is heavier or gains weight is "allowed" to excrete more calcium than someone who is thinner but still below the cutoff point. Second, an individual could have "normal" absolute excretion of calcium but still have a high urinary calcium concentration because of low urine volume. This situation has therapeutic implications, because the goal is to modify the concentration of the lithogenic factors. Finally, the risk of stone formation is a continuum, so the

TABLE 45.1	Commonly Used Definitions of "Abnormal" Values For Lithogenic and Protective Substances in a 24-Hour Urine Sample
Hypercalciuria	≥250 mg/day in women ≥300 mg/day in men
Hyperoxaluria	≥40 mg/day
Hypocitraturia	≤325 mg/day
Hyperuricosuria	≥750 mg in women, ≥800 mg in men
Urine volume	<2 L/day

use of a specific cutoff point may give the false impression that a patient with "high-normal" urinary calcium excretion is not at risk for stone recurrence.

The underlying mechanisms for idiopathic hypercalciuria remain unknown, although hormones and their receptors involved in calcium metabolism, such as 1,25-dihydroxyvitamin D and the vitamin D receptor, likely play contributing roles. The sources of the "excess" calcium in the urine are higher intestinal absorption and higher bone turnover. Hypercalciuria can also be caused by underlying medical conditions, such as primary para hyperparathyroidism or sarcoidosis, and by overdose of vitamin D or calcium-containing supplements.

Higher urinary oxalate concentrations may result from three different sources: high dietary oxalate intake, overabsorption of oxalate in the digestive tract due to an underlying gastrointestinal disorder of the small intestine (secondary or enteric hyperoxaluria [EH]), or increased endogenous production in the liver (primary hyperoxaluria [PH]). These entities will be discussed in more detail later in the chapter.

Purines are metabolized to uric acid. Increased urinary uric acid is the result of higher purine intake and higher endogenous production from purine turnover. In the steady state, urine uric acid excretion is dependent on uric acid generation; thus, the serum uric acid level does not provide any information about 24-hour urine uric acid excretion.

Low urine citrate levels are typically seen in the setting of a systemic metabolic acidosis, such as renal tubular acidoses or excessive gastrointestinal alkali losses from diarrhea. Because citrate is a potential source of bicarbonate, it is actively reclaimed in the proximal tubule after being filtered by the glomerulus.

Dietary Factors

Dietary variables associated with lower risk of incident stone formation include higher dietary intakes of calcium, potassium, and fluid; those associated with higher risk include higher intakes of supplemental calcium, oxalate, animal protein, sodium, and sucrose. Data from observational and randomized, controlled studies support the concept that dietary calcium intake is *inversely* associated with risk of stone formation. The mechanism by which dietary calcium may reduce the risk of stone formation is unknown, but it may involve calcium binding to oxalate in the intestine, reducing oxalate absorption.

Differences in timing of ingestion may explain the apparent contradiction between the protective effect of dietary calcium and the detrimental effect of supplemental calcium. Most people do not consume their calcium supplement with meals containing oxalate; thus, the observed higher risk might rather be a result of increased urinary calcium excretion without any change in urinary oxalate excretion.

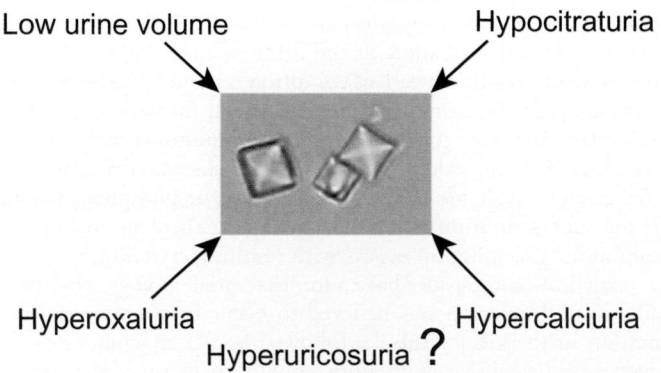

Low urine volume   Hypocitraturia

Hyperoxaluria   Hypercalciuria

Hyperuricosuria ?

• **Fig. 45.2** Urinary risk factors that increase the risk of calcium oxalate stone formation. Calcium oxalate (dihydrate) crystals are shown in the middle.

Many foods contain oxalate, so considerable quantities of oxalate are ingested every day on a standard Western diet, which limits practical implementation of a low-oxalate diet. Table 45.2 provides an overview of foods known to be high in oxalate. However, only 10%-15% of dietary oxalate is absorbed in a healthy gut. Intestinal oxalate absorption can be increased in the setting of an underlying gastrointestinal disorder (enteric hyperoxaluria) or when foods high in oxalate, such as spinach, rhubarb, or beetroot are consumed while maintaining a low calcium diet (dietary hyperoxaluria).

Nondietary Factors

Nondietary factors that increase the risk for kidney stone formation include anatomic genitourinary abnormalities or medical conditions, such as medullary sponge kidney. The latter is a malformative disorder that leads to collecting duct dilatation and is commonly accompanied by hypercalciuria and hypocitraturia. Diabetes mellitus and insulin resistance are associated with hypocitraturia and low urinary pH due to defective ammonium excretion, which favors the formation of uric acid stones. Additionally, diabetes mellitus and obesity are linked to formation of calcium oxalate stones via hyperoxaluria; several mechanisms are currently being discussed, one of them being inflammation-mediated oxalate overabsorption in the gut or altered gastrointestinal oxalate metabolism. The gut-kidney axis is receiving increased attention in the context of kidney stone disease. Disruption of the microbiome and loss of certain bacterial strains in the gut, for example, oxalate-degrading microorganisms, might change the release or production of intestinal metabolites and subsequently induce imbalances in urine composition that favor stone formation, as illustrated in Fig. 45.3. Antibiotics also disturb the microbiome of the gut, which may explain the association between oral antibiotic exposure and an increased risk for nephrolithiasis, as

recently described by several epidemiologic studies. This risk was highest for recent exposure and for exposure at a younger age. Such findings support the hypothesis that the high prescription rate of antibiotics in industrialized countries might also contribute to the increasing prevalence of nephrolithiasis.

Intake of certain drugs can also predispose to nephrolithiasis by either direct crystallization (aztanavir, indinavir, acyclovir, sulfadiazine, methotrexate, triamterene) or by causing alterations in urinary pH (topiramate, acetazolamide, zonisamide).

Clinical Evaluation

There is disagreement in the literature regarding the extent of clinical evaluation necessary of a first-time kidney stone. There is a general consensus that the evaluation of all stone patients should comprise a careful medical, dietary, and family history, including assessment of the total stone burden, residual stones, prior episodes indicating spontaneous stone passage, presence of systemic diseases, and lifestyle habits. Urinalysis and urine sediment evaluation should be performed. An extended metabolic work-up including a serum chemistry panel and identification of urinary risk factors in 24-hour urine collections is recommended for recurrent stone formers and for those presenting with a first stone event who are at high risk for recurrence. The ROKS nomogram might help to identify such high-risk patients. Further, complete evaluation after a first episode should be considered if the patient suffers from unexplained CKD or has a single kidney, for example, after kidney transplantation. Table 45.3 summarizes an approach when evaluating an individual with kidney stones in daily practice.

After having experienced acute renal colic, a patient may attribute a variety of types of chronic back or flank pain to the kidney or to a residual stone. Further questioning may uncover other causes, particularly musculoskeletal. The physical examination may show findings of systemic conditions associated with stone formation, but these signs are uncommon.

Metabolic Evaluation

Retrieval of the stone for chemical analysis is an often overlooked but essential part of the evaluation because treatment recommendations vary by stone type. Urinalysis, comprising a dipstick and urine sediment evaluation, is easy to obtain and cost effective; it can reveal an underlying infection or pathognomonic crystal (e.g., cystine) while also providing urine pH. Similarly, calculi should be submitted for analysis to establish a diagnosis (stone type) and to direct further treatment.

If a metabolic evaluation is pursued, it is identical for first-time and recurrent stone formers. Serum chemistry values that should be measured include electrolytes, kidney function biomarkers, a venous blood gas analysis, and calcium and phosphorus concentrations. The decision to measure parathyroid hormone or vitamin D concentrations is based on the results of serum and urine chemistries. If the patient has high serum calcium, low serum phosphorus, or high urine calcium, then a parathyroid hormone level should be measured. The cornerstone of the evaluation is the 24-hour urine collection. Two 24-hour urine collections should

TABLE 45.2	Oxalate Content of Common Foods High in Oxalate	
Food Item	Serving Size	Oxalate Content (mg)
Spinach, raw	1 cup	656
Rhubarb	½ cup	541
Almonds	1 oz or 22 nuts	122
Miso soup	1 cup	111
Baked potato with skin	1 medium	97
Corn grits	1 cup	97
Beets	½ cup	76
Cocoa powder	4 tsp.	67
French fries	4 oz or ½ cup	51
Cashews	1 oz or 18 nuts	49
Raspberries	1 cup	48
Mixed nuts (with peanuts)	1 oz	39
Potato chips	1 oz	21

Source: https://regepi.bwh.harvard.edu/health/Oxalate/files.

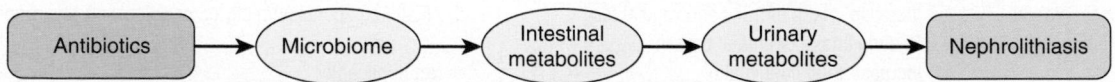

• **Fig. 45.3** Use of antibiotics and the risk of nephrolithiasis are linked via disruption of the microbiome. (Adapted from Tasian G, Miller A, Lange D. Antibiotics and kidney stones: perturbation of the gut-kidney axis. *Am J Kidney Dis.* 2019;74(6):724-726.)

TABLE 45.3   Suggested Stepwise Approach of Metabolic Work-Up in a Patient With Nephrolithiasis

Clinical Situation	Extent of Work-Up
First kidney stone and low risk for recurrence	Complete medical history (risk factors, family history, underlying/concomitant diseases, medications) + Stone analysis + Urinalysis (dipstick including pH, urine sediment)
Recurrent kidney stones + first kidney stone, but moderate or high risk for recurrence or single kidney (e.g., transplant) or patient's preference	Work-up as described above + Serum panel: creatinine, sodium, potassium, chloride, calcium, phosphate, magnesium, uric acid, venous blood gas analysis; if indicated, also PTH, 25-hydroxyvitamin D, and 1,25-dihydroxyvitamin D3 + 24-hr urine (at least two samples): volume, pH, creatinine, sodium, potassium, calcium, oxalate, uric acid, citrate, phosphorus (cystine)

Adapted from Pfau/Knauf, AJKD, 2016

be performed while the patient is consuming his or her usual diet. Because individuals often change their dietary habits soon after an episode of renal colic, a patient should wait at least 6 weeks before carrying out the collections. Two collections are needed because there can be substantial day-to-day variability in the values.

The critical variables that should be measured in the 24-hour urine collections are total volume, calcium, oxalate, citrate, uric acid, sodium, potassium, phosphorus, pH, and creatinine. Some laboratories calculate the relative supersaturation from measurements of the urine factors, which can be used to gauge the impact of therapy.

Medical Treatments

Because stones can remain asymptomatic for years, the actual time of formation of the stone that brought the patient to medical attention is usually unknown. The current metabolic evaluation may, in fact, be completely normal, with no changes to lifestyle needed. Whether the patient is an active stone former influences the decision to treat. The likelihood of recurrence can be estimated but not definitely predicted from the urine chemistry results; a repeat imaging study 1 year later helps determine whether the patient is an active stone former. For patients who are at risk for stone recurrence, lifestyle modification should be attempted first, tailoring the recommendation according to stone type and urine chemistry findings. Lifelong changes are needed to prevent recurrence of this chronic condition. Table 45.4 summarizes the cornerstones of dietary and pharmacologic treatment options of calcium nephrolithiasis based on the urinary abnormalities as obtained during metabolic evaluation.

Dietary Recommendations

The most important measure to prevent kidney stone formation is increased fluid intake with the goal of producing more than 2 L of urine daily. The choice of beverage should be made carefully; sugar-added soft drinks should be avoided as they exert counterproductive effects on stone formation. Additional recommendations include a reduced intake of sodium and animal protein, and instead a diet high in fruits and vegetables (Mediterranean diet). Accordingly, a study on a cohort of more than 16,000 individuals demonstrated that a Mediterranean diet was not only associated with a reduced risk for major cardiovascular events, but also a lower incidence of nephrolithiasis. There is no evidence that dietary calcium restriction is helpful in preventing stone formation. In contrast, a low-calcium diet can increase the risk for calcium oxalate stones as calcium chelates oxalate in the digestive tract and thus can reduce

TABLE 45.4   Dietary and Pharmacologic Treatments to Prevent Calcium Nephrolithiasis, According to Urinary Abnormality

Urinary Abnormality	Dietary Changes	Medication
High calcium concentration	Avoid excessive intake of calcium supplements Maintain adequate dietary calcium intake Reduce intake of animal protein Reduce sodium intake to less than 3 g/day Reduce sucrose intake	Thiazide diuretic
High oxalate concentration	Avoid high-oxalate foods	Pyridoxine, cholestyramine, calcium- or magnesium-containing supplements, if underlying PH or EH
	Maintain adequate dietary calcium intake	—
	Avoid vitamin C supplements	—
High uric acid concentration	Reduce purine intake (i.e., meat, chicken, fish)	Xanthine oxidase inhibitor
Low citrate concentration	Increase intake of fruits and vegetables Reduce intake of animal protein	Alkali (e.g., potassium citrate or potassium bicarbonate)
Low volume	Increase total fluid intake	Not applicable

PH, primary hyperoxaluria; EH, enteric hyperoxaluria.

oxalate absorption from the gut and, subsequently, oxaluria. Further, a low-calcium diet is known to have negative implications on bone health. However, as discussed previously, supplemental but not dietary calcium may increase the risk of kidney stone formation. In someone who has never had a kidney stone, the risk attributable to supplemental calcium is low. For a patient who has had a calcium-containing stone and wishes to continue taking the supplement, 24-hour urine chemistry values should be measured while the patient is taking and not taking the supplement; if the urine calcium is higher while taking the supplement, then it should be discontinued.

For patients with an elevated urine oxalate level, a careful dietary history should be obtained. The benefit of a very low-oxalate diet is less clear because of the previously addressed issues regarding the oxalate content of food; however, spinach and rhubarb should be avoided and intake of nuts moderated. In patients suffering from EH due to oxalate overabsorption in the gut, recommendations are more concrete: diet should be low in oxalate and fat, but high in calcium to reduce gastrointestinal oxalate absorption. In addition, vitamin C supplementation should be avoided since higher vitamin C intake increases urine oxalate excretion.

Pharmacologic Options

The use of medication is indicated if dietary recommendations are unsuccessful in adequately modifying the urine composition. The three most commonly used classes of medications for prevention of calcium-containing kidney stones are (1) thiazide diuretics (e.g., hydrochlorothiazide or chlorthalidone), which reduce urinary calcium excretion; (2) alkalis (e.g., potassium citrate or bicarbonate), which increase urinary citrate excretion; and (3) xanthine oxidase inhibitors (e.g., allopurinol), which reduce urinary uric acid excretion.

For patients who have elevated urinary calcium levels but do not have excessive calcium intake (i.e., <1500 mg/day), a thiazide diuretic has been demonstrated to reduce the likelihood of stone recurrence and to help maintain bone density. Randomized trials of at least 3 years' duration have consistently shown a 50% reduction in the risk of recurrence with thiazide treatment. Yet, the dosages that were implemented in these studies to reduce urinary calcium adequately were higher than those typically used for treatment of hypertension (e.g., hydrochlorothiazide 50 mg or chlorthalidone 25 mg), which might constrain long-term therapeutic management because of side effects, such as low blood pressure or electrolyte disturbances at such doses. In order to clarify which thiazide dosage serves stone patients best, a prospective, randomized, placebo-controlled, multicenter study is being conducted in Europe to compare the effectiveness of different dosages of hydrochlorothiazide (50 vs. 25 vs. 12.5 mg) on risk reduction for calcium nephrolithiasis (NOSTONE trial). Results are expected in 2022. When utilizing thiazides, adequate sodium restriction (<3 g/day) is necessary to achieve maximum benefit; a higher sodium intake leads to greater distal calcium delivery and minimizes or negates the beneficial effect of the thiazide diuretics. For patients who are unable to increase their fluid intake, a thiazide diuretic may be helpful even if the total urine calcium excretion is not high because it will reduce the urinary calcium excretion and, thus, the calcium concentration. In addition, a thiazide diuretic may be more readily prescribed if there is evidence of low bone density.

For patients with low urine citrate levels, any form of alkali will increase urinary citrate excretion. However, citrate is usually the first choice because it is better tolerated than bicarbonate. Potassium salts are preferred to sodium salts because of the potential effect on urinary calcium excretion. The alkali preparations must be taken at least twice daily to maintain adequate citrate levels in the urine. Randomized trials suggest a greater than 50% reduction in risk of recurrence with alkali supplementation.

In one randomized trial, allopurinol reduced the recurrence rate by 50% among individuals with a history of recurrent calcium oxalate stones and isolated high urine uric acid. Given the epidemiologic observation that higher urine uric acid levels do not increase a person's likelihood of being a stone former, it is unclear whether the benefit was caused by the reduction in urine uric acid concentration or by some other mechanism.

Hyperoxaluria-Related Disorders and Systemic Oxalosis

Two rare conditions, primary and enteric (secondary) hyperoxaluria, can cause excessive oxaluria with a high risk of stone recurrence and nephrocalcinosis, resulting in progressive oxalate nephropathy and ESKD. Fig. 45.4 gives an overview over the pathophysiologic mechanisms of both entities. PH is a very rare genetic disease with an autosomal recessive inheritance pattern. Three different subtypes of PH have been described so far, based on the three responsible genes, all of them affecting glyoxylate metabolism and, thus, leading to oxalate overproduction in the liver. PH 1 is the most common (~80% of all PH cases) and most severe subtype with early onset and the highest rate for ESKD. In contrast, EH is caused by oxalate overabsorption in the gut and, therefore, associated with short bowel syndrome, bariatric surgery, Crohn disease, and other malabsorptive disorders in which the colon is intact. With resulting fat malabsorption, calcium is bound in the small bowel to free fatty acids, leaving a lesser amount of free calcium to bind to oxalate. Unabsorbed fatty acids and bile salts further increase the colonic permeability for oxalate. Both mechanisms enhance oxalate absorption in the gastrointestinal tract, which results in hyperoxaluria. Additionally, these patients often lose a significant amount of fluid and alkali from the gastrointestinal tract, so the accompanying low

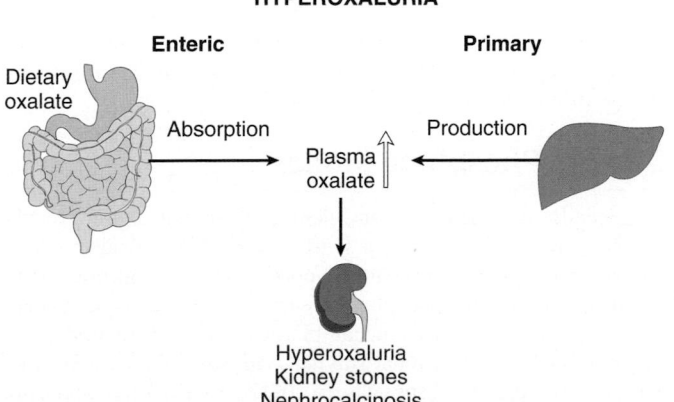

HYPEROXALURIA

• **Fig. 45.4** Pathophysiologic mechanisms in primary (PH) and enteric (EH) hyperoxaluria. Excessive oxaluria can be caused by genetically determined overproduction in the liver (PH) or by overabsorption in the colon due to an underlying gastrointestinal disorder (EH). (Adapted from Ermer T, Eckardt KU, Aronson PS, Knauf F. Oxalate, inflammasome, and progression of kidney disease. *Curr Opin Nephrol Hypertens.* 2016;25:363.)

urine volume presents an additional risk factor. Further, intestinal citrate absorption is increased by metabolic acidosis due to alkali loss, leaving less urinary citrate to serve as a calcium chelator.

In both settings, PH and EH, disease progression and development of CKD have fatal consequences; as GFR declines, urinary oxalate elimination decreases and plasma oxalate concentrations rise. Subsequently, the plasma may be supersaturated and oxalate may deposit in various tissues throughout the body, including the heart, skin, eyes, and joints. This adverse state—termed *systemic oxalosis*—is a life-threatening condition that can already affect patients at young ages. In PH, combined liver-kidney transplantation is the only curative treatment option. As the underlying gastrointestinal disorder in EH is usually a chronic condition and, thus, not completely reversible, EH patients have a high (almost 100%) risk of recurrence after kidney transplantation.

It is, therefore, mandatory to identify individuals with EH and PH from the large pool of patients with a history of calcium oxalate nephrolithiasis to optimize the therapeutic strategy as early as possible and, thus, to improve long-term prognosis.

Until recently, therapeutic possibilities of PH and EH have been restricted despite the often devastating course of disease. Besides citrate supplementation, use of high-dose pyridoxine, a coenzyme of alanine-glyoxylate-aminotransferase, the gene product affected in PH 1, can help to reduce urinary oxalate excretion in 10%-30% of patients with PH 1 (but not PH 2 or 3). For the community of PH patients, it is a great advance that several new treatment options are currently being tested in clinical trials. These strategies include the use of Oxalobacter formigenes, an oxalate-degrading microorganism in the gut, and the implementation of RNA interference (RNAi) therapeutics, which also target oxalate production in the liver by depleting the substrate for oxalate production Lumasiran, one of those RNAi therapeutics, was granted approval by the Food and Drug Administration (FDA) in November 2020, and is now freely available outside of clinical trials..

In EH, citrate supplementation and strict adherence to a diet low in oxalate and fat, but high in calcium, are the cornerstones of therapy. Additionally, intake of calcium or magnesium supplements with meals and—if indicated by the treating gastroenterologist—prescription of bile acid sequestrants (cholestyramine) might lower the extent of gastrointestinal oxalate absorption. However, the total effect of these measures on oxalate load often remains limited in EH, and improvement in therapeutic options is warranted. Oxalate-degrading enzymes as naturally expressed in the bacterium Oxalobacter formigenes are such a promising therapeutic target and currently under investigation.

Calcium Phosphate Stones

In general, the formation of calcium phosphate stones is triggered by the same risk factors as those for calcium oxalate stones, for example, hypercalciuria and hypocitraturia. In contrast, calculi composed of calcium phosphate preferably grow at higher urinary pH (>6.5) and frequently occur in the setting of an underlying disorder, such as distal renal tubular acidosis (dRTA) or primary hyperparathyroidism. Especially in dRTA, marked hypocitraturia might also be present, which makes therapy of calcium phosphate nephrolithiasis challenging. Alkali supplementation increases urinary citrate, but also urinary pH, which is already high. Thus, in this setting, alkali therapy should be stepwise and cautiously titrated to prevent an increase of urinary pH > 7. Further therapeutic measures include implementation of thiazide diuretics to reduce urinary

calcium excretion and treatment of potential underlying disease such as Sjögren syndrome, which is often accompanied by dRTA.

Noncalcium Stones

Uric Acid Stones

Persistently low urine pH is the major driver of uric acid crystal formation. Hence, diabetes mellitus, insulin resistance, and a higher intake of nondairy animal protein are associated with an increased risk of uric acid stone formation. Increased intake of fruits and vegetables, which are high in potential alkali, may raise the urine pH and reduce the risk of uric acid crystal formation.

Alkali supplementation is the most effective treatment of existing uric acid stones. If the urine pH is maintained at 6.5 or higher (which often requires 90 to 120 mEq of supplemental alkali per day), pure uric acid stones will dissolve. Slightly lower doses may be used to prevent new uric acid stone formation. A xanthine oxidase inhibitor is the second-line choice if the patient has marked hyperuricosuria or is unable to maintain a urine pH higher than 6.5.

Cystine Stones

Calculi composed of cystine only form in individuals with the autosomal recessive disorder of cystinuria and are found in 1%-2% of all stone formers, with a higher percentage (5%) among children. A defective transporter in the proximal tubule leads to reduced absorption of dibasic amino acids and urinary wasting of cystine, ornithine, lysine, and arginine (COLA amino acids). Yet only cystine causes stone disease due to its low solubility. Genetic testing is not mandatory, as the evidence of cystine stones and/or the detection of hexagonal-shaped cystine crystals in the urine sediment are sufficient to diagnose cystinuria (Fig. 45.5). A high fluid intake is recommended to increase urine volume to 3-4 L/day, including intake prior to sleep. As solubility of cystine improves at higher pH, constant maintenance of the urinary pH above 7 protects against cystine stones without affecting total cystine excretion. To reach this goal, relatively high dosages of potassium citrate (up to

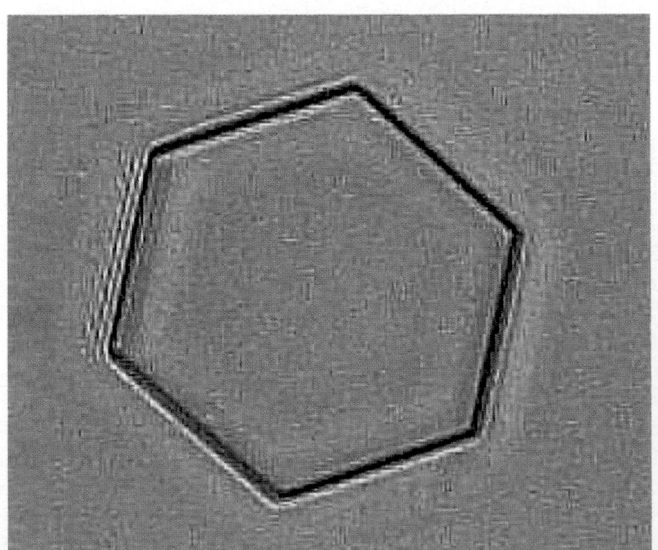

• **Fig. 45.5** Cystine crystal in urine sediment. The typical hexagonal shape is pathognomonic, i.e., identification of a typical cystine crystal allows diagnosis of cystinuria.

3-4 mEq/kg/day if necessary) divided into 3-4 doses are commonly needed. Patients should be further advised to restrict intake of salt, as sodium enhances cystine excretion. Protein intake should also be moderated (0.8-1 g/kg).

If conservative measures fail to reduce the severity of cystine stone disease, medications such as tiopronin and penicillamine might be administered to increase the solubility (but not the total amount) of the filtered cystine. Tiopronin is commonly preferred due to its more favorable side effect profile.

Struvite Stones

Because struvite stones form only in the setting of an infection with urease-producing bacteria in the upper urinary tract, it is unlikely that dietary factors can directly influence struvite stone formation. Instead, recurrent urinary tract infections and predisposing conditions such as a neurogenic bladder, voiding dysfunction, and presence of urinary catheters promote the risk of struvite stone formation, which is based on a unique pathophysiologic mechanism. Urease-producing gram-negative bacteria (*Proteus* spp., *Klebsiella* spp., etc.) metabolize urea in the urine to bicarbonate and ammonium. Subsequently, struvite stones form in the presence of a very high urinary pH (>7) and usually contain magnesium-ammonium-phosphate (struvite). Struvite stones are almost always large and may fill the kidney pelvis, referred to as "staghorn calculi"; complete removal and antibiotic eradication therapy are the cornerstones in the treatment of struvite calculi. As the rate of recurrence is high, urine cultures should be obtained and the choice of the antibiotic regimen should be made in accordance with the resistance pattern of the pathogenic microorganism. Acetohydroxamic acid is the only drug available that inhibits urease; however, it should be used with extreme caution because of its common and serious side effects.

Surgical Management of Stones

In the acute setting, the urologist may assist in the management of kidney stones. If the stone is ≤ 10 mm and does not pass rapidly, the patient can be sent home with appropriate oral analgesics, an alpha-blocker (e.g., tamsulosin 0.4 mg once daily) to increase the likelihood of stone passage, and instructions to return in case of fever or uncontrollable pain. Thus, urologic intervention can be postponed up to 4–6 weeks, except in conditions of sepsis and urinary tract infection, stone size greater than 10 mm, presence of an anatomic abnormality that would prevent passage, acute kidney injury due to obstruction, or intractable pain. Treatment modalities include extracorporeal shockwave lithotripsy (ESWL), ureteroscopy (URS), and percutaneous nephrolithotomy (PNL). More invasive, open techniques are rarely needed. The method of stone removal is determined by stone size, location, stone composition, urinary tract anatomy, the experience of the urologist, and patient's preference. For stones <2 cm in size, ESWL and URS are feasible options. If stone size exceeds 2 cm, PNL, a more invasive approach requiring the placement of a nephrostomy tube, is often unavoidable.

While ESWL is less invasive than other approaches, potential complications include renal colic as a result of a stone fragment entering the ureter, injury to the kidney parenchyma, perirenal hematoma, and possibly a slightly higher risk of hypertension. Furthermore, ESWL should not be used in emergent circumstances, such as urosepsis, and is often ineffective for stones composed of brushite or cystine. URS should be used as first-line therapy in the setting of uncorrected bleeding diatheses or when anticoagulation/antiplatelet therapy cannot be discontinued.

With the increasing prevalence of obesity in the United States, the treatment of existing stones in morbidly obese individuals deserves mention. The ability to image the urinary tract may be limited if the patient's size prohibits access to scanning by CT. ESWL may not be an option, as morbid obesity can interfere with stone localization and the ability of the shock waves to reach the calculus. In those patients, ESWL and PNL have lower success rates, and URS remains the most promising therapeutic approach.

Long-Term Follow-Up

The nephrologist or primary care provider should assume responsibility for the long-term prevention program and should consult with the urologist as needed for further surgical interventions. The plan should include recommendations for prevention based on the evaluation; interventions should be followed by repeat metabolic measurements to assess their success, adjustment of recommendations, and follow-up imaging.

Adherence to recommendations frequently declines with time. In addition, the long-term sequelae of the treatments and the underlying abnormalities may have other implications for the health of the patient. For example, individuals with higher urine calcium excretion typically have lower bone density and are at increased risk for osteoporosis. With appropriate attention and evaluation, the morbidity and cost of recurrent stone disease can be dramatically reduced.

Acknowledgment

We thank Megan Prochaska and Gary C. Curhan for their contributions to the "Nephrolithiasis" chapter of the previous edition.

Bibliography

Asplin JR. The management of patients with enteric hyperoxaluria. *Urolithiasis*. 2016;44(1):33–43.

Brisbane W, Bailey MR, Sorensen MD. An overview of kidney stone imaging techniques. *Nat Rev Urol*. 2016;13(11):654–662.

Cui Y, Chen J, Zeng F, et al. Tamsulosin as a medical expulsive therapy for ureteral stones: A systematic review and meta-analysis of randomized controlled trials. *J Urol*. 2019;201(5):950–955.

Dhondup T, Kittanamongkolchai W, Rule AD, et al. Risk of ESRD and mortality in kidney and bladder stone formers. *Am J Kidney Dis*. 2018;72(6):790–797.

Ferraro PM, Bargagli M, Trinchieri A, Gambaro G. Risk of kidney stones: influence of dietary factors, dietary patterns, and vegetarian-vegan diets. *Nutrients*. 2020;12(3):779.

Pearle MS, Goldfarb DS, Assimos DG, White JR. American Urological Association. Medical management of kidney stones: AUA guideline. *J Urol*. 2014;192(2):316–324.

Pfau A, Knauf F. Update on nephrolithiasis: Core Curriculum 2016. *Am J Kidney Dis*. 2016;68(6):973–985.

Rule AD, Lieske JC, Li X, Melton LJ 3rd, Krambeck AE, Bergstralh EJ. The ROKS nomogram for predicting a second symptomatic stone episode. *J Am Soc Nephrol*. 2014;25(12):2878–2886.

Rule AD, Lieske JC, Pais VM Jr. Management of kidney stones in 2020. *JAMA*. 2020;323(19):1961–1962.

Rule AD, Roger VL, Lieske JC. Kidney stones associate with increased risk for myocardial infarction. *J Am Soc Nephrol*. 2010;21(10):1641–1644.

Shoag J, Tasian G, Goldfarb DS, Eisner B. The new epidemiology of nephrolithiasis. *Adv Chronic Kidney Dis*. 2015;22(4):273–278.

Smith-Bindman R, Aubin C, Cummings SR, et al. Ultrasonography versus computed tomography for suspected nephrolithiasis. *N Engl J Med*. 2014;371(12):1100–1110.

Tangren JS, Powe CE, Thadhani R, et al. Metabolic and hypertensive complications of pregnancy in women with nephrolithiasis. *Clin J Am Soc Nephrol*. 2018;13(4):612–619.

Tasian GE, Jemielita T, Goldfarb DS, et al. Oral antibiotic exposure and kidney stone disease. *JASN*. 2018;29(6):1731–1740.

Taylor EN, Stampfer MJ, Curhan GC. Diabetes mellitus and the risk of nephrolithiasis. *Kidney Int*. 2005;68(3):1230–1235.

Waikar SS, Srivastava A, Palsson R, et al. Association of urinary oxalate excretion with the risk of chronic kidney disease progression. *JAMA Intern Med*. 2019;179(4):542–551.

Weigert A, Martin-Higueras C, Hoppe B. Novel therapeutic approaches in primary hyperoxaluria. *Expert Opin Emerg Drugs*. 2018;23(4):349–357.

PART 9

Special Circumstances

46

Kidney Diseases in Infants and Children

DARCY K. WEIDEMANN, BRADLEY A. WARADY

Kidney Development and Maturation

Nephrogenesis begins in utero at approximately 5 to 6 weeks' gestation and continues until nephron formation is complete at approximately 35 weeks' gestation, although significant functional changes continue in the postnatal period. Fetal urine production commences prior to the end of the first trimester, and by the third trimester becomes the primary component of the amniotic fluid, which is essential for normal pulmonary development. Although the full-term newborn has the same number of nephrons per kidney as an adult (approximately 1 million), the glomeruli and tubules of the infant kidney are relatively immature. Key molecular transcription factors involved with kidney embryogenesis include the Wilms tumor suppressor gene 1 (WT1), fibroblast growth factor 2 (FGF2), vascular endothelial growth factor (VEGF), bone morphogenetic protein 7 (Bmp7), paired-box gene 2 (pax2), and wingless-related (WNT4).

The GFR of a newborn is only around 20 mL/min/1.73 m^2 in the first few days after birth, rising to approximately 40 mL/min/1.73 m^2 near the end of the first week of life, and gradually reaching adult levels of 100 to 130 mL/min/1.73 m^2 by 2 years of age. The changes in GFR that occur after birth are the result of increased cardiac output and mean arterial blood pressure, a decrease in renal vascular resistance, and an increased surface area available for glomerular filtration. Renal blood flow is only 3%–7% of the cardiac output in the fetus, eventually increasing to 25% of cardiac output by 2 years old. Concomitantly, blood flow is redistributed from the cortical-juxtamedullary glomeruli, which are larger but fewer in number than the more numerous glomeruli in the cortex.

In term neonates, the low GFR results in a serum creatinine (sCr) level that reflects the maternal serum creatinine value for the first 24 to 48 hours of life and gradually settles to approximately 0.4 mg/dL at the fifth to seventh day of life. The GFR in preterm infants is significantly lower than in term infants (Table 46.1). The full-term newborn kidney measures 4 to 5 cm in length and continues to grow until reaching 10 to 12 cm by adolescence. Although the glomeruli do grow in size, most of this renal parenchymal expansion results from tubular growth and maturation and from an increased volume of the tubulointerstitial compartment.

The neonatal renal tubules have a limited ability to concentrate or dilute the urine in response to different environmental or dietary conditions. Growing term infants maintain a positive sodium balance; in contrast, preterm infants tend to have a negative sodium balance in the first few weeks after birth due to immature reabsorption capacity in the distal tubules and intestines, and

they require 3–5 mEq of sodium/kg/day for the first several weeks of life. The fractional excretion of sodium (FeNa) is highest during the first week of life, decreasing to adult ranges of <0.4% by 1 month of age. Additionally, the ability of the neonatal proximal tubule to reabsorb filtered HCO_3^- is less than that of adults. As a result, the average serum HCO_3^- concentration in preterm infants (16 to 20 mEq/L) is lower than in term infants (19 to 21 mEq/L) and older children and adults (24 to 28 mEq/L). Newborns also often have higher serum potassium concentrations (6.5 to 7.0 mEq/L) than older children as a result of a decreased glomerular filtration rate (GFR) and a relative insensitivity of the neonatal tubule to aldosterone.

Acute Kidney Injury

Introduction

Information specifically pertaining to pediatric acute kidney injury (AKI) is included in this section; AKI is covered in greater detail in Chapter 31. Despite its widespread use, serum creatinine is a poor marker of kidney function, particularly in the setting of pediatric AKI, as a consequence of its variability due to the influence of age, gender, body habitus, and nutritional status on the level. The use of serum creatinine as a biomarker reflective of kidney function remains particularly challenging in the setting of neonatal AKI, due to the dynamic nature of serum creatinine as a result of physiological changes and the higher prevalence of AKI due to nephrotoxic drug exposures, which tend to manifest as changes in urine output before changes in serum creatinine occur. An ongoing area of research is the study of novel biomarkers useful in the prediction of AKI.

Diagnosis

Substantial variability exists in the reported incidence, morbidity, and mortality estimates for pediatric AKI due to the use of multiple definitions. Significant effort has been made to standardize and validate pediatric AKI consensus definitions, and the most widely used are the Pediatric Risk, Injury, Failure, Loss and End-stage Renal Disease (pRIFLE) and the Kidney Disease: Improving Global Outcomes (KDIGO) consensus classifications (Table 46.2). The RIFLE criteria were developed in 2004 in critically ill adults. RIFLE classifies AKI into five distinct categories based upon the magnitude and direction of change in creatinine, urine output, and duration of kidney replacement therapy (KRT). This classification system was subsequently modified for the pediatric population (pRIFLE) by

<table>
<tr><td colspan="2">

TABLE 46.1 Normal GFR in Premature and Full-Term Neonates, Children, and Adolescents

</td></tr>
</table>

Age	Mean GFR ± SD (mL/min/1.73 m²)
1 week old	Preterm: 15 ± 6 Term: 41 ± 15
2–8 weeks old	Term: 66 ± 25 Preterm: 28.7 ± 14
>8 weeks old	Term: 96 ± 22 Preterm: 51.4 ± 16
2–12 years old	133 ± 27
13–21 years old	Male: 140 ± 30 Female: 126 ± 22

Preterm includes 29–34 WGA (weeks gestational age).
Adapted from Denis F. Geary DF, Schaefer F. *Comprehensive Pediatric Nephrology.* Philadelphia, Elsevier, 2008.

the use of an estimated creatinine clearance based on the original Schwartz formula to quantify the change in GFR (rather than absolute changes in serum creatinine used in the adult version). Notably, the original Schwartz formula was derived based on serum creatinine assayed using the modified Jaffe method rather than the preferred enzymatic methodology, and this definition may also be problematic if a baseline creatinine clearance is unknown. In addition, all children with an estimated creatinine clearance less than 35 mL/min/1.73 m² are placed in the "pRIFLE-F" category (kidney failure class) instead of waiting for the serum creatinine concentration to reach 4 mg/dL, as in adults.

The 2012 KDIGO AKI Consensus Conference definition is recommended for the definition and staging of pediatric AKI and to guide clinical care. The KDIGO definition includes a 0.3 mg/dL

increase in serum creatinine over 48 hours or a urine volume ≤0.5 mg/kg/hr for 6 hours. The diagnostic inclusion criteria of a serum creatinine elevation ≥1.5 times baseline within the prior 7 days allows for the inclusion of patients with late-onset AKI. Similarly, interest in standardizing the definition for neonatal AKI has expanded in the last few years, although, as of yet, there remains no accepted consensus definition for AKI in this patient population. However, modified KDIGO criteria (nKDIGO) for the diagnosis of AKI in neonates have been introduced and are based on increases in the serum creatinine concentration (see Table 46.2). Although epidemiological data vary widely, as discussed above, there is growing awareness that the incidence of pediatric AKI is increasing, particularly in cohorts of critically ill children in the intensive care unit or in those children with comorbid conditions, such as congenital heart disease, cancer, and hematopoietic stem cell transplantation. In all instances, the development of AKI is associated with an increased risk for mortality and adverse outcomes.

At the time of an acute clinical presentation, it may be difficult to distinguish AKI from CKD without imaging studies, evaluation of and laboratory testing for associated complications that are more common in CKD than AKI, or possibly a kidney biopsy. Urine volume in AKI is variable; patients may be anuric, oliguric, or polyuric (especially in neonates). Short stature, CKD-mineral bone disorder (CKD-MBD), delayed puberty, normocytic anemia, and hyperparathyroidism all suggest long-standing CKD rather than AKI.

Kidney function declines when adequate blood supply and oxygenation, parenchymal integrity, and/or patency of the urinary collecting system are interrupted. Consequently, AKI can be viewed as being caused by prerenal, intrinsic kidney, or postrenal factors, although substantial overlap and multifactorial etiologies can exist, particularly in hospitalized children. The most common etiologies of AKI in children are listed in Table 46.3. The likelihood of

TABLE 46.2 Acute Kidney Injury Definitions in Children

pRIFLE		KDIGO		nKDIGOᵃ	
Stage	**Criteria**	**Stage**	**Criteria**	**Stage**	**Criteria**
Risk (R)	eCrCl ↓ 25% UOP <0.5 mL/kg/h × 8 h	1	↑ SCr ≥0.3 mg/dLᵇ or ↑ SCr ≥1.5–2 × ᶜ UOP <0.5 mL/kg/h × 8 h	1	SCr rise ≥0.3 mg/dLᵇ
Injury (I)	eCrCl ↓ 50% UOP <0.5 mL/kg/h × 16 h	2	↑ SCr ≥2–3 × UOP <0.5 mL/kg/h × 16 h	2	Increase in SCr by 150% to <200% from previous trough levelᵈ
Failure (F)	eCrCl ↓ 75% or CrCl<35 mL/min/1.73 m² UOP <0.5 mL/kg/h × 24 h or anuria for 12 h	3	↑ SCr ≥3–4 × or SCr >4 (and meets criteria for AKI) or RRT initiated or eGFR <35 in patients <18 yo UOP <0.5 mL/kg/h × 24 h or anuria × 12 h	3	Increase in SCr by 200% to <300% from previous trough level or SCr ≥ 2.5 mg/dL
Loss (L)	Failure >4 weeks	N/A		NA	
End-stage kidney disease (E)	Failure >3 months	N/A		NA	

ᵃShould be used in children <120 days
ᵇWithin 48 hr
ᶜWithin 7 days
ᵈReference Scr defined as the lowest previous SCr value

AKI, Acute kidney injury; *CrCl,* creatinine clearance; *KDIGO,* Kidney Disease: Improving Global Outcomes; *RRT,* renal replacement therapy; *SCr,* serum creatinine; *UOP,* urine output.
Adapted from Akcan-Arikan A, Zappitelli M, Loftis LL, et al. Modified RIFLE criteria in critically ill children with acute kidney injury. *Kidney Int.* 2007;71:1028–1035; Mehta R, Kellum J, Shah S, et al: Acute Kidney Injury Network: report of an initiative to improve outcomes in acute kidney injury. *Crit Care.* 2007;22:R31; Kidney Disease: Improving Global Outcomes (KDIGO) Acute Kidney Injury Work Group. KDIGO clinical practice guideline for acute kidney injury. *Kidney Int Suppl.* 2012;2:1–138, and Jetton JG, Ashkenazi DJ. *Curr Opin Pediatr.* 2012;24(2):191.

TABLE 46.3	Most Common Etiologies of AKI in Children		

Prerenal AKI	Intrinsic AKI	Postrenal AKI*
Intravascular volume contraction • Dehydration • Hemorrhage • Third-spacing of fluid (sepsis, burns, hypoalbuminemia) **Decreased effective circulating blood volume** • Left-sided heart failure • Cardiac tamponade • Hepatorenal syndrome **Altered intrarenal hemodynamics** • Calcineurin inhibitor toxicity • Hepatorenal syndrome • NSAIDs • ACEI/ARBs	**Prolonged prerenal AKI** **Vascular disease** • Renal artery stenosis • Renal vein thrombosis • Hemolytic uremic syndrome and TTP (microvasculature) **Glomerular disease** • Acute postinfectious glomerulonephritis • Anti-GBM antibody disease • ANCA disease • Lupus nephritis • IgA nephropathy • Henoch-Schönlein purpura nephritis • MPGN **Tubulointerstitial disease** • Proton pump inhibitors, extended-spectrum penicillins, NSAIDs, sulfonamides, rifampin • Infections • Systemic disease • Tumor infiltration	Much rarer cause of AKI (unless patient has a solitary kidney either from renal agenesis, nephrectomy, or transplantation) **Complete urethral or bladder neck obstruction or bilateral ureteral obstruction** • Calculi • Ureteral blood clots • Retroperitoneal fibrosis • Neurogenic bladder • Bladder or pelvic tumors • Urethral stricture

*Postrenal conditions are very rare causes of AKI in children unless the child has a solitary kidney, either from renal agenesis, nephrectomy or transplantation.

recovery from AKI depends, in part, on the presence or absence of urine output, the quantity of urine output, the duration of anuria, and the underlying cause and severity of kidney injury. Quantifying the urine output is essential, as this predicts the clinical course and may aid in identifying the underlying insult. Oliguria is defined as a urine output less than 1 mL/kg/hr in infants and young children and less than 0.5 mL/kg/hr for 6 hours in older children. Children with nonoliguric AKI have lower complication rates and higher survival rates than those with anuric or oliguric AKI.

Treatment

General supportive measures to prevent AKI include restoration of intravascular volume, avoidance of hypotension by providing inotropic support in critically ill children following volume repletion, and careful readjustment of nephrotoxic medications based on close monitoring of drug levels and kidney function. Volume expansion with isotonic saline may reduce the risk of AKI from rhabdomyolysis and associated myoglobinuria, radiocontrast dye, tumor lysis syndrome, and exposure to certain nephrotoxic agents (acyclovir, aminoglycosides, amphotericin B, and cisplatin). Several pharmacologic agents including mannitol, loop diuretics, low-dose dopamine, fenoldopam, and N-acetylcysteine have been studied in children with AKI with no convincing evidence of benefit; accordingly, none are routinely recommended to prevent AKI or its progression.

Management of AKI in children includes relief of obstruction if present, judicious fluid administration to maintain euvolemia, blood pressure management, and treatment of electrolyte abnormalities including hyperkalemia, metabolic acidosis, hypocalcemia, and hyperphosphatemia. Restriction of sodium, potassium, and phosphate intake may be indicated, as may the use of potassium-binding agents to treat hyperkalemia and oral phosphate binders for the management of hyperphosphatemia. Metabolic acidosis should be corrected carefully; the exchange of protein-bound hydrogen ions with calcium can result in a decrease

of the available ionized calcium and result in tetany. Frequent dose adjustment or elimination of potentially nephrotoxic medications is necessary when the GFR is low, and a multidisciplinary approach among intensivists, nephrologists, and specialized pharmacists may be helpful.

The judicious use of nephrotoxic medications and targeted quality improvement measures designed to minimize unnecessary exposure to potentially nephrotoxic medications in hospitalized patients showed remarkable success in the NINJA (Nephrotoxic Injury Negated by Just-in-time Action) collaborative by decreasing hospital-acquired AKI rates by 23.8%. Nutritional support may include enteral or parenteral supplementation and should include the normal maintenance requirements plus additional calories to address the catabolic state associated with AKI. Tight glucose control is recommended. Polyuria and tubular dysfunction (hypokalemia, hypophosphatemia, hypomagnesemia) can be noted in the recovery phase of AKI due to a lag in the tubular reabsorptive capacity, and careful management of fluids and electrolytes during the diuretic phase of AKI is essential.

Kidney replacement therapy (KRT) is indicated when conservative measures fail. Frequent indications include hyperkalemia, severe acidosis unresponsive to pharmacologic therapy, uremia (typically marked by a BUN >100 mg/dL [30 mM] or symptoms of encephalopathy, the latter being particularly challenging to assess in infants and young children), refractory fluid overload (pulmonary edema, heart failure, or hypertension), or an inability to provide adequate nutrition. Volume overload in excess of 10%–20% is increasingly recognized as a predictor of unfavorable outcomes, prompting an overall trend in many centers toward earlier initiation of KRT. Modalities used in AKI include peritoneal dialysis (PD), hemodialysis (HD), and continuous kidney replacement therapy (CKRT) using hemofiltration or hemodiafiltration; the choice is dictated largely by the patient's clinical status, as well as by the availability of equipment and local expertise. Peritoneal dialysis is advantageous in neonates and younger children and in resource-limited countries, with no requirements for systemic/regional anticoagulation, vascular access, or specialized equipment or personnel. Hemodialysis offers the advantage of being able to rapidly correct fluid or electrolyte imbalances but does require patients to tolerate a large extracorporeal volume through an adequate vascular access and mandates specially trained personnel. Finally, where equipment and trained personnel exist, CKRT may be preferred in children with multisystem organ dysfunction or hemodynamic instability; it permits gentler fluid removal rates with less dynamic fluid shifts than HD while allowing full enteral or parenteral nutrition.

Chronic Kidney Disease

Introduction

Although diabetes and hypertension account for the vast majority of chronic kidney disease (CKD) cases in adult patients, approximately two-thirds of childhood CKD is attributed to congenital anomalies of the kidney and urinary tract (CAKUT), including renal hypoplasia/dysplasia and obstructive uropathy (e.g., posterior urethral valves). Environmental (especially cadmium and lead) or drug-related nephrotoxic exposures can increase the risk for CKD or accelerate its progression. Other common causes of CKD include focal segmental glomerulosclerosis (FSGS), chronic glomerulonephritis (lupus nephritis, IgA nephropathy, HSP, or MPGN), ciliopathies (autosomal recessive polycystic kidney disease, nephronophthisis), and HUS. Renovascular thromboembolic disease, Alport syndrome, congenital nephrotic syndrome, primary hyperoxaluria, and cystinosis are rare but important causes of CKD in childhood.

Diagnosis

The determination of GFR is integral to the diagnosis of CKD. Multiple GFR estimating equations have been developed for use in pediatrics (see Table 46.4). The original Schwartz formula to estimate GFR in children was developed in the mid-1970s using serum creatinine, height, and an empiric constant for age/gender. However, the transition from use of the Jaffe chromogen reaction to the enzymatic methodology for serum creatinine determination now used in most centers required a refinement of the pediatric GFR estimating formulas. The Schwartz estimating equation was, in turn, updated in 2009 based on results from the prospective, observational multicenter Chronic Kidney Disease in Children (CKiD) study, in which GFR was measured through the plasma disappearance of iohexol. The CKiD study updated the equation in 2021 to the "U25" creatinine and cystatin C-based equations, which incorporated additional sampling of children younger than 5 years and young adults ages 18-25, as well as calibration of cystatin C to International Federation of Clinical Chemistry approved reference material. The investigators found that the average eGFR using the creatinine and cystatin C estimates was the least biased, more accurate, and more precise than either of the two single-marker estimates. An online calculator is available for public use: https://ckid-gfrcalculator.shinyapps.io/eGFR/

Importantly, a simplified estimating equation was derived—the so-called bedside CKiD equation—which includes an updated constant of 0.413 (36.5 for SI units):

$$eGFR = 0.413 \times height\,(cm)\,/\,serum\,creatinine\,(in\,mg\,/\,dL)$$

While this equation is used most frequently in clinical care, multiple other equations have been published (Table 46.4). For young adults with CKD between the ages of 18–26 years, a simplified average of the bedside CKiD equation or the adult CKD-EPI equation is preferred.

Accurate estimates of GFR are necessary to appropriately stage CKD. In 2002, the National Kidney Foundation's Kidney Disease Outcomes Quality Initiative (NKF-KDOQI) published a CKD classification system based on GFR that was applicable to children and adults (see Chapter 51). The KDIGO 2012 clinical practice guideline revised the 2002 KDOQI classification by defining pediatric CKD in children greater than 2 years old as GFR <60 mL/min/1.73 m^2 for more than 3 months or GFR >60 mL/min/1.73 m^2 that is accompanied by evidence of structural damage or other markers of functional kidney abnormalities including proteinuria, albuminuria, kidney tubular disorders, or pathologic abnormalities as detected by imaging or histopathology (Table 46.5). The current pediatric CKD staging system does not stratify according to albuminuria, in contrast to criteria for adults. For children less than 2 years of age who continue to have physiological maturation of their GFR, the traditional classification system does not apply, and it is recommended to use age-appropriate normative serum creatinine values, with values more than one standard deviation below the mean, indicative of the need to pursue additional investigation.

Several clinical or radiologic elements in the medical history may indicate the presence of early CKD, including abnormal antenatal ultrasound, oligohydramnios or polyhydramnios, polydipsia, polyuria, nocturia, and salt craving. However, many children with CKD are often asymptomatic or have vague, nonspecific complaints, including fatigue, headaches, or gastrointestinal symptoms. Failure to thrive, short stature, delayed puberty, pallor, and difficulty concentrating with poor school performance may occur in more advanced CKD.

Several additional and treatable comorbidities are associated with CKD (Fig. 46.1). A number of clinical assessment tools exist to improve the prediction of children who progress to ESKD (a useful calculator can be accessed at ckdprognosis.com). Hypertension is the most common and often earliest comorbid condition and can arise as a result of a number of factors including sodium retention and extracellular volume expansion, increased activity of the renin-angiotensin system, and enhanced activity of the sympathetic nervous system. Dyslipidemia, particularly elevated triglyceride values, low values of high-density lipoprotein cholesterol (HDL-C), and elevated non-HDL-C are also common. Metabolic derangements are frequent and include hyperkalemia, hyperphosphatemia, hypocalcemia, and metabolic acidosis. CKD-MBD may become evident by CKD stage 3 as a result of reduced urinary phosphate excretion; elevated serum phosphorous, parathyroid hormone (PTH), and FGF23 levels; hypocalcemia; and reduced circulating levels of activated vitamin D (1,25-dihydroxyvitamin D). Anemia typically develops in CKD stage 3 (GFR 30 to 59 mL/min/1.73 m^2) as a result of reduced erythropoietin production along with possible mild iron deficiency. Neurocognitive dysfunction is also noted, with particular deficits in attention and executive functioning.

Treatment

The overall aims of treatment for CKD are fivefold: (1) treat the underlying condition whenever possible, (2) prevent the progression of the disease, (3) treat the complications of CKD, (4) optimize conditions for normal growth and development,

TABLE 46.4	Pediatric Glomerular Filtration Rate Estimating Equations

GFR Marker	GFR (mL/min/1.73 m²) Equation

SCr by alkaline picrate (Jaffe)	*Schwartz equation*[a]
	   eGFR = k × Ht (cm)/Scr
	Counahan-Barratt equation[b]
	   eGFR = 0.43 × Ht (cm)/Scr

SCr by IDMS traceable enzymatic methods	*CKiD bedside equation*[c]
	   eGFR = 0.413 × Ht (cm)/Scr
	Schwartz-Lyon equation[d]
	   eGFR = kL/SCr
	Simple height-independent equation[e]
	   eGFR = 107.3/(SCr/Q)
	CKiD U25 equation, age and sex dependent[f]
	   https://ckid-gfrcalculator.shinyapps.io/eGFR/

CysC	*CKiD cystC equation*[g]
	   eGFR (mL/min/1.73 m²) = 70.69 (CystC)$^{-0.931}$
	Zappitelli et al. cystC equation[h]
	   eGFR (mL/min/1.73 m²) = 75.94 (CystC)$^{-1.170}$
	Filler and Lepage cystC equation[i]
	   eGFR (mL/min/1.73 m²) = 91.62 (CystC)$^{-1.129}$
	CKiD U25 equation[f]
	   https://ckid-gfrcalculator.shinyapps.io/eGFR/

SCr + CysC	*CKiD multivariable equation*[j]
	   eGFR (mL/min/1.73 m²) = 39.8 × Ht (m)/Scr)$^{0.456}$ (1.8/CystC)$^{0.418}$ (30/BUN)$^{0.079}$ (1.076)^{male} (Ht(m)/1.4)$^{0.179}$
	Zappitelli et al. equation[k]
	   eGFR (mL/min/1.73 m²) = 43.82 (1/CystC)$^{0.635}$ (1/Scr)$^{0.547}$ (1.35^{height})
	Bouvet et al. equation[l]
	   eGFR (mL/min/1.73 m²) = 63.2 (1.2/CystC)[(96/88.4)/(Scr)]$^{0.35}$ (weight/45)$^{0.30}$ (age/14)$^{0.40}$

[a]k is a constant, directly proportional to the muscle component of body, and varies with age. The value for k is 0.33 in premature infants through the first year of life, 0.45 for term infants through the first year of life, 0.55 in children and adolescent girls, and 0.7 in adolescent boys. Formula developed against measured inulin GFR [PMID 951142] (Schwartz et al., 1976)

[b]Jaffe reaction after adsorption onto ion exchange to remove noncreatinine chromogens. Recommendations for subtracting 0.14 mg/dL for automated Jaffe creatinine. Formula developed against measured Cr-EDTA GFR [PMID: 1008594] (Counahan et al., 1976)

[c]Formula developed against measured iohexol GFR [PMID: 19158356] (Schwartz et al., 2009)

[d]Formula developed against inulin clearance GFR. K = 0.419 if males > 13 years old, otherwise k = 0.373. [PMID 23285295] (DeSouza et al., 2012)

[e]Formula validated in children and young adults ages 1–25 years. Q = 0.0270 x Age + 0.2329. [PMID: 24046193] (Hoste L et al., 2014)

[f]https://ckid-gfrcalculator.shinyapps.io/eGFR/

[g]CystC by PENIA. Formula developed against single-injection iohexol [PMID: 22622496] (Schwartz et al., 2012)

[h]Formula developed against cold iothalamate [PMID: 16860187] (Zappitelli et al., 2006)

[i]CystC by PENIA. Formula developed against single-injection Tc-DTPA [PMID:12920638] (Filler and Lepage, 2003)

[j]Serum creatinine by IDMS traceable enzymatic method. CystC by PENIA. Formula developed against single-injection iohexol [PMID: 22622496] (Schwartz et al., 2012)

[k]Serum creatinine by enzymatic creatinine. CystC by PENIA. Formula developed against nonradioactive iothalamate steady-state method [PMID: 16860187] (Zappitelli et al., 2006)

[l]Serum creatinine by noncompensated Jaffe method. CystC by PENIA. Formula developed against single-injection Cr-EDTA [PMID: 16794818] (Bouvet et al., 2006)

CKiD, Chronic kidney disease in children; *CystC*, serum cystatin C; *eGFR*, estimated glomerular filtration rate; *GFR*, glomerular filtration rate; *SCr*, serum creatinine.

and (5) avoid further nephrotoxic insults. Hypertension and proteinuria are two modifiable risk factors independently associated with a more rapid progression of CKD. The ESCAPE trial, published in 2009, demonstrated that achieving the 50th percentile for mean arterial blood pressure using an intensified antihypertensive blood pressure regimen including an ACE inhibitor delayed CKD progression in children. In addition, ACE inhibitors reduced protein excretion by approximately 50% within the first 6 months of treatment initiation. Therefore, ACE inhibitors (or angiotensin receptor blockers [ARB]) are considered first-line therapy for hypertension or proteinuria in children with CKD, although hyperkalemia may be dose limiting in very advanced CKD. Successful treatment of metabolic acidosis can also delay CKD progression as well as improve growth. Finally, clinicians and their patients should scrutinize potentially modifiable risk factors that may be associated with slowing of CKD progression, which include smoking cessation or avoidance, maintenance of a healthy body mass index, and avoidance of potential unnecessary nephrotoxins (i.e., NSAIDs).

The anemia of CKD is treated with iron supplementation and erythropoiesis-stimulating agents. CKD-MBD is primarily treated by restricting dietary phosphate intake, providing enteric phosphate binders, ensuring adequate nutritional 25-OH vitamin D stores, and administering calcitriol (synthetic 1,25-dihydroxyvitamin D). These interventions suppress PTH secretion. Calcimimetics (i.e., cinacalcet) bind to the calcium-sensing receptor in the parathyroid gland and lower the threshold for activation by extracellular calcium, thereby decreasing PTH hormone release. Calcimimetics may be used in some children ≥3 years old with persistent and severe hyperparathyroidism despite optimized conventional management (including nutritional and activated vitamin D therapy). Children should target at least their required daily allowance of protein and calories to promote appropriate growth. Recombinant growth hormone therapy may be indicated for short stature once

TABLE 46.5	**Antihypertensive Medications in Children**		
Drug	**Initial Dose**	**Maximum Dose**	**Adverse Effects**
ACE Inhibitors			
Enalapril[a]	0.08 mg/kg/day	0.6 mg/kg/day (max 40 mg/day)	Hyperkalemia, cough, angioedema, ACE fetopathy
Fosinopril[a]	0.1 mg/kg (5 or 10 mg)	0.6 mg/kg (max 40 mg/day)	
Lisinopril[a]	0.07 mg/kg/day (up to 5 mg/day)	0.6 mg/kg/day (max 40 mg/day)	
Benazepril[a]	0.2 mg/kg (up to 10 mg)	0.6 mg/kg (max 40 mg/day)	
Angiotensin-Receptor Blockers			
Losartan[a]	0.7 mg/kg/day (up to 50 mg/day)	1.4 mg/kg/day (max 100 mg/day)	Hyperkalemia, cough (less common than ACE inhibitors)
Valsartan[a]	<6 years: 5–10 mg/day	<6 years: 80 mg/day	
	6–17 years: 1.3 mg/kg/day (up to 40 mg/day)	6–17 years: 2.7 mg/kg/day (max 160 mg/day)	
Aldosterone Receptor Antagonist			
Eplerenone	25 mg/day	100 mg/day	Hyperkalemia, lightheadedness, gynecomastia
Spironolactone[a]	1 mg/kg/day	3.3 mg/kg/day (max 100 mg/day)	
Alpha- and Beta-Adrenergic Antagonist			
Carvedilol	0.1 mg/kg/dose (up to 6.25 mg/day)	0.5 mg/kg/dose (max 25 mg) twice daily	Caution with asthma, heart failure, diabetes; lightheadedness; depression; dry eyes, bradycardia, peripheral edema
Labetalol	1–3 mg/kg/day	1200 mg/day	
Beta Antagonists			
Atenolol	0.5–1 mg/kg/day	2 mg/kg/day (max 100 mg/day)	Caution with asthma, heart failure, diabetes; bradycardia; lightheadedness
Metoprolol[a]	1–2 mg/kg/day	6 mg/kg/day (max 600 mg/day)	
Propranolol[a]	0.5–1 mg/kg/day	8 mg/kg/day (max 640 mg/day)	
Centrally Acting Alpha Agonists			
Clonidine[a]	5–20 µg/kg/day	25 µg/kg/day	Sedation, bradycardia, dry eyes, dry mouth
	OR	OR	
	0.1-mg transdermal patch	0.3-mg transdermal patch	
Calcium-Channel Blockers			
Amlodipine[a]	<6 years: 0.1 mg/kg/day or 5 mg/day	< 6 years: 0.6 mg/kg/day or 5 mg/day	Reflex tachycardia, peripheral edema
	>6 years: 2.5 mg/day	> 6 years: 10 mg/day	
Isradipine[a]	0.05–0.15 mg/kg/dose 3 or 4 times per day	0.8 mg/kg/day (max 20 mg/day)	
Nifedipine, extended release	0.25–0.5 mg/kg/day	3 mg/kg/day (max 120 mg/day)	
Diuretics			
Amiloride	0.4–0.625 mg/kg/day	20 mg/day	Hypokalemia, hypercholesterolemia, hyperglycemia
Chlorthalidone	0.3 mg/kg/day	2 mg/kg/day (max 50 mg/day)	
Furosemide	0.5–2 mg/kg/dose	6 mg/kg/day	
Hydrochlorothiazide[a]	0.5–1 mg/kg/day	3 mg/kg/day (max 50 mg/day)	
Vasodilators			
Hydralazine[a]	0.75 mg/kg/day divided q6–12h	7.5 mg/kg/day (max 200 mg/day)	Tachycardia, edema, hirsutism (minoxidil)
Minoxidil[a]	<12 years: 0.2 mg/kg/day	<12 years: 50 mg/day	
	≥12 years: 5 mg/day	≥12 years: 100 mg/day	

[a]US Food and Drug Administration approved for use in children.
ACE, Angiotensin-converting enzyme.

assured that the child is receiving sufficient calories and the secondary hyperparathyroidism and acidosis of CKD are adequately treated. Meticulous review of medication lists with close attention to appropriate dosing based on kidney function and family and patient education regarding potential exposures to over-the-counter or complementary/alternative medications is an important aspect of prevention of exposure to potential nephrotoxins.

Hypertension

Diagnosis

The American Academy of Pediatrics (AAP) published updated guidelines in 2017 for the screening and management of hypertension in children. A notable update to the guidelines consists of recalculated

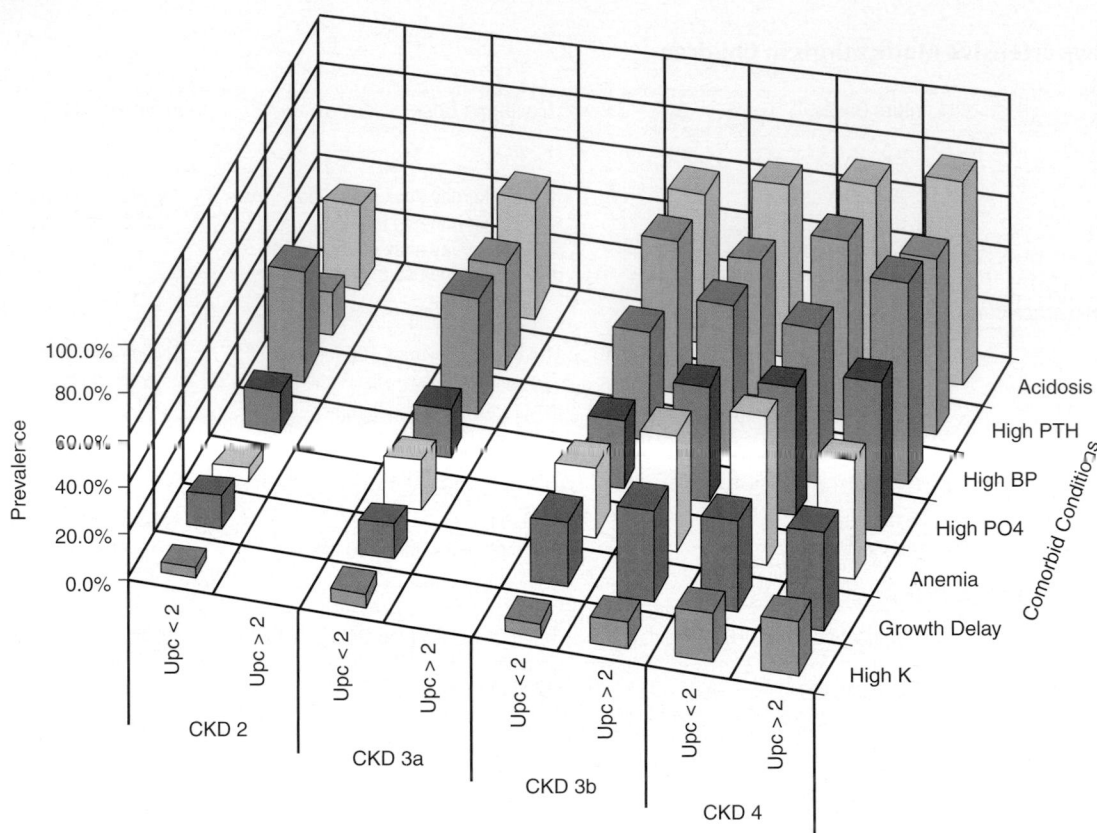

• Fig. 46.1 Chronic kidney disease (CKD) comorb conditions by stage and urine protein-to-creatinine ratio. CKD3 was divided into 3a (GFR 45 to 59 mL/min/1.73 m²) and 3b (GFR 30 to 44 mL/min/1.73 m²) for a more detailed analysis. *BP,* Blood pressure; *GFR,* glomerular filtration rate; *K,* potassium; *PTH,* parathyroid hormone; *Upc,* urine protein-to-creatinine ratio. (Adapted from Furth SL, Abraham AG, Jerry-Fluker J, et al. Metabolic abnormalities, cardiovascular risk factors and GFR decline in children with chronic kidney disease. *Clin J Am Soc Nephrol.* 2011;6:2132–2140.)

normative distribution tables of blood pressure percentiles from healthy children enrolled in the National Health and Nutrition Examination Survey but restricted to those with normal body mass index. Simplification of the definitions of abnormal blood pressure values for children ≥13 years old were included and are consistent with new adult definitions from the American Heart Association and the American College of Cardiology, while recommendations for a more limited initial diagnostic work-up and for an expanded use of ambulatory blood pressure monitoring have been added as well. Elevated blood pressure is now defined as a sustained (on 3 or more occasions) systolic (SBP) or diastolic blood pressure (DBP) ≥90th percentile but <95th percentile for children 1 to <13 years old or a SBP 120 to 129 mm Hg and DBP <80 mm Hg for children ≥13 years old. Stage 1 hypertension is defined as SBP ≥95th percentile to <95th percentile + 12 mm Hg, or 130/80 139/89 mm Hg (whichever is lower) for children aged 1 to <13 years old, and BP between 130/80 to 139/89 mm Hg for children ≥13 years. Stage 2 HTN is defined as a sustained SBP ≥95th percentile + 12 mm Hg, or ≥ 140/90 mm Hg (whichever is lower) for children <13 years old. For children ≥13 years old, stage 2 HTN is defined as BP ≥ 140/90 mm Hg.

Blood pressure is usually measured either through auscultation or with an oscillometric device. Auscultative blood pressure assessment is considered the gold standard, and it has been used for the generation of all pediatric normative data. Oscillometric devices calculate blood pressure by proprietary, unpublished formulas and are known to overestimate blood pressure in children by as much as 5 to

10 mm Hg. Although the use of oscillometric blood pressure assessment has become widespread clinically, caution should be used when diagnosing hypertension with an automated device in children, and elevated readings should always be confirmed by manual auscultation.

Ambulatory blood pressure monitoring (ABPM), discussed in Chapter 64, has recently been introduced into the field of hypertension in children. Individuals with an elevated blood pressure in the clinic but a normal ABPM study are currently designated as having isolated office hypertension, or white-coat hypertension. Those with normal office-based BP and hypertension on ABPM are said to have masked hypertension. Evaluation by APBM over 24 hours offers the advantages of distinguishing white-coat from true hypertension, evaluating for the presence of masked hypertension, and more precisely characterizing changes in blood pressure during daily activities, including while asleep and as a result of anti-hypertensive therapy. Recent data suggest that end-organ changes such as left ventricular hypertrophy are more closely correlated with ABPM-based readings than office-based BP readings. The revised 2017 AAP guidelines recommend confirmation of elevated office-based BP readings with the use of ABPM when possible, and recommend that children with CKD and hypertension should have annual ABPM to assess for possible masked hypertension.

Hypertension may also be classified by etiology. Primary or "essential" hypertension is defined as hypertension without an otherwise identifiable cause. Although this condition used to be considered rare in children, it is now routinely encountered in clinical practice, affecting 3%-5% of US adolescents. Essential hypertension is associated with obesity, a family history of hypertension, sedentary lifestyle, high dietary sodium intake, a history of African ancestry, and a history of prematurity and/or low birth weight. Secondary hypertension is, in contrast, elevated blood pressure due to an identifiable, underlying cause. Kidney parenchymal disorders, including glomerulonephritis, kidney fibrosis, FSGS, renal dysplasia, and polycystic kidney disease, account for the vast majority of secondary causes of hypertension in children. Fibromuscular dysplasia and aortic coarctation are also relatively common causes. Rare but important etiologies include endocrine disorders such as pheochromocytoma or neuroblastoma, Cushing syndrome, and monogenic disorders that affect kidney tubular function. In neonates and premature infants, umbilical artery catheter-associated thromboembolism affecting the renal arteries is the most common cause of hypertension. In general, the likelihood of identifying a secondary cause of hypertension is directly related to the degree of hypertension (i.e., more common in stage 2) and is inversely related to the age of the child.

The evaluation of any child with hypertension largely depends on the likelihood of identifying a secondary cause, and the extent of the evaluation should be individualized. Most younger children with hypertension, adolescents with stage 2 hypertension, and adolescents with stage 1 hypertension without obvious risk factors for essential hypertension should undergo an initial evaluation that consists of a basic metabolic panel, urinalysis, and a kidney ultrasound. An echocardiogram should be considered to exclude the possibility of coarctation of the aorta and to assess for left ventricular hypertrophy. Measurement of fasting lipid profile is also recommended in the new 2017 AAP hypertension guidelines, along with a hemoglobin A1c and liver enzymes in obese children or adolescents to screen for fatty liver.

Treatment

Treatment recommendations are based on the severity of hypertension. For most patients with essential hypertension, a 6- to 12-month trial of nonpharmacologic interventions should be recommended, including the DASH diet (Dietary Approaches to Stop Hypertension, a low-sodium, plant-based diet with whole grains, low-fat dairy, and lean meats), moderate to vigorous exercise on most days of the week, achievement and maintenance of normal body mass index, and limited screen time. Pharmacologic therapy is indicated for treatment of hypertension that persists despite lifestyle changes, secondary hypertension, hypertension associated with end-organ damage, and hypertension associated with chronic disorders, such as diabetes or CKD. Treatment should target a decrease in systolic and diastolic values to <90th percentile or ≤130/80 mm Hg in children 13 years or older. Children with CKD should be treated to a target BP of less than the 50th percentile based on ABPM. In part due to the Best Pharmaceuticals for Children Act, enacted by the FDA in 2002, the number of antihypertensive medications with pediatric-specific indications has increased considerably over the past decade and includes ACE inhibitors, ARBs, beta blockers, calcium channel blockers, and

diuretics (see Table 46.5). The long-term prognosis of pediatric hypertension depends on the underlying etiology. Overall, there is an increased risk for future cardiovascular morbidity and mortality that may be modifiable with prompt recognition and treatment.

Complete bibliography is available at Elsevier eBooks for Practicing Clinicians.

Key Bibliography

Akcan-Arikan A, Zappitelli M, Loftis LL, et al. Modified RIFLE criteria in critically ill children with acute kidney injury. *Kidney Int.* 2007;71:1028–1035.

Flynn J, Daniels S, Hayman L, et al. Update: ambulatory blood pressure monitoring in children and adolescents: a scientific statement from the American Heart Association. *Hypertension.* 2014;63:1116–1135.

Flynn JT, Kaelber DC, Baker-Smith CM, et al. Clinical practice guideline for screening and management of high blood pressure in children and adolescents. *Pediatrics.* 2017;140(3):e2017904.

Furth SL, Abraham AG, Jerry-Fluker J, et al. Metabolic abnormalities, cardiovascular risk factors and GFR decline in children with chronic kidney disease. *Clin J Am Soc Nephrol.* 2011;6:2132–2140.

Furth SL, Pierce C, Hui WF, et al. Estimating time to ESRD in children with CKD. *Am J Kidney Dis.* 2018;71(6):783–792.

Goldstein SL, Dahale D, Kirkendall, et al. A prospective multi-center quality improvement initiative (NINJA) indicates a reduction in nephrotoxic acute kidney injury in hospitalized children. *Kidney Int.* 2020;97(3):580–588.

Hogg RJ, Furth S, Lemley KV, et al. National Kidney Foundation's Kidney Disease Outcomes Quality Initiative clinical practice guidelines for chronic kidney disease in children and adolescents: evaluation, classification, and stratification. *Pediatrics.* 2003;111:1416.

Jetton JG, Boohaker LJ, Sethi SK, et al. Incidence and outcomes of neonatal acute kidney injury (AWAKEN): a multicenter, multinational, observational cohort study. *Lancet Child Adolesc Health.* 2017:184–194.

Kaddourah A, Basu RK, Bagshaw SM, et al. Epidemiology of acute kidney injury in critical ill children and young adults. *N Engl J Med.* 2017;376:11.

Matsell DG, Hiatt MJ. Functional development of the kidney in utero. In: Polin RA, Fox WW, Abman SH, Rowitch DH, Benitz WE, eds. *Fetal and Neonatal Physiology.* 5th ed. Philadelphia: Elsevier; 2017:965–977.

Mitsnefes M, Ho PL, McEnrey PT. Hypertension and progression of chronic renal insufficiency in children: a report of the North American Renal Transplant Cooperative Study (NAPRTCS). *J Am Soc Nephrol.* 2003;14:2618–2622.

Ng DK, Schwartz GJ, Schneider MF, et al. Combination of pediatric and adult formulas yield valid glomerular filtration rate estimates in young adults with a history of pediatric chronic kidney disease. *Kidney Int.* 2018;94:170.

Schwartz GJ, Munoz A, Schneider MF, et al. New equations to estimate GFR in children with CKD. *J Am Soc Nephrol.* 2009;20:629–637.

Selewski DT, Charlton JR, Jetton JG, et al. Neonatal acute kidney injury. *Pediatrics.* 2015;136(2):e463–e473.

The ESCAPE Trial Group. Strict blood-pressure control and progression of renal failure in children. *N Engl J Med.* 2009;361:1639–1650.

Water AM. Functional development of the nephron. In: Geary DF, Schaefer F, eds. *Structural and Functional Development of the Kidney, Part 2: Functional Development of the Nephron.* Philadelphia: Mosby Elsevier; 2008:112.

47

The Kidney in Pregnancy

JESSICA TANGREN, MICHELLE A. HLADUNEWICH

Kidney Anatomy and Physiology During Normal Pregnancy

Pregnancy produces dramatic changes in systemic hemodynamics, leading to alterations in total circulating blood volume, cardiac output, and systemic vascular resistance. The kidney itself undergoes marked changes during gestation, including alterations in kidney size, glomerular hemodynamics, and tubular function. These adaptations are critical for favorable pregnancy outcomes. Although much of our knowledge of kidney anatomic and physiologic changes in human pregnancy is extrapolated from animal models and small studies in healthy pregnant women, understanding the adaptive changes that occur during pregnancy is crucial for differentiating healthy from complicated pregnancies.

Anatomic Changes During Gestation

Kidney size increases during pregnancy from a combination of increased kidney weight and dilatation of the urinary collecting system. In longitudinal studies of kidney size measured by ultrasound, kidney length increases by approximately 1 cm. Dilation of the collecting system is observed as early as the third month of gestation. The right renal pelvis is most often affected. Although traditionally believed to be the result of mechanical compression by the gravid uterus, dilatation occurs well before the uterus is large enough to cause obstruction, arguing for a hormonal contribution as well. Structural changes generally resolve by 12 weeks postpartum. Persistent hydronephrosis beyond 12 to 16 weeks postpartum suggests underlying mechanical obstruction that requires further investigation (Box 47.1).

Physiologic Changes During Gestation

Systemic Hemodynamic Changes

Systemic adaptations to normal pregnancy begin soon after conception, with the development of a low-resistance placental circulation. Changes in maternal systemic vascular resistance and cardiac output can be detected as early as 6 weeks' gestation. Pregnancy leads to systemic vasodilation, increased cardiac output, and plasma volume expansion. Despite the increase in blood volume and cardiac output, systemic blood pressure (BP) decreases over the first half of gestation and reaches a nadir between 18 and 24 weeks of gestation. The mechanisms leading to systemic vasodilation in healthy human pregnancy are not fully understood but likely reflect a balance between vasodilatory and vasoconstrictive mediators, such as the corpus luteum-derived hormone relaxin, nitric oxide (NO), and alterations of the renin-angiotensin-aldosterone system (RAAS). Systemic vasodilation results in venous pooling that triggers volume restorative responses, including increased RAAS activity and a lowered set point for antidiuretic hormone (ADH) release. These changes lead to progressive volume expansion throughout gestation. Despite increases in RAAS activity by 2- to 10-fold, healthy pregnant women are resistant to the vasopressor effects of angiotensin II and systemic BP declines.

Renal Hemodynamic Changes

Similar to the systemic hemodynamic changes seen in healthy pregnancies, renal vascular resistance falls, leading to increased renal plasma flow (RPF) and glomerular filtration rate (GFR). Existing studies in human pregnancy physiology are challenging to interpret because of variations in GFR measurement techniques. In general, GFR and RPF increase by approximately 40%. Increased GFR is noted as early as 4 weeks' gestation, reaches peak level during the first half of pregnancy, and remains elevated until term (Fig. 47.1).

Volume Regulation and Electrolyte Changes

Total body water increases during pregnancy by 6 to 8 L, of which 4 to 6 L are extracellular. Changes in central osmostat regulation result in lower plasma osmolality (10 mOsm/L below normal), represented by a decrease in serum sodium by 4 to 5 mEq/L. Despite decreased plasma sodium concentrations, healthy pregnant women are in positive sodium balance, with a net gain of 3 to 4 mEq/day. Although normal pregnancy results in increased basal metabolic rate and acid generation, plasma pH is more alkaline because of a respiratory alkalosis mediated by elevated progesterone levels. This is accompanied by an appropriate renal metabolic adaptation with reduced serum HCO_3 levels (18 to 22 mmol/L).

Tubular Changes

In the nonpregnant state, kidneys efficiently reabsorb glucose and amino acids. In a small study of euglycemic women who displayed glycosuria, the maximal tubular reabsorption capacity for glucose was significantly decreased. The precise incidence of glycosuria in pregnancy is unclear, with extensive variability noted both between

BOX 47.1

Normal Adaptive Changes During Pregnancy

Structural Changes in the Kidney

Increase in kidney size by approximately 1 cm
Dilation of the urinary collecting system; more prominent on the right

Hormonal Changes

10- to 20-fold increase in aldosterone
8-fold increase in renin
4-fold increase in angiotensin
Resistance to pressor effect of angiotensin
Decreased set point for ADH release
Increased ANP release
Increased production of prostacyclin and nitric oxide

Systemic Hemodynamic Changes

Increased cardiac output by 40%–50%
Increased plasma volume by 40%–50%
Drop in SBP by ≈9 mm and DBP by 17 mm Hg (prominent in second trimester)

Renal Hemodynamic Changes

Increase in GFR and RPF by 50% above normal
Decrease in BUN (to <13 mg/dL) and serum creatinine (to 0.4–0.5 mg/dL)

Metabolic Changes

Increase in total body water by 6–8 L
Net retention of 900 mEq of sodium
Decrease in plasma osmolality by 10 mOsm/L
Decrease in serum sodium by 4–5 mEq/L
Mild respiratory alkalosis with compensatory metabolic acidosis (bicarb of 18–22 mEq/L)
Decrease in serum uric acid levels (to 2.5–4 mg/dL)
Glucosuria irrespective of blood glucose levels

ADH, Antidiuretic hormone; *ANP*, atrial natriuretic peptide; *BUN*, blood urea nitrogen; *DBP*, diastolic blood pressure; *GFR*, glomerular filtration rate; *RPF*, renal plasma flow; *SBP*, systolic blood pressure.

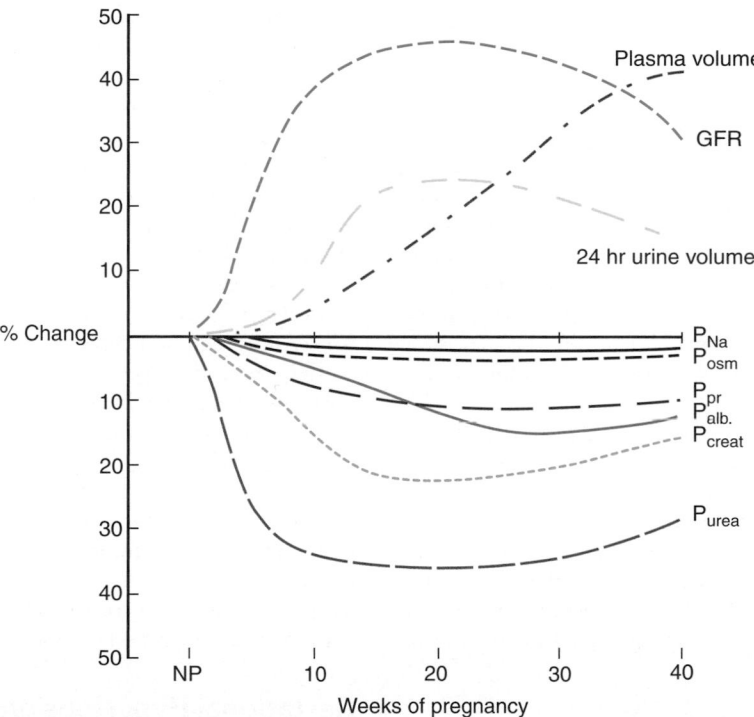

• **Fig. 47.1** Physiologic changes induced in pregnancy. Increments and decrements in various parameters are shown in percentage terms with reference to the nonpregnant baseline. *GFR*, Glomerular filtration rate; *NP*, nonpregnant; P_{alb}, plasma albumin; P_{creat}, plasma creatinine; P_{Na}, plasma sodium; P_{osm}, plasma osmolality; P_{pr}, plasma proteins; P_{urea}, plasma urea. (From Davison JM. The kidney in pregnancy: a review. *J Royal Soc Med.* 1983;76:485–500.)

women and within individual women at different times during pregnancy. There does not appear to be a relationship between glycosuria and clinical diabetes, and the majority of women with glycosuria have normal glucose screening in pregnancy. Uric acid levels drop to 2.5 to 4 mg/dL from the combined effects of increased filtration and decreased tubular reabsorption. Uric acid levels nadir in the second trimester and gradually increase as pregnancy progresses toward term. High renal clearance of uric acid is believed to be necessary to clear the increased production that occurs with fetal growth.

Assessment of Kidney Function

Glomerular Filtration Rate

Serum creatinine-based formulas are not accurate for estimating GFR in pregnancy. Both the Modification of Diet in Renal Disease (MDRD) and Chronic Kidney Disease Epidemiology (CKD-EPI) equations underestimate GFR measured by inulin clearance by approximately 40%. Creatinine clearance (CrCl) measured in a 24-hour urine collection remains one method to estimate GFR during pregnancy, although complete collection can be difficult because of urinary retention. Cystatin C levels have been studied in a variety of clinical settings; however, their use in pregnancy is not established, as cystatin C may be released by the placenta in response to ischemia. Gestational hyperfiltration and subsequent increased GFR result in decreased blood urea nitrogen (BUN) and serum creatinine levels. In a study of over 1 million pregnancies in Ontario, Canada, the mean baseline serum creatinine concentration was 0.68 mg/dL, declining by 4 weeks' gestation, ultimately reaching a nadir of 0.53 mg/dL between 16 and 32 weeks' gestation, and then rising to 0.72 mg/dL within a few weeks postpartum, with gradual return to mean prepregnancy concentrations by 18 weeks' postpartum. Using the 95th percentile as a potential cutoff for abnormal serum creatinine, the authors suggest a mid-trimester creatinine of 0.7 to 0.8 mg/dL or higher is of concern in normal pregnancy and should prompt further investigation.

Proteinuria

Routine prenatal care includes dipstick urine protein assessment at each prenatal visit. While inexpensive, the urine dipstick has high false-positive and false-negative rates. Twenty-four-hour urine protein excretion remains the gold standard for measurement of proteinuria in pregnancy, although, again, it can be difficult to obtain complete collections because of incomplete bladder emptying and urinary stasis. Assessment of the urine protein-to-creatinine ratio (UPCR) or albumin-to-creatinine ratio in spot urine specimens is probably the most practical way to follow protein excretion in pregnancy.

Urinary protein excretion remains below 200 mg/24 hr in normal pregnancy despite glomerular hyperfiltration. Most obstetric guidelines define significant protein excretion as greater than 300 mg in a 24-hour period; however, this cutoff is based on small studies. In one of the largest studies, the mean 24-hour protein excretion was near 100 mg, significantly lower than the established cutoff. As such, even low levels of proteinuria should not be attributed to gestational hyperfiltration and should prompt further evaluation.

Hypertensive Disorders of Pregnancy

Hypertension in pregnancy is defined as BP ≥140/90 mm Hg, measured on at least two separate occasions. Hypertensive disorders complicate up to 10% of pregnancies and are a major cause of maternal morbidity and mortality. Hypertensive disorders in pregnancy are classified into four categories: chronic hypertension, gestational hypertension, preeclampsia, and superimposed preeclampsia. Management of hypertension in pregnancy requires the clinician to balance the effects of treatment on both the mother and developing fetus.

Chronic Hypertension

The diagnosis of chronic hypertension is most often based on essential hypertension diagnosed before pregnancy or a BP greater than 140/90 mm Hg diagnosed before 20 weeks of gestation that does not resolve after delivery. The prevalence of chronic hypertension in pregnancy appears to be increasing because of higher pregnancy rates in women of advanced maternal age and higher rates of maternal obesity. Chronic hypertension is associated with increased risk for preeclampsia (25%), intrauterine growth restriction (IUGR; 17%), and perinatal mortality (4%), compared with the general population.

Management of Hypertension in Pregnancy

The primary management of chronic hypertension in pregnancy includes treatment of high BP and monitoring for superimposed preeclampsia. Nonpharmacologic strategies for hypertension management in nonpregnant populations, including aerobic exercise, weight loss, and dietary sodium restriction, have not been thoroughly evaluated in pregnant women. When hypertension is severe (>160/105 mm Hg), drug therapy is clearly indicated. Until recently, data on specific BP targets in mild to moderate hypertension in pregnancy were sparse. The Control of Hypertension in Pregnancy Study (CHIPS) was a recent multicenter, randomized trial of women with mild to moderate nonproteinuric gestational or chronic hypertension in pregnancy. CHIPS showed no difference in adverse maternal or fetal outcomes in women with chronic hypertension treated to tight (diastolic blood pressure [DBP] target 85 mm Hg) versus less tight (DBP target 100 mm Hg) BP control during pregnancy. Women in the tight control arm did have fewer episodes of severe hypertension during pregnancy. Thus, it appears safe for the fetus to treat women with chronic or gestational hypertension to lower DBP (goal DBP 85 mm Hg), and this may prevent the acceleration of mild/moderate hypertension to severe hypertension during pregnancy. Whether tighter control of BP during pregnancy has a long-term benefit on maternal cardiovascular outcomes is unknown.

Recommended agents used to treat hypertension in pregnancy are summarized in Table 47.1. Medications used for treatment of hypertension in pregnancy include β-blockers, calcium channel blockers, methyldopa, and hydralazine. ACE inhibitors and ARBs cannot be used during pregnancy, as exposure to these agents in the second trimester is associated with fetal renal dysplasia, oligohydramnios, and pulmonary hypoplasia. Diuretics are not first-line agents for chronic hypertension in pregnancy, but can be used, if necessary, to treat volume overload. They should not be used in states like preeclampsia.

Gestational Hypertension

Gestational hypertension is defined as new-onset hypertension without proteinuria after 20 weeks of gestation that resolves within 3 months of delivery. Gestational hypertension and preeclampsia are likely a spectrum of disorders, with 15% to 25% of patients with gestational hypertension developing overt preeclampsia. Gestational hypertension, even in the absence of preeclampsia, is associated with adverse pregnancy outcomes. Offspring of mothers with gestational hypertension are at increased risk for preterm delivery and IUGR. Furthermore, these women are at increased risk for future development of hypertension and cardiovascular disease.

TABLE 47.1	Recommended Oral Antihypertensive Medications in Pregnancy			
Medication	Initial Dose	Maximum Total Daily Dose (mg)		Side Effects
Methyldopa	250 mg twice daily	2000		Fatigue, sedation, hemolytic anemia, increased liver function tests (rare)
Labetalol	200 mg twice daily	1200		Bronchospasm, fatigue
Long-acting nifedipine	30 mg daily	120		Edema, headache
Hydralazine	50 mg three times daily	300		Tachycardia

Preeclampsia

Preeclampsia is a pregnancy-specific multisystem syndrome characterized by development of hypertension and proteinuria occurring after 20 weeks of gestation. It is seen in approximately 5% of pregnancies in the United States. Maternal complications of preeclampsia include liver injury (hepatitis, hepatic hepatoma, or rupture), pulmonary edema, hypertensive encephalopathy, intracerebral edema, kidney failure, and death. Fetal complications include IUGR, placental abruption, and neonatal death. Eclampsia, defined as the occurrence of seizures in a woman with preeclampsia, is now rare in the developed world because of early management of preeclampsia.

Risk Factors

Rates of preeclampsia vary across the globe. It is more common in nulliparous women and multiparous women with a new partner. Other risk factors include a first-degree family member with preeclampsia, multiple gestations, molar pregnancies, extremes of maternal age (<20 and >40 years), prior episodes of preeclampsia, and underlying maternal medical conditions such as hypertension, diabetes, CKD, obesity, and thrombophilias, including antiphospholipid antibody syndrome.

Pathophysiology

Placental abnormalities play a central role in the development of preeclampsia (Fig. 47.2). During pregnancy, trophoblasts migrate into uterine spiral arteries, transforming thick muscular arteries into high-capacity vessels that permit greater blood flow to the uteroplacental unit. In preeclampsia, this process is impaired, and spiral arteries remain high-resistance vessels, leading to inadequate placental oxygen delivery, placental ischemia, and release of factors that induce widespread maternal vascular endothelial dysfunction. Whether placental ischemia alone is sufficient to cause preeclampsia is debatable because IUGR, also characterized by placental insufficiency, does occur without preeclampsia.

There is strong evidence for the role of placental antiangiogenic factors in pathogenesis of preeclampsia. Soluble fms-like tyrosine kinase-1 (sFlt1) is a soluble vascular endothelial growth factor (VEGF) receptor that binds to proangiogenic factors such as VEGF and placental growth factor (PIGF), neutralizing their effects. Excess production of sFlt1 from the placenta results in the widespread endothelial dysfunction characteristic of preeclampsia. Soluble endoglin (sEng) is a truncated tumor growth factor (TGF) β-coreceptor that antagonizes the action of TGF-β and augments the effects of sFlt1 on the endothelium. Both sFlt1 and sEng have been shown to increase before the onset of preeclampsia

and correlate with disease severity. It is believed that preeclampsia occurs as a result of a decrease in growth factors such as VEGF and PIGF, along with overproduction of antiangiogenic factors such as sFlt1 and sEng.

Circulating levels of sFlt1 and PIGF have shown promise as predictive biomarkers of preeclampsia in several studies. Serum PIGF levels are reduced in women who go on to develop preeclampsia as early as the first trimester. In an international study of women presenting with suspected preeclampsia, low sFlt1/PIGF ratio accurately identified women at very low risk for the development of preeclampsia within the next week. A low sFlt1/PIGF had a very strong negative predictive value (99%) in this study. In the future, a negative test may allow for improved risk stratification of women who are at low risk for developing a poor outcome. In a small, open-label study, removal of sFlt1 by dextran apheresis appeared safe to both mother and fetus and prolonged pregnancy in women with early preeclampsia and elevated sFlt1/PIGF ratios. Controlled studies are needed to further investigate dextran apheresis as a therapy for early onset preeclampsia, but this study highlights the potential causative role of sFlt1 in preeclampsia pathogenesis.

Definitions, Diagnosis, and Clinical Features

The definition of preeclampsia differs by region. The American College of Obstetricians and Gynecologists (ACOG) published updated guidelines on the diagnosis of preeclampsia in 2013. Preeclampsia is characterized by a new onset of hypertension (BP of ≥140/90 mm Hg) and proteinuria after 20 weeks of gestation. However, proteinuria is no longer required for the diagnosis of preeclampsia in the most recent guidelines, and the diagnosis can be made based on new-onset hypertension with evidence of other end-organ dysfunction such as thrombocytopenia, impaired liver function tests, reduced GFR, pulmonary edema, or cerebral symptoms. HELLP syndrome is characterized by microangiopathic hemolytic anemia, elevated liver enzymes, and low platelets and occurs in 10% to 20% of patients with preeclampsia.

Management and Prevention

Currently, delivery of the placenta and fetus is the only definitive treatment for preeclampsia. If preeclampsia develops at or near term, immediate delivery is justified. When preeclampsia develops before fetal lung maturity, clinical decisions about delivery timing can be difficult, and a trial of expectant management is justified. Close monitoring of the fetus and mother, treatment of hypertension, and prevention of maternal seizures with intravenous magnesium are all part of expectant management of preeclampsia. In women with underlying kidney disease, magnesium infusion must

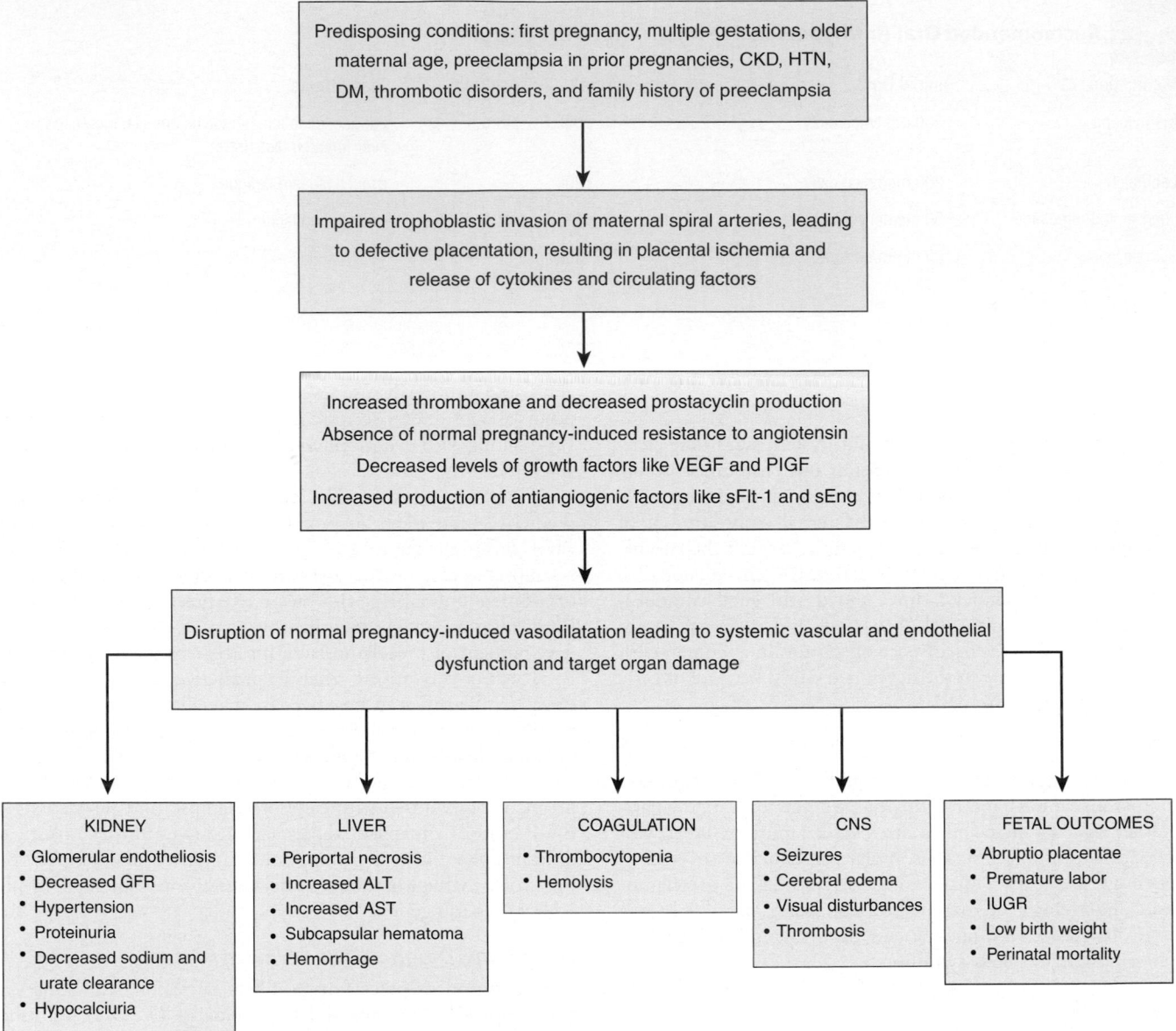

• **Fig. 47.2 Pathogenesis and outcomes of preeclampsia.** *ALT,* Alanine aminotransferase; *AST,* aspartate aminotransferase; *CKD,* chronic kidney disease; *CNS,* central nervous system; *DM,* diabetes mellitus; *GFR,* glomerular filtration rate; *HTN,* hypertension; *IUGR,* intrauterine growth restriction; *PIGF,* placental growth factor; *RPF,* renal plasma flow; *sEng,* soluble endoglin; *sFlt-1,* soluble fms-like tyrosine kinase-1; *VEGF,* vascular endothelial growth factor.

be used cautiously, with frequent monitoring of serum magnesium levels to avoid magnesium toxicity. Dose reductions are also recommended in women with advanced CKD.

Although data from early, multicenter, randomized, controlled trials (RCTs) on low-dose aspirin for the prevention of preeclampsia are conflicting, meta-analyses suggest a benefit, with a Cochrane review of 59 trials demonstrating a 17% reduction of risk for preeclampsia with low-dose aspirin. A recent meta-analysis, aimed at identifying dosage and timing of aspirin use, suggested a 43% reduction in risk for preeclampsia with low-dose aspirin when initiated before 16 weeks of gestation. As such, daily low-dose aspirin is recommended for women at high risk for preeclampsia, started ideally before 16 weeks of gestation. In a recent RCT, 1776 women at high risk for the development of preeclampsia were randomized to 150 mg of aspirin versus placebo between 11 and 14 weeks of gestation. A significant reduction in the incidence of preeclampsia was noted in the women treated with aspirin (odds ratio in the aspirin group, 0.38; 95% CI 0.20–0.74)

Data on the role of calcium in preventing preeclampsia are similarly challenging to interpret because of inconclusive randomized, controlled trials. In a Cochrane review, high-dose calcium supplementation (>1 g/day) was associated with an approximately 50% lower risk of preeclampsia, with the greatest benefit seen in women with low-calcium diets and women at high risk of preeclampsia. However, the authors stress that these data should be interpreted with caution because of the possibility of small-study effect and publication bias. Based on these results, it may be reasonable to use calcium supplements in women with low-calcium intake who are at high risk for preeclampsia.

Long-Term Outcomes After Preeclampsia

Hypertension and proteinuria typically improve shortly after delivery of the fetus and placenta. The majority of women have complete resolution of hypertension and proteinuria within 6 weeks of delivery. Despite this immediate recovery, there is strong evidence for an association between preeclampsia and future risk of cardiovascular and kidney disease, including chronic kidney failure. Large studies, mainly from registry data, have shown increased risk of chronic hypertension (RR 3.6 to 3.7), cardiovascular disease (RR 2.2), stroke (RR 1.8 to 2.0), and chronic kidney failure (RR 4.7 to 16.0) in long-term survivors of preeclampsia. As such, appropriate counseling and postpartum follow-up are critical.

Superimposed Preeclampsia

Women with chronic hypertension who develop new-onset proteinuria after 20 weeks of gestation are diagnosed with superimposed preeclampsia. If patients have proteinuria at baseline, the diagnosis of superimposed preeclampsia is difficult, as proteinuria often increases during pregnancy in women with preexisting kidney disease. Serial fetal surveillance to assess for growth restriction and placental vascular Doppler ultrasonography can provide helpful information when distinguishing between progressive proteinuric kidney disease and superimposed preeclampsia. More centers are utilizing the sFlt1/PIGF ratio as a biomarker to assist with the diagnosis of preeclampsia in these challenging patients.

Secondary Hypertension

While secondary hypertension is a less common cause of hypertension in pregnancy than essential hypertension and gestational hypertensive disorders, secondary causes should be considered in the evaluation of new hypertension in pregnancy. Some studies have shown that up to 25% of women in whom hypertension fails to resolve 6 months after delivery may have a secondary cause of hypertension.

Undiagnosed pheochromocytoma is associated with high maternal and fetal mortality. The diagnosis can be made by 24-hour urine measurements of epinephrine, norepinephrine, and their metabolites because values are unaltered in normal pregnancy or preeclampsia. Diagnosis of primary hyperaldosteronism is difficult because of alterations in renin and aldosterone secretions during pregnancy. Renovascular hypertension from fibromuscular dysplasia can lead to severe hypertension in pregnancy, and successful control of hypertension with angioplasty has been reported but is rarely done. Obstructive sleep apnea is an increasingly common cause of secondary hypertension and should be considered in women with a suggestive clinical history.

Acute Kidney Injury in Pregnancy

Acute kidney injury (AKI) is a rare, but serious complication of pregnancy. The incidence of AKI in low-resource nations is decreasing, in part, because of improvement in management of sepsis (from abortions and childbirth) and postpartum hemorrhage. In high-resource nations, the rate remains very low (2 to 3/10,000 births), but has been slowly increasing because of increasing maternal age and maternal comorbidities. Although any form of AKI that affects adults in the general population can also affect pregnant women, several etiologies are more common in pregnant women (Box 47.2). The most important step in diagnosis of AKI in pregnancy is differentiating among conditions that have overlapping features, such as preeclampsia/HELLP,

---

BOX 47.2

Causes of Acute Kidney Injury in Pregnancy

Volume depletion
  Hyperemesis gravidarum
  Postpartum bleeding
  Placental abruption
Sepsis
  Septic abortion
  Acute pyelonephritis
Severe preeclampsia
Bilateral cortical necrosis
Thrombotic microangiopathies (TTP-HUS)
Acute fatty liver of pregnancy
Urinary tract obstruction from gravid uterus

HUS, Hemolytic uremic syndrome; *TTP*, thrombotic thrombocytopenic purpura.

---

lupus nephritis, thrombotic thrombocytopenic purpura (TTP)/hemolytic uremic syndrome (HUS), and acute fatty liver of pregnancy (AFLP) because management strategies vary dramatically (Table 47.2).

Differential Diagnosis of Acute Kidney Injury in Pregnancy

The timing of AKI in gestation can often help narrow the differential diagnosis. In the first trimester, hemodynamic kidney injury (prerenal azotemia/acute tubular necrosis [ATN]) secondary to hyperemesis gravidarum or septic abortion predominates. However, most cases of AKI develop in the second and third trimesters, including preeclampsia/HELLP syndromes, thrombotic microangiopathies, AFLP, or obstetric hemorrhage. Atypical HUS (aHUS) and other disorders of complement regulation typically occur near term or postpartum. Fig. 47.3 displays the main causes of AKI in pregnancy at different gestational ages. Several pregnancy-specific causes of AKI are discussed as follows.

Hemodynamic Kidney Injury and Bilateral Cortical Necrosis

Hemodynamic-mediated kidney injury is a common cause of AKI in pregnancy. Injury can range from prerenal azotemia to ischemic ATN and, rarely, to bilateral cortical necrosis. Etiologies of hemodynamic AKI in pregnancy vary, but most commonly are seen with catastrophic pregnancy complications such as sepsis, obstetric hemorrhage, AFLP, amniotic fluid embolism, or adrenal failure. Bilateral renal cortical necrosis, the most extreme case of hemodynamic-mediated kidney injury in pregnancy, is a pathologic diagnosis characterized by diffuse cortical necrosis on kidney biopsy, with evidence of intravascular thrombosis. The medulla is usually spared. Pregnant women with severe kidney ischemia are more likely to develop cortical necrosis than the general population. Sudden onset of oliguria/anuria in the setting of hypotension should prompt consideration of renal cortical necrosis. Computed tomography or ultrasound can help establish the diagnosis by demonstrating hypoechoic or hypodense areas in the renal cortex. Most patients require dialysis, and recovery of kidney function is unlikely.

TABLE 47.2 Features of Microangiopathic Syndromes Associated With Pregnancy

Features	HELLP	TTP	HUS	AFLP
Clinical onset	Third trimester	Any time	Postpartum	Third trimester
Unique to pregnancy	Yes	No	No	Yes
Underlying pathophysiology	Abnormal placentation	ADAMTS13 deficiency	Mutations in genes regulating complement function	Defective fetal mitochondrial β-oxidation of fatty acids
Hypertension	Yes	Occasional	Yes	Frequently
Kidney failure	Yes	Yes	Yes	Yes
Thrombocytopenia	Yes	Yes	Yes	Yes
Liver function tests	Abnormal	Normal	Normal	Abnormal
Antithrombin III	Low	Normal	Normal	Low
Management	Delivery	Plasma exchange	Eculizumab	Delivery

AFLP, Acute fatty liver of pregnancy; *HUS,* hemolytic uremic syndrome; *TTP,* thrombotic thrombocytopenic purpura.

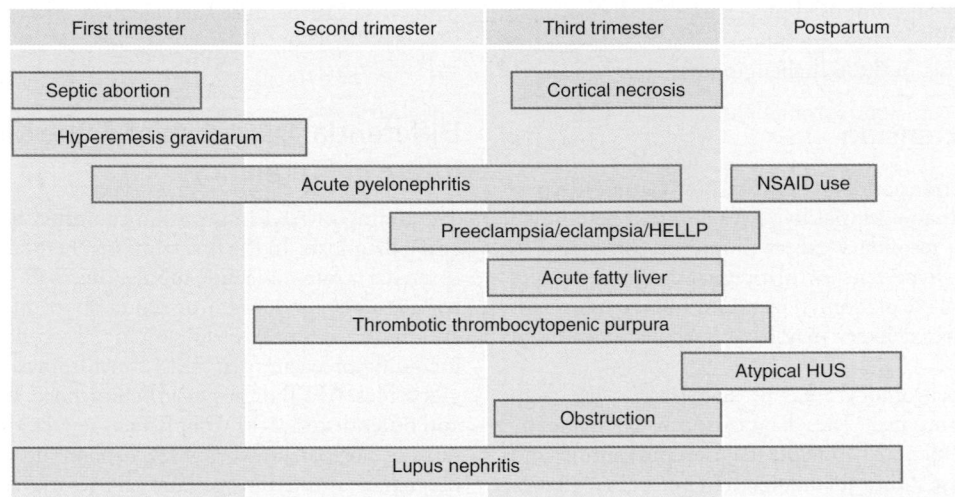

• **Fig. 47.3** Differential diagnosis for pregnancy-associated acute kidney injury based on timing during pregnancy. *HUS,* Hemolytic uremic syndrome; *NSAID,* nonsteroidal antiinflammatory drug.

Preeclampsia/HELLP

Overt AKI is a rare complication of preeclampsia (1%), but is seen more frequently with the HELLP syndrome (7% to 15%). The pathologic kidney lesion seen in preeclampsia is glomerular endotheliosis or widespread glomerular endothelial swelling. Kidney failure in the setting of preeclampsia/HELLP has overlapping clinical features with other pregnancy-associated causes of AKI, including AFLP, lupus nephritis, TTP, and aHUS (see Table 47.2).

Acute Fatty Liver of Pregnancy

AFLP is a rare condition that develops in the third trimester of pregnancy. Pathologically, AFLP is characterized by microvesicular fatty infiltration of maternal hepatocytes, secondary to abnormal oxidation of fatty acids by fetal mitochondria. Fetal deficiency of long-chain 3-hydroxyl CoA dehydrogenase leads to excess fetal free fatty acids that cross the placenta and are hepatotoxic to the

mother. Women often present with symptoms including fatigue, vomiting, and jaundice. Laboratory findings show elevation of serum transaminases, increased bilirubin levels, and thrombocytopenia with or without disseminated intravascular coagulation (DIC). Hypoglycemia, lactic acidosis, and AKI are common. Kidney biopsy findings in AFLP include ATN, fatty vacuolization of tubular cells, and occlusion of capillary lumens by fibrin-like material. Definitive management is prompt delivery of the fetus. Both kidney and liver failure generally resolve postpartum, with few patients requiring liver transplant.

Distinguishing AFLP from HELLP syndrome can be challenging because both are associated with transaminitis. The most common clinical features of AFLP are malaise, nausea, vomiting, abdominal pain, and jaundice. HELLP syndrome more commonly presents with headache, abdominal or epigastric pain, and hypertension. Evidence of synthetic liver dysfunction, such as hypoglycemia and low antithrombin III, are characteristic of AFLP. DIC, AKI, ascites, and encephalopathy are also more common in AFLP.

Thrombotic Microangiopathies

TTP and HUS are important causes of AKI characterized by unexplained thrombocytopenia and microangiopathic hemolytic anemia. Traditionally, TTP is considered when neurologic abnormalities are dominant and HUS when there is profound kidney failure, especially in the postpartum period.

TTP results from a deficiency of von Willebrand factor cleaving protease (ADAMTS13). Most cases of pregnancy-associated TTP occur during the second or third trimester. Pregnancy appears to be a trigger for new onset or relapse of TTP, perhaps because pregnancy is associated with decreases in ADAMTS13 levels. Treatment of TTP in pregnancy is similar to the nonpregnant state with plasma exchange, which should be initiated before the diagnosis is confirmed if TTP is suspected.

Pregnancy-related aHUS, as in the nonpregnant state, is the result of complement dysregulation most often secondary to mutations in genes encoding complement regulatory proteins. Pregnancy can be a trigger for aHUS; however, unlike TTP, it most commonly presents in the peri- or postpartum period. Inhibition of C5 by eculizumab appears safe and effective in pregnant women; thus, a high level of suspicion for aHUS to allow for early diagnosis and treatment is critical. Outcomes are better with shorter duration from diagnosis to treatment, but misdiagnosis is unfortunately common.

Distinguishing TTP/HUS from severe preeclampsia accompanied by HELLP syndrome can be difficult. Thrombocytopenia, microangiopathic hemolytic anemia, AKI, proteinuria, and hypertension occur in both TTP-HUS and HELLP, although elevated liver enzymes are more common in HELLP syndrome.

Pyelonephritis

Although the prevalence of asymptomatic bacteriuria is similar in both pregnant and nonpregnant women, 30% to 40% of pregnant women with untreated asymptomatic bacteriuria develop symptomatic urinary tract infection, including pyelonephritis. Gestational pyelonephritis is a serious condition associated with IUGR, premature labor, and sepsis. AKI occurs in up to 25% of cases. Cephalosporins and penicillins are generally safe and effective. Treatment should be intravenous until the patient is afebrile, and then continued for 14 days. Recurrent pyelonephritis occurs in 6% to 8% of women, so it is reasonable to continue suppressive therapy with low-dose antimicrobial agents for the remainder of the pregnancy.

Obstruction-Related Acute Kidney Injury

Ureteral and bladder outlet obstruction should be considered in the differential diagnosis of AKI in pregnancy, but is overall rare. True obstruction may be difficult to differentiate from physiologic hydronephrosis of pregnancy, which becomes more pronounced as pregnancy progresses to term. Magnetic resonance imaging can help in distinguishing physiologic hydronephrosis from obstruction in pregnancy, while ultrasound is less reliable in such a setting.

Pregnancy in Women With Chronic Kidney Disease

Preexisting CKD increases both maternal and fetal risk. Factors associated with higher risk include CKD stage, comorbid conditions, such as hypertension and diabetes, advanced maternal age, and the use of assisted reproductive technologies. Importantly, women with CKD who enter pregnancy with well-controlled BP, treated proteinuria, and stable kidney function can have excellent outcomes, making preconception kidney care critical.

The potential for pregnancy to accelerate the progression of CKD is of concern. In a recent large-cohort study of women with CKD stage 1, progression to a more advanced stage of CKD during pregnancy occurred in 8% of patients; however, the clinical significance of this change is unclear, as most progressed only to CKD stage 2. Progression is more likely in women with advanced CKD. In a historical study of CKD pregnancies, 40% of women showed significant pregnancy-related loss of kidney function, with 20% of women progressing to kidney failure within 6 months of delivery. More recent studies suggest lower progression rates, with 16% of women with CKD stage 3 and 20% of women with CKD stage 4 to 5 progressing to a more advanced stage of CKD or kidney failure. Predicting which women will experience rapid kidney function decline peri- or postpartum is challenging. Pregnancy termination does not reliably reverse the decline in kidney function.

The risk of adverse pregnancy outcomes increases with lower baseline GFR, although, even when women have preserved kidney function, normal BP, and minimal proteinuria, the risk for pregnancy complications is higher than noted in the general population. In women with advanced CKD, preterm delivery, small-for-gestational-age offspring, and need for neonatal intensive care unit care are common. Many women with advanced CKD have coexisting hypertension and proteinuria, which independently have been shown to increase the risk of adverse outcomes. Because of the detrimental effects that an unplanned pregnancy can have in women with preexisting CKD, contraception should be addressed as part of routine CKD care in reproductive-age women regardless of CKD stage.

Diabetes and Diabetic Kidney Disease

The details of pregnancy management in women with diabetes mellitus complicated by diabetic kidney disease are complex and beyond the scope of this chapter. Women with diabetic kidney disease are at high risk of pregnancy complications because of preexisting vascular disease resulting in poor placental development, and impaired autonomic functioning resulting in inadequate hemodynamic adaptation to pregnancy. There are also numerous maternal and fetal complications secondary to poor glycemic control, including increased rates of fetal malformations. Planning for pregnancy, including optimization of proteinuria with RAAS blockade before pregnancy, is essential for successful outcomes. Multiple small studies have shown that intensive hypertensive and glycemic control in women with diabetic kidney disease before conception improves outcomes. The decision to continue RAAS blockade until women conceive is an individualized decision, but this appears to be a safe approach in women trying to conceive who have regular menses and can stop therapy with their first missed menstrual cycle.

Lupus Nephritis

Lupus predominantly affects women of childbearing age, with clinically significant kidney disease seen in approximately 30% of women with systemic lupus erythematosus (SLE). Pregnancy-related immunologic and hormonal changes can be associated with flares. Predictors of poor pregnancy outcomes include active kidney disease, reduced GFR, hypocomplementemia, and the presence of antiphospholipid antibodies. Preeclampsia is a frequent complication, with a higher incidence in lupus nephritis compared with lupus patients with no kidney involvement and is often difficult to distinguish from a lupus nephritis flare.

A recent multicenter study showed excellent maternal and fetal outcomes in women with minimal or well-controlled kidney disease. Pregnancy may be safely planned in stable patients with quiescent kidney disease, minimal proteinuria, and controlled BP for at least 6 months on pregnancy-safe medications. Mycophenolate mofetil (MMF) is teratogenic and must be changed to azathioprine before conception. All women with SLE should be maintained on hydroxychloroquine during pregnancy because this agent reduces the frequency of lupus flares. A summary of immunosuppressive agents and whether they can be used in pregnancy is shown in Table 47.3. All women with SLE should be screened for the presence of SSA/SSB autoantibodies, which are associated with neonatal heart block and congenital lupus. Low-dose aspirin is recommended for preeclampsia prophylaxis in women with lupus. Women with antiphospholipid syndrome are at high risk for thrombosis and should be anticoagulated with low-molecular-weight heparin.

Other Glomerular Diseases

Immunoglobulin A (IgA) nephropathy is a common glomerular disease in reproductive-age women. In general, the risk of pregnancy is related to CKD stage alone, although the management of women with IgA complicated by kidney dysfunction and heavy proteinuria can be challenging because of the lack of disease-specific therapies. Women with minimal proteinuria (<1 g/day) and normal GFR generally do well in pregnancy, and several studies have shown that GFR 5 years after pregnancy is similar to women who did not conceive.

Data on pregnancy in other glomerular diseases, such as membranoproliferative glomerulonephritis (MPGN), primary focal segmental glomerulosclerosis (FSGS), membranous nephropathy (MN), and antiglomerular basement membrane (anti-GBM) disease, are even more limited. Antineutrophil cytoplasmic antibody (ANCA)-associated vasculitis is uncommon in reproductive-age women compared with older adults, and data on outcomes in pregnancy are limited to case reports. In one of the largest case series, eight out of 21 women with disease in remission relapsed during pregnancy. Induction therapy during pregnancy is challenging because of teratogenicity of many first-line agents. In a study of long-term follow-up in women with primary glomerular disease on

kidney biopsy with preserved GFR, women who became pregnant after clinical onset of disease were no more likely to progress to kidney failure than women who did not conceive, and a general principle is to strive for adequate disease control preconception.

Nephrotic Syndrome

The most common cause of new-onset nephrotic-range proteinuria in late pregnancy is preeclampsia. However, new-onset primary nephrotic syndrome can present during pregnancy. Evaluation for secondary causes of nephrotic syndrome, including serologic testing, should be done in all women with de novo nephrotic syndrome that is not clearly related to preeclampsia. Severe proteinuria, hypoalbuminemia, edema, and hypercoagulability can be especially detrimental during pregnancy. Peripheral volume overload may require the use of diuretics. As pregnancy itself produces a hypercoagulable state, additional urinary losses of antithrombotic proteins in the nephrotic syndrome amplify this risk. Thromboprophylaxis with low-molecular-weight heparin should be considered in women with heavy proteinuria, especially in those with a serum albumin less than 2.0 mg/dL or less than 2.5 mg/dL in the context of other risk factors for thrombosis (e.g., immobility, obesity, membranous nephropathy). Although anticoagulation may be temporarily suspended to reduce peripartum bleeding, it should be continued for at least 6 weeks postpartum.

Autosomal Dominant Polycystic Kidney Disease

Advanced kidney disease in women with autosomal dominant polycystic kidney disease (ADPKD) generally develops after childbearing age. Fertility is normal in women with preserved kidney function. When compared with pregnancies in unaffected family members, women with ADPKD have higher rates of preeclampsia. The presence of preexisting hypertension was the most important risk factor for adverse outcomes. Women with ADPKD and hypertension who had multiple pregnancies (≥4) were at higher risk for CKD progression. Normotensive women with ADPKD, in general, have uncomplicated pregnancies, although pregnant women with ADPKD may experience an increased incidence of asymptomatic bacteriuria, more severe urinary tract infections, and an increase in the size and number of cysts due to estrogen stimulation. Preimplantation genetic testing is available in some centers for at-risk couples.

TABLE 47.3	Immunosuppressive Medications in Pregnancy	
Medication	**Side Effects**	**Dosing Adjustments**
Cyclosporine/tacrolimus	Increased incidence of maternal diabetes, hypertension, and preeclampsia	Higher doses required because of increased metabolism
Sirolimus	Contraindicated in pregnancy	Stopped 6 weeks before conception
Mycophenolic acid	Contraindicated in pregnancy	Stopped 12 weeks before conception
Azathioprine	Widely used despite being category D; low birth weights and leukopenia reported in newborns, but this may reflect risks associated with the underlying disease	No dosing adjustments required
Cyclophosphamide	Increased risk for congenital anomalies and childhood cancer	Should be avoided
Rituximab	Limited human data; crosses placenta; B-cell lymphocytopenia and infections reported in neonates	Limited data

Dialysis

Historically, women dependent on dialysis were unlikely to conceive and often counseled against pregnancy because of the association with poor outcomes. Emerging data suggest that intensive dialysis results in improved outcomes and may be a viable option for women receiving dialysis who are unlikely to receive a kidney transplant during their reproductive years. Early menopause is common in women treated with standard thrice-weekly dialysis regimens. Ovulatory cycles may be restored in women who begin intensified hemodialysis regimens such as home or nocturnal hemodialysis.

Pregnancy outcomes have significantly improved since the report of the first successful pregnancy in a patient undergoing dialysis in 1971. In 1998, only 50% of pregnancies in women conceiving after starting dialysis resulted in surviving infants; however, more recent series note live birth rates in excess of 85%. This improvement likely reflects near universal adaptation of intensified dialysis practices in pregnant women.

Because amenorrhea is common during dialysis, diagnosing pregnancy can be difficult. A pregnancy diagnosis should be confirmed with ultrasound. Medications should be carefully reviewed and teratogenic medications promptly discontinued. Hemodialysis should be intensified to a minimum of 36 hours per week, targeting predialysis BUN less than 50 mg/dL (Box 47.3). Because weight should increase by 0.5 kg/week in the third trimester, weight gain should be expected. Determination of dry weight can be difficult and should be made by clinical examination and assessment of fetal growth. Pregnancy should be managed by a multidisciplinary team that includes high-risk obstetricians and nephrologists.

Kidney Transplantation

Sexual dysfunction and infertility often reverse post transplantation. Ovulation can occur within the first month after transplant. Optimal contraception should be initiated during the peri-transplant period. Oral contraceptive pills are a reasonable choice if BP is adequately controlled. Intrauterine devices (IUDs), previously believed to require an intact immune system, also appear to be a safe and effective option.

The consensus opinion of the American Transplant Society is that pregnancy can be planned when the patient reaches 1 year posttransplantation, as long as the following criteria are met: adequate kidney function on stable, pregnancy-safe immunosuppressive medication, and no evidence of fetotoxic infections, including cytomegalovirus (CMV). The major concerns are the effect of pregnancy on maternal allograft function and potential side effects of medications on fetal growth. Preeclampsia, premature delivery, and low birth weight are more common in transplant recipients than in the general population.

Many studies comparing kidney transplant recipients with and without pregnancies report no difference in long-term allograft survival. In studies from the United States and United Kingdom, women with allograft loss had higher mean prepregnancy creatinine. Recent data from the US Renal Data System (USRDS) showed a 10% incidence of allograft loss at 1 year and a 37% incidence of allograft loss at 5 years in women who conceived after transplant. Conceiving within the first and second year after transplant was a risk factor for accelerated allograft loss, while conceiving during the third posttransplant year was not associated with accelerated allograft loss. These estimates were higher than previously reported in US transplant recipients. Kidney allograft biopsy can be safely performed to evaluate for graft dysfunction during pregnancy.

All immunosuppressive medications cross the placenta; however, steroids, calcineurin inhibitors, and azathioprine have an acceptable safety profile. Much remains to be learned about the pharmacokinetics and pharmacodynamics of immunosuppressive medications during pregnancy and, as expected, most of the available information is from retrospective review and clinical experience (see Box 47.3). Maintenance immunosuppression in pregnant transplant patients generally includes cyclosporine or

---

BOX 47.3

Management of Pregnant Patients Undergoing Hemodialysis

Dialysis Dose

At least 36 hours of dialysis per week; goal predialysis BUN <50 mg/dL

Dialysate Composition

Sodium: 130–135 mEq/L based on serum Na
Potassium: 3.0–4.0 mmol/L
Bicarbonate: 25 mEq/L

Diet/Vitamin Supplementation

Double dose of MVI
Folic acid 5 mg/daily
Unrestricted diet
Protein intake: 1.5–1.8 g/kg/day

Dry Weight

Assess weekly
Increases by 0.5 kg/week in second and third trimesters

Anemia

Increase in ESA and iron doses
Target hemoglobin of 10 g/dL

Hypertension

Target postdialysis BP of 140/90 mm Hg

Diagnosis of Preeclampsia

Difficult to diagnose; must rely on worsening BP control and fetal assessments
Low-dose aspirin daily for prophylaxis of preeclampsia

Metabolic Bone Disease

Vitamin D analogs to maintain PTH levels, as, in general, patients undergoing dialysis
Dialysate calcium: 2.5–3.0 mmol/L
Oral phosphorus binders generally not required

BP, Blood pressure; *BUN*, blood urea nitrogen; *ESA*, erythropoiesis-stimulating agent; *MVI*, multiple vitamin for infusion; *PTH*; parathyroid hormone.

tacrolimus, azathioprine, and prednisone. Mycophenolate should be discontinued in transplant patients planning to become pregnant. Antibodies used to treat rejection, such as thymoglobulin and alemtuzumab, cross the placenta, and there is insufficient experience with these agents in pregnancy.

Kidney Biopsy in Pregnancy

Kidney biopsy in pregnancy is recommended only when there is suspicion of significant disease in which diagnosis will alter therapy. The most common indications are to diagnose unexplained rapid decline in GFR or new-onset nephrotic syndrome in the absence of preeclampsia or other systemic conditions. If necessary, the biopsy should be performed before 32 weeks' gestational age. Kidney biopsies become technically challenging as gestation progresses because the gravid uterus prevents prone positioning. Biopsy is never indicated when preeclampsia is part of the differential diagnosis, as hypertension and abnormal coagulation indices can significantly hamper the safety of the procedure.

Complete bibliography is available at Elsevier eBooks for Practicing Clinicians.

Key Bibliography

American College of Obstetricians and Gynecologists. Task Force on Hypertension in Pregnancy. Report of the American College of Obstetricians and Gynecologists' task force on hypertension in pregnancy. *Obstet Gynecol.* 2013;122:1122–1131.

Bartsch E, Medcalf KE, Park AL, Ray JG. Clinical risk factors for preeclampsia determined in early pregnancy: systematic review and meta-analysis of large cohort studies. *BMJ.* 2016;353:i1753.

Bramham K, Nelson-Piercy C, Gao H, et al. Pregnancy in renal transplant recipients: a UK national cohort study. *Clin J Am Soc Nephrol.* 2013;8:290–298.

Buyon JP, Kim MY, Guerra MM, et al. Predictors of pregnancy outcomes in patients with lupus: a cohort study. *Ann Intern Med.* 2015;163:153–163.

Chapman AB, Johnson AM, Gabow PA. Pregnancy outcome and its relationship to progression of renal failure in autosomal dominant polycystic kidney disease. *J Am Soc Nephrol.* 1994;5:1178–1185.

Fakhouri F, Roumenina L, Provot F, et al. Pregnancy-associated hemolytic uremic syndrome revisited in the era of complement gene mutations. *J Am Soc Nephrol.* 2010;21:859–867.

Harel Z, McArthur E, Hladunewich M, et al. Serum creatinine levels before, during, and after pregnancy. *JAMA.* 2019;321(2):205–207. doi:10.1001/jama.2018.17948.

Hildebrand AM, Liu K, Shariff SZ, et al. Characteristics and outcomes of AKI treated with dialysis during pregnancy and the postpartum period. *J Am Soc Nephrol.* 2015;26:3085–3091.

Hladunewich MA, Hou S, Odutayo A, et al. Intensive hemodialysis associates with improved pregnancy outcomes: a Canadian and United States cohort comparison. *J Am Soc Nephrol.* 2014;25:1103–1109.

Hofmeyr GJ, Lawrie TA, Atallah AN, Duley L, Torloni MR. Calcium supplementation during pregnancy for preventing hypertensive disorders and related problems. *Cochrane Database Syst Rev.* 2014:Cd001059.

Jungers P, Houillier P, Forget D, et al. Influence of pregnancy on the course of primary chronic glomerulonephritis. *Lancet.* 1995;346:1122–1124.

Levine RJ, Maynard SE, Qian C, et al. Circulating angiogenic factors and the risk of preeclampsia. *N Engl J Med.* 2004;350:672–683.

Lindheimer MD, Davison JM. Renal biopsy during pregnancy: "to b … or not to b … ? *Br J Obstet Gynaecol.* 1987;94:932–934.

Magee LA, von Dadelszen P, Rey E, et al. Less-tight versus tight control of hypertension in pregnancy. *N Engl J Med.* 2015;372:407–417.

Odutayo A, Hladunewich M. Obstetric nephrology: renal hemodynamic and metabolic physiology in normal pregnancy. *Clin J Am Soc Nephrol.* 2012;7:2073–2080.

Piccoli GB, Cabiddu G, Attini R, et al. Risk of adverse pregnancy outcomes in women with CKD. *J Am Soc Nephrol.* 2015;26:2011–2022.

Rana S, Powe CE, Salahuddin S, et al. Angiogenic factors and the risk of adverse outcomes in women with suspected preeclampsia. *Circulation.* 2012;125:911–919.

Roberge S, Nicolaides K, Demers S, Hyett J, Chaillet N, Bujold E. The role of aspirin dose on the prevention of preeclampsia and fetal growth restrction: systematic review and meta-analysis. *Am J Obstet Gynecol.* 2017;216:110–120, e6.

Rose C, Gill J, Zalunardo N, Johnston O, Mehrotra A, Gill JS. Timing of pregnancy after kidney transplantation and risk of allograft failure. *Am J Transplant.* 2016;16:2360–2367.

Thadhani R, Hagmann H, Schaarschmidt W, et al. Removal of soluble Fms-like tyrosine kinase-1 by dextran sulfate apheresis in preeclampsia. *J Am Soc Nephrol.* 2016;27:903–913.

Vikse BE, Irgens LM, Leivestad T, Skjaerven R, Iversen BM. Preeclampsia and the risk of end-stage renal disease. *N Engl J Med.* 2008;359:800–809.

48

Management of Kidney Disease in the Elderly

ANTONEY J. FERREY, JOHN E. SY, CONNIE RHEE, ANN O'HARE, KAMYAR KALANTAR-ZADEH

Epidemiology of CKD in the Elderly

The prevalence of chronic kidney disease (CKD) increases markedly with age, and the number of older adults with advanced kidney disease will continue to increase as longevity improves due to medical advances and improved access to healthcare around the world. The prevalence of CKD increases from fewer than 6% in individuals less than 40 years old, to 44% among those age 70 and older. The high prevalence of CKD in older adults partially reflects structural and functional changes that occur in normally aging healthy adults and a higher prevalence of related comorbid conditions (e.g., diabetes and hypertension) at older ages.

Measured and estimated GFR in the general population follow a normal distribution with a median value around 80 to 90 mL/min/1.73 m². The midpoint of this distribution decreases with age and moves closer to 60 mL/min/1.73 m² in some groups. A meta-analysis from published GFR measurements in more than 5000 healthy, Caucasian, potential living kidney donors calculated the expected decrease in mean measured and estimated GFR with age. This change was most pronounced in healthy women, in whom measured GFR decreased from 107 mL/min/1.73 m² in women aged 20 to 30 years old to 69 mL/min/1.73 m² in women over 70 years old. The upper and lower reference limits determined by the study show the anticipated decrease in eGFR by decade (Fig. 48.1). In clinical practice this can roughly be estimated as a decline in eGFR of 0.5 to 1 mL/min/1.73 m²/year.

Urinary protein excretion also increases with age. However, the majority of older adults with CKD have an albumin-to-creatinine ratio (ACR) less than 30 mg/g, such that most older adults with CKD have low eGFR in the absence of significant albuminuria. This contrasts with younger adults with CKD, who are more likely to have albuminuria in the presence of a preserved eGFR (Fig. 48.2).

Prevalence estimates for CKD in older adults vary widely depending on the method used to estimate GFR (see Chapter 3). This specifically affects many elderly patients with eGFR values around 60 mL/min/1.73 m², the threshold used to define CKD. The serum creatinine-based Chronic Kidney Disease Epidemiology Collaboration (CKD-EPI) equation for estimating GFR more accurately estimates GFR in patients older than 65 years of age with eGFR in the 60-89 mL/min/1.73 m² range than the MDRD equation. Newer equations have been developed from populations with a higher representation of older adults and may yield more accurate estimates of CKD. However, due to the substantial variation in the age composition of different clinical practices, equations

validated only in elderly populations, such as the Berlin Initiative Study (BIS1), have not yet been incorporated into routine clinical practice. This may have little clinical impact: Comparisons between the CKD-EPI equation and the BIS1 equation did not show substantial differences from measured GFR values in older adults and the accuracy of estimates of GFR from either equation is likely sufficient to support most clinical decision making.

Non-creatinine-based methods to estimate GFR include formulas that utilize serum cystatin C and β2-microglobulin measurements. Their use was previously limited because these measures are more expensive with a slower turnaround time than serum creatinine. Serum cystatin C in particular is now more readily available and affordable. Ultimately, reliance on more than one filtration marker may be useful when trying to decide whether an older adult meets criteria for CKD, particularly among patients with underlying conditions or characteristics that may influence serum creatinine levels independent of kidney function, such as extremes of muscle mass, prior amputation, and vegetarian diets.

The Clinical Significance of Moderately Reduced Estimated GFR

There is ongoing debate regarding the clinical significance of CKD in older adults because death due to cardiovascular causes is far more common than progression to kidney failure among most older adults who meet criteria for CKD, particularly those with mildly to moderately reduced eGFR (45–59 mL/min/1.73 m²). At lower levels of eGFR the risk of kidney failure eventually exceeds the risk of death for most patient groups, but the threshold level of eGFR at which this transition occurs varies systematically by age (Fig. 48.3).

Although an eGFR below 45 mL/min/1.73 m² is associated with poor outcomes, several studies have demonstrated that, unlike younger adults, those age 65 and older with mild reductions in eGFR in the 50–59 mL/min/1.73 m² range do not have a significantly higher risk of death compared to their age peers with GFR above 60 mL/min/1.73 m². These studies highlight both the measurement issues discussed above and clinical uncertainty about the implications of such modest reductions in eGFR in older adults. The complex relationships among mortality, age, and GFR are likely modified by the presence of other factors including comorbid conditions and socio-demographic differences.

There also are systematic differences in the most common causes of CKD in older versus younger adults. In autopsy studies,

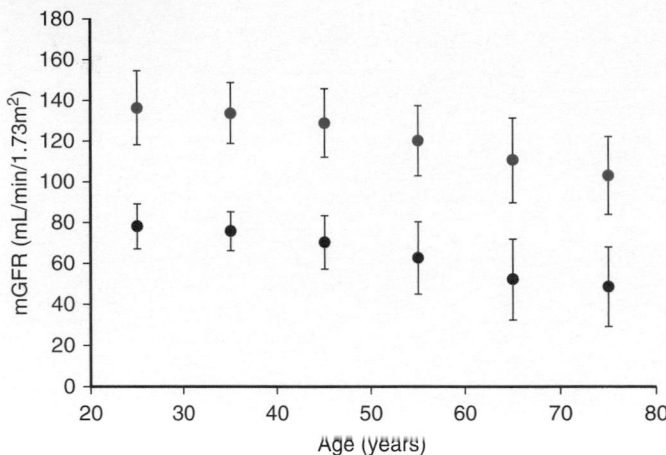

• **Fig. 48.1** A meta-analysis from published glomerular filtration rate (GFR) measurements in healthy, white, potential living kidney donors shows the decrease in mean measured GFR (mGFR) with age. The upper and lower reference limits determined by the study show the anticipated decrease in GFR by decade. (Modified from Pottel H, Delanaye P, Weekers L et al. Age-dependent reference intervals for estimated and measured glomerular filtration rate. *Clin Kidney J*. 2017;10(4):545-551.)

arteriolar sclerosis, global glomerulosclerosis, renal artery stenosis, cholesterol embolization, and tubular atrophy were more common at older ages. While it remains unclear if nephrosclerosis and vascular disease are a normal part of aging, these likely contribute to progression of kidney disease in older adults.

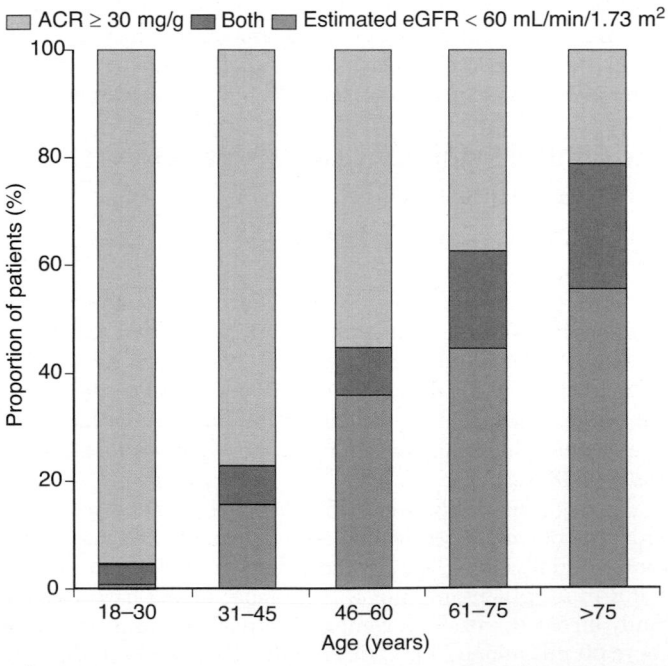

• **Fig. 48.2** Proportions of patients with chronic kidney disease identified by albumin-to-creatinine ratio (ACR), estimated glomerular filtration rate (eGFR), or both in the US population. (From James MT, Hemmelgarn BR, Tonelli M. Early recognition and prevention of chronic kidney disease. *Lancet*. 2010;375:1296–1309. Adapted from McCullough PA, Li S, Jurkovitz CT, et al. CKD and cardiovascular disease in screened high-risk volunteer and general populations: the Kidney Early Evaluation Program [KEEP] and National Health and Nutrition Examination Survey [NHANES] 1999–2004. *Am J Kidney Dis*. 2008;51:S38–S45.)

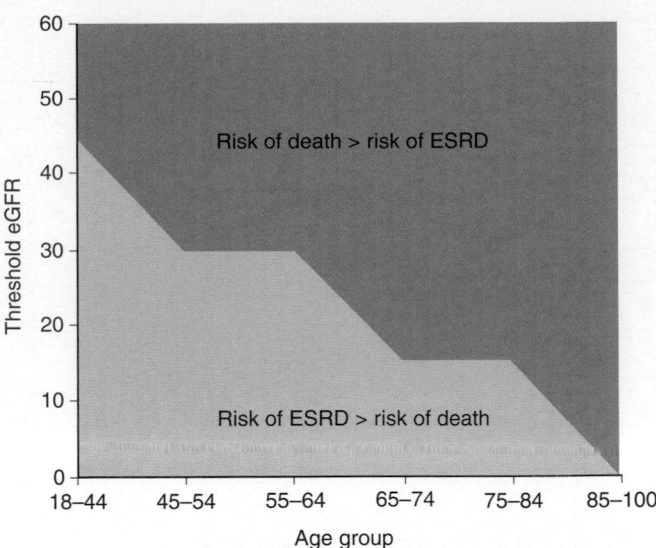

• **Fig. 48.3** Age differences in the threshold level of estimated glomerular filtration rate (eGFR), at which risk of end-stage renal disease (ESRD) exceeds risk of death among a US cohort of veterans. (From O'Hare AM, Choi AI, Bertenthal D, et al. Age affects outcomes in chronic kidney disease. *J Am Soc Nephrol*. 2007;18:2758–2765.)

Progression of CKD and Risk of Developing Kidney Failure

Although the age-adjusted incidence of end-stage kidney disease (ESKD) in the United States has declined slightly since 2010, the prevalence of chronic kidney failure continues to rise. The high prevalence of maintenance dialysis at older ages is likely multifactorial, reflecting the high prevalence of CKD in older adults, increased life expectancy with advances in contemporary medicine, and improvements in dialysis care.

Despite the higher prevalence of CKD in the elderly, older adults more often do not need to start dialysis for kidney failure compared to younger patients with similar levels of kidney function. This is likely due to multiple factors, including greater competing risk of death, slower progression of CKD, and lesser uptake of kidney replacement therapy in older adults. To help predict the risk of kidney failure treated with dialysis, several scores have been developed including the VA risk score by Drawz and colleagues as well as the Kidney Failure Risk Equation. Both models have been widely validated, provide relatively accurate probabilities of requiring maintenance dialysis over 1-5 years, and appear to perform well in older adults with CKD. These scores can be readily incorporated into clinical practice to support discussions with patients and families about prognosis and individualizing care plans. Despite the lower predicted risk of requiring dialysis when compared to younger individuals with similar eGFR, the importance of general advanced care planning should not, however, be downplayed in this population with more comorbid conditions.

Management of Older Adults with Chronic Kidney Disease

In older adults, the presence of multiple comorbid conditions may generate competing health priorities, conflicting treatment recommendations, and polypharmacy (Fig. 48.4). Clinical practice guidelines rarely acknowledge the possibility that a patient may

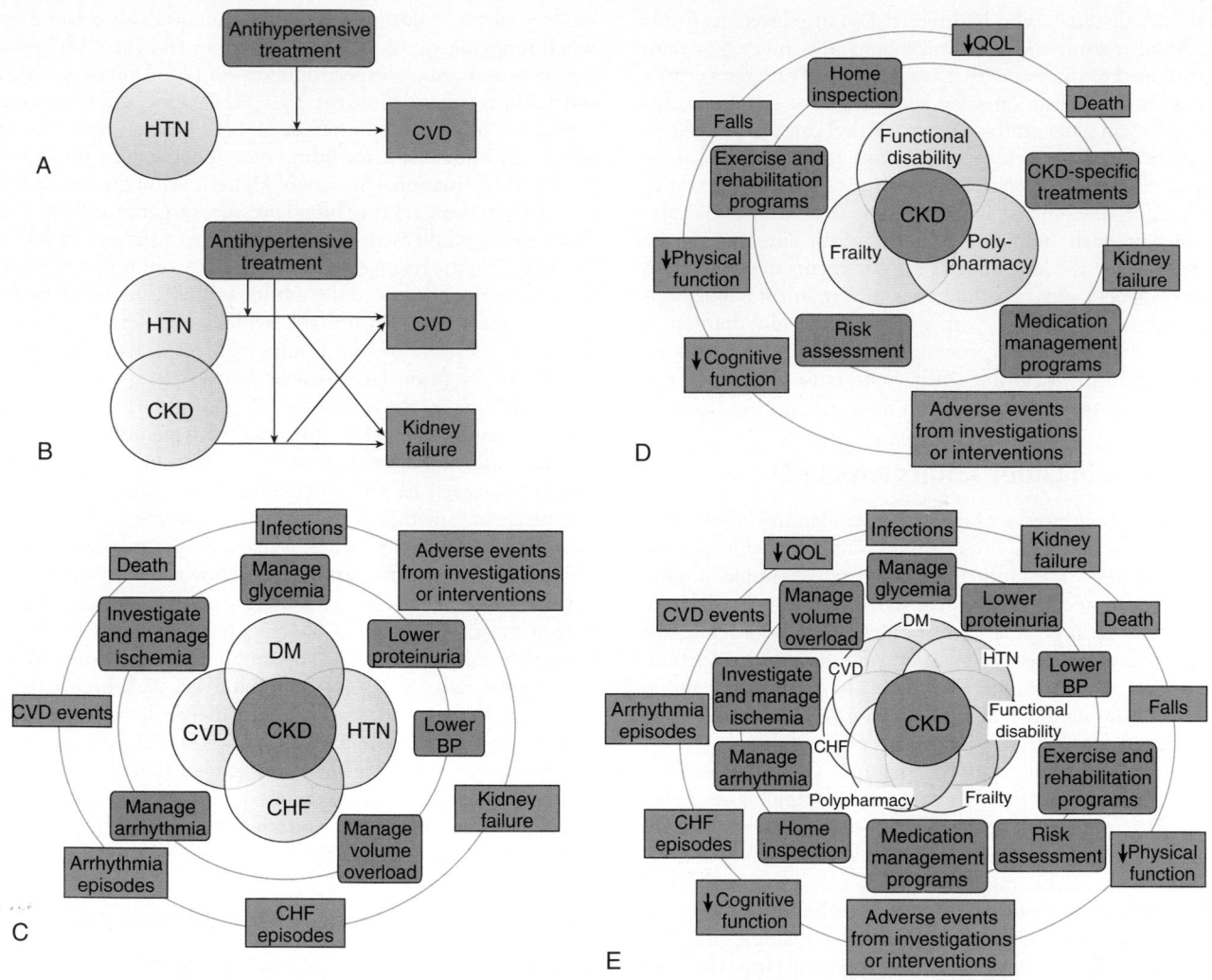

• **Fig. 48.4** Disease models increase in complexity with increasing numbers of disease conditions, treatments, and outcomes considered, such as in patients with chronic kidney disease (CKD) or of older age. *Circles* indicate diseases, *rectangles* outcomes, and *rounded rectangles* treatments. Disease models show treatment of (A) hypertension (HTN) without CKD; (B) HTN in patients with CKD; (C) CKD and a cluster of additional common comorbid conditions; (D) CKD along with a cluster of geriatric syndromes; and (E) CKD in older patients, incorporating clusters of common comorbid conditions, as well as geriatric syndromes (the overlap of C and D). *BP,* Blood pressure; *CHF,* congestive heart failure; *CVD,* cardiovascular disease; *DM,* diabetes mellitus; *QOL,* quality of life. (From Uhlig K, Boyd C. Guidelines for the older adult with CKD. *Am J Kidney Dis.* 2011;58:162–165.)

have more than one condition, nor do they distinguish between patients of different ages. Consequently, many clinical practice guidelines fail to provide guidance on how to manage the multiple competing health priorities that commonly arise in older adults with complex comorbidities. One study modeled the implications of a disease-specific approach to care on a hypothetical older adult with a fairly standard set of comorbid conditions. The onerous pharmacologic and non-pharmacologic treatment regimens that would have been recommended based on existing guidelines for each individual would have resulted in multiple potential drug interactions and competing treatment priorities.

Treatment Effects and Outcomes Among Older Adults

Guidelines for patients with CKD assume a uniform relationship between level of kidney function and clinical outcomes among patients of all ages. However, the relative and absolute frequency

of different clinical outcomes varies systematically among older and younger patients with the same levels of eGFR. Such differences in outcomes can affect the potential benefit of many commonly recommended treatment approaches for individual patients. Interventions intended to reduce cardiovascular disease and risk of kidney failure have the potential to prevent the greatest number of events among high-risk groups (e.g., CKD); however, in individuals with more limited life expectancy (e.g., older patients with CKD) such interventions may provide only modest gains in life expectancy or event-free survival. Given the limited life expectancy of many older adults with CKD, the competing risk of death should be considered when estimating the benefits and harms of recommended interventions. This is particularly true when preparing older adults for dialysis. For example, the morbidity of vascular access placement in a patient who is unlikely to survive long enough to require maintenance dialysis should figure into decision making about preemptive vascular access surgery. One study of octogenarians approaching the need for dialysis found a higher risk of death before initiation of dialysis in individuals who had received an arteriovenous fistula or graft. Another study showed similar outcomes in octogenarians who transitioned to dialysis with a central venous catheter versus a fistula or graft. These data question the wisdom of a uniform "fistula first" policy in older adults. Hence, clinical practice guidelines, quality metrics, and the evidence on which these are based must be interpreted within the context of each patient's life expectancy and risk for the outcome of interest. These decisions should also be grounded in each individual's values, goals, and preferences. Furthermore, given the lack of clear improvements in survival and of improved patient-reported outcomes in certain subpopulations of older adults, such as those with a high comorbidity burden or poor functional status, there is growing interest in conservative non-dialytic management, including greater efforts to preserve kidney function, as viable treatment options in these patients (see below).

Interventions in Older Adults with CKD

Evidence supporting interventions recommended in clinical practice guidelines for CKD are often based on results of clinical trials that failed to enroll (or excluded) a representative sample of older adults. It can be difficult to extrapolate data from younger trial populations to real-world populations of older adults. As a result, the potential benefit versus risk of many recommended interventions remains unclear in older adults. Researchers have recently begun to not only recruit more older individuals into trials but also design and carry out trials specifically focused on older adults.

Historically, preventing the progression of CKD has revolved around the mitigation of risk factors, with an emphasis on diabetes and hypertension management. With the frequent presence of cognitive decline, dementia, sarcopenia, and frailty among older adults with CKD, management of conditions associated with CKD and kidney disease progression, including diabetes and hypertension, becomes more challenging. For example, the current literature is sparse regarding optimal glycemic targets in these individuals. Moreover, patients with CKD are at higher risk for hypoglycemia due to multiple pathways (i.e., reduced renal gluconeogenesis, impaired anti-diabetic medication metabolism and clearance, etc.). While in healthy older adults it is reasonable to continue to aim for similar glycemic targets as in younger adults, in frail older adults with CKD, an HbA1c target less than 8.0% or even 8.5% likely is sufficient and reduces risk of harm from inadvertent hypoglycemia.

With respect to hypertension, two trials, the Hypertension in the Very Elderly Trial (HYVET) and the SPRINT trial, have increased our knowledge of treatment goals for elderly patients. In 2008, the HYVET trial showed that the benefits of reducing mortality and stroke from targeting a blood pressure of less than 150/80 mm Hg extend to patients over 80 years of age with the use of a diuretic and, if needed, an ACE inhibitor. In 2015, the SPRINT trial (which included substantial numbers of adults older than 75 years of age) showed a benefit to targeting a systolic blood pressure of less than 120 mm Hg. In the SPRINT trial, there was a small increase in the risk of some adverse events with lower blood pressure targets including hypotension, syncope, and acute kidney injury. Both trials were discontinued early because the benefit of therapy became evident earlier than anticipated. Neither study enrolled nursing home residents or individuals with estimated GFR below 20 mL/min/1.73 m². Two Japanese trials, the Japan Trial to Assess Optimal Blood Pressure in Elderly Hypertensive Patients (JATOS) and the Valsartan in Elderly Isolated Systolic Hypertension (VALISH) Trial,

did not show major differences in outcomes or adverse events when targeting systolic blood pressure to less than 140 mm Hg. Given mixed results, expert opinion on blood pressure targets in older adults varies. While the 2017 AHA/ACC guidelines recommended a blood pressure target of 130/80 mm Hg or lower for almost all individuals, including most people aged 65 and older, the 2020 International Society of Hypertension guidelines recommend a more conservative blood pressure target of 140/90 mm Hg or lower for adults with CKD who are over the age of 85. Thus, in evaluating the relative benefits and harms of different interventions recommended for older adults with CKD, clinicians should consider the strength of available evidence, trial participant demographics, relevance of trial results with respect to their patients, and the health priorities of individual patients.

In addition to the mitigation of traditional risk factors, there is increasing focus on the nutritional management of CKD. Historically, nutritional management has been under-utilized in the elderly; however, its implementation may reduce the burden of polypharmacy in this population. In resource-limited areas the introduction of dietary measures may be a pragmatic strategy with obvious health benefits. Studies have shown that low protein diets (in the range of 0.6–0.8 g of dietary protein per kg ideal body weight per day, i.e., 50 to 65 g of dietary protein for an 80-kg person) can delay the onset of uremic symptomatology and extend the time to dialysis. A plant-dominant diet with higher fruit and vegetable content can also mitigate metabolic acidosis and the hyperphosphatemia associated with CKD. Additionally, moderate salt restriction (<3 g/day) can reduce the burden of edema and improve hypertension, therefore reducing the need for additional pharmacologic interventions for symptom management in advanced CKD in the elderly.

Comorbid Conditions and Geriatric Syndromes

Chronic kidney disease often coexists with other comorbid conditions in older adults. Patients with CKD are at increased risk for geriatric syndromes such as frailty, cognitive impairment, and functional limitations. These geriatric syndromes can ultimately lead to disability, loss of independence, and death (Table 48.1). The burden of geriatric syndromes and frailty among older adults with CKD is quite high; In several studies, more than 20% of adults with CKD stage 4 had cognitive impairment and frailty, while, among patients undergoing dialysis over the age of 65 years, more than 30% had cognitive impairment and depression and more than 75% were considered frail.

Valuable information regarding the presence of geriatric syndromes can be obtained with the Fried frailty phenotype or the Comprehensive Geriatric Assessment. These tools may not only be helpful in the elderly, but also in younger patients where the presence of CKD is associated with an aged phenotype beyond that expected for a patient's actual age. Understanding these tools can help clinicians and patients with shared decision making by conveying prognostic information to support shared decision making about potential therapeutic interventions.

Chronic Kidney Failure in Older Adults

Outcomes in Elderly Dialysis Patients

There is some evidence that, in complex older adults with advanced CKD, those managed conservatively may have similar survival to those treated with dialysis. This phenomenon likely reflects

TABLE 48.1	Relevance and Significance of Select Geriatric Syndromes in Older Adults With Chronic Kidney Disease	
Geriatric Syndromes	**Relevance and Significance in Older Adults With CKD**
Cognitive impairment	The prevalence and incidence of cognitive impairment is higher with greater albuminuria or at lower levels of eGFR and is common in older adults receiving maintenance dialysis. In both the general population and in dialysis patients, cognitive impairment is associated with higher mortality
Depressive symptoms	Depression is more common in patients with CKD and is associated with worsening kidney function and incident kidney failure. Among patients with depression receiving maintenance dialysis, depression is associated with a higher risk of death
Falls	CKD complications such as neuropathy, muscle weakness, and anemia are associated with falls. CKD patients have higher risk of fractures
Polypharmacy	CKD patients take an average of eight medications and have decreased clearance of many drugs. Among older adults, polypharmacy is associated with higher mortality. Drug dosing is based on creatinine clearance, which may be a poor marker for kidney function in older adults with decreased muscle mass
Poor physical performance	CKD is associated with poor physical performance. In the general population, poor physical performance predicts mortality and functional decline
Frailty	Frailty is more prevalent in older adults with CKD than among those without CKD. Among patients undergoing dialysis, frailty is common even among younger patients and is associated with higher risk of mortality

CKD, Chronic kidney disease; *eGFR*, estimated glomerular filtration rate

greater competing risk of death, the high prevalence of frailty, and the high prevalence of other life-limiting comorbid conditions. Median survival after dialysis initiation for adults ages 75 to 79, 80 to 84, 85 to 89, and ≥90 years is 1.7 years, 1.3 years, 0.9 years, and 0.6 years, respectively. However, considerable heterogeneity in survival exists among patients of similar ages, highlighting the importance of an individualized approach to discussions about prognosis and treatment recommendations.

In addition to advanced age, several negative prognostic factors have been identified in epidemiologic studies of patients with advanced CKD, including frailty or reduced functional status, significant weight loss, low serum albumin concentration, number and severity of comorbidities, late referral, and unplanned dialysis initiation. Given these factors, many providers question whether the benefits of dialysis will outweigh potential harms by extending life or improving quality of life for older adults with high levels of comorbidity and/or disability.

Comparing outcomes among patients who start dialysis versus those who choose conservative and preservative therapies can be challenging, reflecting that most kidney failure registries only include patients treated with kidney replacement therapies and, thus, do not include patients with advanced kidney disease who do not start dialysis either because they make an explicit decision not to or because there are no clinical indications to initiate treatment. Many patients with advanced kidney disease are not referred to a nephrologist, and current studies tend to underestimate the number and percentage of elderly patients who either prefer not to receive or are not offered dialysis. Prediction tools can be helpful in supporting discussions about prognosis and treatment options in patients with advanced kidney disease. The Dialysis Transition Prediction Score for estimating the risk of death in the first year after initiation of dialysis therapy was recently developed (available at www.DialysisScore.com) based on data from US veterans with advanced CKD who transitioned to dialysis and was validated in a diverse population in Southern California. The Dialysis Transition Prediction Scores obtained per patient from this calculator can

help clinicians and patients make more informed decisions and develop individualized care plans.

Much of the research data comparing conservative management versus more aggressive dialysis initiation comes from single-center studies. Available data demonstrate mixed findings with respect to the impact of conservative non-dialytic management vs. dialysis on outcomes in the elderly. One study from Canada found that older adults survived up to 3 years longer from the time they transitioned to dialysis as compared to those who did not receive kidney replacement therapies. Results from French and British studies also suggest higher life expectancy among those starting dialysis versus conservative care. However, other studies suggest that older adults, particularly those aged 80 and over, do not experience a survival benefit from dialysis, highlighting the need for further research in this area.

Regional variations do exist, and the percentage of older patients transitioning to dialysis in the United States is far higher than for other developed countries. In the United States, although an implicit decision not to pursue dialysis was more common in older patients, most older adults with severe CKD had transitioned to dialysis or were preparing to be treated with dialysis at their most recent follow-up. In all studies, those who selected dialysis also spent more days in the hospital and were more likely to die in the hospital. On average, dialysis patients over 80 are hospitalized approximately twice per year, for an average of 25 days.

After transitioning to dialysis, older adults continue to experience a high burden of comorbid conditions and persistent symptoms that may affect their quality of life. Functional decline is common and is especially prominent around the time of dialysis initiation or any hospitalization. In one study of US nursing home residents starting dialysis, fewer than 13% survived for 1 year and maintained their predialysis functional abilities. Similar patterns of functional decline have been noted among ambulatory older adults starting maintenance dialysis and among prevalent dialysis patients after hospitalization.

Despite substantial morbidity and mortality, limited data suggest that many older adults receiving chronic dialysis find their quality of life to be acceptable. In British and American studies, older dialysis-dependent adults had lower physical quality of life but similar mental quality of life (QoL) compared to age-matched peers. Similar results were noted in the international Dialysis Outcomes and Practice Patterns Study (DOPPS). A review of data from the Geriatric Assessment in Older patients starting Dialysis (GOLD) study from the Netherlands found that the trajectory of QoL was slightly better in elderly patients starting dialysis compared to those who opted for maximal conservative care, despite a less frequent need for hospitalization in the latter group. More data are needed to understand which subgroups of older adults are more and less likely to benefit from kidney replacement therapy.

While the decision to transition to dialysis ideally involves a shared decision-making process, the improvements in dialysis care, greater access to home dialysis modalities, and improved longevity in individuals treated with kidney replacement therapies have likely made dialysis a more attractive treatment option for those who remain relatively functional. It is also important to note that, while around 20% of patients who start dialysis also report decisional regret, this was no more frequent in older than in younger patients. Shared decision making should include discussions of anticipated prognosis and outcomes, while clearly delineating treatment alternatives for all patients starting dialysis. Providing estimates of survival and realistic expectations after dialysis transition can better inform the patient decision-making process.

Dialysis Transitions, Palliative Care, and Hospice

While thrice-weekly in-center hemodialysis has been the standard over the last several decades, alternative treatment strategies such as incremental and twice-weekly dialysis may allow for a smoother transition to dialysis and better support the values and goals of some patients. Additionally, peritoneal dialysis may also represent an excellent option for many older adults.

Recognizing the benefits of residual kidney function and gradual transition to dialysis on the health-related quality of life and survival of dialysis patients as well as other relevant outcomes, such as less burden of dialysis vascular access and less frequent transportation to the dialysis facility, there is growing interest in an incremental approach to dialysis initiation, in which hemodialysis frequency and dose are individualized based on patients' native kidney function and concurrent symptoms (Table 48.2). The criteria in Table 48.2 can also be used to make recommendations or decisions to transition patients from twice- to thrice-weekly hemodialysis. The increasing use of incremental and decremental dialysis, for example, palliative dialysis (Fig. 48.5), with a focus on maintaining quality of life and/or palliation of symptoms, may also be more appropriate in cases where neither full thrice-weekly dialysis nor full conservative or preservative care or withdrawal of dialysis are in line with an individual patient's goals for care. In 2015, approximately 23% of patients withdrew from dialysis, and the rate of dialysis withdrawal is almost four times higher among patients over the age of 85 as compared to those aged 20–44 years.

TABLE 48.2	Proposed Decision Support System With 11 Criteria for Initiating and Maintaining Incremental (Twice-Weekly) Hemodialysis (HD) Treatment and for Incremental Adjustment to Thrice-Weekly HD As Indicated

Incremental (Twice-Weekly) Hemodialysis Treatment Criteria

1. Adequate residual kidney function with a urine output >600 mL/day (transition to thrice-weekly if urine output drops to <500 mL/day)[a]

2. Limited fluid retention between two consecutive HD treatments with a fluid gain of <2.5 kg (or < 5% of the ideal dry weight) without HD for 3 to 4 days

3. Limited or readily manageable cardiovascular or pulmonary symptoms without clinically significant fluid overload[b]

4. Suitable body size relative to residual renal function; patients with larger body size may be suitable for twice-weekly hemodialysis if not hypercatabolic

5. Hyperkalemia (K > 5.5 mEq/L) infrequent or readily manageable

6. Hyperphosphatemia (P > 5.5 mg/dL) infrequent or readily manageable

7. Good nutritional status without florid hypercatabolic state

8. Lack of profound anemia (hemoglobin >8 g/dL) and appropriate responsiveness to anemia therapy

9. Infrequent hospitalization and easily manageable comorbid conditions

10. Satisfactory health-related quality of life and functional status

11. Residual urea clearance (KRU) > 3 mL/min/1.73 m^2 (transition to thrice-weekly if KRU < 2 mL/min/1.73 m^2)[c]

Implementation Strategies

1. In order to initiate twice-weekly hemodialysis, the patient should meet the first (urine output >600 mL/day) and the last criteria (KRU > 3 mL/min/1.73 m^2), plus most (five out of nine) other criteria

2. Examine these criteria every 1 to 3 months in all twice-weekly hemodialysis patients and assess outcomes and outcome measures between twice-weekly and thrice-weekly hemodialysis patients

3. Consider transition from a twice-weekly to thrice-weekly hemodialysis regimen if patient's urine output drops <500 mL/day, if KRU declines <2 mL/min/1.73 m^2, or if patient's nutritional status or general health condition shows a deteriorating trend over time

[a]The minimum required urine output to initiate twice-weekly has been changed to 600 mL/day in this adaptation, while >500 mL/day is needed to maintain twice-weekly regimen.

[b]Lack of systolic dysfunction (EF > 40%) and no major coronary intervention over the past 3 months.

[c]Added criterion in this adaptation.

Adapted from Kalantar-Zadeh K, Unruh M, Zager PG, et al. Twice-weekly and incremental hemodialysis treatment for initiation of kidney replacement therapy. *Am J Kidney Dis.* 2014;64(2):181–186.

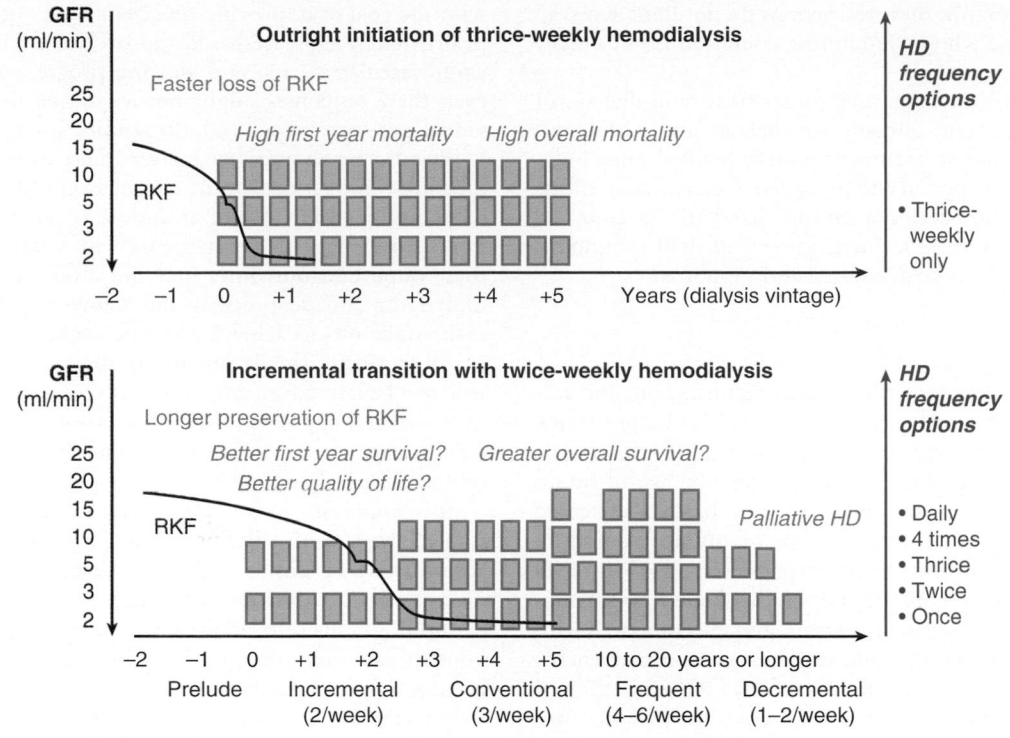

• **Fig. 48.5** Transition from advanced chronic kidney disease to thrice-weekly hemodialysis (upper panel) versus incremental transition to initially twice-weekly hemodialysis followed by thrice-weekly several weeks to month later. Decremental or palliative hemodialysis is depicted on the right side.

Increasing the role of palliative care in caring for patients on dialysis may help address some of the symptoms of kidney failure and dialysis therapy, including fatigue and pain (Fig. 48.6). Strategies commonly used in palliative medicine can also assist in preparing patients for end-of-life decisions while allowing individuals to reconsider the fundamental reasons for choosing dialysis. As shown in the Kidney Care Chart (see Fig. 48.6), conservative management of CKD includes both life-sustaining strategies under the preservative management of CKD and supportive

care including palliative medicine approaches. Critically, effective symptom management should be a focus at all times and not just as patients are approaching the end of life.

Hospice utilization is low among dialysis patients compared to those with other life-limiting conditions such as advanced dementia, heart failure, and cancer. Not only is this likely a result of an "all-or-none" mentality and poor knowledge of hospice as a treatment option, but in the United States this may also be due to restrictions on reimbursement for dialysis, especially among

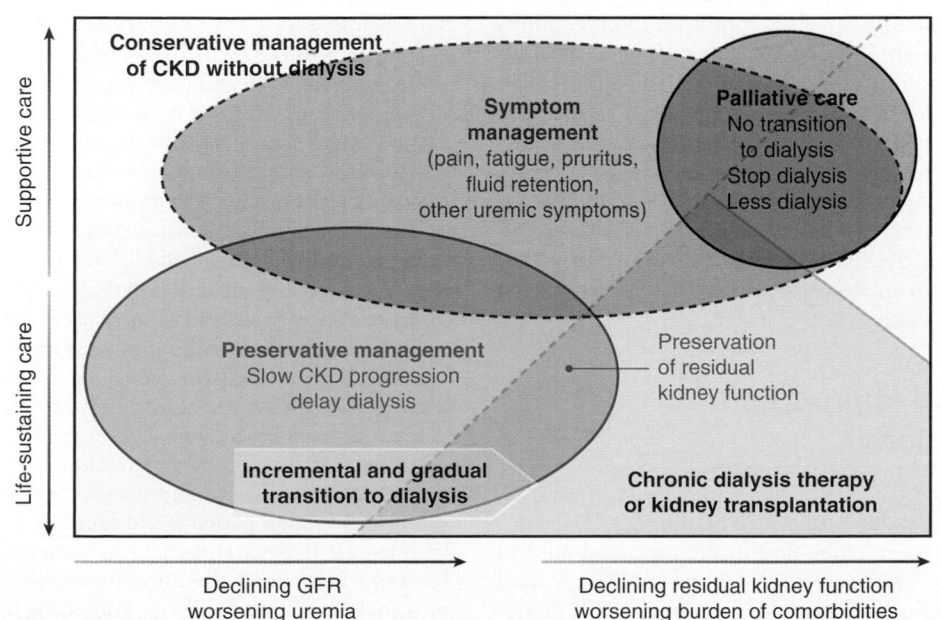

• **Fig. 48.6** Kidney Care Chart highlighting the conceptual model of the conservative management of CKD. (From Kalantar-Zadeh K, Wightman A, Liao S. Ensuring Choice for People with Kidney Failure – Dialysis, Supportive Care, and Hope. *N Engl J Med*. 2020;383(2):99-101.)

hospice patients. Notably, these restrictions do not limit access to hospice among those whose life-limiting condition is not kidney failure.

Overall, the decision to pursue conservative non-dialytic or preservative management, initiation of dialysis, and withdrawal or continuation of dialysis treatment is an individual value judgment that should be respected and protected. Collaborative efforts among healthcare providers can ensure that patients enjoy an improved quality of life, better management of their symptoms, and ultimately have their goals realized and supported.

Transplantation

At the other end of the spectrum of treatment options for kidney failure is transplantation, and the demand for kidney transplantation continues to increase among older adults. Over the last two decades the number of patients over the age of 60 on the United States kidney transplant waiting list has increased 20-fold, such that adults over the age of 60 now comprise approximately 30% of all wait-listed patients and 25% of all kidney transplant recipients. In these individuals, transplantation likely extends life by 1 to 4 years on average compared with remaining on dialysis. More recent studies suggest these benefits extend to selected patients over the age of 75. One study showed that kidney transplantation was cost-effective for patients over the age of 65, but that the attractiveness of transplantation declined as waiting time increased.

The kidney allocation system (KAS) introduced in December 2014 changed the approach to the use of marginal-quality donor kidneys. Particularly relevant to older adults, the KAS introduced the concept of longevity matching, in which better quality kidneys are preferentially given to recipients with longer estimated post-transplant survival. As a result, older recipients are more likely to be offered higher Kidney Donor Profile Index (KDPI) organs (higher KDPI organs are expected to have a higher risk of graft failure). A retrospective review of the Organ Procurement and Transplantation Network (OPTN) and United Network of Organ Sharing (UNOS) databases focusing on adults aged 60 or older who received preemptive transplant with KDPI > 85% kidneys found a similar risk of mortality when compared to older adults who received kidneys with KDPI < 85% after being on dialysis for 1–4 years and a lower mortality risk compared to those who had been on dialysis for 4–8 years. For older patients, particularly those in regions with long waiting times, the benefits of an increased KDPI kidney appears to outweigh the risk of remaining on dialysis. As a result, this option is becoming more common among older transplant recipients. As the demand for transplantation among older adults rises, the selection of candidates and allocation of limited organs has become more complex and has resulted in wide regional variations in practice.

Patient-Centered Approach to Treatment Decisions

The marked heterogeneity in health status, life expectancy, and preferences among older adults may be difficult to accommodate within the practice embodied in disease-based clinical guidelines. The disease-based approach assumes a direct, causal relationship between clinical signs and symptoms and underlying disease pathophysiology. Thus, treatment plans often target pathophysiologic mechanisms relevant to the disease process

with the goal of improving disease-related outcomes. Outcomes prioritized by a disease-based approach to CKD include survival, cardiovascular events, and slowing progression of CKD; however, these outcomes might not always be meaningful to individual patients (Fig. 48.7). In studies surveying patients with kidney disease about what matters most to them, quality of life measures, mitigation and/or elimination of CKD-related symptoms, and maintenance of an independent lifestyle consistently rank above survival. For patients with limited life expectancy, these important outcomes may not always be tied to a specific underlying disease process, and many patients are willing to make trade-offs to achieve those outcomes that are most meaningful to them. This is not to say that older adults with CKD will not benefit from interventions recommended under a disease-oriented approach, but information on prognosis and the comparative effectiveness of different therapies is often helpful in developing an individualized care plan.

It is important to remember that the 1973 Medicare expansion allowed nearly all Americans with terminal kidney failure access to life-sustaining dialysis. It permitted patients to choose dialysis not just to survive, but also to maintain hope: hope of continuing valued relationships, hope for rehabilitation, and hope of achieving life goals and pursuits. However, dialysis has become a powerful default treatment for kidney disease, particularly in the United States, for patients of all ages. This has led to inflexibility in the delivery of dialysis care and has made it difficult to integrate dialysis with other care models of potential relevance to patients with advanced kidney disease such as palliative care, hospice, and conservative care. While many older adults will benefit from dialysis, a default approach to decisions about dialysis initiation and delivery can result in care that is incongruent with the values, goals, and priorities of individual patients. To support a more individualized, patients-centered approach to the care of older adults with advanced kidney disease, a more flexible approach that allows for patients to switch between care pathways and combine different approaches to care to best meet their needs is needed. This might include the following: (1) supporting a conservative approach to the management of advanced kidney disease for patients who do not want to start dialysis, who are not sure if they want to start dialysis, or wish to delay dialysis as long as possible to include use of diet and lifestyle modifications, conventional and new pharmacotherapies, and proactive management of symptoms such as pain and fatigue, as well as mental health issues; (2) offering an opportunity for patients to transition to dialysis gradually when they feel ready to start this treatment, perhaps initiating once- to twice-weekly hemodialysis or less-than-daily peritoneal dialysis at home, each of which may preserve residual kidney function longer than conventional dialysis; (3) supporting an individualized approach to dialysis for all patients that is based on what matters most to them and based on a shared decision-making process about the pros and cons of standard thrice-weekly regimens; (4) integration of palliative care services throughout the continuum of illness, rather than inconsistent opportunity to engage with palliative care specialists; and (5) more patient-centered transitions to end of life to include integration of palliative and hospice services to address terminal symptoms to help patients and families to think about how best to integrate dialysis treatment as patients approach the end of life and whether and when to discontinue treatments. Outcomes prioritized by clinical practice guidelines for CKD may not align with what individual patients value most, and further research on the optimal management approaches for elderly advanced kidney

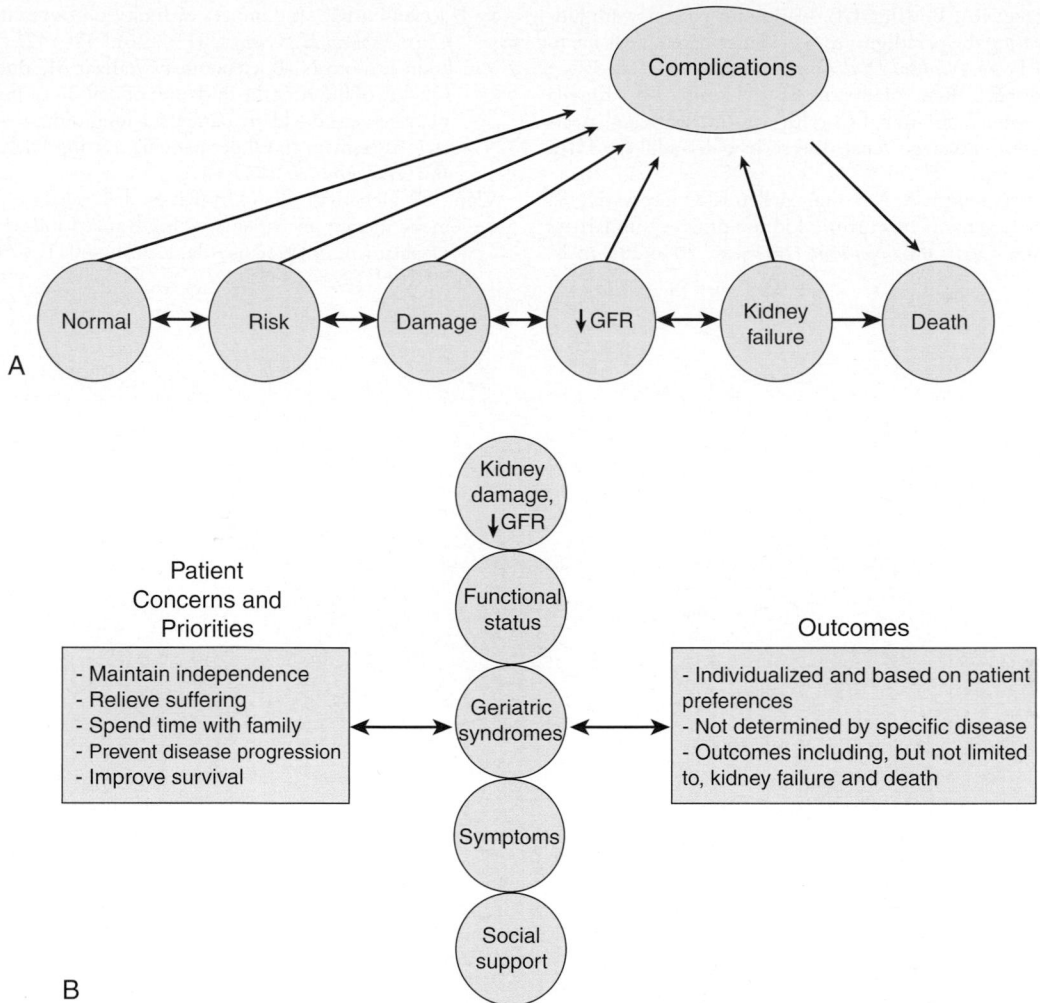

• Fig. 48.7 Conceptualization of (A) disease-based and (B) individualized approaches to chronic kidney disease. *GFR*, Glomerular filtration rate. (From Bowling CB, O'Hare AM. Managing older adults with CKD: individualized versus disease-based approaches. *Am J Kidney Dis*. 2012;59:293–302.)

disease patients is needed. Critically, eliciting individual patient goals and priorities is a crucial step in determining the relevance and potential benefits of guideline-recommended treatment strategies, especially among older adults.

Complete bibliography is available at Elsevier eBooks for Practicing Clinicians.

Key Bibliography

Bowling CB, O'Hare AM. Managing older adults with CKD: individualized versus disease-based approaches. *Am J Kidney Dis*. 2012;59:293–302.

Boyd CM, Darer J, Boult C, Fried LP, Boult L, Wu AW. Clinical practice guidelines and quality of care for older patients with multiple comorbid diseases: implications for pay for performance. *JAMA*. 2005;294:716–724.

Chopra B, Sureshkumar K. Kidney transplantation in older recipients: Preemptive high KDPI kidney vs lower KDPI kidney after varying dialysis vintage. *World J Transplant*. 2018;8(4):102–109.

Hemmelgarn BR, James MT, Manns BJ, et al. Rates of treated and untreated kidney failure in older vs younger adults. *JAMA*. 2012;307:2507–2515.

Hommos M, Glassock R, Rule A. Structural and functional changes in human kidneys with healthy aging. *J Am Soc Nephrol*. 2017;28(10):2838–2844.

Kalantar-Zadeh K, Wightman A, Liao S. Ensuring choice for people with kidney failure — dialysis, supportive care, and hope. *N Engl J Med*. 2020;383(2):99–101.

Ko G, Rhee C, Obi Y et al. Vascular access placement and mortality in elderly incident hemodialysis patients. *Nephrol Dial Transplant*. 2020;35(3):503–511.

Kurella M, Chertow GM, Fried LF, et al. Chronic kidney disease and cognitive impairment in the elderly: the health, aging, and body composition study. *J Am Soc Nephrol*. 2005;16:2127–2133.

Kurella Tamura M, Covinsky KE, Chertow GM, Yaffe K, Landefeld CS, McCulloch CE. Functional status of elderly adults before and after initiation of dialysis. *N Engl J Med*. 2009;361:1539–1547.

Kurella Tamura M, O'Hare A, Lin E, Holdsworth L, Malcolm E, Moss A. Palliative care disincentives in CKD: changing policy to improve CKD care. *Am J Kidney Dis*. 2018;71(6):866–873.

Murray AM, Arko C, SC Chen, Gilbertson DT, Moss AH. Use of hospice in the United States dialysis population. *Clin J Am Soc Nephrol*. 2006;1:1248–1255.

Obi Y, Nguyen DV, Zhou H, et al. Development and validation of prediction scores for early mortality at transition to dialysis. *Mayo Clin Proc*. 2018;93(9):1224–1235.

O'Hare AM, Bertenthal D, Covinsky KE, et al. Mortality risk stratification in chronic kidney disease: one size for all ages? *J Am Soc Nephrol*. 2006;17:846–853.

O'Hare AM, Rodriguez RA, Bowling CB. Caring for patients with kidney disease: shifting the paradigm from evidence-based medicine to patient-centered care. *Nephrol Dial Transplant*. 2016;31:368–375.

O'Hare AM, Rodriguez RA, Hailpern SM, Larson EB, Kurella Tamura M. Regional variation in health care intensity and treatment practices for end-stage renal disease in older adults. *JAMA*. 2010;304:180–186.

Rhee C, Nguyen D, Nyamathi A, Kalantar-Zadeh K. Conservative vs. preservative management of chronic kidney disease: similarities and distinctions. *Curr Opin Nephrol Hypertens*. 2020;29(1):92–102.

Sy J, Johansen KL. The impact of frailty on outcomes in dialysis. *Curr Opin Nephrol Hypertens*. 2017;26(6):537–542.

Van Loon I, Goto N, Boereboom F, Verhaar M, Bots M, Hamaker M. Quality of life after the initiation of dialysis or maximal conservative management in elderly patients: a longitudinal analysis of the Geriatric assessment in OLder patients starting Dialysis (GOLD) study. *BMC Nephrol*. 2019;20(1).

Wong SP, Hebert PL, Laundry RJ, et al. Decisions about renal replacement therapy in patients with advanced kidney disease in the US Department of Veterans Affairs, 2000–2011. *Clin J Am Soc Nephrol*. 2016;11:1825–1833.

49

Global Kidney Disease

VALERIE A. LUYCKX, PABLO GARCIA, SHUCHI ANAND

Introduction

Risk factors for kidney disease span the social determinants of health (poverty, illiteracy, unemployment, pollution, discrimination), infections (HIV/AIDS, tuberculosis, malaria, hepatitis, diarrheal illnesses, pneumonia), and non-communicable diseases (hypertension, diabetes mellitus, cardiovascular disease, chronic liver disease, cancers). It is, therefore, not surprising that as many as 850 million people worldwide may be living with chronic kidney disease (CKD), acute kidney injury (AKI), or kidney failure. Mortality from acute and chronic kidney diseases may reach 5 million per year, in large part due to lack of access to early diagnosis and/or life-saving dialysis and transplantation. Kidney disease is projected to become the world's fifth leading cause of death by 2040, and, globally, kidney disease is the leading cause of catastrophic health expenditure (out-of-pocket payments for healthcare, which further impoverish the household, defined as 10%-40% of household income). Kidney disease is, therefore, an important public health concern, given the numbers affected, the high mortality, and the consequences that extend beyond individual health.

Prevention of kidney disease is possible through public health strategies, such as reducing infection risk or improving nutrition, and a holistic multi-sectoral approach to tackling the social determinants of disease. Natural disasters, the COVID-19 pandemic, and the social justice movement of 2020 all highlight the significant impact of social and structural factors on kidney disease risk and the worse outcomes in those affected. This chapter discusses the epidemiology of and access to care for kidney disease globally, with an emphasis on challenges faced in lower income settings where structural disadvantage is the norm. Awareness of global inequities is important to support advocacy and action to prevent kidney disease, promote innovations and investigations into causes of kidney disease, improve access to kidney care, and ensure global kidney health.

Acute Kidney Injury

In 2013, extrapolations from existing data suggested that around 13.3 million people are affected by AKI each year, of whom 1.7 million (12.8%) die. Most (85%) of these deaths likely occur in low- and middle-income countries (LMICs), although rigorous empiric data are missing and likely underestimate the true AKI burden. In LMICs, laboratory testing necessary for diagnosis is not always accessible, and in many settings the diagnosis may be overlooked or underreported. For example, in a survey from

China, the diagnosis of AKI was missed in 74.2% of patients, and only 16.7% of AKI cases were identifiable by ICD-10 codes. International efforts to standardize diagnosis and raise awareness may slowly be changing the tide.

Causes of Acute Kidney Injury

The spectrum of AKI varies across the globe and is impacted by factors intrinsic to the individual as well as factors reflecting the social determinants of health (Fig. 49.1). AKI is predominantly hospital-acquired in higher-income countries (HICs), where it is associated with multi-morbidity, aging, surgery, cardiac disease, sepsis, and use of nephrotoxic agents. These patients generally have access to the necessary care, including intensive care units and dialysis. In LMICs, community-acquired AKI predominates, women are underrepresented, and adult patients are decades younger with few comorbid conditions. AKI is often associated with volume depletion, sepsis, specific infections (e.g., dengue or malaria), insect/animal bites, pregnancy, and primary kidney diseases. Structural risk factors for AKI that are prevalent in LMICs include poverty, lack of access to clean water, environmental toxin exposure, and natural disasters, often superimposed on inadequate public health measures, poor access to care, and frequent use of traditional remedies. Facilities for diagnosis as well as for intensive care and dialysis care are often limited in LMICs, and access may be further reduced where patients must pay out of pocket. In these settings, the only affordable or accessible means of healthcare may be traditional remedies, some of which may cause or worsen AKI.

Incidence of Acute Kidney Injury

Given the aging world population and increasing multi-morbidity as well as improved awareness and access to diagnosis, global rates of AKI are projected to rise. There is a huge variation in the incidence of reported AKI, consistent with incomplete data collection; estimates of AKI among hospitalized adults and children worldwide range from 0.7% in Northern Africa to 31% in South America. Overall, the global, pooled incidences of AKI were 22% (95% CI 19–24) in adults and 14% (95% CI 9 – 21) in children, suggesting that around one in five adults and one in seven children hospitalized worldwide experience some degree of AKI during admission. A patient group not often captured in the global AKI discourse is preterm neonates, for whom the risk of AKI ranges from 16% to 70%, depending on comorbidities. Globally, around one in 10 infants is born preterm and, therefore, vulnerable to developing AKI. Awareness of neonatal AKI risk in

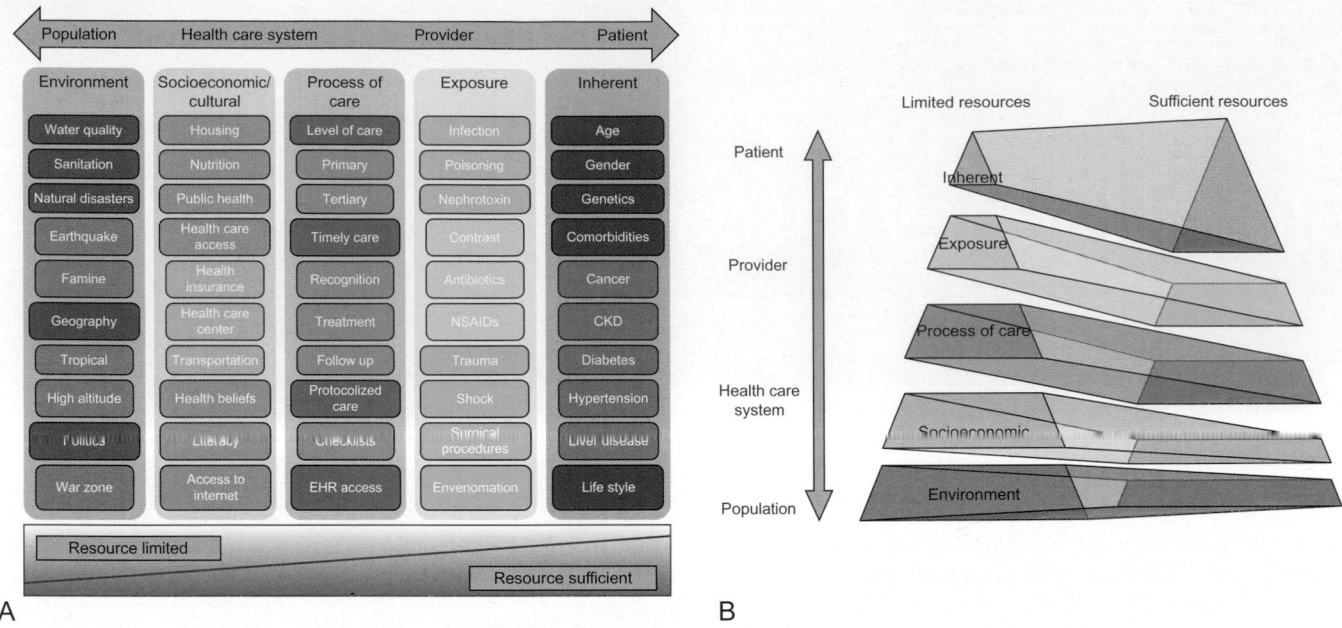

• Fig. 49.1 Social and structural determinants of acute kidney injury (AKI) risk and access to care. Spectrum of risk factors and risk dimensions, relative to country resource capacity, and spanning the patient level, through the health system and the broader population. (From Kashani K, Macedo E, Burdmann EA, et al. Acute kidney injury risk assessment: differences and similarities between resource-limited and resource-rich countries. *Kidney Int Rep.* 2017;2:519-529.)

LMICs is poor, and the contribution of AKI to perinatal mortality in preterm infants is not known.

Mortality in Acute Kidney Injury

Among adults and children admitted to hospitals with AKI, pooled mortality was 24% and 14%, respectively. However, risk of death is significantly associated with severity of AKI (AKI stage), degree of illness (requirement for intensive care), population factors, and access to dialysis. Late presentation and patient inability to pay are important contributors to AKI deaths in LMICs.

Access to Care for AKI

Nephrology consultation is consistently associated with improved patient outcomes in AKI. Knowledge and training about timely and appropriate diagnosis and management of AKI among healthcare workers is, therefore, important. Key elements for sustainable AKI care have been consolidated into the five "Rs": risk, recognition, response, renal support, and rehabilitation. These elements are variably available and/or achievable. Lower-resource settings have the greatest shortage of trained kidney care professionals and the fewest resources in place to manage AKI effectively. An additional "P," for prevention, is likely to be the best solution in resource-limited settings, as many public health interventions such as ensuring access to clean water and sanitation, vaccination, nutrition, infection control, reduction of poverty, and optimization of other social determinants of health (see Fig. 49.1) are likely to reduce AKI incidence.

AKI care is costly, especially when patients require intensive care and/or dialysis. Early diagnosis and action to limit kidney injury, restore kidney perfusion, and treat precipitating diseases can reduce deaths from AKI, improve chances of kidney recovery, and may reduce the likelihood of subsequent CKD. Dialysis may be the only means of survival if AKI is severe. Dialysis was required in 11% of all hospitalized AKI patients in a global meta-analysis, and the need for dialysis tends to be higher in LMICs, likely due to late presentation. Unfortunately, not all who need dialysis in LMICs receive it, as many barriers exist between onset of AKI and access to appropriate care. Survival, therefore, often depends on the availability of affordable dialysis. Reasons why dialysis may not be provided when needed vary across country income strata (Fig. 49.2).

Where resources and infrastructure are limited, acute peritoneal dialysis (PD) is as effective as HD, requires less infrastructure, and can be delivered using less expensive adaptations of fluids and catheters (Table 49.1). However, if kidney recovery does not occur, chronic dialysis costs (usually HD) often are unaffordable, and patients must stop dialysis, often resulting in death.

Chronic Kidney Disease

Causes of Chronic Kidney Disease in LMICs

In high-income countries (HICs), CKD clinics chiefly serve patients over the age of 60 years, many of whom have advanced diabetes mellitus or vascular disease. Less is known about the overall distribution of causes of CKD in LMICs.

Increasing rates of diabetes and aging populations have undoubtedly contributed to CKD as a rising cause of death and disability in LMICs, and over the past 3 decades mortality attributed to kidney disease has climbed by 40%. However, potentially due to the higher vulnerability to infections, environmental or occupational exposures, and use of non-allopathic medications, as well as the possibility of distinct genetic susceptibility factors, 'non-traditional' causes of kidney disease (CKDnt) exist in a greater proportion of residents of low- compared with high-income settings.

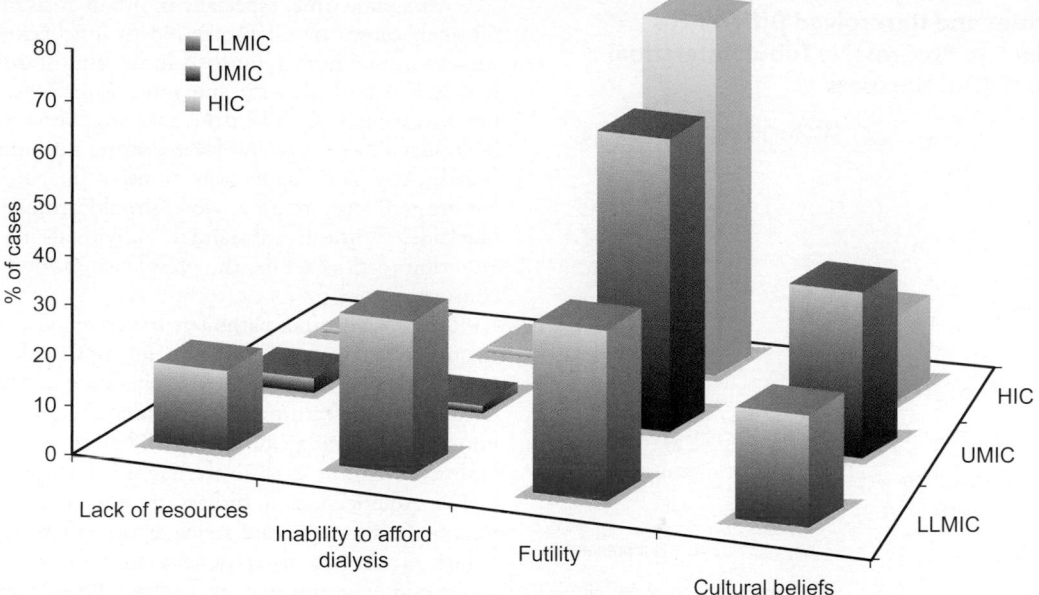

• Fig. 49.2 Reasons for non-receipt of dialysis for AKI across country income categories. Data are derived from the Global Snapshot of AKI (Mehta et al., 2016). Respondents reported reasons why dialysis was not provided in patients in whom a clinical indication existed, and, on average, patients in higher-income countries (*HIC*) were 15 years older than those in low - and lower-middle-income (*LLMIC*) countries. "Futility" was locally defined and likely highly variable. UMIC, upper-middle income countries.

TABLE 49.1	Recommendations for Acute Peritoneal Dialysis for Acute Kidney Injury

As a primary therapy, or if acute hemodialysis is not available, resources are limited, and there is no abdominal or other contraindication:

- Peritoneal dialysis (PD) catheter (flexible preferred over rigid) can be placed at the bedside or in a surgical facility by nephrologists, surgeons, or radiologists if no contraindication exists (e.g., major prior abdominal surgery, coagulopathy, abdominal trauma)

- Alternative catheters can be devised if standard PD catheters are not available, depending on patient size: Foley catheters, intercostal drains, nasogastric tubes, central lines (for babies), rubber tubing. *Any catheter or tubing used must be sterile*

- PD can be performed manually or cycler assisted

- If commercial fluid is not available, fluid usable for PD can be made locally by adding dextrose to Plasmalyte B or Ringer's lactate (both contain potassium) or dextrose, bicarbonate, and hypertonic saline to 0.45% saline (potassium-free) to generate fluid usable for PD with osmolality around 340 mosm/L. Details on exact quantities to be added to which fluid are outlined in Cullis et al. https://doi.org/10.1177/0896860820970834 (adults) https://doi.org/10.1177/0896860820982120 (children)

- Caution: Self-mixing of fluids increases risk of fluid composition errors and infections (a minimum of 8 L/day is required for an average adult)

- PD can be performed carefully in prone patients

Adapted from Cullis B, Abdelraheem M, Abrahams G, et al. Peritoneal dialysis for acute kidney injury. *Perit Dial Int.* 2014;34(5):494–517.

A form of progressive tubulointerstitial disease occurring in agricultural communities (called *chronic kidney disease of unknown etiology (CKDu)* in Sri Lanka, *Mesoamerican nephropathy* in Latin America, and *Uddanam nephropathy* in Andhra Pradesh, India) is the most prominent example of CKDnt. While several similarities exist in the populations affected and the underlying pathology in the first two hotspots, it remains unclear whether CKDnt reflects one disease with a unified cause and different labels or distinct causes with similar downstream pathologies (Table 49.2). Several hypothesized causes are under investigation, including heat stress, poor water quality, trace element or heavy metal exposure, agrochemical exposure, and a kidney-tropic infection.

It is important to point out that two of the diseases mentioned above, Mesoamerican nephropathy and CKDu, have a specific pathologic correlate in that they are recognized to be primary tubulointerstitial processes affecting a high percentage of persons living in rural and agricultural areas in Central America and in Sri Lanka, respectively. However, "CKDnt" is a broader term that could encompass potentially primary glomerular or vascular processes, or even kidney stone burden (Fig. 49.3). The incidence of kidney stones, as an example, is rising worldwide. Despite a recognition that specific dietary habits (e.g., oxalate intake in the form of tea), warming temperatures, and migration to hotter, denser urban areas likely predispose to higher risk for stone formation and subsequent CKD in LMICs, little to no data are available for Asia and Africa, where a majority of the world's population lives. Kidney stone belts have been recognized in the Southeastern United States and Southern China, lending support to the hypothesis that warmer temperatures contribute to higher stone incidence.

The need to study these under-recognized causes of CKD in LMICs is pressing. In the case of aristolochic acid nephropathy, although the singularly recognized hotspot was the Balkan region, other regions of the world, especially China and Taiwan, benefitted from the knowledge unearthed regarding the nephrotoxic and oncogenic potential of this ingredient found in commonly used traditional medication preparations. Taiwan acted by banning all

TABLE 49.2	**Similarities and Unresolved Differences Between Two Progressive Tubulointerstitial Disease (CKDu) Hotspots**	
	Mesoamerica	Sri Lanka
Hot, dry climate	✓	✓
Male predominance	✓	✓
CIN on biopsy	✓	✓
AIN on biopsy in subset	✓	✓
Lack of proteinuria	✓	✓
Rural, agricultural communities	✓	✓
Specific tasks with higher risk	✓	Not present
Low population-based prevalence of diabetes and hypertension	✓	Not present
Heavy use of NSAIDs	✓	Not present
Hyperuricemia	✓	Undefined
Heavy agrochemical application	Under study	✓
Unique water supply through shallow water wells	Undefined	✓
Chewable tobacco	Not present	✓

CIN, Chronic interstitial nephritis; *AIN*, acute interstitial nephritis; *NSAIDs*, nonsteroidal antiinflammatory drugs.

Chronic kidney disease of non-traditional causes

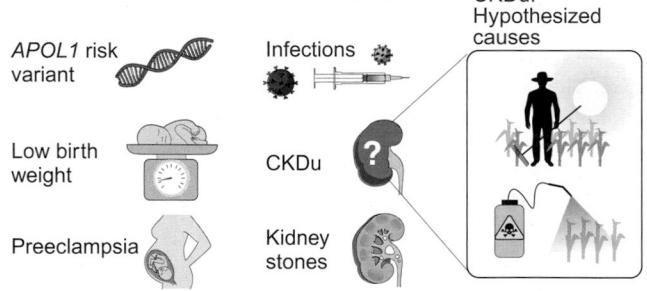

Fig. 49.3 Non-traditional causes of CKD. Non-traditional causes of kidney disease maybe more common in LMICs. Of these, CKDu, a type of tubulointerstitial kidney disease, is occurring in hotspots throughout the world. Some hypothesized causes are heat stress, agrochemical exposure, water-based exposures, and other occupation-based exposures, particularly through agricultural work.

sales of aristolochic acid-containing preparations. Similarly, even if agricultural communities in the U.S. are not seeing the devastating toll of kidney disease recognized in the hotspots of Nicaragua and El Salvador, it is plausible, based on recently reported higher age- and sex-adjusted incidence of ESKD in California's San Joaquin Valley and Texas' Rio Grande Valley compared with the rest of the U.S., that a similar disease exists at a lower level or co-exists with and accelerates other known causes (e.g., diabetes).

At the same time, especially in urban areas of LMICs, the 'traditional' causes of CKD are mostly unchecked. In population surveys from China and urban India, almost 20% of participants with CKD had diabetes and more than 50% had prediabetes; not surprisingly, CKD in these settings most often was marked by moderately or severely elevated urine albumin excretion. Additionally, few participants were aware of their risk (<5%), and few are treated with renin-angiotensin-aldosterone system (RAAS) blockade. Without substantial individual- or population-level attention to risk factors, the prevalence of 'traditional' CKD will continue to rise.

Recently a distinct pathology has emerged among patients who frequently have co-existing diabetes, IgA nephropathy, or hypertension: leukocyte cell–derived chemotaxin (ALECT2) amyloidosis. Clinical features include older age (around 70 years) and non-nephrotic-range proteinuria. Strikingly, this form of amyloidosis is almost exclusively described in persons of Hispanic, Native American, and Indian descent, and currently lacks any treatment, although case series report fast progression to kidney failure. Thus, the heterogeneity in kidney disease progression across ethnic groups may, in a subset, be explained by distinct, as yet undiscovered, pathologies.

How can causes of kidney disease be better elucidated globally? Global studies encompassing diverse cohorts, such as the H3 Africa project, promise to provide broader insights into the clinical presentations and natural history of kidney disease in patients with CKD living in diverse regions of the world. Table 49.3 lists building blocks essential to such investigations, but understanding histology and pathology through performance of kidney biopsies is key. Harnessing increasing healthcare work capacity to enable point-of-care ultrasounds and increasing digital capacity to enable remote pathology review can further facilitate expansion of kidney biopsy capacity. Simultaneously, standardized regional criteria to guide whether a kidney biopsy is appropriate and a robust ethical framework to ensure shared decision making are critical.

In summary, much work is still needed to investigate the differences in types of patients affected by CKD and the varied clinical presentations, causes, and outcomes of CKD globally, but this work is likely to (1) advance scientific knowledge about kidney disease in general and (2) build critical research and infrastructure capacity to address worldwide disparities.

Integrated CKD Screening within Existing or Developing Infrastructure

Cost-effectiveness analyses performed in high-resource settings advise against universal 'screening' for CKD in the absence of risk factors. In many LMICs, insufficient primary care infrastructure results in failure to identify common kidney disease risk factors like diabetes and hypertension with decreasing opportunity to identify kidney disease.

Currently, several international agencies including the World Health Organization and the U.S. Agency of International Development either provide guidelines for and/or sponsor periodic health surveillance in LMICs; while these have provisions for blood pressure and glucose screening, none incorporates recommendations for CKD screening beyond diabetes. In the context of CKDu and Mesoamerican nephropathy, the International Society of Nephrology (ISN) made initial recommendations for CKD screening. However, two-thirds of countries surveyed in the Global Health Kidney Atlas reported inability to assess kidney

TABLE 49.3	Toolkit for Investigations in Chronic Kidney Disease in Low- And Middle-Income Nations		
Type of Study	Potential Uses	Tools Required	Potential Substitutes for "High Cost" Tools
Cross sectional	1. Screening, especially when integrated in community health worker-based efforts 2. Estimating prevalence, awareness, patient-sought treatments, and costs 3. Secular trends in repeated cross sections	1. Questionnaire-based ascertainment of potential correlates (e.g., occupation, environment, family history) 2. Risk assessment for diabetes, vascular disease 3. Laboratory-based assessment of A1c, serum creatinine, and quantified proteinuria/albuminuria	1. Non-laboratory-based risk stratification tools 2. Point-of-care creatinine 3. Urine dipstick 4. Integration into regional or national surveillance strategies
Population cohorts	1. Incidence, risk factors, and outcomes of kidney disease 2. Customized risk prediction tools 3. Infrastructure planning for kidney disease diagnostics, professionals, and health system	1. Field epidemiology 2. Clinical capacity to follow up on findings	1. As above 2. Task-shifting to community health workforce 3. Use of digital technology
Clinic cohorts	1. Demographics and clinical profiles of persons with chronic kidney disease (CKD) 2. Natural history of specific (e.g., diabetic) CKD in diverse cohorts 3. Assessment of management and quality of care 4. Distribution of cause(s)	1. Detailed baseline demographic and clinic information 2. Routine standard follow-up laboratory assessments 3. Standardized protocols for indications of biopsy	1. Open source electronic medical records 2. Point-of-care ultrasounds 3. Virtual pathology

function at the primary care level (Fig. 49.4). Point-of-care creatinine testing offers an attractive strategy to fill the void, but devices with acceptable performance may be cost prohibitive and require venous blood draw.

Urine testing remains underutilized globally. Notably, quantitative proteinuria assessment, specifically urine albumin-to-creatinine ratio screening, is among the most costly screening tests; accordingly, although urine dipstick testing has a lower sensitivity and specificity in detecting proteinuria, its advantages include low cost and easy point-of-care use more adaptable to community healthcare worker-led, home visit-based, screening models being implemented in many LMICs.

In summary, although kidney disease screening is recommended only for high-risk populations in HICs, the lack of primary healthcare in LMICs greatly decreases the likelihood of identifying this high-risk population and/or incidental discovery of abnormal laboratory findings during routine interactions. This context means integrated screening for CKD requires renewed and local evaluation in LMICs. A tiered approach may be required, with "non-laboratory-based" or only "point-of-care" algorithms that step up to referrals for gold-standard testing. Screening programs in LMICs are likely to be fertile ground for innovation in point-of-care kidney disease assessment.

Advancing Management of Chronic Kidney Disease Globally

While CKDnt may exist more commonly in isolation or in combination with traditional causes of kidney disease in LMICs, most cases of CKD worldwide are attributable to non-communicable risk factors, specifically type 2 diabetes and vascular disease. Critically, these conditions are more likely to be unaddressed or undertreated in LMICs, despite substantial opportunity to intervene early with blood pressure control, glycemia management, and kidney-targeted therapies, including RAAS blockade, and, should they be affordable, sodium glucose cotransporter-2 (SGLT-2) inhibitors. Despite widespread availability, fewer than a quarter of patients with cardiovascular disease in LMICs receive standard cardioprotective medications including RAAS blockade, often due to an inability to pay for or obtain these medications, even at a relatively low cost. Given the lack of an acute inciting event, use for CKD is likely even lower.

In this context, even as the treatment for primary glomerular diseases evolve to targeted therapeutics, many therapies will remain unaffordable for decades to come in LMICs. Especially for treatments that are equivalent to or offer an incremental absolute benefit to kidney survival, society guidelines continue to recognize the older, less costly options as reasonable alternatives (e.g., cyclophosphamide versus mycophenolate mofetil for induction in lupus nephritis and ANCA vasculitis). For newer therapies that are clearly superior there is growing awareness that accommodations should be made to increase access in LMICs. With an eye toward generating better evidence for therapies in diverse cohorts and for enabling their use, the ISN recently devised guidelines that pre-specified practical outcome assessments for evaluating therapies in LMICs.

Kidney Failure

The incidence and prevalence of kidney failure vary significantly across the globe. Rates in LMICs are not fully understood because of a lack of data. The global incidence of kidney failure rose from 44 per million population (PMP) in 1990 to 94 PMP in 2010, likely reflecting not only the growing burden of CKD in the setting of increased diabetes and hypertension prevalence but also better access to diagnosis. In countries reporting to the United States Renal Data System (USRDS), the kidney failure incidence

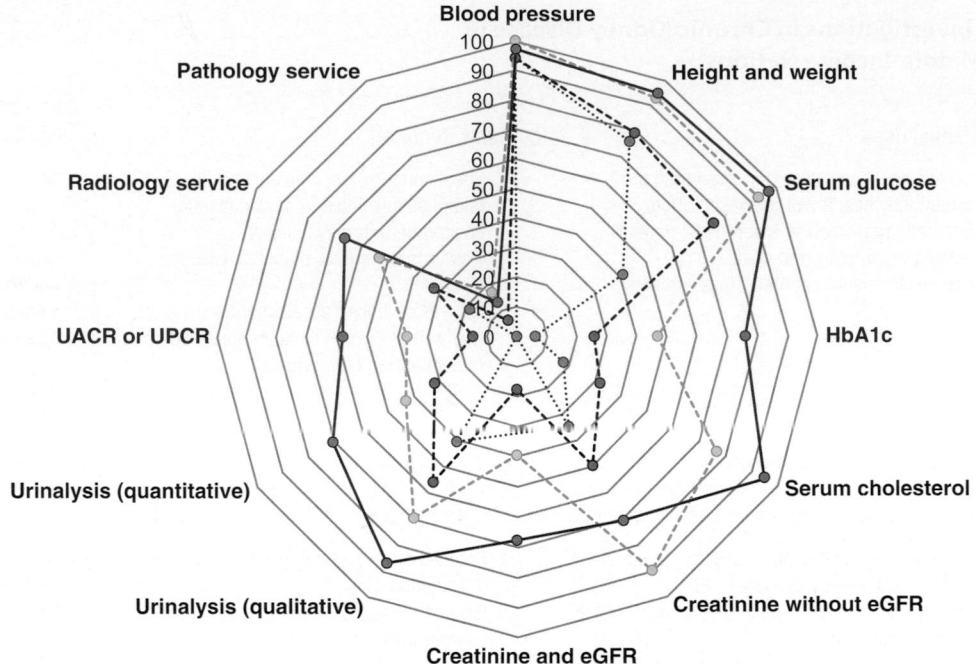

A

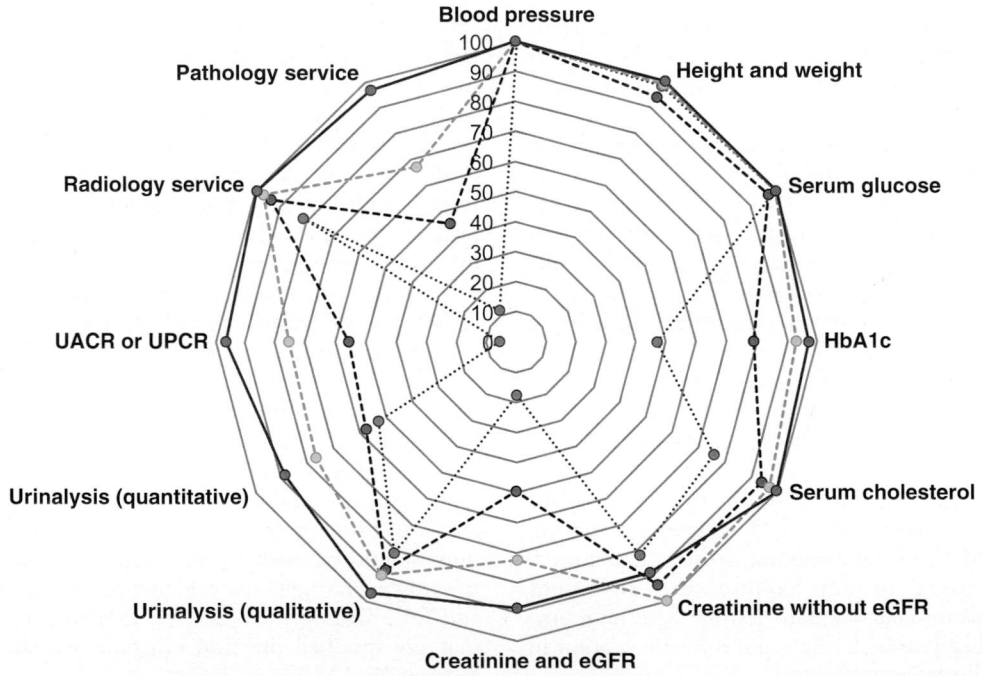

B

• **Fig. 49.4** Inequities in service availability for the identification and management of chronic kidney disease at primary and secondary care across country income groups. Capacities of primary (A) and secondary (B) healthcare services to screen for and monitor chronic kidney disease care are reported as percentages of countries with particular services in each income group. *eGFR,* Estimated glomerular filtration rate; *HbA1c,* glycated hemoglobin; *UACR,* urine albumin-to-creatinine ratio; *UPCR,* urine protein-to-creatinine ratio. (From Htay H, Alrukhaimi M, Ashuntantang GE, et al. Global access of patients with kidney disease to health technologies and medications: findings from the Global Kidney Health Atlas project. *Kidney Int Suppl* 2018;8:64-73.)

in 2016 varied from 22 per million in South Africa to 493 per million in Taiwan. The prevalence of patients receiving treatment for kidney failure range from fewer than one per million in much of Africa to 3392 per million in Taiwan, highlighting major global inequities in access to care (Fig. 49.5).

Disparities in Access to Kidney Failure Therapy Worldwide

In Latin America, there is a significant variation in healthcare coverage in the region; five countries have kidney replacement therapy (KRT) prevalence above 700 per million: Argentina, Brazil, Chile, Jalisco (Mexico), and Uruguay. The rest of the countries have prevalence rates as low as 189 per million (Paraguay). In Africa, prevalence estimates are based on local reports, available registries, and unpublished data. The incidence of patients requiring dialysis in North Africa is around 140 per million and the prevalence is estimated to be around 500 per million. The prevalence of kidney failure due to diabetes and hypertension in sub-Saharan Africa is estimated to be 239 per million, but only around 20 per million have access to KRT. Senegal is currently the only West African country where peritoneal dialysis (PD) is available for kidney failure treatment. The prevalence of KRT in South Africa was 190 per million in 2017; however, this belies the massive inequities between the prevalence in the public sector (84% of the population, 66 per million) and the private sector (14% of the population, 885 per million). In the Middle East and North Africa, the prevalence of patients on dialysis ranges from 83 per million in Iraq to 812 per million in Tunisia. Kidney failure prevalence in India is not known, but over 90% of people requiring KRT in India die because of an inability to afford care, and, among those who initiate dialysis, 60% discontinue for financial reasons. Similar circumstances exist in sub-Saharan Africa.

Access to Kidney Replacement Therapy

Economic prosperity increases access to KRT. In high-income countries, the total number of patients receiving dialysis or transplants is used as a surrogate for prevalence, meaning almost all have access to treatment. In LMICs these numbers generally underestimate kidney failure rates due to under-diagnosis and/or lack of access to KRT, and correlate with gross domestic product. Globally, the number of patients with kidney failure who remain untreated may be 1- to 3-fold higher than the number of patients receiving treatment.

Despite the likely high rates of CKD in LMICs, few individuals receive KRT, reflecting a lack of resources and infrastructure. The ISN Global Kidney Health Atlas of 118 countries notes that all have the capacity to provide maintenance hemodialysis, and 80% have the capacity to provide peritoneal dialysis. However, only 29% of low-income countries (LICs) reported capacity for maintenance PD, rising to 69% and 100% across middle- and high-income countries, respectively. Acute HD services were available in almost all participating countries, with acute PD less common.

Even when LICs and LMICs have the capacity to provide acute and maintenance HD, the quality and sustainability of dialysis remain uncertain, with limitations in dialysis access reported in 17 of the 31 participating countries. Cost is the major limitation even with government funding or subsidies, particularly in settings of high demand where strategies such as limiting HD frequency to once or twice weekly are used to include more patients. This strategy may be feasible among patients with residual kidney function in LMICs: For every two patients who spend their first year of hemodialysis receiving twice rather than thrice weekly therapy, one more patient could receive a year of hemodialysis at no additional cost to the healthcare system.

In HICs, refugees and migrants represent a subpopulation that may have limited access to dialysis or transplantation, leading to high resource use and poor outcomes despite sufficient resources to care for these individuals. Transparent policies are required to ensure that migrants and refugees have access to safe kidney care, spanning the spectrum from prevention to dialysis and transplantation.

Kidney Transplantation

Transplantation may be the most cost-effective form of kidney replacement therapy in most regions, but in LMICs transplant often is inaccessible. Major limiting factors include lack of institutional support for deceased-donation programs, limited resources (surgeons, hospital beds, nurses, radiologists, etc.), geographical barriers, and cost of immunosuppressant medications. Access to kidney transplantation increases with country income level, with services being available in only 23% of LICs, compared to 69% of LMICs, 83% of upper-middle-income countries (UMICs), and 89% of HICs. Donated kidneys in LICs and LMICs come from living donors in 100% and 60% of cases, respectively. The incidence of kidney transplantation using organs from deceased donors is below the global average in Africa, Latin America, the Middle East, North and East Asia, newly independent states, and Russia, and above the global average in Eastern and Central Europe, North America, and Western Europe.

Conclusions

Kidney disease can be considered a barometer for health systems and for health equity. Maintaining kidney health requires addressing the social determinants of health, implementing sound policies to maximize primary prevention, and ensuring sufficient primary care to detect and treat kidney disease early, such that kidney failure can be delayed or prevented, quality of life maximized, and unnecessary mortality reduced. Such holistic strategies are lacking in most lower-income settings. Advocacy is needed by the global nephrology community to strengthen public health policies, to collect and share knowledge and epidemiology of kidney disease within local contexts, and to improve access to quality kidney care across the spectrum, with the goal of preserving global kidney health.

Complete bibliography is available at Elsevier eBooks for Practicing Clinicians.

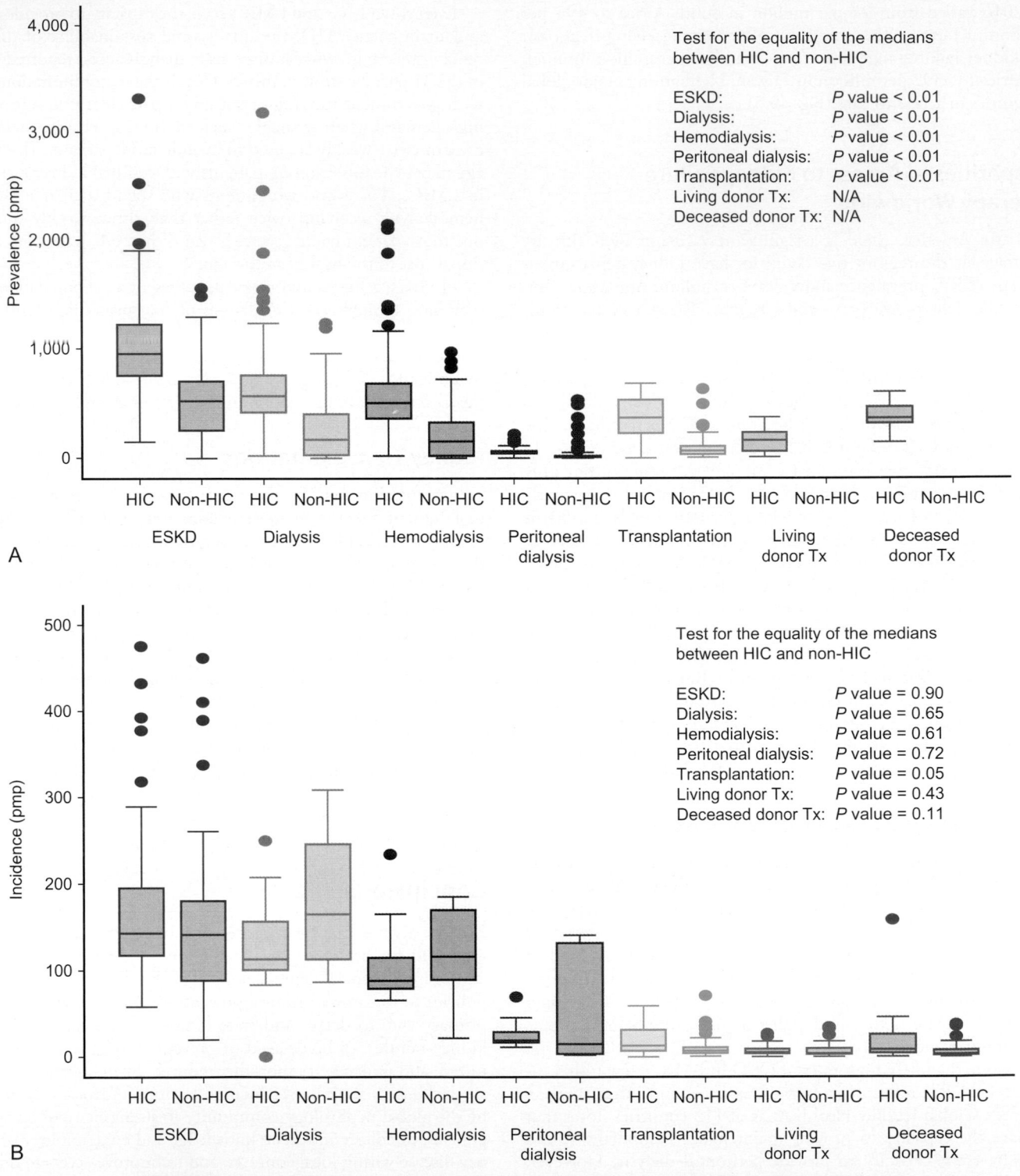

• **Fig. 49.5** Global incidence and prevalence of treated end-stage kidney failure. Variability in incidence and prevalence in end-stage kidney disease (ESKD) treated with various forms of dialysis and transplantation across high-income (HIC) and non-high income (non-HIC) countries is illustrated based on available data. Data from many non-HIC are estimates, given lack of registries. The incidence of untreated ESKD is estimated to be up to threefold higher than that of treated ESKD globally. (From Harris DCH, Davies SJ, Finkelstein FO, et al; Working Groups of the International Society of Nephrology's 2nd Global Kidney Health Summit. Increasing access to integrated ESKD care as part of universal health coverage. *Kidney Int.* 2019;95:S1-S33.)

Key Bibliography

Anand S, Caplin B, Gonzalez-Quiroz M, et al. Epidemiology, molecular, and genetic methodologies to evaluate causes of CKDu around the world: Report of the Working Group from the ISN International Consortium of Collaborators on CKDu. *Kidney Int*. 2019;96(6):1254–1260.

Bradshaw C, Kondal D, Montez-Rath ME, et al. Early detection of chronic kidney disease in low-income and middle-income countries: Development and validation of a point-of-care screening strategy for India. *BMJ Glob Health*. 2019;4(5):e001644.

Cerda J, Mohan S, Garcia-Garcia G, et al. Acute kidney injury recognition in low- and middle-income countries. *Kidney Int Rep*. 2017;2(4):530–543.

Cervantes L, Tuot D, Raghavan R, et al. Association of emergency-only vs standard hemodialysis with mortality and health care use among undocumented immigrants with end-stage renal disease. *JAMA Intern Med*. 2018;178(2):188–195.

Cullis B, Abdelraheem M, Abrahams G, et al. Peritoneal dialysis for acute kidney injury. *Perit Dial Int*. 2014;34(5):494–517.

Essue BM, Laba TL, Knaul F, et al. Economic burden of chronic ill health and injuries for households in low- and middle-income countries. In: Jamison DT, Gelband H, Horton S et al., eds. *Disease Control Priorities. Improving Health and Reducing Poverty*. 3rd ed. Washington, DC: World Bank; 2018:121–143.

GBD Chronic Kidney Disease Collaboration 2020. GBD Chronic Kidney Disease Collaboration. Global, regional, and national burden of chronic kidney disease, 1990-2017: A systematic analysis for the Global Burden of Disease Study 2017. *Lancet*. 2020;395(10225):709–733.

Harris DCH, Davies SJ, Finkelstein FO, et al. Increasing access to integrated ESKD care as part of universal health coverage. *Kidney Int*. 2019;95(4S):S1–S33.

International Society of Nephrology 2017. International Society of Nephrology. Global Kidney Health Atlas: A report by the International Society of Nephrology on the current state of organization and structures for kidney care across the globe. 2017, https://www2.theisn.org/GKHA.

International Society of Nephrology 2019. International Society of Nephrology. Global Kidney Health Atlas: A report by the International Society of Nephrology on the Global Burden of End-stage Kidney Disease and Capacity for Kidney Replacement Therapy and Conservative Care across World Countries and Regions. Brussels, Belgium 2019.

Johnson RJ, Wesseling C, Newman LS. Chronic kidney disease of unknown cause in agricultural communities. *N Engl J Med*. 2019;380(19):1843–1852.

Kashani K, Macedo E, Burdmann EA, et al. Acute Kidney injury risk assessment: differences and similarities between resource-limited and resource-rich countries. *Kidney Int Rep*. 2017;2(4):519–529.

Levin A, Tonelli M, Bonventre J, et al. Global kidney health 2017 and beyond: a roadmap for closing gaps in care, research, and policy. *Lancet*. 2017;390(10105):1888–1917.

Liyanage T, Ninomiya T, Jha V, et al. Worldwide access to treatment for end-stage kidney disease: A systematic review. *Lancet*. 2015;385(9981):1975–1982.

Luyckx VA, Miljeteig I, Ejigu AM, Moosa MR. Ethical challenges in the provision of dialysis in resource-constrained environments. *Semin Nephrol*. 2017;37(3):273–286.

Luyckx VA, Tonelli M, Stanifer JW. The global burden of kidney disease and the sustainable development goals. *Bull World Health Organ*. 2018;96(6):414–422D.

Mehta RL, Burdmann EA, Cerda J, et al. Recognition and management of acute kidney injury in the International Society of Nephrology 0by25 Global Snapshot: A multinational cross-sectional study. *Lancet*. 2016;387(10032):2017–2025.

Norton JM, Moxey-Mims MM, Eggers PW, et al. Social determinants of racial disparities in CKD. *J Am Soc Nephrol*. 2016;27(9):2576–2595.

Van Biesen W, Vanholder R, Ernandez T, Drewniak D, Luyckx V. Caring for migrants and refugees with end-stage kidney disease in Europe. *Am J Kidney Dis*. 2017.

van der Tol A, Lameire N, Morton RL, Van Biesen W, Vanholder R. An International Analysis of Dialysis Services Reimbursement. *Clin J Am Soc Nephrol*. 2019;14(1):84–93.

PART 10

Chronic Kidney Disease

50

Development and Progression of Chronic Kidney Disease

NAVDEEP TANGRI

Chronic kidney disease (CKD) is defined as abnormal measurements of the actual or estimated glomerular filtration rate (GFR) for a minimum of 3 months (Box 50.1), or situations where the GFR is normal but pathology in the kidney is still present, such as radiographically imaged cysts in polycystic kidney disease or isolated proteinuria in early glomerular disease (see Chapter 51). The most commonly reported causes of CKD and end-stage kidney disease (ESKD) (Table 50.1) are diabetic nephropathy (Fig. 50.1) and hypertensive nephrosclerosis, although the diagnosis of "hypertensive nephrosclerosis" has recently been revisited in reference to APOL1 genetic abnormalities (Chapter 36). However, many other conditions can cause CKD, including primary glomerular diseases (e.g., IgA nephropathy, membranous glomerulopathy), secondary glomerular diseases (e.g., lupus nephritis, amyloidosis), and tubulointerstitial, vascular, cystic, and hereditary kidney diseases. Each of these has specific pathophysiologic mechanisms for kidney damage; therefore, the treatments developed for these diseases are unique and aimed at controlling or reversing the underlying disease process.

The idea, then, that CKD could be generalized into one disease process is an oversimplification, because the primary processes causing kidney damage are diverse. However, the pathophysiology of progression of many of these disorders involves similar pathways, and generic treatments aimed at slowing this progression have been applied across a wide variety of kidney diseases effectively and safely. Over the last 20 years, a number of treatments have been developed and proven to delay progression to ESKD. Therefore, early recognition of CKD becomes important to help implement therapy that can alter its trajectory and reduce the associated morbidity and mortality.

Pathophysiologic Mechanisms of Chronic Kidney Disease

The pathophysiology of CKD is complex and in large part dependent on the primary cause. After an acute or chronic insult occurs, such as in diabetic nephropathy or lupus nephritis, many common pathways are activated to perpetuate and exacerbate glomerular and tubulointerstitial injury (Fig. 50.2). These harmful adaptations, occurring because of an initial injury, can be broadly categorized into those that are hemodynamically mediated or those that are nonhemodynamic.

Hemodynamic Injury

Much of the work in hemodynamic-mediated injury stems from the 5/6 nephrectomy animal model. Following unilateral nephrectomy and 2/3 removal of the contralateral kidney in rats, hypertension, proteinuria, and progressive decline in GFR ensue. Pathologic examination of the remaining tissue exhibits hyperfiltration injury, as evidenced by glomerular hypertrophy and focal segmental glomerular sclerosis (FSGS). The process occurs at a linear rate in proportion to the greater reduction in kidney mass. Micropuncture techniques reveal an increase in renal plasma flow and hyperfiltration of the remaining nephrons. Systemic and glomerular hypertension, from activation of the renin-angiotensin-aldosterone system (RAAS), causes progressive glomerular damage and proteinuria. These changes result as efferent arteriolar tone increases more than afferent tone. This net efferent vasoconstriction increases intraglomerular and filtration pressure further, perpetuating hyperfiltration injury. Animal models of other primary kidney diseases, such as that of diabetic nephropathy in the rat, reveal similar pathophysiologic changes of glomerular hypertension, hypertrophy, and hyperfiltration.

These maladaptive hemodynamic effects are mediated by the RAAS (Figs. 50.2 and 50.3). With nephron loss, adaptation leads to release of renin from the juxtaglomerular apparatus because of decreased perfusion pressure and low solute delivery to the macula densa. Renin converts angiotensinogen to angiotensin I, which is converted to angiotensin II (AII) under the influence of angiotensin-converting enzyme (ACE). AII, in addition to increasing aldosterone production from the adrenal gland, is the main perpetrator of glomerular hemodynamic maladaptation. Through an increase in sympathetic activity, AII is a potent vasoconstrictor, especially predominant in the efferent arterioles. It also exhibits a role in salt and water retention, both directly through proximal tubular sodium reabsorption and indirectly through aldosterone-dependent distal sodium reabsorption. Finally, AII stimulates the posterior pituitary to release antidiuretic hormone (ADH).

The net effect of all these mechanisms is an integral component of autoregulation, helping to maintain GFR when perfusion is decreased. However, in the setting of nephron loss through a primary kidney insult or CKD, the effect of continuous AII overactivity is perpetual maladaptation by creating systemic and, notably, glomerular hypertension. This glomerular hypertension increases the filtration fraction, increases the radius of the pores in

BOX 50.1

Important Characteristics of Chronic Kidney Disease

1. Chronic kidney disease (CKD) is currently defined by a reduction in glomerular filtration rate over a period of time or evidence of kidney damage.
2. The most commonly reported causes of CKD are diabetes mellitus and hypertension, and less frequent causes are primary glomerular, tubulointerstitial, and cystic diseases.
3. The pathophysiology of chronic kidney damage is related to the underlying disease, but it is accelerated by glomerular hypertension, systemic hypertension, inflammation, and fibrosis.
4. Risk factors for progression are hypertension, proteinuria, and recurrent acute kidney injury.
5. Treatment for CKD is disease specific, but several generalized methods can be applied to almost all kidney diseases. The goal is slowing or reversing progression with therapies aimed at correcting the pathophysiologic patterns. These involve blocking the renin-angiotensin-aldosterone system (RAAS) with medications, SGLT2 inhibition, controlling blood pressure, and reducing albuminuria when present. This goal is attempted while also targeting cardiovascular risk reduction. Novel methods, which require further study, involve attacking the inflammatory and fibrotic effects of the pathophysiology.

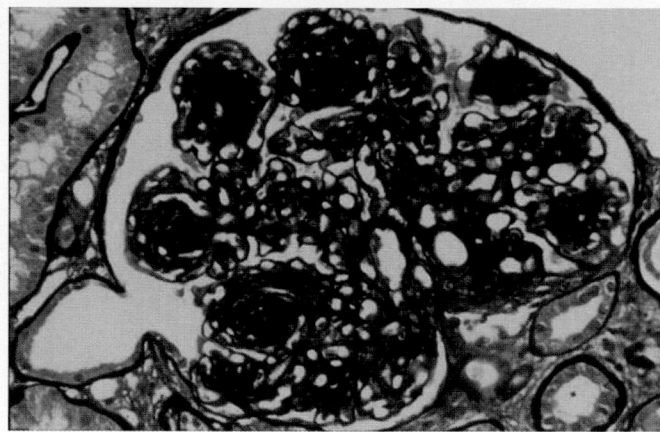

• **Fig. 50.1** Glomerulus from a patient with overt diabetic nephropathy, termed "The Face of the Enemy," by Dr. Edmund J. Lewis. There is marked expansion with nodular glomerular sclerosis, consistent with Kimmelstiel-Wilson nodules. Note the hypertrophied glomerulus, prominent mesangium, and aneurysmal features of the capillary walls, giving the appearance of a daisy flower (methenamine silver stain, ×230).

TABLE 50.1 Frequency of Reported Primary Disease Causing End-Stage Kidney Disease

Disease	Percentage (%)
Diabetes mellitus type 1	3.9
Diabetes mellitus type 2	41.0
Hypertension	27.2
Primary glomerulonephritis	8.2
Tubulointerstitial	3.6
Hereditary or cystic	3.1
Secondary glomerulonephritis or vasculitis	2.1
Neoplasm or plasma cell dyscrasias	2.1
Miscellaneous	4.6
Unknown	5.2

the glomerular basement membrane (GBM) through an increase in hydrostatic pressure, and eventually results in clinical proteinuria and glomerular damage.

The best example of a human model of decreased nephron mass or number is unilateral kidney agenesis. Ashley and Mostofi originally reported 232 patients with unilateral kidney agenesis in the 1960s, and, although the pathology was not described, 16% of the patients died from kidney failure. Later, in the 1980s, autopsy series and case series confirmed the association of unilateral kidney agenesis with hypertension, proteinuria, progressive kidney disease, glomerulomegaly, and FSGS (Fig. 50.4). Besides kidney agenesis, another human example is the condition known as *oligomeganephronia*. This is a form of congenital kidney hypoplasia in which the number of nephrons is reduced. The glomeruli hypertrophy in compensation for the reduced nephron number. The sequelae of this include hypertension, proteinuria, and FSGS related to hyperfiltration and progressive kidney failure. Other

clinical human examples of disease that support this mechanism of kidney injury include obesity-related glomerulomegaly and nephropathy, dysplastic solitary kidney, or partial nephrectomy in the setting of a solitary kidney.

Because animal models and human congenital diseases of reduced nephron mass lead to hemodynamic maladaptation and morphologic evidence of FSGS, it is natural to speculate that a transplant donor would be at risk for this same pathophysiology. Fortunately, the development of hypertension or kidney damage in the remaining kidney in transplant donors is infrequent. This may reflect extensive screening of potential donors, resulting in a sufficiently healthy population with minimal vascular disease, such that the donor can readily compensate for a 50% reduction in kidney mass. Similar results are seen in experimental models where adult rats with unilateral nephrectomy rarely develop hypertension or kidney disease; however, when a single kidney is removed from immature rats, the glomerular lesion FSGS manifests in the remaining kidney. Therefore, hemodynamic injury may be present or clinically apparent only when the kidney is undergoing normal growth. Another explanation of this benign clinical course in patients donating a kidney is that the development of clinical pathology is directly linked to the length of time and degree of reduction of nephron mass. Indeed, there are studies demonstrating an increased risk for hypertension, proteinuria, and progressive kidney disease in patients who have more than a 50% reduction in kidney mass, such as those with bilateral partial nephrectomy for carcinoma, and a greater likelihood of progressive kidney disease with a longer duration of nephron mass reduction.

Nonhemodynamic Injury

Besides the hemodynamic effects of systemic vasoconstriction, sodium retention, and efferent arteriolar vasoconstriction, activation of the RAAS leads to several nonhemodynamic maladaptive pathways (see Fig. 50.2), which, in turn, results in inflammation and fibrosis. AII has been demonstrated in high concentrations in virtually every compartment of the kidney in CKD, including the mesangial cells, endothelial cells, podocytes, the urinary space (Bowman capsule), and the tubulointerstitium.

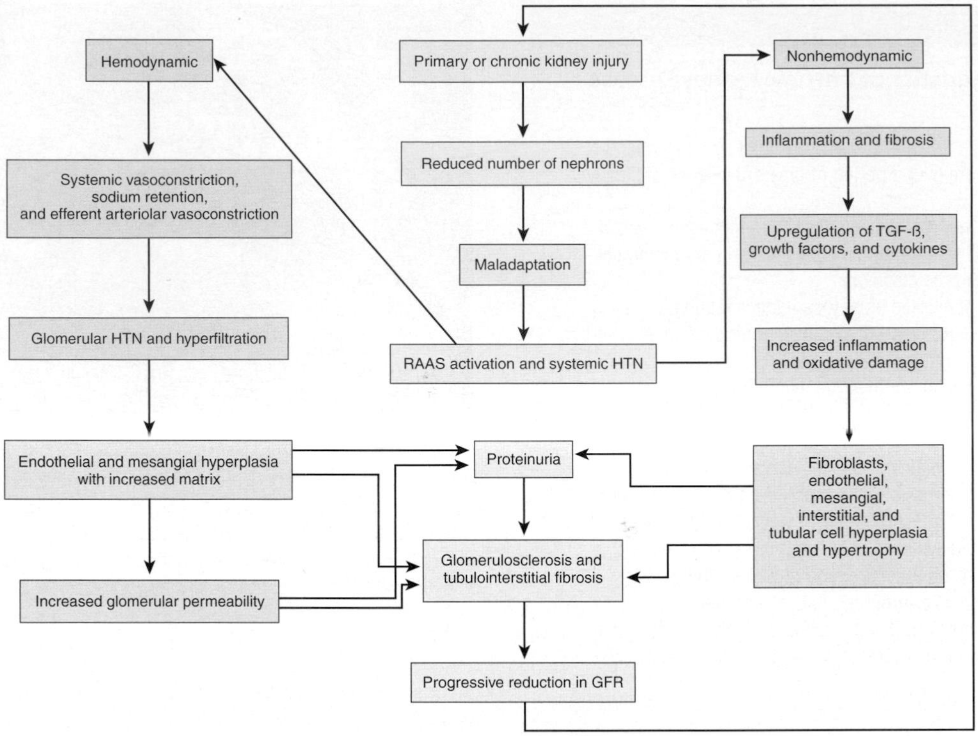

Hemodynamic

Primary or chronic kidney injury

Nonhemodynamic

Systemic vasoconstriction,
sodium retention,
and efferent arteriolar vasoconstriction

Reduced number of nephrons

Inflammation and fibrosis

Maladaptation

Upregulation of TGF-ß,
growth factors, and cytokines

Glomerular HTN and hyperfiltration

RAAS activation and systemic HTN

Increased inflammation
and oxidative damage

Endothelial and mesangial hyperplasia
with increased matrix

Proteinuria

Fibroblasts,
endothelial,
mesangial,
interstitial, and
tubular cell hyperplasia
and hypertrophy

Increased glomerular permeability

Glomerulosclerosis and
tubulointerstitial fibrosis

Progressive reduction in GFR

• **Fig. 50.2** Diagram of the pathogenesis of progressive chronic kidney disease. After a primary or chronic injury occurs, activation of the renin-angiotensin-aldosterone system leads to hemodynamic and nonhemodynamic injury. *GFR*, Glomerular filtration rate; *HTN,* hypertension; *RAAS*, renin-angiotensin-aldosterone system; *TGF*-β, transforming growth factor-β.

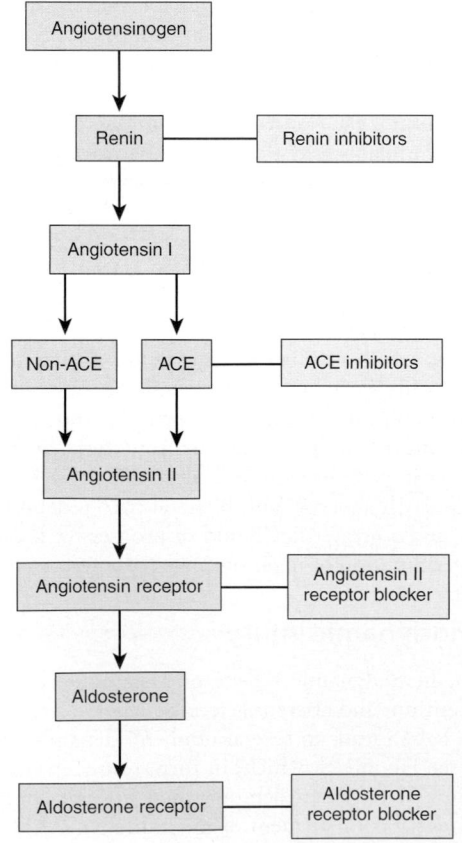

Angiotensinogen

Renin — Renin inhibitors

Angiotensin I

Non-ACE | ACE — ACE inhibitors

Angiotensin II

Angiotensin receptor — Angiotensin II receptor blocker

Aldosterone

Aldosterone receptor — Aldosterone receptor blocker

• **Fig. 50.3** Diagram of renin-angiotensin-aldosterone activation and targeted therapies that interrupt the pathway. *ACE,* Angiotensin-converting enzyme.

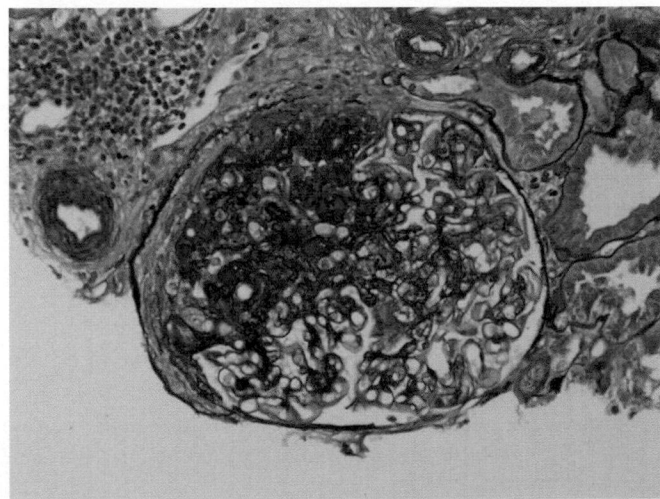

• **Fig. 50.4** Hypertrophied glomerulus with sclerotic segment encompassing almost 50% of the glomerular surface area from a patient with unilateral dysplastic kidney, hypertension, and proteinuria. The uninvolved segment of the glomerulus has patent capillaries and normal architecture. The glomerular diameter was measured to be 270 µm (periodic acid–Schiff stain, ×230). Normal glomerular diameter is 144 ± 11 µm.

Activation of the RAAS eventually results in fibrosis and a progressive decline in GFR. This fibrosis is a consequence of upregulation of several growth factors and their receptors, such as connective tissue growth factor (CTGF), epidermal growth factor (EGF), insulin-like growth factor-1 (IGF-1), platelet-derived growth factor (PDGF), vascular endothelial growth factor (VEGF), transforming growth factor-β (TGF-β), and monocyte chemotactic protein-1 (MCP-1). The activation of these factors by AII and aldosterone leads to cellular proliferation and hypertrophy of glomerular endothelial cells, mesangial cells, podocytes, tubulointerstitial cells, and fibroblasts. AII and TGF-β also upregulate other factors that lead to the overproduction of extracellular matrix, such as type 1 procollagen, plasminogen activator inhibitor 1, and fibronectin. In addition, excess adhesion molecules, such as integrins or vascular cellular adhesion molecule 1, allow the increased extracellular matrix and hypercellularity to accumulate and persist. This leads to cell proliferation, extracellular matrix accumulation, adhesion of these cells, and functional changes with eventual fibrosis (Fig. 50.5).

Inflammation is also a key contributor to the progression of kidney disease (see Fig. 50.2). This may seem obvious in diseases in which inflammation is the primary insult, such as postinfectious glomerulonephritis or severe lupus nephritis, because it is apparent by light microscopy of kidney biopsy specimens. However, inflammation is an important factor in the progression of almost all types of kidney diseases and is mediated in part by the RAAS. AII recruits T cells and macrophages by stimulating endothelin-1 (ET-1) and increases production of nuclear factor κ–light-chain enhancer of activated B cells (NF-κB); these molecules release cytokines, creating more inflammation. Increased expression of TGF-β also induces cellular recruitment. Finally, free radical oxygen species lead to additional injury, which enables further inflammation and fibrosis.

Experimental evidence also supports the idea that proteinuria itself contributes to progressive nephrosclerosis. Through hyperfiltration, the increased glomerular permeability to albumin allows reabsorption of more albumin by the proximal tubular cells. Experimental models show that when this protein becomes prevalent in the interstitium, macrophages and inflammatory mediators, such as ET-1, MCP-1, and other chemokines, are upregulated, which eventually leads to inflammation and subsequent tubulointerstitial and glomerular fibrosis.

Through primary stimulation of the RAAS, predominantly through TGF-β, a cascade of events occurs that begins with inflammation, is perpetuated by accumulation of cells and matrix, is exacerbated by adhesion and persistence of these cells and matrix, and ends with injury, glomerulosclerosis, and tubulointerstitial fibrosis (see Fig. 50.2). This creates a progressive course of CKD, proteinuria, GFR loss, and a vicious cycle of continuous RAAS activation.

Risk Factors for Progression

Risk factors for progression include nonmodifiable characteristics such as older age, male sex, and Black race. One study of younger patients with CKD estimated the lifetime risk for ESKD for a 20-year-old person to be 7.8% for Black women, 7.3% for Black men, 1.8% for White women, and 2.5% for White men. Conversely, other risk factors such as hypertension, proteinuria, and

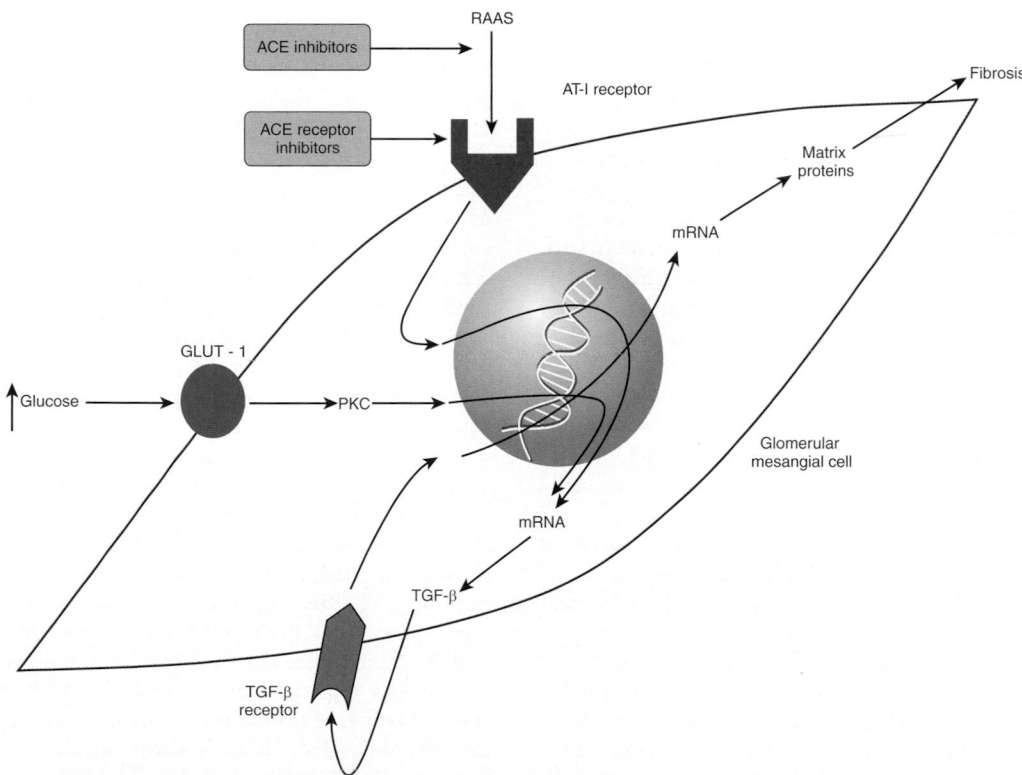

• **Fig. 50.5** Schematic representation of a glomerular mesangial cell in chronic kidney disease due to diabetic nephropathy. Activation of renin-angiotensin-aldosterone system upregulates TGF-β, which leads to matrix accumulation, inflammation, and fibrosis. Hyperglycemia also perpetuates this fibrosis via increased activity of protein kinase C. Through interruption of this cascade, angiotensin-converting enzyme inhibitors and angiotensin receptor blockers are effective treatments, delaying progression of chronic kidney disease in diabetic nephropathy. *ACE,* Angiotensin-converting enzyme; *AT-I,* angiotensin I; *GLUT-1,* glucose transporter; *mRNA,* messenger ribonucleic acid; *PKC,* protein kinase C; *RAAS,* renin-angiotensin-aldosterone system; *TGF-β,* transforming growth factor-β.

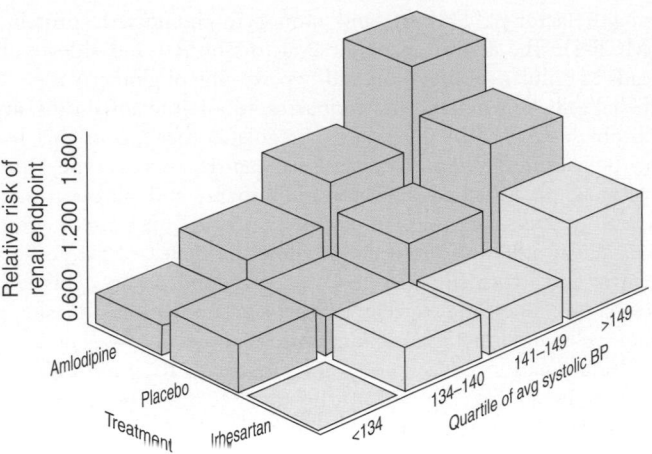

• Fig. 50.6 Simultaneous impact to quartile of achieved systolic blood pressure and treatment modality on the relative risk for reaching a kidney endpoint (doubling of baseline serum creatinine or ESKD, defined as serum creatinine ≥6.0 mg/dL or kidney replacement therapy). *avg,* Average; *BP,* blood pressure. (From Pohl MA, Blumenthal S, Cordonnier DJ, et al. Independent and additive impact of blood pressure control and angiotensin II receptor blockade on kidney outcomes in the irbesartan diabetic nephropathy trial: clinical implications and limitations. *J Am Soc Nephrol.* 2005;16:3031.)

recurrent acute kidney injury (AKI) are all potentially modifiable and deserve attention (Box 50.2).

With increased activity of the RAAS resulting in vasoconstriction and sodium retention, hypertension perpetuates the cycle of progressive CKD. In patients who have diabetic nephropathy from type 2 diabetes mellitus (DM), elevated blood pressure is the most common cause of CKD and a clear risk factor for a progressive decline in GFR, and, notably, treating this hypertension reduces CKD progression. The effect of therapy is even more pronounced in this patient population when treatment is with RAAS blockade (Fig. 50.6). Early in the 1980s, Mogensen established that in patients with diabetic nephropathy, treating elevated blood pressure (mean 162/103 mm Hg) to an achieved level of 144/95 mm Hg reduced the rate of GFR loss from 1.23 mL/min per month to 0.49 mL/min per month. Since that time, other observational studies and well-designed clinical trials have demonstrated that hypertension is clearly a risk factor for ESKD in diabetic nephropathy, and that blood pressure reduction, especially with RAAS blockade, attenuates this risk.

Hypertension is also an established risk factor for progression of nondiabetic kidney disease. The Multiple Risk Factor Intervention Trial (MRFIT), which used various interventions to treat patients with multiple cardiovascular risk factors, such as smoking, hypertension, obesity, and hyperlipidemia, demonstrated that elevated blood pressure was an independent risk factor for the development of kidney failure. Other studies of nondiabetic kidney disease, such as the African American Study of Kidney Disease (AASK), reveal a similar pattern, indicating that patients with nondiabetic CKD benefited from a lower achieved blood pressure, especially if proteinuria was present. Similarly, observational studies suggest slower progression in patients with other causes of CKD, such as polycystic kidney disease, when blood pressure is controlled.

Albuminuria is another well-established risk factor for progression of CKD. In patients with overt diabetic nephropathy, the degree of baseline albuminuria is directly correlated with a more rapid decline in GFR (Fig. 50.7). This is also true in nondiabetic kidney diseases, such as IgA nephropathy or lupus nephritis. In the predominantly nondiabetic patient population recruited for the Modification of Diet in Renal Disease (MDRD) study, those with albuminuria had the highest risk for progressive kidney disease. The Ramipril Efficacy in Nephropathy (REIN) study similarly noted that, in nondiabetic CKD, the baseline level of albuminuria was the strongest predictor of kidney failure, independent of the baseline GFR. Even in patients with earlier stages of CKD, with an estimated GFR of greater than 60 mL/min/1.73 m², those who demonstrate albuminuria by ≥2 + on dipstick or greater than 300 mg albumin/g creatinine are over 3 times more likely to double the serum creatinine over time compared with those with lower levels (30 to 300 mg albumin/g creatinine). This trend is also true when comparing patients who have 30 to 300 mg albumin/g with those who have less than 30 mg/g.

Despite these robust data, controversy exists as to whether albuminuria is truly a pathogenic risk factor or just a marker of kidney disease severity. If albuminuria were a simple manifestation of advanced disease, such as a cough in the setting of pneumonia, then treating the symptom would have minimal to no effect on improving the disease outcome. However, targeting and reducing albuminuria is highly effective at improving kidney outcomes, both in diabetic (see Fig. 50.7) and nondiabetic kidney diseases.

The idea that recurrent or episodic AKI leads to progressive chronic kidney dysfunction is based on the pathophysiology of the disease (see Fig. 50.2). Multiple studies have now shown that in patients with preexisting CKD, AKI is a risk factor for the development of ESKD. The degree of preexisting CKD, severity of AKI, advanced age, presence of DM, and low serum albumin amplify this risk. In a retrospective study by Ishani et al., the hazard ratio of developing ESKD for older adult patients (>67 years) who had CKD without AKI was 8.4, whereas for those patients who had CKD and AKI, the hazard ratio for progressing to ESKD was 41.2.

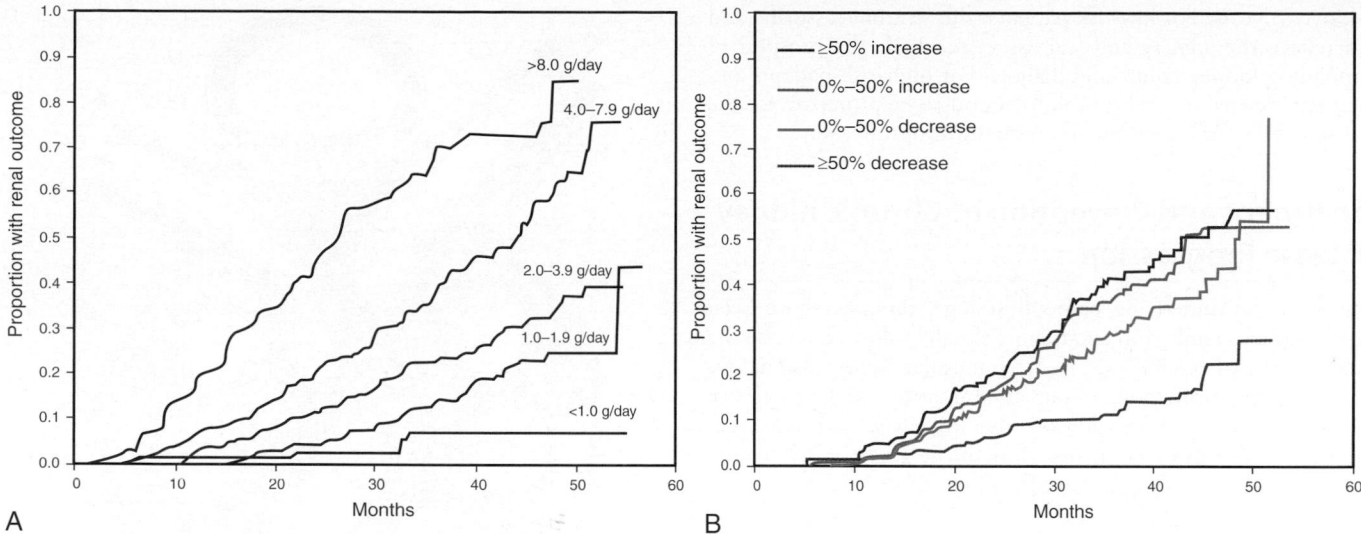

• **Fig. 50.7** (A) Kaplan-Meier analysis of doubling of a baseline serum creatinine level, serum creatinine level of ≥6.0 mg/dL, or the development of ESKD by baseline proteinuria values. (B) Kaplan-Meier analysis of doubling of a baseline serum creatinine level, serum creatinine level of ≥6.0 mg/dL, or the development of ESKD by level of proteinuria change in the first 12 months. (From Atkins RC, Briganti EM, Lewis JB, et al. Proteinuria reduction and progression to kidney failure in patients with type 2 diabetes mellitus and overt nephropathy. *Am J Kidney Dis*. 2005;45:283.)

Knowledge that AKI affects CKD is important so that future therapies can be developed and evaluated in an attempt to retard this progression. It is also relevant as minimizing episodes of iatrogenic AKI in CKD patients can often be achieved. It is sensible to avoid, if possible, situations that may cause AKI, such as iatrogenic hypotension or nephrotoxic injury from polypharmacy, iodinated contrast exposure, atheroemboli, and nonsteroidal anti-inflammatory agents in vulnerable patients.

Many other factors have been associated with a progressive decline in GFR (see Box 50.2). In later stages of CKD, the kidney loses the ability to handle the daily dietary acid load, and metabolic acidosis can occur. Its manifestations include accelerated bone disease, sarcopenia, and faster CKD progression. Multiple randomized, controlled trials and a recent meta-analysis suggest that treatment of metabolic acidosis may slow CKD progression, and new therapies to treat acidosis are on the horizon. Finally, the underlying kidney disease affects the rate of progression, as glomerular diseases and polycystic kidney diseases tend to progress faster than most tubulointerstitial diseases. Evidence exists for the APOL1 genetic mutations as not only a cause of CKD, but also a factor for progression. Elevated levels of the soluble urokinase-type plasminogen activator receptor (suPAR) have also been linked to the development and progression of CKD. Although evidence establishing hyperlipidemia, tobacco dependence, or obesity as risk factors is not as robust as that pointing to hypertension or proteinuria, these associations do exist and targeting these risk factors when present is prudent.

Predicting CKD Progression

Patients with CKD are often focused on two questions: (1) How did I get kidney disease? and (2) Am I going to need dialysis? While the former often requires a careful review of the history and physical examination findings by the nephrologist, the latter can be accurately answered for most patients using the Kidney Failure

Risk Equation (KFRE). The KFRE was developed by Tangri et al. in 2011 in a cohort of patients with CKD stages G3-G5 followed by nephrologists in Ontario, Canada, and has subsequently been validated in more than 720,000 individuals from more than 30 countries and diverse subpopulations.

The four-variable KFRE includes age, sex, estimated GFR, and albuminuria and can predict the 2- and 5-year risk of kidney failure requiring dialysis with accuracy (C statistic ~0.9 in North American and non-North American cohorts). It has been incorporated into electronic health records, health systems, and clinical practice guidelines, and a dedicated website (www.kidneyfailurerisk.com) provides a clinical decision aid, as well as patient education materials to enable its use in shared decision making.

Recently, there have been several independent validation studies of the KFRE, which further establish its accuracy for patients with CKD and identify additional strengths. First, a study from investigators at University of California San Diego found that the KFRE was more accurate than patients and providers in predicting the risk of kidney failure. Second, a recent study from Canada determined that the KFRE was accurate across multiple etiologies of CKD, suggesting its broad applicability regardless of specific glomerular or tubulointerstitial diseases. Finally, two recent reports highlighted the accuracy of the KFRE in kidney transplant recipients and found it to be adequate in discriminating kidney failure outcomes, particularly in patients with reduced eGFR.

In summary, the KFRE is accurate and generalizable, and should be used to predict CKD progression in patients with CKD stages G3-G5. Alternative prediction equations such as the competing risk calculator and the incident CKD equations developed by Grams et al. can supplement the information provided by the KFRE. Trials evaluating a risk-based care paradigm based on the KFRE are underway.

Nevertheless, the prediction from the KFRE can be used in the clinical encounter to provide an accurate estimate of kidney failure risk over 5 years. For low-risk patients, this can be reassuring and can relieve the anxiety and fear associated with the prospect of impending kidney failure and dialysis. For high-risk patients and their care teams, it can be a call to action to help prepare for the real possibility of kidney failure in the most optimal way.

Treatment and Prevention of Chronic Kidney Disease Progression

Based on the underlying pathophysiology, therapies have been developed and studied in an attempt to safely slow or reverse the vicious cycle of RAAS activation, glomerular hypertension, systemic hypertension, proteinuria, inflammation, and progressive fibrosis (Table 50.2). In addition, therapies have targeted other clinically modifiable risk factors, all with the goal of safely reducing or reversing the progression of CKD.

Antagonism of the Renin-Angiotensin-Aldosterone System

Based on the animal models of 5/6 nephrectomy and diabetic glomerulosclerosis, it is plausible that interruption of the RAAS cascade (see Fig. 50.3) could lead to renoprotection. In animal models, AII selectively causes hemodynamic-mediated injury through efferent arteriolar vasoconstriction, whereas the use of ACE inhibitors and angiotensin receptor blockers (ARBs) effectively dilates the efferent arteriole, leading to glomerular relaxation and subsequent reduction in glomerular hypertrophy and injury (Fig. 50.8). RAAS blockade also mediates improvements in systemic hypertension, which further reduces glomerular hypertension. In addition to reducing the hemodynamic impact in glomerular damage, blockade of the RAAS in animals has been shown to disrupt the inflammatory and fibrosing effects of the various cytokines, including TGF-β. The net effect of RAAS antagonism is, therefore, renoprotective on multiple levels: hemodynamic, antifibrotic, and antiproteinuric.

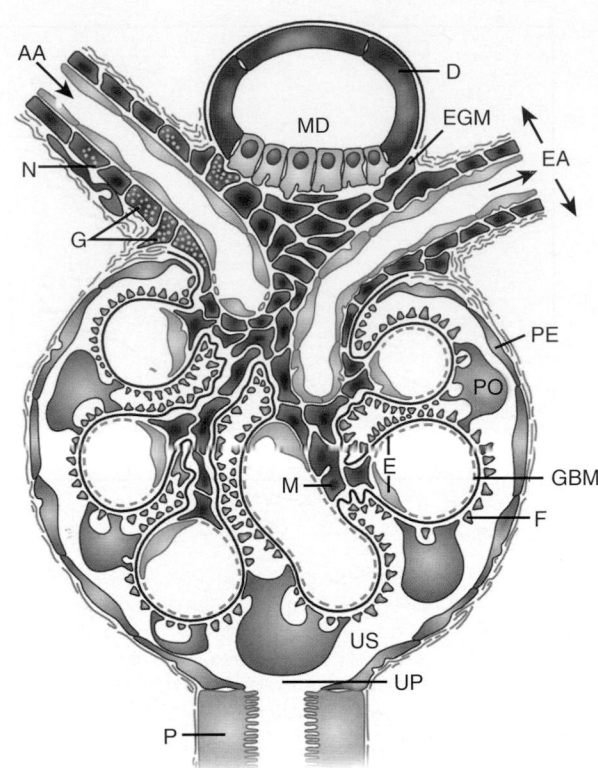

• **Fig. 50.8** Schematic representation of glomerular hemodynamic changes with blockade of the renin-angiotensin-aldosterone system. Angiotensin-converting enzyme inhibitors and angiotensin receptor blockers blunt the intrarenal arteriolar effects of angiotensin II, which leads to net dilation of the efferent arteriole (EA) *(arrows)* and reduction in glomerular hypertension. This reduction in glomerular capillary pressure reduces glomerular hyperpermeability, leading to reduced urinary protein excretion and renoprotection. *AA,* Afferent arteriole; *D,* distal tubule; *E,* endothelial cell; *EGM,* extraglomerular mesangial cell; *F,* foot process; *G,* juxtaglomerular granular cell; *GBM,* glomerular basement membrane; *M,* mesangial cell; *MD,* macula densa; *N,* sympathetic nerve endings; *P,* proximal tubule; *PE,* parietal epithelial cell; *PO,* epithelial podocyte; *UP,* urinary pole; *US,* urinary space.

TABLE 50.2	Therapies for Slowing Progression of Chronic Kidney Disease

Proven Benefit	Preliminary Evidence
Angiotensin-converting enzyme inhibitors	Treatment of metabolic acidosis
Angiotensin receptor antagonists	Dietary measures
SGLT2 inhibitors	Exercise
Blood pressure goal between 120 and 140 mm Hg systolic and 80 and 90 mm Hg diastolic	Weight loss in obesity
	Smoking cessation
	Glycemic control in diabetes mellitus
Selective mineralocorticoid receptor antagonists	Reduction of hyperuricemia, hyperlipidemia, hyperphosphatemia, albuminuria
Aldosterone receptor antagonists	Folate
	Vitamin D
	Acid-base balance
	Endothelin-1 antagonists
	Pirfenidone
	Inhibitors of advanced glycation end products

Lewis and colleagues tested the hypothesis that this could lead to renoprotection in humans in 1993. In a randomized, controlled clinical trial, 409 patients with type 1 diabetic nephropathy received either the ACE inhibitor captopril or placebo with achievement of equivalent systemic blood pressures between the two groups. This study found a dramatic 43% reduction in the doubling of the serum creatinine and a significant reduction in the time to death, dialysis, or transplantation with captopril compared with placebo. Thus, for the first time in human patients, ACE inhibitors established renoprotection by slowing progressive CKD, independent of lowering blood pressure and clinical remission in advanced diabetic nephropathy.

RAAS blockade has also been evaluated in type 2 diabetic nephropathy. In the Irbesartan for Microalbuminuria in Type 2 Diabetes (IRMA-2) trial of patients with type 2 DM, preserved GFR, and low-level albuminuria, irbesartan was more effective at reducing the progression to overt proteinuria from low-level albuminuria than placebo at identical blood pressure levels. Two large, randomized studies subsequently validated the use of ARBs in overt type 2 diabetic nephropathy. In the Irbesartan Diabetic Nephropathy Trial (IDNT), 1715 hypertensive patients with diabetic nephropathy (median baseline serum creatinine

1.67 mg/dL; median baseline urine protein excretion 2.9 g/24 hr) were randomized to receive one of three different treatment regimens: irbesartan 300 mg daily, the calcium channel blocker amlodipine 10 mg daily, or placebo. The achieved blood pressure was not different among the three groups. With irbesartan, the risk for reaching the composite endpoint of doubling of the serum creatinine, ESKD, or death was 20% lower when compared with placebo and 23% lower compared with amlodipine. In addition to use of the ARB, lower systolic blood pressure was also associated with a decreased relative risk in doubling of the serum creatinine or ESKD (see Fig. 50.6). Analogous results were demonstrated with the ARB losartan in the Reduction in Endpoints in non–insulin-dependent diabetes mellitus with the Angiotensin-II Antagonist Losartan (RENAAL) trial. In this randomized, controlled trial, 1513 patients with type 2 diabetic nephropathy were randomized to receive either losartan or placebo. Once again, both groups achieved equivalent blood pressure levels, with losartan reducing the incidence of doubling of the serum creatinine by 25% and the risk for ESKD by 28%. In both trials, there was a significant reduction in albuminuria with use of the ARB. Given the nearly identical results, these trials provide remarkable support for the use of ARBs for renoprotection in diabetic nephropathy.

In addition to systemic and glomerular hypertension, albuminuria is also reduced in patients with diabetic nephropathy treated with RAAS blockade. In both IDNT and RENAAL, baseline albuminuria was directly correlated with the risk of doubling of the serum creatinine or ESKD. More important, those patients who had a decrease in albuminuria experienced improved kidney outcomes (see Fig. 50.7), emphasizing that albuminuria may be an independent risk factor to the development of progressive kidney disease and suggesting that reducing albuminuria might be an appropriate surrogate target for an overall benefit in kidney outcomes.

Similar results are seen in nondiabetic kidney disease, where a meta-analysis by Jafar and colleagues demonstrated that RAAS inhibition slows progression, particularly in individuals with proteinuria exceeding 1000 mg/day. To confirm this finding, investigators for the REIN trial randomized 352 patients with hypertension and albuminuria but without diabetic nephropathy to receive either the ACE inhibitor ramipril or conventional antihypertensive therapy, achieving identical blood pressure control in both groups. Notably, patients randomized to receive ramipril had a 50% lower risk for progression to ESKD during the 3 years of follow-up. Similar to prior findings, patients who had greater degrees of albuminuria and received ramipril had a greater reduction in GFR decline compared with patients receiving conventional antihypertensive therapy.

In nonproteinuric and nondiabetic nephropathy, the data for use of RAAS blockade are not as strong. Primarily in Black patients with kidney disease previously attributed to "hypertensive nephrosclerosis," those without albuminuria have failed to show independent renoprotection with RAAS blockade. The mechanism of progression is linked to APOL1 genetic mutations and the development of focal and global glomerulosclerosis. Treatments targeting this specific mechanism are an area of ongoing research.

It is important to note that RAAS blockade is generally well tolerated, and hyperkalemia is the most common adverse effect. ACE inhibitors can cause a chronic cough, but this is not a concern with the use of ARBs. The management of RAAS blockade-related hyperkalemia in clinical practice often leads to discontinuation or dose reduction, or treatment of the complication with loop diuretics or potassium binders. More recently, new binders (patiromer and sodium zirconium cyclosilicate) have been approved for the treatment of hyperkalemia, and can facilitate RAAS blockade use. Large, randomized trials evaluating the benefit of a binder-enabled RAAS blockade treatment strategy in patients with CKD and heart failure are ongoing.

In summary, clinical trial data reveal that blockade of the RAAS with ACE inhibitors or ARBs provides the strongest renoprotection available to date, especially in patients with diabetic nephropathy or proteinuric CKD not due to DM, and these agents should be first-line therapy in these clinical settings. Critically, advanced CKD does not preclude their use.

SGLT2 Inhibition

In recent years, the introduction of sodium-glucose cotransporter-2 (SGLT2) inhibitors, along with the findings from the outcome trials of these agents, have presented an opportunity to revolutionize CKD care. While these agents were initially developed to treat hyperglycemia, the outcome trials have demonstrated a powerful effect on reducing cardiovascular- and kidney-related morbidity and mortality. Recent trials have demonstrated a >30 % reduction in all-cause mortality with use of these agents in patients with CKD, with or without diabetes, confirming that they are cardiorenal therapeutics and not simply oral hypoglycemics.

SGLT2 inhibitors have multiple mechanisms of action. They reduce plasma glucose level by an amount proportional to the filtered glucose load, and are associated with a 0.6% to 0.9% reduction in HbA1c in a dose-dependent manner. This is primarily accomplished by blockade of the SGLT1 receptor in the proximal tubule leading to a spillover of glucose and sodium beyond the proximal nephron. The resultant effect of these changes is an increased delivery of sodium to the macula densa, restoration of tubuloglomerular feedback, and a fall in the transglomerular pressure and single nephron GFR. This leads to preservation of kidney function and dramatic reductions in the chronic slope of GFR decline and kidney failure events.

In addition, these agents produce a diuretic effect, which leads to a hemoconcentration and a drop of 4-6 mm Hg in systolic blood pressure, independent of baseline volume status and hypertension. Most patients also experience a weight loss of 1-4 kg, additional beneficial effects to metabolic pathways in the liver including positive effects on hepatic glucose output and ketogenesis, and beta cell preservation.

Most importantly, consistent data from multiple, large, outcome trials in patients with CKD, with or without diabetes, has demonstrated that SGLT2 inhibitors reduce cardiovascular morbidity, all-cause mortality, and CKD progression. The effects of CKD outcomes are large in magnitude, ranging from a 30%-50% reduction in event rates, and are additive to RAAS blockade therapy. There does not appear to be any interaction by level of eGFR or albuminuria, and current data suggest that these agents are safe to initiate at eGFR levels above 20-25 mL/min/1.73 m^2 and to continue until patients reach kidney failure. In a typical 60-year-old patient with CKD stage G3 (eGFR 55 mL/min/1.73 m^2) enrolled in the SGLT2 inhibitor outcome trials, the slope of eGFR decline (~5 mL/min/year in the control arm) can be attenuated with treatment (~2 mL/min/year) to potentially delay or prevent the initiation of dialysis by more than a decade. Side effects include a 13/1000 patient-year risk of euglycemic diabetic ketoacidosis and a small but real risk of genital mycotic infections. Nonetheless, for most patients, the benefits greatly outweigh the risks and every effort should be made to initiate and maintain patients on SGLT2 inhibitor therapy.

Selective Mineralocorticoid Receptor Antagonists (MRAs)

Finerenone is a novel nonsteroidal MRA that was recently studied in two large pivotal randomized trials for preventing CKD progression and reducing cardiovascular events in patients with diabetes and chronic kidney disease. The FIDELIO and FIGARO studies randomized more than 13,000 patients to finerenone or placebo and found an 18% relative risk reduction in the CKD endpoint and a 13% relative risk reduction in major adverse cardiovascular events. These trials successfully confirm finerenone as another proven disease-modifying treatment option for patients with diabetes and CKD.

Blood Pressure Control

Blockade of the RAAS exerts its beneficial effect by reducing glomerular hypertension while simultaneously reducing systemic blood pressure. This clearly makes them first-line agents in most patients with hypertension, albuminuria, and CKD. Observational studies and randomized, controlled trials have shown that lowering blood pressure in patients with hypertension and CKD slows the rate of GFR loss. However, the ideal goal blood pressure in patients with CKD remains controversial. Guidelines suggest the target of less than 140/90 mm Hg for patients with CKD or DM. Notably, blood pressure control often requires at least two to four antihypertensive medications, including an agent to block the RAAS and usually a diuretic.

Previous guidelines had recommended a lower goal (<130/80) based on several studies revealing that "intensive" blood pressure control has substantial benefits in CKD for the treatment of nephropathy and/or cardiovascular disease. But how far should blood pressure be lowered, and is there a detrimental effect in lowering blood pressure too much in patients with CKD? This concern was raised in 1988 when the concept of the "J-curve" was introduced. The J-curve implies that lowering blood pressure reduces cardiovascular disease and death to a point, below which a plateau is achieved where lower blood pressure no longer confers a benefit and may result in increased risk for adverse events. A post hoc analysis of the IDNT trial described the J-curve in diabetic nephropathy: Worse outcomes were seen in patients with overt diabetic nephropathy at both high and very low systolic blood pressures. The lowest risk for kidney outcomes was seen at achieved systolic blood pressures between 120 and 130 mm Hg, and the risk for death was increased below an achieved systolic blood pressure of 120 mm Hg. In 2010, investigators for the Action to Control Cardiovascular Risks in Diabetes (ACCORD) trial reported the results of 4733 patients with type 2 DM, relatively preserved kidney function (serum creatinine ≤1.5 mg/dL), and either increased cardiovascular disease risk or a history of cardiovascular disease. These patients were randomized to an intensive systolic blood pressure goal of less than 120 mm Hg compared with a systolic blood pressure goal of less than 140 mm Hg. The achieved blood pressure in the intensive group was 119/64 mm Hg, while in the standard control group it was 134/71 mm Hg. Over an average follow-up of nearly 5 years, there was no difference in cardiovascular disease or stroke between the two groups; however, the intensive-therapy group demonstrated more hypotension, higher serum creatinine, and lower estimated GFR, as well as a tenfold higher rate of hyperkalemia, suggesting that the beneficial effects of hypertension treatment reach a plateau somewhere between a systolic blood pressure of 120 and 140 mm Hg.

Evidence for a plateau also exists in patients without diabetic nephropathy based on data from the AASK trial, where there was no difference in outcomes, including doubling of serum creatinine, ESKD, or death, in patients with the lower achieved mean arterial blood pressure (94.7 mm Hg), unless proteinuria (defined as a urine protein/creatinine ratio of >0.22 g of protein per g of creatinine) was present at baseline. More data on blood pressure goals in nondiabetic patients comes from the Systolic Blood Pressure Intervention Trial (SPRINT). Similar to the ACCORD trial, investigators randomized 9361 patients at high cardiovascular risk but without diabetes mellitus to a systolic blood pressure goal of less than 120 (intensive) versus less than 140 (standard) mm Hg. Although not designed to study hypertension in CKD specifically (mean eGFR 72 mL/min/1.73 m^2; patients with eGFR <20 mL/min/1.73 m^2 and/or proteinuria >1 g/d were excluded), 28% of the patients had CKD (eGFR 20 to 60 mL/min/1.73 m^2). The trial was stopped early (mean duration 3.3 years) because of a benefit of 25% relative risk reduction in the primary outcomes of cardiovascular events, heart failure, and stroke, and a 27% relative risk reduction in mortality in the intensive blood pressure group. Although this benefit extended to patients with CKD (eGFR 20 to 60 mL/min/1.73 m^2), there were more episodes of AKI and electrolyte abnormalities in the intensive group. In addition, the absolute risk reduction of intensive blood pressure lowering was only 0.6% (2.17% to 1.56%), leading to a large number needed to treat of 90. Therefore, in patients without diabetic nephropathy who have nonproteinuric mild to moderate CKD, evidence to target a lower systolic blood pressure goal exists, taking care to monitor for AKI and electrolyte abnormalities.

However, at the present time, lowering blood pressure to less than 120/80 mm Hg in patients with proteinuric CKD or diabetic nephropathy with pharmacologic therapy is not warranted. Consistent blood pressures above 140/90 mm Hg should be treated, and the first-line agent in people with diabetes or with proteinuria should be an ACE inhibitor or ARB. The exact blood pressure goal in patients with CKD remains controversial, but the present guideline of less than 140/90 mm Hg for patients with diabetic nephropathy and/or proteinuria is reasonable.

Management of Risk Factors and Complications

Based on the pathophysiology for CKD, glomerular hyperfiltration due to altered hemodynamics plays a role. Theoretically, decreasing elevated intraglomerular pressure by any means may have a benefit. Dietary protein restriction is a proposed method, and in the animal model of 5/6 nephrectomy, dietary protein restriction demonstrated reduced kidney injury by decreasing afferent arteriolar vasodilation, glomerular hypertension, and oncotic pressure. Unfortunately, contrary to RAAS blockade, human studies on dietary protein restriction have not shown substantial benefits of renoprotection.

The current recommended diet for people with diabetes, consisting of low sodium, low fat, and moderately low protein with high fiber, has been shown to decrease blood pressure in patients with hypertension and type 2 DM in the absence of CKD or albuminuria. Based on available evidence, a prudent diet for a patient with CKD is to limit protein intake to approximately 0.8 to 1.0 g/kg of body weight per day and to limit dietary sodium to less than 2.4 g a day. This is discussed in further detail in Chapter 52. In addition, as discussed in Chapter 26, control of blood glucose levels in patients who have DM is important to reduce microvascular and cardiovascular complications, although few data support intensive glycemic control for reducing the rate of GFR decline in patients with diabetic nephropathy. The method of glucose control may also be important for progressive diabetic nephropathy, as SGLT2 inhibitors, which exert their glucose-lowering effects by inducing glycosuria, have been shown to lower blood pressure and weight and delay progression of CKD compared to placebo.

Obesity and obesity-related glomerulopathy are increasing in prevalence. Obesity is a risk factor for developing CKD and, in patients with CKD, obesity is a risk factor for progression. Preexisting albuminuria is exacerbated by weight gain and decreases with weight loss; in addition, patients achieving sustained weight loss with bariatric surgery have a slower decline in eGFR over time compared to those who have not lost weight. These findings fit well into the model of hyperfiltration and glomerular hypertension with subsequent albuminuria and provide evidence that intervention can be renoprotective.

Hyperlipidemia, similar to obesity, may be a modifiable risk factor to slow progressive CKD. Hyperlipidemia may contribute to CKD progression through proinflammatory and profibrotic mechanisms because low-density lipoproteins (LDL) have these properties. Animal models reveal that rats fed high-cholesterol diets exhibit a greater degree of glomerulosclerosis and interstitial disease compared with those fed a low-cholesterol diet. In the same animal models, 3-hydroxy-3-methyl-glutaryl-CoA (HMG-CoA) reductase inhibitors (statins) have been shown to limit inflammatory cytokines and adhesion molecules and slow the rate of GFR loss. Observational studies in humans also support this hypothesis; however, unlike blockade of the RAAS, human clinical trials investigating the use of statin therapy to decrease the progression of CKD have been discouraging. In the Study of Heart and Renal Protection (SHARP) trial, 6247 patients with moderate to severe CKD were randomized to receive a statin and ezetimibe or placebo, and, although there was a cardiovascular benefit, no difference was seen in the development of kidney failure in the active therapy arm.

Metabolic acidosis is often underrecognized and untreated in patients with CKD, and its consequences can be wide ranging. A randomized trial investigating a novel agent for the treatment of acidosis (veverimer) demonstrated an improvement in physical function and quality of life and a reduction in a composite kidney outcome with 1 year of treatment. These findings require confirmation in a larger study, but combined with previous randomized trials of sodium bicarbonate and dietary interventions for metabolic acidosis, suggest that treatment should be considered for most at-risk individuals.

Hyperkalemia, hyperphosphatemia, and anemia related to CKD have all been linked to CKD progression in observational studies, but, to date, no randomized trials have demonstrated a benefit to treating these complications in patients to prevent GFR loss. As such, these complications require management, but should not be considered disease-modifying.

Other Interventions

Novel therapies attempting to reduce the progression of CKD exist; these target the inflammatory and/or fibrotic effects that occur in the pathophysiology of CKD progression. Pirfenidone is an agent that acts on the fibrosing pathway of CKD and has beneficial effects in animal models of CKD and diabetic nephropathy. However, large, long-term, human clinical trials showing a reduction in the progression of CKD have not yet been completed. Endothelin antagonists are another promising area for the

future as ET-1 contributes to kidney damage via both vasoconstrictive properties and promotion of interstitial fibrosis. Animal models have demonstrated a benefit of endothelin antagonists with a reduction in proteinuria and improvement in creatinine clearance. A recent randomized trial evaluated atrasentan in a subgroup of "responders" and found a 35% relative risk reduction in kidney events, but more frequent fluid retention and anemia-related adverse events. Further analyses to determine the optimal patient population for atrasentan is needed. In patients with polycystic kidney disease, tolvaptan has been shown to slow cyst growth and CKD progression, but its benefit needs to be clearly co-managed with the increased risk of liver injury and polyuria-related side effects.

Another novel medication, pyridoxamine, exerts its effect through antioxidant properties and impairment in advanced glycation end products (AGEs). Pyridoxamine has been evaluated in a multicenter, randomized, controlled trial of patients with overt diabetic nephropathy. In that trial, the drug failed to reduce GFR loss at 1 year, but there was a stabilization noted in the group of patients with the highest baseline level of kidney function. Sulodexide, a glycosaminoglycan, was rigorously tested in clinical trials of patients with diabetic nephropathy and failed to show a benefit. Bardoxolone methyl, an activator of nuclear 1 factor (erythroid derived 2)–related factor 2 (Nrf2), showed a reduction in serum creatinine over a 1-year period in humans, but unfortunately was associated with more cardiovascular events in a randomized, controlled trial.

Treatment of hyperuricemia, hyperphosphatemia, hyperhomocysteinemia, and folate and vitamin D deficiency have been shown in observational studies and/or small clinical trials to be associated with a reduction in albuminuria and/or the progression of CKD. In a large population in China, in an area without folic acid fortification, administration of folate with the ACE-I enalapril was found to slow the rate of eGFR decline compared to enalapril alone. These therapies may hold promise for the future, but validated, long-term, controlled trials are currently lacking.

Cardiovascular Risk Reduction

The leading cause of death in patients with CKD is cardiovascular disease. Hypertension, sodium and volume retention, anemia, hyperphosphatemia, high prevalence of DM and vascular disease, and electrolyte disturbances including hyperkalemia are all reported risk factors for this effect. Consequently, it is prudent to reduce this risk with lifestyle modifications, smoking cessation, use of aspirin, and pharmacologic therapy for hypertension, dyslipidemia, albuminuria, and hyperglycemia (when present), because there appears to be synergy between the development and progression of cardiovascular disease and the development and progression of CKD.

Conclusion

The pathophysiology of CKD is largely dependent on the primary insult, but common pathways exist across almost all subsets of kidney disorders. These include hemodynamic-mediated hyperfiltration and eventual nephron loss and inflammatory and cellular-mediated fibrosis. Much of the pathophysiology arises from maladaptation to autoregulation with hyperactivation of the RAAS. Theoretically, blocking these pathways will interrupt this progression; in fact, the most robust clinical evidence for slowing or reversing the progression is with disruption of the RAAS system. Controlling blood pressure, interrupting the RAAS, avoiding

AKI, and attempting cardiovascular risk reduction are important goals for the physicians treating patients with CKD. SGLT2 inhibitors represent the greatest advancement in slowing CKD progression in decades and should be prescribed whenever indicated and tolerated. New therapies for CKD and its disease-modifying complications are being developed, and large, randomized trials of these agents will be reported in the next 5 years. It is an exciting time to predict and treat CKD progression.

Complete bibliography is available at Elsevier eBooks for Practicing Clinicians.

Key Bibliography

Bakris GL, Agarwal R, Anker SD, et al. for the FIDELIO-DKD Investigators. Effect of finerenone on chronic kidney disease outcomes in type 2 diabetes. *N Engl J Med.* 2020;383(23):2219–2229.

Grams ME, Sang Y, Ballew SH, et al. Predicting timing of clinical outcomes in patients with chronic kidney disease and severely decreased glomerular filtration rate. *Kidney Int.* 2018;93:1442–1451.

Hemmelgarn BR, Manns BJ, Lloyd A, et al. Relation between kidney function, proteinuria, and adverse outcomes. *JAMA.* 2010;303:423–429.

Jafar TH, Stark PC, Schmid CH, et al. Progression of chronic kidney disease: The role of blood pressure control, proteinuria, and angiotensin-converting enzyme inhibition: A patient-level meta-analysis. *Ann Intern Med.* 2003;139:244–252.

Lewis EJ, Hunsicker LG, Bain RP, Rohde RD. The effect of angiotensin-converting-enzyme inhibition on diabetic nephropathy. The Collaborative Study Group. *N Engl J Med.* 1993;329:1456–1462.

Lewis EJ, Hunsicker LG, Clarke WR, et al. Renoprotective effect of the angiotensin-receptor antagonist irbesartan in patients with nephropathy due to type 2 diabetes. *N Engl J Med.* 2001;345:851–860.

Li J, Gong Y, Li C, Lu Y, et al. Long-term efficacy and safety of sodium-glucose cotransporter-2 inhibitors as add-on to metformin treatment in the management of type 2 diabetes mellitus. *Medicine (Baltimore).* 2017;96:e7201.

Mann JF, Schmieder RE, McQueen M, et al. Renal outcomes with telmisartan, ramipril, or both, in people at high vascular risk (the ONTARGET study): A multicentre, randomised, double-blind, controlled trial. *Lancet.* 2008;372:547–553.

Nelson RG, Grams ME, Ballew SH, et al. Development of Risk Prediction Equations for Incident Chronic Kidney Disease. *JAMA.* 2019;322:2104–2114.

Neuen BL, Young T, Heerspink HJL, Neal B, Perkovic V, Billot L, et al. SGLT2 inhibitors for the prevention of kidney failure in patients with type 2 diabetes: A systematic review and meta-analysis. *Lancet Diabetes Endocrinol.* 2019;7:845–854.

Parving HH, Brenner BM, McMurray JJ, et al. Cardiorenal end points in a trial of aliskiren for type 2 diabetes. *N Engl J Med.* 2012;367:2204–2213.

Parving HH, Lehnert H, Brochner-Mortensen J, et al. The effect of irbesartan on the development of diabetic nephropathy in patients with type 2 diabetes. *N Engl J Med.* 2001;345:870–878.

Perkovic V, Jardine MJ, Neal B, et al. Canagliflozin and renal outcomes in type 2 diabetes and nephropathy. *N Engl J Med.* 2019;380:2295–2306.

Pitt B, Filippatos G, Agarwal R, et al. for the FIGARO-DKD Investigators. Cardiovascular events with finerenone in kidney disease and type 2 diabetes list of authors. *N Engl J Med.* 2021;385:2252–2263.

Pohl MA, Blumenthal S, Cordonnier DJ, et al. Independent and additive impact of blood pressure control and angiotensin II receptor blockade on renal outcomes in the irbesartan diabetic nephropathy trial: Clinical implications and limitations. *J Am Soc Nephrol.* 2005;16:3027–3037.

Potok OA, Nguyen HA, Abdelmalek JA, et al. Patients,' nephrologists,' and predicted estimations of ESKD risk compared with 2-year incidence of ESKD. *Clin J Am Soc Nephrol.* 2019;14:206–212.

Torres VE, Chapman AB, Devuyst O, et al. Tolvaptan in patients with autosomal dominant polycystic kidney disease. *N Engl J Med.* 2012;367:2407–2418.

Torres VE, Chapman AB, Devuyst O, et al. Tolvaptan in later-stage autosomal dominant polycystic kidney disease. *N Engl J Med.* 2017;377:1930–1942.

Wesson DE, Mathur V, Tangri N, et al. Long-term safety and efficacy of veverimer in patients with metabolic acidosis in chronic kidney disease: a multicentre, randomised, blinded, placebo-controlled, 40-week extension. *Lancet.* 2019;394:396–406.

Wesson DE, Mathur V, Tangri N, et al. Veverimer versus placebo in patients with metabolic acidosis associated with chronic kidney disease: a multicentre, randomised, double-blind, controlled, phase 3 trial. *Lancet.* 2019;393:1417–1427.

Zelniker TA, Wiviott SD, Raz I, et al. SGLT2 inhibitors for primary and secondary prevention of cardiovascular and renal outcomes in type 2 diabetes: A systematic review and meta-analysis of cardiovascular outcome trials. *Lancet.* 2019;393:31–39.

51

Staging and Management of Chronic Kidney Disease

LESLEY A. INKER, ANDREW S. LEVEY

Chronic kidney disease (CKD) is a growing worldwide public health problem, characterized by increasing prevalence, high cost, and poor outcomes. The poor outcomes include progression of kidney disease leading to kidney failure, increased risk for acute kidney injury (AKI), cardiovascular disease (CVD), and mortality, as well as a wide variety of other complications.

In 2002, the Kidney Disease Outcomes Quality Initiative (KDOQI) of the National Kidney Foundation (NKF) sponsored guidelines for the definition, classification, evaluation, and risk stratification of CKD. The purpose of these guidelines was to create uniform terminology to improve communications among all involved in the care and management of patients with CKD, including patients, physicians, researchers, and policy makers. The guidelines were adopted with minor modification by Kidney Disease: Improving Global Outcomes (KDIGO) in 2005. In response to controversy and accumulation of new data, KDIGO sponsored a Controversies Conference in 2009, followed by an update of the guidelines in 2012, which maintained the definition of CKD but modified the classification. Subsequent reviews by national and international guideline workgroups have endorsed maintaining the CKD definition but expressed reservations about some aspects of the classification. The goals of this chapter are to describe the conceptual model for CKD, the revised 2012 KDIGO guideline recommendations for the definition and stages of CKD, and the associated prevalence and clinical action plan, along with commentary by other national and international guideline workgroups. We also provide an overview of detection, evaluation, predicting prognosis, and management, with comments on the role of nephrologists in the care of these patients.

Course, Definition, Classification, and Prevalence of Chronic Kidney Disease

Course of Chronic Kidney Disease

Fig. 51.1 shows a conceptual model for CKD, and Table 51.1 outlines the outcomes. This model describes the natural history of CKD, beginning with antecedent conditions associated with increased risk for developing kidney disease, followed by the stages of CKD (kidney damage, decreased glomerular filtration rate [GFR], and kidney failure), and associated complications.

Risk factors for the development of CKD include exposure to factors that cause kidney disease, such as hypertension, diabetes, autoimmune diseases, and kidney stones, and characteristics that increase susceptibility to kidney disease, such as older age, minority racial and ethnic status, and reduced nephron mass. The mechanisms underlying increased susceptibility have not been completely described or proven. For example, minority race or ethnicity may imply an underlying genetic tendency or it may be a marker for lack of access to healthcare. Susceptibility factors may explain why a family history of kidney disease, regardless of the cause, places an individual at increased risk for development of kidney disease.

The horizontal arrows in Fig. 51.1 indicate transitions among kidney outcomes. The arrows pointing from left to right emphasize the progressive nature of CKD. However, the rate of progression is variable, and not all CKD progresses; thus, not all patients with CKD develop kidney failure. Early stages of kidney disease may be reversible with treatment, as shown as dashed arrowheads pointing from right to left, and even individuals with kidney failure can revert to earlier stages through kidney transplantation. Studies suggest that CKD is a risk factor for development of AKI and that episodes of AKI may increase the risk for progression of CKD. The earlier stages and the risk factors for progression to later stages can be identified, permitting improvements in outcome by prevention, earlier detection, and initiation of therapies that can slow progression and prevent the development of kidney failure.

The diagonal arrows emphasize complications of CKD other than kidney outcomes. It is well accepted that both decreased GFR and albuminuria are associated with an independent risk of CVD and all-cause mortality. Metabolic and endocrine complications of decreased GFR, including anemia, bone and mineral disorders, malnutrition, and neuropathy, collectively comprising the uremic syndrome, have long been recognized as consequences of kidney failure, but these abnormalities may appear with lesser reduction in GFR. Similarly, nephrotic syndrome occurs in patients with marked albuminuria, but hyperlipidemia and hypercoagulability may be observed with lesser increases in albuminuria. Other complications include threats to patient safety from systemic toxicity from drugs and procedures, as well as an increased risk of infections and impaired cognitive and physical function. Strategies for prevention, early detection, and treatment of CKD complications may prolong survival and improve quality of life, even if there is no effect on kidney disease progression.

Definition of Chronic Kidney Disease

The 2012 KDIGO guideline update defines CKD as abnormalities of kidney structure or function, present for longer than 3 months, with implications for health. Criteria for CKD include

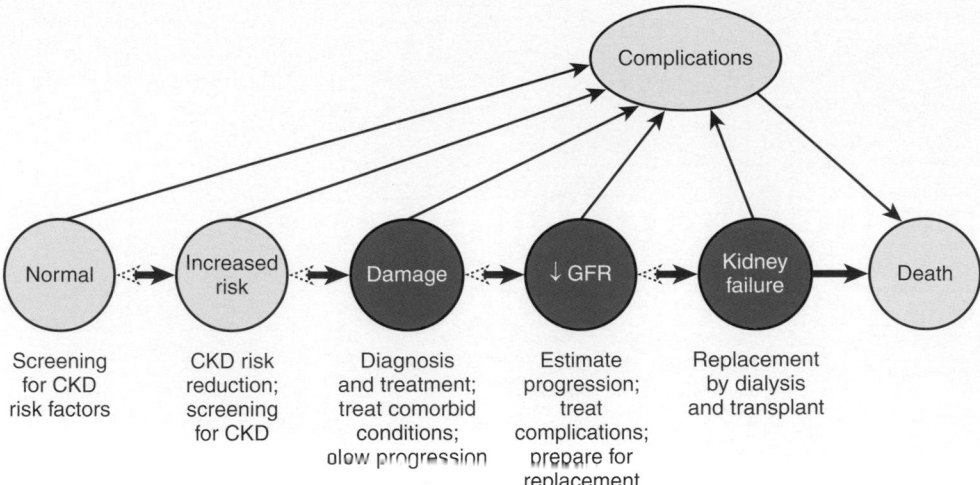

• **Fig. 51.1** Conceptual model for chronic kidney disease. The continuum of development, progression, and complications of chronic kidney disease (CKD) and strategies to improve outcomes. *Dark green circles,* Stages of CKD; *light green circles,* potential antecedents of CKD; *lavender circles,* consequences of CKD; *thick arrows between circles,* development, progression, and remission of CKD. *Complications* refers to all complications of CKD, including cardiovascular disease. Complications may also arise from adverse effects of interventions to prevent or treat the disease. Horizontal arrows pointing from left to right emphasize the progressive nature of CKD. Dashed arrowheads pointing from right to left signify that remission is less frequent than progression. (Modified from the National Kidney Foundation. KDOQI clinical practice guidelines for chronic kidney disease: evaluation, classification, and stratification. *Am J Kidney Dis.* 2002;39:S1–S266; Levey AS, Stevens LA, Coresh J. Conceptual model of CKD: applications and implications, *Am J Kidney Dis.* 2009;53:S4–S16.)

TABLE 51.1	Outcomes of Chronic Kidney Disease and Relationship to Kidney Disease Characteristics		
	KIDNEY DISEASE CHARACTERISTICS		
Outcomes of Chronic Kidney Disease	**Glomerular Filtration Rate**	**Albuminuria**	**Cause**
Kidney Outcomes			
CKD progression (GFR decline and worsening albuminuria)	+	+++	+++
AKI	+++	+	+
Chronic kidney failure	+++	+	+++
Complications (Current and Future)			
CVD and mortality	+++	+++	++
Systemic drug toxicity	+++	+	+
Metabolic/endocrine (anemia, bone and mineral disorders, malnutrition, and neuropathy)	+++	+	+
Infections, cognitive impairment, frailty	++	++	++

Number of + indicates the strength of the risk relationship between the kidney disease characteristic and the outcome.
AKI, Acute kidney injury; *CKD,* chronic kidney disease; *CVD,* cardiovascular disease; *GFR,* glomerular filtration rate.

either kidney damage or GFR of less than 60 mL/min/1.73 m² of body surface area lasting for longer than 3 months (90 days; Table 51.2). Of note, CKD can be diagnosed without knowledge of its cause.

Kidney damage can be within the parenchyma, large blood vessels, or collecting systems, and is usually inferred from markers rather than direct examination of kidney tissue. The markers of kidney damage often provide a clue to the likely site of damage within the kidney and, in association with other clinical findings, the cause of kidney disease. Because most kidney diseases in North America are caused by diabetes or hypertension, persistent albuminuria is the principal marker. Other markers of damage include abnormalities in urine sediment (e.g., blood cells, tubular cells, or casts), abnormal findings on imaging studies (e.g., hydronephrosis, asymmetry in kidney size, polycystic kidney disease, stones, small echogenic kidneys), and abnormalities in blood and urine chemistry measurements (related to altered tubular function, such as renal tubular acidosis). A history of kidney transplantation is also defined as a marker of kidney damage, and patients with a functioning transplant are considered to have CKD, irrespective of the presence of other markers of kidney damage or the level of GFR.

Decreased GFR for more than 3 months, specifically GFR less than 60 mL/min/1.73 m², represents CKD, irrespective of age. The level of GFR is usually accepted as the best overall index of kidney function in health and disease. GFR less than 60 mL/min/1.73 m² represents the loss of half or more of the young adult level of normal kidney function, and it is associated with an increased prevalence of systemic complications. The normal level of GFR varies according to age, sex, and body size. Normal GFR is approximately 120 to 130 mL/min/1.73 m² in a young adult and declines with age by approximately 1 mL/min/1.73 m² per/year after the third decade. More than 25% of individuals aged

70 years and older have GFR of less than 60 mL/min/1.73 m²; whether this results from normal aging or the high prevalence of systemic vascular diseases that cause kidney disease remains controversial. Whatever its cause, GFR less than 60 mL/min/1.73 m² in the elderly is an independent predictor of adverse outcomes such as death and CVD.

Kidney failure is defined either as a GFR less than 15 mL/min/1.73 m² or initiation of kidney replacement therapy (dialysis or transplantation). A number of terms refer to a severe decrease in kidney function, which is not synonymous with kidney failure. *Uremia* is defined as severely elevated concentrations within the blood of urea, creatinine, and other nitrogenous end products of amino acid and protein metabolism that are normally excreted in the urine. The *uremic syndrome,* the terminal clinical manifestation of kidney failure, is the constellation of symptoms, physical signs, and abnormal findings on diagnostic studies that result from the failure of the kidneys to maintain adequate function. *End-stage kidney disease* (ESKD) generally refers to kidney failure treated by dialysis or transplantation, regardless of the level of kidney function, and is used administratively in the United States and elsewhere. The availability of dialysis and transplantation for the treatment of kidney failure varies around the world, and not all patients with kidney failure choose to receive kidney replacement therapy. Therefore, populations defined as having ESKD might not include patients with kidney failure who are not treated with dialysis or transplantation, and the term *kidney failure with replacement therapy* (KFRT) has been suggested as an alternative to ESKD.

Classification of Chronic Kidney Disease

The NKF-KDOQI classification system for stages of CKD was based on the severity of the disease defined only by the level of GFR. The KDIGO classification adds cause of the disease and level of albuminuria to the level of GFR (CGA classification). Because recent epidemiologic data demonstrate strong graded relationships of the level of albuminuria, as well as the level of GFR, with risks of kidney disease progression, CVD, and mortality, this more detailed classification relates more closely to prognosis (see Table 51.1). The cause of disease is generally classified according to the presence or absence of systemic diseases (secondary or primary) and the presumed location of the pathologic-anatomic lesions (glomerular, tubulointerstitial, vascular, cystic, or disease in the kidney transplant; Table 51.3). Categories for GFR and albuminuria levels are shown in Tables 51.4 and 51.5. Fig. 51.2 shows the two-dimensional grid relating the risk of kidney outcomes and mortality to level of GFR and albuminuria. The green, yellow, orange, and red shaded categories represent patients at low, moderate, high, and very high risk of kidney outcomes and mortality, respectively.

TABLE 51.2 Definition of Chronic Kidney Disease

Criteria for Chronic Kidney Disease*	
Markers of kidney damage	• Albuminuria >30 mg/day • Urine sediment abnormalities • Electrolyte and other abnormalities caused by tubular disorders • Pathologic abnormalities • Imaging abnormalities • History of kidney transplantation
Decreased GFR	• GFR <60 mL/min/1.73 m²

*Either of the listed items for more than 3 months.
CKD, Chronic kidney disease; *GFR,* glomerular filtration rate.

TABLE 51.3 Classification of Cause of Chronic Kidney Disease Based on Presence or Absence of Systemic Disease and Location of Pathologic-Anatomic Findings

	Examples of Systemic Diseases Affecting the Kidney	Examples of Primary Kidney Diseases
Glomerular diseases	Diabetes, autoimmune diseases, systemic infections, drugs, neoplasia (including amyloidosis)	Diffuse, focal, or crescentric proliferative glomerulonephritis; focal and segmental glomerulosclerosis; idiopathic membranous nephropathy; minimal change disease
Tubulointerstitial diseases	Systemic infections, autoimmune diseases, sarcoidosis, drugs, urate, environmental toxins (lead, aristolochic acid), neoplasia (myeloma)	Urinary tract infections, stones, obstruction
Vascular diseases	Decreased perfusion (heart failure, liver disease, renal artery disease), atherosclerosis, hypertension, ischemia, cholesterol emboli, vasculitis, thrombotic microangiopathy, systemic sclerosis	ANCA-associated vasculitis; fibromuscular dysplasia
Cystic and congenital diseases	Polycystic kidney disease, Alport syndrome, Fabry disease, oxalosis	Renal dysplasia, medullary cystic disease
Diseases affecting the transplanted kidney	Recurrence of native kidney disease (diabetes, oxalosis, Fabry disease)	Chronic rejection; calcineurin inhibitor toxicity; BK virus nephropathy; recurrence of native kidney disease (glomerular disease)

ANCA, Antineutrophil cytoplasm antibody.
Note: Genetic diseases are not considered separately, because some diseases in each category are now recognized as having genetic determinants.

TABLE 51.4	Categories of Chronic Kidney Disease by the Level of Glomerular Filtration Rate and Corresponding Clinical Action Plan

Category	Glomerular Filtration Rate Levels (mL/min/1.73 m²)	Terms	Clinical Action Plan
G1[a]	>90	Normal or high	Diagnose and treat the cause Treat comorbid conditions Evaluate for CKD risk factors Start measures to slow CKD progression Start measures to reduce CVD risk
G2[a]	60–89	Mildly decreased[b]	Estimate progression
G3a	45–59	Mildly to moderately decreased	Adjust medication dosages as indicated
G3b	30–44	Moderately to severely decreased	Evaluate and treat complications
G4	15–29	Severely decreased	Prepare for kidney replacement therapy (transplantation and/or dialysis) if appropriate
G5	<15	Kidney failure (add D if treated by dialysis)	Start kidney replacement therapy (if uremia present) or continue conservative management

[a]GFR stages G1 or G2 without markers of kidney damage do not fulfill the criteria for CKD.
[b]Relative to young adult level.
CKD, Chronic kidney disease; *CVD*, cardiovascular disease; *GFR*, glomerular filtration rate.
Note: GFR in mL/min/1.73 m² may be converted to mL/s/1.73 m² by multiplying by 0.01667.

TABLE 51.5	Categories of Chronic Kidney Disease by the Level of Albuminuria and Corresponding Clinical Action Plan

Category	Albumin Excretion Rate (mg/day)	APPROXIMATELY EQUIVALENT ALBUMIN-TO-CREATININE RATIO		Terms	Clinical Action Plan
		(mg/mmol)	(mg/g)		
A1	<30	<3	<30	Normal to mildly increased	Diagnose and treat the cause Treat comorbid conditions Evaluate for CKD risk factors Start measures to slow CKD progression Start measures to reduce CVD risk
A2	30–299	3–30	30–299	Moderately increased*	Treatment with renin-angiotensin system blockers and lower blood pressure goal if hypertensive
A3	>300	≥30	>300	Severely increased	Treat nephrotic syndrome (if present)

*Relative to young adult level.
CKD, Chronic kidney disease; *CVD*, cardiovascular disease.

Prevalence

Fig. 51.2 shows the prevalence estimates derived from measurements of serum creatinine to estimate GFR (eGFRcr) and albumin-to-creatinine ratio (ACR) during National Health and Nutrition Examination Surveys (NHANES) from 1999 to 2006. The prevalence of ACR greater than 30 mg/g or estimated GFR less than 60 mL/min/1.73 m² is approximately 11.5% of the US adult population. The proportion of participants with CKD in the groups at moderate, high, and very high risk is about 73%, 18%, and 9%, respectively, representing a prevalence in the general population of about 8.5%, 2%, and 1%, respectively. This prevalence is more than 50 times greater than the prevalence of treated ESKD of approximately 0.2% reported by the US Renal Data System during this interval. Because kidney disease usually begins late in life and progresses slowly, most people in the earlier stages of CKD die of other causes before reaching kidney failure. In these patients, the burden of CKD is reflected in the complications of earlier stages, including increased mortality and morbidity, reduced quality of life, and high cost.

Detection, Evaluation, Predicting Prognosis, and Management

Fig. 51.3 provides a six-step overview of the detection and evaluation of CKD. Care for patients with CKD requires multiple interventions and the coordinated, multidisciplinary effort of primary care physicians, allied healthcare workers, and other specialists, in addition to nephrologists. The KDIGO guidelines can provide a framework for care but cannot be a replacement of the physician's assessment of the needs of individual patients.

Percentage of US Population by eGFR and Albuminuria Category: KDIGO 2012 and NHANES 1999–2006				Persistent albuminuria categories Description and range			
				A1	A2	A3	
				Normal to mildly increased	Moderately increased	Severely increased	
				<30 mg/g <3 mg/mmol	30-300 mg/g 3-30 mg/mmol	>300 mg/g >30 mg/mmol	
GFR categories (mL/min/ 1.73m^2) Description and range	G1	Normal or high	≥90	55.6	1.9	0.4	57.9
	G2	Mildly decreased	60–89	32.9	2.2	0.3	35.4
	G3a	Mildly to moderately decreased	45–59	3.6	0.8	0.2	4.6
	G3b	Moderately to severely decreased	30–44	1.0	0.4	0.2	1.6
	G4	Severely decreased	15–29	0.2	0.1	0.1	0.4
	G5	Kidney failure	<15	0.0	0.0	0.1	0.1
				93.2	5.4	1.3	100.0

• **Fig. 51.2** Prognosis and prevalence of chronic kidney disease in the United States by glomerular filtration rate and albuminuria category. Colors reflect the ranking of relative risk for kidney disease progression and cardiovascular risk. *Green,* low risk (if no other markers of kidney disease, no chronic kidney disease [CKD]); *Yellow,* moderately increased risk; *Orange,* high risk; *Red,* very high risk. Cells show the proportion of adult population in the United States. Data from the NHANES 1999 to 2006, *N* = 18,026. Glomerular filtration rate (GFR) is estimated from a single measurement of standardized serum creatinine with the CKD-EPI 2009 creatinine equation. Albuminuria is determined by one measurement of albumin-to-creatinine ratio, and persistence is estimated. Values in cells do not total to values in margins because of rounding. Category of very high albuminuria includes nephrotic range. *eGFR,* Estimated glomerular filtration rate; *KDIGO,* Kidney Disease: Improving Global Outcomes; *NHANES,* National Health and Nutrition Examination Survey. (From Kidney Disease: Improving Global Outcomes (KDIGO) CKD Work Group. KDIGO 2012 Clinical practice guideline for the evaluation and management of chronic kidney disease. *Kidney Int Suppl.* 2013;3:1–150.)

Detection

Screening for CKD in the general population is not recommended, but case finding is generally accepted in those deemed at high risk. As part of routine checkups, all patients should be evaluated to determine whether they are at increased risk for developing CKD. A reasonable approach to CKD testing in high-risk patients includes, at minimum, eGFRcr and urine ACR. Current guidelines suggest testing in patients with hypertension, diabetes, CVD, cancer, rheumatologic diseases, hepatitis C virus or human immunodeficiency virus (HIV) infection, and before imaging procedures with iodine-based or gadolinium-based contrast. Clinical practice also includes measurement of serum creatinine with GFR estimation as part of the basic metabolic panel for patients with acute illness or before planned invasive procedures. The need for serum cystatin C for GFR estimation or other measures (urinalysis or imaging) to ascertain markers of kidney damage depends on the nature of the risk factors. eGFR less than 60 mL/min/1.73 m^2 or urine ACR greater than 30 mg/g for more than 3 months meet the criteria for CKD. Values

near these thresholds may arouse suspicion for CKD and prompt further testing. At present, there are few data regarding the optimal frequency of testing for CKD in high-risk individuals, although annual testing is recommended in patients with hypertension, diabetes, and HIV. Until evidence is available, it seems reasonable to suggest that others at increased risk be tested at least every 3 years.

Evaluation

The goals of evaluation are to identify the duration and cause of CKD, to assess levels of GFR and albuminuria to determine the severity of disease (stage), to identify the presence of complications, and to determine risk for progression of kidney disease and other outcomes. Evaluation includes a thorough personal and family history, including a review of past laboratory data, and physical examination to detect (1) previous evidence of kidney disease, (2) signs and symptoms that may provide clues to the cause of kidney disease, and (3) any reversible or treatable causes

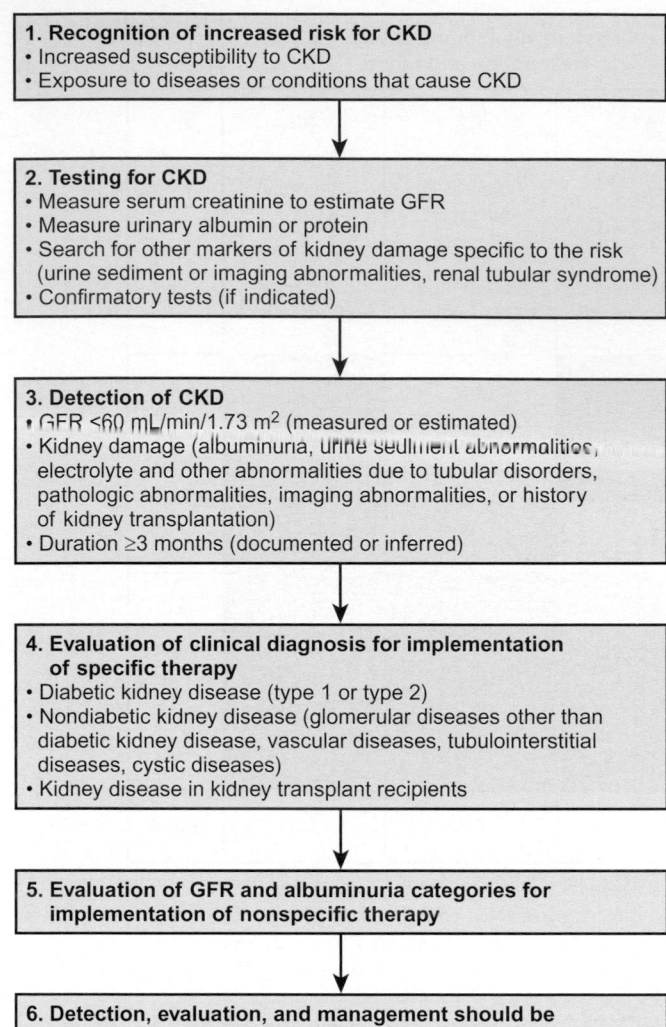

1. Recognition of increased risk for CKD
- Increased susceptibility to CKD
- Exposure to diseases or conditions that cause CKD

2. Testing for CKD
- Measure serum creatinine to estimate GFR
- Measure urinary albumin or protein
- Search for other markers of kidney damage specific to the risk (urine sediment or imaging abnormalities, renal tubular syndrome)
- Confirmatory tests (if indicated)

3. Detection of CKD
- GFR <60 mL/min/1.73 m² (measured or estimated)
- Kidney damage (albuminuria, urine sediment abnormalities, electrolyte and other abnormalities due to tubular disorders, pathologic abnormalities, imaging abnormalities, or history of kidney transplantation)
- Duration ≥3 months (documented or inferred)

4. Evaluation of clinical diagnosis for implementation of specific therapy
- Diabetic kidney disease (type 1 or type 2)
- Nondiabetic kidney disease (glomerular diseases other than diabetic kidney disease, vascular diseases, tubulointerstitial diseases, cystic diseases)
- Kidney disease in kidney transplant recipients

5. Evaluation of GFR and albuminuria categories for implementation of nonspecific therapy

6. Detection, evaluation, and management should be tailored to patient's risk

• **Fig. 51.3** Six-step overview for detection and evaluation of chronic kidney disease (CKD). *GFR,* glomerular filtration rate. (Modified from Levey AS, Coresh J. Chronic kidney disease. *Lancet.* 2012;379:165–180.)

evaluate symptoms of CVD more fully or to detect asymptomatic CVD in patients with multiple risk factors.

Some elderly individuals meet the criteria for CKD solely because of eGFR less than 60 mL/min/1.73 m². There is debate about the importance of a diagnosis of CKD in this setting (see Chapter 48). In the absence of risk factors for CKD, albuminuria, or other markers of kidney damage, patients with isolated decreased GFR may be at low risk for progression to kidney failure but remain at increased risk for CKD complications and for CVD. In such patients, clinicians may elect to defer some parts of the evaluation for CKD; however, a search for reversible causes of decreased GFR, adjustment of medication dosages for decreased GFR, appropriate attention to CVD risk factor management, and subsequent monitoring of GFR are appropriate.

Evaluation of Duration

Kidney diseases and disorders may be acute or chronic depending on their duration. The distinction between "acute" and "chronic" is arbitrary but useful in clinical practice. KDIGO defines chronicity as duration longer than 3 months (90 days); kidney disease with duration less than 3 months, including AKI, is defined as *acute kidney diseases and disorders* (AKD). The duration of kidney disease may be documented or inferred based on the clinical context. For example, a patient with decreased kidney function or kidney damage in the midst of an acute illness, without previous documentation of kidney disease, may be inferred to have AKD. A patient with similar findings in the absence of an acute illness may be inferred to have CKD. In both cases, repeat ascertainment of GFR and markers of kidney damage is recommended for accurate diagnosis. The timing of the evaluation depends on clinical judgment, with earlier evaluation for patients suspected of having AKD and later evaluation for patients suspected of having CKD.

Evaluation of Cause

Identification of the cause of CKD, such as infection, drug toxicity, autoimmune disease, or obstruction of the urinary tract, enables specific, directed treatments. In addition, the cause of kidney disease has implications for the rate of progression and the risk of complications. The cause of the disease is generally established by recognition of the clinical setting and the presence or absence of markers of kidney damage. A simplified system classifies kidney disease by anatomic location: glomerular, vascular, tubulointerstitial, and cystic kidney disorders (see Table 51.3). Clinical judgment is required to determine whether additional methods are necessary to characterize kidney disease, including imaging studies, other urine or serum markers, or biopsy of the kidney. For many patients with CKD (especially older patients with hypertension or diabetes and no evidence of the other mentioned disorders), the cause will be unknown and presumed to be a result of vascular disease. In these cases, management will be based primarily on levels of GFR and albuminuria.

Evaluation of Glomerular Filtration Rate

The KDIGO guideline recommends initial evaluation with eGFRcr, followed by confirmatory tests, if required. The guideline recommends using the Chronic Kidney Disease Epidemiology Collaboration (CKD-EPI) 2009 creatinine equation, or more accurate equations, if available. Confirmatory tests include eGFR based on serum cystatin C with or without serum creatinine, or clearance measurements of exogenous filtration markers or creatinine (more readily available). GFR-estimating equations are discussed in Chapter 3.

(e.g., autoimmune conditions, uncontrolled hypertension, use of nonsteroidal antiinflammatory drugs). Medications should be reviewed to identify those that can cause kidney toxicity and others that must be adjusted based on level of GFR. The physical examination should include particular attention to details such as blood pressure, fundoscopy, and the vascular examination. Laboratory tests should be performed to detect other markers of damage or functional disturbances (e.g., urine specific gravity, urine pH, urine sediment examination, serum electrolytes). Imaging studies should be performed, if indicated, based on clinical clues. Ultrasonography can be used to detect anatomic abnormalities and to exclude obstruction of the urinary tract. It has been recommended that individuals with GFR less than 60 mL/min/1.73 m² should have measurements of hemoglobin, as well as serum calcium, phosphate, albumin, and parathyroid hormone, but these measures are often not abnormal until GFR is less than 45 mL/min/1.73 m². Laboratory evaluation should also include a search for traditional CVD risk factors, such as a lipid profile, and, possibly, tests for nontraditional risk factors such as insulin resistance and inflammation. Additional studies may be necessary to

Evaluation of Albuminuria

The KDIGO guidelines recommend initial evaluation with spot urine ACR, followed by confirmatory tests, if required. Alternative initial evaluation can include spot urine total protein-to-creatinine ratio (PCR) and urine dipstick with automated or manual reading. An early morning specimen is preferred, if possible. Confirmatory tests include a timed urine collection for measurement of albumin excretion rate. Table 51.6 provides a rough guide to measures of urine albumin and total protein in spot and timed urine collections that correspond to the KDIGO albuminuria stages. Conversions from PCR and urine dipstick to ACR are also available. Further discussion of albuminuria and proteinuria is provided in Chapter 5.

Predicting Prognosis

The KDIGO guideline recommends predicting risk for outcomes of CKD with the CGA classification and other risk factors and comorbid conditions specific for the outcome (see Table 51.1 and Fig. 51.2). Risk prediction instruments can be used to provide a numeric risk for specific outcomes, and some have been extensively validated. For example, the Kidney Failure Risk Equation (KFRE) is applicable for patients with eGFR less than 60 mL/min/1.73 m^2 and uses age, sex, and current levels of eGFR and urine ACR to provide an estimate for the risk of developing kidney failure requiring treatment by dialysis or transplantation within 2 or 5 years. Another instrument is available for patients with eGFR <30 mL/min/1.73 m^2 to predict risks for developing kidney failure requiring treatment by dialysis or transplantation, cardiovascular disease, and mortality within 2 or 4 years. It requires additional variables (race, systolic blood pressure, smoking status, diabetes mellitus, and history of cardiovascular disease) in addition to age, sex, eGFR, and urine ACR. Change in eGFR

and ACR can also be used to identify patients at higher risk for adverse outcomes. Recent data suggest a 30% decline in eGFR or a 4-fold increase in urine ACR is associated with substantially increased risk for developing kidney failure, and a lesser increased risk for mortality, compared with patients with a stable eGFR or stable urine ACR. Quantitative risk predictions are not yet available based on changes in eGFR or urine ACR.

Management

Chronic Kidney Disease Care

CKD care is directed by the CGA classification. For all patients, this includes treating specific causes of kidney disease, treating other reversible conditions causing kidney damage or decreased GFR, and prevention and treatment of complications. The action plan for each GFR and albuminuria stage is cumulative (see Tables 51.4 and 51.5). For patients with albuminuria, key aspects include slowing progression of kidney disease by use of ACE inhibitors and ARBs, targeting a lower blood pressure goal, and preventing and treating complications of the nephrotic syndrome. For patients with decreased GFR, key aspects include assuring medication safety by avoiding drugs that are toxic to the kidney and adjusting doses of drugs that are excreted by the kidney, treating metabolic and endocrine complications of decreased GFR, and preparing for kidney replacement therapy or conservative care in patients with severely decreased GFR.

Patient education is central to the management strategy. CKD is often asymptomatic, and patients may not understand the importance of multidrug regimens and laboratory testing without specific education. Complete management requires behavioral change by the patient, which may include lifestyle alterations, dietary adjustments, self-monitoring of blood pressure, and adherence to medication

TABLE 51.6 Albuminuria and Proteinuria Measures

Measure	Normal to Mildly Increased	Moderately Increased	Severely Increased
		CATEGORIES	
AER (mg/24 hr)	<30	30–300	>300
PER (mg/24 hr)	<150	150–500	>500
Albumin-to-Creatinine Ratio			
(mg/mmol)	<3	3–30	>30
(mg/g)	<30	30–300	>300
Protein-to-Creatinine Ratio			
(mg/mmol)	<15	15–50	>50
(mg/g)	<150	150–500	>500
Protein reagent strip	Negative to trace	Negative to positive	Positive or greater

Urine albumin-to-creatinine ratio (ACR) may be divided into more than three categories. The normal urinary ACR in young adults is less than 10 mg/g; ACR 10 to 29 mg/g is high normal. Urine ACR greater than 2000 mg/g is accompanied by signs and symptoms of nephrotic syndrome (low serum albumin, edema, and high serum cholesterol).

Relationships between excretion rates and concentration ratios with urine creatinine are inexact. Excretion of urinary creatinine indicates muscle mass and varies with age, gender, race, diet, and nutritional status and generally exceeds 1.0 g/day in healthy adults; therefore, the numeric value for urinary ACR (mg/g) is usually less than the rate of urinary albumin excretion (mg/day). Rates of 30 to 300 mg/day and greater than 300 mg/day correspond to microalbuminuria and macroalbuminuria, respectively.

Relationships between urinary albumin and total protein are inexact. Normal urine contains small amounts of albumin, low-molecular-weight serum proteins, and proteins that are from renal tubules and the lower urinary tract. In most kidney diseases, albumin is the main urine protein, comprising about 60% to 90% of total urinary protein when total protein is very high. Values corresponding to normal, high-normal, high, very high, and nephrotic-range total protein are approximately less than 50, 50 to 150, 150 to 500, greater than 500, and greater than 3500 mg/g, respectively.

Threshold values for standard international (mg/mol) and conventional units (mg/g) are not exact. Conversion factor for ACR: 1.0 mg/g = 0.113 mg/mmol.

AER, Albumin excretion rate; *PER,* protein excretion rate.

regimens and medical follow-up. Patient education is also important with respect to avoiding medications that are toxic to the kidneys. Patients must be aware that any drug or herbal remedy may be directly nephrotoxic or may require a dosage adjustment for the level of kidney function.

Nephrology Referral

Nephrologists have multiple roles in the care of patients with CKD, including determining the cause of CKD, recommending specific therapy, suggesting treatments to slow progression in patients who have not responded to conventional therapies, identifying and treating kidney disease–related complications, and management in GFR stages 4 and 5 (GFR <30 mL/min/1.73 m²).

Recommendations for referral to a kidney disease specialist are not universal because specific practice patterns are dependent on healthcare systems and the available resources in a geographic region. Table 51.7 lists clinical criteria for referral recommended by the KDIGO guideline. The strongest evidence regarding the importance of referral to a nephrologist is for management of GFR stages 4 and 5. Late referral to a nephrologist (i.e., <3 months before the start of dialysis therapy) has been associated with higher mortality after the initiation of dialysis. It is, therefore, recommended by many organizations, regardless of the healthcare system or geographic region, that all patients with GFR stages 4 and 5 be referred to a nephrologist. During GFR stage 4, it is important to prepare the patient for the possible onset of kidney failure (GFR stage 5). KDIGO recommends beginning preparations when the risk of kidney failure within 1 year is 10% to 20% or higher. Preparation involves estimating the risk of progression to kidney failure, holding discussions regarding kidney replacement therapy (dialysis and transplantation), and instituting conservative therapy for those who choose not to undergo kidney replacement therapy. In patients who elect replacement therapy, timely creation of vascular access for hemodialysis, home dialysis training, and donor evaluation for preemptive transplantation should occur during GFR stage 4. For patients with CKD in GFR stages 1 to 3 (GFR >30 mL/min/1.73 m²), in the absence of a specific treatable cause (e.g., glomerulonephritis), only a subset is likely to require referral to a specialist.

Complete bibliography is available at Elsevier eBooks for Practicing Clinicians.

TABLE 51.7	Recommendations for Referral to Specialists for Consultation and Comanagement of Chronic Kidney Disease

AKI or abrupt sustained fall in GFR

GFR <30 mL/min/1.73 m² (GFR categories G4–G5)

ACR ≥300 mg/g (albuminuria category A3)

Progression of CKD

Urinary red cell casts, RBC >20 per high-power field sustained and not readily explained

CKD and hypertension refractory to treatment with 4 or more antihypertensive agents

Persistent abnormalities of serum potassium

Recurrent or extensive nephrolithiasis

Hereditary kidney disease

ACR, Albumin-to-creatinine ratio; *AKI*, acute kidney injury; *CKD*, chronic kidney disease; *GFR*, glomerular filtration rate; *RBC*, red blood cells.
Adapted from Kidney Disease: Improving Global Outcomes (KDIGO) CKD Work Group. KDIGO 2012 Clinical practice guideline for the evaluation and management of chronic kidney disease. *Kidney Int Suppl.* 2013;3:1–150.

Key Bibliography

Astor BC, Matsushita K, Gansevoort RT, et al. Lower estimated glomerular filtration rate and higher albuminuria are associated with mortality and end-stage renal disease. *Kidney Int.* 2011;79:1331–1340.

Carrero JJ, Grams ME, Sang Y, et al. Albuminuria changes are associated with subsequent risk of end-stage renal disease and mortality. *Kidney Int.* 2017;91:244–251.

Coresh J, Turin TC, Matsushita K, et al. Decline in estimated glomerular filtration rate and subsequent risk of end-stage renal disease and mortality. *JAMA.* 2014;311:2518–2531.

Eckardt KU, Berns JS, Rocco MV, et al. Definition and classification of CKD: the debate should be about patient prognosis—a position statement from KDOQI and KDIGO. *Am J Kidney Dis.* 2009;53:915–920.

Eckardt KU, Coresh J, Devuyst O, et al. Evolving importance of kidney disease: from subspecialty to global health burden. *Lancet.* 2013;382:158–169.

Gansevoort RT, Matsushita K, van der Velde M, et al. Lower estimated GFR and higher albuminuria are associated with adverse kidney outcomes. *Kidney Int.* 2011;80:93–104.

Glassock RJ, Delanaye P, El-Nahas M. An age-calibrated classification of chronic kidney disease. *JAMA.* 2015;314:559–560.

Grams ME, Sang Y, Ballew SH, et al. Predicting timing of clinical outcomes in patients with chronic kidney disease and severely decreased glomerular filtration rate. *Kidney Int.* 2018;93:1442–1451.

Kidney Disease: Improving Global Outcomes (KDIGO) CKD Work Group. KDIGO 2012 clinical practice guideline for the evaluation and management of chronic kidney disease. *Kidney Int Suppl.* 2013;3:1–150.

Levey AS, Becker C, Inker LA. Glomerular filtration rate and albuminuria for detection and staging of acute and chronic kidney disease in adults: a systematic review. *JAMA.* 2015;313:837–846.

Levey AS, Coresh J. Chronic kidney disease. *Lancet.* 2012;379:165–180.

Levey AS, Coresh J, Balk E, et al. National Kidney Foundation practice guidelines for chronic kidney disease: evaluation, classification, and stratification. *Ann Intern Med.* 2003;139:137–147.

Levey AS, de Jong PE, Coresh J, et al. The definition, classification and prognosis of chronic kidney disease: a KDIGO Controversies Conference report. *Kidney Int.* 2011;80:17–28.

Levey AS, Eckardt KU, Dorman NM, et al. Nomenclature for kidney function and disease: executive summary and glossary from a Kidney Disease: Improving Global Outcomes (KDIGO) Consensus Conference. *Kidney Int Rep.* 2020;5:965–972.

Levey AS, Eckardt K, Tsukamoto Y, et al. Definition and classification of chronic kidney disease: a position statement from Kidney Disease: Improving Global Outcomes (KDIGO). *Kidney Int.* 2005;67:2089–2100.

Levey AS, Inker LA, Coresh J. Chronic kidney disease in older people. *JAMA.* 2015;314(6):557–558.

Levey AS, Stevens LA, Coresh J. Conceptual model of CKD: applications and implications. *Am J Kidney Dis.* 2009;53:S4–S16.

Matsushita K, van der Velde M, Astor BC, et al. Association of estimated glomerular filtration rate and albuminuria with all-cause and cardiovascular mortality in general population cohorts. *Lancet.* 2010;375:2073–2081.

National Kidney Foundation. K/DOQI clinical practice guidelines for chronic kidney disease: evaluation, classification, and stratification. *Am J Kidney Dis.* 2002;39:S1–S266.

52

Nutrition and Kidney Disease

MELIS SAHINOZ, T. ALP IKIZLER

Nutrient Metabolism in Kidney Disease

As chronic kidney disease (CKD) progresses, the requirements and utilization of different nutrients change significantly. Protein energy wasting (PEW), defined as a state of decreased body stores of protein and energy fuels, is common in individuals with CKD and has many causes.

Protein Metabolism and Requirements

Amino Acid Metabolism

CKD patients have well-defined abnormalities in their plasma and, to a lesser extent, in their muscle amino acid profiles. Commonly, essential amino acid concentrations are low and nonessential amino acid concentrations high. The etiology of this abnormal profile is complex. The progressive loss of kidney tissue, where metabolism of several amino acids takes place, is an important factor. Specifically, glycine and phenylalanine concentrations are elevated, and serine, tyrosine, and histidine concentrations are decreased. Plasma and muscle concentrations of branched-chain amino acids (valine, leucine, and isoleucine) are reduced in CKD patients, especially in patients treated with maintenance dialysis. In contrast, plasma citrulline, cystine, aspartate, methionine, and both 1- and 3-methylhistidine levels are increased. Although inadequate dietary intake is a possible factor in abnormal essential amino acid profiles, certain abnormalities occur even in the presence of adequate dietary nutrient intake indicating that the uremic milieu has an additional effect. Indeed, it has been suggested that the metabolic acidosis commonly seen in uremic patients plays an important role in increased oxidation of branched-chain amino acids.

Protein Intake in Nondialysis CKD Patients

In general, the minimal daily protein requirement is one that maintains a neutral nitrogen balance and prevents protein wasting; this has been estimated to be a daily dietary protein intake of about 0.8 g/kg. One of the most significant symptoms in advanced CKD is a decrease in appetite. Several studies have indicated that CKD patients spontaneously restrict their dietary protein intake, with levels often less than 0.6 g/kg/day among those with CKD stage 5, suggesting that anorexia predisposes CKD patients to PEW. Accumulation of uremic toxins such as indoxyl sulfate, p-cresyl sulfate, and fibroblast growth factor 23 (FGF-23) may not be the sole cause of decreased dietary nutrient intake. Table 52.1 depicts factors that can cause decreased nutrient intake as well as other potential mechanisms of PEW in CKD patients. Individuals with CKD and coexisting diabetes mellitus are more prone to nutritional abnormalities because of additional dietary restrictions; gastrointestinal symptoms common in diabetes such as gastroparesis, nausea, and vomiting; bacterial overgrowth in the gut; and pancreatic insufficiency. Depression is common in CKD and is also associated with anorexia. CKD patients often are prescribed a large number of medications, particularly sedatives, phosphate binders, and iron supplements, all of which may have gastrointestinal complications. Finally, socioeconomic status, lack of mobility, dependency, and older age may all predispose to decreased dietary protein intake.

Protein Restriction in Nondialysis CKD

Dietary protein restriction, with or without supplementation of ketoanalogues of certain amino acids, has long been considered an attractive intervention to both slow the progression of kidney disease and delay initiation of maintenance dialysis. This is based on earlier studies indicating that excessive dietary protein intake causes vasodilation in the afferent arterioles, resulting in hyperfiltration, which, over time, leads to progression of kidney disease, especially in high-risk populations such as those with coexisting diabetes mellitus and hypertension. Reduced protein intake, however, leads to vasoconstriction in the afferent arterioles and lowers intraglomerular pressure. As suggested by a number of meta-analyses, this dietary protein restriction effect is real, albeit relatively small in the context of progressive kidney disease (0.5 mL/min/year benefit). Notably, patients with certain kidney diseases such as polycystic kidney disease do not seem to benefit from low-protein diets.

Several smaller studies suggest that the favorable effects of dietary protein restriction extend beyond slowing CKD progression. These include amelioration of metabolic acidosis, improvements in the lipid profile and insulin resistance, antioxidant effects, and decreasing dietary phosphorus load. The optimal range of dietary protein restriction to exert the most beneficial outcome is not established, and the applicability of dietary protein restriction is limited by adherence.

In addition to protein restriction alone, a number of studies have also examined the effects of keto acid– or amino acid–supplemented low-protein diets (LPDs) or very-low-protein diets (VLPDs) on certain metabolic and kidney outcome parameters. Since the supplemental keto acids are primarily given to substitute for dietary protein intake, most studies evaluated VLPDs. Accordingly, several meta-analyses indicate that VLPD diets supplemented with keto acids delay the initiation of maintenance dialysis along with a significant decrease in urea production and potential beneficial effects on insulin resistance and oxidative stress in humans.

TABLE 52.1	Factors Leading to Nutritional and Metabolic Abnormalities in Chronic Kidney Disease Patients

Increased Protein and Energy Requirements

Nephrotic syndrome
Losses of nutrients (amino acids and/or proteins) during dialysis
Increased resting energy expenditure
- Acute or chronic inflammation
- Hyperphosphatemia
- Hemodialysis

Decreased Protein and Calorie Intake

Anorexia (uremic toxins)
Frequent hospitalizations
Inadequate dialysis dose
Comorbid conditions
- Diabetes mellitus
- Gastrointestinal diseases
- Heart failure
- Depression
Multiple medications

Increased Catabolism/Decreased Anabolism

Dialysis-induced catabolism
- Amino acid losses
- Induction of inflammatory cascade
Metabolic acidosis
Hormonal derangements
- Growth hormone resistance
- Insulin resistance
- Increased glucocorticoid activity
- Low thyroid hormone levels
- Hyperparathyroidism
- Testosterone deficiency

An important consideration regarding dietary protein restriction in CKD is the potential to adversely affect nutritional status. These concerns are mostly ameliorated by well-designed diets planned by skilled dietitians and followed by motivated and adherent patients, and multiple studies have showed these diets are effective and do not have harmful effects on the nutritional condition. Long-term follow-up of several relatively large cohorts of CKD patients who received 0.47 g/kg/day protein with keto acid supplementation showed no detrimental effect on clinical outcomes. Accordingly, one can conclude that prescribing LPD or VLPD with keto acid or amino acid supplementation with adequate caloric intake and close supervision does not lead to overt PEW.

There are very limited data regarding the optimal level of dietary protein intake in patients with a kidney transplant. In general, these patients should also be considered as having CKD, and the same strategies for dietary protein intake and prescription should be applied. Table 52.2 describes current recommendations for dietary protein and energy intake for patients by CKD stage.

Maintenance Dialysis Patients

Among maintenance dialysis patients, dietary restrictions focus on reducing hyperphosphatemia, hyperkalemia, and metabolic acidosis; however, these restrictions could predispose dialysis patients to an increased risk of PEW, primarily because of the increased metabolic stress associated with dialysis therapies. Nutrient losses through hemodialysis or across peritoneal membranes, loss of residual kidney function due to long-term dialysis treatment, and

increased inflammation due to indwelling catheters, bioincompatible hemodialysis membranes, and peritoneal dialysis (PD) solutions all may lead to an overly catabolic milieu and increase the minimal amount of nutrient intake needed to maintain a neutral nitrogen balance (see Table 52.2). In patients who cannot compensate for this increased need, a state of semi-starvation ensues, resulting in the development or worsening of PEW. Although the current targets for acceptable dialysis dose should be adequate to prevent development of PEW in patients undergoing either hemodialysis or PD, there are limited data suggesting that a substantial increase in dose of dialysis could result in improvement in overall nutrition status in maintenance dialysis patients.

Chronic Inflammation

Systemic inflammation is one of the major contributors to PEW in patients with CKD and is the result of both increased production and reduced kidney clearance of proinflammatory cytokines (Fig. 52.1). Increased levels of proinflammatory cytokines such as interleukin-1 (IL-1), interleukin-6 (IL-6), and tumor necrosis factor-α (TNF-α) play a crucial role in the exaggerated protein and energy catabolism present in individuals with CKD. Proinflammatory cytokines play integral roles in protein breakdown, resulting in muscle atrophy in chronic disease states such as advanced CKD. A plethora of data in maintenance hemodialysis (HD) patients indicates exponentially increased protein catabolism, especially in the skeletal muscle compartment, in the setting of exaggerated systemic inflammation. In addition to increasing protein breakdown, chronic inflammation is associated with reduced physical activity and impairment in both insulin and growth hormone actions; it may also contribute to anorexia due to central effects through the melanocortin system. Small, randomized studies suggest that certain antiinflammatory interventions such as IL-1 receptor blockers, pentoxifylline, and fish oil could improve protein catabolism in maintenance dialysis patients.

Metabolic Acidosis

Metabolic acidosis is associated with increased muscle protein catabolism, promoting muscle wasting in patients with advanced CKD by stimulating the oxidation of essential amino acids. Acidemia also leads to reduced muscle protein synthesis due to insulin resistance and other hormonal derangements. With decline in kidney function, the need for urinary acidification per nephron increases, which may result in further injury in the remaining nephrons. Increased dietary acid load is also associated with hyperfiltration and progression of kidney disease. Multiple studies show improved nutritional status associated with oral bicarbonate supplementation in patients with advanced CKD, while some studies, but not all, suggest that the progression of CKD is slower among individuals treated with oral bicarbonate. Thus, it is suggested that attempts should be made to maintain a steady-state serum bicarbonate level of 23 mmol/L in nondialysis CKD patients. Data on bicarbonate supplementation in hemodialysis are mixed, although epidemiologic data suggest worse outcomes with very high predialysis serum bicarbonate levels, potentially indicating a subset of the HD population with lower dietary protein intake. Dialysate base is covered in more detail in Chapter 56.

Hormonal Derangements

Resistance to the anabolic actions of insulin is a key endocrine abnormality implicated in the loss of muscle mass in chronic disease states including CKD. Enhanced protein catabolism applies to both insulin-deficient and insulin-resistant states. Maintenance HD patients with suboptimally controlled type 2 diabetes have a

TABLE 52.2 Recommended Dietary Intakes of Protein, Energy, and Minerals in Healthy Adults and Kidney Disease

	Protein	Energy	Phosphorus	Sodium
Healthy adults	0.8 g/kg/day	1800–2400 kcal/day for women[a] 2400–3200 kcal/day for men[a]	700 mg/day	<2.3 g/day
Chronic Kidney Disease				
Stages 1–2	No restriction	25–35 kcal/kg/day[b,c]	800–1000 mg/day	≤2.3 g/day
Stages 3–5	0.55–0.60 g/kg/day if non-diabetic[b] 0.6–0.8 g /kg/day if diabetic[b]	25–35 kcal/kg/day[b,c]	800–1000 mg/day[d]	<2.3 g/day
Dialysis				
Hemodialysis	1.0–1.2 g/kg/day	25–35 kcal/kg/day[e]	800–1000 mg/day[d]	<2.3 g/day
Peritoneal dialysis	1.0–1.2 g/kg/day	25–35 kcal/kg/day[e]	800–1000 mg/day[d]	<2.3 g/day
Transplantation				
Posttransplant	CKD 2–3	25–35 kcal/kg/day[a,b]	800–1000 mg/day[d]	<2.3 g/day
Acute Kidney Injury				
No dialysis	1.0–1.2 g/kg IBW/d	30–30 kcal/kg/day	800–1000 mg/day[d]	<2 g/day
Dialysis	1.2–1.4 g/kg IBW/d	30–35 kcal/kg/day	600–800 mg/day[d,f]	<2 g/day

[a]Calculated based on age, weight, and activity level.

[b]If metabolically stable (absence of poorly controlled diabetes, any catabolic state such as cancer, any active inflammatory or infectious disease, significant short-term weight loss, antibiotic or immunosuppressive drug use).

[c]Should be personalized based on sex, age, body composition, physical activity, weight goals, CKD stage, and comorbidities to maintain normal nutritional status and with close supervision and frequent dietary counseling.

[d]Facilitated by phosphate binders, as needed.

[e]30 kcal/kg/day for individuals 60 years and older.

[f]May need to replete if receiving continuous kidney replacement therapy; check PO$_4$ levels daily.

IBW/d, Ideal body weight per day.

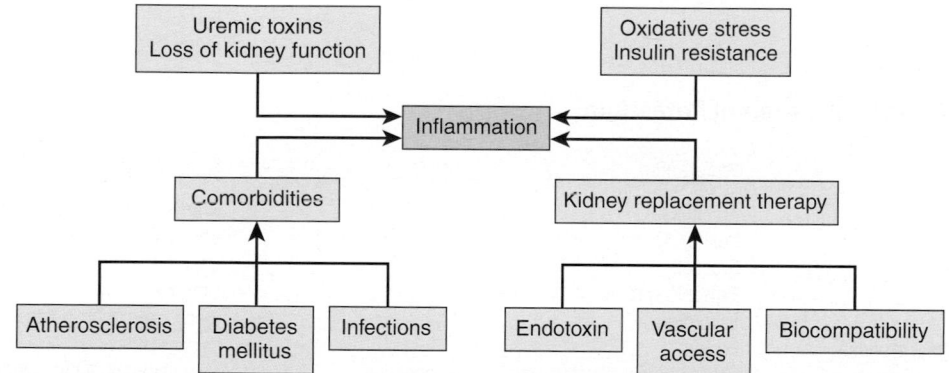

• **Fig. 52.1** Multiple factors can lead to systemic inflammation of patients with chronic kidney disease. Most of these factors are persistent, leading to a persistent inflamed state with short- and long-term adverse consequences.

higher rate of muscle protein loss than HD patients without diabetes, a catabolic state that can be detected even in HD patients with insulin resistance.

Additional metabolic disorders such as increased parathyroid hormone concentration, low levels of testosterone, and several abnormalities in the thyroid hormone profile might also promote hypermetabolism and decrease protein anabolism, leading to excess net protein catabolism in patients with advanced CKD. Acquired resistance to the anabolic actions of growth hormone is a potential cause of increased net protein catabolism in patients with advanced CKD. Growth hormone is the major promoter of growth in children and exerts anabolic actions even in adults, such

as enhancement of protein synthesis, reduced protein degradation, increased fat mobilization, and increased gluconeogenesis, with insulin-like growth factor–1 (IGF-1) being the major mediator of these actions. Studies have shown that recombinant human growth hormone treatment over 6 months improves fat-free mass in maintenance HD patients.

Testosterone levels are also abnormally low among men and women with CKD, especially those treated with maintenance dialysis. Testosterone is an anabolic hormone that induces skeletal muscle hypertrophy by promoting nitrogen retention and stimulating fractional muscle protein synthesis. In dialysis and advanced CKD patients, low testosterone levels are associated with increased mortality risk. In one small, clinical trial, nandrolone decanoate, an androgen analogue of testosterone, was associated with significant improvements in nutritional parameters, body composition, and physical functioning. However, its side effects, such as virilization, voice changes, hirsutism in women and abnormalities in prostate markers in men, and changes in liver enzymes, limit its routine clinical use.

Energy Metabolism and Requirements

The minimum energy requirement of patients with CKD is not well defined (see Table 52.2). An individual's energy requirement is dependent on resting energy expenditure, activity level, and effects of other ongoing illnesses. Resting energy expenditure is higher in maintenance dialysis patients compared with age, sex, and body mass index-matched controls and further increases during the HD procedure, when catabolism is at a maximum due to amino acid losses into the dialysate. Several comorbid conditions also lead to hypermetabolism, including systemic inflammation, uncontrolled diabetes mellitus, and hyperparathyroidism, further increasing energy requirement in patients with CKD. For earlier stages of CKD, energy requirements likely are similar to the general population. The KDOQI Nutrition guidelines recommend that in adults with CKD stages 1-5D and posttransplant who are metabolically stable it is appropriate to prescribe an energy intake of 25–35 kcal/kg ideal body weight per day based on age, sex, level of physical activity, body composition, weight status goals, CKD stage, and concurrent illness or presence of inflammation to maintain normal nutritional status.

Lipid Metabolism and Requirements

Dyslipidemia is common in CKD patients, and abnormalities in lipid profiles can be detected once kidney function begins to deteriorate. The presence of nephrotic syndrome or other comorbid conditions such as diabetes mellitus and liver disease, as well as the use of medications altering lipid metabolism (e.g., thiazide diuretics, beta-blockers), further contributes to the dyslipidemia seen in patients with CKD.

In maintenance HD patients, the most common abnormalities are elevated serum triglycerides and very-low-density lipoproteins (VLDL) and decreased low-density (LDL) and high-density (HDL) lipoproteins. The increased triglyceride component is thought to be related to increased levels of apoCIII, an inhibitor of lipoprotein lipase. A substantial percentage of maintenance HD patients also have elevated lipoprotein (a) (Lp[a]) levels. Patients treated with PD exhibit higher concentrations of serum cholesterol, triglyceride, LDL cholesterol, and apoB, even though the mechanisms that alter the lipid metabolism are similar to patients treated with maintenance HD. This may reflect increased protein losses through the peritoneum, possibly by mechanisms that are operative in the nephrotic syndrome and the glucose load supplied by dialysate causing increased triglyceride synthesis and hyperinsulinemia. Peritoneal dialysis patients also exhibit higher concentrations of Lp(a). Treatment of dyslipidemia is covered in detail in Chapter 54.

Mineral, Vitamin, and Trace Element Requirements

Sodium intake should be restricted in all CKD patients with hypertension and in maintenance dialysis patients regardless of blood pressure. Potassium intake should be less than 2 g/day in patients with CKD stage 4 or 5 and patients receiving HD; many PD patients require more liberal potassium intake. Foods containing high levels of potassium are listed in Table 52.3.

Elevated serum phosphorus levels are associated with increased risk for cardiovascular disease and mortality. Phosphorus is a

TABLE 52.3	Foods Containing High Levels of Potassium	
Fruits	**Vegetables**	**Other Foods**
Apricots	Artichokes	Bran and bran products
Avocado	Beans, dried	Chocolate
Banana	Broccoli	Coconut
Cantaloupe	Brussels sprouts	Granola
Casaba melon	Escarole	Juices from high-potassium fruits and
Dried fruits (dates, figs, raisins, prunes)	Endive	vegetables
Honeydew	Greens (Swiss chard, collard, beet, dandelion,	Low-sodium baking powder or soda
Mango	mustard)	Milk and milk products (ice cream,
Nectarine	Kale	yogurt—2 cups)
Orange	Kohlrabi	Molasses
Papaya	Lentils	Nuts/seeds
Rhubarb	Legumes	Peanut butter
Juice of fruits listed	Lima beans	Salt substitute or "lite" salt (containing
Tangelo	Mushrooms	potassium)
Watermelon	Parsnips	Snuff/chewing tobacco
	Potatoes (French fries, chips, baked, mashed, boiled,	
	sweet potatoes, yams)	
	Pumpkin	
	Rutabaga	
	Spinach, Swiss chard	
	Salt-free vegetable juice (ALL vegetable juices)	
	Tomatoes	
	Winter squash (acorn, butternut, Hubbard)	

TABLE 52.4	Foods Containing High Levels of Phosphorus	
Legumes, Nuts and Seeds, Whole Grains	Meat and Other Foods	Dairy and Beverages
Beans (navy, kidney, lima, pinto)	Chocolate	Beer
Soybeans	Dried fruit	Colas: Coke, Pepsi, Dr. Pepper
Black-eyed peas	Molasses	Eggnog
Lentils	Beef liver, calf liver	Hot chocolate
Peanut butter	Liver sausage	Milk
Nuts	Liverwurst	Casseroles
Coconuts	Beef, bottom round	Cheese
Pumpkin seeds	Pork, fresh	Cream soups
Sunflower seeds	Veal, cubes, rib roast	Custard
Bran, bran flakes, bran muffins		Ice cream
Brown rice		Pudding
Wheat germ		Yogurt
Raisin bran, 100% bran		
100% whole grain		

"hidden" ingredient in most processed foods and often is not listed on nutritional labels; accordingly, nonprocessed food consumption should be emphasized, if affordable. High-phosphorus foods are listed in Table 52.4. In earlier stages of CKD (stages 2 to 3), adjusting the dietary phosphorus intake to maintain the serum phosphate levels within the normal range is recommended. Because further restriction of dietary phosphorus in clinical settings is impractical, phosphate binders in addition to dietary phosphorus restriction are often necessary in advanced CKD, particularly for patients treated with maintenance dialysis. While use of calcium-containing binders can provide supplemental calcium that may be needed in advanced kidney disease, use of non-calcium-containing phosphate binders is generally preferred, especially in patients with a higher burden of vascular calcification, including elderly patients and patients with underlying ischemic heart disease. A detailed review of calcium and phosphorus metabolism can be found in Chapter 53.

Vitamin A concentrations are usually elevated in maintenance dialysis patients, and intake of even small amounts leads to excessive accumulation. There have been several reports of vitamin A toxicity in maintenance dialysis patients and, therefore, it should not be supplemented. Vitamin E levels in patients with advanced stages of kidney disease are not well defined, and there have been reports of increased, decreased, or unchanged concentrations. Therefore, it is not clear whether vitamin E supplementation is required in maintenance dialysis patients. Several randomized, controlled studies suggested that the therapeutic use of pharmacologic doses of vitamin E as an antioxidant does not substantially alter the metabolic profile in advanced CKD patients. Vitamin K supplementation is usually not recommended in maintenance dialysis patients unless they are at high risk for developing vitamin K deficiency, as with prolonged hospitalization, poor dietary intake, or antibiotic therapy, although ongoing research is evaluating whether vitamin K has a role in preventing vascular calcification. Vitamin D (and calcium/phosphorus) metabolism is discussed in detail in Chapter 53.

Serum concentrations of the water-soluble vitamins may be low in maintenance dialysis patients, mainly owing to decreased dietary intake and increased removal during hemodialysis. Multivitamin preparations specifically designed for CKD patients are available and useful for correcting these low concentrations without inducing toxicity.

The concentrations of most of the trace elements are primarily dependent on the stage of CKD. Although there is an extensive list of trace elements that may have altered concentrations in body fluids in maintenance dialysis patients, only a few are thought to be important. Serum aluminum is the most important trace element in maintenance hemodialysis patients because elevated levels are associated with dementia and bone disease. Aluminum intoxication can be caused either by use of inadequately processed water with HD (mostly eliminated with the use of reverse osmosis for water purification) or by use of phosphate binders that contain aluminum hydroxide, which is also very limited currently. Aluminum levels are serially monitored in dialysis patients. Routine supplementation of selenium and zinc, both of which function as antioxidants, are not recommended as the evidence on nutritional and inflammatory benefits is unclear.

Assessment of Nutritional Status in Chronic Kidney Disease Patients

A variety of parameters have been used to determine the nutrition status in CKD patients. Similar to the general population, an approach that incorporates continuous screening combined with more detailed assessment techniques is preferred (Table 52.5). Most screening tests are easy to perform, readily available, and inexpensive, rendering them clinically applicable. More sophisticated and expensive tools, such as dual-energy x-ray absorptiometry (DEXA) and magnetic resonance imaging (MRI), are used more commonly in research. DEXA is the gold standard to assess the body composition of patients with CKD; however, it is affected by fluid status, is expensive, and requires labor. In maintenance HD patients, multi-frequency bioimpedance analysis (BIA) is the preferred method to assess body composition, ideally at least 30 minutes after the hemodialysis session. There is insufficient evidence for the use of BIA in PD. Screening parameters can be collected routinely in clinical practice by any health professional and mostly provide a trigger to conduct a more extensive assessment, confirm or establish the diagnosis, and determine the best course of treatment, if needed. Any of the screening tests are adequate to initiate a more thorough work-up. On the other hand, nutritional assessment generally requires extensive training, provides comprehensive information to make a nutritional diagnosis, and aids in intervention and developing a monitoring plan. This should be performed by qualified individuals, preferably by dietitians. These tests should also be used for guiding nutritional therapies once the patient is deemed to be at risk or has overt PEW. A diagnosis of PEW necessitates confirmation by several tools and usually fits a strict criterion. A number of considerations must be made on the unique situation of CKD patients for appropriate screening and assessment of their nutritional status. Some of these include fluid status, which could alter body composition and biochemical markers; the presence of systemic inflammation, which could change serum concentrations of acute-phase proteins; the presence and extent of proteinuria, a major determinant of serum albumin concentrations; and the level of residual kidney function, which could influence serum concentration of

TABLE 52.5	Suggestions for Monitoring Nutritional Status and Therapy in Kidney Disease	
Simple Assessment (Monthly)	**Findings**	**Possible Interventions**
Body weight	Continuous decline or <85% IBW	Suspect PEW and perform more detailed nutritional assessment
Serum albumin	Below 4.0 g/dL	Consider preventive measures
Serum creatinine	Relatively low predialysis values	No specific intervention needed at this point
Detailed Assessment (as Indicated by Simple Assessment)	**Findings**	**Possible Interventions (Simple)**
Serum prealbumin	Below 30 mg/dL	Dietary counseling to increase DPI ≥1.2 g/kg/day and energy intake 30–35 kcal/day
Serum transferrin	Below 200 mg/dL	Consider timely initiation of maintenance dialysis
LBM and/or fat mass	Unexpected decrease	Assurance of optimal dialysis dose
SGA	Worsening	Upper GI motility enhancer in suitable patients
Repeat Detailed Assessment (2 to 3 Months From Previous)	**Findings (Any of the Markers)**	**Possible Interventions (Moderate to Complex)**
Serum prealbumin	Below 30 mg/dL	Nutritional supplements, including oral supplements, enteric tube feeding, IDPD, AAD
Serum transferrin	Below 200 mg/dL	Anabolic interventions, including anabolic steroids, rhGH (experimental)
Serum creatinine	Relatively low predialysis values	Appetite stimulants, including megestrol acetate, ghrelin (experimental)
LBM and/or fat mass	Unexpected decrease	Antiinflammatory interventions including IL-1ra (experimental), fish oil
C-reactive protein	Above 10 mg/L	

AAD, Amino acid dialysate; *DPI*, dietary protein intake; *IBW*, ideal body weight; *IDPN*, intradialytic parenteral nutrition; *IL1ra*, interleukin 1 receptor antagonist; *LBM*, lean body mass; *PEW*, protein energy wasting; *rhGH*, recombinant human growth hormone; *SGA*, Subjective Global Assessment.
Adapted with permission from Pupim LB, Cuppari L, Ikizler TA. Nutrition and metabolism in kidney disease. *Semin Nephrol.* 2006;26:134–157.

some biochemical markers, such as prealbumin, that are cleared by the kidneys.

Estimation of dietary protein intake can also be used as a marker of overall nutritional status in the CKD patient. Although dietary recall is a direct and simple measure of dietary protein intake, several studies show that this method lacks accuracy in estimating the actual intake. Therefore, other means of measuring dietary protein intake, such as 24-hour urine urea nitrogen excretion in CKD patients or urea nitrogen appearance (UNA) rate calculations derived from urea kinetic modeling in maintenance dialysis patients, have been suggested as useful methods to estimate protein intake. However, these indirect estimations of dietary protein intake are valid only in stable patients and may easily overestimate the actual intake in catabolic patients where endogenous protein breakdown may lead to a high UNA.

Routine nutritional screening should occur in all CKD stages to identify and, when necessary, further evaluate and treat nutritional problems. The main components of a comprehensive nutritional assessment are dietary intake, anthropometric measurements, clinical symptoms, biomarker levels, and medical and psychosocial history. Subjective Global Assessment (SGA) is recommended as a valid tool to assess the nutritional status of patients on maintenance dialysis. Malnutrition Inflammation Score (MIS) is another composite nutritional index that may be used in maintenance dialysis patients or posttransplant to assess nutritional status.

In summary, there are many different methods available for assessing protein and energy nutritional status in CKD patients. Some are easy to perform, readily available, and inexpensive, while others are sophisticated, not available in many centers, and either expensive or carry an unfavorable cost-benefit ratio. For example, a monthly nutritional screening can be easily performed at nearly any clinic or hospital by measuring serum albumin, serum prealbumin, serum transferrin, and bioimpedance values. However, if the goal is to precisely and longitudinally follow changes in body composition, one may want to use anthropometry, dual-energy x-ray absorptiometry, and even more sophisticated methods, if available. For all indirect methods, repeated measures and technical standardization are extremely important to reduce variability of results.

Prevention and Treatment of Protein Energy Wasting

Given the importance of adequate nutritional status and the large number of factors that can result in PEW, especially in later stages of CKD, prevention and therapeutic strategies should involve a multidisciplinary approach to reduce protein and energy catabolism, prevent further losses, and restore negative balance (Fig. 52.2). Prescribing dietary nutrient intake appropriate for the stage of kidney disease (see Table 52.2) is critically important. Many maintenance dialysis patients will continue their predialysis diets while receiving kidney replacement therapy; this is inappropriate, and it is important that dietary protein and calorie intake increase to meet the requirements after dialysis initiation. Critical and often simple and straightforward steps to minimize the risk of developing or worsening PEW include combating the catabolic effects of kidney replacement therapy, treating obvious causes of systemic inflammation, and managing comorbid conditions such as metabolic acidosis, diabetes, and depression. Managing food intake by either dietary counseling or positive reinforcement is crucial, particularly for patients treated on maintenance dialysis.

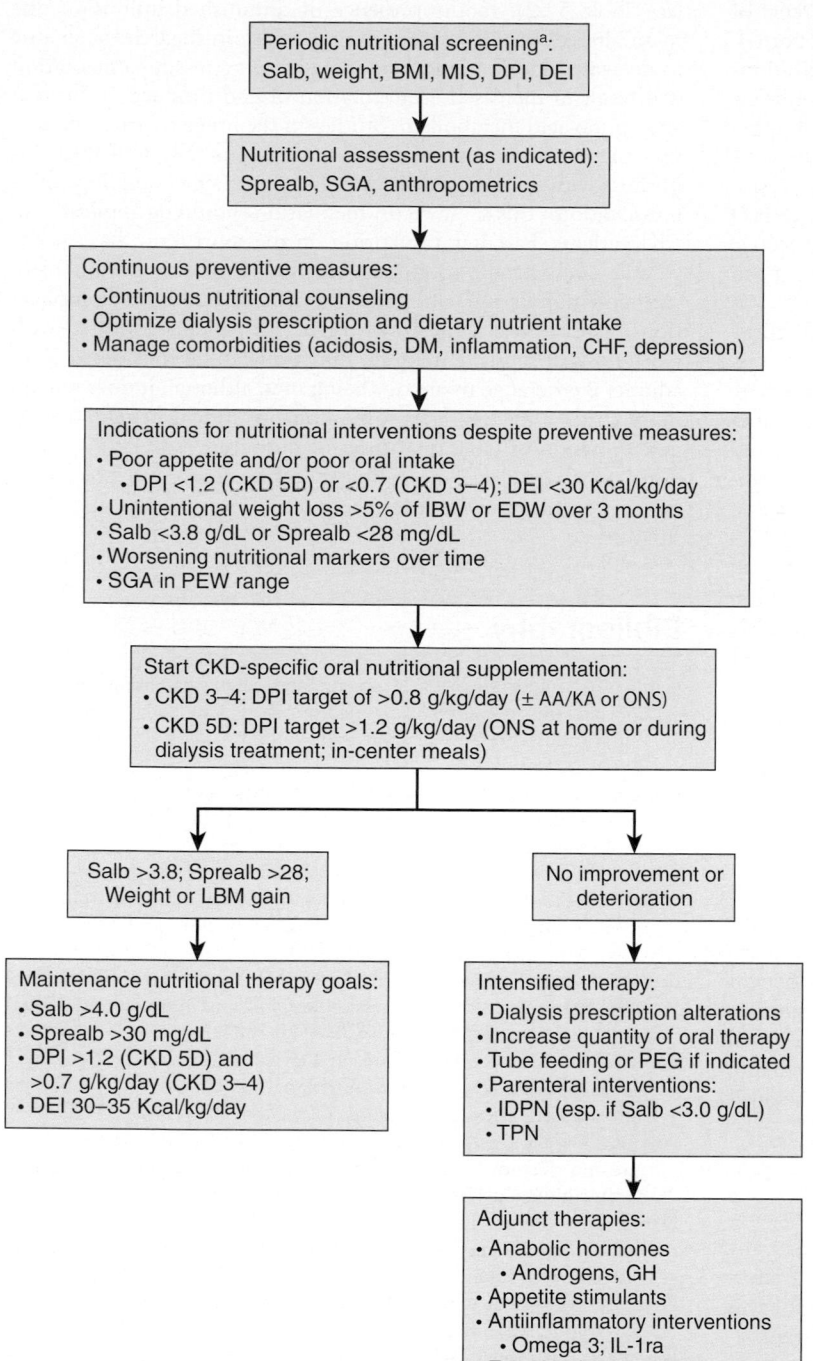

• **Fig. 52.2** Algorithm for nutritional management and support in patients with chronic kidney disease. [a]Minimum every 3 months, monthly screening recommended. Only for end-stage kidney disease (ESKD) patients without residual kidney function. *AA/KA,* Amino acid/keto acid; *BMI,* body mass index; *CHF,* congestive heart failure; *CKD,* chronic kidney disease; *DEI,* dietary energy intake; *DM,* diabetes mellitus; *DPI,* dietary protein intake; *EDW,* estimated dry weight; *GH,* growth hormone; *IBW,* ideal body weight; *IDPN,* intradialytic parenteral nutrition; *IL-1ra,* interleukin-1 receptor antagonist; *LBM,* lean body mass; *MIS,* malnutrition–inflammation score; *ONS,* oral nutritional supplement; *PEG,* percutaneous endoscopic gastrostomy; *PEW,* protein energy wasting; *Salb,* serum albumin (measured by bromocresol green); *SGA,* Subjective Global Assessment; *Sprealb,* serum prealbumin; *TPN,* total parenteral nutrition. (From Ikizler TA, Cano NJ, Franch H, et al. Prevention and treatment of protein energy wasting in chronic kidney disease patients: a consensus statement by the International Society of Renal Nutrition and Metabolism. *Kidney Int.* 2013;84:1096–1107.)

Kidney dietitians play a critical role in providing the majority of educational support and monitoring patient outcomes.

In certain maintenance dialysis patients, where the standard measures are unable to prevent loss of protein and energy stores, nutritional supplementation is a suitable next step. In general practice, the gastrointestinal route is always preferred for nutritional supplementation. Oral supplementation should be given two to three times a day, preferably 2 hours before or after main meals and/or during hemodialysis. Oral supplementation can provide an additional 7 to 10 kcal/kg/day of energy and 0.3 to 0.4 g/kg/day of protein. This requires a minimum spontaneous dietary intake of 20 kcal/kg/day of energy and 0.4 to 0.8 g/kg/day of protein to meet the recommended dietary energy intake and dietary protein intake targets.

It is usually a challenge to determine whether an oral or enteral form of supplementation is necessary and effective if administered in CKD patients not on maintenance dialysis. In these patients, recommendations that are developed for other comorbid conditions such as diabetes mellitus, frailty, and old age should be used while taking into account the implications of the stage of kidney disease, especially in terms of mineral and electrolyte content of the supplementation. The beneficial nutritional effects of these supplements have been reported primarily on serum biomarkers such as albumin, prealbumin, and transferrin, as well as gains in body weight and lean body mass. Improvements in markers of quality of life and physical functioning have also been reported. In prospective, randomized studies examining hospitalizations and death, the statistical power to appropriately assess the efficacy of these interventions is mostly lacking. However, several large-scale, observational studies reported significant survival benefits associated with oral nutritional supplement (ONS) administration during hemodialysis in hypoalbuminemic maintenance HD patients. The limitations of these studies include a retrospective design, convenience sampling, and residual confounding from unmeasured variables.

For patients who are unable to tolerate nutritional supplementation by mouth, nasogastric, percutaneous endoscopic gastrostomy (PEG), or jejunostomy tubes can be considered. When there is evidence of PEW and if nutritional requirements cannot be met by oral or enteral feeding (including oral protein, amino acid, and energy supplementation; nasogastric feeding tubes, PEG, or jejunostomy tubes), total parenteral nutrition (TPN) in CKD 1-5 and intradialytic parenteral nutrition (IDPN) in maintenance HD patients can be considered. Although most of the studies reported beneficial nutritional effects of IDPN administration in maintenance HD patients with overt PEW, a relatively large, prospective, randomized, controlled study comparing IDPN plus ONS versus ONS alone showed similar improvements in nutritional parameters, with no additional benefit on hospitalization or death rates. A recently published, randomized, controlled trial showed that IDPN therapy led to increased prealbumin levels and was superior to nutritional counseling after 16 weeks. Concerns regarding greater fluid volume requirement and high cost remain barriers for the frequent and long-term use of IDPN. Hence, parenteral provision of nutrients should be reserved as an approach for individuals who cannot tolerate oral or enteral administration of nutrients. Studies using amino acid dialysate (AAD) in PD patients have provided conflicting results. In studies that suggested benefit from AAD, serum transferrin and total protein concentrations increased and plasma amino acid profiles trended toward normal with one or two exchanges of AAD per day. On the other hand, exacerbations of uremic symptoms as well as metabolic acidosis are potential complications of AAD.

Nutrition in Acute Kidney Injury

The nutritional hallmark of acute kidney injury (AKI), especially in the setting of critical illness, is excessive catabolism. Factors that have been postulated as the underlying mechanism for this high rate of protein and energy catabolism include concurrent illnesses leading to exaggerated proinflammatory cytokine release, inability to feed patients because of surgical and other reasons, and metabolic derangements predisposing patients to diminished utilization and incorporation of available nutrients. Whether uremic toxin accumulation further exacerbates these abnormalities is questionable because aggressive dialytic clearance does not substantially improve mortality in AKI stage 3 patients.

The nutritional markers that correlate best with efficacy of nutritional therapy and patient outcome are considerably different in AKI patients than in CKD patients. Blood levels of biochemical markers such as serum albumin and prealbumin are influenced by volume status and concurrent inflammatory state. Similarly, utilization of traditional measures of body composition such as anthropometry has limited application in AKI patients owing to major shifts in body water. The actual requirements for protein and energy supplementation in AKI patients are not well defined

(see Table 52.2). In the presence of diminished utilization due to an altered metabolic state as well as diminished clearance due to decreased kidney function, excessive protein supplementation will result in increased accumulation of end products of protein and amino acid metabolism. Studies in the intensive care unit setting suggest that early enteral support is generally well tolerated in those without contraindication (e.g., anatomic, ongoing active resuscitation); this same recommendation should be applicable to AKI patients. Parenteral nutrition, in the short term, has a comparable safety profile to enteral nutrition in the overall intensive care unit population, although the risk of infectious complications increases over time and is higher in patients admitted with a diagnosis of sepsis. Parenteral nutrition can be considered as an adjunct if enteral goals are not being met, although it does remain more costly and may lack some non-nutritional benefits to the gut. Provision of large quantities of nutrients, especially intravenously, may result in more fluid administration and predispose patients to fluid overload, resulting in earlier initiation of dialytic support.

Bibliography

Cano NJ, Fouque D, Roth H, et al. Intradialytic parenteral nutrition does not improve survival in malnourished hemodialysis patients: a 2-year multicenter, prospective, randomized study. *J Am Soc Nephrol.* 2007;18:2583–2591.

Carrero JJ, de Jager DJ, Verduijn M, et al. Cardiovascular and noncardiovascular mortality among men and women starting dialysis. *Clin J Am Soc Nephrol.* 2011;6:1722–1730.

Carrero JJ, Stenvinkel P, Cuppari L, et al. Etiology of the protein-energy wasting syndrome in chronic kidney disease: a consensus statement from the International Society of Renal Nutrition and Metabolism (ISRNM). *J Ren Nutr.* 2013;23:77–90.

de Brito-Ashurst I, Varagunam M, Raftery MJ, Yaqoob MM. Bicarbonate supplementation slows progression of CKD and improves nutritional status. *J Am Soc Nephrol.* 2009;20:2075–2084.

Fontes D, Generoso Sde V, Toulson Davisson Correia MI. Subjective global assessment: a reliable nutritional assessment tool to predict outcomes in critically ill patients. *Clin Nutr.* 2014;33(2):291–295.

Fouque D, Kalantar-Zadeh K, Kopple J, et al. A proposed nomenclature and diagnostic criteria for protein-energy wasting in acute and chronic kidney disease. *Kidney Int.* 2008;73:391–398.

Hanna RM, Ghobry L, Wassef O, et al. A practical approach to nutrition, protein-energy wasting, sarcopenia, and cachexia in patients with chronic kidney disease. *Blood Purif.* 2020;49:202–211.

Ikizler TA. A patient with CKD and poor nutritional status. *Clin J Am Soc Nephrol.* 2013;8:2174–2182.

Ikizler TA, Burrowes J, Byham-Gray L, et al. KDOQI Nutrition in CKD Guideline Work Group. KDOQI clinical practice guideline for nutrition in CKD: 2020 update. *Am J Kidney Dis.* 2020;76(3):S1–107.

Ikizler TA, Cano NJ, Franch H, et al. Prevention and treatment of protein energy wasting in chronic kidney disease patients: a consensus statement by the International Society of Renal Nutrition and Metabolism. *Kidney Int.* 2013;84:1096–1107.

Kalantar-Zadeh K, Fouque D. Nutritional Management of Chronic Kidney Disease. *N Engl J Med.* 2017 Nov;377(18):1765–1776.

Kidney Disease: Improving Global Outcomes (KDIGO) CKD Work Group. KDIGO 2012 Clinical Practice Guidelines for the Evaluation and Management of Chronic Kidney Disease. *Kidney Int Suppl.* 2013;3:1–150.

Kidney Disease: Improving Global Outcomes (KDIGO) CKD-MBD Update Work Group. KDIGO 2017 Clinical Practice Guideline Update for the Diagnosis, Evaluation, Prevention, and Treatment of Chronic Kidney Disease–Mineral and Bone Disorder (CKD-MBD). *Kidney Int Suppl.* 2017;7:1–59.

Lacson E Jr, Wang W, Zebrowski B, et al. Outcomes associated with intradialytic oral nutritional supplements in patients undergoing maintenance hemodialysis: a quality improvement report. *Am J Kidney Dis*. 2012;60:591–600.

Marsen TA, Beer J, Mann H. Intradialytic parenteral nutrition in maintenance hemodialysis patients suffering from protein-energy wasting. Results of a multicenter, open, prospective, randomized trial. *Clin Nutr*. 2017;36(1):107–117.

Naylor HL, Jackson H, Walker GH, et al. Renal Nutrition Group of the British Dietetic Association; British Dietetic Association. British Dietetic Association evidence-based guidelines for the protein requirements of adults undergoing maintenance haemodialysis or peritoneal dialysis. *J Hum Nutr Diet*. 2013;26:315–328.

Pupim LB, Ikizler TA. Assessment and monitoring of uremic malnutrition. *J Ren Nutr*. 2004;14:6–19.

Stenvinkel P. Can treating persistent inflammation limit protein energy wasting? *Semin Dialysis*. 2013;26:16–19.

Stratton RJ, Bircher G, Fouque D, et al. Multinutrient oral supplements and tube feeding in maintenance dialysis: a systematic review and meta-analysis. *Am J Kidney Dis*. 2005;46:387–405.

Tentori F, Karaboyas A, Robinson BM, Morgenstern H, Zhang J, Sen A, Ikizler TA, Rayner H, Fissell RB, Vanholder R, et al. Association of dialysate bicarbonate concentration with mortality in the Dialysis Outcomes and Practice Patterns Study (DOPPS). *Am. J. Kidney Dis.* 2013;62:738–746.

53

Bone and Mineral Disorders in Chronic Kidney Disease

L. DARRYL QUARLES, PIETER EVENEPOEL

Chronic kidney disease (CKD) alters the regulation of calcium, phosphate, and vitamin D homeostasis, leading to secondary hyperparathyroidism, elevations in serum fibroblast growth factor 23 (FGF23), metabolic bone disease, soft tissue calcifications, and other metabolic derangements that have a significant impact on morbidity and mortality. Mineral and bone disorders (MBD) are important targets of therapy in CKD. Earlier interventions and stringent management guidelines to control serum parathyroid hormone (PTH), calcium, and phosphorus concentrations have been proposed by several international foundations and initiatives, including the Kidney Disease: Improving Global Outcomes (KDIGO). Overall, there is lack of consensus regarding the best approach to treat abnormalities in mineral metabolism effectively and safely and to prevent the complications associated with these abnormalities.

Both active vitamin D (analogues) and calcimimetic drugs that target the calcium-sensing receptor (CaSR) in the parathyroid gland are available to suppress PTH, although the specific roles for each remain unspecified. There is similar lack of consensus on other issues, such as the clinical significance of low circulating 25(OH)D levels in people with advanced CKD (which represents vitamin D deficiency in those without CKD); the optimal agent, dose, and route of active vitamin D (analogue) to treat secondary hyperparathyroidism; and the relative role of calcium- and non-calcium-based binders to control serum phosphate. Most recommendations are graded as level 2 (weak), reflecting an important degree of remaining uncertainty.

The importance of vitamin D pathways in regulating innate immunity and cardiovascular function, in addition to its more traditional role in regulating mineral metabolism, is increasingly recognized. However, although low vitamin D levels are associated with increased risk of CVD, infection, and mortality, there are only limited data that nutritional vitamin D supplementation (with cholecalciferol or ergocalciferol) improves clinical outcomes, with recent, large, intervention studies using cholecalciferol in the general population adding further doubts. In addition, treatment with active vitamin D or its analogues does not appear to improve the severity of left ventricular hypertrophy (LVH) in CKD. Another word of caution against indiscriminate use of vitamin D supplements is that this treatment may exacerbate hyperphosphatemia, hypercalcemia, and hyperphosphatinonism (high FGF23).

Finally, emerging knowledge about the endocrine functions of bone (and specifically the role of the phosphaturic- and vitamin D-regulating hormone FGF23 in LVH, cardiovascular mortality, and glomerular filtration rate [GFR] loss) has led to a reexamination of the pathogenesis and treatment of disordered mineral metabolism in CKD.

Pathogenesis of Abnormal Mineral Metabolism and Secondary Hyperparathyroidism in Chronic Kidney Disease

The pathogenesis of secondary hyperparathyroidism is complex and involves many closely intertwined factors. The major metabolic abnormalities leading to the increase in PTH are diminished production of $1,25\text{-}(OH)_2D_3$ (calcitriol, the activated form of vitamin D), decreased serum calcium, and increased serum phosphorus. In normal subjects, PTH is responsible for maintaining the serum calcium concentration within a narrow range through direct actions on the distal tubule of the kidney to increase calcium resorption and actions on bone to increase calcium and phosphate efflux (Fig. 53.1). In addition, some PTH effects are mediated by its role in the production of calcitriol by the kidney via stimulation of Cyp27b1, the enzyme that converts inactive 25 hydroxyvitamin D to active $1,25(OH)_2D$. The net effects of PTH's bone and kidney actions are to create the positive calcium balance that is necessary to maintain calcium homeostasis. To prevent a concomitant positive phosphate balance due to the skeletal effects of PTH and the gastrointestinal actions of calcitriol, PTH acts secondarily to increase urinary phosphorus excretion, mostly by decreasing activity of the sodium phosphate cotransporter in the proximal renal tubule.

Parathyroid disease in CKD is a progressive disorder characterized by both increased PTH secretion and expansion of the number of the PTH-secreting chief cells (hyperplasia). Elevations in serum PTH levels may first become evident when the GFR falls below 60 mL/min/1.73 m^2. This occurs before hyperphosphatemia, reduction in calcitriol levels, or hypocalcemia is detectable by routine laboratory measurements. This delay in detectable serum chemistry abnormalities is presumably caused by the actions of increased PTH to restore homeostasis. PTH levels increase progressively as kidney function declines, such that all untreated subjects reaching CKD stage G5 (GFR <15 mL/min/1.73 m^2 or dialysis) would be expected to have elevated PTH levels.

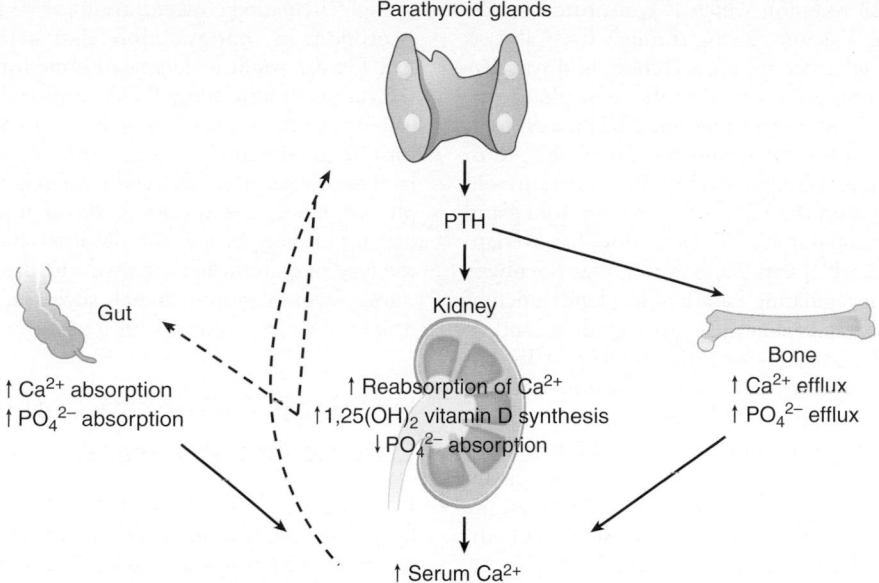

• **Fig. 53.1** Regulation of systemic calcium homeostasis. Parathyroid hormone (PTH) is a calcemic hormone that targets the kidney to promote calcium conservation and the bone to increase efflux of calcium and phosphorus. PTH-mediated production of 1,25(OH)₂D₃ (activated vitamin D) by the kidney increases gastrointestinal calcium and phosphate absorption. The phosphaturic actions of PTH on the kidney cause it to excrete the excess phosphate that accompanies calcium absorption by the intestines and calcium efflux from bone. Changes in calcium, 1,25(OH)₂D₃, and phosphate levels exert feedback on the parathyroid glands *(dashed line)*. In chronic kidney disease (CKD), elevation of serum fibroblast growth factor 23 (FGF23) is an early event leading to suppression of 1,25(OH)₂D production and possibly increased catabolism. FGF23-mediated suppression of 1,25(OH)₂D₃ may be the initiating event leading to secondary hyperparathyroidism. In advanced CKD, elevations of PTH appear to stimulate FGF23 further. Elevated levels of serum phosphate and FGF23 are associated with increased mortality in CKD.

The initial event leading to an incremental rise in PTH has traditionally been attributed to primary reductions in 1,25(OH)₂D levels caused by decreased production by the diseased kidney. More recent data implicate an early role of elevated FGF23 in the genesis of secondary hyperparathyroidism in CKD. In this scenario, increments in FGF23 reduce 1,25(OH)₂D production by suppressing Cyp27b1 activity in the proximal tubule and possibly enhance 1,25(OH)₂D catabolism through increased Cyp24 activity. Cross-sectional studies in humans and serial studies of animal models with CKD suggest that increments in serum FGF23 precede elevations of PTH and correlate with reductions in circulating 1,25(OH)₂D concentrations. This sequence of events, however, is questioned by recent epidemiologic data. Given the multiple, complex, and often reciprocal interactions between the various players (calcium, phosphorus, FGF23, 1,25[OH]₂D), the exact role of each moiety in the pathogenesis of secondary hyperparathyroidism is hard to define. Elevated PTH levels help to maintain normocalcemia and normophosphatemia but are also required to overcome PTH resistance. At a certain stage in the course of CKD, elevated PTH levels may turn maladaptive and cause overall harm.

FGF23, a key regulator of phosphate and vitamin D homeostasis, is perhaps the initial adaptive response in CKD and may also play a role in cardiovascular complications as well as progression of kidney disease. Gene transcription of FGF23 in mouse models is regulated both by systemic factors, such as hyperphosphatemia and elevated 1,25-(OH)₂D₃ levels, and by local bone-derived factors. FGF23 knockout mice are hyperphosphatemic and display soft tissue and vascular calcifications, growth retardation, and bone mineralization abnormalities. FGF23 is expressed mainly in osteocytes in bone and, to a much lesser extent, in the bone marrow, the ventrolateral thalamic nucleus, the thymus, and lymph nodes. FGF23 promotes phosphate excretion by inhibition of sodium-dependent phosphate resorption. It also suppresses kidney and extrarenal calcitriol synthesis. FGF23 may also act in the heart through "off-target effects" to activate FGF receptors (FGFR) in the absence of its coreceptor α-Klotho, or on the kidney through "on-target" effects on FGFR:α-Klotho complexes to regulate genes, such as the suppression of angiotensin-converting enzyme 2 (ACE2). In addition, FGF23 may qualify both as a risk marker and mediator of (cardiovascular) disease. FGF23 production may be lowered by phosphate binders and/or dietary therapy. Whether FGF23 suppression translates to improved intermediate and hard outcomes remains to be proven.

Unless adequately treated, secondary hyperparathyroidism progresses inexorably, with the need for parathyroidectomy proportional to the number of years on dialysis. The difficulty in treating hyperparathyroidism in CKD partly reflects the massive hyperplasia and possibly adenomatous transformation of the parathyroid gland that occurs because of the chronic stimulation of PTH production. Enlarged, hyperplastic parathyroid glands retain some responsiveness to calcium-mediated PTH suppression in secondary hyperparathyroidism. Because this responsiveness is lost with reductions in extracellular CaSR and vitamin D receptor (VDR) expression, as well as autonomous adenomatous transformation of the parathyroid gland, hypercalcemia develops in some patients. This is referred to as *tertiary hyperparathyroidism*.

Three molecular targets have been identified that regulate parathyroid gland function, including the G protein–coupled CaSR, the VDR, and the FGF23 receptor, which is constituted by the FGFR:α-Klotho complex. Calcium, acting through the CaSR, is the major regulator of PTH transcription, secretion, and parathyroid gland hyperplasia. Recent evidence shows that phosphate concentration within the pathophysiologic range for CKD may inhibit CaSR activity via noncompetitive antagonisms. The CaSR, thus, may represent the long-sought phosphate sensor in the parathyroid gland. Calcitriol, which acts on the VDR in the parathyroid gland to suppress PTH transcription but not PTH secretion, has overlapping functions with the CaSR. It appears, however, that the physiologic role of the VDR in regulating parathyroid gland function may be subordinate to that of calcium. In this regard, secondary hyperparathyroidism and bone abnormalities in VDR-deficient mice can be corrected by normalizing the serum calcium concentration. Finally, FGF23 has recently been shown to target the parathyroid gland via FGFR:α-Klotho complexes and to suppress PTH secretion. The actions of FGF23 on the parathyroid gland remain to be further elucidated, because most states of FGF23 excess are associated with elevations of PTH, and stimulation of FGFR pathways would be expected to lead to cell hyperplasia.

Pathogenesis of Bone Disease Associated With Chronic Kidney Disease

Bone is a dynamic tissue that undergoes repetitive cycles of removal and replacement. Osteoclasts, under the influence of paracrine and systemic factors, resorb bone, whereas osteoblasts fill in the resorptive cavities with new extracellular matrix that undergoes mineralization. This process is also regulated by physiochemical properties as well as proteins that either inhibit or promote the mineralization process. A subset of osteoblasts become embedded in the bone matrix to form an interconnected network of cells (osteocytes) that also respond to systemic and local stimuli to secrete factors regulating the bone-remodeling process. During growth, new trabecular bone is added to the long bones beneath the growth plate, and factors that affect bone remodeling can also affect growth plate morphology, leading to rickets. In adults, bone disease can manifest as too little (osteopenia) or too much (osteosclerosis) bone, high or low states of bone turnover, and impaired mineralization.

PTH through PTH receptors, $1,25(OH)_2D$ through VDRs, and calcium and phosphate through effects on mineralization of bone extracellular matrix can all affect bone health. Osteoblast-mediated bone formation entails generation of a collagen matrix that undergoes mineralization controlled by a complex interplay among factors promoting and inhibiting mineralization. Bone formation is coupled to osteoclast-mediated bone resorption through osteoblastic paracrine pathways involving the secretion of a receptor activator of nuclear factor-κB ligand (RANKL), which stimulates osteoclast formation, function, and survival. Osteoblasts also secrete osteoprotegerin (OPG), which bind to RANKL to inhibit bone resorption. Denosumab, a monoclonal antibody that binds to RANKL and mimics the effects of OPG, is used to treat osteoporosis. Osteocytes also regulate bone formation through the production and secretion of sclerostin (SOST), an inhibitor of osteoanabolic Wnt signaling pathways.

The circulating level of PTH is the primary determinant of bone turnover in CKD and is a major determinant of bone disease type. PTH receptors are present in both osteoblasts and osteocytes. PTH suppresses SOST expression and stimulates cyclic adenosine monophosphate (cAMP) as well as other pathways leading to increased osteoblast-mediated bone formation. Long-term exposure to high circulating concentrations of PTH leads to increased bone resorption. In contrast, more short-term, intermittent exposure to PTH can result in increased bone formation in excess of bone resorption. Intermittent PTH administration is the basis for use of teriparatide to treat osteoporosis. In addition, $1,25(OH)_2D$, at least in experimental settings, promotes mineralization and stimulates bone resorption, especially when gastrointestinal calcium supply is limited. The specific types of histologic changes may also depend on patient age, the duration and cause of kidney failure, the type of dialysis therapy used, the presence of acidosis, gonadal status, accumulation of metals such as aluminum, and other conditions affecting mineralization of the extracellular matrix.

Histologic Classification of Bone Disease in Chronic Kidney Disease

Bone disease associated with CKD (Fig. 53.2) has traditionally been classified histologically according to the degrees of abnormal bone turnover and impaired mineralization of the extracellular matrix, although the current classification of bone histology adopted by KDIGO focuses on turnover, mineralization, and volume (TMV) (Fig. 53.3). These histologic changes in bone have been best studied in patients undergoing dialysis. Traditional categories are as follows:

1. Secondary hyperparathyroidism (high-turnover bone disease or osteitis fibrosa).
2. Osteomalacia (defective mineralization).
3. Mixed uremic bone disease (a mixture of high-turnover bone disease and osteomalacia).
4. Adynamic bone disease (decreased rates of bone formation without a mineralization defect).

The 2009 KDIGO MBD guideline initiative recommended the TMV classification. Especially if specific therapies that target each of these characteristics are developed, this classification could prove useful; however, treatments are, at present, directed toward maintaining serum PTH levels in a range that (1) prevents high-turnover osteitis fibrosa and increased cortical porosity on one end of the spectrum and (2) avoids low-turnover (adynamic) bone at the other end.

High-Turnover Bone Disease

High-turnover bone disease caused by excess PTH is characterized by greater number and size of osteoclasts and an increase in the number of resorption lacunae with scalloped trabeculae, as well as abnormally high numbers of osteoblasts. There is an increased amount of osteoid (unmineralized bone), which may have a woven appearance that reflects a disordered collagen arrangement under conditions of rapid matrix deposition. The excess in osteoid surfaces that accompanies increased bone turnover has been described as *mixed uremic bone disease*, but it may reflect a normal response to increased turnover rather than superimposed defective mineralization. Peritrabecular fibrosis (and even marrow fibrosis), reflecting PTH stimulation of osteoblastic precursors, is observed in severe disease.

Osteomalacia

Osteomalacia is characterized by prolongation of the mineralization lag time as well as by increased thickness, surface area, and volume of osteoid. Osteomalacia was formerly linked to

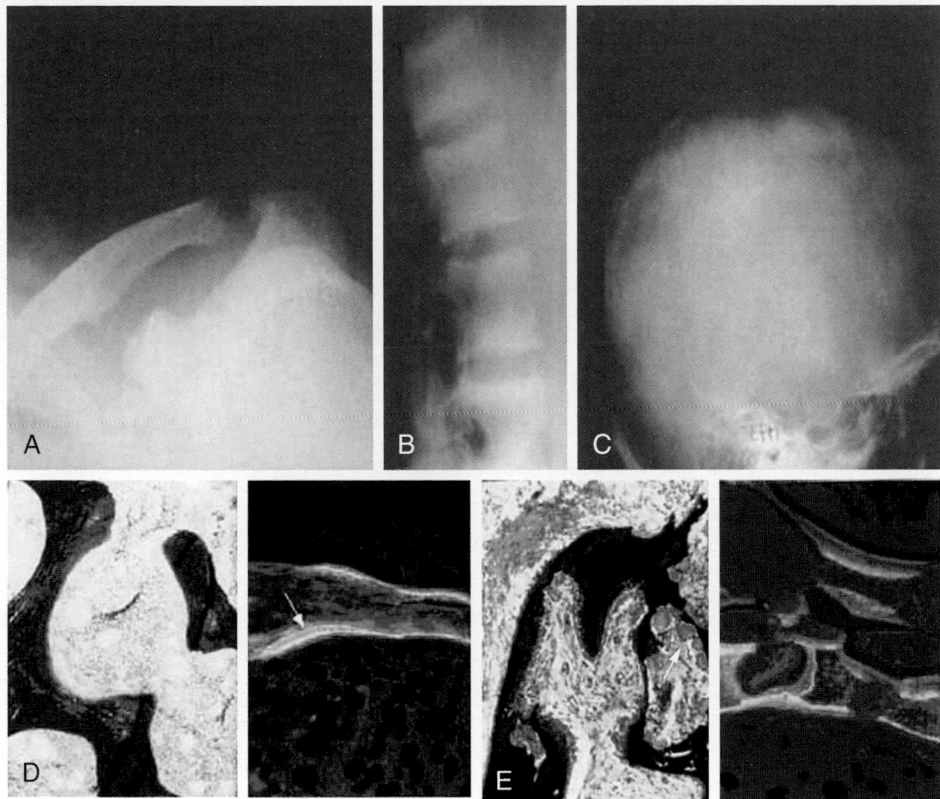

• **Fig. 53.2** Radiographic and histologic features of bone disease associated with chronic kidney disease (CKD). (A) Radiographic findings of severe erosion of the distal clavicle resulting from secondary hyperparathyroidism. (B) Example of "rugger-jersey spine" resulting from sclerosis of the end plates associated with hyperparathyroidism. (C) "Pepper-pot skull" with areas of erosion and patchy osteosclerosis associated with hyperparathyroidism. (D) Histologic appearance of normal bone. On the left, a section stained with Goldner Masson trichrome stain shows mineralized lamellar bone *(blue)* and adjacent nonmineralized osteoid surfaces *(red-brown)*. On the right, a Villanueva-stained section viewed under fluorescent light shows tetracycline labeling of freshly formed bone. Double staining *(arrow)* indicates amount of new bone laid down during the interval between the two periods of tetracycline administration. (E) Histologic appearance of osteitis fibrosa in a patient with CKD stage G5 and elevated parathyroid hormone levels. On the left, Goldner Masson trichrome stain shows increased numbers of multinucleated osteoclasts at resorptive surfaces *(white arrow)* and extensive bone marrow fibrosis *(light-blue staining of marrow)*. On the right, tetracycline labeling shows marked increases in the osteoid *(orange-red staining)* and in sites of new bone formation as measured by the yellow-green bands below the osteoid surfaces. (A–C from Martin KJ, Gonzalez EA, Slatopolsky E. Renal osteodystrophy. In: Brenner BM, ed. *Brenner and Rector's the Kidney.* 7th ed. Philadelphia: Saunders; 2004:2280.)

aluminum toxicity from both contamination of water in dialysates and the use of aluminum-based phosphate binders. Other causes of osteomalacia that may be present in CKD patients include 25-hydroxyvitamin D deficiency (secondary to poor dietary vitamin D and calcium intake, lack of exposure to sunlight because of poor mobility and extended hospitalizations, and urinary losses of vitamin D-binding protein, that is, the major carrier protein for 25-hydroxyvitamin D), metabolic acidosis (which inhibits both osteoblasts and osteoclasts), and hypophosphatemia (e.g., in Fanconi syndrome).

Adynamic Bone Disease

Adynamic bone disease is a low-turnover bone state that has received increased attention. According to recent bone biopsy data, as many as 40% of patients on hemodialysis and 50% of patients on peritoneal dialysis have adynamic bone disease. In this disorder, the amount of osteoid thickness is normal or reduced, and there is no mineralization defect. The main findings are decreased numbers of osteoclasts and osteoblasts and very low rates of bone formation as measured by tetracycline labeling. It is thought that adynamic bone disease in CKD represents a state of relative hypoparathyroidism. Adynamic bone disease is associated with poor outcomes, including increased risk of mortality and progression of vascular calcification. It remains controversial whether the low-turnover bone state per se or the conditions causing suppression of bone turnover account for the association with poor outcomes. These conditions include inflammation, oxidative stress, malnutrition, and diabetes, among others. Pharmacologic therapies that reduce bone turnover, such as calcimimetic and antiresorptive agents, are not associated with increased mortality risk and accelerated vascular calcification, and, contrary to the abovementioned conditions, often result in a positive bone balance, at least transiently.

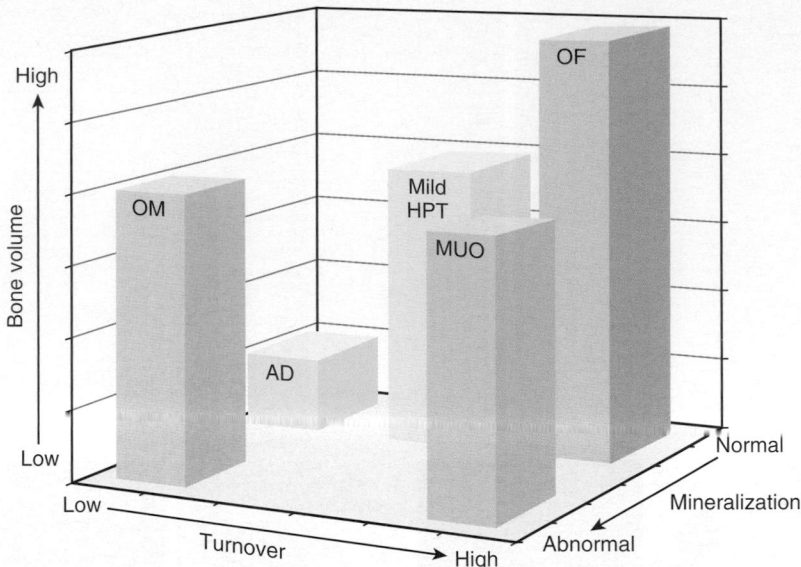

• **Fig. 53.3** The distribution of bone mineral disorders according to the turnover, mineralization, and volume classification system. *AD*, Adynamic bone disease; *HPT*, hyperparathyroidism; *MUO*, mixed uremic bone disease/osteomalacia; *OF*, osteitis fibrosa; *OM*, osteomalacia.

Epidemiology of Bone Disease

Based on limited bone histologic data, approximately 40% of Black and 20% of White subjects with end-stage kidney disease have high turnover disease, with the remainder having normal or low bone turnover in spite of elevated circulating PTH levels. Adynamic bone disease may not be a naturally occurring separate disease, but a consequence of overtreatment of hyperparathyroidism with calcium, calcitriol, and/or calcimimetics. CKD is a state of PTH hyporesponsiveness, most probably caused by downregulation of the PTH receptor and competing downstream signals.

Clinical Manifestations of Bone Diseases Associated With Chronic Kidney Disease

Most patients with CKD and mildly elevated circulating levels of PTH are asymptomatic. When clinical features of bone disease are present, they can be classified into musculoskeletal and extraskeletal manifestations.

Musculoskeletal Manifestations

Fractures, bone pain, muscle pain and weakness, and periarticular pain are the major musculoskeletal manifestations associated with CKD. The most clinically significant effect of metabolic bone disease in CKD is hip fracture, which has a high incidence among CKD stage G5 patients and is associated with an increased risk for death. There is a roughly 4.4-fold increase in hip fracture risk in patients undergoing dialysis compared with the general population. Both high and low serum values of PTH are associated with increased fracture risks. Evidence from prospective cohort studies indicates that measurements of bone mineral density (BMD) may help in predicting fracture risk in CKD as in the general population. The consistency of the risk prediction across stages of disease and degree of PTH control remains unclear. FRAX, a common risk prediction algorithm commonly used in the general population, also predicts fracture probability in patients with CKD. Additional evidence is, however, required to define whether further arithmetic adjustments to conventional FRAX estimates have to be made with knowledge of advanced CKD.

Extraskeletal Manifestations

The most important advance in the understanding of the clinical significance of disordered bone and mineral metabolism in CKD has been the recognition that it is a systemic disorder affecting soft tissues, particularly blood vessels, heart valves, and skin. CVD accounts for approximately half of all deaths of patients on dialysis (see Chapter 54). Prevalence and severity of coronary and peripheral vascular calcifications increase as CKD progresses, especially after initiation of dialysis. Gaining a better understanding of the etiology of vascular calcification and how it may influence clinical cardiovascular events is of critical importance.

Several patterns of vascular calcification have been described. The first occurs as focal calcification associated with lipid-laden foam cells that are seen in atherosclerotic plaques. These calcifications may increase both the fragility and the risk for plaque rupture. Some have questioned the role of calcification in the pathogenesis of the atherosclerotic vascular lesions, raising the possibility that it is an epiphenomenon. The second pattern of vascular calcification is diffuse, is not associated with atherosclerotic plaques, and occurs in the media of vessels. This pattern is seen with aging, diabetes, and progressive kidney failure. Referred to as '*Mönckeberg sclerosis*,' this lesion was initially thought to be of little clinical significance; however, the effects of medial calcification on vascular stiffness and reduced vascular compliance, resulting in a widened pulse pressure, increased cardiac afterload, and LVH, are potential mechanisms that contribute to clinical cardiovascular disease (Fig. 53.4).

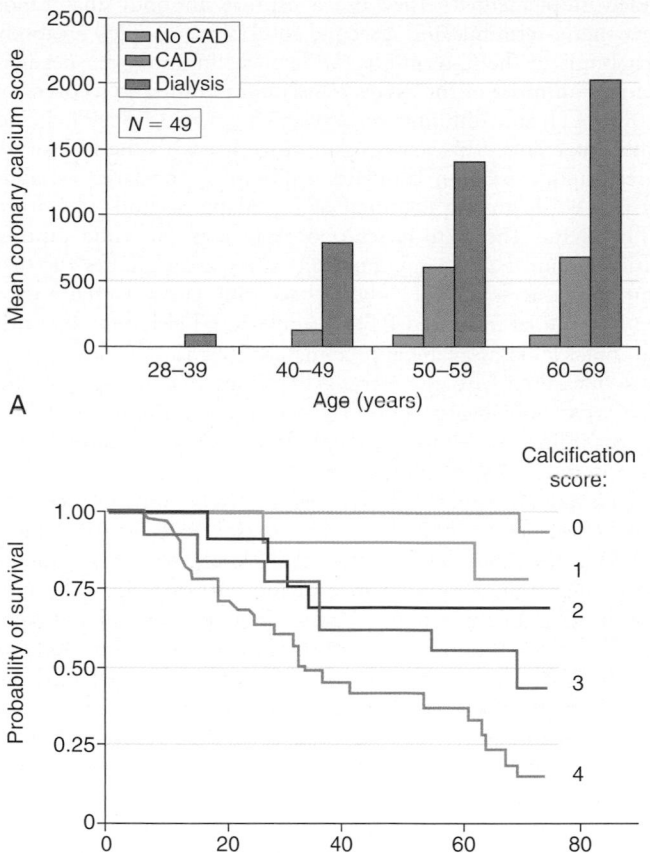

A

B

• **Fig. 53.4** Increased risk of death and cardiovascular calcification in dialysis patients. (A) Calcium score was determined by electron beam computed tomography. The mean coronary artery calcium score was significantly higher in hemodialysis patients than in nondialysis patients with documented cardiovascular disease. (B) Risk of death in patients on hemodialysis increases as a function of a calcification score measured by ultrasound (*P* < .0001 for comparisons among all curves). *CAD*, Calcium artery disease. (A from Braun J, Oldendorf M, Moshage W, et al. Electron beam computed tomography in the evaluation of cardiac calcifications in chronic dialysis patients. *Am J Kidney Dis*. 1996;27:394–401, National Kidney Foundation; B from Blacher J, Guerin AP, Pannier B, et al. Arterial calcification, arterial stiffness, and cardiovascular risk in end-stage renal disease. *Hypertension*. 2001;38:938.)

The mechanisms of vascular medial calcification probably reflect the combined effects of decreased mineralization inhibitors, such as matrix Gla protein (a vitamin K–dependent calcification inhibitor known to be expressed by smooth muscle cells and macrophages in the artery wall) and increased mineralization inducers. Vascular calcification is an active, cell-mediated process resembling osteogenesis. Accumulating evidence suggests that vascular smooth muscle cells undergo a phenotypic transition to an osteoblast-like cell that is important in driving the calcification process. Elevated serum phosphorus causes upregulation of a type III sodium-dependent phosphate cotransporter Pit-1 (POU1F1) in smooth muscle cells. The resulting increased intracellular phosphorus upregulates core binding factor alpha 1 (Cbfa1/RUNX2), a transcription factor believed to be critical in mediating this phenotypic switch to osteoblast-like cells. Concomitantly, bone matrix proteins, such as osteopontin and osteocalcin, are found only in calcified vessels.

An emerging area of study concerns how the kidney failure milieu may affect the vascular calcification process, independent of its effects on serum phosphorus. Numerous uremic toxins have been shown to initiate or accelerate vascular calcification though a multitude of mechanisms, with increased oxidative stress often playing a central role. The glycoprotein fetuin-A, which is down-regulated during the acute-phase response and is also reduced among dialysis patients, is an important inhibitor of calcification and may be associated with cardiovascular risk.

The contribution of vitamin D to vascular calcification is controversial and debated. Some studies suggest that calcitriol can modulate vascular smooth muscle growth and influence vascular calcification by upregulation of the VDR and increased calcium uptake into smooth muscle cells. Vitamin D treatment enhances the extent of arterial calcification in animals that are also given warfarin to inhibit γ-carboxylation of the matrix Gla protein. On the other hand, low doses of both calcitriol and paricalcitol seem to be protective, probably through restoration of α-Klotho and osteopontin expression. A U-shaped dose response of active vitamin D can thus be postulated with regard to vascular calcification. A consistent survival benefit of treatment with active vitamin (analogues) in patients undergoing hemodialysis has been described in several retrospective studies and a recent meta-analysis, and the benefit seemed to be more pronounced in the low-dose range. Data from a 2018 randomized, controlled trial, however, failed to confirm these findings, with investigators observing no reduction of cardiovascular events and mortality in hemodialysis patients without secondary hyperparathyroidism receiving 0.5 μg of oral alfacalcidol per day.

Calcemic Uremic Arteriolopathy

Calcemic uremic arteriolopathy (CUA), or calciphylaxis, is another form of vascular calcification that is observed primarily, although not exclusively, in CKD stage G5, likely in 1% to 4% of dialysis patients. CUA manifests with extensive calcifications of the skin, muscles, and subcutaneous tissues. Most often, skin lesions occur on the breast, abdomen, and thighs. Unusual presentations, such as necrosis of the tongue and of the penis, as well as visceral involvement of the lungs, pancreas, and intestines, have been described. Examination may not only show a violaceous rash, skin nodules, skin firmness, and eschars, but also livedo reticularis and hyperesthesia of the skin. Nonhealing ulcerations of the skin and gangrene resistant to medical therapy often lead to amputation, uncontrollable sepsis, and death. Histologically, there is extensive medial calcification of small arteries, arterioles, capillaries, and venules, as well as intimal proliferation, endovascular fibrosis, and sometimes thrombosis. Whether the molecular pathogenesis of CUA is due to medial calcification is not clear. Cases reported to be associated with very high PTH levels improved after parathyroidectomy. However, there are other cases in which the PTH levels were only mildly elevated. Interestingly, in the EVOLVE (Evaluation of Cinacalcet Therapy to Lower Cardiovascular Events) study, the use of cinacalcet in addition to standard therapy for secondary hyperparathyroidism reduced the incidence of CUA. Other risk factors for CUA are obesity, advancing age, female sex, diabetes mellitus, warfarin use, recent trauma, hypotension, and calcium ingestion. Anecdotal reports suggest that sodium thiosulfate, bisphosphonate therapy, daily hemodialysis, hyperbaric oxygen treatment, vitamin K, and normalization of serum phosphate levels may improve outcomes.

Disordered Mineral Metabolism and Mortality in Chronic Kidney Disease

Cardiovascular and all-cause mortality are high in CKD. In addition to traditional cardiovascular risk factors associated with underlying diseases leading to CKD and inflammation associated with CKD, abnormalities of bone and mineral metabolism are linked to increased mortality. In particular, hyperphosphatemia and elevated FGF23 concentrations show the most consistent and robust association with increased mortality.

Observational studies suggest that elevation of serum phosphorus is an independent risk factor for increased mortality in dialysis and advanced CKD patients, resulting in a guideline statement that recommends "lowering elevated phosphate levels toward the normal range." Some studies also advise that use of noncalcium compared with calcium-based phosphate binders to control hyperphosphatemia, leading the KDIGO 2017 guideline to "suggest restricting the dose of calcium-based phosphate binders." In addition, PTH in the 400- to 600-pg/mL range, hypercalcemia, and elevated alkaline phosphatase are associated with increased mortality in observational studies of maintenance hemodialysis patients. However, the EVOLVE study, which compared the use of cinacalcet with standard therapy with active vitamin D analogues and phosphate binders, only showed a 7% nonsignificant survival benefit.

Elevated serum FGF23 is associated with increased LVH and mortality in CKD and dialysis. The increased mortality risk is independent of concomitant hyperphosphatemia in ESRD. Of interest, in the EVOLVE study, treatment-induced reductions in serum FGF23 were found to be associated with lower rates of cardiovascular death and major cardiovascular events. Because high-dose active vitamin D analogues increase serum phosphate, calcium, and FGF23 concentrations, associative studies indicating that treatment with active vitamin D analogues impart a survival advantage need to be reexamined. Indeed, the PRIMO and OPERA studies failed to show an effect of paricalcitol on left ventricular mass in CKD patients not yet on dialysis, but demonstrated increased risk of hypercalcemia.

Diagnosis of Bone Diseases Associated with Chronic Kidney Disease

Biochemical Parameters

Full-length circulating PTH has a half-life of 2 to 4 minutes. PTH is cleaved into an inactive C-terminal fragment, an active N-terminal fragment, and inactive midregion fragments in the peripheral tissues. These PTH fragments are normally excreted by the kidney and have a prolonged half-life in kidney failure. Circulating PTH, thus, is a heterogeneous mixture of full-length hormone and fragments, with (7-84)PTH accounting for up to 50% of overall PTH. The (7-84)PTH fragment may lack biologic activity or may potentially have distinct biologic actions. It may have hypocalcemic effects in vivo, and it has been shown to inhibit osteoclastic bone resorption in vitro.

Increasingly specific immunoreactive PTH assays have been developed, and second-generation assays are currently most widely implemented. They use a capture antibody that binds near the N-terminus and a second solid phase-coupled antibody that binds to the C-terminus. Differences in antibody specificities and affinities of the assays translate into differing recovery of (1-84)PTH and differing cross-reactivity with (7-84)PTH and other fragments. This may explain, together with the lack of an agreed-upon common standard (calibrator), the large variability that exists among commercially available second-generation PTH assays. The third-generation assay uses the same capture antibody, but the detection antibody is more specific for the first four amino acids of PTH, thereby avoiding cross-reactivity with the N-terminal truncated PTH fragments. PTH levels using this bio-intact PTH assay are approximately 50% to 60% lower than those measured with the intact PTH assay. A fourth-generation PTH assay only measures nonoxidized (biologically active) PTH, but according to preliminary data offers no or very limited added value in discriminating bone turnover.

Defining the target PTH level in the setting of CKD remains a challenge. Because of end-organ hyporesponsiveness (resistance) to PTH, the recommended target PTH levels in dialysis patients are greater than the upper limit of the normal range. The previously recommended target ranges for serum intact PTH, specifically 35 to 70 pg/mL, 70 to 110 pg/mL, and 150 to 300 pg/mL for CKD stages G3, G4, and G5, respectively, reflected the progressive resistance to PTH as CKD progresses (Table 53.1). Because of the lack of standardization of PTH assays, KDIGO preferred to define the target in terms of times the upper normal limit. In dialysis patients, KDIGO suggests "maintaining intact PTH levels in the range of approximately 2 to 9 times the upper normal limit for the assay." The long-term impact of this more conservative management strategy remains to be determined. While this approach may minimize oversuppression of PTH and low-turnover bone disease, it includes the risk of undersuppression of parathyroid gland hyperplasia leading to progression of secondary to tertiary hyperparathyroidism.

PTH levels are a direct measure of parathyroid gland function and an indirect and crude measure of bone remodeling. The utility of PTH levels as an indicator of bone turnover can be increased, albeit modestly, by assessment of bone-specific alkaline phosphatase levels, which correlate with the degree of osteoblastic activity. In the absence of liver dysfunction, total alkaline phosphatase activity can be used as a surrogate. Other biochemical markers of bone turnover are being developed that may provide a more accurate assessment of osteoblast and osteoclast activity in bone in CKD, including intact procollagen type I N-propeptide for

TABLE 53.1	Kidney Disease: Improving Global Outcomes and Japanese Society of Dialysis Therapy Clinical Practice Guidelines for Bone Metabolism and Disease in Chronic Kidney Disease		
	Phosphorus (mg/dL)	Calcium (Corrected, mg/dL)	Intact PTH (pg/mL)
KDIGO	Normal range	Normal range	150–600 (2–9 × normal)
JSDT	3.5–6	8.4–10	60–180

JSDT, Japanese Society of Dialysis Therapy; *KDIGO*, Kidney Disease: Improving Global Outcomes; *PTH*, parathyroid hormone.

bone formation and tartrate-resistant acid phosphatase 5b for resorption. Defining the diagnostic accuracy of these and other biomarkers, including miRNA signatures, for bone turnover as determined by histomorphometry (gold standard) is an area of ongoing research both in dialysis and nondialysis CKD patients. Furthermore, prospective studies are required to determine whether evaluating trends in biomarker concentrations could guide therapeutic decisions.

Bone Biopsy

The gold standard for assessing and diagnosing the various types of bone disease in patients with CKD is an iliac crest bone biopsy with double tetracycline labeling. Histomorphometric analysis of the biopsy specimen includes assessment of bone and fibrosis volumes, amount of osteoid and mineralization, and number of osteoblasts and osteoclasts seen on bony surfaces. Bone biopsies should be considered in the setting of atraumatic fracture with no other clear underlying cause, suspected aluminum toxicity (although rare today) to confirm the presence of osteomalacia before chelation therapy, before parathyroidectomy in patients with severe musculoskeletal symptoms and/or hypercalcemia with intermediate (100 to 500 pg/mL) intact PTH levels, and to exclude adynamic bone disease before the initiation of antiresorptive therapy.

Imaging

In general, radiographic studies are not indicated in the diagnosis of the bone disorders associated with CKD, although certain radiographic changes can be seen (see Fig. 53.2A-C). Increased osteoblast function, especially in the setting of severe elevations of PTH, can lead to increased trabecular bone volume and accounts for the sclerotic changes that manifest as a "rugger-jersey spine" on radiography. Osteoclast-mediated bone resorption of secondary hyperparathyroidism results in cortical thinning and the classic radiographic evidence of subperiosteal, intracortical, and endosteal bone resorption. Subperiosteal erosions are best seen at the distal ends of the phalanges and clavicles and at the sacroiliac joints. Radiographically, expansile lytic lesions (brown tumors) can be seen in severe osteitis fibrosis. Pseudofractures, which appear as wide, radiolucent bands perpendicular to the bone long axis, can be seen in osteomalacia.

Osteoporosis is defined as a BMD that is at least 2.5 standard deviations lower than the mean BMD of a young adult of the same sex. Although patients with CKD typically have lower BMDs than the general population, the interpretations of dual-energy X-ray absorptiometry (DEXA) scans are complicated in secondary hyperparathyroidism because of focal areas of osteosclerosis, the presence of extraskeletal calcifications, and the variable presence of osteomalacia. Despite these limitations, DEXA BMD predicts fractures in CKD as evidenced by recent cohort studies. Current guidelines suggest BMD testing to assess fracture risk in patients with CKD stages G3a-5D with evidence of CKD-MBD and/or risk factors for osteoporosis if results will affect treatment decisions. While vertebral fracture assessment and/or lateral spine imaging may be recommended to detect asymptomatic fractures, trabecular bone score and alternative imaging techniques need further clinical evaluation before clinical implementation. Importantly, there is no accurate correlation between BMD as measured by DEXA and the type of CKD-associated bone disease present.

Treatment of Mineral and Bone Disorder in Chronic Kidney Disease

The treatment of disordered mineral metabolism in CKD is directed toward normalizing serum calcium, phosphate, PTH, and metabolic acidosis while minimizing the risks associated with therapies. In the United States, the types of treatments chosen for dialysis patients are influenced by the bundled payment system that limits the frequency of hemodialysis in most patients to three treatments per week and includes calcimimetics and vitamin D analogues in the dialysis payment bundle. Clinical practice guidelines for bone metabolism and disease in CKD have been developed by several organizations and are outlined in Table 53.1.

These recommendations are influenced by observational data linking an elevated serum phosphorus concentration or an elevated calcium concentration to increased mortality, and by the growing concern that excessive calcium exposure may increase the risk of cardiovascular calcification. Of note, there are no clinical trial data demonstrating that any current treatments available for CKD-MBD reduce mortality, and achieving these targets with current treatment regimens is difficult. Nonetheless, these guidelines are a first step toward standardizing the approach to this difficult disorder.

The various tools for treating hyperphosphatemia and secondary hyperparathyroidism include dietary phosphorus restriction, calcium-based and noncalcium-based phosphate binders, calcitriol or other active vitamin D analogues, calcimimetic agents, daily or nocturnal hemodialysis, and parathyroidectomy.

Controlling Serum Phosphorus

Dietary phosphorus restriction (800 to 1000 mg/day) is difficult to attain but should be initiated for all subjects with CKD stage G5 (see Chapter 52). There are three major sources of exogenous phosphorus to be considered: natural phosphate (as cellular and protein constituents) contained in raw or unprocessed foods, phosphate added to foods during processing (daily exposure may be as high as 1000 mg), and phosphate in dietary supplements and medications. For patients who are undergoing thrice-weekly dialysis and are receiving adequate nutrition, dietary phosphate restriction usually will be inadequate to correct the positive phosphate balance, especially in the presence of concurrent active vitamin D therapy, which increases phosphorus absorption from the gut. More frequent and prolonged hemodialysis and hemodiafiltration (see Chapter 56) are associated with lower serum phosphorus levels, but with conventional thrice-weekly hemodialysis, phosphate binders are typically needed.

The choice of phosphate binder (i.e., calcium containing vs. noncalcium containing) depends on many considerations, including the binder's efficacy, side effects, and cost. For many years, calcium-based phosphate binders were the mainstay of therapy to control serum phosphate levels. Commonly used calcium-based phosphate binders include calcium carbonate and calcium acetate. Calcium carbonate contains 500 mg of elemental calcium in a 1250-mg tablet (40%), whereas calcium acetate contains 169 mg of elemental calcium in one 667-mg tablet (25%). Calcium-based phosphate binders should be taken with meals to maximize binding of ingested phosphorus in the gut. When they are taken in the fasting state, more calcium is absorbed systemically and less phosphorus is bound. The concomitant use of active vitamin D sterols increases calcium absorption and the risk of hypercalcemia. The recent KDIGO update cautions against excessive intake of calcium without defining a specific safe limit. Calcium acetate has greater phosphorus-binding capacity than calcium carbonate, potentially allowing the use of lower doses of calcium binder. However, various small trials have not shown significant differences in the prevalence of hypercalcemia between these two compounds.

Vascular calcification has been documented by electron beam computed tomography in the coronary arteries of dialysis patients before 30 years of age. This, taken with growing concern about the possible clinical consequences of vascular calcifications, has led to the greater use of noncalcium binders. Sevelamer is a noncalcium phosphate binder containing cross-linked polyallylamine hydrochloride. It acts as an ion exchange polymer to bind phosphorus in the gut but is less effective than calcium on a weight basis. However, in human trials, sevelamer, when titrated to meet serum phosphorus goals, appeared equal in efficacy to the calcium-containing binders. Sevelamer also has a cholestyramine-like effect, decreasing serum total and low-density lipoprotein cholesterol in CKD stage G5 patients. Sevelamer is associated with fewer arterial calcifications than calcium-based phosphate binders in dialysis patients, but is more costly than calcium binders and may be associated with gastrointestinal side effects at higher doses, potentially limiting its use in some individuals. In addition, sevelamer may exacerbate vitamin K deficiency.

The effect of sevelamer on cardiovascular mortality remains a critical question. Prospective trials comparing the effect of sevelamer versus calcium-containing phosphate binders on mortality produced equivocal results. One small, randomized trial with 127 incident hemodialysis patients monitored for a mean of 44 months demonstrated a significant overall survival advantage for sevelamer, although specific cardiovascular mortality was not assessed. The larger, open-labeled Dialysis Clinical Outcomes Revisited (DCOR) trial, which randomly assigned 2103 patients to either sevelamer or calcium-containing binders with a mean follow-up of 20.3 months, failed to show a difference in cardiovascular mortality between the two groups. In subgroup analysis of the DCOR results, patients older than 65 years who were treated with sevelamer had a lower all-cause mortality but not lower cardiovascular mortality. In addition, patients who remained in the study for longer than 2 years on treatment with sevelamer had a decrease in all-cause mortality. The short duration of follow-up, the high dropout rate, and the fact that the study was not powered statistically to detect differences in specific causes of death are limitations of this study. More recently, significant survival benefits were demonstrated for patients treated with sevelamer versus calcium-containing binders in a multicenter Italian study (INDEPENDENT Study). This study suffers, however, from a moderate risk of bias and, therefore, should be interpreted with caution. Together with data from formal calcium balance studies, this new evidence supported a more general recommendation to restrict calcium-based phosphate binders in hyperphosphatemic patients of all CKD stages.

Although they are the most effective binders, aluminum-containing phosphate binders are not often used because of the potential for systemic aluminum absorption and subsequent neurologic, hematologic, and bone toxicity. Absorption of aluminum is increased by the concomitant use of sodium citrate for metabolic acidosis. Because of the potential for long-term toxicity, aluminum-containing antacids should be used only for a short period (<4 weeks) and only for severe hyperphosphatemia that is refractory to other treatments.

Another noncalcium-based phosphate binder is lanthanum carbonate. Lanthanum, like aluminum, is a trivalent cation with an ability to chelate dietary phosphate and low systemic absorption. Mild gastrointestinal symptoms were the most common side effect in the lanthanum group. Lanthanum, unlike sevelamer, is an effective binder even in the acidic environment of the gut and does not bind bile acids. Adherence may be better than with calcium-based binders or sevelamer as a result of a lower pill burden. Because there is accumulation of small amounts of lanthanum over time, safety concerns have been raised. However, it is reassuring that, after more than 850,000 person-years of worldwide patient exposure, there is no evidence that lanthanum is associated with adverse safety outcomes in patients with ESRD.

An increasing body of experimental and clinical evidence linking magnesium to improved (cardiovascular) outcomes has revived interest in magnesium-containing phosphate binders. Most recently, sucroferric oxyhydroxide and ferric citrate have become available on the market. These phosphate binders have promising results with regard to biochemical endpoints. Data on patient-centered outcomes are limited. In a small, randomized, controlled trial in patients with advanced CKD, ferric citrate treatment resulted in significantly fewer annualized hospital admissions, fewer days in hospital, and a lower incidence of the composite end point of death, provision of dialysis, or transplantation. The armamentarium to lower the phosphate continues to expand, with other phosphate binders and drugs targeting intestinal phosphate transport approaching clinical use.

Activating the Calcium-Sensing and Vitamin D Receptors to Suppress Parathyroid Hormone

Secondary hyperparathyroidism is a common complication of CKD that, if left untreated, may result in considerable morbidity and mortality. Current guidelines suggest to maintain PTH levels in the range of approximately 2 to 9 times the upper normal limit of the assay. Overall, there is no consensus on what should be the first-line treatment option to correct secondary hyperparathyroidism in CKD stage G5D patients: calcimimetics, calcitriol, or vitamin D analogues; a combination of calcimimetics and calcitriol; or vitamin D analogues. The individual choice should be guided by considerations about concomitant therapies, availability, and the serum calcium and phosphate levels.

Vitamin D Analogues

Treatment with $1,25-(OH_2)D_3$ (calcitriol) or an active vitamin D analogue (paricalcitol, doxercalciferol, alfacalcidol, or 22-oxacalcitol) is a means of controlling secondary hyperparathyroidism. By binding to the VDR on parathyroid tissues, the vitamin D analogue suppresses PTH production. There is no uniform agreement about the route, dose, or type of active vitamin D analogue that should be given. Some of the available vitamin D analogues may cause less hypercalcemia than calcitriol, possibly because of decreased intestinal effect on calcium absorption. The "second-generation" analogue paricalcitol has generated interest because studies suggest that it leads to less elevation of serum calcium and phosphorus, as well as a greater PTH suppression, than calcitriol. When paricalcitol was compared with calcitriol in a large observational study of hemodialysis patients, its use was associated with significantly lower mortality. Although this study initially raised questions about the extent to which efforts to control secondary hyperparathyroidism with vitamin D analogues might cause harm, subsequent retrospective studies suggested improved survival in dialysis patients treated with active vitamin D analogues compared with patients who did not receive vitamin D at all. However, a recent analysis of a large international dialysis database supported the possibility that the effect of vitamin D may represent a patient selection bias. Prospective clinical trials are needed to determine whether vitamin D therapy offers a survival advantage in dialysis patients. At least in hemodialysis patients with controlled secondary hyperparathyroidism, calcitriol (0.5 µg with dialysis) offers no survival benefit.

Calcitriol and vitamin D analogues can be administered intravenously and orally. Equipotent intravenous doses of calcitriol, paricalcitol, and doxercalciferol for PTH suppression are approximately 0.5, 2.5, and 5.0 µg, respectively, for PTH suppression. While it remains to be established which approach is most effective in lowering serum PTH and reducing toxicity, oral administration is gaining rapid popularity. Of note, in Europe, the oral route has been the preferential route of administration for years.

CKD stage G5 patients whose PTH levels drop to less than 2 times the upper normal limit for the assay during treatment for secondary hyperparathyroidism should have a reduction in their active vitamin D analogue or phosphate binders.

Current guidelines suggest to correct vitamin D deficiency and insufficiency, defined by $25(OH)D_3$ levels below 20 and 30 ng/mL, respectively, with treatment strategies recommended for the general population. Clinical evidence in favor of vitamin D supplementation is limited. In a double-blind, placebo-controlled, randomized, controlled trial, 6 months of supplementation with ergocalciferol increased serum 25(OH)D levels in patients on hemodialysis with vitamin D insufficiency or deficiency but had no effect on erythropoietin utilization or secondary biochemical and clinical outcomes. Vitamin D supplementation may improve vascular health, but optimal thresholds for vitamin D replacement and preferred formulations and doses remain ill defined. Negative results from a recent, large, randomized, controlled trial in the general population may dampen enthusiasm to supplement nutritional vitamin D, but should be interpreted cautiously as vitamin D stores were sufficient in more than half of participants at enrollment.

Since the cost and risk of adverse side effects of nutritional vitamin D supplementation are small, and given the potential beneficial effects of 25(OH)D on innate immunity and other cellular functions, hormonal replacement therapy in patients with low circulating 25(OH)D levels may still be warranted pending further evidence.

Calcimimetics

Calcimimetics offer a novel approach for treating secondary hyperparathyroidism without using active vitamin D analogues or raising serum calcium levels. Calcimimetics are CaSR agonists that act on the parathyroid gland by allosterically increasing the sensitivity of the receptor to calcium. Cinacalcet, the first available drug of this group, was approved by the US Food and Drug Administration (FDA) in 2004 to treat secondary hyperparathyroidism in patients with CKD stage G5. Treatment with cinacalcet causes significant decreases in PTH without elevating serum calcium or phosphorus concentrations (Fig. 53.5). In fact, there is usually a reduction in serum calcium and a tendency toward reduced serum phosphorus with calcimimetics. In one study, the use of cinacalcet resulted in approximately 41% of patients attaining the PTH and calcium-phosphorus product goals recommended by the K/DOQI guidelines at the time, compared with fewer than 10% achieving these targets in the group treated with

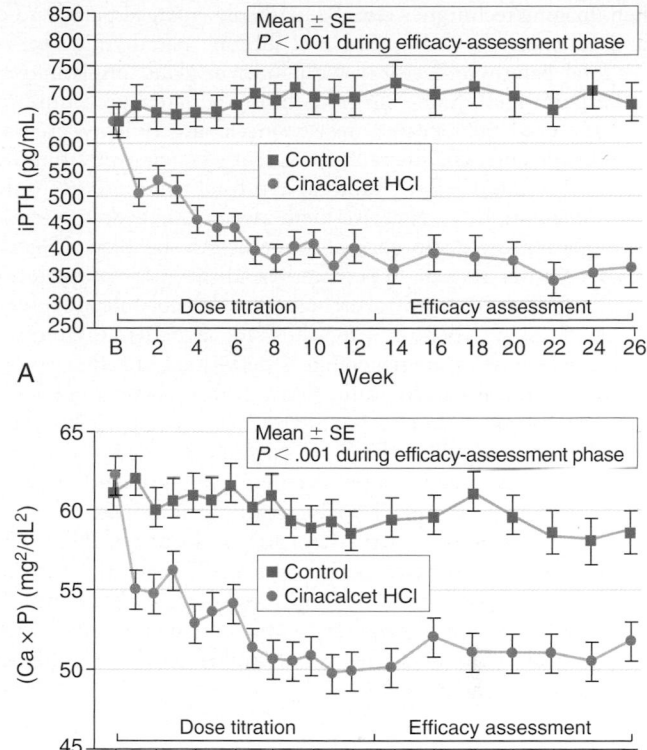

• **Fig. 53.5** Suppression of serum parathyroid hormone levels (A) by cinacalcet without elevation of the serum calcium-phosphorus product and (B) in patients on hemodialysis with secondary hyperparathyroidism not adequately controlled by treatment with phosphate binders and vitamin D analogues. *HCl,* Hydrochloride; *iPTH,* intact parathyroid hormone; *SE,* standard error. (From Block GA, Martin KJ, de Francisco AL, et al. Cinacalcet for secondary hyperparathyroidism in patients receiving hemodialysis. *N Engl J Med.* 2004;350:1516–1525.)

phosphate binders and vitamin D analogues alone. Additional studies are needed to evaluate the effect of cinacalcet in altering the natural history of parathyroid gland hyperplasia. Prospective trials examining the impact of lowering the calcium-phosphorus product with calcimimetics in combination with active vitamin analogues, however, did not reduce vascular calcifications. The EVOLVE study also failed to meet its primary endpoint that cinacalcet reduces the risk of death or clinically important vascular events in CKD stage G5D patients. However, the results of secondary analyses suggest that cinacalcet may yet be beneficial in this population or a subset. These studies reflect the difficulty in demonstrating survival benefits from interventions directed at correcting (individual) abnormalities of mineral metabolism in CKD.

Most recently, another calcimimetic, etelcalcetide, has been approved by FDA and European Medicines Agency (EMA). This intravenous calcimimetic proved to be superior to cinacalcet in reducing serum PTH concentration among patients receiving hemodialysis with moderate to severe secondary hyperparathyroidism. Intermediate or hard endpoint clinical trials with etelcalcetide are currently lacking.

Parathyroidectomy

As a remaining option for patients with uncontrolled hyperparathyroidism, parathyroidectomy should be considered, especially when imaging techniques reveal a markedly enlarged parathyroid gland (diameter > 1 cm). Either a subtotal parathyroidectomy or a total parathyroidectomy with forearm gland implantation can be performed. Some surgeons favor the latter procedure to avoid the need for repeated invasive neck surgery if hyperparathyroidism recurs. Glands can subsequently be removed from the forearm if necessary. Both subtotal and total parathyroidectomy with implantation are effective methods, and there are no studies comparing these approaches. Nonetheless, there is a 15% to 30% recurrence rate of hyperparathyroidism after complete or partial parathyroidectomy. Percutaneous ethanol injection into the gland as an ablation procedure for hyperparathyroidism refractory to medical management is performed in some centers in lieu of surgical parathyroidectomy. *Hungry bone syndrome* is a frequent complication of parathyroidectomy, especially when markedly elevated PTH values are acutely reduced. This syndrome is characterized by hypocalcemia, hypophosphatemia, and hypomagnesemia secondary to increased bone uptake of these three ions after removal of the resorptive influence of PTH. For unclear reasons, hyperkalemia is occasionally seen. If severe or symptomatic hypocalcemia develops, treatment with a continuous calcium infusion is necessary. Concomitant treatment with oral calcitriol before and after parathyroidectomy may mitigate the hungry bone syndrome.

Chronic Kidney Disease Stages G3 and G4

Treatment of patients with CKD stages G3 and G4 has not been well studied; however, the early development of parathyroid gland hyperplasia caused by chronic stimulation suggests that treatment should focus on prevention of parathyroid gland hyperplasia. Phosphate restriction and calcium supplementation are the mainstays of treatment in CKD stages G3 and G4, with phosphate binders sometimes also needed to lower serum phosphorus toward the normal range. Metabolic acidosis causes an efflux of calcium from bone as bone buffers hydrogen ions with carbonate release. Chronic metabolic acidosis should also be addressed.

CKD patients are at increased risk for low levels of 25-hydroxyvitamin D for several potential reasons, including lack of sunlight if chronically ill or bedridden, poor oral intake of foods containing vitamin D, lower skin production of vitamin D_3 in elderly patients secondary to lower skin content of 7-dehydrocholesterol, and the presence of nephrotic syndrome causing loss of 25-hydroxyvitamin D and vitamin D–binding protein in the urine. Although the level of 25-hydroxyvitamin D in CKD that is diagnostic of hypovitaminosis D has not been firmly established, levels less than 30 ng/mL are associated with rising PTH levels. CKD stages G3 and G4 patients with vitamin D levels lower than 30 ng/mL should be supplemented with ergocalciferol (vitamin D_2) or cholecalciferol (vitamin D_3). In patients without CKD, correction of vitamin D deficiency increases BMD and decreases the incidence of fractures.

The need for and timing of therapy with active vitamin D analogues in CKD stages G3 and G4 have not been firmly established. The demonstration of a significantly increased risk of hypercalcemia in patients treated with paricalcitol compared with placebo, in the absence of beneficial effects on surrogate cardiac endpoints (PRIMO and OPERA study), combined with the opinion that moderate PTH elevations may represent an appropriate adaptive response, urged KDIGO to recommend a more restricted use of active vitamin D (analogues) in the setting of predialysis CKD. In the revised guidelines, it is stated that the use of calcitriol or

vitamin D analogs in patients with CKD stages 4G to 5G should be reserved for only severe and progressive secondary hyperparathyroidism.

Cinacalcet has not been well studied in patients with CKD stages 3G and 4G and is not approved by the FDA for these patients. Of note, the suppression of PTH in predialysis CKD patients goes along with an undesired increase of serum phosphate levels.

Osteoporosis

The management of osteoporosis in patients with CKD stages G1-G3 is the same as for the general population, as long as there are no biochemical abnormalities suggesting the presence of CKD-MBD. Bisphosphonates and denosumab, the most commonly used anti-osteoporosis drugs in the general population, are poorly studied in the setting of advanced CKD (stages G4-G5D), and, at present, are not widely prescribed in this setting mainly because of doubts about their efficacy and concerns about their safety. Evolving evidence, however, suggests that antiresorptive agents may be effective in advanced CKD and that vascular and skeletal risks are not excessively high. Kidney risks of bisphosphonates are poorly explored in patients with CKD stages G4-G5D and call for caution. Denosumab has no risk of worsening CKD, but the risk of severe hypocalcemia with denosumab is increased in CKD and needs to be addressed by concomitant vitamin D and calcium supplementation. Withdrawal of denosumab therapy may be associated with an increased risk of vertebral fracture rate. At all times, risks and benefits of available pharmacologic interventions need to be balanced at the individual level and discussed with the patient. Formal, informed consent may be required when considering off-label use.

Kidney Transplantation

The bony changes of secondary hyperparathyroidism improve after transplantation; however, in patients with severe hyperparathyroidism before transplantation, elevated serum levels of PTH can persist for as long as 10 years. The incidence of parathyroidectomy remains high after kidney transplantation, probably reflecting the irreversible hyperplasia of parathyroid tissue that occurs during the course of CKD. It is not uncommon for patients to develop hypophosphatemia after kidney transplantation. This reduction in serum phosphorus may be mediated by persistent hyperparathyroidism and by other variables unrelated to PTH, such as increased levels of FGF23 that also reduce tubular reabsorption of phosphate. Typically, phosphate supplementation is reserved for severe hypophosphatemia (<1.5 mg/dL). More aggressive use of phosphate supplementation may exacerbate secondary hyperparathyroidism. Transplantation also prevents, but does not reverse, bone damage from amyloidosis caused by β_2M deposition. Symptoms of amyloidosis frequently abate after transplantation, perhaps because of concomitant steroid therapy.

Although successful kidney transplantation corrects many of the conditions that lead to disordered mineral metabolism associated with kidney failure, the glucocorticoids used to prevent rejection result in increased bone fragility, osteoporosis, and increased fracture rates. Other risk factors for fractures in this population include the presence of pretransplantation fracture, diabetes mellitus, vitamin K deficiency, and older age. In fact, the risk of fractures is greater in kidney transplant recipients than in patients on dialysis, at least in the first years after transplantation. While older studies demonstrated significant BMD loss, often exceeding 5% during the first year after transplantation, more recent cohort studies reported no or only minimal losses. Steroid minimization most probably accounts, to a large extent, for this favorable trend. DEXA scans have been recommended in kidney transplant patients at the time of transplantation and then yearly, at least for the next several years. Mounting evidence indicates that low BMD by DEXA correlates with increased fracture risk in kidney transplant recipients, as in CKD patients and the general population. Calcium and vitamin D supplementation may be effective in counteracting the effects of glucocorticoids to reduce gastrointestinal calcium absorption. Studies have shown that calcium supplementation used with active vitamin D compounds preserves BMD at least early in the posttransplant period, but data showing that such treatment reduces fracture incidence are lacking. Bisphosphonates and denosumab appear to decrease the rate of bone loss as measured by BMD. However, given the concern for antiresorptive treatment-induced adynamic bone disease in this population and the lack of data on reduced facture incidence with this approach, there are currently no consensus recommendations on the use of this therapy in kidney recipients. Decisions should be individualized, and caution should be maintained.

Avascular necrosis is another complication of kidney transplantation. It most typically occurs in the femoral heads or other weight-bearing joints and is characterized by the collapse of surface bone and cartilage. The pathogenesis of this disorder is not clear, but it is probably related to corticosteroid therapy. Magnetic resonance imaging is the most sensitive technique to evaluate patients with hip pain after transplantation for the presence of avascular necrosis. Surgical therapies include core decompression and hip replacement.

Complete bibliography is available at Elsevier eBooks for Practicing Clinicians.

Key Bibliography

Block GA, Klassen PS, Lazarus JM, et al. Mineral metabolism, mortality, and morbidity in maintenance hemodialysis. *J Am Soc Nephrol.* 2004;15:2208–2218.

Block GA, Martin KJ, de Francisco AL, et al. Cinacalcet for secondary hyperparathyroidism in patients receiving hemodialysis. *N Engl J Med.* 2004;350:1516–1525.

Block GA, Raggi P, Bellasi A, et al. Mortality effect of coronary calcification and phosphate binder choice in incident hemodialysis patients. *Kidney Int.* 2007;71:438–441.

Brown EM, Gamba G, Riccardi D, et al. Cloning and characterization of an extracellular Ca^{2+}-sensing receptor from bovine parathyroid. *Nature.* 1993;366:575–580.

Chertow GM, Burke SK, Raggi P, et al. Sevelamer attenuates the progression of coronary and aortic calcification in hemodialysis patients. *Kidney Int.* 2002;62:245–252.

D'Haese PC, Spasovski GB. A multicenter study on the effects of lanthanum carbonate (Fosrenol) and calcium carbonate on renal bone disease in dialysis patients. *Kidney Int.* 2003;85:S73–S78.

Evenepoel P, Cunningham J, Ferrari S, et al.; European Renal Osteodystrophy (EUROD) workgroup, an initiative of the CKD-MBD working group of the ERA-EDTA, and the committee of Scientific Advisors and National Societies of the IOF. European Consensus Statement on the diagnosis and management of osteoporosis in chronic kidney disease stages G4-G5D. *Nephrol Dial Transplant.* 36(1):42–59. doi:10.1093/ndt/gfaa192.

Faul C, Amaral AP, Oskouei B, et al. FGF23 induces left ventricular hypertrophy. *J Clin Invest.* 2011;121:4393–4408.

Gutierrez OM, Mannstadt M, Isakova T, et al. Fibroblastic growth factor 23 and mortality among patients undergoing hemodialysis. *N Engl J Med.* 2008;359:584–592.

J-DAVID Investigators; Shoji T, Inaba M, Fukagawa M, et al. Effect of oral alfacalcidol on clinical outcomes in patients without secondary hyperparathyroidism receiving maintenance hemodialysis: the J-DAVID randomized clinical trial. *JAMA.* 2018;320(22):2325–2334. doi:10.1001/jama.2018.17749.

Kidney Disease: Improving Global Outcomes (KDIGO) CKD-MBD Work Group. KDIGO clinical practice guideline for the diagnosis, evaluation, prevention, and treatment of chronic kidney disease-mineral and bone disorder (CKD-MBD). *Kidney Int Suppl.* 2009;(113):S1–S130. doi:10.1038/ki.2009.188.

Kidney Disease: Improving Global Outcomes (KDIGO) CKD-MBD Update Work Group. KDIGO 2017 clinical practice guideline update for the diagnosis, evaluation, prevention, and treatment of chronic kidney disease–mineral and bone disorder (CKD-MBD). *Kidney Int Suppl.*, 2017;7:1–59.

Malluche HH, Mawad HW, Monier-Faugere MC. Renal osteodystrophy in the first decade of the new millennium: analysis of 630 bone biopsies in black and white patients. *J Bone Miner Res.* 2011;26:1368–1376.

Manson JE, Cook NR, Lee IM, et al. Vitamin D supplements and prevention of cancer and cardiovascular disease. *N Engl J Med.* 2019;380(1):33–44.

Nigwekar SU, Thadhani R, Brandenburg VM. Calciphylaxis. *N Engl J Med.* 2018;378(18):1704–1714. doi:10.1056/NEJMra1505292.

Raggi P, Chertow GM, Torres PU, et al. The Advance study: a randomized study to evaluate the effects of cinacalcet plus low-dose vitamin D on vascular calcifications in patients on hemodialysis. *Nephrol Dial Transplant.* 2011;26:1327–1339.

Sugarman JR, Frederick PR, Frankenfield DL, et al. Developing clinical performance measures based on the Dialysis Outcomes Quality Initiative Clinical Practice Guidelines: process, outcomes and implications. *Am J Kidney Dis.* 2003;42:806–812.

Suki WN, Zabaneh R, Cangiano JL, et al. Effects of sevelamer and calcium-based phosphate binders on mortality in hemodialysis patients. *Kidney Int.* 2007;72:1130–1137.

Teng M, Wolf M, Lowrie E, et al. Survival of patients undergoing hemodialysis with paricalcitol or calcitriol therapy. *N Engl J Med.* 2003;349:446–456.

Thadhani R, Appelbaum E, Pritchett Y, et al. Vitamin D therapy and cardiac structure and function in patients with chronic kidney disease: the PRIMO randomized controlled trial. *JAMA.* 2012;307:674–684.

The EVOLVE Trial Investigators. Effect of cinacalcet on cardiovascular disease in patients undergoing dialysis. *N Engl J Med.* 2012;367:2482–2494.

Weisinger JR, Carlini RG, Rojas E, et al. Bone disease after renal transplantation. *Clin J Am Soc Nephrol.* 2006;6:1300–1313.

54

Cardiac Function and Cardiovascular Disease in Chronic Kidney Disease

DANIEL E. WEINER, MARK J. SARNAK

Cardiovascular disease is the leading cause of death across the spectrum of chronic kidney disease (CKD), with increased risk seen in individuals with reduced glomerular filtration rate (GFR) and in those with even minimally elevated urine albumin excretion. There is a high incidence and prevalence of atherosclerotic disease and nonatherosclerotic disease, ischemic heart disease, heart failure and left ventricular hypertrophy (LVH), valvular diseases, and arrhythmia in individuals with CKD, with prevalence increasing as GFR declines, and the interplay among these contributes to heightened overall cardiovascular disease risk among those with CKD. The risk of cardiovascular disease outcomes increases as kidney function declines, with the risk of cardiovascular death in patients undergoing dialysis 10 to 20 times that of the general population. This chapter focuses largely on individuals with reduced GFR, acknowledging that albuminuria both identifies individuals with CKD and is a very strong predictor of cardiovascular disease risk at all levels of kidney function, including individuals with CKD stages G1 through G3a where metabolic sequelae of reduced GFR are not yet clinically apparent.

Epidemiology of Cardiovascular Disease in Chronic Kidney Disease

Chronic Kidney Disease Stages G3 to G4

Manifesting with cardiac ischemia, heart failure, and arrhythmia, cardiovascular disease is overwhelmingly the leading cause of morbidity and mortality in individuals with CKD. Among individuals with reduced GFR, there is a progressive increase in the age-standardized incidence of cardiovascular disease events as kidney function declines, such that, compared with an age-standardized baseline rate of 21 cardiovascular events per 1000 person-years in individuals with estimated glomerular filtration rate (eGFR) greater than 60 mL/min/1.73 m², rates increase to 37, 113, 218, and 366 events per 1000 person-years among people with eGFR of 45 to 59 (CKD stage G3a), 30 to 44 (CKD stage G3b), 15 to 29 (CKD stage G4), and less than 15 mL/min/1.73 m² (CKD stage G5), respectively. Even in analyses that adjust for demographic factors as well as cardiovascular risk factors such as diabetes, hypertension, albuminuria, and dyslipidemia, the risk of cardiovascular death is dramatically increased at lower GFR levels (Fig. 54.1).

The risk relationship between eGFR and cardiovascular disease events is independent of a person having preexisting cardiovascular disease.

These associations also are seen in individuals with functioning kidney transplants. Among kidney transplant recipients, each 5 mL/min/1.73 m² higher eGFR at levels below 45 mL/min/1.73 m² is independently associated with a 15% lower risk of both CVD. Similarly, the presence of albuminuria, independent of the eGFR level, is also associated with a higher risk of cardiovascular disease events among kidney transplant recipients.

The prevalence of cardiovascular disease in people with CKD is similarly high. Using Medicare data from the United States, after adjustment for age, sex, and race, CVD was present in 37.5% of patients without CKD compared with 63% of patients with diagnostic codes for CKD stages G1-G2 CKD, 67% of patients with CKD stage G3, and 75% of patients with CKD stages G4-G5 (Fig. 54.2). Critically, both reduced eGFR and moderately increased albuminuria with preserved eGFR (urine albumin-to-creatinine ratio [UACR] 30 to 300 mg/g, indicating CKD stages G1 to G2) are independently associated with prevalent cardiovascular disease.

Cardiovascular disease may be subclinical in CKD populations; in Chronic Renal Insufficiency Cohort (CRIC) participants undergoing cardiac computed tomography, there was a graded increased risk of coronary artery calcification (CAC) with both lower eGFR and higher levels of albuminuria, even in individuals with no known history of cardiovascular disease, although the utility of CAC for identifying an atherosclerotic process in advanced CKD is uncertain. Similarly, in the elderly, the frequency of advanced atherosclerotic lesions on autopsy specimens increased as eGFR decreased (33.6% for eGFR ≥60 mL/min/1.73 m², 41.7% for CKD stage G3a, 52.3% for CKD stage G3b, and 52.8% for CKD stage G4).

Vascular calcification likely has an important role in the pathogenesis of cardiovascular disease in people with CKD, with medial calcification increasingly prevalent in large arteries as GFR declines, although, even in individuals with longstanding kidney failure, it appears unusual to have medial coronary artery calcification. Medial calcification is particularly common in individuals with CKD and diabetes, and results in a process distinct from typical atherosclerotic mechanisms of vascular disease. Calcification likely reflects the interplay of multiple factors, including a procalcific milieu due to hyperphosphatemia and other factors as well

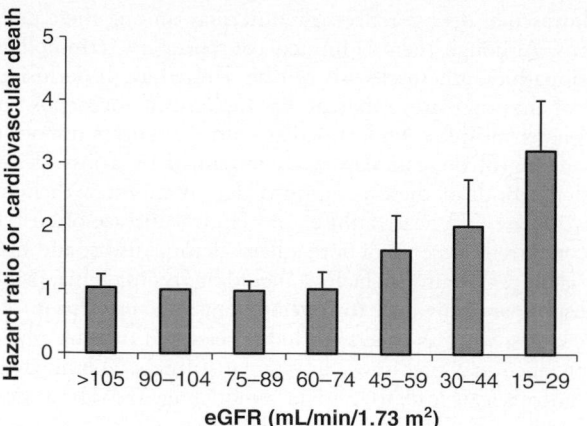

• **Fig. 54.1** Hazard ratios for cardiovascular events according to the baseline estimated glomerular filtration rate (eGFR). Adjusted for age, sex, race, cardiovascular disease history, smoking status, diabetes mellitus, systolic blood pressure, serum total cholesterol, and urine albumin-to-creatinine ratio. (Plotted with data from van der Velde M, Matsushita K, Coresh J, et al. Lower estimated glomerular filtration rate and higher albuminuria are associated with all-cause and cardiovascular mortality. A collaborative meta-analysis of high-risk population cohorts. *Kidney Int.* 2011;79:1341–1352.)

respectively. These findings contrast with a prevalence of LVH of less than 20% in older adults in the general population.

Both incident and prevalent heart failure are common in people with CKD. Among adult members of a large group-model health maintenance organization in the northwestern United States, 6.0% of individuals with predominantly early CKD stage G3 had a diagnostic code for heart failure versus 1.8% in an age- and sex-matched population, while, in the Atherosclerosis Risk in Communities (ARIC) study, individuals with eGFR less than 60 mL/min/1.73 m^2 at baseline were at twice the risk of incident heart failure hospitalization and death compared with those with eGFR of ≥90 mL/min/1.73 m^2, regardless of the presence of baseline coronary disease.

Other structural heart diseases seen commonly in CKD include aortic valve, mitral valve, and mitral annular calcification. Mitral valve or mitral annular calcification was present in 20% of individuals with reduced kidney function (roughly CKD stage G3 to G4) in the Framingham Offspring Study. In CRIC, lower eGFR was strongly associated with increased likelihood of mitral annular calcification, with risk increased by 50%, 130%, 226%, and 278% for eGFR categories 50 to 60, 40 to 50, 30 to 40, and less than 30 mL/min/1.73 m^2, respectively, when compared with eGFR

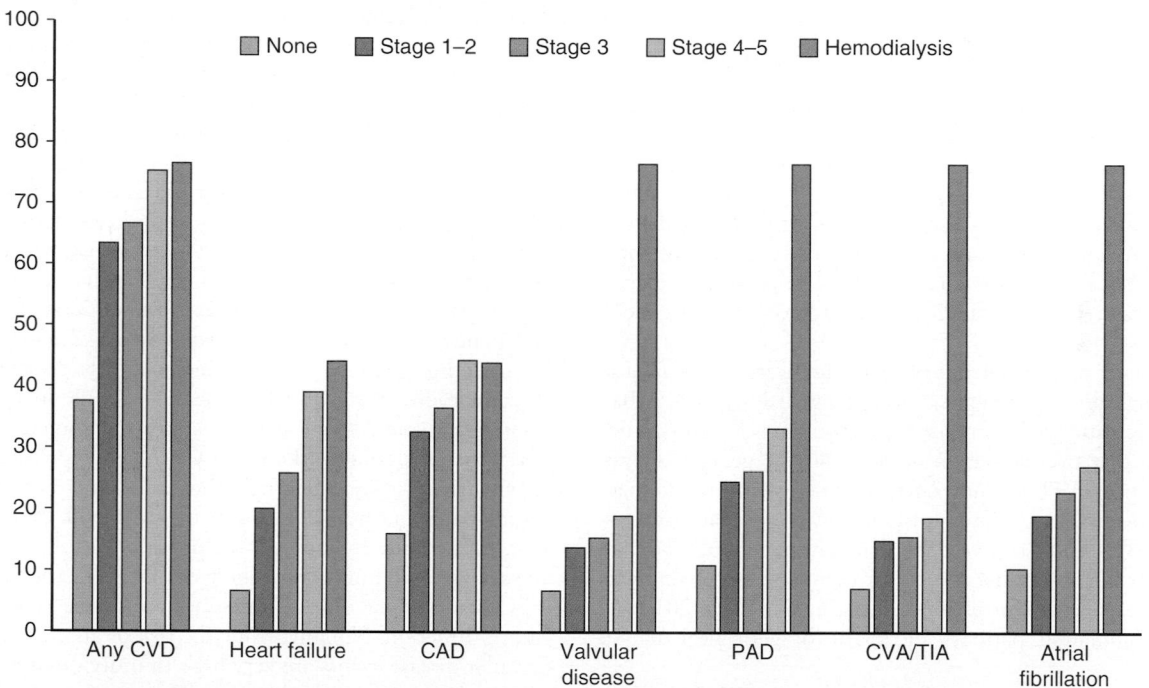

• **Fig. 54.2** Age-, sex-, and race-adjusted prevalence of cardiovascular disease (*CVD*) and its subtypes in individuals with chronic kidney disease (CKD). *CAD,* Coronary artery disease; *CVA,* cerebrovascular accident; *PAD,* peripheral artery disease; *TIA,* transient ischemic attack. (Data from the USRDS 2020 Annual Data Report, Volume 1, Chapter 4 and Volume 2, Chapter 8. https://adr.usrds.org/2020/chronic-kidney-disease/4-cardiovascular-disease-in-patients-with-ckd. Accessed January 19, 2021.)

as lower levels of calcification inhibitors, such as γ-carboxylated matrix gla protein and fetuin-A. This is discussed further in Chapter 53.

LVH is also common in CKD stages G3 and G4, likely reflecting pressure and volume overload. In CRIC, the prevalence of LVH assessed by echocardiography was 32% for eGFR above 60 mL/min/1.73 m^2, rising to 48%, 57%, and 75% for eGFR categories 45 to 59, 30 to 44, and less than 30 mL/min/1.73 m^2,

≥60 mL/min/1.73 m^2. Similar results were seen from a large echocardiography database from Duke, where mitral annular calcification was present in 24% of individuals with eGFR below 30 mL/min/1.73 m^2. The Framingham Heart Study and other studies also show a high prevalence of aortic valve calcification in individuals with CKD, with CRIC demonstrating a "dose-dependent" association between lower eGFR and greater aortic valve calcification that was independent of traditional cardiovascular risk factors.

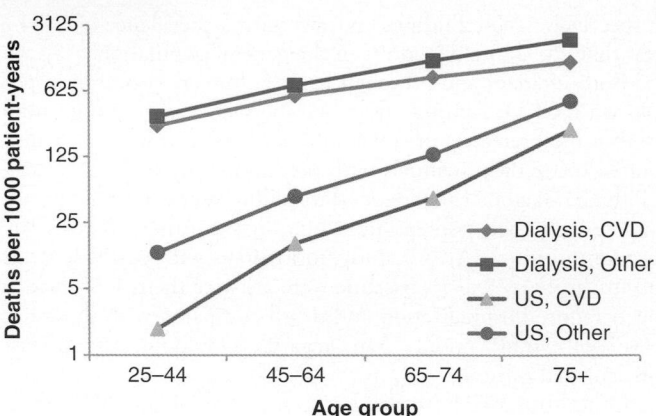

• Fig. 54.3 Cardiovascular disease and noncardiovascular disease mortality in the general United States (US) population (2014) compared with patients with chronic kidney failure treated by dialysis (2012–2014). Cardiovascular disease (CVD) death in the US population includes "Diseases of the heart" (I00–I09, I11, I13, I20–I51) and "Cerebrovascular diseases" (I60–I69). CVD death in dialysis includes myocardial infarction, pericarditis, atherosclerotic heart disease, cardiomyopathy, arrhythmia, cardiac arrest, valvular heart disease, congestive heart failure, and cerebrovascular disease. The youngest general population group is 22 to 44 years old.

Chronic Kidney Disease Stage G5/Dialysis

In patients undergoing dialysis, incident cardiovascular disease is common, with similar cardiovascular mortality rates in a 30-year-old patient undergoing dialysis and an 80-year-old individual from the general population (Fig. 54.3). This likely reflects a high prevalence of cardiovascular disease (~43% of prevalent dialysis patients in the United States in 2018 carried a diagnosis of coronary artery disease and ~43% had a congestive heart failure diagnosis) as well as a high case-fatality rate compared with the general population.

The incidence and prevalence of LVH and heart failure are also extremely high among patients undergoing dialysis. More than 30% of participants in the Frequent Hemodialysis Network studies (a group that overall was healthier than the general dialysis population) had LVH at study entry, assessed with cardiac magnetic resonance imaging. Based on United States Renal Data System (USRDS) administrative data that rely on billing codes to identify heart failure events, the 2-year cumulative probability of developing heart failure for patients initiating dialysis in 2016 was 50% for hemodialysis patients and 36% for peritoneal dialysis patients.

Patients undergoing hemodialysis also have a high prevalence of valvular calcification. In one study, 45% of participants had calcification of the mitral valve, and 34% had calcification of the aortic valve; this compares with expected prevalence of 3% to 5% in the general population. Studies have demonstrated rates of mitral annular calcification ranging from 30% to 50% in patients undergoing hemodialysis.

Types of Cardiovascular Diseases

Cardiovascular disease in individuals with CKD has a variety of manifestations, broadly conceptualized as atherosclerotic disease and nonatherosclerotic disease, with the latter incorporating increased vascular stiffness, cardiomyopathy, valvular disease, and arrhythmia (Table 54.1). In most cases, clinically apparent

cardiovascular disease reflects the interplay among these manifestations. Although there is limited consensus on terminology for arteriopathies, atherosclerosis can be defined as an occlusive disease of the vasculature that occurs because of the deposition of lipid-laden plaques, while vascular stiffness reflects nonocclusive remodeling of the vasculature accompanied by a loss of arterial elasticity. Both of these conditions may manifest with ischemic heart disease and heart failure, and clinical disease often reflects the concurrent presence of both atherosclerotic disease and vascular remodeling. Certain risk factors, including dyslipidemia, primarily predispose an individual to development and progression of atherosclerosis, whereas others, including elevated calcium-phosphorus product, may predispose to vascular stiffness. Volume overload and anemia can lead to cardiac remodeling and LVH, whereas hypertension, which is common at all stages of CKD, is associated with all of these disease manifestations. Over time, the interplay among these manifestations may yield both segmental perfusion defects due to disease affecting larger coronary arteries and insufficient subendocardial perfusion secondary to cardiac hypertrophy (causing increased demand) and capillary dropout. The end result is myocyte death, heart failure, and increased risk of arrhythmia.

Risk Factors for Cardiovascular Disease

Much of the increased burden of cardiovascular disease in CKD is a result of increased prevalence of both traditional and nontraditional cardiovascular disease risk factors. Traditional risk factors were identified in the Framingham Heart Study as conferring increased risk of cardiovascular disease in the general population. Nontraditional risk factors were not defined in the initial reports of the Framingham Heart Study but increase in prevalence as kidney function declines and are hypothesized to be cardiovascular disease risk factors in individuals with CKD (Table 54.2). All CKD stages, even stages G1 and G2 where GFR is preserved but urine albumin excretion is at least moderately elevated, are independently associated with cardiovascular disease in epidemiologic studies. Although CKD, particularly late-stage CKD, may directly cause cardiovascular disease through mechanisms that include fluid retention, anemia, abnormal mineral metabolism, and hypertension, it is likely that CKD also represents a risk state in which factors associated with the development of CKD (including diabetes and hypertension) account for the enhanced cardiac risk. In the latter hypothesis, the presence of CKD is a marker of the severity and duration of these other risk factors.

Cardiovascular disease outcomes are worse at lower levels of kidney function. Notably, while the risk of atherosclerotic cardiovascular disease events are very high in individuals with advanced CKD, the markedly higher risk likely represents the influence of a dramatic rise in the contribution of nonatherosclerotic cardiovascular events (Fig 54.4).

Ischemic Heart Disease

Prediction of Ischemic Heart Disease

The 2013 American College of Cardiology/American Heart Association (ACC/AHA) Guideline on the Assessment of Cardiovascular Risk recommends use of a calculator based on the traditional risk factors incorporated into the Framingham coronary heart disease prediction equations, including age, sex, diabetes, blood pressure, and lipid levels, plus race and smoking status to estimate cardiovascular risk and guide statin use, aspirin use, and blood

TABLE 54.1 Types of Cardiac Diseases in Chronic Kidney Disease

Cardiovascular Disease Type	Pathologic or Structural Manifestation	Risk Factors	Indicators/Diagnostic Test	Clinical Sequelae
Arterial disease	Atherosclerosis: Luminal narrowing of arteries because of plaques	Dyslipidemia Diabetes mellitus Hypertension Other traditional and nontraditional risk factors	Inducible ischemia on nuclear imaging Cardiac catheterization	Myocardial infarction Angina Sudden cardiac death Heart failure
	Vascular stiffness: Diffuse dilatation and wall hypertrophy of larger arteries with loss of arterial elasticity	Hypertension Volume overload Hyperparathyroidism Hyperphosphatemia Other factors predisposing to medial calcification	Vascular calcification Increased pulse pressure Aortic pulse wave velocity Cardiac computed tomography Other arterial imaging	Myocardial infarction Angina Sudden cardiac death Heart failure LVH
Cardiomyopathy	LV hypertrophy: Adaptive hypertrophy to compensate for increased cardiac demand	Pressure overload Increased afterload because of hypertension, valvular disease, and arteriosclerosis Volume overload Volume retention because of progressive kidney disease ± anemia	Echocardiography Cardiovascular magnetic resonance imaging	Myocardial infarction Angina Sudden cardiac death Heart failure
	Decreased LV contractility	Ischemic heart disease Hypertension LVH Other traditional and nontraditional risk factors	Echocardiography	Cardiorenal syndrome[a] Sudden cardiac death Heart failure Myocardial infarction Angina
	Impaired LV relaxation	Hypertension Anemia and volume overload Abnormal mineral metabolism Other arteriosclerosis risk factors Other traditional and nontraditional risk factors	Echocardiography	Heart failure Myocardial infarction Angina Sudden cardiac death
Structural disease	Pericardial effusion	Delayed or insufficient dialysis	Echocardiography	Heart failure Hypotension
	Aortic and mitral valve disease	CKD stages G3b through G5 Abnormal calcium/phosphate/PTH metabolism Aging Dialysis vintage	Echocardiography	Aortic stenosis Endocarditis Heart failure
	Mitral annular calcification	CKD Stages G3b through G5 Abnormal calcium/phosphate/PTH metabolism	Echocardiography Uniform echodense rigid band located near the base of the posterior mitral leaflet	Arrhythmia Embolism Endocarditis Heart failure
	Endocarditis	Valvular disease Central venous catheters	Echocardiography	Arrhythmia Heart failure Embolism
Arrhythmia	Atrial fibrillation	Ischemic heart disease Cardiomyopathy	Electrocardiography	Hypotension Embolism
	Ventricular arrhythmia	Ischemic heart disease Cardiomyopathy Electrolyte abnormalities	Electrocardiography Electrophysiology study	Sudden cardiac death

[a]Cardiorenal syndrome is reviewed in Chapter 29.

CKD, Chronic kidney disease; *LV*, left ventricle; *LVH*, left ventricular hypertrophy; *PTH*, parathyroid hormone.

TABLE 54.2	Traditional and Nontraditional Cardiac Risk Factors in Chronic Kidney Disease	
Traditional Risk Factors	**Nontraditional Factors**	
Older age	Albuminuria
Male sex	Lipoprotein (a) and apo (a) isoforms
Hypertension	
Higher LDL cholesterol	Lipoprotein remnants
Lower HDL cholesterol	Anemia
Diabetes	Abnormal mineral metabolism
Smoking	Extracellular fluid volume overload
Physical inactivity	
Menopause	Electrolyte abnormalities
Family history of cardiovascular disease	Oxidative stress
	Inflammation
Left ventricular hypertrophy	Malnutrition
	Thrombogenic factors
	Sleep disturbances
	Altered nitric oxide/endothelin balance
	Sympathetic overactivity

HDL, High-density lipoprotein; *LDL*, low-density lipoprotein.
Revised from Sarnak MJ, Levey AS, Schoolwerth AC, et al. Kidney disease as a risk factor for development of cardiovascular disease: a statement from the American Heart Association Councils on Kidney in Cardiovascular Disease, High Blood Pressure Research, Clinical Cardiology, and Epidemiology and Prevention. *Circulation.* 2003;108:2154–2169.

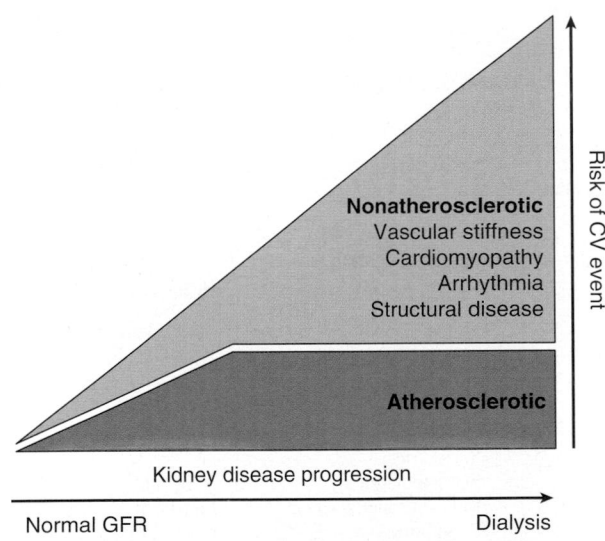

• **Fig. 54.4** The relative contributions of cardiovascular disease types across CKD stages. CVD mechanisms are further detailed in Table 54.1. (Adapted from Wanner C, Amann K, Shoji T. The heart and vascular system in dialysis. *Lancet* 2016;388: 276–84.) *CV,* Cardiovascular; *GFR,* glomerular filtration rate.

pressure targets in the general population. In the general population, the addition of kidney measures, particularly albuminuria, to traditional risk factors appears to improve cardiovascular event prediction.

Use of the ACC/AHA risk equation to assign cardiac risk to individuals with advanced CKD (particularly those receiving dialysis) may be problematic, as risk factors that are at least in part dependent on intact nutrition (e.g., serum cholesterol) and cardiac health (e.g., systolic and diastolic blood pressure) appear to have different relationships with adverse outcomes. Accordingly,

although many of the traditional risk factors that predict coronary heart disease in the general population are important risk factors in the late-stage CKD population, the relative importance of each risk factor may be different.

In patients undergoing dialysis, risk equations geared to the general population fail altogether, although older individuals and those with diabetes do have higher cardiovascular event rates. For example, in patients undergoing maintenance hemodialysis, there is little increase in mortality risk at even markedly elevated systolic blood pressures, whereas lower systolic blood pressures (<120 mm Hg) are associated with the highest risk of mortality. These altered relationships do not speak to pathophysiology but rather likely reflect underlying health status and cardiac and nutritional reserve.

Diagnosis

No single diagnostic test is optimal for identifying ischemic heart disease in individuals with CKD, and each has pitfalls specific to CKD that may affect sensitivity and specificity. Currently, a functional assessment of perfusion that includes cardiac imaging is likely the best initial option to identify cardiac ischemia. Options include exercise or pharmacologic nuclear stress tests as well as exercise or pharmacologic stress echocardiography. Importantly, the ability to perform exercise stress testing is often limited by comorbid conditions in the CKD population. Overall, dobutamine stress echocardiography, assuming adequate institutional expertise and based on limited data, may have higher specificity and at least equivalent or higher sensitivity than pharmacologic nuclear stress tests for detecting angiographically apparent coronary lesions, although both myocardial perfusion scintigraphy and dobutamine stress echocardiography have only moderate accuracy for detecting obstructive coronary lesions in advanced CKD. Another advantage of stress echocardiography is that it simultaneously provides additional information on valvular and other structural disease.

Coronary artery calcium assessment and coronary computed tomography angiography (CTA) have become increasingly popular for noninvasive assessment of cardiovascular risk in the general population. Coronary artery calcium score may be able to offer prognostic information, as higher scores are associated with worse outcomes in all CKD stages; however, its role in guiding treatment decisions in the advanced CKD population remains uncertain. Of note, there is no absolute contraindication to iodinated contrast administration, either for CTA or cardiac catheterization in patients with CKD, including those already receiving maintenance dialysis, although preservation of existing kidney function is an important consideration in all stages of kidney disease, including those receiving hemodialysis and especially those treated with peritoneal dialysis. Given this, the risks and benefits associated with contrast-based diagnostic tools must be carefully weighed, although with careful management and conservative use of iodinated contrast, many individuals with advanced CKD can safely receive iodinated contrast.

Prevention and Treatment

Chronic Kidney Disease Stages G3 to G4

In the earlier stages of CKD, there is a moderate body of data, predominantly derived from subgroup analyses of larger clinical trials, demonstrating benefits with many interventions that are favorable in the general population. Therefore, currently accepted strategies for primary and secondary prevention of cardiac disease in individuals with CKD stages G3 to G4 typically mirror those seen in the general population, while exercising caution to minimize therapies with increased risk in patients with CKD.

In individuals with CKD stages G3 to G4, dyslipidemia (Table 54.3), hypertension, and diabetes likely should be treated according to current general population guidelines. Based on AHA/ACC joint guidelines, beta-blockers remain the first-line agent for stable symptomatic ischemic heart disease, for ischemic cardiomyopathy, and for immediate and up to 3 years of postmyocardial infarction care, regardless of left ventricular function. There are limited data regarding benefits of longer-term beta-blocker use in ischemic heart disease, but they can be considered for patients with coronary or other vascular disease. Specific indications for angiotensin-converting enzyme (ACE) inhibitors and angiotensin receptor blockers (ARBs) include ischemic cardiomyopathy, coexistent proteinuric kidney disease, and diabetes. Current blood pressure targets for nondialysis CKD are systolic pressures below 130 mm Hg based on high-quality data, including from the SPRINT trial, and diastolic pressures below 80 mm Hg based largely on expert opinion. Blood pressure management is discussed in detail in Chapter 65, and diabetes and diabetic kidney disease in Chapter 26.

Individualized care is important, given the challenges associated with therapies. For example, there is an increased risk of

TABLE 54.3 Randomized, Controlled Studies of Statin Treatment Specifically in Chronic Kidney Disease

Study	Intervention	Population	Median Follow-Up	Primary Outcome	Risk of Primary Outcome	Risk of All-Cause Mortality
4D	Atorvastatin 20 mg daily (vs. placebo)	1255 participants Age 18–80 years Type 2 diabetes Hemodialysis for <2 years LDL 80–190 mg/dL	4.0 years	Composite of death from cardiac causes,[a] fatal stroke, nonfatal MI, or nonfatal stroke	HR = 0.92 (0.77–1.10)	RR = 0.93 (0.79–1.08)
AURORA	Rosuvastatin 10 mg daily (vs. placebo)	2776 participants Age 50–80 years Hemofiltration or hemodialysis for more than 3 months	3.8 years	Composite of death from cardiovascular causes, nonfatal MI, or nonfatal stroke	HR = 0.96 (0.84–1.11)	HR = 0.96 (0.86–1.07)
ALERT	Fluvastatin 40 mg daily with dose increase permitted (vs. placebo)	2102 participants Age 30–75 years More than 6 months from transplant Stable kidney graft function No recent MI Total cholesterol 155–348 mg/dL	5.4 years	Major adverse cardiac event, defined as cardiac death, nonfatal MI, or coronary revascularization procedure	RR = 0.83 (0.64–1.06)	RR = 1.02 (0.81–1.30)
SHARP	Simvastatin 20 mg daily + ezetimibe 10 mg daily (vs. placebo)	9270 participants Age 40+ years No previous MI or coronary revascularization Creatinine more than 1.7 mg/dL (men) or more than 1.5 mg/dL (women)	4.9 years	Composite of coronary death,[b] nonfatal MI, ischemic stroke, or any revascularization procedure	RR = 0.83 (0.74–0.94)	RR = 1.02 (0.94–1.11)
	Subgroups within SHARP[c]	Nondialysis (n = 6247)	Not reported	As above	RR = 0.78 (0.67–0.91)	Not reported
		Hemodialysis (n = 2527)			RR = 0.95 (0.78–1.15)	
		Peritoneal dialysis (n = 496)			RR = 0.70 (0.46–1.08)	

Data in parentheses represent 95% confidence intervals. HR and RR report the relationship between treatment versus placebo, with values below 1 favoring treatment and above 1 favoring placebo.

[a]In 4D, death from cardiac causes comprised fatal myocardial infarction (death within 28 days after a myocardial infarction), sudden death, death due to congestive heart failure, death due to coronary heart disease during or within 28 days after an intervention, and all other deaths ascribed to coronary heart disease. Patients who died unexpectedly and had hyperkalemia before the start of the three most recent sessions of hemodialysis were considered to have had sudden death from cardiac causes.

[b]In SHARP, the original primary outcome included cardiac death, defined as death due to hypertensive heart disease, coronary heart disease, or other heart disease; the analytic plan was modified before data analysis to focus on death due to coronary heart disease rather than cardiac death.

[c]In SHARP, there was no statistically significant difference in the risk of the primary outcome between dialysis and nondialysis patients (P = 0.25) or between hemodialysis and peritoneal dialysis patients (P = 0.21).

4D, German Diabetes Dialysis Study; *ALERT*, Assessment of Lescol in Renal Transplantation; *AURORA*, a study to evaluate the use of rosuvastatin in subjects in regular hemodialysis: an assessment of survival and cardiovascular events; *HR*, hazard ratio; *LDL*, low-density lipoprotein; *MI*, myocardial infarction; *RR*, risk ratio; *SHARP*, Study of Heart and Renal Protection.

hyperkalemia with blockade of the renin-angiotensin-aldosterone system that needs to be balanced against the benefits of this therapy in the individual patient. Hypotension and reduced kidney perfusion may limit the ability to use multiple medications concurrently (such as ACE inhibitors, beta-blockers, and diuretics), although each may have reasonable clinical and evidence-based data supporting their use. Other concerns include an increased risk of rhabdomyolysis seen with dual statin and fibrate therapy, and this combination should be avoided in advanced CKD.

Statins are among the best studied medications in the CKD population, with the Study of Heart and Renal Protection (SHARP) demonstrating a significant benefit for primary prevention of cardiovascular disease events in individuals with CKD stage G3b to G4 (see Table 54.3). The 2013 Kidney Disease: Improving Global Outcomes (KDIGO) Clinical Practice Guideline for Lipid Management in CKD recommended statin or statin/ezetimibe treatment for all adults 50 years old or older with CKD stages G3a to G5 (nondialysis) and for all younger adults with CKD and diabetes, known coronary disease or stroke, or high cardiovascular disease risk. Critically, the KDIGO workgroup stressed a "fire-and-forget" approach to statin use in CKD rather than treating to a specific low-density lipoprotein (LDL)-cholesterol target. Recommended statin doses from this guideline are in Table 54.4 and reflect that there may be increased side effects, particularly involving muscle, in individuals with severely reduced kidney function.

The benefits of other common interventions are less certain. For example, low-dose aspirin use in individuals with known cardiovascular disease or a high burden of cardiac risk factors is likely beneficial; however, data on more aggressive antiplatelet therapy with agents including glycoprotein IIb/IIIa inhibitors or clopidogrel following myocardial infarction or in the setting of acute coronary syndromes suggest that there may be a substantial risk of bleeding in individuals with advanced CKD, resulting in greater equipoise regarding use in many situations.

Choosing between medical management and invasive management of coronary disease in advanced CKD remains uncertain, and interventions for acute management remain inadequately studied. The ISCHEMIA-CKD trial randomized 777 patients with moderate or severe ischemia on stress testing and CKD stages G4-G5D, including 344 receiving maintenance hemodialysis and 60 receiving peritoneal dialysis, to an initial invasive strategy consisting of coronary angiography and revascularization (if appropriate) added to medical therapy or an initial conservative strategy consisting of medical therapy alone, with angiography reserved for those whom medical therapy had failed. The primary outcome, a composite of death or nonfatal myocardial infarction, was similar between groups. Of note, the invasive strategy was associated with a higher incidence of stroke and, among the subset not receiving dialysis at baseline, shorter time to the composite of all-cause death or dialysis initiation, suggesting an important role for conservative, noninvasive medical management for stable angina in the advanced CKD population, particularly among those with moderate ischemia on stress testing.

Given the existing data, including the results from ISCHEMIA-CKD, an individualized approach appears optimal for CKD stage G3b and G4 patients with coronary artery disease, with options including intensive medical therapy as a first-line treatment, particularly if symptoms are manageable. Percutaneous interventions and coronary artery bypass grafting may be deferred to a later time or used as part of a more aggressive first-line approach based on an individual patient's symptom burden and disease severity, anatomic characteristics, longer-term prognosis, and lifestyle values.

A radial artery approach as compared to a femoral artery approach has gained favor for percutaneous cardiac interventions in the general population due to fewer complications. This represents an important option for advanced CKD patients, although, prior to intervention, communication should occur between kidney and cardiology providers to ensure that future vascular access plans are accounted for when determining the approach in order to maximize likelihood of hemodialysis access success.

Chronic Kidney Disease Stage G5/Dialysis

To date, clinical trial data demonstrating a significant survival benefit with accepted cardiovascular disease therapies in the dialysis population are lacking, although data from the United States suggest that the rates of cardiovascular disease death in patients undergoing dialysis continue to decrease, albeit for reasons that remain uncertain. The overall failure to find specific interventions that significantly reduce the cardiovascular disease burden in individuals treated with maintenance dialysis most likely reflects the fact that there are numerous competing causes of death in these patients, and addressing single risk factors may be insufficient to reduce mortality. As noted above, the ISCHEMIA-CKD trial demonstrated that, particularly for dialysis patients with moderate ischemia, a conservative, noninterventional strategy may be preferable for managing stable ischemic heart disease.

Statin treatment is the best studied medical therapy, particularly among hemodialysis patients, with two large, adequately powered clinical trials both showing no benefit in patients undergoing hemodialysis, and a third trial, SHARP, showing no benefit in the subgroup receiving hemodialysis at trial initiation (see Table 54.3); individuals receiving peritoneal dialysis remain inadequately studied. Based on these results, KDIGO did not recommend routinely

TABLE 54.4	Recommended Doses of Statins in Adults with Chronic Kidney Disease	
Agent	Intensity in General Population	Advanced Chronic Kidney Disease and Dialysis
Atorvastatin	High at 40–80 mg Moderate at 10–20 mg	20 mg
Rosuvastatin	High at 20–40 mg Moderate at 5–10 mg	10 mg
Simvastatin	Moderate at 20–40 mg Low at 10 mg	20 mg
Pravastatin	Moderate at 40–80 mg Low at 10–20 mg	40 mg
Lovastatin	Moderate at 40 mg Low at 20 mg	Not evaluated
Fluvastatin	Moderate at 80 mg Low at 20–40 mg	80 mg
Pitavastatin	Moderate at 2–4 mg Low at 1 mg	2 mg

High-potency statins lower LDL cholesterol by at least 50% while lower potency statins lower LDL by 30% to 50% on average. Dosing recommendations are from the KDIGO guideline, and most are derived from medication doses safely used in trials. Statin metabolism is not affected by kidney function; however, the risk of side effects, particularly affecting muscle, is more common in individuals with low GFR.

KDIGO, Kidney Disease: Improving Global Outcomes; LDL, low-density lipoprotein.

initiating statin therapy in patients undergoing hemodialysis, although the guideline suggests continuing statins in those who were receiving them prior to dialysis initiation. In patients with longer life expectancies, such as patients expected to receive a kidney transplant, we suggest individualized decision making, and, consistent with the KDIGO guideline, continue statins in those currently prescribed these agents. Of note, KDIGO recommends statin therapy in transplant recipients.

Current practice for other cardiovascular risk-modifying therapy is chiefly based on observational data and extrapolations from the non-CKD population. In individuals receiving dialysis, interventions directed at blood pressure and diet are challenging, given the difficulty of maintaining blood pressure in a narrow range as well as the catabolic nature of the dialysis milieu. In addition, some risk factors associated with adverse events in the general population appear to be protective in the dialysis population. For example, higher blood pressure and obesity both are associated with better survival in patients undergoing dialysis, probably because they reflect greater cardiac and nutritional reserves, respectively. Other challenges with risk-factor management include difficulty with ascertainment. For example, blood pressure measurements are often unreliable because of the presence of dialysis access and arterial calcification, home and ambulatory blood pressure measurements are infrequently used for clinical care, and glycated hemoglobin measurements may not accurately reflect glycemic control.

Despite a lack of definitive supporting evidence, the following targets could be reasonable, based predominantly on evidence from the nondialysis population. A predialysis blood pressure goal of less than 140 to 150/90 mm Hg should be targeted if achievable without hypotension-limiting ultrafiltration, ideally through optimization of dry weight before initiation of pharmacologic therapy. Modest glycemic control requires frequent blood glucose assessments, assuming that hypoglycemia can be avoided. In some patients, tighter control of cardiovascular disease risk factors, if achievable safely, may be advisable and cost effective, although tools to identify patients undergoing dialysis who are most likely to benefit from these interventions remain insufficient. Finally, smoking cessation efforts are essential in all stages of CKD. As with earlier stages of CKD, ischemic heart disease can be treated successfully with invasive therapies in patients undergoing dialysis; however, the risk of complications is higher in patients with CKD. Accordingly, the optimal strategy remains unknown, and a policy of shared decision making is suggested.

Left Ventricular Hypertrophy and Heart Failure

Diagnosis

Diagnosis of LVH is readily accomplished with echocardiography, an inexpensive, noninvasive, and widely available test. Cardiac function should be assessed in the euvolemic state, as both significant volume depletion and overload may reduce cardiac inotropy. Accordingly, in patients undergoing dialysis, two-dimensional echocardiography is likely to be most informative if performed on the interdialytic day, and, notably, is less vulnerable to volume fluctuation than one-dimensional echocardiography methods. Although three-dimensional echocardiography may be useful to assess left ventricle (LV) structure because it avoids the use of

geometric assumptions of LV shape that are required to estimate LV mass and volume, increasing availability likely makes cardiac magnetic resonance imaging (MRI) the modality of choice if highly accurate assessment of LV structure is needed. It additionally offers better assessment of cardiac fibrosis. Cardiac positron emission tomography (PET) remains insufficiently evaluated in individuals with kidney failure. Screening echocardiography was recommended for incident patients undergoing dialysis in an early guideline that has not been revisited; however, there is no evidence that routinely obtaining echocardiograms improves clinical outcomes.

Heart failure and cardiorenal syndromes are extensively discussed in Chapter 29. Heart failure is a clinical syndrome characterized by specific symptoms, including dyspnea and fatigue, and signs, including edema and rales. Although this constellation of symptoms and signs may be consistent with heart failure, these symptoms also occur in many individuals with CKD and may simply reflect volume overload. Regardless of the specific cause, individuals with persistent or recurrent volume overload have poor clinical outcomes overall. Importantly, in patients undergoing hemodialysis, in whom preload is rapidly changing and fluid overload is managed with ultrafiltration, hypotension may be the only manifestation of heart failure.

Treatment

Potentially modifiable risk factors for LVH include anemia, hypertension, extracellular volume overload, abnormal mineral metabolism including hyperphosphatemia and secondary hyperparathyroidism, and, on rare occasions, arteriovenous fistulas causing high-output heart failure. Definitive clinical trials evaluating whether modifying these risk factors reduces mortality are not currently available, leading to reliance on surrogate outcomes. Some data suggest that ACE inhibitor and ARB therapy may result in favorable effects on a putative surrogate outcome (left ventricular mass reduction). In contrast, randomized trials in CKD patients targeting normalization of hemoglobin levels with recombinant human erythropoietin had no effect on the similar surrogate outcome of LVH or left ventricular mass. Critically, no trials in CKD stages G3 to G4 have demonstrated a reduction in cardiac outcomes or mortality with these interventions when they are used for the purpose of treating or preventing LVH. In patients undergoing hemodialysis enrolled in the Frequent Hemodialysis Network study, those who received more frequent hemodialysis experienced a significant improvement in LV mass, suggesting a critical role for consistent volume control.

Heart failure therapy differs by CKD stage because diuretics are a mainstay of therapy in advanced CKD, whereas fluid overload in patients undergoing dialysis is treated primarily with ultrafiltration. As discussed previously, ACE inhibitors and ARBs may have cardiac benefits independent of their blood pressure-lowering effects in systolic heart failure patients with CKD stage G1 to early stage G4, with limited data suggesting some improvement in LV geometry as well as cardiovascular outcomes. Potential further benefits associated with mineralocorticoid receptor blockade, including spironolactone and eplerenone, are currently being studied, with a potential limitation of hyperkalemia, especially when used in conjunction with ACE inhibitors or ARBs. Notably, recent data evaluating use of the mineralocorticoid receptor blocker finerenone in individuals with diabetic kidney disease showed a significant reduction in the composite of death, kidney failure, or a 40% reduction in GFR. Importantly, there was also a significantly lower risk of the key secondary outcome of CVD death, nonfatal MI, nonfatal stroke, or heart failure hospitalization among those randomized to finerenone.

Beta-blocking agents, another mainstay of heart failure therapy in the general population, are also likely beneficial in patients with nondialysis CKD, and evidence from one small trial supports carvedilol use to reduce mortality risk in patients undergoing dialysis with left ventricular dysfunction. Cardiac glycosides (e.g., digoxin) are occasionally used in heart failure in the general population where they decrease morbidity but not mortality. Although there are no specific studies of cardiac glycosides in CKD, they should be used judiciously if at all in these patients, with careful attention to dosage, drug levels, and potassium balance.

Initially viewed as glycemic agents, SGLT2 inhibitors, mostly in trials of individuals with type 2 diabetes but increasingly in trials that include individuals without diabetes but with heart failure or albuminuric kidney disease, have shown substantial cardiovascular benefits that are largely driven by reductions in heart failure and cardiovascular death. Notably, two CKD-focused SGLT2 inhibitor trials recruited patients with proteinuric kidney disease at GFR levels as low as 25 mL/min/1.73 m². Based on very favorable trial results, SGLT2 inhibitors should be early-line agents in individuals with albuminuric kidney disease, regardless of diabetes status, while their role in nondiabetic, nonalbuminuric kidney disease remains uncertain.

Arrhythmia and Sudden Cardiac Death

Arrhythmias are extremely common in individuals with CKD, likely reflecting a high prevalence of structural heart disease, ischemic heart disease, and electrolyte abnormalities. Atrial fibrillation is the most common arrhythmia, with prevalence estimates for paroxysmal and permanent atrial fibrillation as high as 30% in individuals with advanced CKD, including patients undergoing dialysis. Bradycardia, asystole, and ventricular arrhythmias are probably also exceedingly common, although true rates cannot be determined; one small study of hemodialysis patients described bradycardia as the most common arrhythmia and noted that arrhythmia was most common at the end of the long interdialytic interval and during the first hemodialysis session of the week. Prevalent dialysis patients have cardiovascular disease mortality rates of more than 80 deaths per 1000 person-years, with cardiac arrest/arrhythmia accounting for 34% and 31% of all deaths (and 44% and 40% of deaths with a known cause) among hemodialysis and peritoneal dialysis patients, respectively, in 2018, highlighting arrhythmia as a critical issue for this population.

There are few data on prevention and treatment of arrhythmia and sudden cardiac death in the nondialysis CKD or dialysis population, with most current treatment recommendations for individuals not treated with dialysis mirroring those seen in the general population. Among hemodialysis patients, the temporal relationship of arrhythmia to the dialysis cycle suggests that volume status and electrolytes as well as rapid fluctuation of electrolyte levels may be modifiable factors to reduce the risk of arrhythmia and sudden cardiac death. Although an increasing number of late-stage CKD patients and patients undergoing dialysis are receiving implantable cardioverter-defibrillators (ICDs) to prevent sudden cardiac death, there are no trial data that have shown a survival benefit or demonstrated cost effectiveness. Of note, ICD and other cardiac device wires typically traverse the left subclavian vein and may predispose to central stenosis, adversely affecting hemodialysis vascular access options. Newer, leadless devices may be particularly good options for the advanced CKD and dialysis populations, where vein preservation is paramount. Given the high incidence of sudden cardiac death, one key preventative strategy for ambulatory settings where CKD patients are treated, including clinics and dialysis facilities, is to ensure the presence of an automated external defibrillator (AED) and trained clinic personnel.

Stroke and Stroke Prevention

Cerebrovascular disease is also common in individuals with CKD (see Fig. 54.2), with a higher incidence of both ischemic and hemorrhagic events than seen in the general population. Critically, even in the absence of clinically evident strokes, both silent lesions and substantial brain white matter disease may be present. Not surprisingly, the presence of cardiovascular disease is associated with cerebrovascular manifestations in individuals with CKD, including worse cognitive function.

Although not specifically studied, stroke prevention and treatment strategies for patients with earlier stages of CKD likely should follow general population guidelines, including management of traditional risk factors and the use of antithrombotic agents as indicated. For example, among individuals with CKD stage G3 participating in the Stroke Prevention in Atrial Fibrillation 3 trials, warfarin use based on general population recommendations was associated with a considerable reduction in the incidence of embolic stroke without a substantial increase in adverse events. Newer trials using direct oral anticoagulants (DOACs) rather than warfarin suggest that these agents are safe and effective in individuals with CKD stage G3, albeit with careful selection and attention to kidney function.

Two major evidence gaps exist in dialysis patients with atrial fibrillation, where the risk of bleeding complications and falls is substantially higher than in the general population: (1) Does anticoagulation for primary prevention improve outcomes? and (2) What is the optimal agent for anticoagulation? In dialysis cohorts, data on the value of warfarin for primary thromboembolism prevention in atrial fibrillation are mixed, with some observational data suggesting an increased risk of death in patients treated with warfarin. If true, this may reflect not only an increased risk of bleeding events but also the relationship between warfarin and increased vascular calcification, mediated by preventing vitamin K-dependent carboxylation of matrix Gla protein, a calcification inhibitor. Given the frequency with which atrial fibrillation occurs in individuals with kidney failure, the lack of trial data on anticoagulation in patients undergoing dialysis, and the many competing risks of death in this population, optimal management of primary and secondary stroke prevention with anticoagulants urgently requires an adequately powered clinical trial to inform management decisions. Unfortunately, this is unlikely to occur.

Clinical trial data examining DOAC use, compared to warfarin and to placebo, currently are absent in patients undergoing dialysis. Limited safety and efficacy data exist for DOACs in CKD stage G4, stage G5, or dialysis. Apixaban is specifically approved by the US Food and Drug Administration (FDA) for use in dialysis, albeit based on no safety data from clinical trials. The current AHA/ACC guideline highlights the ongoing equipoise, stating that: *For patients with AF who have a CHA2DS2-VASc score of 2 or greater in men or 3 or greater in women and who have (CKD stage G5) or are on dialysis, it might be reasonable to prescribe warfarin (INR 2.0 to 3.0) or apixaban for oral anticoagulation.* Despite this lack of data, apixaban has been widely adopted in the dialysis population, with additional uncertainty regarding whether the appropriate dose is 2.5 mg or 5 mg twice daily, although limited data suggest that the 2.5-mg twice-daily dose may be reasonable. Overall, given the lack of high-quality data, including the lack of validated thrombosis risk scores and bleeding risk scores in dialysis, individual decision making incorporating informed patient input and multidisciplinary clinician input is critical for management.

Recently, left atrial appendage occlusion has emerged as a mechanical alternative to systemic anticoagulation for preventing atrial fibrillation-associated thromboembolism in the general population. Results from several smaller studies suggest that this procedure is safe and diminishes the need for long-term systemic anticoagulation, although anticoagulation is used for 1-2 months following the procedure followed by 6 months of dual antiplatelet therapy prior to transition to aspirin monotherapy.

Complete bibliography is available at Elsevier eBooks for Practicing Clinicians.

Key Bibliography

Baigent C, Landray MJ, Reith C, et al. The effects of lowering LDL cholesterol with simvastatin plus ezetimibe in patients with chronic kidney disease (Study of Heart and Renal Protection): a randomised placebo-controlled trial. *Lancet.* 2011;377:2181–2192.

Bakris GL, Agarwal R, Anker SD, et al.; FIDELIO-DKD Investigators. Effect of finerenone on chronic kidney disease outcomes in type 2 diabetes. *N Engl J Med.* 2020;383(23):2219–2229. doi: 10.1056/NEJMoa2025845. PMID: 33264825.

Bangalore S, Maron DJ, O'Brien SM, et al.; ISCHEMIA-CKD Research Group. Management of coronary disease in patients with advanced kidney disease. *N Engl J Med.* 2020;382(17):1608-1618. doi: 10.1056/NEJMoa1915925. PMID: 32227756; PMCID: PMC7274537.

Chronic Kidney Disease Prognosis Consortium. Association of estimated glomerular filtration rate and albuminuria with all-cause and cardiovascular mortality in general population cohorts: a collaborative meta-analysis. *Lancet.* 2010;375:2073–2181.

Fox CS, Larson MG, Vasan RS, et al. Cross-sectional association of kidney function with valvular and annular calcification: the Framingham heart study. *J Am Soc Nephrol.* 2006;17:521–527.

Fox CS, Muntner P, Chen AY, et al. Use of evidence-based therapies in short-term outcomes of ST-segment elevation myocardial infarction and non-ST-segment elevation myocardial infarction in patients with chronic kidney disease: a report from the National Cardiovascular Data Acute Coronary Treatment and Intervention Outcomes Network registry. *Circulation.* 2010;121:357–365.

Go AS, Chertow GM, Fan D, et al. Chronic kidney disease and the risks of death, cardiovascular events, and hospitalization. *N Engl J Med.* 2004;351:1296–1305.

Hart RG, Pearce LA, Asinger RW, et al. Warfarin in atrial fibrillation patients with moderate chronic kidney disease. *Clin J Am Soc Nephrol.* 2011;6:2599–2604.

Heerspink HJL, Stefánsson BV, Correa-Rotter R, et al.; DAPA-CKD Trial Committees and Investigators. Dapagliflozin in patients with chronic kidney disease. *N Engl J Med.* 2020;383(15):1436–1446. doi:10.1056/NEJMoa2024816. PMID: 32970396.

Kidney Disease: Improving Global Outcomes (KDIGO) Lipid Work Group. KDIGO clinical practice guideline for lipid management in chronic kidney disease. *Kidney Int Suppl.* 2013;3:259–305.

Lentine KL, Costa SP, Weir MR, et al. Cardiac disease evaluation and management among kidney and liver transplantation candidates: a scientific statement from the American Heart Association and the American College of Cardiology Foundation: endorsed by the American Society of Transplant Surgeons, American Society of Transplantation, and National Kidney Foundation. *Circulation.* 2012;126:617–663.

Matsushita K, Coresh J, Sang Y, et al. Estimated glomerular filtration rate and albuminuria for prediction of cardiovascular outcomes: a collaborative meta-analysis of individual participant data. *Lancet Diabetes Endocrinol.* 2015;3:514–525.

Ohtake T, Kobayashi S, Moriya H, et al. High prevalence of occult coronary artery stenosis in patients with chronic kidney disease at the initiation of renal replacement therapy: an angiographic examination. *J Am Soc Nephrol.* 2005;16:1141–1148.

Palmer SC, Di Micco L, Razavian M, et al. Effects of antiplatelet therapy on mortality and cardiovascular and bleeding outcomes in persons with chronic kidney disease: a systematic review and meta-analysis. *Ann Intern Med.* 2012;156:445–459.

Perkovic V, Jardine MJ, Neal B, et al.; CREDENCE Trial Investigators. Canagliflozin and renal outcomes in type 2 diabetes and nephropathy. *N Engl J Med.* 2019;380(24):2295–2306. doi:10.1056/NEJMoa1811744. PMID: 30990260.

Raggi P, Boulay A, Chasan-Taber S, et al. Cardiac calcification in adult hemodialysis patients: a link between end-stage renal disease and cardiovascular disease? *J Am Coll Cardiol.* 2002;39:695–701.

Roberts MA, Polkinghorne KR, McDonald SP, et al. Secular trends in cardiovascular mortality rates of patients receiving dialysis compared with the general population. *Am J Kidney Dis.* 2011;58:64–72.

Sarnak MJ, Amann K, Bangalore S, et al.; Conference Participants. Chronic kidney disease and coronary artery disease: JACC state-of-the-art review. *J Am Coll Cardiol.* 2019;74(14):1823-1838. doi: 10.1016/j.jacc.2019.08.1017. PMID: 31582143.

Sarnak MJ, Levey AS, Schoolwerth AC, et al. Kidney disease as a risk factor for development of cardiovascular disease: a statement from the American Heart Association Councils on Kidney in Cardiovascular Disease, High Blood Pressure Research. *Clinical Cardiology, and Epidemiology and Prevention. Circulation.* 2003;108:2154–2169.

Wanner C, Amann K, Shoji T. The heart and vascular system in dialysis. *Lancet.* 2016;388:276–284.

55

Anemia and Other Hematologic Complications of Chronic Kidney Disease

JONATHAN W. BAZELEY, JAY B. WISH

Anemia

Epidemiology and Pathogenesis

Anemia is defined by the World Health Organization as a hemoglobin (Hb) concentration less than 13.0 g/dL in adult men and nonmenstruating women and less than 12.0 g/dL in menstruating women. The incidence of anemia in patients with chronic kidney disease (CKD) increases as the glomerular filtration rate (GFR) declines. Population studies, including the United States National Health and Nutrition Examination Survey (NHANES) and the Prevalence of Anemia in Early Renal Insufficiency study, suggest that the incidence of anemia is less than 10% in CKD stages 1 and 2, 20% to 40% in CKD stage 3, 50% to 60% in CKD stage 4, and more than 70% in CKD stage 5.

The pathogenesis of anemia in patients with CKD is multifactorial (Box 55.1), but the contribution of erythropoietin (EPO) deficiency becomes greater as GFR declines. Hypoxia inducible factor (HIF), which is produced in the kidneys and other tissues, is a substance whose spontaneous degradation is retarded in the presence of decreased oxygen delivery because of anemia or hypoxemia. The sustained presence of HIF leads to signal transduction and the synthesis of EPO. In normal patients, plasma EPO levels increase dramatically in response to anemia. Because of alterations in their functioning mass, the kidneys in patients with CKD fail to increase EPO production in response to anemia or other conditions that decrease oxygen delivery. This is due both to impaired hypoxia sensing and a decreased population of EPO-producing cells.

The kidneys produce about 90% of circulating EPO, and loss of EPO production in the setting of CKD is the primary cause of anemia in these patients. EPO binds to receptors on erythroid progenitor cells in the bone marrow, specifically the burst-forming units (BFU-E) and colony-forming units (CFU-E). The absence of EPO causes these cells to undergo programmed death or apoptosis, which is mediated by Fas ligand. In the presence of EPO, these erythroid progenitors differentiate into reticulocytes and red blood cells (RBCs).

Fig. 55.1 demonstrates the complex interactions among EPO; proinflammatory cytokines such as interleukin 1 (IL-1), tumor necrosis factor-α (TNF-α), IL-6, and interferon-γ (IFN-γ); hepcidin; and iron in the production of RBCs. Hepcidin is a peptide produced by the liver that interferes with RBC production by decreasing iron availability for incorporation into erythroblasts. Hepcidin gene expression is upregulated by IL-6 and iron overload and downregulated by TNF-α and iron deficiency. Hepcidin clearance is substantially reduced in CKD. At the cell surface of macrophages and proximal intestinal cells (and probably other cells), hepcidin binds to ferroportin, the membrane-embedded iron exporter, resulting in internalization and degradation of the complex. This inhibits iron transport across the cell membrane, trapping it in macrophages and preventing it from being absorbed from the intestine. Hepcidin activity is probably the basis for most "anemia of chronic disease" syndromes and contributes to the anemia in patients with CKD when inflammation and infection are present. However, in anemic CKD patients without inflammation or infection, EPO deficiency plays a much greater role than hepcidin excess.

The evidence for inhibition of RBC production by uremic toxins in patients with CKD is poor, as most CKD patients have an appropriate erythropoietic response to exogenously administered EPO if they are iron replete and free of inflammation or infection. It has been demonstrated that RBC survival is decreased from 120 days in normal individuals to 60 to 90 days in patients with CKD not yet receiving dialysis. This may be a result of RBC trauma from microvascular disease, as well as decreased resistance to oxidative stress.

Clinical Manifestations

The major clinical manifestations of anemia in patients with or without CKD are fatigue (both with exercise and at rest), decreased cognitive function, loss of libido, and decreased sense of well-being. These symptoms tend to occur when the Hb is less than 10 g/dL and are more severe as Hb levels fall further. More insidious are the cardiac complications of anemia, which may occur when the patient is otherwise asymptomatic and contribute to the adverse cardiovascular morbidity and mortality observed among patients with CKD. In patients with underlying coronary artery disease, anemia may lead to an exacerbation of angina because of decreased myocardial oxygen delivery. Decreased oxygen delivery to tissues because of anemia leads to peripheral vasodilation, increased sympathetic nervous system activity, increased

Factors That Cause or Contribute to Anemia in Patients with Chronic Kidney Disease

Insufficient production of endogenous EPO
Iron deficiency
Acute and chronic inflammatory conditions
Severe hyperparathyroidism
Aluminum toxicity
Folate deficiency
Decreased survival of RBCs and RBC loss

EPO, Erythropoietin; *RBCs,* red blood cells.

heart rate and stroke volume, and, ultimately, left ventricular hypertrophy (LVH). LVH strongly correlates with adverse outcomes, including hospitalization and mortality, in patients with CKD. Each decrease in Hb of 0.5 g/dL is associated with a 32% increased risk of LVH over the course of a year; in contrast, each 5-mm Hg increase in systolic blood pressure correlates with only an 11% increase in LV mass. Many anemic CKD patients treated with erythropoiesis-stimulating agents (ESAs) report a decrease in subjective symptoms and improved quality of life (QoL), but evidence supporting regression of LVH, fewer clinical cardiac events, or decreased mortality with ESA treatment is not compelling (see later discussion).

Laboratory Evaluation

Because anemia is common in CKD, the consequences of anemia are severe, and treatment is available, the 2012 Kidney Disease: Improving Global Outcomes (KDIGO) clinical practice guidelines for anemia in CKD recommended screening all patients with

CKD stage 3 at least annually and more frequently in those with more advanced CKD; in those with diagnosed anemia not receiving treatment, Hb concentration should be measured at least every 3 months in patients with CKD stage 3 to 5 and monthly in patients on maintenance dialysis. If anemia is present (defined as Hb <13.0 g/dL in adult men and Hb <12.0 g/dL in adult women), further evaluation should be undertaken to determine the cause. This evaluation should include a complete blood count including RBC indices, reticulocyte count, serum ferritin concentration, and transferrin saturation (TSAT) or reticulocyte Hb content (CHr). The anemia of EPO deficiency is normocytic (normal mean corpuscular volume [MCV]) and normochromic (normal mean corpuscular Hb concentration [MCHC]). A low MCV (microcytosis) is suggestive of iron deficiency but may be seen in hemoglobinopathies such as thalassemia. A high MCV (macrocytosis) is suggestive of vitamin B_{12} or folate deficiency. If the MCV is elevated, vitamin B_{12} and folate levels should be assessed.

The serum ferritin level correlates with iron bound to tissue ferritin in the reticuloendothelial (RE) system. Serum ferritin does not carry or bind to iron, and its function is unknown. Serum ferritin is also an acute phase reactant that increases in the setting of acute or chronic inflammation independent of tissue iron stores. TSAT is a measure of circulating iron available for delivery to the erythroid marrow and is calculated by dividing the serum iron concentration by the total iron binding capacity (TIBC). The TIBC correlates with the serum level of transferrin, which is the major iron-carrying protein in the blood. TSAT less than 20% in an anemic patient with CKD is consistent with absolute or functional iron deficiency, both of which are characterized by decreased delivery of iron to the erythroid marrow.

Absolute iron deficiency occurs in the setting of decreased total body iron stores and is accompanied by serum ferritin level less than 25 ng/mL in men and less than 12 ng/mL in women. Functional iron deficiency is seen in patients with low TSAT and normal or elevated serum ferritin. It may be a result of the pharmacologic stimulation of RBC production by ESAs, which causes

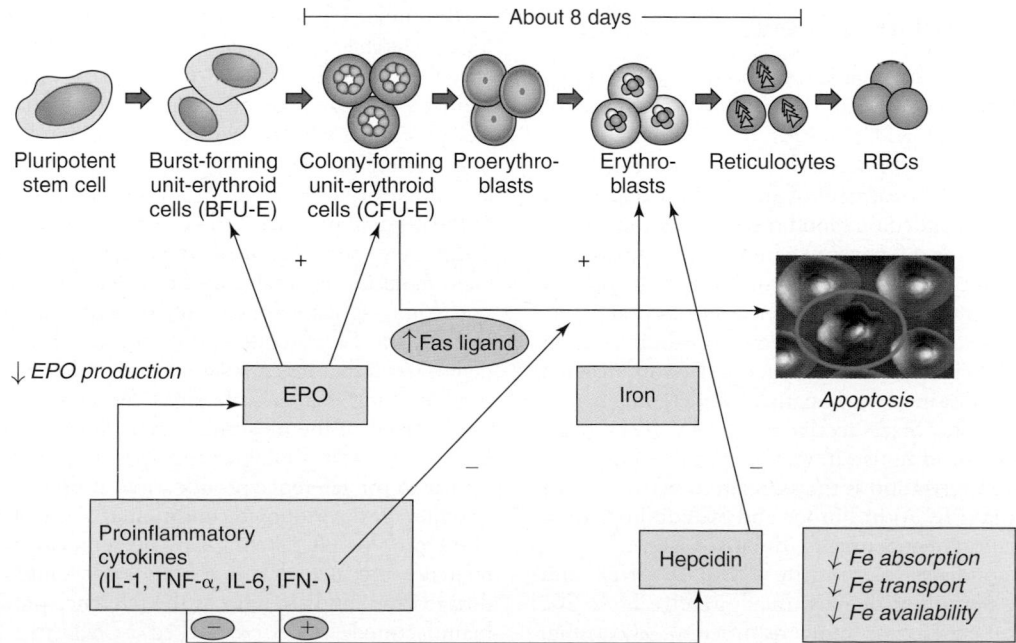

• **Fig. 55.1** Erythropoiesis in chronic kidney disease. *EPO,* Erythropoietin; *Fe,* iron; *IFN,* interferon; *IL,* interleukin; *RBCs,* red blood cells; *TNF,* tumor necrosis factor. (Courtesy Iain Macdougall, MD.)

iron demand by the erythroid marrow in excess of the ability of the RE system to release iron to circulating transferrin. Functional iron deficiency may also result from the action of hepcidin in the setting of inflammation or infection. The hallmark of functional iron deficiency anemia is that it responds to the administration of intravenous (IV) iron supplements, with increase in Hb level and/or decrease in ESA requirements despite the normal or elevated serum ferritin concentration. If the anemic patient with low TSAT and normal or high serum ferritin level does not respond to IV iron, the presumptive diagnosis is RE blockade, meaning that hepcidin has completely prevented the release of iron from macrophages to circulating transferrin. It should be noted that, although the diagnosis of iron depletion is based on serum ferritin concentration less than 25 ng/mL, and that of iron-deficient erythropoiesis is based on TSAT less than 16%, anemic CKD patients with considerably higher serum ferritin and TSAT levels often respond to iron supplementation (see Iron Therapy, later).

The reticulocyte count is a useful and inexpensive test to distinguish anemia caused by underproduction of RBCs from that caused by RBC loss or destruction. In the setting of EPO deficiency, RBC production is decreased, and most anemic patients would be expected to have decreased absolute reticulocyte count (<40,000 to 50,000 cells per milliliter of whole blood). Elevated reticulocyte count is inconsistent with EPO deficiency, and an evaluation for hemolysis and blood loss should be undertaken.

Although it would seem that demonstration of decreased blood EPO level would secure the diagnosis of EPO deficiency, routine testing for EPO levels in anemic patients with CKD is not recommended. The reason is that patients who respond to exogenous ESAs may have normal or even elevated EPO concentration, which, nevertheless, may be inappropriately low for the severity of their anemia. Furthermore, the test is expensive. Therefore, it is recommended that EPO deficiency be a diagnosis of exclusion (i.e., negative evaluation for other treatable causes of anemia) in the anemic CKD patient. However, a cause other than EPO deficiency should be considered if anemia severity is disproportionate to the GFR or if leukopenia and/or thrombocytopenia are present.

Erythropoiesis-Stimulating Agents

After other treatable causes of anemia have been excluded and a diagnosis of EPO deficiency inferred, the treatment of choice for many anemic patients with CKD is an ESA. Recombinant human erythropoietin (rHuEPO, or epoetin) has been available since 1989 and revolutionized the treatment of anemia in patients with CKD who previously depended on blood transfusions and androgens. Although absorption of epoetin administered subcutaneously (SC) is incomplete with degradation of some of the protein before it reaches the circulation, the slower absorption and sustained serum epoetin levels may make this route of administration 20% to 30% more efficient than a comparable IV-administered dose. Nonetheless, the vast majority of patients undergoing hemodialysis (HD) in the United States receive an ESA by the IV route because of convenience of administration. One possible additional motivation for IV administration is the association between cases of pure red cell aplasia (PRCA) in Europe and SC administration of the Eprex formulation of epoetin alfa (discussed later).

Patients with nondialysis-dependent (NDD) CKD and patients undergoing peritoneal dialysis usually receive ESAs SC. The package insert for epoetin recommends thrice-weekly dosing, because the clinical trials submitted for approval by the US Food and Drug Administration (FDA) involved patients undergoing

HD who received the drug with each treatment. For NDD-CKD patients and patients on peritoneal dialysis, thrice-weekly SC dosing is painful and not practical. Further, it is not necessary because clinical trials in these patients have shown epoetin administered every 1 to 2 weeks to be equally effective. Epoetin is effective in maintaining target Hb levels in 76% of NDD-CKD patients when administered as infrequently as every 4 weeks.

Darbepoetin alfa is a bioengineered epoetin molecule with two additional N-linked carbohydrate side chains. It has a longer half-life and duration of action than epoetin. As with epoetin, studies have demonstrated that darbepoetin is effective in maintaining target Hb levels when administered as infrequently as every 4 weeks in selected patients. There appears to be no difference in SC versus IV administration in terms of efficacy. The side effect profile of darbepoetin is virtually identical to that of epoetin; both agents are associated with the development or exacerbation of hypertension in 20% to 30% of patients. The mechanism for hypertension is multifactorial and related to increased RBC mass, attenuation of the peripheral vasodilation associated with anemia, and, perhaps, a direct inhibitory effect on vascular endothelial vasodilatory mediators such as nitric oxide and prostaglandins. The existence or exacerbation of hypertension is not a contraindication to ESA therapy; rather, the hypertension should be treated with more aggressive pharmacologic therapy, increased ultrafiltration on dialysis, and/or a decrease in the ESA dose to slow the rate of Hb rise and to allow for physiologic vasomotor adaptation. There is no evidence that the rate of vascular access thrombosis is increased in patients undergoing HD when ESA treatment is used to maintain Hb levels within the currently recommended target range. All other side effects reported with ESA therapy are no greater than with placebo.

Mircera (methoxy polyethylene glycol-epoetin beta) has been extensively used in other parts of the world for a number of years and was introduced into the US market following the expiration of patents on epoetin in 2014. The pegylation of the molecule retards its metabolism and allows for once-monthly IV or SC dosing. Mircera carries the same FDA warnings as epoetin and darbepoetin.

Biosimilar ESAs, which are lower-cost versions of the originator or reference ESAs, have become available in the United States after being extensively used in other parts of the world. The FDA defines a biosimilar agent as one that is "highly similar to the reference product with no clinically meaningful differences in terms of the safety profile, purity, or potency." Because of the molecular complexity of biologic drugs, biosimilars are not exact copies of the original product, unlike generic versions of small molecule drugs. Since the clinical safety and efficacy of an originator biologic molecule have already been demonstrated, the FDA does not require sponsors of biosimilar agents to repeat these studies. Instead, the FDA requires the sponsor of a biosimilar agent to demonstrate that it is not significantly different from the reference product using smaller-scale direct comparisons and extrapolation. The sponsor of the biosimilar agent must provide evidence demonstrating that its biologic product is structurally and functionally similar to the reference product; that it uses the same mechanism of action for the proposed condition(s) of use; that the condition(s) of use proposed in labeling have been previously approved for the reference product; that it has the same route of administration, dosage form, and strength as the reference product; and that it is manufactured, processed, packed, or held in a facility that meets standards designed to assure that the biologic product continues to be safe, pure, and potent. Epoetin alfa-ebpx, a biosimilar of epoetin alfa, was first approved by the FDA in 2018 for use in the United States and is marketed under the trade name Retacrit. The pharmacologic properties of ESAs approved in the United States as of 2020 are summarized in Table 55.1.

Pure Red Cell Aplasia

PRCA is a form of aplastic anemia caused by the production of anti-EPO antibodies induced by administration of exogenous ESAs. The diagnosis of PRCA should be suspected in a patient with a sudden weekly drop in Hb of approximately 1 g/dL, or a weekly transfusion requirement and low reticulocyte count (<20,000 cells/μL), despite a high dose of ESA for several months. In contrast to classic aplastic anemia, the white blood cell and platelet counts are preserved in PRCA. A definitive diagnosis of PRCA is made by the demonstration of anti-EPO antibodies in the blood or a bone marrow examination showing normal cellularity and less than 4% erythroblasts. Treatment includes discontinuation of the ESA and immunosuppressive therapy (e.g., cyclophosphamide); most patients respond after several months and do not relapse after the immunosuppressive therapy is discontinued. A cluster of PRCA cases in Europe was traced almost exclusively to subcutaneous administration of a form of epoetin alfa stabilized with Tween 80. This additive was never used in the United States where PRCA has always been rare. With removal of this preparation from the European market, the incidence of PRCA fell dramatically. An additional small cluster of PRCA cases was reported with one of the biosimilar ESAs approved in Europe. That cluster was traced to interaction of the agent with tungsten used in the manufacturing of the needles of prefilled syringes. Once the root cause was identified and eliminated, no further clusters of PRCA with that agent have been reported.

Target Hemoglobin Level

The target Hb level for anemic patients with CKD treated with ESAs has been controversial because observational studies disagree with the results of interventional trials. Based on studies of epoetin efficacy in the early 1990s that compared outcomes in untreated patients with hematocrit (Hct) values in the mid-20s with those in treated patients with Hct values in the mid-30s, the first iteration of the NKF-DOQI anemia guidelines (1997) had an opinion-based recommendation that the target Hct for epoetin-treated patients should be 33% to 36%. However, observational studies from the United States Renal Data System (USRDS) and large dialysis chain databases suggested that the benefits of higher

Hct or Hb levels extend to levels greater than 39% and 13 g/dL, respectively, with QoL increasing directly across the spectrum of Hct/Hb levels. In 1998, results from the Normal Hematocrit Study (NHS), which randomized 1223 patients undergoing HD with underlying cardiac disease receiving epoetin to target Hct 30% versus target Hct 42%, became available. The study was terminated early because of the low likelihood that the patients randomized to the higher Hct would show better outcomes. The patients in the higher target Hct group had a relative risk of 1.3 (confidence interval, 0.9 to 1.9) for the primary endpoints of death or myocardial infarction. Furthermore, patients in the higher target Hct group had a significantly greater incidence of vascular access thrombosis.

The Cardiovascular Risk Reduction by Early Anemia Treatment with Epoetin Beta (CREATE) study randomly assigned 603 patients with GFRs between 15 and 35 mL/min/1.73 m² and a baseline Hb of 11 to 12.5 g/dL to one of two groups. High target patients were immediately treated with epoetin beta to target Hb 13 to 15 g/dL, while low target patients were treated only when their Hb fell to less than 10.5 g/dL with target Hb 10.5 to 11.5 g/dL. There was no difference between the two groups in the primary endpoint (time to first cardiovascular event). Although there was no difference in the rate of decline in GFR between the two groups, more patients in the higher Hb target group required dialysis. There was no difference between the two groups in combined adverse events.

The Correction of Hemoglobin and Outcomes in Renal Insufficiency (CHOIR) study randomized 1432 patients with CKD stage 4 to target Hb 11.3 g/dL versus 13.5 g/dL. The average follow-up period was 16 months, and the study was terminated early because of safety concerns in the higher target Hb group. The primary endpoint was a composite of death, myocardial infarction, hospitalization for congestive heart failure (without kidney replacement therapy), and stroke. The patients in the higher target Hb group had a significantly higher incidence of the composite endpoint, congestive heart failure, death, and hospitalization (cardiovascular and all-cause). There was no difference between the groups in rates of stroke, myocardial infarction, kidney replacement therapy, or QoL.

The Trial to Reduce Cardiovascular Events with Aranesp Therapy (TREAT) study was published in 2009. TREAT examined the use of darbepoetin in anemic patients with type 2 diabetes and NDD-CKD. Unlike the CHOIR and CREATE studies, the TREAT study had a placebo arm. Important outcomes that were considered included death, cardiovascular events, progression of

TABLE 55.1	Erythropoiesis-Stimulating Agents Available in the United States, 2020		
Generic Name	Brand Name	Dosing Frequency	Starting Dose
Epoetin	Epogen, Procrit, Retacrit (biosimilar)	Three times weekly IV in HD patients; every 1–2 weeks SC in NDD-CKD and PD patients	50 units/kg based on three times weekly dosing
Darbepoetin	Aranesp	Every 1–2 weeks IV or SC in ESKD patients; every 4 weeks SC in NDD-CKD patients	0.45 μg/kg weekly or 0.75 μg/kg every 2 weeks in ESKD patients; 0.45 μg/kg every 4 weeks in ND-CKD patients
Methoxy polyethylene glycol-epoetin beta	Mircera	Initiation: every 2 weeks; maintenance: monthly. IV in HD patients, SC in NDD-CKD and PD patients	0.6 μg/kg every 2 weeks; monthly when Hb is stable at twice the every-2-weeks dose

CKD, Chronic kidney disease; *ESKD*, end-stage kidney disease; *Hb*, hemoglobin; *HD*, hemodialysis; *IV*, intravenous; *NDD*, nondialysis-dependent; *PD*, peritoneal dialysis; *SC*, subcutaneous.

kidney disease, and QoL. One group received darbepoetin to target Hb of 13 g/dL, and the other was not administered any ESA unless the Hb level decreased to less than 9 g/dL. Other than a higher incidence of stroke in the higher target Hb group, cardiovascular events and deaths were similar in both arms. Unsurprisingly, there were more blood transfusions in the placebo group. A finding of some concern was that patients with a history of cancer were more likely to die of cancer if randomized to the higher Hb target. The findings of the NHS, CHOIR, CREATE, and TREAT studies are summarized in Table 55.2.

In 2011, the FDA substantially changed the product information for ESAs, eliminating a prior target Hb range of 10 to 12 g/dL and adding a new boxed warning regarding the risk of death, myocardial infarction, stroke, venous thromboembolism, thrombosis of vascular access, and tumor progression and recurrence. Other elements of the 2011 FDA guidelines are summarized in Box 55.2. The elimination of a target Hb range for ESA therapy, which had generally driven the development and use of standardized ESA dose titration protocols, and the substitution of a recommendation for "individualization" of ESA therapy with the goal of transfusion avoidance led to considerable confusion and controversy within the nephrology community. Especially challenging is the FDA recommendation that ESA therapy in NDD-CKD patients not be initiated until the Hb is less than 10 g/dL, and that the dose be reduced or interrupted if Hb rises to greater than 10 g/dL. Given the stated goal of minimizing transfusions, it is the authors' opinion that the FDA should have given more direction and recommended Hb target ranges of 9 to 10 g/dL and 9 to 11 g/dL in the NDD- and dialysis-dependent (DD) CKD populations, respectively.

The concept of individualization in therapy is appropriate to properly balance the risk and benefit. Transfusion avoidance is a higher priority to avoid allosensitization in patients who are candidates for kidney transplantation. The QoL benefits of ESA therapy and higher Hb levels vary with patients' comorbidities, psychologic structures, functional levels, and expectations. Furthermore, QoL is intrinsically more difficult to quantify and track than is hemoglobin level. Ideally, the goals of ESA therapy should incorporate the effect of treatment on patients' perception of their QoL with instruments that focus attention on the specific domains that are affected by anemia. The improvement in each of these domains, including fatigue, energy level, sense of vitality, and physical functioning, should be assessed on an individual basis to determine the Hb target range for each patient.

In 2012, the KDIGO Clinical Practice Guideline for Anemia in CKD was published. The KDIGO recommendations regarding target Hb level for patients receiving ESA therapy are summarized in Box 55.3. It should be noted that the KDIGO guideline acknowledges a QoL benefit from ESA therapy, which the FDA does not. This guideline replaces the 2006 to 2007 KDOQI anemia guidelines as the most current evidence basis for treatment of anemia in patients with CKD in the United States.

HIF-Prolyl Hydroxylase Inhibitors

Novel anemia treatments include agents that potentiate HIF activity by inhibiting the prolyl hydroxylase (PH) enzyme that normally leads to HIF degradation in proteosomes. In the absence of prolyl hydroxylation, HIF-α translocates to the nucleus and forms a heterodimer with HIF-β that promotes transcription of proteins that upregulate erythropoiesis (Fig. 55.2). Among three subtypes of HIF-α, HIF-2α has the greatest effects on erythropoiesis. This stimulates the production of endogenous EPO, even in patients with end-stage kidney disease (ESKD), suggesting that significant extrarenal EPO

TABLE 55.2	Large, Randomized Studies of Erythropoiesis-Stimulating Agents in Chronic Kidney Disease Patients with Anemia			
	NHS	CHOIR	CREATE	TREAT
Year published	1998	2006	2006	2009
Location	United States	United States	Europe	International
ESA	Epoetin alfa	Epoetin alfa	Epoetin beta	Darbepoetin alfa
CKD stage and comorbidity	Dialysis with cardiac disease	Nondialysis	Nondialysis	Nondialysis with type 2 diabetes
Number of patients	1223	1432	603	4038
High Hb target (g/dL)	14 (Hct 42)	13.5	13–15	13
Low Hb target (g/dL)	10 (Hct 30)	11.3	10.5–11.5	9
CV endpoints	RR 1.3 (CI 0.9–1.9)	Higher in high Hb group	No difference	No difference except higher stroke in high Hb group
Progression of CKD	Not applicable	No difference	More in high Hb group	No difference
Cancer deaths	Not noted	Not noted	Not noted	Higher in high Hb group among patients with previous cancer
QoL	Better in high Hb group	No difference	Better in high Hb group	No difference except less fatigue in high Hb group

CHOIR, Correction of Hemoglobin and Outcomes in Renal Insufficiency; *CI*, confidence interval; *CKD*, chronic kidney disease; *CREATE*, Cardiovascular Risk Reduction by Early Anemia Treatment with Epoetin; *CV*, cardiovascular; *ESA*, erythropoiesis-stimulating agent; *Hb*, hemoglobin; *Hct*, hematocrit; *NHS*, Normal Hematocrit Study; *QoL*, quality of life; *RR*, risk ratio; *TREAT*, Trial to Reduce Cardiovascular Events with Aranesp Therapy.

BOX 55.2

US Food and Drug Administration Guidelines on Use of Erythropoiesis-Stimulating Agents in Patients with Chronic Kidney Disease

General Guidance

In controlled trials, patients experienced greater risks for death, serious adverse cardiovascular reactions, and stroke when administered ESAs to target a Hb level of greater than 11 g/dL.

No trial has identified a Hb target level, ESA dose, or dosing strategy that does not increase these risks.

Use the lowest ESA dose sufficient to reduce the need for RBC transfusions.

Physicians and patients should weigh the possible benefits of decreasing transfusions against the increased risks of death and other serious cardiovascular adverse events.

For All Patients With CKD

When initiating or adjusting therapy, monitor Hb levels at least weekly until stable, then monitor at least monthly. When adjusting therapy, consider Hb rate of rise, rate of decline, ESA responsiveness, and Hb variability. A single Hb excursion may not require a dosing change. Do not increase the dose more frequently than once every 4 weeks. Decreases in dose can occur more frequently. Avoid frequent dose adjustments.

If the Hb rises rapidly (e.g., more than 1 g/dL in any 2-week period), reduce the dose of ESA by 25% or more, as needed to reduce rapid responses.

For patients who do not respond adequately (Hb increase <1 g/dL after 4 weeks of therapy), increase the dose by 25%.

For patients who do not respond adequately over a 12-week escalation period, increasing the ESA dose further is unlikely to improve response and may increase risks.

Evaluate other causes of anemia.

Discontinue ESA if responsiveness does not improve.

For Adult Patients Not on Dialysis

Consider initiating ESA treatment only when the Hb level is less than 10 g/dL, AND

The rate of Hb decline indicates the likelihood of requiring RBC transfusion, AND

Reducing the risk of allosensitization and/or other RBC transfusion related risks is a goal.

If the Hb level exceeds 10 g/dL, reduce or interrupt the dose of ESA.

For Adult Patients on Dialysis

Initiate ESA treatment when the Hb level is less than 10 g/dL.

If the Hb level approaches or exceeds 11 g/dL, reduce or interrupt the dose of ESA.

The intravenous route is recommended for patients on hemodialysis.

CKD, Chronic kidney disease; *ESA,* erythropoiesis-stimulating agent; *Hb,* hemoglobin; *RBC,* red blood cell.

BOX 55.3

Key KDIGO Recommendations Regarding Target Hemoglobin Level in Patients Receiving ESA Therapy

For adult CKD nondialysis patients with Hb less than 10 g/dL, it is suggested that the decision to initiate ESA therapy is individualized based on the rate of fall of Hb, previous response to iron therapy, risk of needing transfusion, risks related to ESA therapy, and presence of symptoms attributable to anemia.

For adult CKD patients on dialysis, it is suggested that ESA therapy is used to avoid having the Hb concentration fall below 9 g/dL by starting ESA therapy when the Hb is 9 to 10 g/dL. Individualization of therapy is reasonable, as some patients may have improvements in QoL at higher Hb concentration, and ESA therapy may be started above 10 g/dL.

In general, it is suggested that ESAs are not used to maintain Hb concentration above 11.5 g/dL in adult patients with CKD.

Individualization of therapy will be necessary, as some patients experience improvements in QoL at Hb concentrations above 11.5 g/dL and will be prepared to accept the risks.

In all adult patients, it is recommended that ESAs not be used intentionally to increase the Hb above 13 g/dL.

CKD, Chronic kidney disease; *ESA,* erythropoiesis-stimulating agent; *Hb,* hemoglobin; *KDIGO,* Kidney Disease Improving Global Outcomes; *QoL,* quality of life.

production can be induced. These agents also downregulate hepcidin production, which may make them more effective than conventional ESAs for treating patients with underlying inflammation. Moreover, the HIF-PH inhibitors can be taken orally, which makes them potentially attractive to NDD-CKD patients and those on home dialysis who would otherwise have their ESA administered SC. There are three HIF-PH inhibitor agents undergoing or completing analysis of phase 3 studies in the United States. Table 55.3 summarizes the properties of HIF-PH inhibitors under development in the United States. The most common side effects noted with HIF-PH inhibitors have been gastrointestinal effects of nausea, vomiting, and diarrhea. Some patients developed hyperkalemia. Because HIF effects are not limited to erythropoiesis, potential safety concerns include protumorigenic effects, proangiogenic effects (affecting diabetic retinopathy or pulmonary hypertension), thromboembolism, worsened systemic hypertension, effects on CKD progression, and cyst growth. These concerns have not been validated to a statistically significant degree in animal or premarketing studies to date. The publication of phase 3 studies involving thousands of patients, as well as postmarketing surveillance will be needed to put these concerns to rest or incorporate them into a risk-benefit analysis in the use of this class of agents. HIF-PH inhibitors offer a promising new therapeutic option for treatment of anemia of CKD. Time will tell if the safety issues related to higher target Hb levels with ESAs also hold true with these agents.

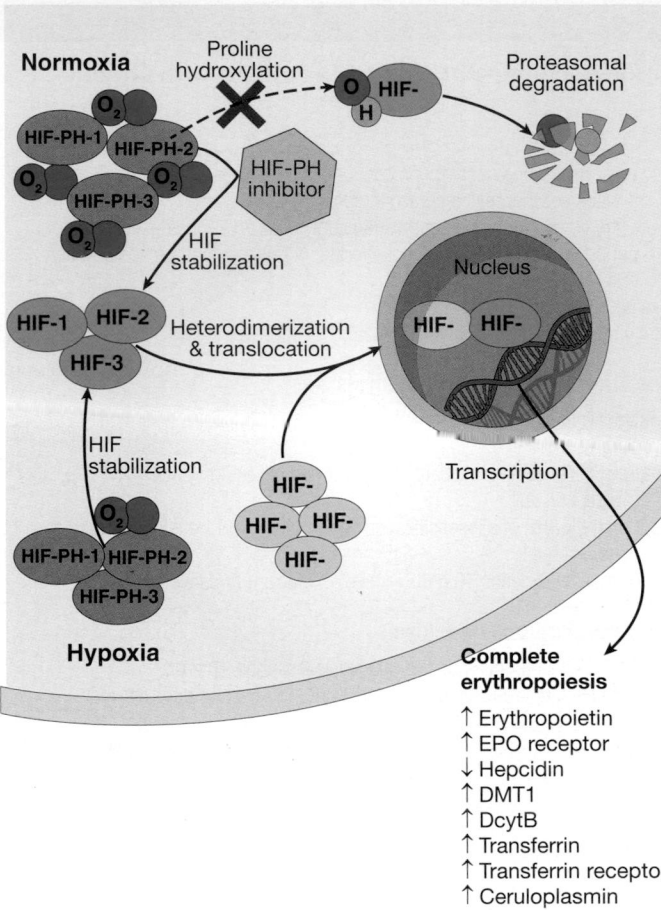

Normoxia

Proline hydroxylation

Proteasomal degradation

HIF-PH-1 HIF-PH-2

HIF-PH inhibitor

HIF-PH-3

HIF stabilization

HIF-1 HIF-2

Heterodimerization & translocation

HIF-3

Nucleus

HIF- HIF-

HIF stabilization

HIF-

HIF- HIF-

HIF-PH-1 HIF-PH-2

HIF-

HIF-PH-3

Hypoxia

Transcription

Complete erythropoiesis

↑ Erythropoietin
↑ EPO receptor
↓ Hepcidin
↑ DMT1
↑ DcytB
↑ Transferrin
↑ Transferrin receptor
↑ Ceruloplasmin

• **Fig. 55.2** Hypoxia inducible factor pathway. *HIF,* Hypoxia inducible factor; *PH,* prolyl hydroxylase; *EPO,* erythropoietin; *DMT1,* divalent metal transporter 1; *DcytB,* duodenal cytochrome B. (Adapted from Gupta N, Wish JB. Hypoxia-inducible factor prolyl hydroxylase inhibitors: a potential new treatment for anemia in patients with CKD. *Am J Kidney Dis.* 2017;69:815–826.)

Iron Therapy

Iron deficiency frequently coexists with EPO deficiency as a cause of anemia in NDD-CKD patients, and it almost universally develops in patients treated with HD because of blood losses in the extracorporeal circuit, frequent blood testing, oozing from vascular access sites after dialysis needles are withdrawn, and vascular access procedures. NDD-CKD patients may develop absolute iron deficiency because of inadequate oral iron intake resulting from dietary protein restriction or loss of a taste for red meat. Even if iron deficiency is not present at the time of initial anemia evaluation, it often develops after initiation of ESA therapy because the stimulation of new RBC production exhausts existing iron stores. Therefore, it is important to monitor iron status with serum ferritin and TSAT levels monthly during initiation of ESA therapy and every 3 months after stable Hb level has been achieved. The target serum ferritin and TSAT levels for patients receiving ESAs are higher than those used to diagnose iron deficiency in the general population because of the phenomenon of functional iron deficiency.

Supplemental iron can be administered orally or intravenously. Oral iron may be sufficient to achieve target iron parameters in non-HD CKD patients because they do not have the ongoing blood losses of patients undergoing HD. However, even in non-HD CKD patients, oral iron may be ineffective because of incomplete adherence, impaired absorption, side effects, and the magnitude of iron deficit. Commonly prescribed oral ferrous iron salts (sulfate, fumarate, gluconate) must be oxidized by stomach acid to the ferric form before they can be absorbed by the small intestine. This step may be impaired if stomach acid is buffered by food or an antacid or if the patient is taking a histamine-2 blocker or proton pump inhibitor. Therefore, these oral iron salts should be administered 1 hour before or 2 hours after a meal. The minimal effective oral iron dose to repair iron deficiency is 200 mg of elemental iron daily, but each 325-mg tablet of ferrous sulfate

TABLE 55.3 Hypoxia Inducible Factor Stabilizers Under Clinical Development

Compound	Effective Daily Oral Doses in Phase II Trials	Dosing Schedule	Half-life	Plasma EPO (IU/L)	Under Development for Use in the United States
Daprodustat	5–25 mg	Daily or 3 times weekly	1–7 hr	24.7 (5 mg DD-CKD) 34.4 (5 mg NDD-CKD) 82.4 (10 mg DD-CKD)	Yes
Desidustat	100–200 mg	Every alternate day	6–14 hr	20.9 (100 mg NDD-CKD) 39.6 (150 mg NDD-CKD) 42.71 (200 mg NDD-CKD)	No
Enarodustat	2–6 mg	Daily	9 h (mean)	18.4 (2 mg DD-CKD) 22.5 (4 mg DD-CKD) 23.7 (6 mg DD-CKD)	No
Molidustat	25–150 mg	Daily	4–10 hr	39.8 (50 mg NDD-non-CKD)	No
Roxadustat	0.7–2.5 mg/kg	3 times weekly	12–15 hr	113 (1 mg/kg NDD-CKD) 397 (2 mg/kg NDD-CKD) 130 (1.3 mg/kg DD-CKD)	Yes
Vadadustat	150–600 mg	Daily or 3 times weekly	4.7–9.1 hr	32	Yes

EPO, Erythropoietin; *IU,* international units; *DD,* dialysis-dependent; *NDD,* nondialysis-dependent. Modified from Sanghani NS, Haase VH. Hypoxia-inducible factor activators in renal anemia: current clinical experience. *Adv Chronic Kidney Dis.* 2019;26:253–266.

contains only 65 mg of elemental iron, requiring an iron-deficient patient to take at least three tablets daily in divided doses. A 325-mg tablet of ferrous fumarate contains approximately 100 mg of elemental iron, requiring an iron-deficient patient to take two tablets daily in divided doses. A 325-mg tablet of ferrous gluconate contains 39 mg of elemental iron, requiring five to six tablets daily in an iron-deficient patient. Oral polysaccharide-iron complex contains 150 mg of elemental iron in each 150-mg capsule, requiring one tablet twice daily to provide greater than 200 mg elemental iron. The bioavailability of oral iron salts is only 1% to 2% of the administered dose in patients with elevated serum ferritin, so even an adherent patient may be unable to repair an iron deficit with an oral agent. Frequently, oral iron salts are associated with gastrointestinal side effects such as epigastric pain and constipation that may further limit adherence.

Newer oral iron preparations have become available which may offer an improved efficacy and side effect profile. Ferric citrate initially gained FDA approval as a phosphate binder in 2014, but further studies resulted in an additional FDA-approved indication in 2017 for treating anemia due to iron deficiency in NDD-CKD patients. Studies have suggested effectiveness in raising hemoglobin and decreasing ESA and IV iron requirements in DD-CKD patients, but this is an off-label use. Ferric maltol is another agent that is FDA approved for treatment of iron deficiency anemia in adults including those with NDD-CKD. Gastrointestinal effects remain the most common adverse events with these newer agents but may be less prominent than with older ferrous iron formulations because the ferric ion is less reactive. Sucrosomial iron consists of ferric pyrophosphate encased in a phospholipid bilayer and sucrose ester. This configuration protects the iron from an acidic stomach and allows direct endocytosis by microfold cells (M cells) in Peyer's patches of the small bowel. This formulation has been well tolerated in studies of patients with celiac disease, bariatric surgery, and malignancy. Safety and efficacy data for this preparation in CKD patients are limited to date.

For non-HD patients with iron deficiency unresponsive to oral iron, and for all patients undergoing HD receiving ESAs whose iron parameters are at or below target levels, IV iron therapy is recommended. Six forms of IV iron are available in the United States (in order of FDA approval): iron dextran, iron sucrose, iron gluconate, ferumoxytol, ferric carboxymaltose, and ferric derisomaltose (iron isomaltoside). Iron dextran is the least expensive, but it has been associated with fatal anaphylactic reactions leading to a "black box" warning by the FDA and the need for a test dose of 25 mg at the time of first administration. The absence of a reaction to the test dose makes it less likely, but it does not guarantee that the patient will not have an anaphylactic reaction to a therapeutic dose of iron dextran. An advantage of iron dextran is that it can be administered in dosages as high as 1000 mg in a single session. This may be a consideration for non-HD patients with limited access to a healthcare facility to receive IV iron, and it preserves veins for future HD vascular access because fewer infusions are required. Iron sucrose and iron gluconate have never been associated with a fatal anaphylactic reaction and do not require a test dose. However, they can be administered to a maximum of only 250 to 300 mg per session, so a non-HD patient with severe iron deficiency will require several infusions to replete iron stores. Iron sucrose and iron gluconate are preferred in patients undergoing HD whose regular visits and access to the circulation through the extracorporeal circuit make smaller and more frequent dosing appropriate. Iron sucrose and iron gluconate have been associated with nonfatal anaphylactic reactions, hypotension, and nausea/vomiting. For iron dextran, sucrose, and gluconate, slower infusion rates and smaller doses in a single session are associated with a lower incidence of side effects.

Ferumoxytol, ferric carboxymaltose, and ferric derisomaltose can be given in infusion doses of 510, 750, and 1000 mg, respectively. Ferumoxytol is approved by the FDA for administration of 510 mg over at least 15 minutes. A second dose can be administered 3 to 8 days later in a patient with TSAT less than 20%. Ferumoxytol has been associated with a small number of fatal anaphylactic reactions and received a strengthened warning from the FDA in 2015 due to anaphylaxis risk. Ferric carboxymaltose is given in a dose of 750 mg administered as an infusion over at least 15 minutes or a slow IV push over at least 7.5 minutes. A second 750-mg dose of ferric carboxymaltose can be administered at least 7 days later. In 2021 the FDA approved a single 1000 mg dose of ferric carboxymaltose. Iron isomaltoside is FDA approved for administration of a single dose of 1000 mg over 20 minutes. These agents have potential appeal to non-HD CKD patients with iron deficiency because they allow decreased frequency and duration of clinic visits to receive IV iron therapy, and they preserve veins for future HD vascular access. The safety profiles of ferumoxytol, ferric carboxymaltose, and iron isomaltoside appear to be similar to those of iron sucrose and gluconate, with serious adverse events occurring in 0.4% to 0.6% of treatments. More recently, the risk of "6H syndrome" (high FGF-23, hypophosphatemia, hyperphosphaturia, hypovitaminosis D, hypocalcemia, and secondary hyperparathyroidism) has been noted with some agents, most commonly ferric carboxymaltose. Characteristics of available IV iron preparations are summarized in Table 55.4.

The Dialysis Patients' Response to IV Iron with Elevated Ferritin (DRIVE) study examined the efficacy of IV iron administration in patients undergoing HD who had Hb less than 11 g/dL on adequate ESA therapy, TSAT less than 25%, and serum ferritin 500 to 1200 ng/mL. The study showed that administration of eight 125-mg doses of iron gluconate resulted in more efficient erythropoiesis, a more rapid rise in Hb levels, a decrease in ESA requirements, and adverse events similar to those in a control group that received no IV iron. These findings suggest that there is a spectrum of responsiveness to IV iron that extends to patients with serum ferritin levels as high as 1200 ng/mL.

The PIVOTAL trial compared proactive high-dose IV iron sucrose (400 mg monthly; held for ferritin >700 µg/L) to a reactive strategy (0–400 mg monthly administered when ferritin was <200 µg/L or transferrin saturation <20%) in 2141 hemodialysis patients with a median follow-up of 2.1 years. The primary outcome was a composite of myocardial infarction, stroke, heart failure hospitalization, or death assessed in a time-to-first event analysis. Fewer patients in the high-dose group experienced the primary outcome (320 vs. 338 patients; HR 0.85, 95% CI 0.73–1.0, p = 0.04). These results suggest relative safety of a more aggressive IV iron repletion strategy as long as ferritin levels are <700 µg/L in this population. Patients in the proactive iron group achieved the same average Hb levels but required 19% less ESA at year one than the reactive iron group.

Concerns have been raised about the potential toxicity of IV iron supplements, including cellular and vascular damage from oxidative stress and impaired white blood cell function based on in vitro studies. There has been evidence of increased urinary excretion of markers of tubular injury, but not increased albuminuria, in CKD patients receiving IV iron sucrose. However, observational studies have not demonstrated increased hospitalizations or mortality in patients undergoing HD receiving an average of

TABLE 55.4	Intravenous Iron Preparations Available in the United States			
Generic Name	Brand Name	Labeled Dosing for Iron Deficiency	IV Administration Time	Test Dose Required?
Iron dextran	DexFerrum, INFeD	1000 mg in 10 divided doses or total dose as a single IV infusion	Infusion rate should not exceed 500 mL/hr	Yes
Iron sucrose	Venofer	1000 mg in 10 divided doses (hemodialysis) 1000 mg in 5 divided doses (nondialysis) 1000 mg in 2 doses of 300 mg and 1 dose of 400 mg (peritoneal dialysis)	5 min undiluted; 15 min if diluted in saline Undiluted over 5 min or infused over 30–60 min 300 mg infused over 1.5 hr 400 mg infused over 2.5 hr	No
Iron gluconate	Ferrlecit, Nulecit	1000 mg in 8 divided doses (hemodialysis only)	60 min diluted in saline	No
Ferumoxytol	Feraheme	510 mg × 2 doses	Undiluted or infused over ≥15 min, 5–8 days apart	No
Ferric carboxymaltose	Injectafer (US), Ferinject	750 mg × 2 doses 1000 mg × 1 doses	Slow IV push over ≥7.5 min or infused over ≥15 min, ≥7 days apart Slow IV push or infusion ≥15 min	No
Ferric derisomaltose (iron isomaltoside)	Monoferric (US), Monofer	<50 kg: 20 mg/kg as a single dose ≥50 kg: 1000 mg as a single dose	Infused over ≥20 min	No

less than 400 mg of IV iron per month, and IV iron therapy was not identified as a risk factor for bacteremia in patients undergoing HD in a multivariate analysis.

The REVOKE single-center trial of oral ferrous sulfate vs. IV iron sucrose in 136 NDD-CKD patients followed for an average of 2.2 years identified an adjusted incident rate ratio of 2.51 (95% CI 1.56–4.04) higher serious cardiovascular events and 2.12 (1.24–3.64) higher infections resulting in hospitalization in the IV iron arm, leading to early trial cessation. In contrast, the FIND-CKD study of 626 NDD-CKD patients receiving oral ferrous sulfate vs. IV ferric carboxymaltose with 1 year of follow-up found no such concerns. Differences in study design and safety reporting preclude full reconciliation of these findings. Concerns about higher rates of adverse events with IV iron formulations in non-HD CKD patients persist, while the need to effectively manage iron deficiency anemia often necessitates utilizing IV iron.

The 2012 KDIGO anemia guidelines recommend a trial of IV iron (or a 1- to 3-month trial of oral iron in NDD patients) for adult CKD patients with anemia not on iron or ESA therapy if an increase in Hb concentration without starting ESA therapy is desired, TSAT is ≤30%, and ferritin is ≤500 ng/mL. For those CKD patients receiving ESA therapy not receiving iron supplementation, a trial of IV iron (or a 1- to 3-month trial of oral iron in NDD patients) is recommended if an increase in Hb concentration or decrease in ESA dose is desired, TSAT is ≤30%, and ferritin is ≤500 ng/mL. More recent UK guidelines acknowledge a high prevalence of CKD patients with ferritin >500 ng/mL and endorse repleting iron up to ferritin levels of 800 ng/mL.

Another product is available that provides lower doses of iron on a more continuous basis for patients undergoing HD and may thereby decrease the risk of excessive iron storage. Ferric pyrophosphate citrate (FPC) is added to the hemodialysate and provides the 5 to 7 mg of iron estimated to be lost during each dialysis treatment due to blood remaining in the dialysate circuit, oozing from needle sites, and phlebotomy. Phase 3 studies with FPC demonstrated stable serum ferritin and TSAT levels with decreased IV iron and ESA requirements. FPC is added to the bicarbonate central delivery system or to individual bicarbonate concentrate containers.

Resistance to Erythropoiesis-Stimulating Agents and Adjuvant Therapy

ESA resistance has been defined as failure to achieve Hb greater than 11 g/dL despite an epoetin dose of greater than 300–450 units/kg/week or the equivalent of another ESA. The causes of ESA resistance are the same as the causes of anemia in CKD (see Box 55.1), with the obvious exception of EPO deficiency and with the addition of PRCA. After iron deficiency, the most common cause of ESA resistance in patients with CKD is inflammation or infection. This is often associated with high levels of acute phase reactants such as serum ferritin, C-reactive protein (CRP), and erythrocyte sedimentation rate (ESR), but the source of the inflammation or infection may not be readily apparent. It has been demonstrated that patients undergoing HD, who use catheters for vascular access, have lower mean Hb levels and higher mean ESA doses, which probably reflects the inflammatory state induced by the presence of the catheter and its biofilm. Occult periodontal disease has also been recognized as a cause of ESA resistance.

Although the intention-to-treat analyses of the CHOIR and TREAT studies conclude that higher target Hb levels are associated with increased cardiovascular events, secondary analyses of these studies implicate the higher ESA doses received by the patients in the higher Hb target arms. The conclusion is that ESA doses should not be uptitrated indefinitely in patients who fail to achieve target Hb levels because the risk of ESA therapy far exceeds the benefit in patients who do not respond readily to ESAs. For patients who have not responded adequately over a 12-week escalation period, the FDA recommends that increasing the dose further is unlikely to improve response and may increase risks. For NDD-CKD patients, an epoetin dose ceiling of 300 units/kg/week (or the equivalent of another ESA) should be considered, whereas the dose ceiling for patients undergoing dialysis should be 450 units/kg/week (or equivalent dose of another ESA).

There is insufficient evidence to support the use of adjuvants to ESA therapy, such as L-carnitine and vitamin C, in the management of anemia in patients with CKD. Although androgens were widely used to increase Hb levels in patients undergoing dialysis in the pre-ESA era, their use is not recommended because of insufficient evidence to support their efficacy in patients receiving adequate doses of ESAs and because of the potential for long-term toxicity.

Despite the use of adequate doses of ESA and iron therapy, transfusions with RBCs are sometimes required in the setting of ESA resistance or acute blood loss. Transfusions are considered a last resort because of the potential development of sensitization affecting future transplantation candidacy and the small risk of blood-borne infections. There is no single Hb concentration that necessitates transfusion, and the decision of whether and when to transfuse should be made based on the patient's individual situation, including comorbid illnesses, symptoms, acuity of Hb decrease, and potential for future transplantation, as well as the Hb level.

Other Hematologic Manifestations of Kidney Disease

Abnormalities of Hemostasis

Patients with advanced CKD typically have normal results on coagulation studies and normal platelet counts, but they exhibit an increased bleeding tendency because of defects in platelet function. This is manifested by prolonged bleeding time and abnormal studies of platelet aggregation and adhesiveness. There may also be an abnormal interaction between platelets and the vascular endothelium, mediated by decreased activity of GbIIb-IIIa binding to von Willebrand factor (vWF), as well as increased release of endothelial nitric oxide related to accumulation of guanidosuccinic acid and methylguanidine. Thrombocytopenia has been reported to rarely occur in patients undergoing hemodialysis with polysulfone membranes sterilized by electron beam technology. The clinical manifestations of these abnormalities include an increased tendency to and increased duration of bleeding after trauma and in the setting of serosal inflammation. This often manifests as epistaxis, bleeding with tooth brushing, and easy bruisability, but it can result in life-threatening gastrointestinal hemorrhage or hemorrhagic pericarditis. The bleeding diathesis is only partially corrected by dialysis, and larger molecules that accumulate in the setting of kidney failure, such as parathyroid hormone, have also been implicated. Anemia may also contribute to the bleeding diathesis of uremia, as higher RBC counts push platelets closer to the vessel wall, making them more effective. Treatment of anemia with RBC transfusion and/or ESAs to Hb greater than 10 g/dL improves the bleeding diathesis. Platelet function improves after the initiation of ESA therapy but before the Hb rises, suggesting that ESAs may improve platelet function directly.

The treatment of choice for bleeding episodes in uremic patients is to provide adequate dialysis with minimal or no anticoagulation and to initiate ESA therapy. If bleeding continues or if the patient is at risk for bleeding from an invasive procedure, then treatment with desmopressin (DDAVP) should be considered. DDAVP is a synthetic form of antidiuretic hormone that has minimal vasopressor activity and is used in the treatment of diabetes insipidus. The mechanism of its action in the setting of uremic bleeding is thought to be related to the release of vWF from endothelial cells and platelets. The dose of DDAVP is 0.3 µg/kg IV or 3 µg/kg intranasally, and it can be repeated 1 to 2 times before tachyphylaxis develops. The onset of action is immediate, and the duration of action is 4 to 8 hours. More than half of patients treated with DDAVP respond with an improvement in bleeding time, and the reason for the lack of response in other patients is unknown. Because of tachyphylaxis, it is recommended that DDAVP be administered only once, immediately before an invasive procedure (and not the day before). DDAVP tachyphylaxis appears to abate after 48 hours, and twice-weekly therapy has been shown effective in some patients with chronic bleeding.

Conjugated estrogens (Premarin) act to reduce bleeding for up to 14 days, but the onset of action takes 6 hours. The dose is 0.6 mg/kg daily for 5 consecutive days, and this regimen has been effective in controlling gastrointestinal bleeding associated with arteriovenous malformations in uremic patients. The mechanism of action may be related to inhibition of vascular nitric oxide production.

Like DDAVP, cryoprecipitate provides vWF, but is less convenient to use and carries the risk of blood-borne infections. The onset of action of cryoprecipitate is 1 hour, and its effect peaks at 12 hours. The dose is 10 units and can be repeated as necessary. The response to cryoprecipitate is highly variable, and it should be reserved for life-threatening hemorrhage.

The platelet hemostatic defect in uremia does not appear to protect against vascular access thrombosis, which is a common problem in patients on hemodialysis. The use of antiplatelet agents such as aspirin and clopidogrel to preserve vascular access may be associated with an unacceptably high rate of bleeding and is not typically recommended. Use of these agents for conventional indications, such as coronary artery and cerebrovascular disease, is not contraindicated in patients with CKD, although the benefit must be weighed against risk. Similarly, heparin and warfarin are frequently needed for conventional indications in patients with CKD, but the use of these agents superimposes a risk of bleeding on the underlying abnormalities of platelet function. It is estimated that the incidence of venous thrombotic and thromboembolic disease (exclusive of vascular access thrombosis) in patients with CKD is twice that of the general population. This is attributed to the complications of nephrotic syndrome with increased plasma fibrinogen and decreased plasma antithrombin III levels, the presence of systemic lupus with circulating "anticoagulants" such as antiphospholipid antibodies, elevated levels of homocysteine, venous injury from previous catheter placement, and the continued presence of intravascular "foreign bodies," such as dialysis catheters and arteriovenous grafts.

Increased experience with enoxaparin in patients with CKD has simplified anticoagulation in certain settings because monitoring of the partial thromboplastin time is not required. The dose of enoxaparin for CKD patients with GFR less than 30 mL/min/1.73 m² including those on dialysis is 1 mg/kg subcutaneous daily for deep venous thrombosis (DVT) and acute coronary syndromes or 30 mg daily subcutaneous for DVT prophylaxis. When given in prophylactic doses, enoxaparin has not been shown to increase the risk of bleeding complications irrespective of the degree of impairment of kidney function. In patients with CKD at high risk for bleeding receiving therapeutic doses of enoxaparin, anti-Xa monitoring is recommended with a target peak level to 1 to 2 IU/mL if enoxaparin is administered q24 hours and 0.6–1 IU/mL if enoxaparin is administered q12 hours.

The direct oral anticoagulants (DOACs) are excreted by the kidneys to varying degrees, and dosing recommendations for most agents are available for mild CKD (creatinine clearance [CrCl] >30 mL/min). DOACs have not been well studied in patients with advanced CKD, limiting the ability to give firm recommendations. However, some retrospective studies have not shown an increased risk of bleeding with apixaban, as compared to warfarin in patients with CrCl <25 mL/min, including those on dialysis. In nonvalvular atrial fibrillation, a reduced dose of 2.5 mg twice daily is recommended by some experts when CrCl is less than 30 mL/min. Anti-Xa monitoring is an option to balance safety and efficacy, though this approach has not been studied rigorously. Consultation with an updated dosing reference is recommended.

Abnormalities of Leukocytes

Except for a transient decrease in circulating granulocytes during the first 15 to 30 minutes of hemodialysis with older, unmodified cellulosic membranes, the white blood cell count of patients with uremia tends to be normal. The decrease in circulating granulocytes during unmodified cellulosic membrane hemodialysis is caused by alternative complement pathway activation, which leads to microleukoagglutination and margination of granulocytes in the pulmonary circulation. This may be responsible for the transient hypoxia that is sometimes observed during hemodialysis, and it is completely reversed by the end of the dialysis treatment. The function of granulocytes, including chemotaxis, adherence, phagocytosis, and production of reactive oxygen species, is altered in uremia; these changes may also be exacerbated by exposure to unmodified cellulosic membranes. Impaired granulocyte function is associated with increased susceptibility to infection with encapsulated bacteria, such as *Staphylococcus,* contributing to the high incidence of these infections in patients undergoing dialysis.

Monocyte and lymphocyte function are also impaired in uremia, leading to a decrease in cellular-type immunity. This may manifest as an increased susceptibility to viral infections, such as influenza, decreased response to vaccinations, and anergy to immunologic skin testing. The activity of autoimmune diseases, such as systemic lupus erythematosus may be attenuated after uremia supervenes. An impairment of cytokine release decreases the febrile response to pathogens in uremic patients so that infections may go unnoticed and may become more serious before diagnosis. The clinical implication is that symptoms suggestive of infection must trigger an aggressive diagnostic and therapeutic response in this vulnerable population.

Complete bibliography is available at Elsevier eBooks for Practicing Clinicians.

Key Bibliography

Agarwal AK, Yee J. Hepcidin. *Adv Chronic Kidney Dis.* 2019;26:298–305.

Agarwal R, Kusek JW, Pappas MK. A randomized trial of intravenous and oral iron in chronic kidney disease. *Kidney Int.* 2015;88:905–914.

Agarwal R. Iron deficiency anemia in chronic kidney disease: uncertainties and cautions. *Hemodial Int.* 2017;21:S78–S82.

Bailie GR, Larkina M, Goodkin DA, et al. Data from the Dialysis Outcomes and Practice Patterns Study validate an association between high intravenous iron doses and mortality. *Kidney Int.* 2015;87:162–168.

Batchelor EK, Kapitsinou P, Pergola P, et al. Iron deficiency in chronic kidney disease: updates on pathophysiology diagnosis, and treatment. *J Am Soc Nephrol.* 2020;31:456–468.

Besarab A, Bolton WK, Browne JK, et al. The effects of normal as compared with low hematocrit values in patients with cardiac disease who are receiving hemodialysis and erythropoietin. *N Engl J Med.* 1998;339:584–590.

Coyne DW, Kapoian T, Suki W, et al. DRIVE Study Group. Ferric gluconate is highly efficacious in anemic hemodialysis patients with high serum ferritin and low transferrin saturation: results of the Dialysis Patients' Response to IV Iron with Elevated Ferritin (DRIVE) Study. *J Am Soc Nephrol.* 2007;18:975–984.

Drueke TB, Locatelli F, Clyne N, et al. Normalization of hemoglobin level in patients with chronic kidney disease and anemia. *N Engl J Med.* 2006;355:2071–2984.

Gupta N, Wish JB. Hypoxia-inducible factor prolyl hydroxylase inhibitors: a potential new treatment for anemia in patients with CKD. *Am J Kidney Dis.* 2017;69:815–826.

Kidney Disease Improving Global Outcomes (KDIGO) Anemia Work Group 2012. Kidney Disease Improving Global Outcomes (KDIGO) Anemia Work Group. KDIGO clinical practice guideline for anemia in CKD. *Kidney Int Suppl.* 2012;2:1–335.

Kshirsagar AV, Li X. Long-term risks of intravenous iron in end-stage renal disease Patients. *Adv Chronic Kidney Dis.* 2019;26:292–297.

Lewis EF, Pfeffer MA, Feng A, et al. Darbepoetin alfa impact on health status in diabetes patient with kidney disease: a randomized trial. *Clin J Am Soc Nephrol.* 2011;6:845–855.

Lewis JB, Sika M, Koury MJ, et al. Ferric citrate controls phosphorus and delivers iron in patients on dialysis. *J Am Soc Nephrol.* 2015;26:493–503.

Macdougall IC, Bock AH, Carrera F, et al. FIND-CKD: a randomized trial of intravenous ferric carboxymaltose versus oral iron in patients with chronic kidney disease and iron deficiency anaemia. *Nephrol Dial Transplant.* 2014;29:2075–2084.

Macdougall IC, White C, Anker SD, et al. Intravenous iron in patients undergoing maintenance hemodialysis. *N Engl J Med.* 2019;380:447–458.

Pergola PE, Fishbane S, Ganz T. Novel oral iron therapies for iron deficiency anemia in chronic kidney disease. *Adv Chronic Kidney Dis.* 2019;26:272–291.

Pfeffer M, Burdmann E, Chen C, et al. A trial of darbepoetin alfa in type 2 diabetes and chronic kidney disease. *N Engl J Med.* 2009;361:2019–2032.

Sanghani NS, Haase VH. Hypoxia-inducible factor activators in renal anemia: current clinical experience. *Adv Chronic Kidney Dis.* 2019;26:253–266.

Shah HH, Fishbane S. Biosimilar erythropoiesis-stimulating agents in chronic kidney disease. *Adv Chronic Kidney Dis.* 2019;26:267–271.

Singh AK, Szczech L, Tang KL, et al. Correction of anemia with epoetin alfa in chronic kidney disease. *N Engl J Med.* 2006;355:2085–2098.

PART 11

Treatment of Kidney Failure

56

Hemodialysis and Hemofiltration

MADHUKAR MISRA

Hemodialysis (HD) is an extracorporeal therapy that is prescribed to reduce the signs and symptoms of uremia and to partially replace a number of the key functions of the kidneys when kidney function is no longer sufficient to maintain an individual's well-being or life. Although HD is one of several kidney replacement therapies (along with peritoneal dialysis, hemofiltration [HF]/hemodiafiltration [HDF], and transplantation) that can be used for the treatment of end-stage kidney disease (ESKD), this chapter focuses primarily on HD. Peritoneal dialysis and transplantation are covered in detail elsewhere in the *Primer*.

Principal Functions of Hemodialysis

HD for the treatment of kidney failure is effective in (1) reducing the concentration of uremic toxins, particularly small- and medium-sized molecules, primarily by diffusion, (2) removing excess fluid volume by convection, and (3) correcting some of the metabolic abnormalities, such as acidosis and hyperkalemia, by the use of dialysate solutions with variable solute concentrations. The two major components of the HD procedure that will be discussed are the dialyzer and the dialysate.

Dialyzer

Structure

The most commonly used device for the performance of HD is the hollow fiber dialyzer, composed of several thousand hollow fibers made of thin, semipermeable membranes. These fibers are encased in a plastic tubing device that allows blood to be pumped from the patient through the hollow fibers while an aqueous solution, the dialysate, is pumped outside the fibers, typically in the opposite direction of the blood flow (countercurrent), to maximize the diffusion gradients across the membranes and along the length of the dialyzer.

There are generally two types of dialysis membranes (Fig. 56.1). The first are called "low-flux" membranes and are made up of fibers with small pore sizes. These allow the diffusion of small solutes such as urea and water but not the passage of larger molecules such as β2-microglobulin. "High-flux" membranes, the second type, have larger pore sizes that allow the passage of larger molecules such as β2-microglobulin. Because of these larger pores, the rate of water transfer (ultrafiltration coefficient) is much higher than that for low-flux membranes. "Low-flux" dialyzers currently are infrequently used for maintenance hemodialysis.

The manufacturing process of these membranes is such that, regardless of whether it is a low-flux or a high-flux membrane, the pore sizes are not uniform, and there is a distribution of pore sizes that allows the diffusion or removal of differently sized molecules at different rates (Fig. 56.2). It is important to note that the distribution of pore sizes for high-flux membranes is such that it does not allow for the passage of very large molecules like albumin.

Principal Functions of the Dialyzer

Diffusion

Diffusion describes the movement of solutes from a milieu with high concentrations across a semipermeable membrane into a milieu where they are in lower concentration. The rate and amount of solute that diffuses across the membrane in either direction depend on the difference in concentration between the blood and dialysate compartments; the molecular size of the solute; the characteristics of the membrane including its surface area, thickness, and porosity; and the conditions of flow (e.g., turbulent or smooth). These membrane characteristics are generally labeled *mass transfer characteristic* or *coefficient of diffusion* and are specific for the membrane used and the solute under consideration.

Using urea as an example of a small molecular solute, HD allows the movement of urea from the blood compartment, where it is in high concentration, to the dialysate compartment across the hollow fiber membranes. Thus, as blood is pumped and traverses through the dialyzer inside the hollow fibers, the urea concentration of the blood is reduced; concurrently, the urea concentration of the dialysate increases as it flows outside the hollow fibers in the opposite direction. If the blood and dialysate were to flow in the same direction, then the urea concentration gradient between the blood and dialysate compartments would be considerably reduced at the exit site of the dialyzer, whereas a countercurrent flow ensures a maximum difference in concentration along the entire dialyzer length and, therefore, higher flux of solute from the blood compartment into the dialysate compartment.

The principles of diffusion apply not only to urea and other solutes that have a higher concentration in the blood than dialysate, but also to the diffusion of substances that have a higher concentration in the dialysate than blood. An example of the latter is the diffusion of bicarbonate from the dialysate into the blood compartment. The rate of diffusion (R) of a small blood solute like urea across the dialyzer membrane is proportional to the blood solute concentration (C) and is governed by laws of first-order kinetics. Based on this concept, R is proportional to C, or R = KC and therefore K = R/C, where K is a constant referred to as *clearance*. K of any solute across the dialyzer membrane is an

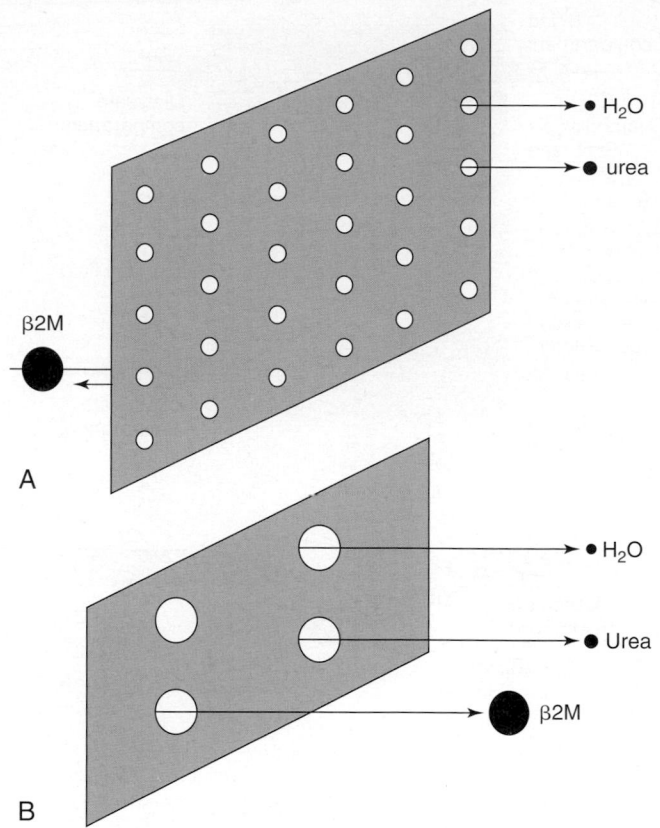

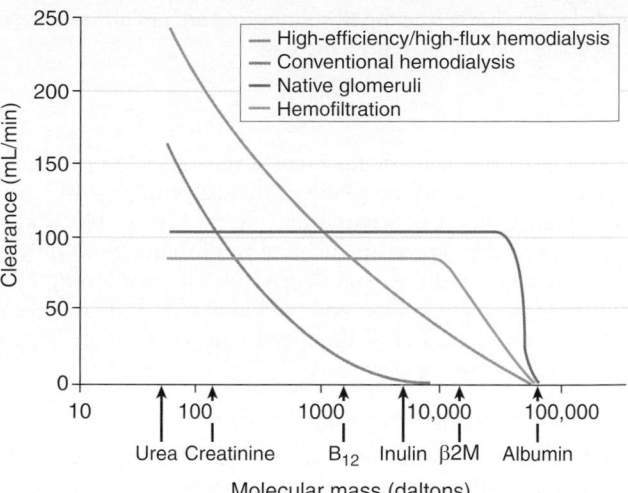

• **Fig. 56.2** Solute clearance profile of various membranes. The curves are constructed based partially on data and partially on theoretical projection. The actual values may vary depending on the surface area of the membrane and operating conditions (e.g., blood flow rate). The curve for native glomeruli represents the summation of all the glomeruli in two normal kidneys. "Glomeruli" instead of "kidneys" are used because tubular reabsorption substantially lowers the kidney clearance of certain solutes, such as urea and glucose. Clearance of solutes by diffusion (via either conventional or high-efficiency/high-flux dialysis) deteriorates rapidly with increases in the molecular mass of the solute. In contrast, clearance by convection (hemofiltration or glomeruli) remains constant over a wide range of molecular mass. B_{12}, Vitamin B_{12}; *β2M*, β2-microglobulin.

• **Fig. 56.1** Schematic diagrams of low-flux and high-flux membranes. (A) Low-flux membranes have small pores that are highly permeable to small solutes such as water and urea (60 Da) but restrict the transport of middle molecules such as β2-microglobulin (β2M). Because of their small pores, they also tend to have low ultrafiltration coefficients, although the ultrafiltration coefficient can be increased by increasing the surface area of the membrane. A low-flux membrane can be either high-efficiency or low-efficiency for urea transport, depending on its surface area and, to a lesser extent, its thickness. (B) High-flux membranes have large pores that facilitate the transport of middle molecules such as β2M in addition to small molecules. Their ultrafiltration coefficients are high. A high-flux membrane can be either high-efficiency or low-efficiency, depending on its surface area and, to a lesser extent, its thickness.

expression of the effectiveness of dialysis. It remains constant during intermittent treatments as both blood concentrations of small solutes (C) and solute removal rates (R) decrease simultaneously. A useful way to express K is:

$$K = \frac{Q_B (C_A - C_V)}{C_A}$$

K of a solute from the blood compartment (in mL/min) is expressed as the difference in the amount of a solute at the inlet ($Q_B \times C_A$, where Q_B is the blood flow rate in mL/min and C_A is the concentration in mg/mL at the inlet or "arterial" side of the dialyzer) and the amount of solute at the outlet ($Q_B \times C_V$, where C_V is the concentration at the outlet or "venous" side of the dialyzer), divided by the concentration at the inlet (C_A).

Convection

The simple equation for solute clearance mentioned above does not include convective clearance of solutes. Convection refers to the mass transport of solutes along with the fluid it is dissolved in (plasma water) and is driven by the higher hydrostatic pressures in the blood compartment generated by the blood pump. The amount of solute removed by convection is not dependent on the concentration gradient of the solute, but rather on the difference in hydrostatic pressure between the blood and dialysate compartment and a specific membrane characteristic, termed the "sieving coefficient." The sieving coefficient (S) represents the ratio of the concentration of the solute in the ultrafiltrate and the concentration in plasma water, with values ranging from 0 (membrane impermeable to solute) to 1 (membrane freely permeable to the solute).

The relative contribution of convective transport to overall clearance depends on the pore size of the membrane, as well as the size and charge of the solute. In general, the relative contribution of convective transport to the overall clearance for small molecules, such as urea, is minor, but it is more substantial for larger molecules (e.g., β2-microglobulin) because of the low diffusive clearance.

Therefore, a more complete representation of solute clearance incorporating both diffusion and convection is:

$$K = \frac{Q_{Bi} \times C_A - Q_{Bo} \times C_V}{C_A} \approx \frac{Q_{Bo} (C_A - C_V)}{C_A} + Q_{uf}$$

where Q_{uf} is the difference between Q_{Bi} (inlet blood flow) and Q_{Bo} (outlet blood flow) and is termed the *ultrafiltration rate (UFR)* in mL/min. However, the overall combined diffusive and convective clearance does not represent an exact sum of both individual clearances. This is because diffusion and convection mutually interact, each dynamically interfering with the efficiency of the other process. Because any solute removed from the blood compartment appears in the dialysate, another expression of solute clearance (K) that includes both convective and diffusive removal is based on the measurement of the concentration of that solute at the outlet of the dialysate; this is true for all solutes that are not already present in dialysate and can be represented as:

$$K = \frac{Q_{DO} \times C_{DO}}{C_A}$$

where Q_{DO} is the dialysate flow rate at the outlet (mL/min), C_{DO} is the concentration of the solute in the dialysate (mg/mL) at the outlet, and C_A is the concentration (mg/mL) in the blood at the inlet. Because this represents the net loss of solute (both diffusive and convective), and does not depend on the partitioning of the solute between plasma water and red blood cells or on calculation of the sieving coefficient of the membrane, it is a more accurate measurement of solute clearance.

Hemofiltration and Hemodiafiltration

A technique that allows for the removal of solutes, as well as plasma water, primarily or solely by convection (i.e., without diffusion) is called *hemofiltration* (*HF*). In this technique, there is no dialysate flow, and the ultrafiltrate has the same composition as plasma water. Conceptually, this technique mirrors the clearance mechanism that occurs across the native glomerulus (Fig. 56.3). However, in the absence of fluid reabsorption mediated by the renal tubules in the native kidney, the HF technique relies on infusion of large amounts of fluids to replace the large convective fluid losses. In convective removal techniques, the removal of small molecules is limited by their sieving coefficient "S," as well as the total volume of the ultrafiltrate. In contrast, diffusive removal is dependent on the concentration gradient and, therefore, diffusion is more efficient for the removal of small solutes. HF is particularly effective for removal of larger molecules that depend on convective removal.

HDF incorporates both diffusive and convective removal. Simply put, including the dialysate component in the HF circuit adds a diffusive component to the convective removal achieved by pure HF. A typical HDF procedure uses high-flux dialyzers, blood and dialysate flow rates of 300 and 500 mL/min, respectively, and a predefined amount of substitution fluid to achieve a minimum convection volume of 20% of total processed blood volume. Owing to the requirement of large volumes of sterile substitution solutions (infusate) to replace the ultrafiltrate, the infusate is prepared "online" (from the incoming dialysate), followed by further purification to render the fluid sterile and pyrogen free, before being infused directly into the patient's blood stream. Only one FDA-approved HDF device is currently available for use in the United States. Therefore, unlike in Europe, online HDF is not a commonly available modality option for dialysis patients in the United States.

Net Clearance

Although the previous equations predict that the clearance of a substance will increase as blood flow (Q_B) and/or dialysate flow (Q_D) increase, in reality the clearance of solutes increases linearly with increases in blood and/or dialysate flow only up to a point before leveling off (Fig. 56.4). This plateau is reached at different clearance values depending on the size of the solute and the specific membrane characteristics (porosity, thickness, surface charge, the chemical composition of the membrane, etc.). These summative membrane characteristics are called the *mass transfer coefficient* (*Ko*). The mass transfer coefficient is specific for the membrane used and the solute being considered; for dialyzers, this is usually represented as KoA, where A is the effective surface area of the specific dialyzer. Manufacturers generally provide the KoA of the different solutes for the specific dialyzer, and the clearance of

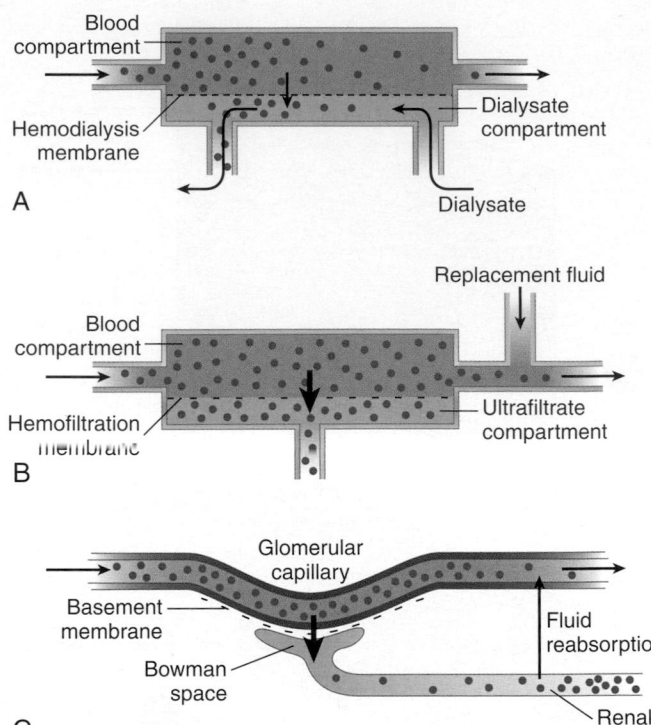

• **Fig. 56.3** Schematic representation of solute and fluid transport across the semipermeable artificial membranes and glomerular basement membrane. (A) Hemodialyzer. The plasma concentration of solutes *(solid circles)* in the blood inlet is high. Because of diffusive loss across the semipermeable hemodialysis membrane *(dotted line)*, the plasma concentration in the blood outlet is much lower. The thin arrow across the dialysis membrane represents a small amount of fluid loss (which is not necessary for solute removal). A high dialysate flow rate is used to maintain the concentration gradient across the dialysis membrane for solute removal. (B) Hemofilter. Plasma concentrations of solutes in the blood compartment remain unchanged, as blood travels the length of the fiber, and are similar to their concentrations in the ultrafiltrate. The hemofiltration membrane *(dashed line)* has relatively large pores, which allow the necessary removal of a large volume of fluid *(heavy arrow)*. Replacement fluid is infused into the blood outlet to lower the plasma concentration of solutes and compensate for the fluid loss. (C) Glomerulus. Analogous to hemofiltration, plasma concentration of solutes remains unchanged throughout the length of the glomerular capillary and is similar to that in Bowman space. Fluid removal across the glomerular basement membrane *(dashed curve)* is large *(heavy arrow)*. Reabsorption of fluid from the renal tubules lowers the plasma concentration of the solutes.

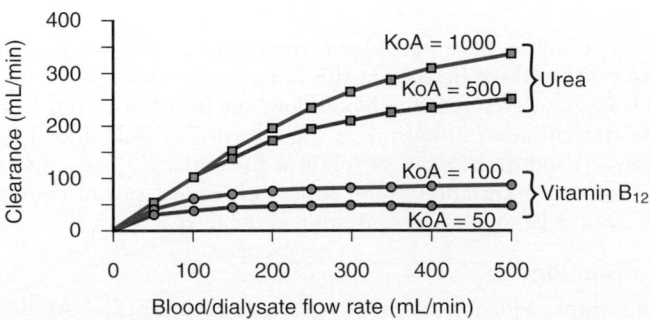

• **Fig. 56.4** The relationship between blood flow, dialysate flow, and membrane characteristics. The mass transfer coefficient is usually represented as KoA, where A is the effective surface area of the specific dialyzer.

specific solutes at different blood and dialysate concentrations can be calculated from such values. However, it is important to keep in mind that these KoA values are determined by manufacturers in aqueous solutions, and the actual clearance obtained in vivo is typically lower than that supplied by the manufacturer.

Another important feature in the relationship between higher clearance and higher blood flow rate is the fact that, in the clinical setting, blood flow rate measured by the blood pump may not accurately represent the actual blood flow rate flowing through the hollow fibers of the dialyzer. For example, in cases where the size of the needle used in the inlet bloodline (arterial fistula needle) is too narrow or the HD vascular access is malfunctioning because of an inlet stenosis, it is possible that the volume of blood that is delivered by each rotation of the blood pump may be less than predicted, and therefore the blood flow rate noted on the dialysis machine, which is calculated from the number of rotations of the blood pump, as well as the diameter of the intrapump segment of the dialysis tubing, may overestimate both the blood flow rate and the resultant solute clearance. Thus, the use of higher blood flow rates can only improve clearance up to a certain point. In addition, at increasing blood flow rates, the prepump pressure (Fig. 56.5) may become excessively negative (greater than –250 mm Hg). This, in turn, leads to a higher risk of red blood cell lysis, presumably from the sudden change between the negative pressures in the blood tubing before the blood pump and the rapid rise in hydrostatic pressures after the pump.

Finally, there are practical limits to increasing the dialysate flow rate; not only is there cost associated with preparing water for dialysate preparation, but, because of the limitation of the mass transfer coefficient for specific solutes and specific dialysis membranes, the optimal combination of dialysate flow is approximately 1.5 to 2.0 times the true blood flow rate inside the hollow fibers. Therefore, if the maximum blood flow rate (above which the negative arterial pressure prepump exceeds –250 mm Hg) is 350 mL/min, then the optimal dialysate flow rate is around 600 mL/min. Further increase in the dialysate flow rate from 600 to 800 mL/min may not lead to a substantial increase in clearance.

Assessing the Dialysis Dose

The total amount of solute removed during a dialysis procedure can be calculated from Kt (where K, the clearance in mL/min, is multiplied by the time [t] of the procedure in minutes); this assumes that the clearance (K) remains constant throughout the time of the procedure. The other variable that determines the net impact of solute removal from the patient with HD is the volume of distribution of the solute. The dose of dialysis is usually defined as Kt/V, where V is the volume of distribution of that particular solute. Urea has been the index molecule used to define the dose of dialysis as it is easily measured, is small and therefore diffuses readily across a dialysis membrane, and, importantly, its volume of distribution (total body water) can be calculated from the weight of the patient. Therefore, the dose of dialysis traditionally is defined in terms of urea, rather than other solutes, and the K in the earlier equation typically refers to *urea clearance*.

A simpler but conventional measure of dialysis dose is the urea reduction ratio (URR). The URR is also based on urea but avoids the need to define or measure clearance or determine the volume of distribution. The URR usually is expressed as percent reduction, defined as:

$$\text{URR} = \frac{\left(C_{pre} - C_{post}\right)}{C_{pre}} \times 100$$

where C_{pre} is the urea concentration before the start of dialysis, and C_{post} is the urea concentration at the completion of dialysis. The URR is traditionally expressed as a percentage.

Solute Clearance Other Than Urea

Although solute clearance by diffusion is dependent on the size of the solute molecule, other considerations, such as the electrical charge of the molecule and its *effective size*, also affect the net transfer of uremic solutes across the membrane. One example is the clearance of phosphate. Phosphate (PO_4) is a uremic toxin that accumulates as kidney failure progresses. Although phosphate has a low molecular weight and, based on its molecular size, would be expected to be easily cleared by high-flux dialysis membranes, in reality, phosphate is cleared rather poorly during dialysis because of its highly negative charge and the large number of water molecules that circulate with it; in addition, because of the large intracellular reservoirs of phosphate and slow transfer from the intracellular to the plasma compartment, net phosphate clearance by dialysis is poor. This results in a time-dependent clearance during conventional dialysis, with moderate clearance and declining removal during the first 2 hours of standard HD, and negligible removal afterward. However, as discussed later, the removal of phosphate is higher during longer dialysis treatments, such as with nocturnal dialysis (~8 hours), since the longer sessions allow the time-dependent transfer of phosphate from the intracellular to the plasma compartment; accordingly, patients treated with nocturnal dialysis often require fewer or no phosphate binders.

Extracellular Volume Control (Ultrafiltration)

Another important function of HD is the removal of excess fluid that accumulates in the absence of effective urine output. The major driving force that determines the rate of ultrafiltration or convective flow is the difference in hydrostatic pressure between the blood compartment and the dialysate compartments across the dialysis membrane; this is called the *transmembrane pressure (TMP)*. Modern dialysis equipment adjusts this hydrostatic pressure gradient by varying the negative ("suction") pressure in the dialysate compartment rather than increasing the pressure in the blood compartment; this avoids the potential for increased lysis of red blood cells. Although the traditional low-flux dialysis membrane exhibited a linear relationship between the TMP and the amount of fluid removed, the commonly used high-flux membranes have much larger pore sizes, allowing more rapid UFRs and more rapid transfer of plasma water. However, because this rapid transfer of plasma water occurs at the inlet of the dialyzer, the concentration of

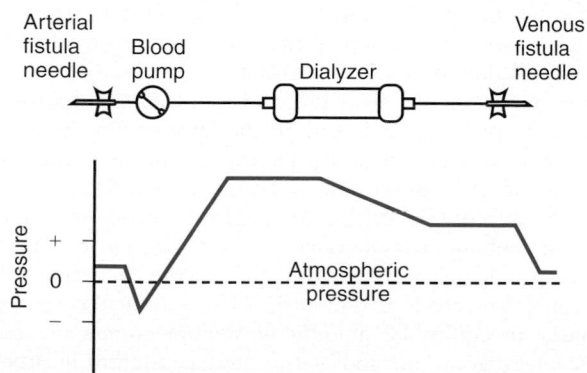

• **Fig. 56.5** The dialysis circuit, with positive and negative pressures at different points in the circuit.

protein (oncotic pressure) rapidly rises in the blood compartment, and, because these proteins are also negatively charged, there is a corresponding development of a "concentration polarization" due to a rapid increase in negatively charged plasma protein concentration at the membrane surface (inside the blood compartment). This has the effect of disproportionately increasing the oncotic pressure at the interface between the blood compartment and the surface of the membrane. The high oncotic pressure at the surface of these high-flux membranes inhibits further ultrafiltration to the extent that, toward the blood outlet of high-flux dialysis membranes, "reverse filtration" may occur with dialysate solutions moving across the membrane into the blood compartment. This reverse filtration phenomenon is more likely to occur in membranes with large pore sizes (high-flux membranes) that allow more rapid ultrafiltration than in low-flux membranes, and it also results in a nonlinear relationship between the rate of ultrafiltration and TMP in dialysis with a high-flux membrane as shown in Fig. 56.6.

Because of this nonlinear relationship, the UFR is currently determined by accurately measuring the dialysate inflow and outflow rates in a closed-loop circuit rather than manually adjusting the TMP. An accurate fluid pump is used to remove fluid at the desired UFR; as fluid is removed from this closed-loop circuit, a negative pressure is generated in the dialysate loop that allows the ultrafiltration of exactly the same amount of fluid from the blood compartment. In this way, the rate of ultrafiltration is no longer dependent on the high-flux ultrafiltration characteristics of the membrane but rather the UFR set by the operator (Fig. 56.7).

Dialysate

In addition to removal of uremic solutes by diffusion and extracellular volume removal by ultrafiltration, a third function of HD is to address a number of metabolic abnormalities that result from the absence of kidney function. Although there are numerous abnormalities in the concentration of various metabolites that result from kidney failure, acid-base (bicarbonate) balance and potassium concentration are examples of the use of various dialysate solutions to correct such abnormalities.

Bicarbonate

In the absence of kidney function, the acidic moieties produced during metabolism accumulate in the blood and, after exhausting other available buffers, are neutralized by ambient serum bicarbonate

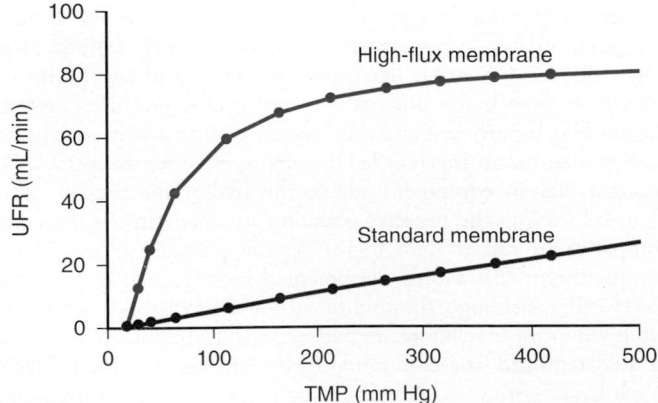

• **Fig. 56.6** The relationship between ultrafiltration rate (UFR) and transmembrane pressure (TMP) for different types of dialysis membranes.

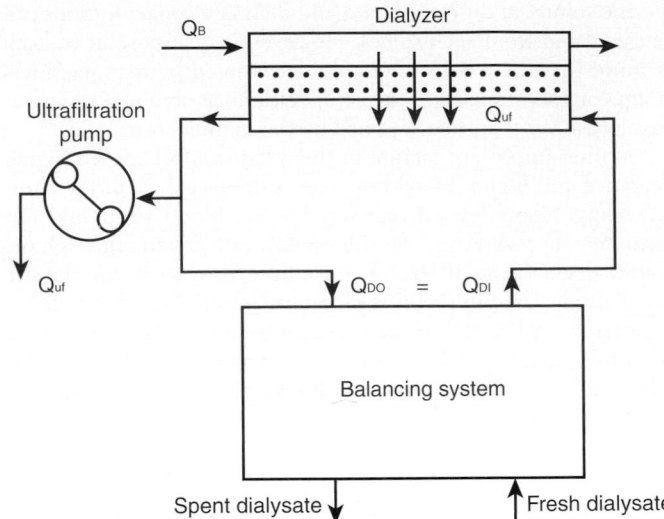

• **Fig. 56.7** Schematic diagram of the "closed-loop" ultrafiltration control used with high-flux membranes.

molecules. This results in a metabolic acidosis with serum bicarbonate levels often ranging from 16 to 18 mEq/L in patients with advanced chronic kidney disease (CKD) before initiation of dialysis.

One of the functions of dialysis is to compensate for metabolic acidosis by replenishing blood bicarbonate. Most often, this is accomplished using dialysate formulations with bicarbonate concentrations above 30 mEq/L. This "higher than normal" bicarbonate concentration is needed to provide a concentration gradient from the dialysate to the blood compartment to replenish consumed bicarbonate and allow the patient to have an interdialysis bicarbonate "reserve." Thus, the patient on dialysis cycles from a state of mild metabolic acidosis with respiratory compensation at the beginning of dialysis to a state of mild metabolic alkalosis (and compensatory hypoventilation) at the end of dialysis.

Sodium bicarbonate is used as the source of alkali in the dialysate. However, this product cannot simply be added as a component of dialysate, as the presence of other electrolytes needed in the dialysate (specifically calcium and magnesium) would result in their precipitation as crystals, thereby reducing the concentration of all three components. Current dialysate delivery technology requires the preparation of two separate dialysate streams, one called "*acid concentrate*," which combines all the ingredients of dialysate except sodium bicarbonate, and a second that contains sodium bicarbonate and sodium chloride. These two concentrates are then separately diluted with treated water (a third stream) and combined just before reaching the dialysate inlet, resulting in a modestly alkaline (pH = 7.8) dialysate solution.

One important detail in the choice of dialysate bicarbonate levels is the presence of acetate in the formulation of the "acid concentrate" mentioned earlier. Depending on the manufacturer and whether the concentrate is liquid or powder, most "acid concentrates" contain organic acid (glacial acetic acid or citric acid) to maintain an acidic milieu and thus prevent precipitation of calcium and magnesium salts. The reaction between sodium bicarbonate and acetic acid or citric acid (in the acid concentrate) generates an equimolar amount of sodium acetate or sodium citrate ions that are metabolized to produce sodium bicarbonate in the body. The equimolar conversion does not change the total buffer base available to the patient.

The disodium acetate present in the acid concentrate (Granuflo) contains acetic acid and sodium acetate. The acetic acid reacts with sodium bicarbonate to generate 4 mmol/L of sodium acetate, while the sodium acetate component of sodium diacetate provides an additional 4 mmol/L of sodium bicarbonate in the body. If the dialysate sodium bicarbonate is 35 mEq/L to begin with based upon the prescribed sodium bicarbonate stream, the final buffer base available to the patient may reach 43 mEq/L (35 + 4 + 4 = 43), representing a significant contribution of alkali (8 mEq/L) from the acid concentrate. There are ongoing studies about the optimal concentration of total buffer, but most observational data suggest that a total buffer of around 35 to 37 mEq/L is optimal; ideally, such a concentration should be adjusted for each patient, depending on his or her dietary intake, protein catabolic rate, and the resulting predialysis and postdialysis bicarbonate level.

Potassium

Similar therapeutic considerations apply to the prescription of dialysate potassium levels. In the absence of kidney function, potassium (and other electrolytes such as magnesium) accumulates in the blood; accordingly, an important function of dialysis is to reduce the potassium concentration during dialysis episodes to a level that prevents significant predialysis hyperkalemia during the interdialytic period, while avoiding significant hypokalemia after dialysis.

As potassium removal depends on the difference in potassium concentration between the blood and the dialysate, the simplest way by which potassium removal can be maximized is to use a dialysate potassium concentration of 0 mEq/L. However, "0 Potassium" dialysate results in an early and very rapid decline in serum potassium concentrations, exceeding the rate at which serum potassium can be replenished from intracellular stores, potentially predisposing to cardiac arrhythmias or cardiac arrest. In the opinion of the author, the optimal dialysate potassium for almost all patients is 2 or 3 mEq/L, and, for patients with a high predialysis potassium level, the safest option likely is to use a dialysate potassium of 2 or 3 mEq/L, while extending the dialysis duration to remove more potassium but at a slower rate. The use of a low-potassium diet and newer gastrointestinal cation exchangers like patiromer and zirconium cyclosilicate are important adjuvants.

Preparing Patients for Maintenance Hemodialysis

Patient Education and Choice of Therapy

It is important to emphasize that the selection of HD therapy should be a joint decision by the patient and the physician that follows a full discussion about other available kidney replacement therapy options (peritoneal dialysis, home HD, deceased- or living-donor transplantation), as well as the option of conservative management. Such a discussion provides the nephrology team with an opportunity to advise the patient about the medical aspects and the advantages and disadvantages of each modality, accounting for individual patient factors, including patient age, underlying kidney diagnosis and other medical conditions, family and social conditions, and patient life goals. Active management of patients' symptoms without dialytic support (comprehensive conservative care) is an option that may be recommended to patients, particularly the elderly and those with extensive comorbidity. Although the final decision should always consider the patient's preferences, the nephrologist has the responsibility not only to discuss fully the therapeutic options available but also to offer advice and recommendations about the available choices.

If the patient is competent to make decisions, and the patient and physician are in agreement, there is little that should stand in the way of carrying out their choice, be it for or against the initiation of dialysis. Anecdotally, some patients refuse to consider dialysis treatment while in the office, but they seldom refuse it when confronting acute pulmonary edema or pericarditis; thus, the relationship between the CKD patient and the nephrology team ideally should be longstanding to allow full discussion of the therapeutic options, the necessary time for the psychological acceptance of the therapy before dialysis is urgently needed, and sufficient time for the creation of a functional native arteriovenous (AV) fistula for repetitive blood access or placement of a peritoneal dialysis catheter.

30-20-10 Program for Dialysis Preparation

In the United States, more than 40% of patients who initiate dialysis do so without previous nephrology care, even though most patients have had some interaction with the healthcare system before kidney failure. Even for patients who are followed by nephrologists, there may be reluctance by the patient and even by the nephrologist to fully discuss the therapeutic options for treating kidney failure. Unless such discussion occurs, the patient will typically end up on HD ill prepared, resentful, and depressed.

Several publications have highlighted the advantages of using a 30-20-10 "rule-of-thumb" for an orderly process of patient referral to a nephrologist and initiation of kidney replacement therapy. According to this rubric, at a glomerular filtration rate (GFR) of 30 mL/min, patients should be referred for active follow-up with a nephrologist, preferably jointly with the referring physician. When the patient's GFR is around 20 mL/min, an AV fistula should be placed in patients who have not already elected an alternative kidney replacement modality. Finally, at a GFR of around 10 mL/min, an informed choice of kidney replacement modality (including conservative care) should be in place for initiation when medically indicated.

Psychological Factors in Dialysis Initiation

Patients who are informed about the probable need to initiate dialysis often undergo the same reactions as those patients being informed about any life-threatening illness; most proceed through the stages of grief that have been described by Kübler-Ross—denial, anger, bargaining, depression, and finally acceptance of this lifelong chronic hardship.

It is essential to allay the anxiety and fear common in patients nearing kidney failure. Whenever possible, family members should be included in the decision-making process, and all members of the nephrology team, including the nephrologist, nurses, social workers, transplant coordinators, and dietitians, should participate in this process. If possible, patients and interested family members should visit the dialysis unit well before requiring treatment, as this simple exercise may help alleviate many of their fears and misconceptions. Because most patients also anticipate much pain during dialysis, it should be stressed that almost no pain is involved. This can be accomplished by introducing prospective patients to those already on dialysis. The need for adherence with diet, fluid intake, medications, and dialysis schedules should be stressed, and the patient should be empowered to participate in his or her own care, helping to ensure compliance and improve satisfaction. For patients presenting with an acute need to start dialysis, a trial can be presented, stressing that the decision to perform is not binding and can be reconsidered if individual goals are not met. This is especially relevant in older and frailer patients with multiple comorbidities.

Choice of Treatment Modalities

The cause of kidney failure and comorbid conditions are elements that should be integrated into the selection of treatment options; for example, patients with brittle diabetes or previous abdominal surgery may benefit from thrice-weekly, in-center HD, whereas those with cirrhosis or severe cardiomyopathy may be treated more successfully with peritoneal dialysis or daily HD regimens. When different dialysis modalities are equally possible from a medical standpoint, practical issues such as the presence of a supportive family environment, work habits, and socioeconomic factors (e.g., availability of transportation, housing issues, and distance from dialysis centers) often favor one modality over another.

Vascular Access

Preparation and Timing of Vascular Access

Whichever option the patient chooses (except in cases of well-matched, living-related transplantation that can be preplanned), it is recommended that all patients approaching the need for HD initiation have an AV fistula created at a GFR around 20 mL/min.

Native AV fistulas have a significantly lower incidence of infection, and their half-life, if they are well developed before their use, is much longer than that of synthetic grafts. In some medical centers, access-related problems account for 30% to 40% of all nephrology admissions, representing a medical, emotional, and economic burden to the patient; thus, the presence of either rapidly progressing or already advanced kidney disease should prompt AV fistula creation well before the expected date of dialysis initiation. Central vein catheters, even if placed for a short time, are associated with a high risk of infection and may adversely affect the longevity of any subsequent AV fistula or graft.

The following recommendations are useful guidelines:

1. A vascular access surgeon should evaluate patients with progressive GFR loss at the earliest opportunity to determine the best sites for vascular access (this should occur no later than at a GFR of around 20 mL/min, according to the 30-20-10 rubric). Early placement of AV fistulas not only allows for the development of the fistula (primary patency typically takes at least 6 to 8 weeks and perhaps longer) but also allows for needed interventions, including placement of a second fistula if the initial fistula does not mature. Studies show that in approximately 50% of cases of AV fistula creation, a second procedure is required before the fistula is usable for HD. This is often due to central venous stenoses, particularly in patients who previously had central venous catheters.

2. Although access should be planned first in the nondominant arm, sites also should be preserved in the other arm. The use of the nondominant arm is preferred, particularly for self-dialysis, as it facilitates self-cannulation. Radial arteries and cephalic veins should be preserved except in life-threatening situations. In particular, use of radial arteries for nonessential "arterial lines", as well as the use of peripherally inserted central catheter (PICC) lines should be discouraged. Whenever possible, phlebotomy should be limited to veins over the dorsum of the hand and the ulnar side of the forearm. If

absolutely necessary, median antecubital veins may be punctured with small butterfly needles. Intravenous lines should spare the cephalic vein. If long-term outpatient infusions are required, consider using small bore tunneled internal jugular catheters rather than PICC lines.

3. In hospitalized patients, sites being preserved should be marked with a black felt-tipped pen as a reminder to all. A notice on the wall above the patient's bed is also helpful.

4. Patients should be educated to preserve their own vasculature. Rubber wrist bands identifying an arm to be spared from phlebotomy IV access can be effective.

Types of Arteriovenous Fistulas

Radiocephalic Arteriovenous Fistulas

A standard vascular access now preferred by most access surgeons is a distal cephalic vein to radial artery end-to-side anastomosis near the wrist. Again, the preservation of both cephalic veins from the time of kidney disease diagnosis is critical, because the radiocephalic fistula is the optimal first option. This preserves upper-arm veins for later use (Fig. 56.8).

Brachiocephalic and Brachiobasilic Fistulas

The next best approach is a more proximal fistula also using the patient's own vasculature, as described in Fig. 56.8. Upper-arm fistulas tend to have higher flow and, therefore, are more vulnerable to aneurysmal dilation; in addition, patients may have more difficulty self-cannulating an upper-arm access. Nevertheless, in patients without adequate forearm cephalic veins, brachiocephalic or brachiobasilic AV fistulas should still be placed approximately 6 months in advance of the time when dialysis is anticipated.

Percutaneous Endovascular Arteriovenous Fistulas

Surgically placed AV fistulas involve significant vessel trauma and manipulation during access placement. These factors may contribute to acute thromboses, as well as poor maturation rates of AV fistulas. Percutaneous endovascular AV fistula creation (endo AVF) is an emerging technique that utilizes minimally invasive technology for creating AV fistulas. This involves catheterizing a forearm artery (radial/ulnar) and vein using ultrasound or fluoroscopic guidance and subsequently "fusing" the artery to the vein by radio frequency or thermal resistance. Early results using such techniques show promise and offer an alternative technique to reduce the frequency of complications seen in surgically created AV fistulas.

Alternative Accesses

Grafts

In patients who cannot receive either a forearm or an upper-arm fistula using their own vasculature, a synthetic graft may be placed in the forearm. Either a distal radial artery to basilic vein (straight) graft or a loop from the brachial artery to the basilic vein could be considered. Synthetic grafts are more prone to infection and clotting than fistulas with endogenous vessels. Therefore, synthetic grafts should not be placed in anticipation of future dialysis need until generally 1 to 2 months before initiation of dialysis, with the understanding that optimal timing can be a challenge.

Catheters

Because kidney disease is often "silent," it is inevitable that some patients will present with clear indications for initiation of dialysis

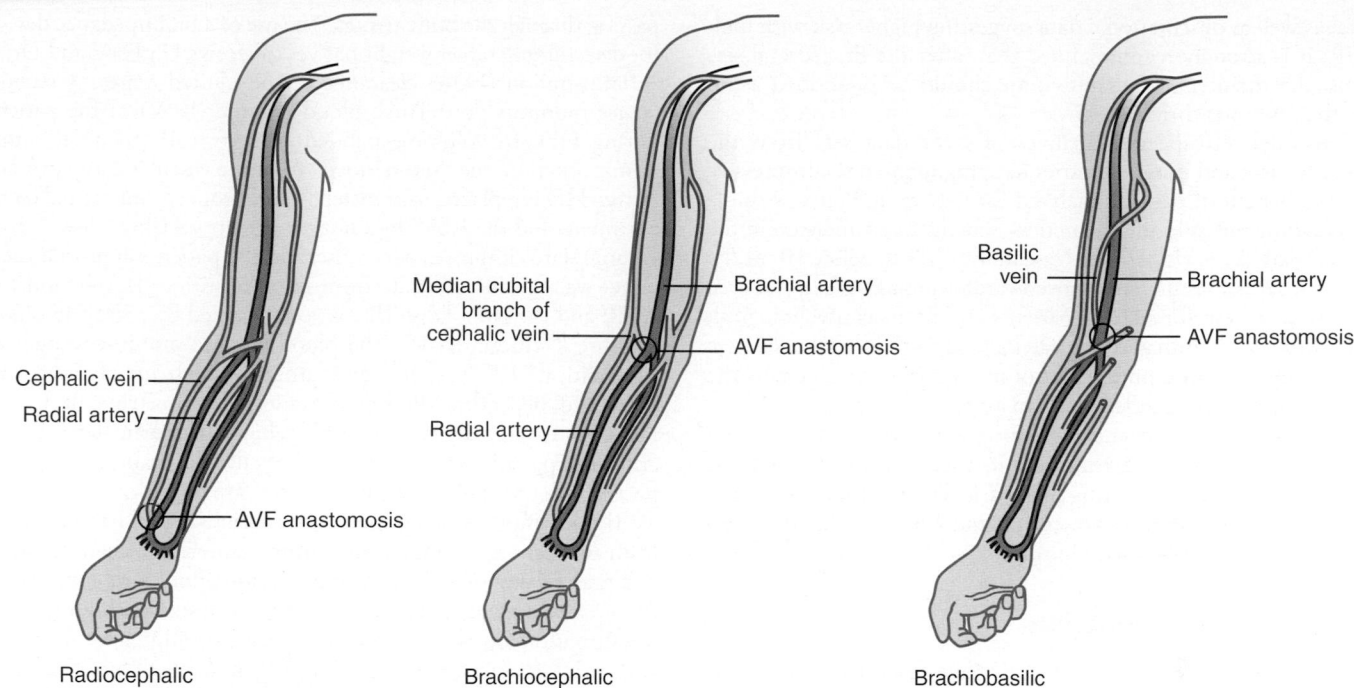

• **Fig. 56.8** Anatomy of the upper extremity vasculature. Vessels named are instrumental for the creation of hemodialysis fistula and grafts for vascular access. *AVF*, Arteriovenous fistula. (Adapted from Allon M, Robbin ML. Increasing arteriovenous fistulas in hemodialysis patients: problems and solutions. *Kidney Int.* 2002;62:1109–1124.)

without a permanent access. In such cases, if HD is elected, dialysis initiation requires the placement of a catheter, preferably in the internal jugular vein. Because of the much higher propensity for infections, catheter malfunction, inadequate blood flow, and progressive vein stenosis along the path of the catheter, it is critical that a permanent access plan be developed and implemented as soon as it is determined that the patient has chronic (and not acute) kidney failure. Ideally, the placement of permanent access, preferably an AV fistula, should take place during the hospital admission for dialysis initiation.

Initiation and Prescription of Hemodialysis

Assuming that HD is the modality of choice, what is the optimal dialysis prescription? This section briefly discusses different dialysis techniques, including short, daily HD, and nocturnal HD, with a focus on conventional, thrice-weekly, in-center dialysis, as this remains the most common HD strategy. The dialysis dose, the time needed to optimize kidney replacement therapy, and strategies for accomplishing this are reviewed. To place common HD strategies into context, current in-center HD regimens average approximately 3.5 hours per procedure and tend to provide less than 10 mL/min of creatinine clearance for the patient on an intermittent basis. Considering that this level is below the level at which HD is initiated, it is clear that the delivery of dialysis is inadequate and likely allows for shortened survival. Despite a significant decline in adjusted relative mortality rates on HD in recent years, the annual mortality rate of patients on such therapy remains unacceptably high. The 5-year survival of ESKD patients is less than many forms of cancer. Several factors should be considered in the prescription of dialysis to optimize outcomes.

Dialysis Time

It is possible to estimate the minimum dialysis time that a patient may need to achieve a specific target Kt/V or URR, taking into consideration the patient's residual kidney function (RKF). The first step is to calculate the volume of urea distribution, which is total body water. For the hypothetical 70-kg person, this is assumed to be 60% of body weight for men (42 L), whereas in women, it is assumed to be 55% of body weight (38.5 L). The next step is to determine the clearance of the dialyzer at specific blood and dialysate flow rates. An in vitro evaluation of urea clearance is usually included in the package insert of the dialyzer, accounting for the surface area of the dialyzer, the dialysate flow rate, and other dialyzer factors. However, since this is an in vitro assessment based on an aqueous solution (rather than blood), it is reasonable to assume that the in vivo urea clearance is approximately 80% of the reported in vitro clearance. Accordingly, assuming the in vitro urea clearance at a "blood flow" of 300 mL/min and dialysate flow of 500 mL/min is 250 mL/min, then the presumed in vivo urea clearance is 250 × 0.8 = 200 mL/min.

If the goal of therapy is to achieve a minimum single pool Kt/V of 1.2, as recommended by Kidney Disease Outcomes Quality Initiative (K/DOQI) guidelines, then the minimum time needed for this hypothetical 70-kg man to achieve a Kt/V of 1.2 can be derived as below:

$$Kt/V = 1.2$$

$$t = 1.2 \times V/K = 1.2 \times (42{,}000 \text{ mL})/(200 \text{ mL}/\text{min}) = 252 \text{ min}$$

Although larger surface area dialyzer and higher blood flow rates are means of reducing the dialysis duration, based on these data, as well as observational data suggesting higher risk with high UFR, it is strongly recommended that, after the first several sessions, the maintenance dialysis time should be prescribed at no less than 4 hours thrice weekly.

Recently, retrospective analyses of large data sets from the United States and other countries have highlighted the impressive survival benefit of patients dialyzed for 4 or more hours. Possible explanations include the theoretical benefits of an increase in the dose of dialysis, as well as a decrease in the UFR to below 10 mL/kg per hour with a resultant improved cardiovascular stability. A final important reason for starting patients at 4 hours is psychological; after a patient is initiated on dialysis for less than 4 hours, there is a strong reluctance on the part of many patients to increase the dialysis duration, regardless of the reason.

For stable CKD patients with progressive kidney failure who may have their initial HD in the outpatient setting, it would be reasonable to consider starting such patients for 2 hours in the first session, 3 hours in the second session, and 4 hours in the third session to avoid possible disequilibrium.

Residual Kidney Function

Almost all patients initiating dialysis have some RKF and urine output. RKF correlates strongly and consistently with patient survival. Although residual function provides additional (and continuous) clearance of solutes and water, the initiation of HD may lead to a more rapid loss of RKF, possibly reflecting dialysis-associated hypotension and ischemic kidney injury, progression of the underlying kidney disease, or the inflammatory burden associated with the dialysis procedure itself. Although it is important to preserve RKF, the mere presence of some RKF (native kidney urea clearance greater than 2 mL/min) cannot justify shorter dialysis duration and/or reduced dialysis frequency. This is due to the fact that, after the initiation of dialysis, not only does RKF decline fairly rapidly, but there may also be strong resistance from patients to extend treatment time once RKF is lost.

Target or "Dry" Weight and Rate of Ultrafiltration

A critical item for patients initiating dialysis is the establishment of a target weight, defined as the weight that the patient needs to achieve at the end of dialysis and at which the patient is close to euvolemia—the so-called "*dry weight*." Although patients who present with dependent peripheral edema or pulmonary edema have excess fluid volume that can be easily targeted, often it is difficult to determine the target dry weight on clinical examination since fluid overload can be present even in the absence of edema.

For the rare patient not prescribed antihypertensive medications, the achievement of near-normal blood pressure may be one sign of achieving target weight; however, most CKD patients receive multiple blood pressure medications, complicating the use of blood pressure readings as an index of euvolemia. Blood pressure medications also complicate the achievement of the target weight, because these medications may predispose patients to hypotension during fluid removal. Accordingly, achievement of target weight based on clinical assessment is often a process of trial and error that may lead to frequent hypotensive episodes in some patients.

Several devices exist to help in determining target weight. The first, bioimpedance, can be used on the patient during dialysis by applying electrodes to the skin and estimating hydration status by measuring the resistance encountered by the electrical current passing through the body tissues. The use of a bioimpedance device for determining target weight has yet to receive US Food and Drug Administration (FDA) clearance in the United States. A second device monitors the relative blood volume (RBV) of the patient during HD. In volume-expanded patients with adequate autonomic function, the fluid removed from the vascular compartment during HD is replaced by transfer of fluid from the interstitial compartment, and the RBV does not change appreciably. However, as volume status improves with time, and the patients approach their target weight, the refill rate from the interstitium lags behind the UFR, and the RBV falls. This is accompanied by a drop in blood pressure ("critical" RBV). The blood volume monitor recognizes the "critical" RBV as the value around which hypotension can occur and, depending on the integration of the instrument, lowers the UFR to keep RBV above this value. This particular value of critical RBV varies from patient to patient. Clinical trial data supporting the use of either of these devices are mixed.

The attempt to determine target weight should not distract from another important consideration, namely, the determination and prescription of UFRs, the rate at which fluid is removed from the total body water. Recent literature suggests that high rates of ultrafiltration are associated with higher morbidity and mortality, with risk highest at rates exceeding 13 mL/kg per hour. Strategies to address high fluid removal rates should include extra dialysis sessions or increasing dialysis time. Additional measures in such situations may include an enhanced focus on dietary salt restriction and the use of diuretics to increase urine output in patients with significant RKF.

Dose of Delivered Dialysis

As discussed earlier, the dose of delivered dialysis is traditionally determined by changes in urea concentration before and after dialysis. Although urea is no longer considered the principal "uremic toxin," urea concentration in the blood and subsequent urea clearance with dialytic therapy correlate reasonably well with observed clinical changes. Furthermore, urea is easily measured in the blood and dialysate, is evenly distributed in total body water, and rapidly diffuses from intracellular to extracellular and vascular spaces. Therefore, it is reasonable to assume that changes in urea concentration during dialysis represent a reasonable measure of the dose of dialysis.

Using urea as the accepted marker of the dose of dialysis, the K/DOQI guidelines established by the National Kidney Foundation recommend that achievement of a urea single pool Kt/V of at least 1.2 represents the minimum accepted dose of thrice-weekly HD. On the basis of limited, long-term studies and no clinical trial data, the best patient outcomes appear associated with Kt/V values of 1.2 to 1.4, to be achieved in no less than 4 hours (as discussed previously) and at UFRs that do not exceed 13 mL/kg per hour. The determination of URR or Kt/V depends critically on the accurate measurement of pre- and postdialysis urea and the accurate determination of dialysis time. It is, therefore, important to be aware of the potential errors that could be introduced in determining each of these measures.

Potential Errors in Predialysis Urea Measurement

Blood for measurement of predialysis urea is generally collected after insertion of the needle in the patient's vascular access or is drawn directly from the catheter. If the blood sample is drawn from a catheter or a recently flushed bloodline, there is a strong likelihood that the blood sample will be diluted with residual saline solution. To address this, approximately 5 mL of blood should be drawn and discarded before the blood sample for urea measurement is obtained.

Potential Errors in Postdialysis Urea Measurement

The postdialysis urea blood sample must be drawn from the "arterial" (intake) needle at least 2 minutes after dialysis is terminated (preferred), the UFR is set to 0, and the blood pump has been stopped (after slowing it to 100 mL/min for at least 10 to 20 seconds before stopping) to avoid recirculation. *Recirculation* of blood not only refers to the possibility of mixing the inlet (arterial) blood with the outlet (venous) blood that occurs when access malfunction results in blood flow that is lower than the blood pump speed (access recirculation) but also to a phenomenon called *cardiopulmonary recirculation*. Cardiopulmonary recirculation occurs whenever the arterial blood feeds the dialyzer inlet (AV access). The dialyzed blood from the dialyzer outlet (relatively poor in urea) subsequently reaches the right heart (and mixes with urea-rich blood coming from other tissues) and passes through the lungs before finally reaching the aorta. The blood in the aorta (consisting of urea-"poor" and urea-"rich" components) is then pumped back to the AV access and to other tissues. The "urea-poor" component of the blood supply feeding the AV access lowers the overall concentration of blood urea in the AV access. This phenomenon does not occur when the access is fed via a venous catheter. This process occurs throughout a dialysis session and can be illustrated by the following observation: when tested, the urea concentration of the blood entering the dialyzer is often different from the urea concentration of the blood in distant peripheral tissues. Cardiopulmonary recirculation is more pronounced in patients dialyzed with high-efficiency dialysis (large dialyzer surface area or rapid blood flow) and in patients with low cardiac output. In many patients, the solute (urea) concentration at the arterial (inlet) bloodline rises by approximately 10% over a 3-minute period after dialysis is discontinued, and blood samples drawn immediately after termination of dialysis will have artificially lower urea concentration, resulting in overestimation of urea reduction and Kt/V compared with blood samples drawn after the urea concentration is uniformly distributed throughout the patient. It is, therefore, important to emphasize the need for prescribing exactly how the postdialysis urea sample needs to be drawn.

Potential Errors in Treatment Time

Although treatment time is generally considered to be the difference between the dialysis start time and termination time, actual treatment time may be significantly lower than "clock time," reflecting factors such as the time taken to reach maximum blood flow, alarm stoppages, and other interruptions, such as time for patients to use bathrooms. Modern dialysis machines report either actual dialysis time or blood volumes processed, the latter based on the rotation of the blood pump (with its attendant caveat mentioned earlier).

Anticoagulation Prescriptions

The contact of the blood with "foreign" surfaces such as the dialyzer membrane triggers the coagulation cascade. In the absence of anticoagulants, this results in blood clotting inside the dialyzer hollow fibers, leading initially to loss of dialyzer surface area and eventually to possible loss of appreciable volumes of patient blood in the clotted dialyzer. Because the coagulation cascade is triggered as soon as blood is in contact with foreign surfaces, anticoagulation must be effective before such blood–membrane contact. The most commonly used anticoagulant is unfractionated heparin; initial dosing is most often weight based (approximately 50 units/kg), administered as a bolus immediately following needles insertion and establishment of access patency. Because it is important to allow the heparin to reach the systemic circulation, an interval of approximately 3 minutes following the administration of heparin should elapse before the blood is allowed to reach the extracorporeal circuit via the blood pump. If blood reaches the dialyzer membrane before full anticoagulation, it is likely that local clotting inside the fibers will occur, reducing the available dialyzer membrane surface area and, therefore, the clearance of uremic toxins.

Because of the steady decline in heparin concentration and level of anticoagulation during dialysis (via both heparin metabolism and adsorption on the extracorporeal surface), it is recommended that a continuous infusion of low doses of heparin be administered throughout most of the treatment at a rate of approximately 1000 units/h. For patients with permanent accesses (AV fistula or graft), it is also recommended that this continuous heparin be discontinued approximately 30 minutes before the end of dialysis to facilitate timely hemostasis of the vascular access after the withdrawal of the needles at the termination of dialysis. For patients dialyzed with a catheter, continuous heparin may be prescribed until the end of the treatment to reduce the risk of clotting of the catheter tips, because "hemostasis" of the catheter at the termination of dialysis is not required.

Although these recommendations are not based on extensive studies, they are clinically effective in most patients. In patients who may be using warfarin anticoagulation for other reasons, the dose of heparin should be reduced, although not eliminated, as heparin and warfarin have different mechanisms of action on the coagulation cascade. In a small fraction of patients, heparin results in significant thrombocytopenia, and alternative methods of anticoagulation need to be considered. Very limited safety data exist supporting direct oral anticoagulant (DOAC) use in dialysis, with only the factor Xa inhibitor, apixaban, carrying an indication for use in kidney failure patients. Dosing of apixaban remains uncertain in the dialysis population, although likely should be lower than that in the general population.

Frequency of Dialysis and Alternative Modalities

Thrice-weekly dialysis, with each session lasting a few hours, was established as the standard for maintenance HD in the 1970s, primarily for practical reasons including patient and staff convenience. Because of technologic advances in the delivery of dialysis, the dialysis procedure has become much safer, with greater availability of equipment suitable for home use. Accordingly, regimens with different frequencies and different times of day are being explored. Nevertheless, thrice-weekly, daytime, in-center HD remains by far the most common regimen.

Nocturnal Dialysis

Reflecting dialysis facility capacity issues, nephrologists who wanted to prescribe dialysis times of 6 to 8 hours implemented nocturnal dialysis. Patients begin their dialysis treatment in the evening, spending 6 to 8 hours receiving dialysis (generally while sleeping). This can be performed either in-center or at home. Such prolonged dialysis allows for an increase in the total dose of dialysis with much slower rates of ultrafiltration and diffusive clearance. Despite extensive observational data supporting the putative benefits of "more intensive dialysis" (extra session length, frequency, or both), when tested in the Frequent Hemodialysis Network (FHN) Nocturnal trial, nocturnal dialysis did not show any benefits on prespecified outcomes of composite of mortality and either change in left ventricular mass or the physical component score of the Short Form (SF)-36. This trial, however, did demonstrate improvement in secondary outcomes of interdialytic weight gain, blood pressure, and predialysis phosphorous levels.

Although the concept of nocturnal dialysis is theoretically attractive, patient acceptance, nurse recruitment, and the need for physician visits at night are some of the barriers for this therapy. Nocturnal dialysis can be performed at home, but the fear of catastrophic events, such as severe hypotension and needle dislodgement while the patient is asleep, has limited this strategy. Of note, remote hemodynamic monitoring and devices that are activated by red blood cells and awaken the patient if there is a blood leak are now available; these may improve the safety of nocturnal dialysis procedure, both in-center and at home.

Short Daily Hemodialysis

An alternative to nocturnal dialysis that still increases the weekly number of dialysis hours is short, daily HD, which is most often performed 5 or 6 times weekly for approximately 3 hours per session. The FHN Daily trial showed improvements in prespecified primary composite outcome of mortality and change in left ventricular mass. Secondary outcomes, specified above for nocturnal dialysis, also improved.

Regardless of the above discussion, it is clear that more attention needs to be paid to dialysis duration if patient outcomes are to continue to improve. Recent data clearly demonstrate that the adequacy of HD should not be solely based on small molecule clearance (which can be accomplished in shorter times with large surface-area dialyzers) but also consider the cumulative weekly dialysis time, as well as the rate of ultrafiltration.

Bibliography

Chertow GM, Levin NW, Kliger AS, et al. In-center hemodialysis six times per week versus three times per week. *N Engl J Med.* 2010; 363:2287–2300.

Culleton BF, Walsh M, Klarenbach SW, et al. Effect of frequent nocturnal hemodialysis vs conventional hemodialysis on left ventricular mass and quality of life: a randomized controlled trial. *JAMA.* 2007;298:1291–1299.

Eknoyan G, Beck GJ, Cheung AK, et al. Hemodialysis (HEMO) Study Group. Effect of dialysis dose and membrane flux in maintenance hemodialysis. *N Engl J Med.* 2002;347:2010–2019.

El Ters M, Schears GJ, Taler SJ, et al. Association between prior peripherally inserted central catheters and lack of functioning arteriovenous fistulas: a case-control study in hemodialysis patients. *Am J Kidney Dis.* 2012;60:601–608.

Finkelstein FO, Story K, Firenek C, et al. Perceived knowledge among patients cared for by a nephrologist about chronic kidney disease and end-stage renal disease therapies. *Kidney Int.* 2011;58:235–242.

Foley RN, Gilbertson DT, Murray T, et al. Long interdialytic interval and mortality among patients receiving hemodialysis. *N Engl J Med.* 2011;365:1099–1107.

Goldstein MB, Jindal KK, Levin A, et al. The adequacy of hemodialysis: assessment and achievement. In: Jacobson HR, Striker GE, Klahr S, eds. *The Principles and Practice of Nephrology.* St. Louis, MO: Mosby; 1995.

Grootman MP, Van den Dorpal MA, Bots ML, et al. Effect of online hemodiafiltration on all cause mortality and cardiovascular outcomes. *J Am Soc Nephrol.* 2012;23:1087–1096.

Jones RG, Morgan RA. A Review of the current status of percutaneous endovascular arteriovenous fistula creation for haemodialysis access. *Cardiovasc Intervent Radiol.* 2019;42:1–9.

Lacson E Jr., Brunelli SM. Hemodialysis treatment time: a fresh perspective. *Clin J Am Soc Nephrol.* 2011;6:2523–2530.

Lacson E, Lazarus JM, Himmelfarb J, et al. Balancing fistula first with catheters last. *Am J Kidney Dis.* 2007;50:379–395.

Lacson E Jr., Wang W, DeVries C, et al. Effects of a nationwide predialysis educational program on modality choice, vascular access, and patient outcomes. *Am J Kidney Dis.* 2011;58:235–242.

Lacson E Jr., Wang W, Zebrowski B, et al. Outcomes associated with intradialytic oral nutritional supplements in patients undergoing maintenance hemodialysis: a quality improvement report. *Am J Kidney Dis.* 2012;60:591–600.

Mavrakanas TA, Samer CF, Nessim SJ, et al. Apixaban pharmacokinetics at steady state in hemodialysis patients. *JASN.* 2017;28(7): 2241–2248.

McIntyre CW, Rosensky SJ. Starting dialysis is dangerous. *Kidney Int.* 2012;82:382–387.

Mehrotra R, Agarwal R. End stage renal disease and dialysis: nephrology re-assessment. *NephSAP, volume.* 2012. Available at http://www.asn-online.org/education/nephsap/active.aspx. Accessed May 24, 2013.

Owen WF, Lew NL, Liu Y, et al. The urea reduction ratio and serum albumin concentration as predictors of mortality in patients undergoing hemodialysis. *N Engl J Med.* 1993;329:1001–1006.

Rocco MV, Lockridge RS Jr, Beck GJ, et al. The effects of frequent nocturnal home hemodialysis: the Frequent Hemodialysis Network Nocturnal Trial. *Kidney Int.* 2011;80:1080–1091.

Shen JI, Winkelmayer WC. Use and safety of unfractionated heparin for anticoagulation during maintenance hemodialysis. *Am J Kidney Dis.* 2012;60:463–486.

Spiegel DM. Avoiding harm and achieving optimal dialysis outcomes—the dialysate component. *Adv Chronic Kidney Dis.* 2012;19:166–170.

Suri RS, Nesrallah GE, Mainra R, et al. Daily hemodialysis: a systematic review. *Clin J Am Soc Nephrol.* 2006;1:33–42.

Ward RA, Idoux JW, Hamdan H, et al. Dialysate flow rate and delivered Kt/V$_{urea}$ for dialyzers with enhanced dialysate flow distribution. *Clin J Am Soc Nephrol.* 2011;6(9):2235–2239.

57

Peritoneal Dialysis

NIKHIL SHAH, JEFFREY PERL

Introduction

In peritoneal dialysis (PD), a chronically indwelling catheter is placed into the peritoneal space. A peritoneum enriched in a vascular capillary network is the dialysis membrane. Introduction of dialysis fluid into the peritoneum (glucose [or dextrose monohydrate] based) creates an osmotic pressure gradient across the membrane promoting fluid removal, and movement of uremic solutes across the membrane occurs by both diffusion and convection. Unique to PD (and arguably its major advantage over other dialysis modalities) is that it is performed by the individual at home, allowing treatment flexibility and autonomy over dialysis treatments compared to center-based dialysis. This may occur with or without assistance of a care partner. Two PD modalities exist: manual exchanges throughout the day (typically continuous ambulatory PD [CAPD]) or automated PD (APD), performed with the aid of a machine (cycler) that instills and drains dialysis fluid at the bedside, typically via repeated overnight intervals. True absolute contraindications to PD are rare and center around conditions that either preclude successful PD catheter placement, or those that significantly compromise bowel integrity (i.e., active inflammatory bowel disease), thereby creating an unacceptably high risk of intraabdominal infection. In contrast, relative contraindications to PD center largely around physical, cognitive, and psychosocial challenges in the ability to perform PD at home, particularly in the absence of a care partner. Another key requirement for PD is having a suitable environment in which to perform PD treatments with aseptic technique. The major complications of PD include infections (peritonitis, exit site, and tunnel infections), noninfectious complications (i.e., PD catheter dysfunction, PD fluid leaks, hernias), and deleterious changes to the peritoneal membrane, leading to impairments in either solute and/or fluid removal. Impaired peritoneal solute and/or water removal tends to occur more frequently over time and may be more clinically significant in the face of the loss of residual kidney function (RKF).

Current State

Globally, less than 20% of patients receiving maintenance dialysis are treated with PD, with substantial variation in PD utilization between countries. Between-country variation is a complex interplay between cultural, educational, and financial differences and policies related to dialysis reimbursement, as well as the relative local costs of various treatment modalities. For example, in the United States, the new ESRD prospective payment system has created a more favorable reimbursement structure, likely resulting in increasing use of PD in the United States after decades of ongoing decline. In 2017, according to the United States Renal Data System, 10.1% of incident ESRD patients began kidney replacement therapy with PD, while on December 31, 2017, 7.1% of all prevalent ESRD patients (denominator including transplant patients) were receiving PD therapy.

The lack of provider education and comfort with PD, the lack of adequate exposure to PD during nephrology fellowship training, and the lack of awareness and education of patients and their care partners regarding PD as a viable dialysis modality treatment option remain major ongoing challenges that may be further limiting the use of PD. Perceptions of more stringent PD-eligibility criteria by providers, coupled with a higher risk of treatment-related failure, are further challenges. In a recent study of over 29,000 incident PD patients in the United States, who were followed for a median of over 21 months, over 41% of patients who initiated PD transferred from PD to center-based hemodialysis (HD), suggesting that premature transition to HD among patients receiving PD remains a major and ongoing challenge that is limiting its use.

Anatomy of the Peritoneal Membrane

The peritoneal membrane is a serous semi-permeable membrane that lines the abdominal wall (parietal peritoneum, 40% of peritoneal surface area) and, in a contiguous fashion, also envelops the intraabdominal viscera (visceral peritoneum, 60% of peritoneal surface area) (Fig. 57.1). The parietal peritoneal blood supply is derived from the abdominal wall and intercostal and epigastric regions draining into the inferior vena cava, while the visceral peritoneum receives its blood supply from the mesenteric artery draining into the portal vein circulation. In animal models of PD, the parietal peritoneum plays a greater role in peritoneal solute and water removal compared to the visceral peritoneum. The anatomical surface area of the peritoneal membrane ranges from 1.6 to 2 m². It roughly approximates body surface area but is greatly augmented by the presence of microvilli. The semi-permeable membrane is made up of several layers, which together form the barrier to solute and fluid transport in PD. The potential barrier is made up of layers, as shown in Fig. 57.1. The capillary endothelium forms the most important barrier to the solute and water transport. Peritoneal capillary blood flow is approximately 50–150 mL/min.

Physiology of PD

In PD, one mode by which uremic toxins and small solutes are removed is diffusion. For each solute, diffusive removal is a function of the concentration differences across the peritoneal membrane.

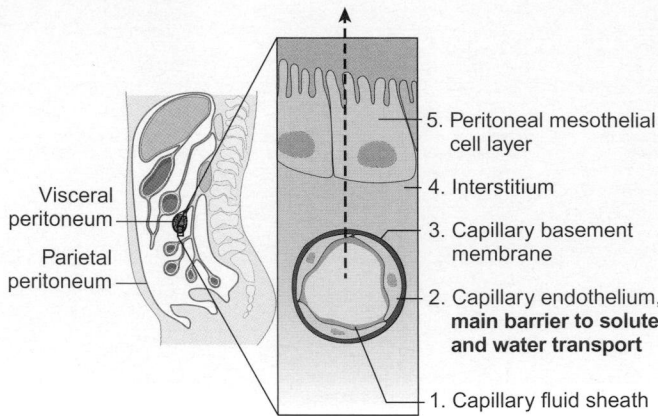

5. Peritoneal mesothelial cell layer

4. Interstitium

3. Capillary basement membrane

2. Capillary endothelium, **main barrier to solute and water transport**

1. Capillary fluid sheath

Visceral peritoneum

Parietal peritoneum

• **Fig. 57.1** Sagittal section through the abdomen to demonstrate the visceral and parietal peritoneum and layers forming the barrier to movement of solute and water during PD.

For example, solutes such as urea and creatinine will move from an area of higher concentration (the peritoneal capillaries) to an area of lower concentration (the dialysate), where, initially, in the dialysis solution, there is no urea or creatinine. Solute transfer will continue until equilibrium has been achieved, such that the peritoneal capillary and dialysis concentrations are equal. Diffusion can be bidirectional across the peritoneal membrane (capillary to dialysis fluid and vice versa). For example, medications such as antibiotics can be instilled into the PD fluid and reach therapeutic serum concentrations by moving along their concentration gradients from the peritoneal fluid to the peritoneal capillaries until antibiotic concentrations have equalized. To maximize diffusive removal of solutes, new dialysis solution can be instilled repeatedly, and old dialysis fluid can be drained after diffusive equilibrium has been reached for most small solutes. Therefore, the greater the total dialysis volume exchanged per day, the greater the degree of solute removal. Moreover, the lower the molecular weight of a solute, the faster it will diffuse across the peritoneal membrane. Larger solutes may require more time and, in turn, longer dialysis exchange times to equilibrate. Clearance of larger solutes rely more on convective than diffusive clearance (Fig. 57.2).

Glucose is the most commonly used osmotic agent in PD solutions, resulting in "crystalloid osmosis" (see PD Solutions). Osmosis is defined as the movement of a solvent, in this case water, from lower solute concentration to higher solute concentration across a semi-permeable membrane. In PD, the crystalloid osmotic gradient generated by glucose drives water across the peritoneal membrane. Because glucose is absorbed as it freely moves via diffusion from the instilled PD fluid to the peritoneal capillaries over the course of an exchange, ultrafiltration (UF) is greatest at the beginning of a PD exchange. Eventually, osmotic equilibrium is reached, defined as the peak UF volume achievable during an exchange. Thereafter, UF diminishes and, if PD fluid is left dwelling long enough, net absorption will occur. Therefore, the duration of an exchange is a key determinant of UF volume. There is also lymphatic absorption of fluid from the peritoneal cavity, typically occurring at a rate of 90 mL/hour. Therefore, net UF in PD is the result of transcapillary UF minus the fluid that is absorbed via the lymphatic system.

Another determinant of fluid removal in PD is glucose concentration (Fig. 57.3). The higher the initial glucose concentration that is used, the greater the amount of UF that can be achieved, and the longer the time until fluid is reabsorbed. A final determinant of fluid removal is the rate at which glucose is absorbed across the peritoneal membrane; this will vary among individuals. The faster that glucose is absorbed, the faster the osmotic gradient will dissipate, leading to lower UF (see Assessment of Peritoneal Solute and Water Transport). As water moves across the peritoneal membrane, dissolved solutes move along with water in a process called *convection*. Therefore, solute removal can occur via convection in addition to diffusion. Convective clearance of solutes is, therefore, directly proportionally to the amount of fluid that is removed via PD.

Three-Pore Model of Peritoneal Solute Transport

Based on the physiologic principles described above, the clinical observation that the dialysate sodium drops during the initial part of the PD exchange led to the postulation that "water only" transport channels existed in the peritoneal membrane, leading to free water movement into the peritoneal cavity, and, as a result, a drop in the dialysate sodium concentration occurs. This led to the description of the three-pore model of peritoneal solute transport, which states that in addition to ultrasmall water-only pores (aquaporin-1, unlike aquaporin-2 that is in the kidney), the capillary wall has two additional pore types through which solute and fluid transport occurs in PD (Fig. 57.4, Table 57.1).

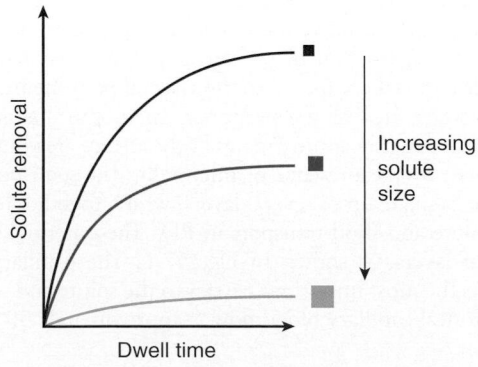

■ Small size solutes (e.g., urea)
■ Medium size solutes (e.g., creatinine, phosphate)
■ Large size solutes (e.g., β2 microglobulin, albumin)

• **Fig. 57.2** Rate of solute transfer depends on the size of the solute.

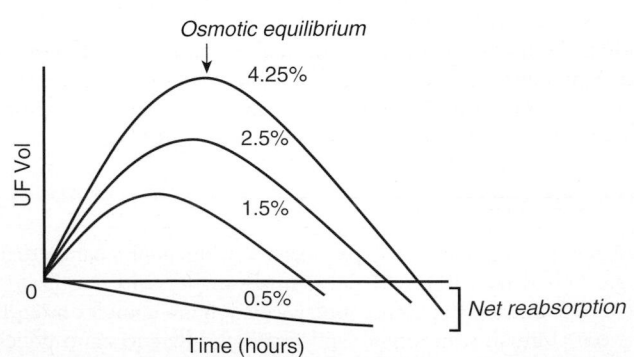

• **Fig. 57.3** Ultrafiltration (UF) volume is a function of dwell time and dextrose concentration of the fluid. (From Perl J, Bargman JM. Peritoneal dialysis: from bench to bedside and bedside to bench. *Am J Physiol Renal Physiol*. 2016;311:F999-F1004.)

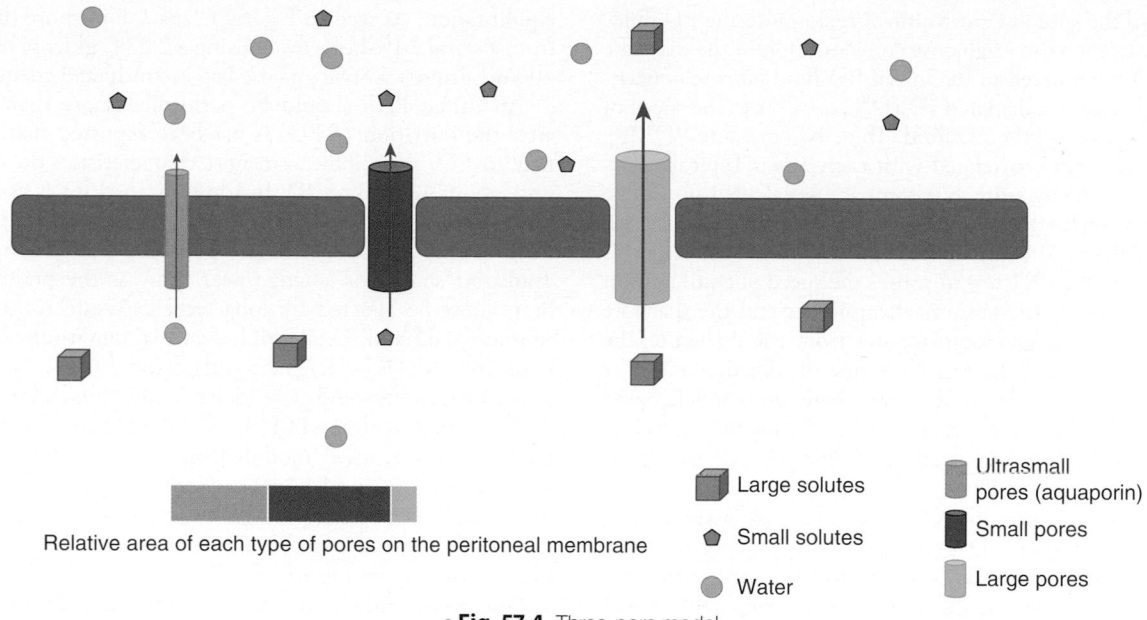

Relative area of each type of pores on the peritoneal membrane

Large solutes

Small solutes

Water

Ultrasmall
pores (aquaporin)

Small pores

Large pores

• **Fig. 57.4** Three-pore model.

TABLE 57.1	Peritoneal Membrane Pore Types	
Pore	Size	Note
Ultrasmall pores (aquaporins)	2.5 Å	These are small, intracellular, water channels presumably AQP1, which exclusively transport free water and are impermeable to solutes.
Small pores	40-50 Å	Form the bulk of the pores and are the major sites of solute and fluid transport.
Large pores	250 Å	Few, predominant sites of middle molecules' transfer and major sites of protein loss.

UF that occurs early in the exchange is mediated predominantly by the ultrasmall pores (AQP1) present within the capillary endothelium followed by the small pores; there is a much smaller contribution to UF mediated by the large pores, which, though large, are far fewer in number. Later in the exchange, there is greater sodium-coupled water transport via the small pores. If PD exchanges are too rapid, particularly using high concentrations of glucose, there is a risk that aquaporins will be overrecruited relative to the small pores, leading to excessive water-only transport in a phenomenon known as *sodium sieving*. The clinical consequences of sodium sieving are impairments in sodium removal and hypernatremia, stimulating thirst and excessive fluid intake. Because fluid and solutes move via the small and large pores exclusively, these pores are the site of convective and diffusive clearance of solute, with small pores predominant due to their sheer number relative to the comparatively sparse large pores.

There have been further refinements to the three-pore model including the distributed model, which introduced the concept of effective vs. anatomic peritoneal surface area. The distributed model dictates that the degree and speed of diffusion of solutes is a function of capillary density and proximity to the peritoneal surface. The greater the vascularity of the membrane, the greater the area for diffusion.

Assessment of Peritoneal Solute and Water Transport

Hemodialysis uses an artificial semi-permeable membrane for solute and fluid removal with consistent and reliable specifications. In contrast, PD uses a naturally occurring semi-permeable peritoneal membrane subject to variability between individuals. It is common practice to test and identify an individual's membrane characteristics initially and longitudinally in an effort to personalize the PD prescription and assess changes to peritoneal membrane function over time.

Peritoneal Equilibration Test (PET) and Modifications

The peritoneal equilibration test (PET) is the most widely used assessment tool for solute and water transport in patients on PD and requires following a standardized protocol to obtain reliable and comparable results. The key steps include performing a long, overnight exchange (8–12 hours), full drainage of the overnight dwell (20 minutes, sitting position), and correct volume and concentration of the test dwell (2 L, 2.5% dextrose) instilled at 200 mL/min over 10 minutes, with a dwell time of 240 minutes. The dialysate sample is collected at 0, 30, 60, 120, 180, and 240 minutes, while the blood is sampled 120 minutes into the test. Dialysate (4 hours) to plasma (2 hours) creatinine (D/P$_{creat}$) is calculated and is a measure of the speed of creatinine diffusion into the PD fluid. Simultaneously, the ratio of glucose concentration in the dialysate at 4 hours (D_4) compared to the initial PD fluid glucose concentration (D_0 glucose) is calculated (D_4/D_0) and assesses the speed of glucose diffusing out of the PD fluid. These two measures (D/P_{creat} and D_4/D_0) are highly correlated with each other. Typically, creatinine is used as the measure, but comparable calculations can be made for other small solutes such as urea. At the end of the 4-hour period, the dialysate is completely drained, and net effluent volume is recorded. The PET test measures the speed of equilibration of creatinine between the peritoneal capillaries and the dialysate and the rate at which glucose dissipates from the dialysate. The higher the D/P_{creat} ratio, the faster the rate of diffusive transport of solutes. D/P_{creat} has a theoretical range between 0 and 1. Based on the speed of solute transfer, the peritoneal membrane solute transport characteristics are classified as *Fast, Fast Average, Slow Average*, and *Slow* (Fig. 57.5).

Membrane solute transport characteristics may assist in formulating an appropriate PD prescription. The membrane type describes how quickly osmotic equilibrium is reached within the peritoneum. The glucose in the PD fluid is a small solute and undergoes diffusion into the peritoneal capillaries. The osmotic equilibrium occurs when the concentration gradient of glucose is lost, and effective UF stops. Slow transporters preserve the glucose gradient the longest and enjoy higher UF, while the osmotic gradient dissipates much faster in fast transporters, resulting in lower UF during the PET. Whereas fast transporters sometimes struggle with fluid removal, small solute clearance is preserved, and shorter, more frequent exchanges, such as those offered in APD, play an important role in facilitating adequate fluid removal. Slow transporters, by virtue of enhanced UF, have greater total convective solute removal compared to fast transporters (Fig. 57.6).

Depending on the membrane type, osmotic equilibrium occurs at various time points and, thus, provides information regarding the most appropriate prescription. In addition to the membrane type, the concentration of the glucose in the instilled bag also affects the UF profile by having different times of osmotic equilibration. As seen in Fig. 57.6, net UF of more than 200 mL from a standard 4-hour dwell using a 2.27% glucose or more than 400 mL from a 3.86% glucose bag is considered adequate UF.

An initial PET should be performed more than 4–6 weeks after the initiation of PD. It has been reported that, in patients new to PD, membrane transport characteristics do not stabilize until about 4 weeks of PD. In addition, the PET is not performed during an episode of peritonitis, as peritoneal inflammation often leads to transient increases in solute transport during this time. Transport status can change over time, as the peritoneal membrane may be affected by long-term exposure to glucose-based solutions and additional insults, and in longitudinal evaluation, many individuals experience a progressive increase in solute transport characteristics and potentially a reduction in UF capacity.

There are several modifications of the test that have been developed over the years. A modified PET uses a 4.25% dextrose bag with a dwell time of 4 hours. In addition to the identification of membrane type, a 4.25%-based PET identifies the UF capacity of the membrane and can also allow for measurement of aquaporin function by measuring the degree to which the drop in dialysate sodium occurs early in the exchange. Impaired UF on the PET test is defined as a UF volume of <200 mL during a standard PET using a 2.5% solution or a UF volume of <400 mL during a modified PET with 4.25% solution. It is important to note that if the suboptimal UF is due to peritoneal membrane dysfunction, this may be the result of (1) increased peritoneal solute transport rate, leading to impaired UF due to the loss of the glucose osmotic gradient (in which case solute transport characteristics will also be increased); (2) a reduction in the osmotic conductance to glucose (OCG, defined as the ability of glucose to exert enough osmotic pressure to cause UF) that is often accompanied by the presence of peritoneal fibrosis; or (3) a combination of both increasing solute transport rates and a simultaneous reduction in OCG. Lymphatic absorption of peritoneal fluid tends to remain constant over time; accordingly, excessive lymphatic absorption of PD fluid remains an uncommon cause of peritoneal UF impairment and usually presents as impaired UF at the start of PD in a small minority of individuals.

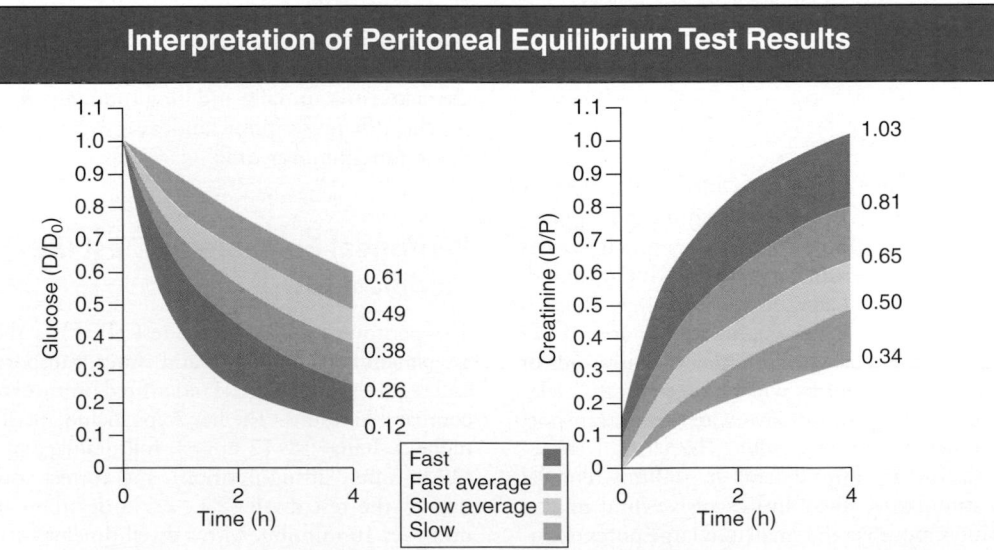

• **Fig. 57.5** Interpretation of peritoneal equilibration test (PET) results. (Modified from Twardowski ZJ, Nolph DK, Khanna R, et al: Peritoneal equilibration test. *Perit Dial Bull* 1987;7:138-147. In: Feehally J. *Comprehensive Clinical Nephrology*, ed 6, Elsevier, 2019.)

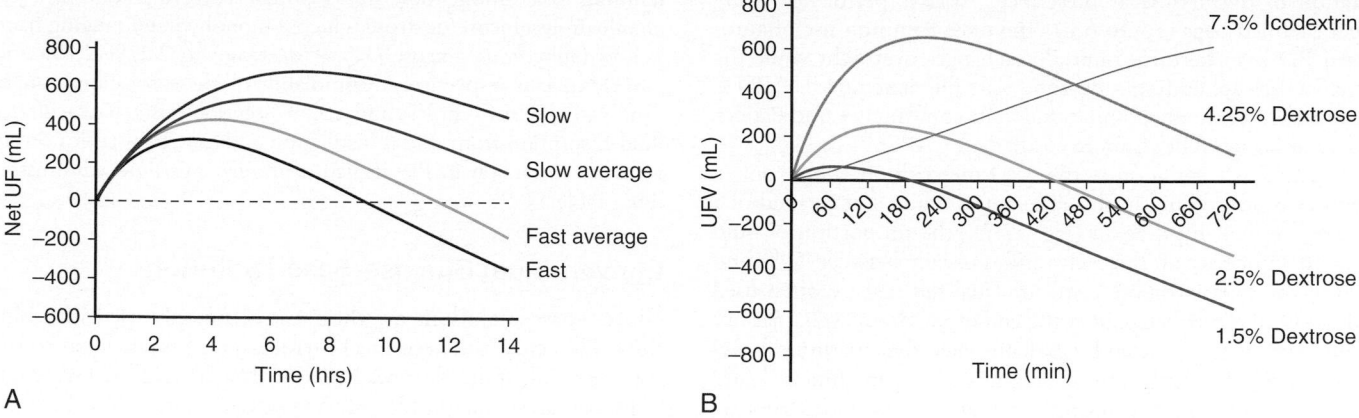

• **Fig. 57.6** Ultrafiltration (UF) by transport types and ultrafiltration profiles depend on the osmotic concentration of the dialysate and dwell time.

PD Access

Access to the peritoneal cavity requires a permanent, safe, and reliable PD catheter. The International Society for Peritoneal Dialysis (ISPD) publishes guidelines at regular intervals for selection of types of catheters, as well as catheter-placement methods.

PD Catheter Type and Configuration

Most PD catheters are made of polyurethane or silicone and come in various sizes and configurations. Catheters have an intraperitoneal section, a tunnel section, and an extraperitoneal section. The intraperitoneal catheter tip can be straight or coiled and has numerous side holes to facilitate fluid flow. Catheters typically have 1 or 2 polyester/Dacron cuffs along the tunnel section. The deep cuff is placed into the rectus sheath (ideally secured with a purse string suture) or at the parietal peritoneal entry site. The second cuff, if present, is usually placed 3 to 5 cm from the exit site. A two-cuff catheter may be beneficial over a one-cuff catheter by providing extra tensile strength to the catheter and a potential reduction in infection risk. The intraperitoneal section can be either straight or precurved (swan-neck configuration). Extended two-piece catheter systems can be used, if necessary, to increase the catheter length and to bring the exit site to a more desirable and accessible location, depending on the body habitus and the status of the lower abdomen (i.e., the presence of scars or a stoma). The exit site itself is placed either facing laterally (if using a straight catheter configuration) or downward (if using a swan-neck configuration).

Methods of PD Catheter Placement

PD catheters can be placed by surgeons, interventional radiologists, or interventional nephrologists/nurse practitioners. Catheters can be inserted in operating rooms, interventional radiology suites, or at the bedside, depending on the operator experience and resources available. Mini-laparotomy, basic and advanced laparoscopy, and the percutaneous Seldinger technique are various methods of catheter insertion by surgeons and interventionalists. While no method has been demonstrated to be superior to another, advanced laparoscopic PD catheter insertion is considered the gold standard. With this technique, there is an ability to directly visualize the PD catheter placement and perform ancillary procedures to assist

with better PD catheter function, such as lysis of bowel adhesions, omentopexy, hernia repair, etc. Local expertise and availability of resources typically dictates catheter insertion methods.

The extraperitoneal section can be embedded in the subcutaneous space (Moncrief/Popovich method) for the advantage of being placed electively far in advance of requiring PD, thus keeping the patient committed to starting PD. Embedded catheters do require a small outpatient procedure to exteriorize the catheter at the time of PD initiation. For routine PD catheters (nonembedded), optimally a period of 2 to 4 weeks is needed for healing of the PD catheter insertion site. After this, PD training can start with smaller volumes initially, building up to full-volume dialysis in a week or so. However, for the use of PD for acute kidney injury (as seen during the COVID-19 pandemic) and in patients who start dialysis urgently (see section on urgent start PD), successful reports of PD have been described with the use of the PD catheter within 24 hours after placement, accepting a higher risk of pericatheter fluid leaks that can be reduced by using low dialysate volumes and prescribing PD in the supine position (see section on noninfectious complications of PD).

PD Modalities

The instillation and drainage of PD fluid in the peritoneal cavity at regular intervals is carried out either manually using gravity, typically referred to as *CAPD*, or with the assistance of a cycler, typically referred to as *APD*. CAPD is the most common method of performing PD worldwide. It involves instillation of PD fluid (0.5–3 L) from prefilled bags into the abdomen by gravity. In the same manner, the used or spent dialysate from the previous exchange is drained by gravity into a drain bag. This manual process is repeated for each exchange (1–5 manual exchanges per day). The innovative "Y" connection between the PD catheter and the dialysis fluid and drain bags, with the drain bag and dialysate bag sharing a single connection to the PD catheter, reduces the number of manipulations needed and, in turn, has reduced the risk of touch contamination-related infection and peritonitis over the last two decades. The Y connection also enables a flush-before-fill technique, further reducing the risk of infection. Manual exchanges are typically performed every 2–5 hours during the day, with a long overnight dwell.

APD is facilitated by a machine called the *cycler* that instills fluid. The machine can control the volume of fluid instilled and duration of dwell time as prescribed. APD is performed using larger prefilled bags (1.5 to 6 L). The most common use of automated PD is to perform multiple exchanges overnight while the patient is asleep, adding a daytime "last fill" if required. APD is becoming increasingly popular due to its convenience and patient choice, although APD is more costly than CAPD.

Tidal PD is a variation in the APD prescription, where only a proportion of the fluid in the abdomen is drained at the end of a cycle before it is filled again (Fig. 57.7). The proportion of fluid removed can be set on the cycler and is usually between 50% and 85% of the initial volume instilled. Tidal settings are often used with APD to remediate pain at the end of the drain cycle that not infrequently is experienced by patients when their peritoneal cavity is completely empty and to prevent catheter malfunction and alarms mediated by the challenges in draining low intraperitoneal volumes toward the end of cycler drainage of intraperitoneal fluid.

Each modality has drawbacks. For example, CAPD requires multiple connections and disconnections, and sufficient UF in fast transporters may be difficult. APD has greater potential for increased drain pain and alarms, sodium sieving, increased costs, and more sleep disruption. Both may be associated with burnout. Across studies, rates of peritonitis, transition to HD, and mortality do not differ between these modalities; accordingly, modality choice is driven largely by patient preference and available resources.

PD Solutions

A PD solution consists of an osmotic agent to facilitate UF, a buffer, and a combination of electrolytes to maintain acid-base and electrolyte balance in the patient. The most used conventional PD fluids contain sodium (132–135 mmol/L), calcium (1.25–1.75 mmol/L), magnesium (0.5 mmol/L), chloride (95–103.5 mmol/L), and lactate (35–40 mmol/L). Lowering the dialysate sodium further is currently under investigation as a means to increase diffusive sodium

removal. In addition, these fluids contain a varying concentration of anhydrous glucose/dextrose (glucose monohydrate) ranging from 1.36% (anhydrous glucose)/1.5% (dextrose) to 2.27%/2.5% and 3.86%/4.25%, respectively. Osmolality of these solutions ranges from 344–486 mOsmol/L, and a 0.5% solution exists that facilitates fluid absorption from initial instillation and may be used for severe volume contraction in PD in lieu of intravenous fluid administration (Table 57.2).

Conventional Glucose-Based Solutions

Glucose-based solutions are the most commonly used PD solutions. UF across the peritoneal membrane is proportional to the concentration of the glucose. Traditional lactate-buffered PD solutions have an acidic pH (usually 5.0–5.8). Lactate is absorbed and is converted by the liver to bicarbonate. The low pH may clinically lead to infusion pain, particularly in patients new to PD; this may be remedied with the use of bicarbonate supplementation in the PD fluid or the use of a neutral pH PD solution, discussed below. Traditional PD solutions also undergo heat sterilization, which may lead to caramelization of the glucose during this process. Heat sterilization of glucose-based fluids generates glucose degradation products (GDPs) that have the potential to generate advanced glycation end products (AGEs). These GDPs and AGEs have been implicated in structural and functional abnormalities of the PD membrane over time and nephrotoxicity based largely on animal and *in vitro* studies.

Neutral-pH, Low-GDP Solutions

Using multiple-chambered bags allows for the sterilization and storage of glucose solution at lower pH, leading to lower GDPs in production and storage. These chambers are mixed right before instillation to create a solution with a (neutral) pH of 7.0.

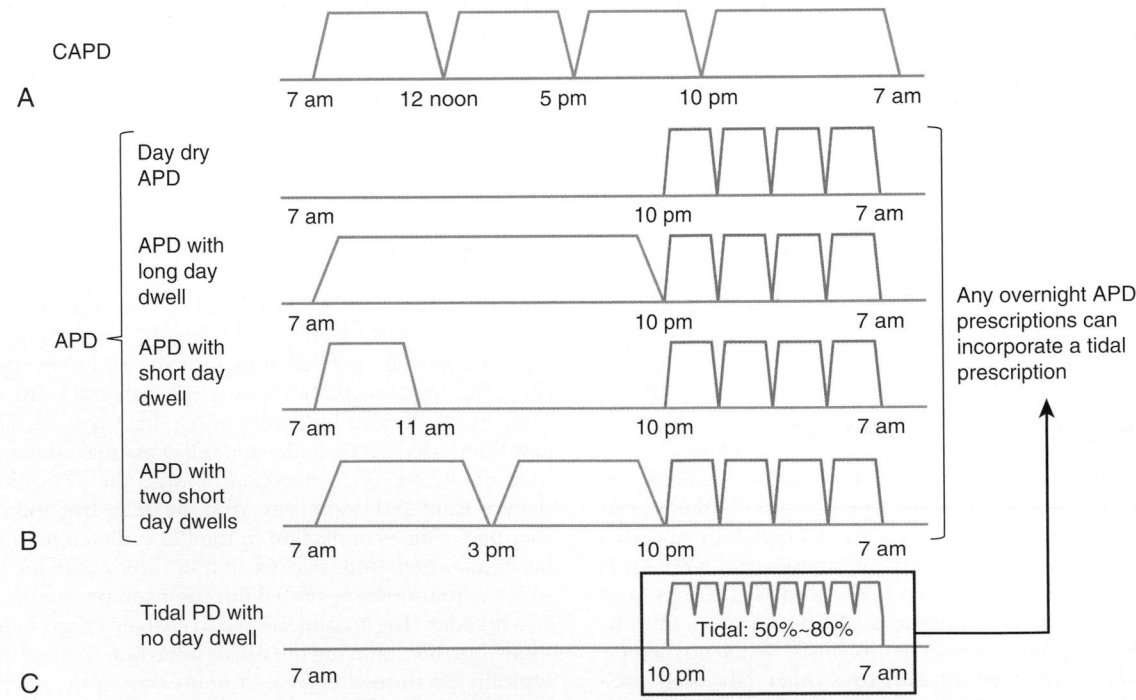

• **Fig. 57.7** (A–C) Examples of various peritoneal dialysis prescriptions including Tidal peritoneal dialysis (PD). (Dialysis exchange schedule provided here is for illustrative purposes only and can be adapted to individual patient needs.) *APD,* Automated peritoneal dialysis; *CAPD,* continuous ambulatory peritoneal dialysis.

TABLE 57.2 Composition of Various Currently Available Peritoneal Dialysis Solutions

	Dianeal Standard Glucose PD Solutions	Physioneal	Icodextrin or Extraneal or 7.5% Solution	Amino Acid or Nutrineal or 1.1% Solution	StaySafe Standard Glucose PD Solutions	StaySafe Balance	Bica Vera
Sodium (mmol/L)	132	132	133	132	134	134	134
Calcium (mmol/L)							
Low	1.25 (PD-2)	1.25	—	1.25	1.25	1.25	—
Standard	1.75 (PD-4)	1.75	1.75	—	1.75	1.75	1.75
Ultralow	1.00 (PD-1)	—	—	—	—	—	—
Magnesium (mmol/L)	0.25	0.25	0.25	0.25	0.5	0.5	0.5
Chloride (mmol/L)	96	95 (Physioneal-40) 101 (Physioneal-35)	96	105	103.5	100.5 for 1.25 mmol Ca 101.5 for 1.75 mmol Ca	104.5
Lactate (mmol/L)	40	15 (Physioneal-40) 10 (Physioneal-35)	40	40	35	2	0
Bicarbonate (mmol/L)	—	25	0	0	0	35	35
Glucose (mmol/L)	1.36%, 76 2.27%, 126 3.86%, 214	1.36%, 75.5 2.27%, 126 3.86%, 214	0	0	1.5%, 83.2 2.3%, 126.1 4.25%, 235.8	1.5%, 83.2 2.3%, 126.1 4.25%, 235.8	1.5%, 83.25
Icodextrin (g/L)	0	0	75	0	0	0	0
Amino acids (mmol/L)	0	0	0	87[a]	0	0	0
Overall pH	5.5	7.4	5.2	6.6	7	7	7.4
Approximate osmolality	PD-2 1.36%, 346 mOsm 2.27%, 396 mOsm 3.86%, 485 mOsm PD-4 1.36%, 345 mOsm 2.27%, 395 mOsm 3.86%, 483 mOsm PD-1 1.36%, 344 mOsm 2.27%, 394 mOsm 3.86%, 484 mOsm	1.36%, 344 mOsm 2.27%, 395 mOsm 3.86%, 483 mOsm	284 mOsm	365 mOsm	1.25 mmol/L Ca solution 1.5%, 356 mOsm 2.3%, 399 mOsm 4.25%, 509 mOsm 1.75 mmol/L Ca solution 1.5%, 358 mOsm 2.3%, 401 mOsm 4.25%, 511 mOsm	1.25 mmol/L Ca solution 1.5%, 356 mOsm 2.3%, 399 mOsm 4.25%, 509 mOsm 1.75 mmol/L Ca solution 1.5%, 358 mOsm 2.3%, 401 mOsm 4.25%, 511 mOsm	358 mOsm

[a]The 1.1% solutions consist of a combination of amino acids, including histidine, valine, isoleucine, alanine, leucine, arginine, lysine, glycine, methionine, proline, phenylalanine, serine, threonine, tyrosine, and tryptophan.

(From Himmelfarb J, Ikizler TA: Chronic Kidney Disease, Dialysis, and Transplantation, A Companion Guide to Brenner and Rector's the Kidney, ed 4, Elsevier, 2019.)

Another advantage of using multi-chambered bags is the ability to use bicarbonate as a buffer. Traditionally, bicarbonate cannot be used alongside calcium- and magnesium-containing solutions due to risk of precipitation. However, in these multi-chambered bags, bicarbonate, either as the sole buffer or in combination with lactate, can be mixed immediately prior to instillation. Taken together, the most significant benefit of neutral-pH, low-GDP solutions appears to be superior preservation of RKF. No significant difference is observed in peritonitis rates, patient survival, or technique survival compared to glucose-based PD solutions. These solutions are not currently available in the United States.

Glucose Polymer Solutions

Icodextrin is a large, starch-derived glucose polymer with a MW of 13,000–19,000 Da. The currently available concentration is a 7.5% solution with a sodium of 133 mmol/L and lactate of 40 mml/L; it is isosmotic at 284 mOsm/L. Icodextrin is not significantly metabolized in the peritoneum and only slowly absorbed into the blood stream via the peritoneal lymphatics. It is metabolized by circulating alpha-amylase into oligosaccharides and maltose. Slow, steady ultrafiltration is achieved compared to glucose via colloid osmosis as opposed to crystalloid osmosis with glucose-based solutions (see Fig. 57.6).

Several RCTs, observational studies, and systematic reviews show that icodextrin has significantly better UF and sodium removal compared to the conventional glucose solutions when used for the long dwell (overnight in CAPD), daytime dwells in APD), and in rapid transporters. Rapid transporters experience greater UF with icodextrin than glucose-based solutions, compared to their slow transporter counterparts. Patients have a lower incidence of uncontrolled fluid overload and better metabolic profile with icodextrin as compared to glucose. Icodextrin can cause a skin rash in a minority of patients, often described as a mild or moderate psoriasiform macular rash. This may include desquamation of the skin over the palms of the hands and soles of the feet, which often disappears after cessation of icodextrin. Lymphatic reabsorption of icodextrin and its metabolites can interfere with glucometers that use the *glucose dehydrogenase-pyrroloquinoline quinone* method of blood glucose estimation, resulting in overestimates of the blood glucose. This has resulted in excess treatment of glucose, leading to significant hypoglycemia and several deaths. Therefore, patients receiving icodextrin and institutions treating PD patients using icodextran solution should exclusively employ the use of glucose-specific test strips. Of note, several point-of-care chemistry and blood gas analyzers do not have glucose-specific testing and can result in inaccurate glucose estimation in patients treated with icodextrin.

Amino Acid Solutions

PD patients lose 3–4 g/day of amino acids and 4–15 g/day of total proteins. These numbers can increase substantially when the peritoneum is inflamed, as occurs during peritonitis. Amino acid-based solutions were designed to replace some of these losses without the additional phosphorus burden that may occur with dietary protein intake. The commercially available amino acid solution is a 1.1% containing 87 mmol/L of amino acids. This exerts a similar osmotic force as a 1.36% glucose solution. There is a slight tendency to increased urea levels and metabolic acidosis in patients using these products, limiting their use. There are several observational studies and RCTs exploring the utility of these solutions, but a clear indication is not identified yet.

Prescribing PD

Residual Kidney Function

The Canada-USA (CANUSA) cohort study reported that, for every 5 L per week per 1.73 m^2 residual creatinine clearance, there was a 12% lower relative risk of death; in contrast, no relationship was identified between higher peritoneal urea clearance and death. This landmark finding clarified that the kidney clearance provides advantages as compared to solely peritoneal clearance of solutes, as RKF provides enhanced middle molecule removal, volume control, and metabolic benefits by obviating the need for additional glucose to achieve similar fluid removal. It is clear from several studies over the last few decades that RKF is independently associated with lower mortality for PD patients. (Table 57.3)

Attention to maintaining RKF should incorporate the same intensity as preservation of GFR in CKD stages 3–5. Intensifying PD after the loss of RKF is important but does not fully compensate for the permanent loss of the clearance of many uremic solutes. Diuretics are useful in controlling the volume status in a patient on PD with urine output of more than a cup (~250 mL) per day; however, diuretics do not play a role in preserving RKF.

TABLE 57.3	Benefits of and Strategies for Preserving Residual Kidney Function	
Benefits of Preserving Residual Kidney Function	**Strategies to Preserve Resident Kidney Function**	
• Maintenance of euvolemia • Improved blood pressure control • Better nutritional status • Reduced erythropoietin requirements • Lower risk of peritonitis • Less systemic inflammation • Possibility of incremental dialysis • Improved survival and technique failure	• Consider starting patients on peritoneal dialysis instead of hemodialysis • Consider incremental dialysis • Use of biocompatible PD solutions • Preferential use of ACE inhibitor/ARB as antihypertensive medications on PD • Prevent intravascular volume depletion and hypotension • Avoid nephrotoxic agents	

Determining an Initial PD Prescription

1. Determine the initial modality. Employing shared decision making, the individual and the prescriber assess the patient's lifestyle and determine if they prefer all manual exchanges (CAPD) or automated overnight exchanges (APD). Typically, patients working during the day may prefer APD, while those not comfortable with the idea of being tethered to a machine at night or those who are light sleepers may prefer CAPD. Crafting the prescription to accommodate patients' and care partners' lifestyles is important for success. APD may be advantageous in patients at risk for noninfectious PD complications, such as leaks, hernias, or back pain, who may not tolerate daytime exchanges (see section on noninfectious complications of PD) (Table 57.4).
2. Determine the volume of each exchange. Patients typically tolerate dwell volumes from 1.25 - 1.5 L/m^2, varying with position (average 2–3 L). Larger volumes are tolerated, while

TABLE 57.4	Benefits and Concerns of Automated Peritoneal Dialysis and Continuous Ambulatory Peritoneal Dialysis Modalities for Peritoneal Dialysis	
	APD	**CAPD**
Cost	$$$$	$$
Training	Less confident with twin bags	More confident with twin bags
Mechanical complications	Lower risk of hernia, leaks, back pain (if start with dry day)	Higher risk of hernia, leaks, back pain
Catheter complications	Drain pain, alarms	May be easier for "fussy" catheter
Special patient population Assisted PD (elderly)	Easier (one or two visits per day)	More challenging
Cirrhosis/ascites	More challenging	Can control volume of drain
Urgent start PD	Lower risk of leaks	Higher mechanical complications

supine and higher dwell volumes provide better small solute clearance. Patients with recent PD catheter insertion, a known hernia or a recent hernia repair, back pain, or are at a higher risk for leaks may benefit from lower dwell volumes and potentially supine dialysis, including using APD with a dry day to reduce these risks.

3. The number of exchanges in CAPD. Manual regimens typically have one to four exchanges during the daytime and a longer overnight exchange. Early on, patients may require fewer exchanges in the presence of significant RKF (see section on incremental PD). CAPD beyond four daily exchanges may be cumbersome, and those patients may favor a switch to APD.

4. The number of exchanges in APD. The duration of total cycler length should be dictated by the number of hours that a patient sleeps (e.g., over 8-9 hours, the number of exchanges is typically 3–5). More exchanges may be necessary in rapid transporters; however, if too many exchanges are prescribed during this period, there may be excessive time spent filling and draining the PD fluid and shorter dialysis dwell times, thereby decreasing the efficiency of the therapy.

5. Consider incremental dialysis. Patients with significant RKF can be considered for incremental dialysis, which may entail fewer exchanges, lower dialysate volumes to start, and less than 7 days of dialysis per week. Incremental PD allows for personalization of PD prescription to reduce initial workload, allowing patients to build confidence in performing the therapy. In addition, incremental PD results in lower costs, less exposure to glucose solutions, and fewer mechanical side effects, especially when the patient newly transitions to PD and potentially may slow the decline in RKF. Over time, there must be an intention to increase the peritoneal clearance as required, particularly in the face of RKF loss. Some typical incremental PD prescriptions are outlined in Box 57.1.

6. Urgent start PD. PD catheters placed surgically or percutaneously need 2–4 weeks for the healing to complete. If PD needs to be started before that, urgent start protocols can be used for initiation. This typically entails low-volume, supine dialysis on the cycler, typically with dry abdomen when the patient is upright. Once the healing is complete, the dwell volume can be gradually increased to full volume. Similar principles can be employed in the use of PD for acute kidney injury.

BOX 57.1

Typical Incremental Peritoneal Dialysis Prescriptions

CAPD	APD
3 × 2 L daily	APD with no day dwell
2 × 2 L daily (single or both icodextrin)	APD five nights a week
1 × 2 L icodextrin long dwell daily	APD three nights a week
4 × 1.5 L daily	APD with 1.5 L dwell volumes
CAPD 4–6 days a week	APD for 6 h each night

PD: peritoneal dialysis; APD, automated peritoneal; CAPD, continuous ambulatory peritoneal dialysis.

From Blake PG, Dong J, Davies SJ. Incremental peritoneal dialysis. Perit Dial Int. 2020;40(3):320–326.

A prescription entails modifications of the variable components to arrive at a regimen that provides for adequate solute and fluid removal to meet clinical needs and maintain reasonable quality of life. The most common prescriptions for CAPD and APD were reported by the Peritoneal Dialysis Outcomes and Practice Patterns Study (PDOPPS) registry; in North America, this is CAPD with four exchanges per day and 2–2.5 L volume per exchange. Similarly, most patients on APD perform 4–5 exchanges per treatment with the daytime dwell volumes <2 L, while the overnight cycler exchanges between 2 and 2.5 L.

PD Adequacy and Goal-Directed Dialysis

For several years, "adequacy" of PD was conceived as measures and targets for small solute/urea clearance or creatinine clearance achieved on PD. Recently published ISPD guidelines encourage a more individualized PD prescription with focus on (1) maintenance of a patient's quality of life, (2) minimization of symptoms of ESRD, and (3) provision of high-quality dialysis.

"Adequacy of dialysis" is better conceptualized as "goal-directed dialysis," defined as "using shared decision making between the patient and care team to establish realistic care goals that allow patients to make their own life goals and allow the clinician to provide individualized high-quality dialysis care." This is outlined in Table 57.5.

Optimizing Solute Clearance and Fluid Removal

Patients who present with symptoms of uremia and lab results suggestive of poor solute clearance (e.g., low albumin, high phosphorus, etc.) should have their PD prescription evaluated (Table 57.6). Changes to the initial, empiric PD prescription are often needed to account for change in the patient condition and symptoms or signs that may represent poor dialysis. Small solute clearance is commonly monitored in patients, but it is only one of the many markers of a good dialysis prescription and adaptation. Increasingly, remote monitoring of patients on PD enables assessment of volume and blood pressure on a regular basis. This is in addition to the ability to monitor a patient's individual therapy details online and identify issues that can be preemptively managed.

Small solute clearance in PD has traditionally been quantified by the weekly total Kt/V_{urea}. This measure sums weekly peritoneal (PKt/V_{urea}) and kidney (RKt/V_{urea}) urea clearance, standardized to the volume of distribution of urea (Table 57.7); hence, it is dimensionless. Many guidelines state the minimum weekly Kt/V_{urea} in dialysis should be 1.7, but, in our opinion, a patient should also demonstrate symptoms of inadequate dialysis to warrant a change in the prescription. Prescription changes may be most necessary when RKF is declining. Strategies to improve the solute clearance include doing dialysis continuously (avoiding dry periods), increasing the dwell volume to the maximum tolerated volume, and increasing the total drain volume (including UF) by manipulating dwell volumes and/or the number of exchanges. Volume management can be optimized by considering dietary sodium and fluid restriction and by adding or optimizing the diuretic doses, preserving RKF, avoiding negative UF by optimizing dwell times and fluid concentration, and increasing the osmotic gradient.

Nutrition

Nutrition is discussed in more detail in Chapter 52. The recommended targets for protein intake for PD patients are ≥1.2 g/kg/day and energy intake are ≥30–35 kcal/kg/day. The prevalence of protein

TABLE 57.5	International Society for Peritoneal Dialysis Recommendations for Providing Goal-Directed Peritoneal Dialysis
Shared decision making	Patient, caregiver, and the peritoneal dialysis team should aim for maximizing the quality of life, satisfaction, reduction of symptoms, and provide quality of care together to align with the patient's life goals
Local resources	Peritoneal dialysis prescription should account for local resources at program level and patient/caregiver level, and should remain aligned with the patient's goals of care
High-quality PD	• HRQoL: Assess symptom burden, impact of PD prescription on life participation and psychosocial status • Volume status: Maintain euvolemia considering the residual kidney function and ultrafiltration • Blood pressure: No clear targets have been defined, however; suggested range is SBP ≥110 to ≤150 mm Hg • Nutritional status: Appetite and protein intake monitoring. Electrolyte targets include bicarbonate ≥24 mmol/L; albumin ≥38 g/L; potassium 4–5.4 mmol/L; sodium ≥135 mmol/L • Urea-based small solute clearance: Should be measured. However, caveats related to estimation of urea distribution of volume (V) must be considered. A certain minimum small solute clearance may improve uremia-related symptoms, but its impact on quality of life, technique survival, and mortality are uncertain • Incremental peritoneal dialysis: Adapting to the residual kidney function can be considered • Modification: Peritoneal dialysis prescription does not need to be changed if patient's nutrition volume and symptoms are well controlled
Residual kidney function	Preservation of RKF is key to managing patients on peritoneal dialysis, and all efforts must be made to slow the loss of RKF
Treatment burden	Peritoneal dialysis prescription should be aligned with patient's life goals, especially for the old and frail

TABLE 57.6 Dialysis-Related Reasons for Potentially "Insufficient" Peritoneal Dialysis

Cycles and concentration of prescribed solutions are in sufficient for the patient

Nonadherence, inaccurate, or missed PD cycles

Actual dwell times differ from prescribed times

Loss of residual kidney function

Incomplete drainage

Hypercatabolic state

Adapted from Yee-Moon Wang A. Peritoneal Dialysis Solutions, Prescription and Adequacy. In: Chronic Kidney Disease, Dialysis, and Transplantation. Elsevier; 2019:480–508.e9. doi:10.1016/B978-0-323-52978-5.00031-8.

TABLE 57.7 Kt/V$_{urea}$ (Small Solute Clearance) and Its Calculation

Kt/V – Fractional clearance of urea is expressed as Kt/V, which is the clearance of urea (K) per unit of time (t) in relation to its volume of distribution of total body water (V).

Peritoneal Kt/V = [24 hour PD effluent urea divided by plasma urea concentration (D/P urea)] / Volume of distribution of urea OR total body water (V)

Kidney Kt/v = [24 hour urine urea divided by plasma urea (U/P urea)]/ volume of distribution of urea OR total body water (V)

Daily total Kt/V = peritoneal Kt/V + kidney Kt/V

Weekly Kt/V = daily Kt/V x 7

energy wasting (PEW) in PD patients ranges from 18%–55%. This reflects losses of amino acids and protein in the dialysate, with protein loss approximating 8 to 12 g/day. In addition to factors common in kidney failure, PD-specific factors include peritonitis, which markedly increases dialysate protein losses, and appetite suppression by the absorbed dialysate glucose. While lower serum albumin level is associated with both mortality and hospitalization in PD patients, albumin is greatly influenced by inflammation and is a poor marker of nutritional status when used alone.

The use of amino acid dialysate (in which amino acids replace the glucose) has been tried on a limited basis as a means of correcting protein malnutrition, but proof of its long-term nutritional benefit is lacking. The number of calories absorbed from dialysate glucose depends on the dextrose concentration used (1.5, 2.5, or 4.25 g/dL) and on the membrane permeability of the patient. The development of obesity is not unusual in patients undergoing PD, especially in those who were already overweight at the start of dialysis. In addition, glucose absorption frequently results in dyslipidemia, which may contribute to atherosclerotic cardiovascular disease.

Complications of PD

Infection

PD-related infections are broadly divided into PD-related peritonitis and catheter-related infections (CRI), which include both exit site infections (ESI) and tunnel infections. Each infection type may occur in isolation, but any combination is also possible in a given patient. PD-related infections (and, in particular, peritonitis) are the major cause of catheter loss, premature transition to HD, and hospitalization. Exit site infection and tunnel infection may increase the risk for future peritonitis. The ISPD has published guidelines for prevention of PD-related infections (Table 57.8).

Peritonitis

Peritonitis remains a major complication of PD despite improvements over time reflecting advances in connections and aseptic technique. Peritonitis accounts for 15% to 35% of hospital admissions in patients on PD and is the major cause of PD catheter loss and premature transfer to HD. Postulated routes of infection

TABLE 57.8	Prevention of PD-Related Infections

- Prophylactic systemic antibiotics administered at the time of PD catheter insertion; antibiotic choice depends on the local microbiology profile and is often a glycopeptide or a first-generation cephalosporin

- PD catheter and PD bag "connectology" with a "flush-before-fill" Y-connection design

- Extensive and continuous training of the staff and patients with periodic reviews

- Daily exit-site care using topical antimicrobials including mupirocin or gentamicin

- Prophylactic antifungal use for secondary prevention of fungal peritonitis when PD patients receive antibiotic courses (for any indication)

- Prompt treatment of ESI and tunnel infections with systemic antibiotics

- Prophylactic antibiotic use when patients undergo invasive procedures including colonoscopy, urogynecological procedures, and, at some centers, dental procedures

- Establishment of a continuous quality improvement process for identifying and monitoring exit site/tunnel infection rate and peritonitis rate

- Detailed and meticulous patient technique review and retraining undertaken after each episode of ESI or peritonitis

include (1) entry of bacteria into the catheter during an exchange procedure (touch contamination); (2) entry of bacteria along the external surface of the catheter with or without the development of a PD catheter biofilm; (3) migration into the peritoneum from the abdominal viscus (transudation of organisms across the bowel wall) even in the absence of overt bowel compromise; (4) transient bacteremia seeding the peritoneal cavity; (5) entry of organisms via the female reproductive tract; and (6) fungal peritonitis in immunocompromised individuals and/or patients exposed to prolonged courses of antibiotics (particularly broad-spectrum). PD peritonitis most often presents with abdominal pain and cloudy PD effluent, although not all cloudy effluent is due to an infection. Other noninfectious causes of cloudy PD effluent include chemical peritonitis, hemoperitoneum, malignancy, and chylous effluent.

Diagnosis of peritonitis requires the presence of any two of the following:
- Organisms identified on gram stain or subsequent culture
- Cloudy fluid (white cell count >100/mm³, >50% neutrophils)
- Symptoms and signs of peritoneal inflammation (i.e., cloudy fluid, abdominal pain)

Cloudy dialysate effluent is almost invariably present, and abdominal pain is present in 80% to 95% of peritonitis cases. Gastrointestinal symptoms, chills, and fever are present in as many as 25% of cases, and abdominal tenderness in 75%. Concomitant bacteremia is rare and usually signifies that the peritoneum is a metastatic site of infection. In many centers, up to 20% of peritonitis episodes result in a "no growth" culture result (culture-negative), predominantly because of suboptimal sample collection, transportation, inadequate culture techniques (optimal techniques described in the ISPD guidelines), antibiotic exposure prior to obtaining a PD effluent culture, or a combination of these. *Culture-negative peritonitis* usually responds to conventional antimicrobial therapy. In culture-negative peritonitis that does not respond to conventional

antimicrobial therapy, it is important to consider organisms such as mycobacteria and obtain special cultures for these and other atypical organisms.

The rate of peritonitis with coagulase-negative staphylococcal (CoNS) species has decreased since the introduction of the Y-set and the "flush-before-fill" technique; accordingly, *Staphylococcus aureus* and enteric organisms now account for a larger proportion of peritonitis episodes than in the past. Because outcomes including catheter removal are higher with these organisms compared to infections caused by CoNS, peritonitis has become a less frequent but more severe complication, often requiring hospital admission. Peritonitis rates, originally extremely high in the late 1970s and early 1980s, have decreased, and a recent PDOPPS publication reported a rate of 0.24–0.40 episodes per patient year across various countries.

The initial treatment of peritonitis is empiric and covers both gram-positive and gram-negative organisms (including antipseudomonal coverage). Intraperitoneal administration of antibiotics is the preferred route. The ISPD guidelines published in 2016 recommend center-specific empiric therapy based on the local history of sensitivities of organisms causing peritonitis. Gram-positive organisms may be covered by vancomycin or a first-generation cephalosporin if methicillin resistance is rare, and gram-negative organisms by a third- or fourth-generation cephalosporin or aminoglycoside while dialysate effluent culture report is awaited; subsequent therapy is tailored to the sensitivity results. When used, serum vancomycin trough levels should be monitored to ensure adequate dosing. In addition, aminoglycoside levels should be monitored to avoid accelerated loss of RKF and vestibulo-ototoxicity.

Factors to be considered in treating peritonitis include:
- Route of administration. While IP administration of antibiotics has been recommended by the ISPD guidelines, evidence is limited, and prompt treatment likely is more important than the route of antibiotic administration
- RKF. Patients with significant RKF (>5 mL/min GFR) are more likely to be underdosed due to increased clearance of administered antibiotics and may require augmentation of the standard doses, particularly in relapsing and repeat peritonitis episodes
- PD modality. Most of the antibiotic dosing data are based on studies on CAPD. Extrapolation of CAPD-based pharmacokinetics data to APD patients may not be appropriate. APD reportedly has higher antibiotic clearance and can result in inadequate level of antibiotics and potential treatment failure
- Intraperitoneal intermittent vs. continuous dosing. Dosing differs for intermittent (in once-daily exchange x 6 hours) and continuous (every exchange) administration of antibiotics. Some studies have suggested that once-daily administration could potentially lead to subtherapeutic antibiotic drug levels. Duration of therapy depends on the organisms and the severity of the peritonitis; it is usually 14 days for *S. epidermidis* infections and 21 days for most other infections. Some antibiotics have been studied with both intermittent and continuous dosing, while some can only be administered continuously (i.e., ampicillin)

Episodes of peritonitis can also be characterized as refractory, relapsing, recurrent, or repeat (Table 57.9). ISPD guidelines recommend that PD catheters should be removed for refractory, relapsing, or fungal peritonitis. Refractory exit site and/or tunnel infections may need catheters to be moved to different sites or removed. Catheter removal may also be considered for peritonitis with multiple enteric organisms, mycobacterial infections, and repeat peritonitis.

TABLE 57.9	Terminology for Peritonitis
Recurrent	An episode that occurs within 4 weeks of completion of therapy of a prior episode but with a different organism
Relapsing	An episode that occurs within 4 weeks of completion of therapy of a prior episode with the same organism or culture-negative
Repeat	An episode that occurs more than 4 weeks after completion of therapy of a prior episode with the same organism
Refractory	Failure of the effluent to clear after 5 days of appropriate antibiotics
Catheter-related	Peritonitis in conjunction with an exit-site or tunnel infection with the same organism or with no growth from either the exit site or peritoneal fluid

Adapted from Li PK-T, Szeto CC, Piraino B, et al. ISPD Peritonitis Recommendations: 2016 Update on Prevention and Treatment. Perit Dial Int. 2016;36(5):481–508.

Refractory peritonitis is defined when there is a failure of the effluent to clear after 5 days of appropriate antibiotics and/or persistent positive culture of the PD effluent. Relapsing peritonitis occurs in about 10% to 15% of episodes. Relapsing infections, especially those due to CoNS, suggest colonization of PD catheter with biofilm. PD catheter removal is necessary in as many as 15% of these cases, and death has been reported in 1% to 3%. For fungal peritonitis, it is now standard practice to remove PD catheters emergently in addition to giving antifungal treatment post-PD catheter removal.

Peritonitis results in a marked increase in acute peritoneal protein losses and a transient decrease in UF due to the increased peritoneal permeability with inflammation. Peritoneal fibrosis may ensue in severe episodes or as a cumulative effect of multiple episodes of peritonitis (see later discussion).

Peritoneal Catheter Exit-Site and Tunnel Infection

Peritoneal catheter infections can involve the exit site (erythema or purulent drainage), the tunnel (edema, erythema, or tenderness and collections along the subcutaneous pathway), or both simultaneously. *S. aureus* is the most common cause of exit-site and tunnel infections, with *Pseudomonas species* being the next most frequent organism. *S. aureus* exit-site infections are difficult to treat and can commonly progress to tunnel infections and peritonitis, in which case, catheter removal is required for resolution. *S. aureus* nasal carriage is associated with an increased risk of *S. aureus* catheter infection. Treatment of nasal carriers with intranasal mupirocin twice daily for 5 days each month, mupirocin applied daily to the exit site regardless of carrier status, or oral rifampin 600 mg/day for 5 days every 12 weeks has been effective in reducing *S. aureus* catheter infections.

ISPD guidelines strongly recommend daily topical application of antibiotic cream or ointment to the exit-site. Several options are available for application with various degrees of evidence supporting their use. Topical exit-site mupirocin or gentamicin cream/ointment are the most commonly used agents.

Noninfectious

PD Catheter Malfunction

PD catheter malfunction often occurs early where PD cannot be reliably started; less often, PD catheter malfunction is a late complication. Common causes include both intraluminal factors (clots, fibrin), which would present with inflow and outflow obstruction, and extraluminal factors (constipation [most common], catheter tip dislodgement out of the true pelvis), which may present as outflow obstruction with preserved inflow (Table 57.10). Occlusion of catheter holes by omental wrapping is a common finding at the time of laparoscopic revision of a nonfunctioning catheter and can be prevented by omentopexy at the time of PD catheter insertion. Omental wrap may present as either inflow or outflow obstruction. A kidney, ureter, and bladder (KUB) radiographic study is useful in localizing the PD catheter tip for malposition and assessing the intraabdominal stool burden. Depending on the cause, appropriate therapy may entail laxatives and heparinized saline flushes. The Bristol Stool Chart provides good visual clues for the severity of constipation. Sometimes urokinase or tissue plasminogen activator (TPA) instillation into the catheter to relieve blockages or manipulation under fluoroscopic guidance (using a stiff wire or stylet with a "whiplash" technique) can be attempted, although the latter often has limited success. Advanced laparoscopic revision or catheter exchange may yield the greatest opportunity for restoration of PD catheter function.

Leaks

Dialysate leak occurs when the PD fluid tracks around the PD catheter (pericatheter leak) or into another body compartment (pleural, genital, etc.). Extraperitoneal fluid leak of the dialysate can occur in 5%–10% of all PD patients. Leaks are typically investigated using contrast studies, either with enhanced CT scan or nuclear scan, and management is discussed in Table 57.11.

Hernias

Instilled PD fluid increases the intraabdominal pressure. Intraabdominal pressure is a function of the dwell volume and the position of the patient, with maximum intraabdominal pressure occurring in the sitting position. In addition to leaks, hernias are also common. Preexisting hernias should be assessed before catheter insertion and repaired either at the time of catheter insertion or earlier. Multiparity, obesity, and polycystic kidney disease are risk factors for hernias in patients receiving PD, and umbilical hernias

TABLE 57.10	Causes of Inflow- and Outflow-Related Catheter Dysfunction	
Inflow Obstruction		**Outflow Obstruction**
Inadvertent extraperitoneal/ subcutaneous placement of PD catheter		Omental wrap
Fibrin plug or sheath with complete lumen obstruction		Occlusion of side holes by viscus and other abdominal organs
Catheter kink		Catheter tip migration
Clotting of PD catheter due to perioperative bleeding		Constipation

TABLE 57.11 Peritoneal Dialysis–Related Leaks

	Pathogenesis/Risk Factors	Diagnosis	Management
Pericatheter leak	**Patient Risk Factors** • High BMI • Diabetes • Immunosuppression • Increased intraabdominal pressure • Poor tissue healing **Catheter Risk Factors** • Malposition of deep cuff • Absence of purse-string suture at deep cuff • Median (vs. paramedian) incision **Therapy-Related Risk Factors** • Early start (<2 weeks after catheter insertion) • Predominantly upright position of patient • Large volume instilled	Persistent wetness around the PD catheter exit site	PD interruption to allow for complete healing usually resolves the problem
Genital leaks	• Poor tissue healing/tensile strength • Straining • Infections • Hernias • Patent processus vaginalis	Progressive genital edema after starting PD	PD interruption may be tried; definitive management involves surgical intervention; may need transition to HD
Pleural leaks	• Poor tissue healing/tensile strength • Straining • Infections • Hernias • Congenital defects in the diaphragm	Dyspnea, pleural effusion on imaging studies	Surgical intervention to close diaphragmatic ports is rarely successful; may need transition to HD

BMI, Body mass index; *HD*, hemodialysis; *PD*, peritoneal dialysis. Adapted from Jones CB et al: Noninfectious complications of peritoneal dialysis. In: Himmelfarb J: *Chronic Kidney Disease, Dialysis, and Transplantation*, ed 4, Elsevier; 2019.

are most common. For those patients already using PD, most hernias can be managed by surgical correction and a period of peritoneal rest. In some cases, there is a possibility, after a brief period of holding PD, to restart the patient with low-volume, supine PD posthernia repair in the absence of interim HD, particularly in patients with significant RKF, and if the hernia was repaired using an extraperitoneal mesh with no exposure of the mesh to the peritoneum and little concern of mesh infection should peritonitis develop. However, if the mesh is used as part of the hernia repair and is placed intraperitoneally, we recommend a period of healing with possible bridging HD until such time as the mesh heals and is no longer exposed to the peritoneum. With regard to hernias, the smaller the hernia, the greater the risk of incarceration; accordingly, smaller hernias ideally should be repaired to reduce the risk of incarceration. Patients should be warned about the risk of incarceration and monitored for an irreducible hernia. Incarcerated hernias should be considered in any PD patient with a known or unknown hernia presenting with abdominal pain (particularly localized) and/or signs or symptoms of peritonitis.

Encapsulating Peritoneal Sclerosis (EPS)

Encapsulating peritoneal sclerosis (EPS) is defined as "a clinical syndrome continuously, intermittently, or repeatedly presenting with symptoms of intestinal obstruction due to adhesions of a diffusely thickened peritoneum." It is the most serious and devastating noninfectious complication of PD. One series reported a 60% mortality within 4 months from diagnosis. Thankfully, it is also rare, observed in less than 1% of PD patients. Diagnosis of EPS requires signs and symptoms of repeated bowel obstruction with weight loss and malnutrition, new ascites, combined with typical

CT scan features (peritoneal membrane thickening and calcification, thick-walled bowel loops tethered to the mesentery) and/or demonstration of fibrous cocoon.

In many patients, EPS may manifest as development of ascites after they have stopped PD and transitioned to HD. In North America, there are limited data on EPS incidence, although incidence may be low because of less time on PD for the average patient compared to countries like Japan. For the minority of patients who have been undergoing PD for more than 5 years, it is prudent to discuss the risks of EPS and be vigilant for signs of a sudden increase in peritoneal permeability, development of hemoperitoneum, bowel obstruction, or cloudy effluent, particularly in association with raised inflammatory markers or gastrointestinal symptoms of intermittent obstruction. Treatment consists of resting the bowel with total parenteral nutrition and surgical enterolysis for obstructive symptoms, which is best undertaken at specialist centers. Some advocate for cessation of PD and conversion to HD, but others suspect that such a change may exacerbate the fibrotic process. There are anecdotal reports of the use of prednisone early in the course of EPS and long-term antifibrotic agents such as tamoxifen or adjunct immunosuppressive agents with limited success.

PD in Special Populations

Frail and Elderly

Frailty is common in older patients and is characterized by a combination of poor physical function and exhaustion, with increased vulnerability to and inability to cope with day to day stressors.

These patients are prone to falls, hospitalization, and death, and coincident cognitive impairment is common. This population may require more care partner assistance with PD than those with higher physical function. The Frail Elderly Patient Outcomes on Dialysis (FEPOD) study suggested that, while there were no differences in the QoL or physical function of patients receiving assisted PD versus those receiving HD, assisted PD was associated with better treatment satisfaction.

Assisted PD can be provided by trained members of the family, paid nursing or technical help, health aides, or others, and can occur in patients' homes, nursing homes, or long-term care and palliative care facilities. Assisted PD avoids regular, scheduled, in-center dialysis visits and may preserve quality of life.

Obesity

Many choose to avoid PD in patients who are obese. The main concerns are metabolic complications from the obligate peritoneal glucose absorption, infectious complications, as some reports suggest a relationship between BMI and peritonitis risk, PD fluid leaks, lower dialysis solute clearance, and worse survival. While these certainly pose challenges to the prescriber, these are not absolute contraindications. The approximately 100–200 g of dextrose in the bags used for CAPD can constitute nearly 20% of daily caloric intake and, hence, can account for increasing weight. In these situations, a nondextrose solution like Icodextrin lowers the total glucose load and may improve ultrafiltration efficiency per gram of carbohydrate absorbed. Measurements of Kt/V_{urea} in the obese patients are fraught with challenges. Calculating the precise volume of urea distribution ("V") in an obese patient is difficult, as using actual body weight may overestimate the volume of distribution of urea, which does not distribute in the fat tissue. Increasing the dwell volume and using cycler-assisted therapy to facilitate larger volumes can result in higher achieved Kt/V_{urea}. Patients with obesity may have a significant abdominal pannus, and an exit site located within these folds poses a higher risk of infection. PD catheters with remote exit sites facilitated by a two-piece extended PD catheter can be used to bring the exit site to the upper abdominal or presternal region for optimal exit site location and care.

Anuria

RKF predicts survival in PD patients. Anuric patients are often not offered PD out of fear of suboptimal dialysis, poor fluid balance, and worse mortality. However, there are several studies demonstrating acceptable survival in anuric PD patients, particularly with the use of APD. An anuric patient will often require one or more additional daytime exchanges, and peritoneal membrane function should be closely monitored along with the development of uremic symptoms, with HD transition planning including a vascular access creation where appropriate.

Polycystic Kidney Disease

Patients with polycystic kidney disease tend to be younger and typically enjoy improved survival on PD compared to other patient populations. Additionally, the benefits of PD in these patients include avoidance of the need for heparin, as required in HD. This may reduce the risk of bleeding into kidney cysts or worsening sequelae from an intracranial hemorrhage (due to aneurysm rupture).

Concerns about PD in ADPKD stem from the perception that the large kidneys and/or a polycystic liver lead to increased intraabdominal pressure, preventing adequate dwell volume and resulting in poorer clearance. Occasionally, patients may need a nephrectomy for transplant preparation, and this results in time off PD and reduces the RKF. Other complications thought to be related to ADPKD are mechanical, including leaks due to raised intraabdominal pressure and higher risks of hernias. Patients with ADPKD frequently have diverticulosis, and transmigration of gut bacteria into the PD fluid can predispose to PD peritonitis. Notably, a large, retrospective trial showed that ADPKD patients on PD have similar or better outcomes compared to other PD patients, with no higher risk of peritonitis due to enteric organisms.

Diabetes

Patients with diabetes are offered PD less often due to fears of a presumed higher risk of peritonitis, longer wound healing post-catheter insertion, UF failure, and metabolic and nutritional consequences. Older data suggest worse outcomes in individuals with diabetes treated with PD compared to center-based HD; however, several newer studies report improving outcomes with PD. Advantages include less HD-induced hypotension (particularly advantageous with significant autonomic neuropathy), better preservation of RKF, and avoidance of heparin. There does not appear to be a consistently increased risk of technique failure, UF failure, or peritonitis when compared to nondiabetics. Icodextrin should be considered, especially for the long dwell, as it is associated with less weight gain, higher achieved UF, and potentially improved lipid profile.

Kidney Transplant Failure

There is no significant difference in the outcomes of postkidney transplant patients starting on PD or HD. In observational studies using national Canadian Organ Replacement Registry (CORR) data and USRDS data, researchers found no difference in overall survival by dialysis modality and highlighted that PD is underused in this group.

Ascites

Dialysis in patients with liver cirrhosis and kidney failure presents several challenges for both HD and PD. With HD, hemodynamic instability and bleeding risk may be barriers, while, with PD, infection and malnutrition are major considerations (Table 57.12). In several small, observational studies, the overall mortality, infectious, and mechanical complications rates appear to be similar in PD patients with or without liver cirrhosis. PD appears to be safe in patients with liver cirrhosis and ascites, but experience and reports in North American cohorts remain limited.

PD also may be successful in patients with cardiac-mediated ascites. PD has been used successfully, particularly as an adjunct therapy to diuretic-resistant heart failure, reducing the risk of heart failure-related hospitalization. In particular, PD may have a much more favorable hemodynamic profile than hemodialysis in this population.

Complete bibliography is available at Elsevier eBooks for Practicing Clinicians.

Considerations for Peritoneal Dialysis in Patients with Liver Cirrhosis and Ascites	
Concerns with PD	**Advantages of PD**
Excessive intraabdominal pressure	Better hemodynamic tolerance to dialysis
Difficult healing of the PD catheter due to tense ascites	Easier management of ascites (avoids repeated paracentesis)
Excessive protein loss (10–30 g/day)	No need for vascular access
Excessive drainage of ascitic fluid	Additional caloric load of dialysate
Added risk of PD-related peritonitis over preexisting risk of spontaneous bacterial peritonitis	No heparin exposure

TABLE 57.12

Key Bibliography

Bargman JM, Thorpe KE, Churchill DN. Relative contribution of residual renal function and peritoncal clearance to adequacy of dialysis: A reanalysis of the CANUSA Study. *JASN*. 2001;12(10):2158–2162.

Brown EA, Van Biesen W, Finkelstein FO, et al. Length of time on peritoneal dialysis and encapsulating peritoneal sclerosis: position paper for ISPD. *Perit Dial Int*. 2009;29(6):595–600.

Crabtree JH, Shrestha BM, Chow K-M, et al. Creating and maintaining optimal peritoneal dialysis access in the adult patient: 2019 update. *Perit Dial Int*. 2019;39(5):414–436.

Devuyst O, Rippe B. Water transport across the peritoneal membrane. *Kidney Int*. 2014;85(4):750–758.

Flessner MF. Peritoneal transport physiology: insights from basic research. *JASN*. 1991;2(2):122–135.

Lee MB, Bargman JM. Myths in peritoneal dialysis. *Curr Opin Nephrol Hypertens*. 2016;25(6):602–608.

Li PK-T, Szeto CC, Piraino B, et al. ISPD peritonitis recommendations: 2016 update on prevention and treatment. *Perit Dial Int*. 2016;36(5):481–508.

Milia VL, Limardo M, Virga G, Crepaldi M, Locatelli F. Simultaneous measurement of peritoneal glucose and free water osmotic conductances. *Kidney Int*. 2007;72(5):643–650.

Paniagua R, Amato D, Vonesh E, et al. Effects of increased peritoneal clearances on mortality rates in peritoneal dialysis: ADEMEX, a prospective, randomized, controlled trial. *JASN*. 2002;13(5):1307–1320.

Perl J, Bargman JM. Peritoneal dialysis: from bench to bedside and bedside to bench. *Am J Physiol-Renal Physiol*. 2016;311(5):F999–F1004.

Perl J, Fuller DS, Bieber BA, et al. Peritoneal dialysis-related infection rates and outcomes: Results from the Peritoneal Dialysis Outcomes and Practice Patterns Study (PDOPPS). *Am J Kidney Dis*. 2020.

Shamy OE, Sharma S, Winston J, Uribarri J. Peritoneal dialysis during the coronavirus disease-2019 (COVID-19) pandemic: acute inpatient and maintenance outpatient experiences. *Kidney Med*. 2020;2(4):377–380.

Szeto C-C, Li PK-T, Johnson DW, et al. ISPD catheter-related infection recommendations: 2017 update. *Perit Dial Int*. 2017;37(2):141–154.

Teitelbaum I. Crafting the prescription for patients starting peritoneal dialysis. *CJASN*. 2018;13(3):483–485.

Twardowski Z j, Nolph KO, Khanna R, et al. Peritoneal equilibration test. *Perit Dial Int*. 1987;7(3):138–148.

Yee-Moon Wang A. Peritoneal dialysis solutions, prescription and adequacy. In *Chronic Kidney Disease, Dialysis, and Transplantation*. 9th ed. Elsevier; 2019:480–508.

58
Conservative Kidney Management

SAMANTHA L. GELFAND, AMAR D. BANSAL, JANE O. SCHELL

Introduction

Dialysis extends and improves the lives of many patients with advanced kidney disease. It frequently serves as an effective bridge to kidney transplantation. However, for some patients, dialysis does not add meaningful time and negatively impacts quality of life. Conservative kidney management (CKM) is a holistic, team-based approach to treating end-stage kidney disease (ESKD) without dialysis. CKM includes medical management of chronic kidney disease (CKD), symptom management, psychosocial and spiritual support, advance care planning, and end-of-life care. Through shared decision making and patient-centered care, CKM emphasizes quality of life and an individualized care plan that adapts to the evolving needs of the patient over time.

Elective CKM Versus Choice-Restricted Care

In low-income countries, kidney replacement therapy may not be available for a variety of reasons and a nondialytic approach is not chosen but occurs by default. This is called "choice-restricted conservative care." In most high-income countries, kidney replacement therapy is widely available and patients who develop kidney failure have the option of electing dialysis or CKM. The principles reviewed in this chapter pertain to resource-rich settings, where there is no scarcity of dialysis access and patients can select the therapy that best fits their values and priorities.

Why Patients Choose CKM

CKM is an ideal treatment approach whenever the burdens of dialysis are likely to outweigh the benefits. CKM may be appropriate for those of advanced age, patients residing in long-term care facilities, and patients with a serious illness other than kidney disease such as heart failure, cirrhosis, dementia, advanced cancer, or advanced vascular disease. These patients generally have limited survival and often have goals and values that do not align with their anticipated trajectory on dialysis. With CKM, patients and clinicians focus on quality-of-life, whereas the traditional focus of dialysis is on biochemical optimization. Evidence shows that patients with kidney disease and other serious illnesses often prioritize relief from pain and other symptoms, preservation of functional status, and maximizing time at home with loved ones. Therefore, when discussions of dialysis and CKM highlight the different emphasis of each pathway, some patients choose CKM for its deliberate and systematic focus on quality of life.

Discussing CKM with Patients and Families

Shared Decision Making

Shared decision making (SDM) is the cornerstone of CKM. SDM can be conceptualized as the meeting of two experts—the patient as expert on their life and values, and the clinician as expert on medical prognosis and options—with the goal of working together to make the best healthcare decision for the patient. This highly collaborative approach contrasts traditional paternalistic and informative models. In paternalism, the clinician is viewed as the expert who "knows best" and accordingly dictates the course of action based on the patient's medical condition. In an informative approach, the clinician provides information and then expects the patient to make his or her own choice. SDM overcomes the limitations of both of those models by empowering both clinician and patient to explore treatment options together in the context of a relationship where both parties' input is valued and applied.

SDM is useful in any conversation about treatment options for kidney failure. For example, clinicians might use SDM to help patients pick between in-center hemodialysis and peritoneal dialysis. The goal of SDM is to have patients choose a treatment that best fits their preferences and lifestyle. Similarly, with regards to CKM, SDM is used to explore whether initiating dialysis is a fitting choice for the individual patient. In one qualitative study of US dialysis patients over the age of 65, patients overwhelmingly felt they had not made the choice to initiate dialysis. Rather, they believed that the alterative to dialysis was imminent death, or that their doctor had made the decision for them. Initiating dialysis should be a choice, and the alternative is not always imminent death. SDM ensures that choosing a therapy for kidney failure is an active and explicit process, not a default. For these reasons, the Renal Physicians Association (RPA) and Choosing Wisely Campaign recommend clinicians and patients engage in SDM for this complex deliberation.

SHARE Approach

The SHARE Approach is a five-step process for SDM framework endorsed by the Agency of Healthcare Research and Quality (Fig. 58.1). Steps include (1) Seek the patient's participation;

Seek patient's participation	What would be helpful for me to know about you and your life? What is your understanding of your kidney disease? How much involvement have you had in other medical decisions? How much do you want? Who should we include in these discussions and decisions?
Help patient compare treatment options	**Option 1** Trial of dialysis: For patients who are older with other advanced conditions, dialysis may add more time, but the extra time will likely include setbacks such as decreasing independence and more hospitalizations. **Option 2** CKM: For patients similar to you, choosing conservative kidney management may give you less time; however, all care is focused on managing your symptoms and quality of life without dialysis.
Assess patient's values and preferences	Given this news, what is most important to you? As you think about the future, what are you hoping for? What are you worried about? If you become sicker, how much are you willing to go through for the possibility of gaining more time?
Reach a decision together	From our discussion, I have a sense of what matters most to you. Would it be OK if I make a recommendation?
Evaluate the decision together	It's been two months since we started [dialysis or CKM], what has been your experience? When we started [dialysis or CKM], we hoped _____. Has this become a reality? What concerns do you have moving forward?

• **Fig. 58.1** SHARE approach to shared decision making using Ask-Tell-Ask. *CKM*, Conservative kidney management.

(2) Help the patient explore and compare treatment options; (3) Assess the patient's values and preferences; (4) Reach a decision with the patient; and (5) Evaluate the patient's decision. One of the key communication techniques in SDM is the skill of Ask-Tell-Ask, in which the clinician ensures a two-way exchange that starts and ends with eliciting the patient's perspective, sandwiched around medical information or recommendations from the clinician. Ask-Tell-Ask is useful during every step of the SHARE Approach outlined below. Fig. 58.1 shows an example of this technique.

Seek the Patient's Participation

SDM should begin with an exploration of the patient's illness understanding, prognostic awareness, and desired level of involvement in the decision-making process. Open-ended questions such as "What is your understanding of your kidney disease and overall health?," provide a helpful foundation for the rest of the conversation, in which the clinician attempts to gain an understanding of the patient's experience, culture, and expectations. Some patients may defer the decision making to a loved one or may request a clinician-led approach that is more directive.

Help the Patient Compare Treatment Options

After seeking the patient's participation, a discussion of his or her anticipated clinical trajectory with and without dialysis is useful. Helping patients understand the risks and benefits of a treatment option involves sharing prognostic information. Prognostication and important considerations in CKM such as survival, quality of life, and intensity of end-of-life care are discussed below.

Prognostication in Advanced Kidney Disease

Nephrologists may feel uncomfortable or unprepared for discussing prognosis. However, most patients report that they would make different care decisions if they knew that time may be short. Evidence shows that patients with kidney disease tend to overestimate their survival and, yet, the vast majority want accurate prognostic information from their providers.

Since prognostication can be challenging, validated prognostic models have been developed for patients with kidney disease. A recent meta-analysis and systematic review including 36 studies and nearly 300,000 patients identified several validated indices for predicting survival in incident ESKD. Most had c-statistics between 0.7 and 0.79, indicating good discrimination. The Charlson Comorbidity Index (CCI) was the most commonly used and showed the best and most consistent performance. For older patients, a Renal Epidemiology and Information Network (REIN) score greater than or equal to 9 predicted over 70% mortality at 6 months after the start of dialysis. These estimates are intended to supplement a clinician's general gestalt of how an individual patient might do. It is important to remember that survival prediction tools do not provide individualized information.

Patient decision aids (PDAs) may help guide patients and families compare treatment options. One free, online, interactive CKM PDA (ckmcare.com) was developed in part from a study of 70,000 patients in the United States Renal Data System (USRDS) and Medicare claims database. This tool integrates patient-specific prognostic markers such as age, comorbidities, functional status, cognitive function, and living situation with patient values, preferences, and overall goals of care. Although this tool is designed for patients, providers can use it to guide their discussions with patients and their loved ones in a systematic and patient-centered way.

Survival with CKM or Dialysis

There may not be a significant difference in survival between CKM and dialysis among patients who develop ESKD over 80 years of age. In a study from the Netherlands, mean survival in both groups was 1 to 2 years. This held true when measuring survival from multiple starting points, including an estimated glomerular filtration rate (eGFR) <20 mL/min/1.73 m², eGFR <15 mL/min/1.73 m², eGFR <10 mL/min/1.73 m², and time of treatment decision.

In patients 70 to 79 years old, there was a statistically significant survival advantage with dialysis, although the added survival time was substantially reduced among patients with multiple comorbidities or cardiovascular disease. The septuagenarian patients without cardiovascular comorbidities had a mean survival of 7.3 years on dialysis and 1.9 years on CKM ($P < .001$), whereas patients in the same age range with cardiovascular disease had a mean survival of 2.3 years with dialysis and 1.5 years with CKM ($P < .003$).

Comparative survival studies have limited generalizability since they are typically retrospective or observational and have a small number of patients. Due to variability in the starting point from which survival is measured, they are prone to lead-time bias. Additionally, CKM is a heterogeneous entity that is resourced differently in different countries. Results from these studies should be interpreted with these caveats in mind.

Quality of Life with CKM or Dialysis

In survey studies, most patients with kidney disease associate quality of life with relief from pain and other symptoms, independence, and quality time with loved ones.

Symptoms are common in patients living with kidney failure, regardless of whether they are treated by dialysis or CKM. Among patients receiving dialysis, symptoms are often underreported, underrecognized by providers, and may be directly related to dialysis treatment (such as muscle cramping, access-related pain, and postdialysis fatigue). Among patients treated with CKM, uremic symptoms are common, including pruritus, nausea, and fatigue. Patients who elect CKM are more likely to receive high-quality symptom management compared to those who opt for dialysis. In one study from Australia, 57% of patients receiving CKM had stable or improved symptoms over 12 months and 59% reported stable or improved overall quality of life.

Independence, which is often measured by activities of daily living scores (e.g., ability to bathe, dress, transfer independently), is another aspect of quality of life that is highly prioritized by patients. Functional status in these domains has been shown to decline rapidly among frail patients who initiate dialysis. In a study of nearly 4000 nursing home residents, only 13% maintained their predialysis functional status during the year after dialysis initiation. Knowing this data is helpful when guiding treatment decisions because it means that a trial of dialysis will rarely be successful if the intention is to restore strength or mobility. On the contrary, among patients receiving CKM, some evidence suggests that functional status may remain quite stable during most of the last year of life, with a precipitous decline during the month before death. Reasons for this are not clear, though it may be that recurrent hospitalizations for dialysis complications lead to an accelerated loss of muscle mass and function.

End of Life with CKM or Dialysis

Lastly, some patients define a high quality of life as avoidance of hospitalizations and procedures with maximal time at home, especially at the end of life. If this is a top priority for an older patient, CKM appears to be more likely to achieve these goals than dialysis. In one study, a cohort of older patients who elected dialysis spent approximately 50% of their survived days (173 days/patient/year) either receiving dialysis or in the hospital. Patients who elected CKM spent less than 5% (16 days/patient/year) of their time in the hospital (Fig. 58.2). When engaging in SDM about dialysis, it can be very helpful for older patients and their families to know that a significant proportion of the added time will likely be occupied by dialysis treatment and hospitalizations. At end of life,

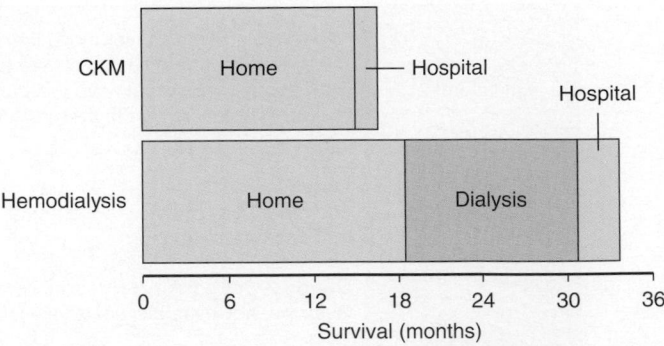

• **Fig. 58.2** Location and median survival of conservative kidney management (CKM) versus hemodialysis in the elderly. Median survival in CKM (mean age, 82 years) and hemodialysis (76 years) in a cohort of 141 patients. Data shown are how many days were spent hospital-free compared with days spent at dialysis or admitted to the hospital. (Adapted from Carson RC, Juszczak M, Davenport A, Burns A. Is maximum conservative management an equivalent treatment option to dialysis for elderly patients with significant comorbid disease? *Clin J Am Soc Nephrol* 2009;4:1611-1619.)

patients on CKM are more likely to receive hospice services and die in a home-like place (their own home or a hospice facility). This experience is in stark contrast to the end-of-life experience of most patients on dialysis, who have more frequent hospitalization (often with intensive care) and undergo more frequent invasive procedures during the last 6 months of life. Patients receiving dialysis are also less likely to receive hospice care at the end of life compared to those on CKM.

Assess Patient's Values and Preferences

In the SHARE framework, after sharing prognostic information and helping the patient compare treatment options, the focus of the conversation should shift toward eliciting how this information fits in with the individual's goals and values. This ensures that the ultimate decision is patient centered and goal concordant.

Evidence shows that clinicians do not always know the top priority of their patients. One way to elicit this information is to ask open-ended questions about what the patient is hoping for or worried about in the future given their condition. Hopes for regaining strength, spending quality time with family, and reaching family milestones (such as birthdays or weddings) are common, as are worries about suffering, loss of control, being a burden, and having a painful death.

Sometimes it is difficult for patients to articulate what matters most to them. They may never have been asked this before. It can be helpful to contextualize the questions within the treatment options at hand by saying, "Some people want to live as long as possible and choose dialysis even at the risk of frequent hospitalizations and less independence. Others wish to receive treatment focused on reducing symptoms without dialysis, even if this means life could be shorter. Do you have a sense of how you feel about this?"

Another aspect of this part of SDM is a thorough psychosocial and spiritual assessment, which can uncover important aspects of the patient's outlook and value system. Culture, religion, experience, and family dynamics may all influence a patient's approach to medical decision making. Social workers and chaplains can therefore be extremely helpful during SDM. For example, patients who are religious may worry that not starting dialysis is akin to suicide and therefore a sin. Chaplains can explore this worry, offer counseling, and, if necessary, connect with community religious leaders for additional guidance.

Reach a Decision with the Patient

After learning a patient's priorities, the clinician should offer a treatment recommendation that incorporates the prognostic data and the patient's goals and values. Most patients desire a direct recommendation from clinicians. It is therefore helpful to *ask permission* to provide a recommendation. If the patient or family member agrees, the clinician can proceed with delivering a goal-concordant treatment recommendation.

For patients with debility related to advanced age or serious illness, relevant treatment options include a trial of dialysis or CKM. It is important to frame the choice of dialysis in this population as a "trial" because it suggests a flexible approach and eliminates the idea that starting dialysis is a permanent commitment that is never revisited or reevaluated. In a trial of dialysis, the clinician and patient start by outlining the intended goals of therapy. Goals may include "bridging" to kidney recovery, an important life event, symptomatic relief, or functional improvement. When discussing a trial of dialysis, it is important to outline specific milestones that convey success or progress, such as getting stronger or staying out of the hospital. In addition, outlining setbacks that indicate the trial of dialysis is not achieving goals should also be discussed. For example, worsening frailty or increased hospitalization might prompt a discussion of whether dialysis should be stopped. A parallel in oncology is the stopping of palliative chemotherapy that has not provided intended symptom relief to a patient with incurable cancer.

Evaluate the Decision

Once the patient and clinician agree on a treatment path—either CKM or trial of dialysis—the final step of evaluating the decision might take place over the following weeks to months. For patients who elect a trial of dialysis, evaluating the decision means checking in with the patient and his or her family to reassess how treatment is going, whether milestones have been met, and whether reassessment of the decision is warranted. For patients who elect CKM, evaluating the decision may involve checking in during times of transition, like major clinical change. This often involves revisiting the previous discussion rather than starting from the beginning ("With this news about your condition, I'd like to check in on our previous discussions about managing your kidney disease").

Treatment preferences may evolve over time as patients' health status changes. Despite adequate SDM, patients may change their minds about CKM and request dialysis. This is normal and does not necessarily reflect an ineffective SDM conversation. Rather, values and priorities may evolve. Starting dialysis after a decision to do CKM is only concerning if it results from poor management of a symptom crisis or inadequate SDM rather than a true shift in a patient's priorities or goals.

It is not uncommon for patients or families to ask about dialysis after the decision to elect CKM. Rather than interpreting this as a request to do dialysis, we encourage clinicians to respond with curiosity and exploration. There are numerous factors that can influence preference stability of patients on CKM including fear around death, lack of knowledge about CKM, family pressure to choose dialysis, or mixed messages from other healthcare providers. Open-ended questions such as "Tell me what you've been thinking" or "What's worrying you the most?" can uncover these unmet information or emotional needs. In addition, how SDM is documented in the electronic health record can impact how these discussions go when a patient presents to providers outside of nephrology, such as primary care clinicians, geriatricians, and emergency medicine clinicians. It is essential that the goals and values that informed the decision are documented and communicated to other clinicians involved in the patient's care.

It is important to distinguish patients whose values are most consistent with CKM from those whose main motivation is to avoid initiating dialysis for as long as possible. The latter is a normal impulse that should be validated as part of general CKD care, particularly since delaying dialysis initiation until absolutely necessary aligns with best-practice, evidence-based guidelines. Asking about values through some of the questions outlined in step 3 above can help distinguish between these groups of patients.

PROVIDING CKM

CKM consists of medical management of CKD, symptom management, and advance care planning (Table 58.1). The expected trajectory of the patient dictates the focus of care, which usually evolves over time and often depends on the patient's prognosis. For example, in a patient with slowly deteriorating kidney function who has decided on CKM well before the onset of uremia or volume overload, CKM bears a strong resemblance to conventional CKD care with most interventions focused on reducing the rate of disease progression. On the other hand, CKM for a patient with more rapid progression of their kidney disease or other conditions will focus heavily on symptom management, psychosocial support, and advance care planning. This personalized approach helps ensure that the specific needs of each patient and family are met.

Quality metrics for CKM are in development. In 2015, the KDIGO Controversies Conference on Supportive Care in Chronic Kidney Disease outlined recommendations for clinical, educational, and research initiatives to help define standards of care in CKM.

Medical Management of CKD

CKD management in CKM involves weighing the burdens and benefits of each medical intervention for each individual patient. At present, all of the following recommendations are based on expert opinion rather than quality or outcome data. The benefit of many conventional medical therapies is uncertain in this

TABLE 58.1	Domains of Quality Care in Conservative Kidney Management

Medical Management of chronic kidney disease (CKD)
- Delaying kidney function loss
- Treatment for symptomatic anemia and hypertension
- Patient-centered management to electrolyte abnormalities

Symptom Management
- Physical symptoms
- Psychological symptoms
- Spiritual or existential distress

Advance Care Planning
- Assigning a healthcare proxy
- Crisis planning: anticipating symptoms or hospitalizations
- Discussing hopes, worries, and end-of-life preferences

population, as most are studied in trial subjects whose risk, comorbidity burden, and life expectancy differ greatly from those who choose CKM. Additionally, in all of the following care domains, clinicians should inquire about patient and caregiver stress related to polypharmacy and adjust the care plan to reduce the number of medications and the frequency of administration when possible.

- **Delaying kidney function loss:** Most interventions that have been shown to slow progression of kidney disease have been studied in younger populations at high risk for ESKD. Most people who elect CKM are older and either already have ESKD or are at higher risk of death than ESKD. Therefore, benefit related to use of certain medications, such as ACE inhibitors/ARBs, is uncertain. In fact, stopping renin-angiotensin-aldosterone system blockers is often advisable in CKM both for the increase in GFR due to efferent arteriolar constriction and the decreased risk of hyperkalemia.

- **Access planning:** For patients whose values align with CKM, one aspect of the treatment decision is to forego creation of an arteriovenous fistula or placement of an arteriovenous graft. For the subset of patients who choose CKM and then opt for a trial of dialysis, insertion of a tunneled dialysis catheter is often the most patient-centered approach, especially when the patient's prognosis is expected to be short.

- **Hypertension:** Tight blood pressure control may not confer the same benefit to the CKM population as those in the large studies that have informed our conventional targets. The objective of blood pressure control in CKM is to avoid symptoms and acute end-organ damage. Decisions about specific medication classes will depend on the patient's comorbidities and severity of hypertension. In general, blood pressure goals are usually liberalized from conventional targets.

- **Anemia:** Management of anemia in CKM should be entirely symptom-driven. Fatigue, malaise, and breathlessness are all common symptoms of profound anemia and should improve with pharmacotherapy. Erythropoiesis-stimulating agents (ESAs) and iron supplementation remain the mainstay of therapy and should be titrated to symptom improvement. Iron deficiency may also exacerbate restless leg syndrome, although supplementation does not always provide relief. Monitoring complete blood counts and iron stores every 3 months is a common practice in CKM, although frequency of monitoring should be adjusted based on patient and family preference. Additionally, choice of oral versus intravenous iron and at-home versus clinic-based ESA administration should be determined together with patients and their families.

- **Acidosis:** Conventional targets for serum bicarbonate may not confer the same benefit to the CKM population as those observed in studies of younger patients. Potential benefits of bicarbonate supplementation include improved potassium control and avoidance of respiratory distress. Potential risks include polypharmacy, adverse drug reactions like nausea, and worsening edema due to sodium loading with bicarbonate supplementation. Therefore, the decision to use supplemental bicarbonate will depend on the patient's prognosis and preferences.

- **Mineral bone disease:** The benefit of controlling hyperphosphatemia and secondary hyperparathyroidism is accrued over years; therefore, the prognosis of the patient will determine the utility of monitoring and intervening on mineral derangements in CKM. For many patients, the pill burden and uncertain benefit of tight control result in a decision not to follow these parameters at all. Bone pain and myalgias may result

from severe hyperparathyroidism and may merit a trial of pharmacotherapy. Additionally, despite traditional teaching to the contrary, pruritus is inconsistently correlated with hyperphosphatemia and secondary hyperparathyroidism, and interventions do not always result in symptom relief.

- **Hyperkalemia:** Management of hyperkalemia in CKM depends largely on whether the burden of laboratory monitoring and therapy is acceptable to the patient and family. In most cases, even if there will be no regular laboratory monitoring, it is reasonable to discuss medications and dietary modifications. Potassium-binding resins such as sodium polystyrene sulfonate (Kayexalate), patiromer (Veltassa), or sodium zirconium cyclosilicate (Lokelma) may be used if tolerated. Supplemental bicarbonate and high-dose oral diuretics are also helpful, ideally, with once-daily dosing. Restricting dietary potassium is controversial, as it takes away a wide range of flavorful and nutritious foods and is not necessarily appropriate in CKM.

- **Hyperlipidemia:** There is no evidence that statins, which confer benefit in cardiovascular outcomes over months to years, are useful in patients with serious life-limiting illnesses with prognoses of weeks to months. There is evidence from a pragmatic, randomized, controlled trial that stopping statins is safe and can improve quality of life. Lipid-lowering therapy is, therefore, often discontinued in CKM.

- **Diet modification:** Liberalizing dietary sodium intake can increase pleasure and options in eating, although these benefits must be balanced with risks of hypertension, risk of symptomatic peripheral or pulmonary edema, and patient preference. Some patients have had decades of medical advice to the contrary and may not be comfortable with liberalizing their salt intake. There is also growing interest in the effect of low-protein diet (LPD) and very-low-protein diet (VLPD) on kidney function and uremic symptoms. Plant-based diets with minimal animal protein (i.e., meat) may reduce CKD progression through decreased intraglomerular pressure and nitrogenous waste production. However, these diets are not always fitting for patients on CKM, who are often malnourished. Additionally, restricting meat may not align with a patient's culture or social life. All dietary advice in CKM should be as patient centered and culturally competent as possible.

Symptom Assessment and Management

Systematic symptom assessment is an integral part of CKM. Although data are subjective, they are still amenable to standardized and reproducible measurement using validated symptom assessment tools. Several symptom assessment tools have been studied in patients receiving CKM including the Integrated Palliative Care Outcome Scale-Renal (IPOS-renal) and the Edmonton Symptom Assessment Scale (ESAS).

Symptoms should be assessed during every clinical visit, whether in person or by virtual means, and may be tracked over time. A key part of symptom assessment is not only to identify symptoms but to gauge the degree of related distress, such that a prioritized intervention plan can be developed and adjusted over time. Some symptom tools, such as the IPOS-renal, also include a functional assessment, though this information may be collected separately.

The most prevalent symptoms in patients on CKM include fatigue, poor sleep, pruritus, poor appetite, nausea/vomiting, pain, restless legs, shortness of breath, edema, and anxiety. Therapies for each symptom include pharmacologic agents, integrative approaches, and lifestyle adjustments. Table 58.2 outlines first-line therapies for the most common symptoms.

In addition to physical symptoms, psychological distress is common. Anxiety, depression, spiritual distress, and existential angst are possible. Ideally, CKM is provided by an interdisciplinary team that includes or has access to social workers, chaplains, psychiatrists, or integrative medicine specialists. In the absence of such a team, nephrology clinicians can screen for depression with the Patient Health Questionnaire-9 (PHQ-9) and anxiety with the Generalized Anxiety Disorder-7 (GAD-7) tools and refer to specialists as needed. Alternative therapies such as acupuncture, music therapy, massage therapy, and dignity therapy may be useful but have not yet been studied in this population.

Advance Care Planning

It is important to prepare CKM patients for end of life. This process is called *advance care planning* (ACP) and involves identifying a medical decision maker (proxy) and outlining end-of-life care preferences. ACP also entails completion of advance directives and medical orders for life-sustaining treatment (POLST/MOLST) forms.

Another important part of ACP is crisis planning, which is a proactive discussion about anticipated setbacks, such as hospitalizations and acute symptom crises that may occur among patients on CKM near end of life. This is an essential part of CKM because many patients are asymptomatic when they elect a nondialytic approach and become sicker and more symptomatic over time. In a prospective observational cohort study, symptom burden and functional status remained stable in conservatively managed patients until the last 2 months before death, during which time, symptoms became profound. Without adequate preparation for end of life, patients and families may elect emergency medical services and acute dialysis initiation rather than end-of-life care that meets their symptoms and goals of care needs. Therefore, crisis planning involves patient and family education about what to expect as time goes on.

Clinicians should normalize end-of-life care as part of the CKM path ("I hope that things continue to remain stable, but I'd also like to talk with you about how we will care for you when symptoms do occur in the future. Would that be ok?"). They should also explore potential worries or stressors that may serve as a barrier to preparing for end of life. Patients often have specific hopes, worries, and priorities related to the end of life including fear of losing independence or continence, fear of being a burden on one's family, or preference for a certain location of death. Clinicians should explicitly introduce the option of hospice services as a way to ensure the patient's symptoms are managed in a home-like place that includes services,

TABLE 58.2 Approach to Common Symptoms in Conservative Kidney Management

Symptom	Evaluation	Potential Interventions
Fatigue/weakness	• History and physical exam • Functional status assessment • Medication review • Sleep and mood assessment	• Reduce polypharmacy • Sleep hygiene • Integrative therapies • Normalize symptoms
Pruritus	• History and physical exam • Labs: CBC, LFTs, phosphorus, PTH	• Lifestyle changes: avoid extreme heat and cold • Topical emollients • Trial calcium channel alpha-2-delta ligands (gabapentin, pregabalin) • For refractory symptoms, consider UV light, other topical agents, and dermatology referral

Nausea/vomiting	• History and physical exam
	• Medication review
	• Imaging if indicated
	  • If distended, abdominal radiograph
	  • If diabetic, gastric motility studies
		• Trial small regular meals, avoid skipping meals
		• Avoid strong smells
		• Address constipation
		• Trial antiemetic medications

Dysgeusia/anorexia	• History and physical exam • Medication review • Dietician and social work assessments • Mood assessment	• Maintain oral hygiene • Rinse with sodium bicarbonate mouthwash • Encourage spices and tart flavors to reduce bitter taste • Avoid metal cutlery
Restless legs syndrome	• History and physical exam • Labs: CBC, iron studies • Medication review	• Replete Iron • Trial calcium channel alpha-2-delta ligands (gabapentin, pregabalin) • Trial dopamine agonist (pramipexole, ropinirole)
Shortness of breath	• History and physical exam • Medication review • Anxiety assessment	• Diuretics • Low-dose opioids • Crisis planning
Depression /Anxiety	• History and physical exam • Psychosocial and spiritual assessment • Medication review	• Cognitive behavioral therapy • SSRIs • Supervised exercise
Pain	• History and physical exam • Imaging if indicated • Functional assessment • Psychosocial assessment	• Analgesics • Meaning making • Goal setting • For refractory symptoms, specialty palliative care referral

TABLE 58.3	Hospice Eligibility and Levels of Care

HOSPICE ELIGIBILITY	
All Patients	**Kidney Patients**
In order to elect hospice care under Medicare, an individual must be: 1. Entitled to Medicare Part A 2. Certified as having a terminal illness, defined as expected survival of 6 months or less if illness takes usual course	Individual has 1 *and* either 2 or 3: 1. The patient is not planning dialysis or transplantation 2. Creatinine clearance <10 mL/min (<15 mL/min in diabetes) 3. Serum creatinine >8.0 mg/dL (>6.0 mg/dL in diabetes)

HOSPICE LEVELS OF CARE		
Routine Hospice	**General Inpatient Hospice**	**Inpatient Respite Care**
• Usually at home, sometimes in nursing home • At home, family or loved one acts as caregiver • Average 1 hour of visiting services 3–4 times/week in the patient's home • Patient and family taught how to administer medications • Most medications and custodial care provided by family or private-pay aids • 24/7 phone support (instead of 911)	• Provision of hospice services in a hospice or hospital • Eligible if pain or other symptoms are refractory to oral therapy at home	• Designed to provide a break for family or other caregivers • Brief admission to inpatient hospice for patients receiving routine hospice care at home • Admission limited to 5 days

such as chaplaincy and bereavement support for the patient's loved ones after death. Table 58.3 summarizes basic information about hospice, including eligibility criteria and options for different types (or "levels") of hospice services. This information can be useful to share with patients who are nearing the end of life.

Global Trends and Care Models for CKM

CKM Availability

There is marked variability between countries in the management of ESKD among patients with advanced age and debility. A majority of countries report some kind of CKM availability, but only a minority have robust CKM programs and accessibility. Evidence regarding the number of patients who choose CKM, or would choose it if offered, is limited. In an observational study from Australia of patients with kidney failure and a mean age of 80, 65% were offered CKM and 14% ultimately chose it.

In the United States, numerous barriers and disincentives have kept CKM availability and use very low. The diagnosis of ESKD itself is still defined by Center for Medicare and Medicaid (CMS) as the need for kidney replacement therapy, which consists of dialysis or transplantation. Reimbursement for CKM visits is the same as for less advanced CKD and much less than dialysis treatments. With respect to education and skill building, nephrologists have classically received little communication training during fellowship, with less than half reporting explicit teaching about how to lead a decision-making conversation with patients and families. Qualitative analyses suggest that many nephrologists still equate not using kidney replacement therapy with "giving up," and may not offer CKM or accept a patient's preference not to start dialysis. Lastly, access to specialty palliative care in the United States is often limited or restricted to patients who have cancer. These cultural, financial, and health systems-related differences may account for the much higher rates of dialysis among those over 85 in the United States (41%) compared to Canada (7%) and Australia and New Zealand (5%).

CKM Care Models

CKM care models vary markedly in size, scope, and resources. Three main care delivery systems have been described: primary kidney palliative care, embedded specialty kidney palliative care, and mobile/home-based kidney palliative care.

In primary kidney palliative care models, nephrology clinicians (nephrologists, nurses, social workers) provide CKM. This is individualized CKD care plus routine palliative care to manage basic symptoms, engage in shared decision making, and assist with advance care planning. In the United States, increased training in primary palliative care skills will facilitate growth of this model of CKM, which does not require fellowship training in palliative care or access to palliative medicine specialists.

In embedded specialty kidney palliative care models, nephrologists do additional formal training in palliative medicine or partner with palliative medicine specialists to provide CKM. Specialists trained in palliative medicine can manage refractory symptoms, complex goals of care, and conflict within families or between staff and families. This is the most common model in countries with the most rigorous CKM programs, including Australia, New Zealand, the United Kingdom, and Canada. This model most closely resembles specialty palliative care delivery in oncology and cardiology.

Both primary and specialty palliative care models can have a mobile/home-based kidney care delivery option. This may include home visits and/or virtual visits through videochat platforms. Since the start of the COVID-19 pandemic, the virtual component of CKM programs has become particularly useful and in demand.

Challenges and Opportunities in CKM

CKM is an area of growth, innovation, and research in nephrology. Challenges in developing CKM include heightening awareness among patients and providers, deepening communication and symptom management skills among nephrologists, and advocating for multidisciplinary teamwork within kidney care delivery models. If provided in a patient-centered way, CKM has the potential to maximize autonomy for patients, bring satisfaction and pride to nephrologists, and avoid low-value, nonbeneficial care at the end of life.

Bibliography

Bansal AD, Schell JO. Strategies to address clinician hesitancy toward conservative care. *Nephrol Dial Transpl.* 2019;34(8):1286–1288.

Couchoud C, Hemmelgarn B, Kotanko P, et al. Supportive care: time to change our prognostic tools and their use in CKD. *Clin J Am Soc Nephrol.* 2016;11(10):1892–1901.

Dahlerus C, et al. Patient perspectives on the choice of dialysis modality: results from the Empowering Patients on Choices for Renal Replacement Therapy (EPOCH-RRT) study. *Am J Kidney Dis.* 2016;68(6):901–910.

Davison SN, Jassal SV. Supportive care: integration of patient-centered kidney care to manage symptoms and geriatric syndromes. *Clin J Am Soc Neph.* 2016;11(10):1882–1891.

Davison SN, et al. Recommendations for the care of patients receiving conservative kidney management: focus on management of CKD and symptoms. *Clin J Am Soc Neph.* 2019;14(4):626–634.

Gelfand SL, Scherer JS, Koncicki HM. Kidney supportive care: core curriculum 2020. *Am J Kidney Dis.* 2020;75(5):793–806.

Kurella TM, Covinsky KE, Chertow GM, et al. Functional status of elderly adults before and after initiation of dialysis. *N Engl J Med.* 2009;361(16):1539–1547.

Ladin K, Lin N, Hahn E, et al. Engagement in decision-making and patient satisfaction: a qualitative study of older patients' perceptions of dialysis initiation and modality decisions. *Nephrol Dial Transplant.* 2017;32(8):1394–1401.

Lam DY, Scherer JS, Brown M, et al. A conceptual framework of palliative care across the continuum of advanced kidney disease. *Clin J Am Soc Neph.* 2019;14(4):635–641.

Murphy EL, et al. Understanding symptoms in patients with advanced chronic kidney disease managed without dialysis: use of a short patient-completed assessment tool. *Nephron. Clin Prac.* 2009;111(1):c74–c80.

Murtagh FEM, et al. Symptoms in advanced renal disease: a cross-sectional survey of symptom prevalence in stage 5 chronic kidney disease managed without dialysis. *J Pall Med.* 2007;10(6):1266–1276.

O'Hare AM, et al. Interpreting treatment effects from clinical trials in the context of real-world risk information: the example of end-stage renal disease prevention in older adults. *JAMA Internal Medicine.* 2014;174(3):391–397.

Paladino J, Lakin JR, Sanders JJ. Communication strategies for sharing prognostic information with patients: beyond survival statistics. *JAMA.* 2019;322(14):1345–1346.

Schell JO, Lam D. Steps toward sustainable change in advance care planning. *Am J Kidney Dis.* 2017;70(3):307–308.

Thamer M, Kaufman JS, Zhang Y, et al. Predicting early death among elderly dialysis patients: development and validation of a risk score to assist shared decision making for dialysis initiation. *Am J Kidney Dis.* 2015;66(6):1024–1032.

Wachterman MW, Marcantonio ER, Davis RB, et al. Relationship between the prognostic expectations of seriously ill patients undergoing hemodialysis and their nephrologists. *JAMA Intern Med.* 2013;173(13):1206–1214.

Williams AW, Dwyer AC, Eddy AA, et al. Critical and honest conversations: the evidence behind the "Choosing Wisely" campaign recommendations by the American Society of Nephrology. *Clin J Am Soc Nephrol.* 2012;7(10):1664–1672.

Wong SPY, Yu MK, Green PK, et al. End-of-life care for patients with advanced kidney disease in the US Veterans Affairs Health Care System, 2000-2011. *Am J Kidney Dis.* 2018;72(1):42–49.

Wong SPY, et al. Experiences of US nephrologists in the delivery of conservative care to Patients with advanced kidney disease: a national qualitative study. *Am J Kidney Dis.* 2020;75(2):167–176.

Wong SPY, et al. Decisions about renal replacement therapy in patients with advanced kidney disease in the US Department of Veterans Affairs, 2000–2011. *Clin J Am Soc Neph.* 2016;11(10):1825–1833.

59

Selection of Prospective Kidney Transplant Recipients and Donors

GREG KNOLL, TODD FAIRHEAD

Kidney transplantation is the treatment of choice for most patients with end-stage kidney disease (ESKD) because it prolongs survival, improves quality of life, and is less costly than the alternative therapy of dialysis. However, less than 20% of ESKD patients will be wait-listed or receive a transplant. Many patients are not suitable candidates because of coexisting illness that may affect perioperative risk and survival after transplantation, but many eligible patients lack access to or are not appropriately referred for transplant evaluation. For those patients who are eligible, waiting times are long, as there are simply not enough organs available. As the primary contact for patients with advanced chronic kidney disease (CKD), as well as for those already on dialysis, nephrologists are in a unique position to counsel and guide patients through the transplantation process. Transplantation should be considered the first option for kidney replacement therapy. A thorough understanding of who is suitable for transplantation and the required evaluation process is essential to maximize patient access.

Who Should Be Considered for Kidney Transplantation?

There are very few absolute contraindications for kidney transplantation. In most populations studied, including the elderly and patients with diabetes with ESKD, kidney transplantation confers a survival advantage. All patients should be assessed by their nephrologist for transplant suitability and potentially referred to a transplant center for further evaluation. Eligibility should not be based on age, sex, race, or socioeconomic status. Given that donor kidneys are a rare and limited resource, a patient must be expected to survive beyond current waiting times for transplantation. In the United States, the median waiting time for a deceased donor kidney transplant is 4 years, although there is substantial variation due to region and patient characteristics. Careful evaluation of physiologic age, medical comorbidities, and functional status will help determine whether a patient may be eligible for transplantation. Box 59.1 lists the contraindications for transplantation.

Timing of Referral

Both mortality and graft outcomes are improved with early transplantation. Patients who receive a preemptive kidney transplant have a superior outcome compared with patients who undergo dialysis treatments before receiving a transplant. Similarly, the length of exposure to dialysis affects transplant outcomes and mortality. Improved outcomes are inversely related to the duration of dialysis. Thus, to allow adequate time to complete the required medical tests before transplantation and to facilitate potential preemptive transplantation, patients with CKD should be referred to a kidney transplant center early in their disease course. Many potential transplant recipients are medically complex. Determining their suitability for transplantation may require multiple specialist visits and medical tests. This process may take 6 to 12 months to complete and should be factored into the overall referral time. For patients with potential living donors, appropriate time should be allocated for donor workup as well.

In the United States, the United Network for Organ Sharing (UNOS) allows listing for transplantation when a patient's estimated glomerular filtration rate (eGFR) falls below 20 mL/min, whereas organizations in other countries have established stage 5 CKD (eGFR below 15 mL/min) as the upper limit for listing. Therefore, patients should be referred for transplantation evaluation when they have stage 4 CKD (eGFR below 30 mL/min) that is progressing. In some regions, transplantation assessment is initiated with referral to a multidisciplinary kidney replacement therapy planning clinic. In these clinics, transplant eligibility is considered and teaching is provided alongside planning for dialysis initiation. Education and identification of potential living kidney donors should be prioritized. It is important to recognize that certain barriers to transplant referral have been identified. Access to transplantation may be decreased for patients of certain ethnicities, those with lower socioeconomic status and/or education level, or those living a greater distance from a transplant center. Communication between a patient's primary nephrologist and the transplant program is essential to ensure eligible recipients are efficiently evaluated and wait-listed.

Medical Evaluation for Transplantation

A complete medical, surgical, and psychosocial history is required upon consideration for transplantation. A thorough physical examination may identify underlying systemic diseases that could affect transplant suitability, such as poor dentition or diminished arterial pulses. Table 59.1 lists the minimum investigations required before transplantation. Additional testing based on medical comorbidities may be necessary. Each coexisting illness should be evaluated for its potential effect on transplant outcome. In addition, total disease burden and functional capacity must be factored

BOX 59.1

Contraindications to Kidney Transplantation

Chronic illness with life expectancy <1 year
Active malignancy with short life expectancy
Active infection
Poorly controlled psychosis
Medical nonadherence or active substance abuse

TABLE 59.1 Elements of the Evaluation for Potential Kidney Transplant Candidates

Test	Comments
Physical examination	Attention to cardiovascular exam, arterial pulses, and evidence of chronic infection including poor dentition and cutaneous ulcers
Tissue typing	ABO blood type, HLA identification, PRA
Viral serology	CMV, EBV, VZV, HSV, HCV, HBV, HIV, HTLV, VDRL
Cardiac testing	ECG Echocardiogram Risk stratification if high risk
Imaging	Chest radiograph Abdominal ultrasound or imaging equivalent Arterial vascular imaging if high risk (Doppler ultrasound, CT scan, angiogram)
Female specific	Breast examination and mammogram Pap smear
Male specific	Prostate examination
Consultations	Transplant surgeon Cardiologist (if high risk) Social worker

CMV, Cytomegalovirus; *CT,* computed tomography; *EBV,* Epstein-Barr virus; *ECG,* electrocardiogram; *HBV,* hepatitis B virus; *HCV,* hepatitis C virus; *HIV,* human immunodeficiency virus; *HLA,* human leukocyte antigen; *HSV,* herpes simplex virus; *HTLV,* human T-lymphotropic virus; *PRA,* panel-reactive antibody; *VDRL,* Venereal Disease Research Laboratory (test); *VZV,* varicella-zoster virus.

into a final decision. Patient frailty is increasingly recognized as a strong predictor of waitlist eligibility and transplant outcome. The international guideline group Kidney Disease: Improving Global Outcomes (KDIGO) published comprehensive clinical practice guidelines for the eligibility of kidney transplant recipients in 2020, building on prior guidelines from the American Society of Transplantation (2001), the Canadian Society of Transplantation (2005), and the European Renal Best Practice group (2015).

General Considerations

Advanced age is not a contraindication to transplantation. At present, patients over 65 years of age are the fastest growing group of wait-listed potential recipients. Death-censored graft outcomes are similar or better in these older adult recipients. With advanced age, special attention should be paid to pretransplant medical comorbidities, functional status, and quality of life. The cost of maintaining a proposed recipient on the waiting list is not insignificant. A patient's capacity to survive beyond current waiting list times to transplantation and beyond must be considered. Standardized tests of frailty, history of falls, and hospital admission days while wait-listed predict wait-list and posttransplant mortality. The technical aspects of the transplant surgery limit transplantation in extremely young children. However, this should not delay transplant work-up, and preemptive transplantation should be considered when possible.

Obesity

Patients with extreme obesity are susceptible to an increased risk for transplant-related complications, including delayed graft function, wound complications, and infections, as well as an increased risk for new-onset diabetes after transplantation. In some studies, long-term graft failure rates and mortality are higher among obese recipients when compared with otherwise comparable recipients. There is variability among transplant programs in the willingness to transplant extremely obese individuals, and individual programs may limit transplantation to individuals under a certain body mass index (BMI), usually 40 kg/m². In patients with a BMI between 30 and 39 kg/m², weight-loss counseling should be provided, and bariatric surgery may be considered in individuals with a BMI greater than 40 kg/m².

Kidney Disease Etiology

Many kidney diseases recur after transplantation. Recent analyses suggest that allograft failure secondary to recurrent disease is now the third most common reason for graft failure, behind rejection and death with a functioning graft. In an analysis of the Australia and New Zealand Dialysis and Transplant Registry (ANZDATA), allograft loss due to recurrent disease occurred in 8.4% of patients with biopsy-proven glomerulonephritis who received a kidney transplant. Similarly, when the Mayo Clinic retrospectively analyzed specific causes of kidney allograft loss, recurrent disease was diagnosed in 14.3% of all lost allografts. An additional 6.5% of graft loss was due to glomerular pathology that could not be classified as recurrent because of incomplete clinical information. Despite this, the risk for recurrence rarely precludes transplantation, and allograft failure from recurrence is rare in the first 5 years posttransplant. In the ANZDATA analysis, the overall 10-year incidence of allograft loss was similar among transplant recipients with glomerulonephritis versus those with other causes of kidney failure, and no risks were identified that would preclude transplantation. It is important to counsel prospective transplant recipients about the risk for recurrent disease. Table 59.2 shows the incidence of recurrence of different forms of kidney disease.

Immunoglobulin A (IgA) nephropathy may recur in up to 60% of allograft biopsies; however, clinically significant recurrence (with elevated creatinine or proteinuria) develops in only 30% of kidney transplants. Furthermore, clinical recurrence tends to be late, and graft loss due to IgA nephropathy occurs in only 10% of patients. Focal segmental glomerulosclerosis (FSGS) can recur in up to 30% of transplant recipients and is more common in those with primary FSGS. In patients with a previously failed allograft due to recurrent FSGS, the risk for recurrence rises to as high as 50%–80%. In many cases, recurrence appears to be secondary to a circulating permeability factor that affects podocyte foot process and glomerular

TABLE 59.2	Risk for Recurrence and Graft Loss After Transplantation	
Type of Glomerulonephritis	Risk for Clinically Relevant Recurrence (% of Patients)	Risk for Graft Failure 5–10 Years Posttransplant (% of Patients)
IgA nephropathy	15–50	10
FSGS	30	20
Membranous nephropathy	40	15
MPGN (immune complex)	30–50	15
MPGN (dense deposit disease or C3-dominant)	80	50
ANCA glomerulonephritis	10–15	5
SLE	5	3
Anti-GBM	<5	Rare
Fibrillary/ immunotactoid glomerulopathy	>50	Unknown

ANCA, Antineutrophil cytoplasmic antigen; *FSGS*, focal segmental glomerulosclerosis; *GBM*, glomerular basement membrane; *MPGN*, membranoproliferative glomerulonephritis; *SLE*, systemic lupus erythematosus.

slit diaphragm integrity. Plasma exchange may reduce proteinuria and prolong the life of the allograft. Membranous nephropathy can recur in up to 40% of cases posttransplant. Unlike in the nontransplanted kidney, spontaneous remission is rare, and graft failure can occur in as many as 50% of cases by 10 years. Anti-phospholipase A2 receptor (anti-PLA2R) antibody titer can be used to inform the risk of recurrence, and anti-CD20 therapy may limit proteinuria and allograft damage after recurrence.

Membranoproliferative glomerulonephritis (MPGN) has a variable rate of recurrence posttransplantation depending on the underlying etiology. Monoclonal immune complex-mediated (IC-) MPGN, even in the absence of a detectable paraprotein, has a high risk of recurrence and poor graft outcome, whereas treated polyclonal IC-MPGN has a much lower rate of recurrence and improved outcome. Complement C3 glomerulopathy (C3G), including dense deposit disease and C3 glomerulonephritis, has a high rate of recurrence (~75%) and a 5-year graft survival of only 50%. The presence of serum monoclonal proteins and low complement levels at the time of transplantation are risks for MPGN recurrence. Recurrence of MPGN is usually early in the transplant course and is associated with proteinuria. Recurrence of rapidly progressive glomerulonephritis is rare if disease is quiescent at the time of transplantation. In patients with anti-glomerular basement membrane (anti-GBM) disease, the absence of circulating anti-GBM antibodies should be confirmed before considering transplantation. Although the presence of antineutrophil cytoplasmic antibodies (ANCA) does not preclude transplantation, patients should achieve a period of clinical remission in which they are not taking immunosuppressive medications before transplantation. Similarly, a positive serostatus in patients with systemic lupus

erythematosus (SLE) does not preclude transplantation; however, disease should be quiescent. Recurrence of lupus nephritis is rare (<20%), possibly because of protection from immunosuppressive transplant medications. Glomerular diseases with organizing deposits, such as amyloidosis, fibrillary, and immunotactoid glomerulonephritis, can all recur with rates greater than 50%. With both primary and secondary forms of amyloidosis, transplantation is often limited by severe cardiac disease; early death from cardiovascular disease or infection is quite high. Patients with AL-amyloidosis should be excluded from transplantation unless they have minimal extrarenal disease and have undergone potentially curative therapy. Patients with AA-amyloidosis can be considered if the underlying cause of amyloidosis has been adequately treated.

Genetic forms of kidney disease may affect the transplanted allograft. Rarely, patients with Alport disease can develop antibodies against type IV collagen leading to a condition similar to anti-GBM disease. Patients with primary oxalosis are highly susceptible to rapid oxalate deposition in the transplanted kidney without treatment. These patients are best managed with concurrent liver transplantation and supplementation with orthophosphate and pyridoxine. Patients with atypical hemolytic uremic syndrome (aHUS) due to complement mutations have a rate of recurrent disease and graft failure of up to 60% to 70% at 2 years posttransplantation. Treatment with the complement C5 inhibitor, eculizumab, should strongly be considered. Patients with kidney failure secondary to sickle cell nephropathy can be safely transplanted with good results, providing their overall health allows transplantation.

Infection

The presence of an active infection—bacterial, fungal, or viral—is a contraindication for transplantation. All potential recipients should be screened for chronic infections during the transplant evaluation and assessed for acute infection at the time of transplantation. Clinical and occult dialysis access-related infections in indwelling peritoneal dialysis catheters and tunneled hemodialysis catheters need to be fully treated before transplantation.

Efforts to protect immunosuppressed recipients should occur before transplantation. Transplant candidates should be immunized against seasonal influenza, hepatitis B virus (HBV), and pneumococcal pneumonia. In addition, vaccination against human papillomavirus and primary (chickenpox) and secondary (shingles) varicella-zoster infection and repeat vaccination with the measles, mumps, rubella (MMR) vaccine should be considered in appropriate recipients. Although efficacy of immunization is notably poor in the ESKD population, risk for infection posttransplant is high.

Cytomegalovirus (CMV) can be transmitted via kidney transplant, and commonly leads to disease if untreated. Measuring a potential recipient's CMV serostatus is important before transplantation, but a negative serostatus does not preclude receipt of a kidney transplant from a CMV-positive donor. In addition, potential recipients and donors should be screened for Epstein-Barr virus (EBV) and herpes simplex virus (HSV) before transplant. Those recipients with an EBV-mismatched kidney transplant should undergo EBV virus surveillance for posttransplant lymphoproliferative disorder (PTLD), whereas HSV-mismatched patients may be offered acyclovir for prophylaxis.

Screening for nonviral infections should be tailored to local infection risk. Syphilis, Strongyloides, Chagas disease, and malaria should be screened for and treated in endemic areas. Tuberculosis

(TB) infection is common in immunosuppressed kidney transplant patients, and may approach 15% in TB-endemic areas. Risk factors for developing TB after transplant include a positive tuberculin skin test reaction before transplant, prior residence in a TB-endemic area, a chest radiograph suggestive of prior TB, and older age. Before transplantation, all potential recipients should undergo tuberculin skin testing or interferon-gamma release assay and a chest radiograph. High-risk patients should undergo prophylactic TB treatment before or immediately after transplantation in the absence of documented prior treatment.

Kidney transplantation of human immunodeficiency virus (HIV)–positive recipients is possible in the current era of antiretroviral therapy (ART). In general, patients should be compliant with ART therapy, HIV RNA should be undetectable, and the CD4 count should be greater than 200 mm³ before consideration for transplant. Patient and allograft survival in this population is acceptable, although the incidence of acute rejection is increased. Patients with HIV should be referred to a transplant center with experience managing this infection.

In the modern era of immunosuppression, allograft loss due to BK (polyoma) virus has emerged as an important threat to graft survival. Polyoma virus infection is ubiquitous in the general population, with over-immunosuppression thought to be responsible for clinically evident disease. Limited evidence suggests that retransplantation in patients who have suffered a previous allograft failure from the BK virus may be successful; thus, the BK virus should not preclude retransplantation.

Malignancy

The immune system plays a role in suppressing malignancy, and immunosuppression may promote tumor growth and increase the risk for cancer recurrence. This is best illustrated by the potent antitumor response after administration of immune checkpoint inhibitors, medications that nonspecifically enhance immune responses. As allograft survival lengthens, death from malignancy increases. Thus, active malignancy is an absolute contraindication to transplantation, with the exception of superficial squamous cell and basal cell skin cancers or low-grade prostate cancers (Gleason score ≤6). In patients with a history of malignancy, a waiting period between successful treatment of cancer and transplantation is recommended. The length of this waiting period should be made collaboratively with the patient's oncologist and depends on the type of malignancy and the risk of recurrence. Previously, a waiting period of 2 years was recommended for most types of cancers, while a 5-year waiting period for high-risk cancers was recommended. With improved knowledge of cancer biology and new cancer therapies, many cancers now have an improved prognosis and survival. Genomic profiling assays can now be used to provide a more individualized granular assessment of cancer recurrence risk. In cases with low-risk profiles, a wait of 2 years may not be necessary after completion of potentially curative therapy. Small, incidentally discovered renal cell cancers, in situ cervical cancer, DCIS breast cancer, superficial bladder cancers, and low-grade thyroid cancers do not require any waiting period. Multiple myeloma is a contraindication for transplantation unless considered concurrently with an allogeneic bone marrow transplant.

Although life expectancy is shortened in dialysis-dependent prospective kidney transplant recipients, most programs perform pretransplant malignancy screening. This screening should be based on clinical practice guidelines for the general population as part of a periodic health examination. All patients should receive a chest radiograph, abdominal ultrasound, and age-appropriate colon cancer screening as part of their work-up. Women should undergo breast examination, pelvic examination, and Pap smear as dictated by their age. Men should receive a prostate examination and prostate-specific antigen (PSA) screening as dictated by their age or if symptomatic. Patients with a heavy smoking history should undergo a chest CT. In addition, patients who have received cyclophosphamide in the past should be considered for urine cytology and cystoscopy to rule out bladder malignancy.

Prospective transplant recipients should be counseled about the risk of malignancy posttransplant. The risk of nonmelanoma skin cancer and lymphoma is much higher than similarly matched dialysis controls. The risk of squamous cell cancer increases with advancing age, lighter skin tones, a prior history of skin cancer, and cumulative lifetime sun exposure. Recipients should be counseled to avoid prolonged direct sun exposure and should wear ultraviolet A (UVA) and ultraviolet B (UVB) sunscreens along with protective clothing. The posttransplant lymphoma risk is much higher in EBV-naïve recipients. Transplant recipients should continue to receive ongoing cancer screening as per clinical practice guidelines.

Cardiovascular Disease and Risk Factors

Cardiovascular disease is the leading cause of death in patients on dialysis and in kidney transplant recipients, with diabetics at particular risk. Therefore, all potential transplant recipients should be carefully assessed for the presence of heart disease before listing. Evaluation for cardiac disease helps risk-stratify perioperative risk as well as informing life expectancy and transplant outcome. At a minimum, patients should be assessed for signs and symptoms of cardiovascular disease and undergo an electrocardiogram (ECG) and an echocardiogram. Patients with progressive anginal symptoms should not be offered transplantation without additional evaluation and treatment. Transplantation should be delayed in patients following recent myocardial infarction or revascularization, as recommended by the patient's cardiologist. In patients with severe and irreversible coronary artery disease, projected life expectancy must be balanced against the risks of transplant surgery. It is worth noting that left ventricular dysfunction due to uremic cardiomyopathy is not a contraindication to transplantation and frequently improves after surgery. In patients at high risk for underlying coronary disease (including men over age 40, women over age 50, patients with diabetes, patients with multiple traditional cardiovascular risk factors), noninvasive testing may be performed to identify underlying disease. Patients with positive noninvasive stress test results may be referred for angiography and potential revascularization before transplantation.

At present, cardiac risk stratification of potential kidney transplant candidates is guided by little supporting evidence. Although data demonstrate that noninvasive testing can accurately diagnose coronary artery disease in patients with diabetes and in CKD patients without diabetes, subsequent management varies widely from center to center. Current guidelines from the American College of Cardiology (ACC)/American Heart Association (AHA) recommend revascularization only in symptomatic patients with high-risk cardiac lesions. In two clinical trials that examined preoperative revascularization versus medical management in moderate- to high-risk individuals, perioperative event rates and mortality did not differ. The recent ISCHEMIA-CKD trial did not show a reduction in myocardial infarction or death after revascularization in patients with advanced CKD and moderate-to-severe ischemia on stress testing. Therefore, preoperative revascularization should only be considered in symptomatic individuals, or in selected high-risk individuals in collaboration with cardiology. The question of life expectancy after organ transplant in individuals with a significant burden of coronary artery disease has not been directly addressed. With prolonged waiting times, cardiovascular disease in high-risk individuals may progress. Many programs perform periodic noninvasive rescreening in wait-listed patients; however, the value of this practice is unknown, and current evidence suggests that revascularization of asymptomatic individuals should not be performed. Trials to address this strategy are ongoing.

Modifiable risk factors for cardiovascular disease should be managed appropriately in prospective kidney transplant recipients. Physical activity and dietary modification should be encouraged. Blood pressure potentially should be treated to a target of at least 140/90 mm Hg if tolerated without significant intradialytic hypotension, and smoking cessation should be encouraged. The utility of treating dyslipidemia in patients undergoing dialysis has recently come into question (see Chapter 54); however, control of low-density lipoprotein (LDL) cholesterol should be considered in high-risk individuals. Maintenance anti-ischemic medication, including aspirin and beta-blockers, should be continued while on the waiting list and perioperatively.

Peripheral Arterial Disease

There is a high prevalence of peripheral arterial disease (PAD) in ESKD patients due to the high prevalence of traditional cardiac risk factors and altered calcium and phosphorus balance. The presence of PAD may predict patient survival of potential kidney transplant recipients, but may also increase perioperative surgical complications and limit graft arterial blood flow. Patients with symptomatic PAD or at high risk of PAD should undergo noninvasive vascular testing. Patients with nonhealing extremity ulcers or extensive aorto-iliac arterial disease should not be offered transplantation.

Cerebrovascular Disease

After transplantation, recipients are at an increased risk for cerebrovascular disease when compared with pretransplant patients or the general population. Patients with symptomatic transient ischemic attacks or a recent stroke should be symptom free for 6 months before transplantation. Consideration of carotid endarterectomy should be given to those individuals with known carotid stenosis. The screening of asymptomatic patients is unclear. Again, modifiable risk factors, including smoking and blood pressure, should be addressed before transplant.

Liver Disease

Because progressive liver disease causes significant morbidity and mortality in transplant patients, all prospective recipients should be screened. In patients with liver disease not caused by viral hepatitis, liver function testing and a liver biopsy should be considered to assess the severity of disease. The patient's immunosuppressed state in the posttransplantation period permits viral replication that can accelerate chronic viral hepatitis. Therefore, all patients should be screened for HBV and hepatitis C virus (HCV) infection. In patients with significant liver disease and/or cirrhosis, consideration of combined liver-kidney transplant may be an option. All patients with viral hepatitis or chronic liver disease should be regularly screened for hepatocellular carcinoma.

Transplant outcomes are generally worse in patients who are HBsAg-positive compared with those who are negative. Patients with positive hepatitis B surface antigen (HBsAg) should undergo testing for hepatitis B viral load by polymerase chain reaction (PCR), hepatitis B early antigen (HBeAg), and hepatitis D virus (HDV). Patients with evidence of active viral replication (HBeAg-positive or hepatitis B viral load–positive) or hepatitis D infection should forgo transplantation until consultation with a liver disease specialist and a plan for antiviral treatment and monitoring is established. In patients with chronic active hepatitis and elevated liver enzymes, imaging to assess for cirrhosis and/or hepatocellular carcinoma should be performed, and posttransplant antiviral therapy (e.g., lamivudine) should be considered.

HCV infection can lead to accelerated liver disease after transplantation. All prospective transplant recipients who have serologic evidence of HCV exposure should undergo HCV viral load testing by PCR and imaging to assess for cirrhosis and/or hepatocellular carcinoma. Although patients with HCV have worse outcomes after transplantation when compared with those without infection, the outcomes are improved over remaining on dialysis. Treatment outcomes of HCV infection in ESKD patients, including posttransplantation, have significantly improved after the introduction of direct-acting antivirals (DAAs). If there is active hepatitis C infection, treatment with direct acting antivirals should be considered before or immediately after transplant. Physicians should be aware of drug interactions with calcineurin inhibitors posttransplantation. Use of HCV-positive donor organs is discussed in more detail below and in Chapter 62.

Pulmonary Disease

Patients with pulmonary disease are at increased risk for perioperative respiratory complications. Thus, patients with severe, irreversible lung disease, including severe chronic obstructive pulmonary disease (COPD), cor pulmonale, and those needing supplemental oxygen, should not be offered kidney transplantation. Patients with known lung disease should be referred to a pulmonary specialist and undergo pulmonary function testing as necessary. Smokers who undergo transplantation are at risk for increased perioperative events and have poor long-term outcomes compared with nonsmokers. All smokers should undergo lung cancer screening with a chest CT and be offered smoking cessation aids and counseling as necessary to encourage smoking cessation.

Thrombotic Risk

Patients with a history of venous or arterial thromboembolic disease may be at risk for perioperative graft loss due to thrombosis. Screening for genetic risks of thrombosis should be considered in those individuals with a positive medical history, and a plan for perioperative anticoagulation should be constructed. Patients with a history of SLE should be screened for antiphospholipid antibodies.

Urologic Evaluation

Patients with a history of lower urinary tract abnormalities, bladder dysfunction, or recurrent urinary tract infections (UTIs) require urologic investigation and voiding cystourethrogram. In addition, high-risk patients, such as those with diabetes, should be screened with a postvoid residual. Efforts should be made to preserve the native bladder, and self-intermittent catheterization is preferable to urinary diversion with ureteroileostomy. Patients with significant exposure to cyclophosphamide should be screened with cystoscopy to rule out malignancy. Pretransplant nephrectomy should be considered in patients with severe reflux or recurrent nephrolithiasis with infection, difficult-to-control hypertension, severe nephrotic syndrome, and symptomatic polycystic kidneys.

Psychological Evaluation

All prospective transplant recipients should undergo screening to identify cognitive or psychologic impairments that may alter their ability to provide informed consent or their ability to follow medical protocols after transplantation. Medication nonadherence remains a major cause of graft loss. However, identification of individuals at risk is difficult and not often apparent during the transplant work-up. In general, one should be cautious in restricting access to transplantation in those at risk for nonadherence. Patients with addiction or a history of chemical dependency should be offered counseling and rehabilitation. Many programs require a period of abstinence before a patient is put on the waiting list. Those individuals with major psychiatric illness should receive appropriate psychiatric care with the recognition of potential medication interactions and side effects.

Immunologic Considerations Before Transplantation

Tissue compatibility between donor and recipient is determined by matching ABO blood type and human leukocyte antigen (HLA), or major histocompatibility complex (MHC). Blood and HLA tissue typing is performed on all suitable transplant candidates at the time of wait-listing. For the most part, the donor kidney must be ABO compatible with the recipient. In North America, ABO B blood type recipients have a longer waiting period as compared with other blood types. Many programs now allocate ABO A2 kidneys to ABO B recipients to improve equity.

Although HLA matching is desired, it is rarely achieved because of the tremendous allelic polymorphisms present in the MHC genes. Traditionally, HLA-A, B, and DR were thought to be most important for kidney transplant histocompatibility, but HLA-C, DQ, and DP are now increasingly implicated in tissue compatibility. Both early rejection and long-term allograft survival are affected by HLA matching, with a well-matched kidney having a decreased risk for rejection and better long-term survival as compared with a poorly HLA-matched kidney. A zero-antigen mismatched kidney carries a significantly improved long-term graft survival.

A major barrier to transplantation is the development of antibodies against HLA epitopes, called *sensitization*. Anti-HLA antibodies are formed during exposure to foreign HLA through blood transfusions, pregnancy, and prior transplantation. The presence of anti-HLA antibodies against a donor HLA type precludes transplantation in most circumstances because of the extreme risk for hyperacute rejection and graft failure. Thus, all candidates on the waiting list are screened for the presence of anti-HLA antibodies at least every 3 months.

Screening for anti-HLA antibodies is performed through serologic testing (by mixing donor lymphocytes with recipient serum) or, now more routinely, through solid-phase assays, such as flow cytometry or the Luminex platform. Historically, an estimate of a recipient's anti-HLA antibody burden was assessed by mixing recipient serum with a panel of lymphocytes representing random donors from the general population. The percentage of lymphocytes that reacted to recipient antibodies was called *panel-reactive antibody (PRA)* and provided an estimate of the likelihood of finding a suitable donor within the population. A high PRA means it will be more difficult to find a compatible donor. In addition, a high PRA is associated with worse graft survival, even if the final cross-match against the donor is negative. Currently, most transplant centers use solid-phase assays to determine the specificity of a recipient's anti-HLA antibodies. A list of unacceptable HLA antigens can then be compiled for a recipient based on anti-HLA antibody specificities. The calculated PRA (cPRA) is an estimate of the percentage of donors in a population to whom a transplant candidate has at least one HLA antibody directed against. Pretransplant, a list of a recipient's anti-HLA antibodies can be compared to the donor's HLA type to assess tissue histocompatibility, termed a *virtual cross-match*. Solid-phase assays to detect anti-HLA antibodies are much more sensitive than serologic detection and can often identify low-titer antibodies that were previously undetectable. Even with a negative cross-match, presence of low-titer antibodies against donor HLA is associated with antibody-mediated rejection and higher rates of graft loss.

At the time of transplantation, a final cross-match is completed to ensure tissue compatibility. Recipient serum is mixed with donor tissue. A positive cross-match indicates the presence of donor-specific anti-HLA antibodies (DSAs) and predicts hyperacute rejection. Because not all positive cross-match results are due to antibodies that cause hyperacute rejection, further laboratory tests may be necessary before transplantation. In patients with a high PRA, the cross-match is often performed with historical sera that have the highest PRA value. Recipients with a current negative cross-match but a historical positive cross-match may undergo transplantation, but they are at a higher risk for antibody-mediated rejection.

Patients with a high PRA are disadvantaged and often have prolonged waiting times because of the limited number of compatible donors. Strategies to lower a patient's PRA to increase the probability of finding a suitable donor are constantly evolving. Noninvasive strategies, such as enrollment in a living donor–paired exchange program, have increased access for mismatched living donor pairs (see later). Strategies to decrease or eliminate anti-HLA or anti-ABO antibodies may include targeting of either the antibodies or the B cell/plasma cell clones that produce the antibodies. Plasmapheresis and high-dose intravenous immunoglobulin (IVIG) have been used successfully to greatly reduce or eliminate anti-HLA antibodies. Rituximab and bortezomib (and, rarely, splenectomy) target B cells and plasma cells. Although these strategies have allowed successful transplantation with ABO-incompatible or positive cross-match donors, the risk for antibody-mediated rejection and graft loss remains increased.

Deceased Donor Organs

Because of the shortage of deceased donor organs, novel sources of kidneys for transplantation continue to be explored. In North America, the majority of organs are removed from deceased donors following the neurologic determination of death (NDD). More recently, organs have been removed from donors not meeting the criteria for brain death but whose death is determined by cardiac criteria (donation after cardiocirculatory death, or DCD). Organ procurement in DCD donors can be controlled or uncontrolled. In controlled DCD donation, consent for donation is obtained before death, and life support is withdrawn in a controlled fashion. An uncontrolled donor dies before consent for organ donation, and attempts are made to preserve the organs until consent can be obtained. DCD kidneys have a higher rate of delayed graft function; however, long-term outcomes are similar to recipients who received a kidney from an NDD donor. In the United Kingdom, DCD donors now account for approximately 40% of all deceased organ donors. Hepatitis C-infected deceased donors are routinely utilized for hepatitis C-positive patients, accompanied by concomitant direct-acting antiviral administration.

There is substantial variability in the quality of donor kidneys. Most obviously, a kidney from a donor with a decreased glomerular filtration rate (GFR), older age, or significant medical comorbidities might be expected to have a shorter graft survival as compared with a kidney from a young, healthy donor. Attempts have been made to evaluate donor organ quality and allocate donor kidneys based on expected outcomes. The concept of marginal donor kidneys affecting transplant outcome was formalized in 2002 with the definition of expanded criteria donors (ECDs). ECD kidneys include those from donors over the age of 60 or from donors between 50 and 59 years old with two of the following: cerebrovascular accident as the cause of death, hypertension, or terminal serum creatinine greater than 1.5 mg/dL. ECD kidneys have a 1.7-fold higher probability of graft failure 2 years after transplantation as compared with standard criteria donor (SCD) kidneys; however, early access to transplantation may benefit potential transplant recipients. In patients over the age of 65 or patients over the age of 40 with diabetes and prolonged deceased donor transplant wait times, receipt of an ECD kidney confers a survival advantage over waiting for an SCD kidney. Younger, healthier kidney transplant candidates may be better served by waiting for an SCD kidney.

In the United States, donor kidney quality is now assessed and quantified on a continuous scale by calculating the Kidney Donor Risk Index (KDRI), which estimates donor kidney quality based on 10 donor characteristics including age, ethnicity, creatinine, and specific donor health comorbidities. The Kidney Donor Profile Index (KDPI) converts the KDRI into a percentile used to express the quality of the donor kidney relative to other kidneys. A higher KDRI or KDPI indicates a lower expected graft survival. By using the KDPI, healthy donor kidneys (<20%) can be allocated to recipients with the longest life expectancy, while higher KDPI kidneys can be allocated to older recipients, similar to ECD recipients. Fig. 59.1 shows the expected half-life of donor kidneys based on KDPI.

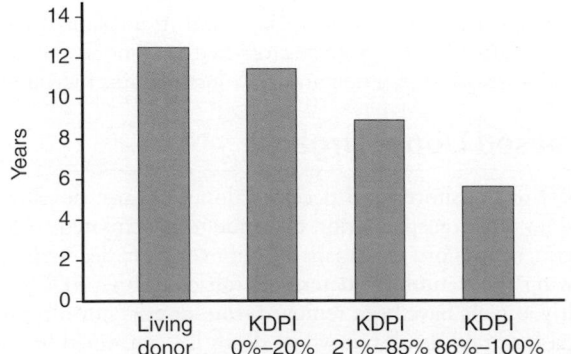

• **Fig. 59.1** Estimated graft half-lives (years). KDPI, Kidney donor profile index. (Organ Procurement & Transplantation Network. https://optn.transplant.hrsa.gov/. Accessed August 26, 2016.)

Allocation of Deceased Donor Organs in the United States

UNOS and the Organ Procurement and Transplant Network (OPTN) allocate donated kidneys in the United States. Patients who are medically ready for transplantation may be placed on the UNOS waiting list for a deceased donor kidney. Kidneys are allocated by policies designed to balance equity and efficacy. Only a brief overview of this process will be provided; policies can be viewed in more detail online (https://optn.transplant.hrsa.gov/learn/professional-education/kidney-allocation-system/).

Deceased donor kidneys are generally allocated by ABO blood type—thus, blood type O donor kidneys are available only to O recipients. This allocation is followed for A, B, and AB kidneys also. Donor kidneys are first offered regionally and then nationally. All potential recipients on the UNOS waiting list are allocated points, which determine their priority for transplantation. Patients with more points receive higher priority. Points are awarded for length of waiting time, degree of sensitization (PRA), medical urgency, and special recipient status (including pediatric patients, prior kidney donors, and liver transplant recipients). Details of the point system for kidney allocation can be reviewed at the OPTN website (see earlier).

In 2015, a new kidney allocation policy was introduced, which attempts to account for factors associated with allograft and recipient survival to increase the efficiency of organ utilization and to increase access for certain underrepresented recipient candidates. Policy changes attempt to increase access to patients with a high PRA, those of ABO blood type B, and those who are referred late for transplant assessment. An estimated posttransplant survival score (EPTS) is calculated for all adult candidates on the waiting list and is based on recipient age, time on dialysis, presence or absence of diabetes, and history of a prior transplant. Those candidates with a high probability of long-term survival (EPTS <20%) are eligible to receive kidneys from donors with a KDPI of <20%. In this manner, kidneys are matched to the recipient based on the expected survival of the kidney and the recipient. While the new policy has improved access, certain groups continue to be disproportionately disadvantaged. Analysis of outcomes and iterative adjustments continue to be made to the current allocation system.

Living Kidney Donation

Although the number of deceased donors has increased significantly since 1990 (Fig. 59.2), this has not kept pace with the increased number of patients being added to the kidney transplant waiting list. As of 2020, approximately 91,000 patients were wait-listed for kidney transplantation in the United States. Encouragingly, the number of wait-listed patients has been declining since 2014; nevertheless, the waiting time for kidney transplantation remains significant. The median waiting time for a deceased donor kidney nationwide is 4 years, but can be significantly longer for certain age groups, blood types, and highly sensitized patients. The lack of access to deceased donor organs, as well as the superior outcomes with live donors, has resulted in the increased usage of living kidney donors for transplantation. After a dramatic increase in living donation that peaked in 2004, living donation stagnated (see Fig. 59.2). Encouragingly, living kidney donation has slightly increased in recent years, and there were more than 6500 living kidney donors used for transplantation in 2018 alone.

Living kidney donation offers several potential advantages over deceased donor transplantation. First, the procedure is elective

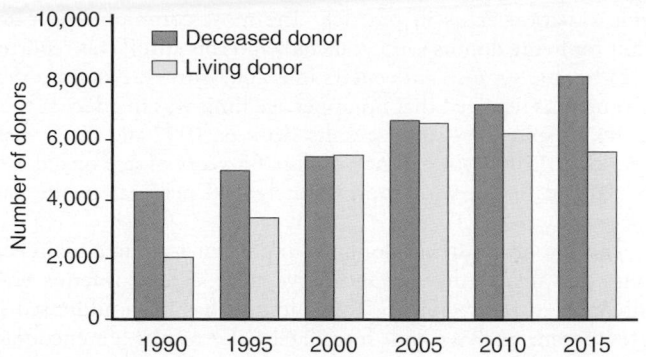

• **Fig. 59.2** Living and deceased organ donors in the United States. (Organ Procurement & Transplantation Network. https://optn.transplant.hrsa.gov/. Accessed August 26, 2016.)

and scheduled, thus ensuring that both donor and recipient are in optimal medical condition. The planned nature of the operation also facilitates the use of preemptive transplantation (i.e., kidney transplantation without prior dialysis), which has been associated with both improved patient and allograft survival. Second, the incidence of delayed graft function (the need for dialysis in the first week posttransplantation) is much lower for recipients of living donor kidneys. In 2016, less than 5% of living donor kidney recipients had delayed graft function, compared with 25% of deceased donor transplant patients. Finally, patient and allograft survival rates are superior for living donor kidneys compared with deceased donors. In the most recently available data, patients who received a living donor kidney transplant in 2017 had a 1-year allograft survival of 97%, compared with 93% for deceased donor recipients. The 5-year patient survival in living donor recipients was 88%, compared with only 80% for deceased donor recipients. Similarly, for those who received a living donor transplant in 2015, the 5-year allograft survival was 85%, compared with only 77% for recipients of deceased donor kidney transplant. Despite the advantages of living donation, it remains an underutilized option for many ESKD patients. Kidney donors continue to be predominantly Caucasian and female. Barriers to living kidney donation include inadequate patient education and health literacy as well as the financial burden to the donor.

Prospective recipients with a willing, living donor who is ABO-incompatible or possesses an incompatible HLA antigen may consider registering in a local, regional, or national paired exchange program. Incompatible donor pairs are entered into a computer registry that compares the medical information on all registered pairs and identifies pairs that might be able to exchange donors. Proposed matches can identify a single matching pair or may identify a series of pairs that may exchange donors in a chain-like or domino fashion. Living donor paired exchange increases access to transplantation and offers the benefits of living donor transplantation to those recipients with an incompatible living donor.

Living Donor Evaluation Process

Living donation is a unique medical situation in which the patient (donor) undergoes an operation with risk, yet receives no direct medical benefit from the procedure. Living kidney donation carries small but measurable risks of perioperative complications and adverse long-term health outcomes including ESKD. However, many donors do report benefits, such as an improved sense of well-being from seeing a friend or relative thrive after transplantation.

Given the exceptional circumstances surrounding living donation, it is crucial that informed consent be obtained in an open and thoughtful manner. Consent should be obtained for both the evaluation process and the surgical procedure itself. The potential donor needs to understand that the evaluation process requires a series of tests, and that the results of some of these tests may be abnormal. Certain test results may prompt disclosure to another agency (e.g., HIV-positive test results reported to public health) or may affect future insurability (e.g., significant proteinuria). In general, kidney donors enjoy better health outcomes as compared to the general population, but living donation does carry a small risk of long-term health outcomes when compared to matched nondonors. Donors need to be counseled on the lifetime risk of kidney failure. This can be estimated at http://www.transplantmodels.com/esrdrisk/. Other points that should be fully discussed as part of the informed consent process are outlined in Box 59.2.

After informed consent, the evaluation consists of a psychosocial and medical assessment. The psychosocial assessment must be conducted by an appropriate professional with experience in living kidney donation. This person will vary from site to site, but is most often a social worker, clinical psychologist, or psychiatrist. Important components of the psychosocial assessment are outlined in Box 59.3. Significant concerns with any of these factors may preclude donation or require further assessment by other health care professionals (e.g., psychiatrist).

The medical assessment should be conducted by a surgeon or physician (ideally both) with expertise in living kidney donation. The OPTN requires that all donors have a designated, independent, living donor advocate. The goal of the medical evaluation is to determine (1) the overall health of the potential donor and whether he or she is fit for surgery; (2) the current kidney health of the potential donor and his or her risk for kidney disease or medical complications in the future; (3) the presence of any conditions that may result in disease transmission (e.g., infection) to the recipient; and (4) the immunologic compatibility of the potential donor with the intended recipient. The tests required to

---

BOX 59.2

Key Points of Informed Consent Process for Living Kidney Donors

Living kidney donors should understand the following items as part of the informed consent process:

- Consent may be withdrawn at any time.
- The evaluation process and operation both involve risk.
- Abnormalities discovered during the evaluation might affect future insurability or may require reporting to another agency (e.g., positive HIV test).
- There is a small but real risk for death with live donor nephrectomy (3.1 per 10,000 donors).
- Perioperative risks include hemorrhage, ileus, infections, and wound complications including hernia
- All donors will lose kidney function postoperatively, but the actual amount is difficult to predict.
- The risk of ESKD in living donors is no greater than the general population but is higher than comparatively healthy nondonors (attributable risk 26.9 per 10,000 donors).
- There is an increased risk of hypertension, gestational hypertension, preeclampsia, and gout among kidney donors.

ESKD, End-stage kidney disease; *HIV*, human immunodeficiency virus.

Key Points to Be Addressed in the Psychosocial Assessment of Living Kidney Donors

Capacity suitable for informed consent
No evidence of coercion to donate
Social support network adequate to assist with recovery from surgery
Financial stability to take time off from work and cover expenses
High-risk behavior (e.g., IV drug use) that might increase risk for disease transmission to the recipient
Current or previous psychiatric disorders that might influence decision making or response to adverse outcomes

address these components of the medical evaluation are listed in Box 59.4. In 2017, KDIGO published clinical practice guidelines on the evaluation and follow-up care of living kidney donors. The guidelines can be found at http://kdigo.org/home/guidelines/.

Before proceeding with specific testing, a medical history and physical examination is required for all living donors. The history should focus on conditions related to overall health and fitness for surgery, such as the presence of cardiovascular disease, liver disease, pulmonary disease, or hematologic conditions (bleeding disorders or thrombosis). Significant abnormalities in any of these areas may preclude donation or require more specialized testing and/or referral to another consultant.

Age of the Living Kidney Donor

Age is an important consideration when assessing living kidney donors. Most programs will not allow living donors younger than 18 years of age, and 15% of transplant centers require donors to be at least 21 years old. On the opposite end of the age spectrum,

wide variation exists in practice. The most common upper age limit for living donors is 65 years old, and this cutoff was reported at 21% of US transplant centers in a 2007 survey. Notably, 59% of programs reported that no upper age limit was in effect at their center. Despite these survey results, between 1992 and 2011, there were only 1200 living kidney donors 65 years of age or older in the United States, with approximately 100 per year in the past few years.

The age of the living donor is important for three main reasons. The first is that advanced age may lead to inferior graft outcomes in the recipient. This question has been addressed in a few recent analyses and, fortunately, the results are encouraging. A large analysis using the United States Renal Data System (USRDS) registry showed that transplant patients who received a kidney from a living donor older than 55 years of age had a risk for graft loss similar to those who received a kidney from a living donor 55 years of age or younger (adjusted relative risk 1.00; 95% confidence interval [CI] 0.47 to 2.13). It is important to note that graft survival from these older living donors was actually superior to younger standard criteria *deceased* donors. A subsequent analysis showed that recipients of live kidneys from donors above the age of 70 had similar graft survival to those who received standard criteria allografts from 50- to 59-year-old deceased donors (hazard ratio 1.19; 95% CI 0.87 to 1.63).

A second reason for the importance of the age of living donors is related to comorbidity. Advanced age is often associated with increased comorbidity, which may lead to more perioperative complications at the time of the donor nephrectomy. Other than a longer hospital stay (median difference, 1 day), living donors older than 60 years of age do not have a significant difference in minor complications (e.g., UTI), major complications (e.g., reoperation), or even death following nephrectomy. In an analysis of 80,347 live donors, the 90-day mortality rate was 3.1 per 10,000 donors, and this rate was not significantly different for donors above or below 60 years of age. In addition, the long-term survival

Medical Assessment of Living Kidney Donors

1. General donor health and immediate surgical risk
   - Complete blood count, prothrombin time or INR, partial thromboplastin time
   - HCG for women of childbearing potential
   - Electrolytes, transaminases, bilirubin, calcium, phosphorus, albumin
   - Chest radiograph and electrocardiogram
2. Current kidney health and future disease risk
   - Serum creatinine
   - Fasting blood glucose, total cholesterol, HDL-cholesterol, LDL-cholesterol, triglycerides
   - Urinalysis, urine culture
   - Proteinuria measurement: ACR, PCR, or 24-hour urine collection for total protein and/or albumin
   - Kidney function measurement: 24-hr urine collection for creatinine clearance or measured GFR using an exogenous marker (inulin; radioactive or cold iothalamate, iohexol, DTPA, or EDTA)
   - CT or MR angiogram

3. Potential disease transmission to recipient
   - CMV, HSV, and EBV antibody
   - HIV
   - HTLV
   - HBV surface antigen, core antibody, and surface antibody
   - HCV virus antibody
   - Rapid plasma reagin test for syphilis
   - Emerging/geographic-specific infections (e.g., West Nile virus, Zika virus)
   - Papanicolaou test for women
   - Mammogram for women over 40 years
   - Prostate-specific antigen for men over 50 years (40 years if Black or positive family history)
   - Colon cancer screen for donors over 50 years (fecal occult blood testing or visualization with colonoscopy, virtual colonoscopy, or flexible sigmoidoscopy)
4. Immunologic compatibility with recipient
   - ABO blood type
   - HLA typing

ACR, Albumin-creatinine ratio; *CMV,* cytomegalovirus; *DTPA,* diethylenetriaminepentaacetic acid; *EDTA,* ethylenediaminetetraacetic acid; *EBV,* Epstein-Barr virus; *GFR,* glomerular filtration rate; *HBV,* hepatitis B virus; *HCV,* hepatitis C virus; *HCG,* human chorionic gonadotropin; *HIV,* human immunodeficiency virus; *HLA,* human leukocyte antigen; *HSV,* herpes simplex virus; *HTLV,* human T lymphotropic virus; *INR,* international normalized ratio; *PCR,* protein-creatinine ratio.

to 12 years was actually greater for donors older than 60 years compared with an age-matched cohort of nondonors who did not have contraindications to live donation.

The third reason is that age is important when considering live donors because it influences the amount of time that the donor is at risk to develop ESKD or other complications that might negatively affect someone with a solitary kidney. For example, a 22-year-old overweight man with prediabetes has a significant risk for developing overt diabetes and ESKD given the many potential years of life ahead of him. Although being overweight and having prediabetes are not absolute contraindications to donation on their own, this young man may not be an appropriate donor because of his future risk for disease. In contrast, a 63-year-old woman with well-controlled hypertension on one medication might be a suitable donor given that her lifetime risk for kidney failure is much lower than that for a younger patient with risk factors.

Kidney Function

Ninety percent of programs in the United States use a 24-hour urine collection for creatinine clearance as the measure of kidney function, with the remainder using a direct measure of GFR, such as a radioisotopic clearance. The threshold for declining donors based on GFR or creatinine clearance is somewhat controversial with varied practice. Approximately two-thirds of US centers exclude donors with a creatinine clearance less than 80 mL/min/1.73 m^2, whereas 25% require the value to be within two standard deviations of the mean creatinine clearance for the donor age. See Table 59.3 for creatinine clearance values in the normal population.

From the perspective of the transplant recipient, it is crucial to ensure that kidney mass and function are adequate to prevent premature graft loss. Although a kidney donor loses 50% of nephron mass with nephrectomy, the GFR returns to 70% of baseline by 2 weeks and 75%-85% of baseline in long-term follow-up. When the donor's creatinine clearance is above 80 mL/min/1.73 m^2, postnephrectomy kidney mass is usually adequate. Lower values can provide adequate kidney mass and may be appropriate for certain recipients (e.g., older adults). However, from the perspective of the living donor, the appropriate clearance threshold might be somewhat different. It is well known

that GFR declines with age and, thus, a creatinine clearance of 80 mL/min/1.73 m^2 in a 20 year old is very different from a clearance of 80 mL/min/1.73 m^2 in a 65-year-old donor. For 20 year olds, this cutoff is well below two standard deviations of the mean for their age, and nephrectomy (with a further loss of GFR) may put them at increased risk for ESKD given their long potential lifetime. For 65-year-old donors, a clearance of 80 mL/min/1.73 m^2 is within the normal range for their age, and the risk for ESKD is much less given that they have fewer years of life remaining. For these reasons, it is preferred to individualize donor acceptance with age-based creatinine clearance or GFR values, with consideration also given to the intended recipient, rather than with rigid cutoffs.

Blood Pressure

Sitting blood pressure should be measured rigorously on at least two different occasions in any potential living donor. Ambulatory blood pressure monitoring should be considered if the assessment of hypertension is indeterminant, or if isolated office hypertension is suspected. Hypertension was previously considered a contraindication to donation, but practice is now quite varied. Only 47% of programs exclude donors with controlled blood pressure on one antihypertensive medication while 36% continue to exclude only those with persistently borderline blood pressure values. The increased acceptance of hypertensive donors is based on favorable data from select, mostly White, patients with well-controlled hypertension who have undergone living donation. Limited outcome data are available from hypertensive donors in other populations who may be at higher risk. The Amsterdam forum and the KDIGO guideline on the care of the live kidney donor suggest that patients with easily controlled blood pressure who meet other criteria (i.e., age >50 years, GFR >80 mL/min, no proteinuria) may be acceptable as live kidney donors. Apolipoprotein L1 (APOL1) risk alleles may substantially modify the risk of ESKD in affected individuals with hypertension. Genetic screening for APOL-1 risk alleles should be considered for at-risk living kidney donors.

Proteinuria

The 24-hour urine collection is still used by most programs (75%) to assess for proteinuria, but spot urine protein or albumin (protein-creatinine or albumin-creatinine ratios) measurements are becoming more commonly used. Mildly abnormal values should be repeated, especially if patients were acutely ill with fever or were exercising before testing. The threshold for excluding donors based on proteinuria is not consistent among centers. Whereas 36% of programs exclude donors with greater than 150 mg/day of total protein, 44% require proteinuria to be greater than 300 mg/day before exclusion. The KDIGO guideline recommends using albuminuria (albumin excretion rate, AER), rather than proteinuria. Albuminuria more closely reflects glomerular disease and is a better predictor of cardiovascular events. Given the strong link with proteinuria and kidney disease, it seems prudent to exclude any donor with abnormal albuminuria (>30 mg/day) or total proteinuria greater than 300 mg/day. A lower threshold may be needed in cases of familial kidney disease, borderline blood pressure, or other abnormalities, such as microscopic hematuria.

Hematuria

Isolated microscopic hematuria should be confirmed with repeat urinalysis including microscopy to verify the presence of red blood cells as the cause of dipstick hematuria. Infection, nephrolithiasis,

TABLE 59.3	Measured Creatinine Clearance According to Age			
Age (Year)	Mean Creatinine Clearance (mL/min/1.73 m^2)	SD	Mean—SD	Mean—2 SD
17–24	140	12	128	116
25–34	140	21	119	98
35–44	133	20	113	93
45–54	127	17	110	93
55–64	120	16	104	88
65–74	110	16	94	78
75–84	97	16	81	65

Used with permission of the American Society of Nephrology; previously published in Kher A, Mandelbrot DA. The living kidney donor evaluation: focus on renal issues. *Clin J Am Soc Nephrol.* 2012;7:366–371.

malignancy, and glomerulonephritis need to be ruled out in potential donors with hematuria. Urine culture should be performed to rule out infection, and menstrual contamination should always be considered in premenopausal women. Imaging will rule out a structural kidney cause, but most donors must undergo cystoscopy to rule out local bladder causes. Finally, glomerular hematuria from IgA nephropathy, hereditary nephritis, or thin basement membrane nephropathy must be considered in an otherwise healthy donor. These conditions can only be diagnosed by kidney biopsy, and this test should be considered if the donor understands the risks and is motivated to continue the evaluation. The most common practice (43% of programs) is to accept donors with hematuria only if urologic evaluation and kidney biopsy are both normal. However, 21% of programs would exclude patients with hematuria (>10 red blood cells/high-power field) regardless of these investigations.

Diabetes

Given the risk for diabetic nephropathy, established diabetes is a contraindication to donation. All donors should have a fasting blood glucose performed to rule out undiagnosed diabetes, impaired fasting glucose, or prediabetes. Patients at increased risk for diabetes (e.g., history of gestational diabetes, first-degree relative with diabetes, BMI >30) should have an oral glucose tolerance test or glycated hemoglobin test. Potential donors with impaired fasting glucose need to be assessed on a case-by-case basis; young patients or those with other risk factors, such as obesity, hypertension, or dyslipidemia, should be excluded from donation.

Obesity

Obesity (BMI >30 kg/m^2) is associated with short-term surgical complications following nephrectomy, as well as an increased risk for future medical conditions, such as diabetes, hypertension, and dyslipidemia. Fifty-two percent of programs exclude donors with a BMI greater than 35 kg/m^2 and an additional 20% exclude those with BMI above 40 kg/m^2. A recent study found that obesity was associated with more hypertension and dyslipidemia after a mean follow-up of 11 years, but was not significantly different from an obese control group that did not donate. A meta-analysis of United States obese donors found an increased 20-year, postdonation risk of ESKD. Not all patients with an elevated BMI have central obesity, and potential donors should be examined for body habitus and muscle mass before exclusion based on BMI alone. Obese donors may also lose weight to a certain target before proceeding with surgery, with appropriate support and counseling to prevent immediate weight gain postnephrectomy.

Nephrolithiasis

Kidney stones are a very common occurrence, with as many as 19% of men and 9% of women having a symptomatic kidney stone in their lifetime. As such, nephrolithiasis is not an uncommon problem in potential living donors. The major concern for the living donor is recurrence postnephrectomy, leading to obstruction of the single remaining kidney. The majority of programs (53%) accept donors with a history of kidney stones as long as the metabolic work-up is normal. Another consideration is age at onset and time since the symptomatic episode of nephrolithiasis. Younger patients are at an increased risk for recurrence, given their long projected lifespan. Patients whose stone episode was remote (>10 years) are at lower risk for recurrence. Patients with a history of stone disease or stones on imaging should have a metabolic work-up done, including serum calcium and bicarbonate to rule out metabolic acidosis. A 24-hour urine collection (preferably on two occasions) should be performed to assess calcium, oxalate, uric acid, and citrate excretion. Patients who should be excluded as donors include those with recurrent stones and those at high risk for recurrence, such as those with metabolic abnormalities (e.g., hypercalciuria), chronic diarrhea/malabsorption, gout, cysteine, uric acid, or struvite stones.

Conclusion

Historically, limited data were available to guide the selection of living kidney donors; studies were often single-center analyses with small sample size or a relatively short duration of follow-up. Recent improvements in large database research and renewed interest in living kidney donor outcomes has led to improved national (OPTN) standards and international guidelines (KDIGO) for living kidney donation. Contraindications to living donation have been published and are presented in Table 59.4. It is important to assess potential donors individually and to use the information available as a guide. When evaluating younger donors, the higher lifetime risk for developing complications, such as diabetes or ESKD should be recognized and incorporated into the assessment. Similarly, older donors have a much lower lifetime risk for complications and may be appropriate for donation with certain conditions (e.g., hypertension). Further research focusing on complete and long-term follow-up, especially involving those with medical abnormalities, is needed to enrich the data available to make evidence-based decisions in living kidney donation.

Complete bibliography is available at Elsevier eBooks for Practicing Clinicians.

TABLE 59.4	Absolute and Relative Contraindications to Living Kidney Donation
Absolute Contraindications	**Relative Contraindications**
Age <18 years	Age 18–21 years
Mentally incapable of making informed decision	Creatinine clearance <2 SD below mean for age (see Table 59.3)
Uncontrolled hypertension, or hypertension with end-organ damage	Albuminuria or proteinuria
Diabetes	Hypertension in non-White race
BMI >35 kg/m^2	Hypertension in young donor
Untreated psychiatric conditions	Prediabetes in young donor
Nephrolithiasis with high likelihood of recurrence	Two apolipoprotein L1 (APOL1) risk alleles
Evidence or suspicion of donor coercion or illegal financial exchange between donor and recipient	BMI >30 kg/m^2
	Bleeding disorder
	History of thrombosis or embolism
	Nephrolithiasis
Active malignancy or incompletely treated malignancy	History of malignancy, especially if metastatic
Persistent infection	Significant cardiovascular disease

BMI, Body mass index.
Used with permission of the American Society of Nephrology; previously published in Kher A, Mandelbrot DA. The living kidney donor evaluation: focus on renal issues. *Clin J Am Soc Nephrol.* 2012;7:366–371.

Key Bibliography

Abramowicz D, Cochat P, Claas FH. et al. European Renal Best Practice Guideline on kidney donor and recipient evaluation and perioperative care. *Nephrol Dial Transplant*. 2015;30:1790–1797.

Chadban SJ, Ahn C, et al. Summary of the Kidney Disease: Improving Global Outcomes (KDIGO) Clinical Practice Guideline on the evaluation and management of candidates for kidney transplantation. *Transplantation*. 2020;104:708–714.

Cosio FG, Cattran D. Recent advances in our understanding of recurrent primary glomerulonephritis after kidney transplantation. *Kidney Int*. 2017;91:304–314.

Dew MA, Jacobs CL, Jowsey SG, et al. Guidelines for the psychosocial evaluation of living unrelated kidney donors in the United States. *Am J Transplant*. 2007;7:1047–1054.

Doshi MD, Ortigosa-Goggins M, et al. *APOL1* genotype and renal function of Black living donors. *J Am Soc Nephrol*. 2018;29:1309–1316.

Fairhead T, Knoll G. Recurrent glomerular disease after kidney transplantation. *Curr Opin Nephrol Hypertens*. 2010;19:578–585.

Gill J, Bunnapradist S, Danovitch GM, et al. Outcomes of kidney transplantation from older living donors to older recipients. *Am J Kidney Dis*. 2008;52:541–552.

Goldberg DS, Abt PL, et al. Trial of transplantation of hcv-infected kidneys into uninfected recipients. *N Engl J Med*. 2017;376:2394–2395.

Hart A, Smith JM, et al. OPTN/SRTR annual data report 2018: kidney. *Am J Transplant*. 2020;20(s1):20–130.

Kher A, Mandelbrot DA. The living kidney donor evaluation: focus on renal issues. *Clin J Am Soc Nephrol*. 2012;7:366–371.

Kidney Disease 2017. Kidney Disease. Improving Global Outcomes (KDIGO) Living Kidney Donor Work Group. KDIGO clinical practice guideline on the evaluation and care of living kidney donors. *Transplantation*. 2017;101(8S):S1–S109.

LaPointe Rudow D, et al. Consensus conference on best practices in live kidney donation: recommendations to optimize education, access, and care. *Am J Transplant*. 2015;15:914–922.

Lentine KL, Costa SP, Weir MR, et al. Cardiac disease evaluation and management among kidney and liver transplantation candidates: a scientific statement from the American Heart Association and the American College of Cardiology Foundation: endorsed by the American Society of Transplant Surgeons, American Society of Transplantation, and National Kidney Foundation. *Circulation*. 2012;126:617–663.

Locke JE, Reed RD, et al. Obesity increases the risk of end-stage renal disease among living kidney donors. *Kidney Int*. 2017;91:699–703.

Mukhtar RA, Piper ML, Freise C, Van't Veer LJ, Baehner FL, Esserman LJ. The novel application of genomic profiling assays to shorten inactive status for potential kidney transplant recipients with breast cancer. *Am J Transplant*. 2017;17:292–295. doi:10.1111/ajt.14003.

Muzaale AD, Massie AB, Wang MC, et al. Risk of end-stage renal disease following live kidney donation. *JAMA*. 2014;311:579–586.

O'Keeffe LM, Ramond A, et al. Mid- and long-term health risks in living kidney donors: a systematic review and meta-analysis. *Ann Intern Med*. 2018;168:276–284.

Patel SI, Chakkera HA, et al. Peripheral arterial disease preoperatively may predict graft failure and mortality in kidney transplant recipients. *Vasc Med*. 2017;22:225–230.

Segev DL, Muzaale AD, Caffo BS, et al. Perioperative mortality and long-term survival following live kidney donation. *JAMA*. 2010;303:959–966.

60

Posttransplantation Monitoring and Outcomes

BRITTANY L. SCHREIBER, TANUN NGAMVICHCHUKORN, ANIL CHANDRAKER

Introduction

Kidney transplantation is the kidney replacement modality of choice for most patients with end-stage kidney disease (ESKD). Evidence shows that most kidney transplant recipients (KTRs) experience a higher quality of life and improved long-term survival compared to wait-listed patients receiving dialysis. However, the risk of death in KTRs compared to wait-listed dialysis patients is actually higher during the early posttransplant period due to the operative risk as well as increased risks of procedure-related complications, allograft rejection, and complications of induction immunosuppression (IS), particularly infection. Thus, the natural course of kidney transplantation is complex and dynamic, with evolving risk profiles and complications, which require various approaches for risk mitigation to optimize patient and allograft outcomes. While the immediate and early posttransplant phases of care focus primarily on postsurgical management, monitoring of allograft function, and optimization of IS to balance toxicity, immunologic risk, and infectious risk, later phases of care strategize to minimize and manage long-term complications of IS such as posttransplant malignancy, cardiovascular disease (CVD), posttransplant diabetes mellitus (PTDM), and more. This chapter reviews the salient features of the general management of the KTR from immediately posttransplant to beyond, including novel methods for monitoring allograft function and minimizing the risk of infections, malignancy, CVD, and other complications affecting patient and allograft outcomes.

Routine Follow-Up

Given the complexity of care and higher infectious and immunologic risk in the immediate and early posttransplant period, patients are followed by a transplant nephrologist at a minimum for the first 3 to 6 months after transplant. Frequency of follow-up is highest in the early posttransplant period (first 3 months), though it varies among centers and often depends on the stability of the patient and individual risk factors. A typical follow-up schedule for KTRs entails clinic visits twice weekly for the first 2 to 4 weeks, then weekly for 1 month, followed by every 2 weeks for 1 month, then once every 3 months for the first year posttransplant. Patients with stable allograft function and maintenance IS regimens may then be followed by an internist or general

nephrologist in consultation with a transplant nephrologist as the risk of rejection and infection decrease. However, KTRs still require close monitoring to maintain optimal graft function and assess for complications of IS including infection, malignancy, CVD, and PTDM, as well as complications from reduced kidney function such as anemia and mineral and bone disorder.

While frequency and type of laboratory monitoring vary from center to center, most institutions follow protocols similar to those proposed in the 2009 Kidney Disease: Improving Global Outcomes (KDIGO) clinical practice guidelines; Table 60.1 is an example. In addition to basic serum and urine chemistries, this table also includes whole blood IS levels and common preemptive viral monitoring. Follow-up should also include a routine history and physical exam.

Monitoring Allograft Function

Allograft dysfunction, if left unaddressed, may lead to irreversible allograft injury and eventual allograft failure. Early recognition, diagnosis, and treatment of allograft dysfunction is paramount as most causes of allograft dysfunction are reversible if treated promptly. While outcomes vary across institutions, the 1-year unadjusted survival rate of a kidney allograft in the United States (US) is approximately 93.2% and 97.5% for cadaveric and living donor kidneys, respectively. Despite dramatic improvements in 1-year allograft survival, late allograft loss remains a significant challenge. Fortunately, long-term allograft and patient survival for both deceased-donor and living-donor KTRs is gradually improving with advancements in healthcare. Both short- and long-term allograft survival are dependent on a variety of factors, many of which are interdependent and relate to donor and recipient characteristics as well as immunologic and nonimmunologic factors (Table 60.2). It is important to consider the time frame when evaluating allograft dysfunction as the causes vary dramatically over the immediate, early, and late posttransplant periods.

Assessment of Allograft Dysfunction

Monitoring allograft function includes the evaluation of urine output, serum creatinine levels and estimated glomerular filtration rate (eGFR), urine protein levels, kidney allograft ultrasound, and, if indicated, kidney allograft biopsy. In patients with high immunologic risk or if there is concern for rejection, additional

TABLE 60.1 Suggested Frequency of Laboratory Test Following Kidney Transplantation	
Test	**Frequency**
Basic chemistry panel (including eGFR), magnesium and phosphorus	Every visit
Complete blood count with differential	Every visit
CNI or mTOR inhibitor trough level (or C2*)	Every visit
Urinalysis with sediment examination	Every visit
Spot urine protein-to-creatinine ratio (or dipstick urine protein)	Every visit
Fasting blood glucose	Weekly for the first 4 weeks, then at 3 and 6 months, then yearly[†]
Hemoglobin A1c[‡]	Every 3 months or every visit if less frequent
Complete fasting lipid profile	At 3 and 12 months, then yearly
PTH and 25-hydroxyvitamin D level	At 3 and 12 months
BK polyoma virus blood and/or urine NAT	Monthly for the first 6 months, and then at 9, 12, 18, and 24 months
Cytomegalovirus blood NAT (if not on antiviral prophylaxis)	Weekly for the first 3 months
Epstein-Barr virus NAT (in high risk individuals)	Immediately posttransplant, then monthly for the first 3 months, then at 6, 9, and 12 months

eGFR, Estimated glomerular filtration rate; *CNI*, calcineurin inhibitor; *mTOR*, mammalian target of rapamycin; *PTH*, parathyroid hormone; *NAT*, nucleic acid testing.
*C2, Whole blood concentration at 2 hours after drug administration reflecting peak level.
[†]May be substituted for Hemoglobin A1c after month 3.
[‡] If fasting or nonfasting blood glucose abnormal.

TABLE 60.2 Factors Affecting Short-Term and Long-Term Allograft Survival	
Donor Factors	**Recipient Factors**
Age	Age
Donor type (living vs deceased)	Ethnicity
KDPI	Gene polymorphisms
Comorbidities and illness	Comorbidity
Inadequate kidney mass	Drug noncompliance
Brain death status	Dialysis vintage and type prior to transplant
	Geography
Immunologic Factors	**Nonimmunologic Factors**
Degree of sensitization (DSA and non-DSA)	Delayed graft function
Degree of HLA mismatching	Center effect
ABO blood group incompatibility	Infection (CMV, BKV, etc.)
Number of rejection episodes	Tissue injury
Recurrent or de novo glomerular disease	Immunosuppression type and toxicity
	Posttransplant hypertension
	Hyperlipidemia
	Hyperhomocysteinemia
	Ultrasonographic resistive index
	Proteinuria

KDPI, Kidney Donor Profile Index; *DSA*, donor-specific antibody; *HLA*, human leukocyte antigen; *CMV*, cytomegalovirus; *BKV*, BK polyomavirus.

laboratory work-up should include evaluation of donor-specific antibodies (DSA) and/or novel validated biomarkers such as molecular-based diagnostics. DSAs are routinely evaluated prior to kidney transplant as sensitized patients are at higher risk of subclinical and clinical active antibody-mediated rejection (ABMR) early posttransplant; thus, high levels of DSA are generally a contraindication to successful transplantation. Similarly, the appearance of *de novo* DSA posttransplant often precedes clinical allograft dysfunction and portends poor outcomes with higher rates of allograft failure. However, the positive predictive value of DSA (both by cytotoxic cross match and single-bead assay) for developing active ABMR is low, calling into question the utility of posttransplant DSA monitoring in diagnosing ABMR or predicting graft outcomes.

With the advent of "omics" molecular methods, including genomics, transcriptomics, proteomics, and metabolomics, many noninvasive molecular diagnostics have been developed to detect subclinical and acute rejection. In fact, the 2017 Banff classification system incorporated the use of validated molecular assays as part of the diagnostic criteria for ABMR, and in 2019 launched the Banff Human Organ Transplant (B-HOT) discovery gene panel, a consensus-based, standardized molecular assay. In addition to B-HOT, there are many other novel biomarkers under investigation including functional cell-based immune monitoring, molecular blood biomarkers such as mRNA and DNA gene panels and donor-derived cell-free DNA assays, urine biomarkers, and advanced imaging modalities. While several of these biomarkers provide good diagnostic and/or prognostic utility, few have been incorporated into the clinical setting and it is unknown whether their use translates to improved allograft outcomes. Molecular methods are also being applied to developing surrogate endpoints for clinical trials. Currently, the only FDA/EMA-approved surrogate endpoint is biopsy proven rejection, the accuracy of which was challenged by the results of the BENEFIT trial where the incidence of acute T cell-mediated rejection (TCMR) did not correlate with long-term allograft loss in the arm receiving belatacept. To address this concern, the 2017 Banff conference commissioned a new working group to build a validated scoring system that would integrate histopathology and novel biomarkers to establish a surrogate endpoint for clinical trials. A recent multicenter, prospective, cohort study by Loupy et al. developed and validated an accurate practical risk stratification score for predicting long-term allograft failure, which incorporated functional, histologic, and immunologic allograft parameters, called the *iBox*. Not only did the iBox demonstrate accuracy and generalizability in stratifying patients into clinically meaningful risk groups, but it also fulfilled Prentice criteria, potentially making it a satisfactory surrogate endpoint that may open opportunities for improved clinical trial design and therapeutic development in the future. Other novel advancements on the horizon include the incorporation of machine learning into the digital automation of pathology to optimize diagnostic accuracy and decrease inter-observer variability. While still in development, the use and standardization of machine learning algorithms may better combine biopsy findings with clinical and laboratory data and molecular methods to provide a more comprehensive clinical picture and facilitate cross-center collaboration.

Immediate (<1 Week) Posttransplant

Kidney transplant recipients who develop immediate allograft dysfunction commonly present with low urine output and/or failure of the serum creatinine to decrease after transplantation. Frequent evaluation of serum creatinine (every 12-24 hours) and urine volume are integral in assessing immediate graft function. It is important to consider the patient's baseline daily urine output prior to transplant as this will affect interpretation of urine output as it relates to allograft function. Kidney allograft ultrasound with Doppler should also be considered early to detect complications such as vascular thrombosis, urinary obstruction, and fluid collections. Prompt recognition is critical as immediate allograft dysfunction may be indicative of catastrophic vascular complications, which require immediate intervention for graft salvage. Other causes in the immediate and early posttransplant period that mandate rapid intervention for effective amelioration include acute rejection, urinary obstruction, urine leak, and certain recurrent native diseases such as focal segmental glomerulosclerosis (FSGS).

Surgical Complications

Surgical complications are unique to the immediate and early posttransplant period and may represent transplant emergencies. These commonly include vascular and urologic complications such as vascular thrombosis, fluid collections, and urinary obstruction.

Vascular thrombosis is a rare complication that often results in loss of the allograft without emergent thrombectomy. It is well known to be associated with rejection and other hypercoagulable states (secondary), though may occur as a primary entity. Patients typically present with an abrupt, painless cessation of urine output, which is commonly followed by a sudden elevation in serum creatinine and sometimes thrombocytopenia and hyperkalemia. While extremely limited, there is evidence to suggest that prophylactic low-dose aspirin is beneficial in decreasing the incidence of vascular thrombosis, and individuals at high risk of thrombosis may benefit from continued anticoagulation after kidney transplantation.

The most common fluid collections occurring posttransplant include urinary leaks (urinomas), perinephric hematomas, and lymphoceles. Most are diagnosed by ultrasound and confirmed by cell count or chemistries of the fluid aspirate. Urinary leaks usually occur at the site of the ureteroneocystostomy and can result from distal ureteric ischemia. They typically present with increased wound drainage, decreased urine output, and significant pain over the allograft within the first few days after transplant or onset of diuresis. A diagnosis is established when the creatinine concentration of the fluid aspirate is significantly elevated above serum levels. Postsurgical perinephric hematomas are often small and do not require intervention. However, in cases of significant bleeding, hematoma expansion can lead to compression of the allograft, ureter, or vascular supply and may require operative evacuation. Lymphoceles are fluid collections consisting mainly of lymph and lymphocytes caused by extravasation of severed lymphatics. Like perinephric hematomas, most are small and do not require intervention unless symptomatic. If indicated, large lymphoceles can be managed with drainage, sclerotherapy, or surgery, with surgical intervention having the lowest rate of recurrence.

Urinary obstruction can be precipitated by several common causes including extrinsic ureteric compression by fluid collections as mentioned above, bladder dysfunction, ureteral stricture, catheter blockage, blood clots, stones, and later by prostatic hyperplasia. Low-grade obstruction may also be seen in the setting of immediate graft function from ureteral edema associated with vigorous posttransplant diuresis and is usually self-resolving. Obstruction is often associated with a rise in serum creatinine and increasing hydronephrosis on ultrasound. In the case of ureteric stricture, urologic intervention with nephrostomy tube placement, stenting, or sometimes ureteric excision and reimplantation may be required.

Nonsurgical Complications

Once surgical emergencies have been ruled out, medical etiologies for allograft dysfunction should be considered. These include prerenal factors such as volume depletion and supratherapeutic calcineurin inhibitor (CNI) levels as well as intrinsic kidney etiologies including postischemic acute tubular necrosis (ATN), early acute rejection, recurrence of primary glomerular disease, thrombotic microangiopathy (TMA), and, less commonly, oxalate nephropathy and atheroemboli. Patients with severe allograft dysfunction that requires dialysis within the first week after transplantation are defined as having delayed graft function (DGF), a major risk factor for allograft failure.

The most common cause of DGF is postischemic ATN. DGF is more prevalent among deceased-donor recipients compared to living-donor recipients, particularly if the kidney donor profile index (KDPI) is above 85. KDPI is a measure of donor quality comprised of 10 characteristics used to provide an estimation of relative allograft survival compared with kidneys transplanted in the US in the previous year. For example, a donor kidney with a KDPI of 85% would reflect an allograft that is expected to survive longer than only 15% of all kidneys transplanted and indicates the donor kidney is of marginal quality. The increased rate of DGF in this cohort likely reflects the significant contribution of inherent donor vascular disease to ischemic susceptibility and graft injury. Other factors known to be associated with DGF include several premorbid donor factors, recipient factors, operative factors, and perioperative factors, which are summarized in Table 60.3. If DGF persists beyond 1 week or rejection is suspected, an allograft biopsy should be performed to evaluate for immune-mediated injury. In cases of prolonged DGF, biopsy should be repeated every 7 to 10 days to monitor for acute rejection.

Hyperacute ABMR, typically caused by preformed cytotoxic DSA to human leukocyte antigen (HLA), is an important historic cause of allograft loss within 24 hours, which was commonly diagnosed by the surgeon immediately upon engraftment. While advancements in histocompatibility testing have virtually eliminated the incidence of hyperacute ABMR, it is important to consider the limitations of the virtual crossmatch (a prediction of immunologic compatibility based on donor HLA genotype and recipient alloantibody profile) in predicting hyperacute ABMR in the event a cytotoxic crossmatch cannot be immediately performed.

Early (1 Week to 3 Months) and Late (>3 Months) Posttransplant Complications

As kidney transplant recipients progress beyond the first week from transplantation, the causes for acute allograft dysfunction evolve from ones of procedure-related complications to ones that encompass alloantigen-dependent and -independent injury, complications of IS, and the traditional spectrum of native kidney disease. While there is no definitive consensus, acute allograft

TABLE 60.3	Risk Factors Associated With Delayed Graft Function in Deceased Donor Kidney Transplantation*	
Premorbid Donor Factors	**Recipient Factors**	
Kidney Donor Profile Index (KDPI) >85%[†]	Age	
Donor macro- or microvascular disease	Black race (compared to white)	
	Peripheral vascular disease	
Brain death status	Dialysis vintage and modality	
Prolonged use of vasopressors	Prior sensitization (PRA >50%)	
Preprocurement ATN	Repeat transplant	
Nephrotoxic agent exposure	Obesity (body mass index >30 kg/m²)	
	Hypercoagulable state[‡]	
Operative Factors (Procurement and Transplant)	**Perioperative and Postoperative Factors**	
Intraoperative hemodynamic instability	Hypotension, shock	
Laparoscopic donor nephrectomy	Recipient volume contraction	
Traction on kidney vasculatures	Early high-dose CNI	
Cold storage flushing solutions	mTOR inhibitors[¶] (sirolimus and everolimus)	
Cold storage vs. machine perfusion		
Prolonged warm and cold ischemia time		
Prolonged rewarmed time (anastomotic time)		

CVA, Cerebrovascular accident; *CNS*, central nervous system; *ATN*, acute tubular necrosis; *PRA*, panel reactive antibodies; *CNI*, calcineurin inhibitors; *mTOR*, mammalian target of rapamycin.

* Contributory role of some risk factors may vary across studies.

[†]This calculation includes age, height, weight, ethnicity, history of hypertension, history of diabetes, cause of death (CVA/stroke, head trauma, anoxia, CNS tumor, other), serum creatinine, HCV status, donation after cardiac death status.

[‡] Factor V Leiden mutation, antiphospholipid syndrome, etc.

[¶] May prolong delayed graft function and should be avoided immediately posttransplant.

dysfunction can be characterized by (1) an increase in serum creatinine ≥25% from baseline in less than a 3-month period, (2) failure of the serum creatinine to decrease following transplantation (i.e., <2.0 mg/dL), or (3) new proteinuria. Proteinuria, even mild proteinuria between 0.25 and 1.0 g/day, is associated with worse long-term allograft function and increased CVD and mortality.

Alloantigen-Dependent Injury

Acute Rejection

One of the hallmark complications in the early posttransplant period is acute rejection. While the incidence of acute rejection has dramatically decreased since the advent of CNIs and antiproliferative agents, acute rejection remains a significant risk factor for late allograft failure and reduced allograft survival, occurring with an incidence in the first year posttransplant of approximately 8%. Patients at high immunologic risk for acute rejection include those with the following risk factors: pre-sensitization (either with DSA or a high panel reactive antibody), increased number of HLA mismatches, pediatric recipient, Black race, ABO-incompatibility, prolonged cold ischemia time, DGF, multiple prior transplants, and medication nonadherence or inadequate immunosuppression. It is important to note that while data have consistently shown that kidneys from Black donors are associated with lower rates of graft survival, the contribution of high-risk ApoL1 allele expression to allograft outcomes has not been fully elucidated and is currently undergoing investigation in the nationwide APOL1 Long-term Kidney Transplantation Outcomes Network (APOLLO) study. Acute allograft rejection typically presents with a sudden rise in serum creatinine and may be accompanied by worsening hypertension and new proteinuria >1.0 g/day. In the era of potent IS regimens, patients are typically asymptomatic, though, rarely, they may present with the classic symptoms of fever, malaise, oliguria, and allograft tenderness.

The gold standard for the diagnosis of acute rejection remains a kidney allograft biopsy. The Banff classification criteria, initially published in 1993 and most recently revised in 2019, can be used to classify acute rejection into two histologic forms: acute TCMR and active ABMR. While these two forms may coexist, it is important to identify the presence of active ABMR as it is often refractory to treatment for acute TCMR and can result in graft loss if left untreated. Acute TCMR is characterized by infiltration of the allograft by T cells, which react to donor histocompatibility antigens, resulting in interstitial inflammation, tubulitis, and arteritis. Active ABMR is caused by inflammation and tissue damage induced by binding of DSA to their molecular targets on vascular endothelium, which include HLA classes I and II, incompatible ABO antigens, and other non-HLA alloantigens. To make the diagnosis of active ABMR, three components are required: histologic evidence of tissue injury, evidence of current/recent antibody interaction with vascular endothelium, and serologic evidence of circulating DSA. According to the Banff 2017 and 2019 updates, if patients meet the first two criteria but have no evidence of circulating DSA, the presence of peritubular C4d staining or the expression of validated gene transcripts can substitute for DSA, though extensive DSA testing, including testing for non-HLA antibodies, is still strongly recommended.

Chronic Allograft Nephropathy

Chronic allograft dysfunction and late allograft loss remain challenges in kidney transplantation despite significant improvements in short-term allograft survival. Insidious decline of allograft function, indicated by a gradual rise in serum creatinine, progressive proteinuria, and worsening hypertension, is an incompletely understood, multifactorial phenomenon that often precedes allograft loss. Historically, this entity has been termed *chronic rejection, chronic allograft nephropathy*, or *transplant nephropathy*, but the preferred nomenclature when a specific cause cannot be identified is *interstitial fibrosis and tubular atrophy without evidence of any specific etiology* to encourage diagnostic effort. The exact mechanisms for this process are not well understood, and both immune and nonimmune factors are thought to play a role. However, it is becoming increasingly clear that inflammation, particularly early immune injury, subclinical rejection, and chronic allograft inflammation, is predictive of chronic histologic findings and allograft failure.

Interstitial fibrosis and tubular atrophy (IFTA) is a term established in the 2005 Banff revision used to describe nonspecific histologic findings associated with chronic injury in the absence of active rejection or CNI toxicity occurring at least 3 months posttransplant. These findings include duplication of arterial basement membrane, thickening of arterial intima, capillary rarefaction, and glomerulosclerosis. Transplant glomerulopathy (TG) is another characteristic morphologic lesion in chronic allograft dysfunction defined by reduplication of the glomerular basement membrane in the absence of electron-dense immune deposits associated with chronic, repetitive glomerular endothelial cell injury. TG occurs in up to 20% of KTRs and is associated with a 5-year graft survival rate of less than 50% from the time of diagnosis. It is thought to be immune-mediated via alloantibodies, autoantibodies, cell-mediated injury, TMA, and/or hepatitis C viral (HCV) infection. Another histologic finding associated with poor allograft outcomes is inflammation within areas of interstitial and tubular atrophy (i-IFTA). Adopted as an elementary lesion in the 2015 Banff revision, i-IFTA has been found to be closely associated with TCMR and insufficient immunosuppression and was, therefore, officially included in the diagnostic criteria for chronic active TCMR in the 2017 Banff revision. Despite its close association with chronic active TCMR, i-IFTA is a nonspecific lesion that may also be present in BK polyomavirus (BKV) nephropathy, pyelonephritis, ABMR, recurrent glomerulonephritis, and urinary obstruction.

Chronic active ABMR is an entity characterized histologically by evidence of chronic tissue injury, such as TG, current/recurrent antibody interaction with vascular endothelium, and serologic evidence of current or prior posttransplant circulating DSA (not remote) or a validated surrogate (C4d staining or positive molecular ABMR assay). Circulating DSA in conjunction with histologic changes herald shortened allograft survival even in the absence of an acute rejection episode. The largest risk factor for chronic active AMR is medication nonadherence. Chronic active ABMR is more difficult to treat than acute active ABMR. While there is currently no high-quality evidence to guide management, some studies have shown limited efficacy with rituximab as well as anti-IL-6 therapy. Conversely, bortezomib and eculizumab have not shown clinical efficacy.

Alloantigen-Independent Injury

Calcineurin Inhibitor Toxicity

CNIs are the mainstay of maintenance immunosuppression regimens in the US, used in over 90% of KTRs. There is significant overlap between the range of therapeutic and toxic CNI levels with considerable inter- and intrapatient variability. Consequently, CNI nephrotoxicity represents one of the most common causes of both acute and chronic allograft dysfunction. Acute CNI nephrotoxicity is largely due to the potent vasoconstrictive effect of CNIs on the afferent arteriole, which is usually dose dependent and reversible within 24–48 hours of dose adjustment. Long-term CNI use is a well-known cause of chronic allograft injury thought to be provoked by stimulation of endothelin synthesis and prolonged microvascular vasoconstriction. Pathologic findings consistent with chronic CNI toxicity include striped fibrosis, tubular vacuolization, arteriolar hyalinosis, and endotheliosis. Management may include CNI minimization, conversion to extended-release CNI formulations, or a CNI-free regimen. It is important to note that while CNI minimization may decrease long-term toxicity, immune-mediated injury contributes significantly to the development of chronic allograft dysfunction, thereby calling into question the safety of minimization approaches. Optimal strategies for CNI dosing, therefore, remain a topic of debate.

Viral Infections

Viral infections, especially BKV and cytomegalovirus (CMV) infection, constitute an important cause of allograft dysfunction and can precipitate interstitial nephritis, glomerulopathy, and inflammatory cytokine release. BKV nephropathy, in particular, is a common cause of allograft dysfunction and graft loss and presents a difficult therapeutic challenge. It is discussed further in Chapter 62.

Thrombotic Microangiopathy

Posttransplant TMA may be caused by several etiologies including ABMR, medications (CNIs, mTOR inhibitors, and valacyclovir), viral infections (CMV, parvovirus B19, and human immunodeficiency virus [HIV]), and recurrence of native disease such as atypical hemolytic uremic syndrome (aHUS), thrombotic thrombocytopenic purpura (TTP), antiphospholipid syndrome, and other hypercoagulable states. Treatment entails addressing the underlying cause and may require transition of CNI or mTOR inhibitor therapy to a co-stimulation blocking agent, such as belatacept.

Recurrent and De Novo Glomerular Disease

The incidence of recurrent primary glomerular disease in the allograft is often variable, depending on the etiology, and can be difficult to distinguish from de novo glomerular disease, particularly in patients who did not have a specific tissue diagnosis of their native kidney disease. Clinical presentation is similar to that of the native disease and typically requires an allograft biopsy for diagnosis. Glomerular diseases that commonly occur after transplantation include FSGS, IgA nephropathy, diabetic nephropathy, membranoproliferative glomerulonephritis (MPGN), primary membranous nephropathy, aHUS, C3 glomerulopathy, and dense deposit disease. FSGS is the primary glomerular disease most notoriously associated with recurrence and loss of the allograft; it is important to recognize it early as therapeutic interventions such as plasmapheresis may improve outcomes.

Immunosuppression

To prevent allograft rejection, KTRs receive immunosuppressive therapy consisting of induction and/or maintenance regimens. This section presents an overview of basic principles of immunosuppression and approaches to drug monitoring. Chapter 61 provides further details regarding specific immunosuppressive agents, including mechanisms of action, adverse effect profiles, and common drug-drug interactions.

Induction Therapy

Induction immunosuppressive therapy refers to the potent immunosuppression regimens administered at the time of transplantation. The goals of induction therapy are to reduce the risk of acute rejection and to allow for delayed initiation, minimization, or avoidance of maintenance agents known to cause toxicity. For instance, depleting induction agents can be used to provide adequate IS to reduce the risk of rejection and allow for the delayed initiation of CNIs in the setting of DGF or with corticosteroid avoidance or early withdrawal protocols. The agents used for induction therapy include high-dose glucocorticoids in conjunction with an antibody therapy (either monoclonal or polyclonal) directed against receptor targets on lymphocytes, most of which are lymphocyte depleting.

Lymphocyte-depleting agents are very potent and often take months or sometimes years for immune reconstitution. These agents, anti-thymocyte globulin (ATG) or alemtuzumab, are recommended for individuals at high risk of rejection. For individuals at lower immunologic risk, the decision to use depleting induction agents remains controversial, though current trends show depleting agents are preferred for the vast majority of kidney transplants. Individuals without high immunologic risk or who have a contraindication for depletion therapy, such as hypotension, leukopenia, or thrombocytopenia, may receive an anti-CD25 antibody (basiliximab), which abrogates IL-2 activity and subsequent T cell proliferation. Antibody induction therapy may be waived in select patients, such as recipients of another functioning solid organ transplant already on maintenance IS or Caucasian recipients of a two-haplotype-identical, living-related donor kidney.

Maintenance Therapy

Maintenance IS is usually initiated at the time of transplant and continued throughout the duration of the allograft. Maintenance regimens typically consist of a primary and secondary agent plus or minus glucocorticoids. Primary agents include CNIs (tacrolimus or cyclosporine), mammalian target of rapamycin (mTOR) inhibitors (sirolimus or everolimus), or costimulatory blockade agents (belatacept). Secondary agents are usually an antiproliferative agent (azathioprine or mycophenolate preparations [MPA]) or mTOR inhibitor. Most KTRs in the US are maintained on a regimen of tacrolimus and MPA with or without steroids (57.8% and 37.5%, respectively). A stable maintenance IS regimen is ideally established within the first 6 months posttransplant, though many patients require modification of the initial regimen to mitigate complications such as infection, malignancy, or drug toxicity. Therefore, it is important to be familiar with the advantages and disadvantages of each maintenance agent, including potency, adverse effect profile, and potential drug interactions, when individualizing a patient's maintenance regimen.

As rates of acute rejection have fallen dramatically, optimization of maintenance regimens has focused on strategies that minimize long-term toxicity, particularly that of prolonged CNI and glucocorticoid exposure. Given the numerous adverse effects of glucocorticoids, exposure should be safely reduced whenever possible. Most centers will rapidly taper maintenance prednisone doses down to 5 to 10 mg daily within the first 4 to 6 weeks posttransplant. Avoidance or complete withdrawal of glucocorticoids, however, remains controversial. Studies have shown that while early steroid withdrawal and avoidance regimens may have a beneficial impact on blood pressure, hyperlipidemia, bone disease, and glycemic control, there is an increased risk of acute rejection and recurrent glomerulonephritis. However, it is unclear if this increased risk of rejection translates to worse outcomes. A Cochrane systematic review on 7803 randomized patients showed that, while there was a significantly increased risk of acute rejection, there was no significant difference in patient mortality or graft loss up to 5 years posttransplant. Given the lack of clarity, corticosteroid withdrawal or avoidance protocols should only be considered in patients with low immunologic risk with close follow-up and the potential benefits of IS minimization should always be weighed against the risk for chronic immune-mediated injury.

Treatment of Acute Rejection

In assessing a patient's cumulative IS exposure, it is important to include the IS administered for episodes of acute rejection as these regimens are often potent and differ depending on the type and severity of immune injury. Acute TCMR is the most common form of rejection within the first 6 months posttransplant with incidence gradually decreasing over time. If suspected, findings should be confirmed on biopsy prior to initiating therapy. In addition to intensification of maintenance IS, treatment of acute TCMR should include a short course of intravenous pulse corticosteroids and, in severe cases, polyclonal ATG. In contrast, therapy for active ABMR aims to reduce DSA-mediated injury directly by removal or inactivation of circulating DSA or indirectly via B cell depletion or inhibition. Plasmapheresis and high-dose intravenous immune globulin (IVIg) are utilized to remove and inactivate DSA, respectively, and are, therefore, the cornerstone of therapy for active ABMR. Many protocols will also target B cell maturation with anti-CD20 agents (rituximab) and, in cases of refractory ABMR, DSA production with proteasome inhibitors (bortezomib). Another therapeutic, which has shown some promise in reducing the rate of acute ABMR among positive crossmatch recipients, is eculizumab, an anti-C5 complement inhibitor.

Drug Dosing and Monitoring

Due to the wide variability in the bioavailability and absorption seen in CNI therapy, whole-blood drug concentration monitoring is essential to ensure proper dosing and avoid over-immunosuppression and drug toxicity. Trough levels correlate well with drug exposure and clinical events and are most commonly used in tacrolimus therapy. While target therapeutic levels of CNI may differ depending on prior IS and induction therapy, higher levels are typically targeted in the first 3 months after transplant with gradual reduction over the following 6 months. When evaluating abnormal CNI drug levels, it is important to consider dose timing and drug formulation as well as common drug-drug interactions that may alter the metabolism of CNIs. Other drug-specific conditions, such as increased concentrations of tacrolimus in the setting of bowel wall inflammation and diarrhea, should also be considered. Unlike CNIs, routine drug level monitoring is not necessary with MPA as trough levels do not correlate with clinical efficacy. Instead, drug dosing is titrated to a target dose found to correlate with efficacy in clinical trials (2 g daily for mycophenolate mofetil and 1440 mg daily for mycophenolate sodium, typically in divided doses). Temporary dose reduction or discontinuation of MPA is often required in cases of significant gastrointestinal symptoms or profound leukopenia; however, full doses should be resumed, as tolerated, as prolonged dose reductions or discontinuation are associated with inferior graft survival.

Nonadherence to immunosuppressive medications may occur any time after kidney transplantation and is associated with a high risk of acute and chronic immune-mediated allograft injury and graft loss. Nonadherence to long-term immunosuppression is incredibly common, occurring in as many as 35.6 cases per 100 person-years in KTRs. Consequently, assessment of medication nonadherence and subsequent measures to reduce nonadherence are important aspects of IS management. Risk factors for nonadherence encompass four interrelated domains: patient/environment, caregiver, disease, and medication-related factors.

Common risk factors include a history of nonadherence prior to transplantation, psychiatric/psychologic disorders, substance abuse, cognitive impairment, poor social support, young age, time from transplantation, lack of adequate follow-up, adverse effects, medication cost, and complexity of medical regimen. A multidisciplinary approach focused on education, monitoring, recognition, and intervention should be individualized and updated continuously to optimize adherence and patient outcomes. Strategies may include simplified drug regimens, blister packaging of medications, electronic compliance alarms, and increased frequency of follow-ups.

Adverse Effects and Drug Interactions

Many of the commonly used maintenance immunosuppression agents have well-described adverse effects. Given the relatively narrow therapeutic window of many of these agents, it is important to screen for signs and symptoms of drug toxicity at each follow-up visit. Many of these significant side effects are summarized in Table 60.4 and is discussed in Chapter 61. As CNIs constitute the backbone of most maintenance regimens, it is important to recognize common drug-drug interactions that may interfere with cytochrome 450 (CYP450) metabolism and thereby affect CNI

TABLE 60.4	Adverse Effects of Common Maintenance Immunosuppressants
Immunosuppression Class	Adverse Effect
Calcineurin Inhibitors	Hirsutism and gingival hyperplasia (cyclosporine), alopecia (tacrolimus), neurologic disturbances (i.e., tremor), insomnia, hypertension, acute and chronic kidney dysfunction, electrolyte abnormalities (i.e., hypomagnesemia, hyperkalemia), NODAT (tacrolimus), HLD, hyperuricemia, malignancies, anemia and rarely thrombotic microangiopathy
Antiproliferative agents	GI disturbances, particularly diarrhea (MPA), bone marrow toxicity (i.e., leukopenia, anemia), pancreatitis and hepatitis
Corticosteroids	Cataracts, bone loss and fractures, avascular necrosis, hypertension, weight gain, dyslipidemia, glucose intolerance, mood lability, and acne
mTOR inhibitors	Pulmonary edema, hypertension, poor wound healing, joint pain, anemia, edema, hypertriglyceridemia/hypercholesterolemia
Co-stimulation blockade	Peripheral edema, hypertension, headache, electrolyte abnormalities, fever, infections (i.e., UTI, nasopharyngitis, URI), GI disturbances (i.e., diarrhea, constipation, nausea, vomiting), anemia, leukopenia, and proteinuria

NODAT, New-onset diabetes after transplantation; HLD, hyperlipidemia; MPA, mycophenolic acid; UTI, urinary tract infection; URI, upper respiratory tract infection.

TABLE 60.5	Selected Common Drug Interactions with Calcineurin Inhibitors
Increase CNI Level (Inhibits Enzyme)	Decrease CNI Level (Stimulates Enzyme)
Calcium channel blockers • Diltiazem • Verapamil	Antibiotics • Rifabutin • Rifampin
Antiarrhythmics • Amiodarone	Antiepileptics • Phenobarbital • Phenytoin • Carbamazepine
HIV protease inhibitors • Ritonavir • Saquinavir • Indinavir	Herbal substances • St. John's wort
Azole antifungal agents • Ketoconazole • Clotrimazole • Itraconazole • Voriconazole	
Antibiotics • Erythromycin base • Synercid (quinupristin and dalfopristin)	
Antidepressants • Fluvoxamine	
Other agents • Grapefruit juice	

Listed drugs interact with the calcineurin inhibitors, cyclosporine, and tacrolimus because they are metabolized by the cytochrome P450 CYP3A4 isoenzyme.
CNI, Calcineurin inhibitors; HIV, human immunodeficiency virus.

levels. Agents that interfere with CYP450 metabolism should be avoided if possible or introduced cautiously with frequent CNI drug level monitoring. Common CYP450 drug inhibitors and inducers are outlined in Table 60.5. While MPA does not undergo CYP450 metabolism and has fewer drug-drug interactions than CNIs, it is important to consider its effects on bone marrow toxicity and avoid any drugs that may potentiate leukopenia.

Infectious Complications

Basic Principles

Infection is a major cause of death in the early posttransplant period. Transplant recipients are highly susceptible to both opportunistic and community-acquired infections and may develop infection upon exposure to a lower inoculum. Additionally, the inflammatory response to infection is suppressed in transplant recipients, making presentation with attenuated signs and symptoms more difficult to recognize. Taken together, this often leads KTRs to present with a high burden of organisms and firmly established infection, which is more difficult to treat and may require surgical intervention. When evaluating infectious risk, it is important to consider the net state of immunosuppression—a conceptual measure of the factors contributing to host susceptibility, which encompasses dose and duration of immunosuppression, underlying comorbidities, presence of invasive devices (indwelling venous catheter), and concomitant immunocompromising infections (CMV, Epstein-Barr virus [EBV], human herpes virus

[HHV]-6 and -7, hepatitis B [HBV], HCV, and HIV), as well as biologic or target therapy. It is also important to assess a patient's exposure risk, which may include both new and potentially reactive remote epidemiologic exposures (*Mycobacterium*, coccidiomycosis, herpes simplex virus [HSV], varicella zoster [VZV], CMV, and HBV) as well as the risk for donor-derived infection. The risk of infection by specific pathogens varies over time after transplantation and corresponds to procedure-related factors and the potent induction IS regimens used. Therefore, considering the timing of infection posttransplant is an essential step in forming a differential diagnosis (Table 60.6). It is also important to note that serologic testing is generally not useful for the diagnosis of acute infection posttransplant as seroconversion is often delayed or fails to develop in the immunocompromised recipient. A detailed approach to and management of infectious complications posttransplant, including CMV, BKV, and urinary tract infections, are further discussed in Chapter 62.

Vaccination, Prophylaxis, and Preemptive Therapy

Given the high prevalence, morbidity, and mortality associated with infectious complications, strategies to minimize infection risk are employed including vaccination, universal prophylaxis, and preemptive therapy. Standard, age-appropriate vaccines along with those recommended for immunocompromised hosts should be given prior to transplant and beginning at 3 to 6 months posttransplant, avoiding the early posttransplant period where IS is highest. KTRs should not receive live or live-attenuated vaccines, though inactivated vaccines are generally considered safe. It is also important for close contacts and healthcare providers of KTRs to be fully immunized, receiving inactivated vaccines when possible to avoid the theoretical risk of transmission of attenuated viruses.

Universal antimicrobial and antiviral prophylaxes are routinely given to KTRs for the first 6 to12 months posttransplant, though prophylaxis may be extended depending on patient-specific factors. While prophylaxis protocols may differ among institutions, most centers use a combination of trimethoprim-sulfamethoxazole (TMP-SMX) and valganciclovir or ganciclovir for universal antimicrobial and antiviral prophylaxes, respectively. TMP-SMX is the preferred antimicrobial for prevention of *Pneumocystis jirovecii* pneumonia as it also provides broad antimicrobial coverage against common urinary, respiratory, and gastrointestinal pathogens as well as *Toxoplasma gondii*, *Listeria*, and many *Nocardia* species. Valganciclovir or ganciclovir are often used as prophylaxis against CMV reactivation in at-risk KTRs (seropositive recipients and recipients with seropositive donors), though some centers prefer a preemptive approach to reduce drug exposure, costs, and antiviral toxicity. Patients who do not receive CMV prophylaxis should receive antiviral prophylaxis against HSV and VZV during the first 3 to 6 months posttransplant or in the setting of lymphodepleting therapy.

Preemptive therapy involves routine viral load monitoring with sensitive assays and initiation of treatment upon evidence of reactivation and early infection. It is commonly used for CMV, EBV, and BKV in at-risk KTRs. While still investigational, some centers use nonpathogen-specific and pathogen-specific immune monitoring assays to identify at-risk KTRs for a more targeted approach to prophylaxis or preemptive therapy. For instance, recent studies have shown absolute lymphocyte count and CMV-specific T-cell interferon-gamma release assays are adequate markers for risk assessment of CMV infection and may be helpful in guiding clinical decision making.

Malignancy

The incidence of de novo malignancies is two- to fourfold higher in organ transplant recipients than in the general population. Driving this increased risk is the use of potent immunosuppression, high prevalence of oncogenic viral infections (particularly human papillomavirus, EBV, CMV, and HHV-8), and prevalence of native kidney-related cancer such as renal cell carcinoma. Cumulative IS dose is an important risk factor as IS impairs immune-mediated tumor surveillance. Consequently, the cornerstone of posttransplant malignancy management is vigilant screening, early detection, and IS minimization, if indicated.

The most common malignancies in KTRs are dermatologic. Risk factors include cumulative IS, sun exposure, fair skin, geographic area, ethnicity, genetic factors, human papilloma virus infection, and prior or precancerous skin lesion. Over 90% of skin malignancies after transplantation are squamous cell carcinomas and basal cell carcinomas, with a 250-fold and 10-fold increased incidence, respectively, compared with the general population. Other types of skin cancer including melanoma, Merkel cell carcinoma, and Kaposi sarcoma are also more common in KTRs. Key strategies for risk mitigation include counseling patients to avoid sun exposure and to regularly use sunscreen and protective clothing. Routine self-skin and lip examinations as well as annual total skin examination performed by a dermatologist are also recommended. Suspicious lesions should be biopsied; if malignancy is confirmed, IS adjustment should be considered. While there is no consensus on optimal IS management, strategies include discontinuation of antiproliferative agents, CNI minimization, or conversion to an mTOR inhibitor. Evidence suggests that mTOR inhibitors are beneficial in skin cancer and Kaposi sarcoma in KTRs due to their antiproliferative and antitumoral effects. However, the role of mTOR inhibitors in other malignancies is still not clear.

TABLE 60.6	Timing of Infection After Transplantation
Time after Transplantation	**Type of Infection**
0–1 month	Nosocomial: mostly bacterial or candida, CAUTI, CLABSI, PNA Procedure-related: mostly bacterial or *Candida*, wound infection, perinephric abscess Donor derived (rare)
1–6 months	Opportunistic: viral (CMV, BK polyomavirus, VZV), bacterial (*Nocardia*, *Listeria*), fungal (PJP, *Aspergillus*), parasitic (*Strongyloides*, *Toxoplasma*)
>6 months	Community-acquired: viral (influenza, Norovirus, COVID-19), bacterial (*Streptococcus pneumoniae*, *Listeria*, *Salmonella*), fungal (*Cryptococcus*, endemic fungi), parasitic (*Cryptosporidium*).

CAUTI, Catheter-associated urinary tract infection; *CLABSI,* central line-associated blood stream infection; *PNA,* pneumonia; *CMV,* cytomegalovirus; *VZV,* varicella zoster; *PJP, Pneumocystis jirovecii; COVID-19,* coronavirus disease 2019.

While relatively rare, one of the most serious complications of transplantation, carrying a mortality rate of over 50%, is posttransplant lymphoproliferative disease (PTLD). PTLD is predominantly an EBV-associated lymphoid or plasmacytic proliferation, which occurs in the setting of marked IS and impaired T cell immunosurveillance, typically arising within the first year after transplantation when immunosuppression is most intensive, particularly T cell suppression. Numerous studies have found that lymphocyte-depleting induction immunosuppression is associated with a higher risk of PTLD. One study found that the standardized incidence ratio of lymphoma compared with a similar nontransplant population was 21.5, 4.9, 29.0, 21.6, 7.8, and 9.4 for patients administered OKT3, ATG, ATGAM, thymoglobulin, IL-2 receptor antagonists, and no induction, respectively. PTLD occurs in 1% 2% of KTRs and may present along a spectrum of clinical syndromes, ranging from acute mononucleosis to various forms of B cell and T/NK cell lymphoma. EBV serostatus plays an important role in risk stratification as EBV-negative recipients of EBV-positive donors are at highest risk and may benefit from antiviral prophylaxis. Preemptive therapy is another preventative strategy for at-risk groups; high EBV viral loads often precede clinical presentation of PTLD, thereby allowing clinicians to intervene with IS reduction and antiviral drugs. Treatment of PTLD typically involves IS reduction and administration of an anti-CD20 antibody with or without adjunctive cytotoxic therapies, depending on clonality, subtype, and aggressiveness.

Diabetes Mellitus

Diabetes mellitus, both preexisting and posttransplant diabetes mellitus (PTDM), is associated with an increased risk of posttransplant CVD and infection, the leading causes of mortality among KTRs. Development of PTDM has significant adverse effects on both patient and long-term allograft survival, conferring up to a three fold increased relative risk for CVD-related death. Reported incidence of PTDM has been variable over time, depending on the context of the definition that was used, population assessed, immunosuppression regimen investigated, and time from transplant, though recent data from OPTN/SRTR have shown that the prevalence of PTDM at 1-year posttransplant has decreased from around 10% in 2007 to under 4% in 2018. Many of the traditional risk factors for diabetes mellitus are also applicable to the posttransplant setting, including older age >40, obesity, African ancestry, Hispanic ethnicity, prior history of impaired glucose tolerance, and a family history of diabetes. Transplant-specific factors include IS regimen (glucocorticoids, CNIs, and mTOR inhibitors), chronic viral infections (HCV and CMV), perioperative hyperglycemia, hypomagnesemia, increasing HLA/DR mismatching, and, possibly, native polycystic kidney disease.

Glucocorticoids are known to cause hyperglycemia through multiple mechanisms, and higher doses of glucocorticoids have been associated with new onset diabetes after transplant (NODAT). While rapid reduction and minimization of glucocorticoids have been shown to decrease glucose intolerance, complete steroid withdrawal is not recommended due to the risk of rejection. Rejection episodes are often treated with pulsed high-dose glucocorticoids, which, in turn, increase the risk of PTDM. Calcineurin inhibitors, particularly tacrolimus, are known to cause reversible toxicity to pancreatic islet cells and may impair insulin granule formation and secretion directly via transcriptional dysregulation. While tacrolimus has been shown to be more diabetogenic than cyclosporine, it is unknown whether reduced tacrolimus dosing or

cyclosporine-based regimens confer better outcomes. However, switching from tacrolimus to cyclosporine may be considered for patients whose diabetes remains difficult to control on low-dose tacrolimus. Conversion of CNIs to mTOR inhibitors is not recommended for the indication of PTDM as there is evidence that conversion may worsen insulin resistance and glycemic control. Similarly, conversion from CNI to belatacept for the indication of PTDM alone is not generally recommended, though patients converted for other indications have demonstrated improved glucose control.

PTDM is typically managed in a stepwise approach to achieve and maintain glycemic control. The optimal glycemic goal in PTDM is not known, though the American Diabetes Association recommends a hemoglobin (Hgb) A1c target of <7% for most patients with PTDM without extensive comorbid conditions while KDIGO recommends HgbA1c of 7% to 7.5%. Lifestyle modifications, including dietary changes, exercise, and weight reduction, are recommended for all patients with PTDM as an initial step. If hyperglycemia persists, pharmacologic therapy is considered, starting with oral hypoglycemic agents and escalating to insulin therapy if needed. There are limited data to support a first-line agent for the treatment of PTDM and clinicians should consider the adverse-effect profile and metabolism of each drug in relation to concurrent immunosuppression regimen and allograft function. For instance, metformin is often avoided due to the increased risk of lactic acidosis in patients with significantly reduced kidney function. Strategies to improve glucose tolerance by adjusting immunosuppression may also be considered; however, the potential benefits must always be weighed against the risk of allograft rejection.

Cardiovascular Disease

As mentioned previously, kidney transplantation confers a survival advantage over remaining on dialysis. Mechanisms underlying this observed survival advantage remain unclear, though likely reflect improved cardiovascular health and a reduction in major adverse cardiovascular events (MACE) with improved kidney function. Improved volume control, cessation of hemodialysis-induced repetitive myocardial injury, and improved clearance of uremic toxins and advanced glycosylation end products with resultant reduction of inflammation, oxidative stress, and microvascular disease are all proposed mechanisms. While transplant recipients have a lower risk of MACE compared to wait-listed patients on dialysis, they are still at a significantly higher risk for MACE compared with the general population. Cardiovascular disease is the leading cause of death and allograft loss among KTRs, constituting up to as much as 60% of posttransplant mortality. Many traditional and nontraditional risk factors for cardiovascular disease affect transplant recipients, including preexisting CVD, older age, dyslipidemia, hypertension, PTDM, smoking, inflammation, anemia, and obesity, particularly in the setting of metabolic syndrome. Many KTRs will also have significantly reduced GFR and elevated levels of albuminuria, both of which are also associated with CVD events in this population. Many of these factors are exacerbated by immunosuppression. CVD is further discussed in Chapter 54.

Hypertension

Posttransplant hypertension is common, occurring in up to 50%-80% of kidney transplant recipients, and is associated with higher rates of allograft failure. While blood pressure often rises immediately posttransplant, many of the factors that contribute to hypertension in this setting, such as hypervolemia and salt retention, will resolve with improving allograft function. Many immunosuppression agents, most notably CNIs and glucocorticoids, may exacerbate hypertension through various mechanisms including vasoconstriction, salt retention, weight gain, and a mineralocorticoid effect.

It is important to recognize transplant renal artery stenosis (RAS) in cases of refractory posttransplant hypertension as it is correctable with intervention. RAS typically presents 3 months to 2 years posttransplant with refractory hypertension, persistent erythrocytosis, reversible allograft dysfunction upon initiation of an angiotensin-converting enzyme (ACE) inhibitor or angiotensin receptor blocker (ARB), and sometimes flash pulmonary edema or hypertensive urgency. Risk factors for transplant RAS include organ procurement complications, atherosclerotic disease, CMV infection, and DGF. It is most commonly diagnosed through imaging modalities, arteriography being preferred.

Given the risks of worsened CVD and hypertensive injury to the allograft, posttransplant hypertension should be closely monitored and treated diligently. Optimal blood pressure goals are variable between societies and depend on the presence of proteinuria as well as comorbid conditions, such as PTDM. The 2021 KDIGO clinical practice guideline on the management of blood pressure in chronic kidney disease continues to recommend maintaining a blood pressure of less than 130/80 mmHg. While antihypertensive regimens should be tailored to patient-specific factors, dihydropyridine calcium channel blockers (CCBs) and ARBs are generally recommended as the first-line antihypertensive agents in adult KTRs as their use is associated with superior allograft survival. Although a 2009 meta-analysis of randomized trials showed that ACE inhibitors were more effective at reducing proteinuria, only CCBs reduced graft loss. Similarly, a recent update for this Cochrane systematic review showed that dihydropyridine CCB use was associated with a 38% reduction in graft loss and ARB use was associated with a 65% reduction in graft loss. However, due to their effects on reduced eGFR, anemia, and hyperkalemia, ACE inhibitors and ARBs are typically deferred for the first 6 months posttransplant but may be considered in patients with proteinuria ≥1 g/day with stable graft function and normal potassium levels. While thiazide diuretics are common first-line agents in the general population, there is sparse evidence studying their effects in a transplant population. A recent study comparing chlorthalidone to amlodipine found that chlorthalidone use was associated with a 32% reduction in proteinuria compared to only 4% reduction with amlodipine; however, chlorthalidone treatment was associated with lower eGFR and increased serum levels of uric acid and HgbA1c.

Dyslipidemia

Dyslipidemia is common in the posttransplant population, occurring in over 50% of recipients in the first year after transplant. Many immunosuppressants, including mTOR inhibitors, CNIs, and glucocorticoids, are known to directly cause and contribute to lipid abnormalities. As CVD is highly prevalent among KTRs and is the leading cause of mortality in this population, lipid modification may be an important intervention for improving cardiovascular outcomes based on data extrapolated from the general population and heart transplant recipients. However, it is important to note that, while there is some suggestive evidence, there are no definitive data demonstrating the benefits of statin

therapy on CVD outcomes among KTRs. The Assessment of Lescol in Renal Transplantation (ALERT) trial is the only randomized, controlled trial that investigated the effects of statin therapy on CVD outcomes after kidney transplantation. After 5 years of follow-up, the group receiving statins achieved a 32% reduction in LDL levels and had significantly fewer cardiac deaths or MIs compared to placebo. However, the primary composite outcome of cardiac death, nonfatal MI, or coronary interventions only showed a trend towards reduction that failed to meet statistical significance. Based on data in heart and lung transplant recipients, statins have also been suggested to reduce rates of acute rejection. However, after multiple conflicting clinical trials, there is inadequate evidence to support the use of statins to reduce rates of acute rejection in KTRs.

Obesity and Metabolic Syndrome

Obesity, defined by a body mass index (BMI) >30, is a highly prevalent complication among KTRs, with older age, female sex, Black race, and increased comorbidity being associated risk factors. Metabolic syndrome, consisting of central obesity, dyslipidemia, hypertension, and fasting hyperglycemia, is also highly prevalent in KTRs with one study reporting up to 63% of transplant recipients meeting criteria at 6 years posttransplant. Weight gain after kidney transplant is quite common and may reflect improved appetite after uremia reversal, use of glucocorticoids, particularly high-dose in the peritransplant period, and physical inactivity. As in the general population, obesity in KTRs is associated with an increased risk of adverse cardiovascular events, including cardiac death after transplantation, heart failure, and atrial fibrillation.

Diet and exercise are the mainstays in weight management for KTRs. Pharmacologic management of obesity is generally not recommended as many of these medications, including antidepressants, herbal remedies, and orlistat, may interfere with CYP450 metabolism or absorption of CNIs. While safety and efficacy data are still limited, there is some evidence to suggest SGLT2 inhibitor therapy may result in modest weight reduction in diabetic KTRs. Bariatric surgery can also be considered as a safe and effective weight-loss intervention in patients with severe obesity. A recent study in 38 solid organ transplant recipients showed that bariatric surgery was associated not only with significant weight loss and improvement in comorbidities, but also increased stability in tacrolimus blood trough levels from 39% to 47%. While the study showed blood trough levels slightly declined after bariatric surgery, all levels remained within therapeutic range and none of the subjects required dose adjustment, suggesting that bariatric surgery did not significantly impact immunosuppressant absorption or pharmacokinetics. However, bariatric surgery may exacerbate several nutritional deficiencies and has, in case reports, been associated with enteric hyperoxaluria and subsequent oxalate nephropathy in the kidney allograft.

Hematologic Complications

Leukopenia

Leukopenia, either neutropenia or lymphocytopenia, is a frequent adverse drug effect commonly attributed to IS, antivirals, and/or TMP-SMX. Many viral entities are also known to contribute to leukopenia including CMV, EBV, parvovirus B19, HHV-6, and influenza. While dose adjustment or withdrawal of offending medications is often the first step in managing leukopenia, immunosuppression reduction may increase the risk of allograft rejection and must be done with caution. One important exception is in the setting of active CMV infection where antiviral dose reduction may promote drug resistance. In that circumstance and in cases of severe leukopenia or neutropenia with an absolute neutrophil count of <1500 cells/μL, granulocyte colony-stimulating factors are the favored therapeutic strategy.

Anemia

Anemia occurs in up to 40% of KTRs and is found in nearly all patients prior to transplant due to iron deficiency and decreased erythropoietin (EPO) synthesis and responsiveness, commonly observed in CKD. Despite a robust, early increase in EPO production by the allograft, anemia may persist or even worsen due to intraoperative volume expansion, surgical blood loss, inflammation, abrupt cessation of EPO-stimulating agents, initiation of induction and maintenance immunosuppression, and/or DGF. Anemia often improves within the first few months after transplantation, though may recur upon development of iron deficiency, allograft dysfunction, acute rejection, viral infection, or as an adverse drug effect from commonly used medications including immunosuppression, antivirals, ACE inhibitors and ARBs, and TMP-SMX. In the presence of low reticulocyte count and refractory isolated anemia, parvovirus B19 should be considered. Other etiologies of refractory anemia include occult gastrointestinal tract bleeding, tertiary hyperparathyroidism, and chronic inflammation.

Erythrocytosis

Posttransplant erythrocytosis (PTE) is defined by elevated Hgb (>17 g/dL) and/or hematocrit (>51%) that develops after transplant, typically between 8 and 24 months, and persists for more than 6 months in the absence of thrombocytosis, leukocytosis, and other potential causes. Patients often present with malaise, headache, plethora, lethargy, and dizziness, and are at high risk of thromboembolic complications. The pathogenesis of PTE involves the uncontrolled stimulation of erythroid progenitor cells due to dysregulated EPO metabolism, angiotensin II, insulin-like growth factor, and high serum-soluble stem cell factor. Risk factors include presence of native kidneys, male sex, robust allograft function, absence of rejection, elevated hemoglobin prior to transplant, and polycystic kidneys. Patients with persistent erythrocytosis, particularly in conjunction with hypertension, edema, and allograft bruit, should undergo evaluation for transplant RAS. Other causes of nontransplant erythrocytosis, including renal cell carcinoma in the native and transplant kidney, should also be excluded. Once confirmed, ACE inhibitor or ARB therapy is the preferred initial treatment as these induce erythroid precursor apoptosis and reduce insulin-like growth factor. Phlebotomy may also be considered when ACE inhibitor or ARB therapy is contraindicated or ineffective.

Thrombocytopenia

Thrombocytopenia is often found in the first year posttransplant and usually arises in combination with leukopenia and anemia as a result of bone marrow suppression from IS, antivirals, or viral infections. When associated with anemia, with or without allograft dysfunction, clinicians should also consider TMA and pursue further work-up to identify the underlying etiology.

Mineral Bone Metabolism and Disease

Chronic kidney disease-mineral bone disorder (CKD-MBD) is common in individuals with CKD, including after kidney transplantation despite markedly improved kidney function. It is defined as a systemic disorder of mineral and bone metabolism due to CKD manifested by either one or a combination of the following: (1) abnormalities of calcium, phosphorus, parathyroid hormone (PTH), or vitamin D metabolism, (2) abnormalities in bone turnover, mineralization, volume, linear growth, or strength, or (3) vascular or other soft tissue calcification. As kidney function improves posttransplant, posttransplantation bone disease typically evolves from a spectrum of preexisting CKD-MBD to one of overlapping osteoporosis due to a variety of posttransplant factors. As the clinical consequences of bone fracture and vascular calcification may have important ramifications on morbidity and mortality among KTRs, it is important to identify and address mineral bone disease early. Factors predisposing KTRs to bone disease, particularly bone loss, include immunosuppression drugs (CNIs and glucocorticoids), preexisting abnormal bone histology due to CKD (also known as *renal osteodystrophy*), and persistent hyperparathyroidism posttransplant. Patients should undergo regular monitoring of biochemical parameters including serum calcium, phosphate, PTH, and 25-hydroxyvitamin D levels as well as bone mineral density assessment.

Persistent Hyperparathyroidism

Persistent hyperparathyroidism posttransplant is an independent risk factor for allograft loss, MACE, and all-cause mortality, and affects up to 50% of KTRs. Secondary hyperparathyroidism is found in maintenance dialysis patients and many progress to tertiary hyperparathyroidism with loss of PTH calcium-dependent autoregulation and structural parathyroid changes. Consequently, when eGFR and kidney PTH responsiveness are restored upon transplantation, persistent unregulated hyperparathyroidism results in hypercalcemia and hypophosphatemia. This may persist for years after transplant, contributing to allograft nephrocalcinosis and dysfunction, fracture risk, vascular calcification, and increased risk of MACE. The risk factors for persistent hyperparathyroidism posttransplant are long duration of dialysis, severity of pretransplant hyperparathyroidism, vitamin D insufficiency, and allograft dysfunction. In KTRs with persistent hyperparathyroidism posttransplant and mild to moderate hypercalcemia, calcimimetics (cinacalcet) are used to correct hypercalcemia and hypophosphatemia and improve PTH levels. However, subtotal parathyroidectomy has been shown to be superior to cinacalcet in correcting hypercalcemia and improving MBD and should be considered in patients who have refractory hyperparathyroidism, persistent severe or progressive hypercalcemia (serum calcium >12mg/dL), clinical effects of hypercalcemia (nephrolithiasis, nephrocalcinosis), and osteoporosis.

Osteoporosis

The major bone diseases affecting KTRs are osteoporosis and osteonecrosis, both of which can contribute significantly to morbidity and mortality. Bone loss occurs rapidly in the initial posttransplant period and then tends to stabilize by the end of the first year. In addition to traditional risk factors, transplant-specific risk factors include persistent hyperparathyroidism, preexisting CKD-MBD-related bone abnormalities, and the use of glucocorticoids and

CNIs. Corticosteroid-induced suppression of bone formation is the most significant risk factor for osteoporosis, even overriding the effects of age, sex, and PTH. Dual-energy X-ray absorptiometry (DEXA) is recommended in the first 3 months posttransplant in patients with eGFR over 30 mL/min/1.73m² receiving corticosteroids or at high risk of osteoporosis. Osteoporosis is managed in a stepwise fashion, with the first step being lifestyle modification and the minimization of corticosteroids. The next step involves correction of persistent hyperparathyroidism and/or hypophosphatemia, if present. If not present or successfully treated, antiresorptive agents, such as bisphosphonates, should be considered in patients with an eGFR >30 mL/min without evidence of adynamic bone disease (assessed by PTH and bone alkaline phosphatase). The novel drugs such as denosumab and teriparatide have been used for osteoporosis treatment in KTRs though data are limited and their use is currently not endorsed by guidelines.

Electrolyte and Acid-Base Disorders

Electrolyte and acid-base disturbances commonly occur after kidney transplantation and typically include hypomagnesemia, hyperkalemia, hypercalcemia, hypophosphatemia, and metabolic acidosis. Many of these disturbances are secondary to posttransplant medication regimens, particularly CNIs, as well as PHP upon restored kidney function. Hypomagnesemia is very common posttransplant and has been identified as an independent risk factor for development of NODAT and CNI nephrotoxicity. CNIs are thought to be directly responsible via CNI-induced downregulation of a kidney magnesium channel, TRPM6, resulting in magnesium wasting. Hyperkalemia posttransplant is often multifactorial and can result from impaired allograft function and metabolic acidosis along with concomitant use of medications known to precipitate hyperkalemia, including CNIs, TMP-SMX, beta-blockers, and ACE inhibitors and ARBs. Excepting hyperkalemic emergency, the first step in management of hyperkalemia is to discontinue or reduce potentially offending medications in consultation with a transplant nephrologist. Metabolic acidosis should also be corrected if present. If hyperkalemia is persistent, addition of a loop diuretic may be considered to facilitate urinary potassium excretion. Posttransplant metabolic acidosis is often mild and indicative of impaired allograft function, reduced nephron mass with impaired kidney acid handling, and/or CNI nephrotoxicity. CNIs can impair tubular acid secretion and precipitate a type 4 renal tubular acidosis. Posttransplant acidosis may exacerbate mineral and muscle metabolism derangements as well as posttransplant anemia. Treatment is similar to that seen in CKD, consisting mainly of alkali therapy.

Hyperuricemia and Gout

Hyperuricemia and gout are common after kidney transplantation, largely as a result of a CNI-induced reduction of uric acid excretion. Pharmacologic management of hyperuricemia and gout in KTRs is complicated by reduced kidney function, risk of infection, and the increased risk for complex and potentially serious adverse drug interactions, either due to immunosuppression regimens or pharmacologic management of other highly prevalent comorbid conditions, including PTDM, hypertension, and CVD. Complicating this further is the dearth of high-quality evidence to guide the optimal pharmacologic management of gout flares or urate-lowering therapy in this population. Consequently, the use of antiinflammatory drugs and urate-lowering therapy is only recommended for patients with complications (i.e., gout, tophi, or uric acid stones) and should be guided by an experienced transplant clinician, individualized to patient-specific factors, and monitored closely on follow-up.

Sexual Function and Fertility

Impaired sexual function and infertility are common among patients with CKD and ESKD and are usually improved within the first few months after transplantation and restoration of the hypothalamic-pituitary-gonadal axis. This improvement may be impacted by impaired allograft function, comorbidities (i.e., PTDM, hypertension, and CVD), psychological factors, and possibly IS regimen as there is some evidence to suggest sirolimus may impair spermatogenesis. Consequently, both men and women should be counseled on the potential improvements in sexual and reproductive function posttransplant and associated risks.

Pregnancy

Pregnancy after transplantation is considered high risk in nature and requires multidisciplinary management with a high-risk obstetrician and transplant nephrologist. In women of childbearing age, preconception counseling should begin prior to transplant to discuss posttransplant pregnancy outcomes, maternal risk (including risk to the allograft), contraceptive methods, timing of conception, and management of immunosuppression. Despite the improvement in fertility, pregnancy rates among KTRs are markedly lower compared with that of the general population. This difference may be partially explained by the intentional avoidance of pregnancy in this population given the added risks to the mother, fetus, and allograft. While the risks of pregnancy and childbirth are higher for KTRs, most pregnancies in uncomplicated KTRs with good allograft function, no significant proteinuria, and well-controlled blood pressure have good outcomes with comparable live birth rates. Stability of allograft function, infection risk, and immunosuppression play significant roles in pregnancy outcomes, making timing of conception paramount in minimizing risks to the mother, fetus, and allograft. General consensus by the American Society of Transplantation (AST) in 2005 recommends delaying pregnancy until at least 1 year posttransplant and to consider conception only in patients with optimal allograft function with no or minimal proteinuria, no episodes of rejection in the previous year, no concurrent fetotoxic infections such as CMV, no concurrent fetotoxic/teratogenic medications, and stable maintenance IS levels.

Modification of IS regimen is often necessary prior to conception as all immunosuppression agents carry some risk and a few, namely, MPA and mTOR inhibitors, are contraindicated in pregnancy. It is also important to consider the changes in pharmacokinetic factors such as metabolism, volume of distribution, and increased filtration that occur during pregnancy, which may affect IS levels and subsequently require more frequent monitoring. After counseling on the risks of rejection with IS adjustment, conversion to a regimen of a CNI, azathioprine, and low-dose prednisone is most often recommended. Allograft function should be closely monitored for a few months on the new IS regimen prior to conception to ensure allograft stability. After conception, patients should be closely monitored for maternal complications including hypertension, preeclampsia, allograft dysfunction, rejection, gestational diabetes, infection (particularly bacterial urinary tract infections and CMV), and anemia.

Contraception

As sexual and reproductive function is restored rapidly post-transplant in women, contraceptive planning should start prior to transplant and be initiated prior to resuming sexual activity. Estrogen-containing contraceptives are not advised in women with complicated transplants and should be delayed until 6 weeks after transplantation due to the increased thrombotic risk perioperatively. Additionally, mycophenolate is known to reduce serum estrogen levels and may theoretically reduce the effectiveness of estrogen-containing contraceptives. Bearing this in mind, the optimal form of contraception in KTRs is unknown and contraception should be individualized to side-effect profile and patient-specific factors including comorbidities and concomitant medication use.

Mental Health

Mental health in the KTR population remains a poorly studied entity despite the inordinately high prevalence of anxiety and depression among ESKD patients and the known effects of anxiety and depression on medication nonadherence. Studies of depression and anxiety in KTRs have shown conflicting results regarding the benefit of transplantation on mental health, likely reflecting the superimposition of the complex nature of transplantation and its risks of complications onto a population rife with psychiatric trauma, anxiety, and depression. Adding to the complexity is the reciprocal nature of mental and allograft health; mental health has a significant effect on allograft outcomes and allograft outcomes have a significant effect on mental health. One study found that return to hemodialysis after transplant, particularly after only a short duration of graft function, was associated with severe depression. Further studies are needed to identify risk factors as well as determine optimal approaches to patient screening and interventions, especially in patients with preexisting mental health disorders, medical comorbidities, and high-risk KTR subgroups.

Complete bibliography is available at Elsevier eBooks for Practicing Clinicians.

Key Bibliography

Allen UD, Preiksaitis JK. Post-transplant lymphoproliferative disorders, Epstein-Barr virus infection, and disease in solid organ transplantation: guidelines from the American Society of Transplantation Infectious Diseases Community of Practice. *Clin Transplant.* 2019;33(9):e13652.

Altuğ Y, Liang N, Ram R, et al. Analytical validation of a single-nucleotide polymorphism-based donor-derived cell-free DNA assay for detecting rejection in kidney transplant patients. *Transplantation.* 2019;103(12):2657–2665.

Crespo E, Roedder S, Sigdel T, et al. Molecular and functional noninvasive immune monitoring in the ESCAPE study for prediction of subclinical renal allograft rejection. *Transplantation.* 2017;101(6):1400–1409.

Djamali A, Kaufman DB, Ellis TM, Zhong W, Matas A, Samaniego M. Diagnosis and management of antibody-mediated rejection: current status and novel approaches. *Am J Transplant.* 2014;14(2):255–271.

Engels EA, Pfeiffer RM, Fraumeni Jr JF, et al. Spectrum of cancer risk among US solid organ transplant recipients. *JAMA.* 2011;306(17):1891–1901.

Fishman JA. Infection in solid-organ transplant recipients. *N Engl J Med.* 2007;357(25):2601–2614.

Haas M, Loupy A, Lefaucheur C, et al. The Banff 2017 Kidney Meeting Report: Revised diagnostic criteria for chronic active T cell-mediated rejection, antibody-mediated rejection, and prospects for integrative endpoints for next-generation clinical trials. *Am J Transplant.* 2018;18(2):293–307.

Hart A, Smith JM, Skeans MA, et al. OPTN/SRTR 2018 Annual Data Report: kidney. *Am J Transplant.* 2020;20(suppl 1):S20–S130.

Hartmann EL, Gatesman M, Roskopf-Somerville J, Stratta R, Farney A, Sundberg A. Management of leukopenia in kidney and pancreas transplant recipients. *Clin Transplant.* 2008;22(6):822–828.

Humar A, Matas AJ. Surgical complications after kidney transplantation. *Semin Dial.* 2005;18(6):505–510.

Kalantar-Zadeh K, Molnar MZ, Kovesdy CP, Mucsi I, Bunnapradist S. Management of mineral and bone disorder after kidney transplantation. *Curr Opin Nephrol Hypertens.* 2012;21(4):389–403.

Kasiske BL, Snyder JJ, Gilbertson D, Matas AJ. Diabetes mellitus after kidney transplantation in the United States. *Am J Transplant.* 2003;3(2):178–185.

KDIGO 2009. KDIGO clinical practice guideline for the care of kidney transplant recipients. *Am J Transplant.* 2009;9(suppl 3):S1–S155.

Kotton CN, Kumar D, Caliendo AM, et al. The third international consensus guidelines on the management of cytomegalovirus in solid-organ transplantation. *Transplantation.* 2018;102(6):900–931.

Loupy A, Aubert O, Orandi BJ, et al. Prediction system for risk of allograft loss in patients receiving kidney transplants: international derivation and validation study. *BMJ.* 2019;366:l4923.

Loupy A, Haas M, Roufosse C, et al. The Banff 2019 kidney meeting report (I): updates on and clarification of criteria for T cell- and antibody-mediated rejection. *Am J Transplant.* 2020;20(9):2318–2331.

McKay DB, Josephson MA, Armenti VT, et al. Reproduction and transplantation: report on the AST Consensus Conference on reproductive issues and transplantation. *Am J Transplant.* 2005;5(7):1592–1599.

Pallardó Mateu LM, Sancho Calabuig A, Capdevila Plaza L, Franco Esteve A. Acute rejection and late renal transplant failure: risk factors and prognosis. *Nephrol Dial Transplant.* 2004;19(suppl 3):iii38–iii42.

Rangaswami J, Mathew RO, Parasuraman R, et al. Cardiovascular disease in the kidney transplant recipient: epidemiology, diagnosis and management strategies. *Nephrol Dial Transplant.* 2019;34(5):760–773.

Schinstock CA, Mannon RB, Budde K, et al. Recommended treatment for antibody-mediated rejection after kidney transplantation: the 2019 Expert Consensus From the Transplantation Society Working Group. *Transplantation.* 2020;104(5):911–922.

61

Immunosuppression in Transplantation

SINDHU CHANDRAN, FLAVIO G. VINCENTI

The central issue in organ transplantation remains the prevention of allograft rejection. Understanding the physiology of the immune response to a transplanted organ, developing targeted immunosuppressive drugs, and devising the best combinations to maintain safety and improve efficacy are key for successful graft function and long-term graft survival.

Physiology of Immunorecognition

The immune system evolved to discriminate self from non-self, and this response against non-self consists of an array of receptor-mediated sensing and effector mechanisms broadly described as innate and adaptive. *Innate immunity* is primitive, does not require priming, and is of relatively low affinity but broadly reactive. *Adaptive immunity* is antigen-specific, depends on antigen exposure or priming, and can be of very high affinity. The major effectors of innate immunity are complement, granulocytes, monocytes/macrophages, natural killer (NK) cells, mast cells, and basophils. The major effectors of adaptive immunity are B and T lymphocytes.

A transplant between genetically distinct individuals of the same species is called an *allogeneic graft,* or an *allograft.* The immune response to an allograft requires three elements: recognition of foreign antigens, activation of antigen-specific lymphocytes, and the effector phase of graft rejection. The recognition of antigens as peptide fragments bound to major histocompatibility complex (MHC) molecules, known as *human leukocyte antigens* (HLAs), is the central event in the initiation of an alloresponse. HLA molecules (Fig. 61.1) are highly polymorphic, follow Mendelian codominant inheritance, and constitute the principal antigenic barrier to transplantation. The degree of HLA matching between the donor and the recipient has been long recognized to play an important role in graft survival, and HLA matching has been incorporated into kidney allocation. More recently, mismatched "eplets," or patches of polymorphic residues within a radius of 3.0–3.5 Å, which form essential components of HLA epitopes recognized by antibodies, have been found to be a significant risk factor for the development of de novo donor-specific antibody, chronic humoral rejection, and graft loss. In addition, non-HLA molecules, such as MHC class I–related chain A (MICA), are recognized as playing a significant role in rejection, particularly in recipients of well–HLA-matched kidneys.

There are two types of HLA molecules: class I and class II. Class I HLA molecules are expressed on all nucleated cells, whereas class II molecules are usually expressed only on antigen-presenting cells (APCs), which include dendritic cells, B lymphocytes, and macrophages. Cytokines such as interferon-γ (IFN-γ) induce, upregulate, and broaden HLA expression, so that all cells in a graft can become potential targets of the immune response. Ischemia-reperfusion injury in the graft leads to the production of inflammatory cytokines and recruitment of macrophages, and acute rejection episodes are more common in grafts with prolonged ischemia times. Recipient T cells may respond directly to peptides/HLA complexes presented by donor APCs in the graft or to donor HLA peptides presented on the recipient's own APCs (Fig. 61.2). Acute rejection of an allograft is believed to be primarily dependent on direct allorecognition, whereas the indirect pathway may play a larger role in chronic rejection.

T cells are critically important in the rejection of allogeneic grafts. CD4 T cells (helper T cells) are thought to mediate the initial recognition of an allograft as well as amplify and coordinate the subsequent immune response, including providing help to CD8 (effector) T cells. T cell recognition of the alloantigen occurs via binding of the T cell receptor (TCR)/CD3 complex on the T cell's surface to the peptide/MHC complex on APCs. This is referred to as *signal 1* and leads to phosphorylation of TCR-associated proteins and downstream activation of several pathways, including calcineurin, protein kinase C, and mitogen-activated protein (MAP) kinase pathways. The calcineurin pathway is the most well characterized, and it involves the activation of calcineurin (a phosphatase) by an increase in cytosolic calcium. Calcineurin dephosphorylates nuclear factor of activated T cells (NFAT), allowing NFAT to translocate from the cytoplasm to the nucleus. The NFAT binds to regulatory sequences and increases gene transcription of several cytokines, including interleukin (IL)-2, a T cell growth factor, as well as IL-4, IFN-γ, and tumor necrosis factor-α (TNF-α).

Although the specificity of the immune response is determined by *signal 1*, a costimulatory signal, *signal 2,* which occurs though accessory molecules, is essential for T cell activation. The most potent of these signals regulating T cell clonal expansion and differentiation is provided by the B7/CD28 family of molecules (Fig. 61.3). B7-1 (CD80) and B7-2 (CD86) are ligands on APCs that bind to CD28, expressed on most T cells. Engagement of CD28 increases the production of IL-2 and other cytokines, resulting in T cell proliferation. CD80 and CD86 also regulate T cells by binding another antigen on T cells called cytotoxic *T-lymphocyte antigen-4 (CTLA-4),* which inhibits T cell proliferation. A costimulatory interaction between CD40 on APCs and CD40 ligand (CD154, CD40L) on T cells is also critical for activation of APCs and upregulation of B7 expression on T cells. One way to induce T cell anergy in vitro is to provide the T cell

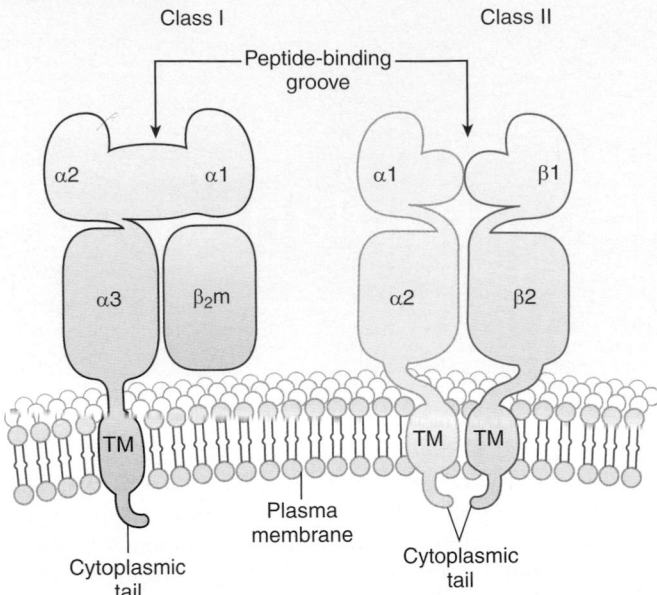

• **Fig. 61.1** Structure of human leukocyte antigens class I and class II molecules. Beta$_2$-microglobulin (β_2m) is the light chain of the class I molecule. The α chain of the class I molecule has two peptide-binding domains (α1 and α2), an immunoglobulin-like domain (α3), the transmembrane (TM) region, and the cytoplasmic tail. Each of the class II α and β chains has four domains: the peptide-binding domain (α1 or β1), the immunoglobulin-like domain (α2 or β2), the transmembrane region, and the cytoplasmic tail. (From Klein J, Sato A. The HLA system. *N Engl J Med*. 2000;343:702–709.)

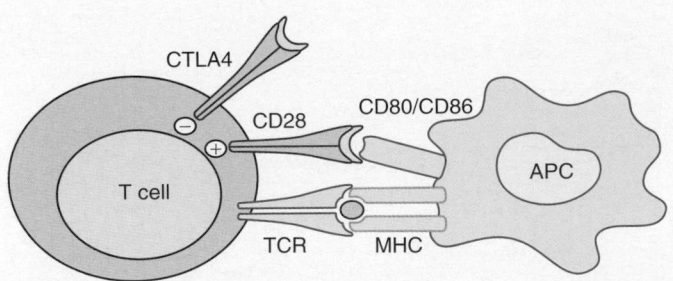

• **Fig. 61.3** Signal 1 and signal 2. *APC*, Antigen-presenting cell; *MHC*, major histocompatibility complex; *TCR*, T-cell receptor. (From Vincenti F. Costimulation blockade in autoimmunity and transplantation. *J Allergy Clin Immunol*. 2008;121:299–306.)

with an antigen-specific signal through the TCR (signal 1) in the absence of CD28 engagement (signal 2). However, in most in vivo models of B7 blockade, anergy has been difficult to demonstrate, which is possibly due to the complexity of costimulation that involves multiple stimulatory and inhibitory signals.

Antigen-specific activation of T cells, particularly CD4 T cells, leads to the production of cytokines, the recruitment of monocytes, and the proliferation of CD8 T cells, NK cells, and B cells. CD8 T cells cause cell death in the graft through the release of soluble cytotoxic factors (granzymes and perforin) as well as upregulated Fas ligand on T cells that bind to Fas (CD95) on target cells and trigger apoptosis.

In addition to T cells, B cells and the humoral arm of the immune system play a major role in acute and chronic graft injury. Antibodies produced by the differentiation of B cells into plasma cells cause cell injury through complement fixation or antibody-dependent cellular cytotoxicity. Hyperacute rejection occurs when preformed recipient antibodies to donor HLA antigens or ABO blood group antigens result in complement activation, intravascular coagulation, and graft necrosis within 24 hours of transplantation. Although cross matching and ABO blood typing have virtually eliminated hyperacute rejection, B cells and plasma cells continue to play an important role in subsequent antibody-mediated rejection (AMR) and may be important mediators of chronic graft injury and late graft loss.

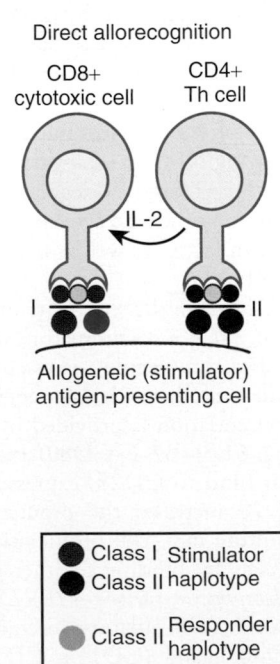

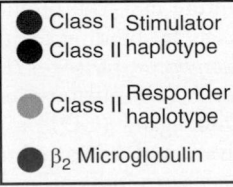

• **Fig. 61.2** Diagrammatic representation of the direct and indirect pathways of allorecognition. *IL*, Interleukin; *MHC*, major histocompatibility complex. (From Rogers NJ, Lechler RI. Allorecognition. *Am J Transplant*. 2001;1:97–102.)

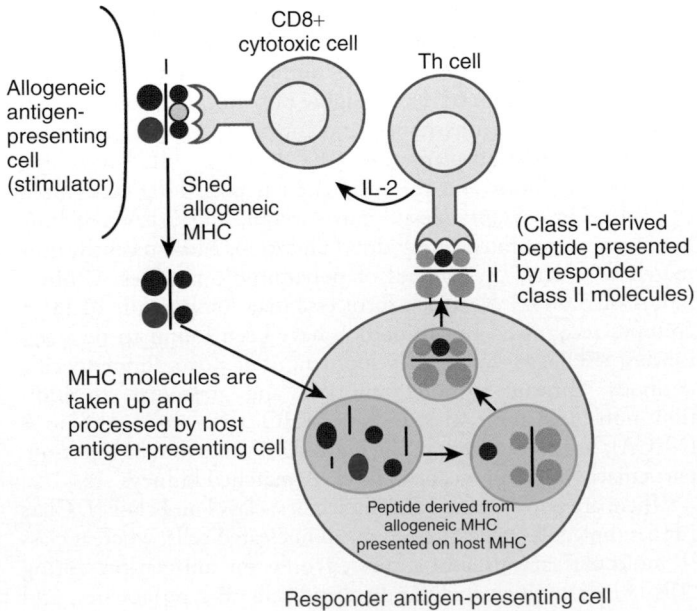

Strategies for Immunosuppression

The first attempts at immunosuppression used total-body irradiation. Azathioprine was introduced in the early 1960s, and soon thereafter was routinely accompanied by prednisolone in an immunosuppressive regimen. The polyclonal antilymphocyte antibody preparations became available in the mid-1970s. The introduction of cyclosporine in the early 1980s dramatically improved 1-year graft survival rates from 50% to over 80%, and in 1985, OKT3, a monoclonal antibody to CD3, was introduced for the treatment of acute rejection. In the 1990s, tacrolimus and mycophenolate mofetil (MMF) emerged as alternatives to cyclosporine and azathioprine, anti–IL-2 receptor antibodies were approved for induction, and sirolimus became available. Everolimus was approved in 2010 for use in kidney transplant recipients in combination with calcineurin inhibitors. In 2011, belatacept was approved as the first biologic agent for use in maintenance immunotherapy. Commonly used immunosuppressants and their mechanisms of action are listed in Table 61.1.

Transplant immunosuppression is guided by three key principles: (1) multiple agents directed at different molecular targets within the alloimmune response are used simultaneously to maximize synergy and efficacy while minimizing toxicity; (2) greater immunosuppression (induction) is needed for early engraftment or to treat established rejection rather than for long-term graft maintenance; and (3) continuous vigilance is essential to identify rejection, drug toxicity, and infection so that the immunosuppressive regimen can be modified appropriately.

Mechanisms of Action of Immunosuppressive Drugs

T cells have historically been the major target of immunosuppression. The three-signal model of T cell activation and subsequent cellular proliferation provides a useful guide to the sites of action of the major immunosuppressive agents (Fig. 61.4). Signal 1 is the antigen-specific signal provided by the interaction of the MHC/peptide complex on APCs with the TCR/CD3 complex. Signal 2 is a non-antigen-specific costimulatory signal provided by the engagement of B7 on APCs with CD28 on the T cell. These two signals activate intracellular pathways, leading to the production of IL-2 and other cytokines. Stimulation of the IL-2 receptor (CD25) leads to activation of mammalian target of rapamycin (mTOR), a protein kinase, and provides signal 3, which triggers

TABLE 61.1 Commonly Used Induction and Maintenance Immunosuppressive Agents

Drug	Phase of Use	Mechanism of Action	Side Effects
Glucocorticoids: methylprednisolone (Solu-Medrol), prednisone (Deltasone)	Induction and maintenance	Binds cytosolic receptors and heat shock proteins, and blocks transcription of IL-1, IL-2, IL-3, IL-6, TNF-α, and IFN-γ	Hypertension, hyperglycemia, dyslipidemia, osteoporosis, impaired wound healing, cosmetic effects
Calcineurin inhibitors: cyclosporine (Sandimmune, Neoral, Gengraf), tacrolimus (Prograf)	Maintenance	Forms a complex with cyclophilin or FK-binding protein, which binds to calcineurin, preventing dephosphorylation of regulatory proteins and decreasing transcription of IL-2, IL-4, IFN-γ, and TNF-α; also increases TGF-β, which inhibits IL-2	Tremor, nephrotoxicity, hypertension, hyperglycemia, hyperuricemia, hyperlipidemia (CsA), hirsutism (CsA), gingival hyperplasia (CsA), hair loss (tacrolimus)
Antiproliferative Agents			
Azathioprine (Imuran, Azasan)	Maintenance	Purine analog that blocks DNA, RNA, and protein synthesis	Marrow suppression, pancreatitis
Mycophenolate mofetil (Cellcept), mycophenolic acid (Myfortic)	Maintenance	Inhibits IMPDH, preventing de novo guanosine nucleotide synthesis	Diarrhea, marrow suppression, teratogenic
mTOR inhibitors: sirolimus (Rapamune), everolimus (Zortress)	Maintenance	Forms a complex with FK-binding protein-12, which blocks p70 S6 kinase, causing G1 cell cycle arrest	Hyperlipidemia, hyperglycemia, thrombocytopenia, impaired wound healing, interstitial pneumonitis, embryotoxic
Biologics			
Basiliximab (Simulect)	Induction	Monoclonal antibody to CD25 (IL-2 receptor α chain), which blocks IL-2 engagement	Rare infusion reactions
Rabbit antithymocyte globulin (Thymoglobulin)	Induction	Polyclonal antithymocyte antibody, which depletes T cells	Cytokine release syndrome, serum sickness, thrombocytopenia, prolonged lymphopenia
Alemtuzumab (Campath)	Induction	Monoclonal antibody to CD52, which depletes T cells, B cells, and NK cells	Cytokine release syndrome, prolonged lymphopenia
Belatacept (Nulojix)	Maintenance	CTLA-4-Ig fusion protein, which competes with CD28 for CD80/86 binding, inhibiting T-cell costimulation	Rare infusion reactions

CSA, Cyclosporine A; *IFN,* interferon; *IL,* interleukin; *IMPDH,* inosine monophosphate dehydrogenase; *mTOR,* mammalian target of rapamycin; *NK,* natural killer; *TGF-β,* transforming growth factor-β; *TNF-α,* tumor necrosis factor-α.

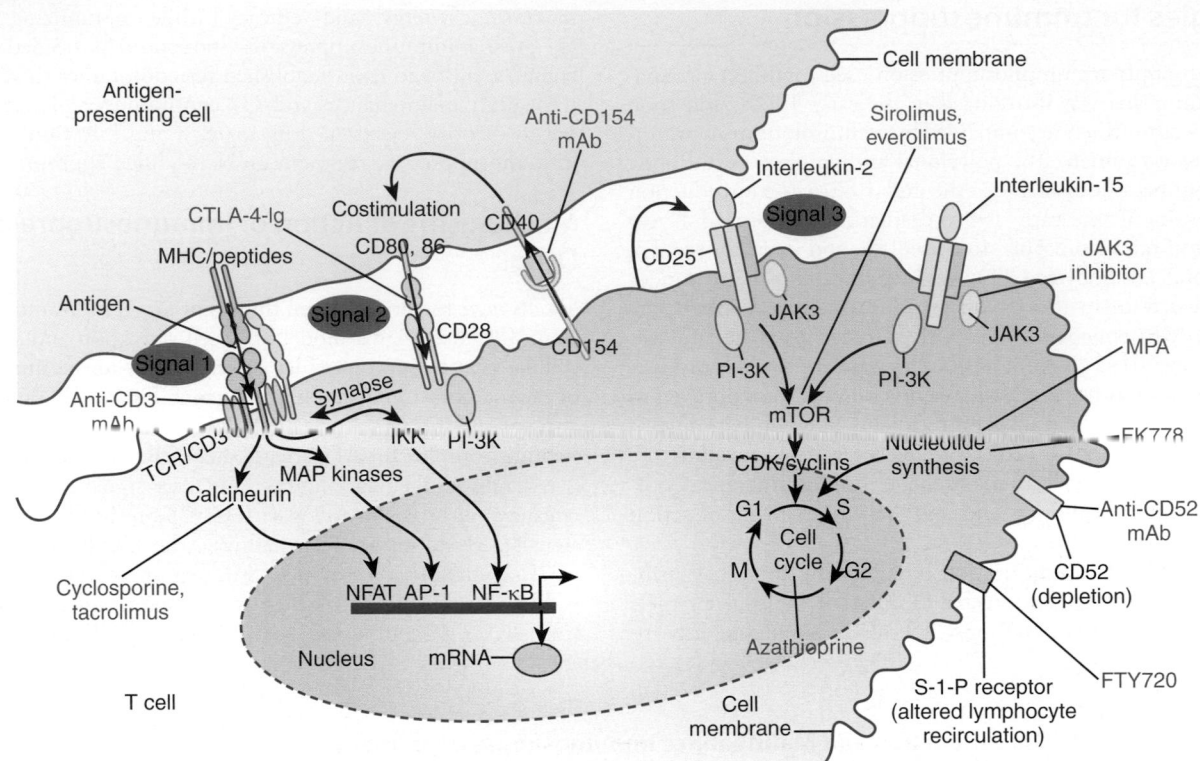

• **Fig. 61.4** Individual immunosuppressive drugs and sites of action in the three-signal model. *CDK*, Cyclin-dependent kinase; *IKK*, IκB kinase; *MAP*, mitogen-activated protein; *MHC*, major histocompatibility complex; *MPA*, mycophenolic acid; *NFAT*, nuclear factor of activated T cells; *TCR/CD3*, T-cell receptor. (From Halloran PF. Immunosuppressive drugs for kidney transplantation. *N Engl J Med.* 2004;351:2715–2729.)

cell proliferation. Therapies targeting antibody-mediated injury are directed against B cells, plasma cells, and complement activation. In general, all drugs in current clinical use have been more effective at suppressing primary rather than memory immune responses.

Induction Immunosuppression

High intravenous doses of corticosteroids are used as part of nearly all induction immunosuppression protocols. Induction therapy with antibodies is used to delay the use of nephrotoxic calcineurin inhibitors (CNIs) and/or to intensify the initial immunosuppressive therapy in patients at high immunologic risk (i.e., broadly sensitized, high immunologic risk, children, or individuals with a prior transplant). Antibody induction is currently used in over 90% of kidney transplant recipients and consists of either T cell-depleting agents or IL-2 receptor antagonists.

Depleting agents diminish the recipient's lymphocyte population at the time of transplantation, and induction with these agents has been shown to improve graft survival. Antithymocyte globulin (ATG), a polyclonal antilymphocyte preparation directed against T cells, is the most common induction agent in kidney transplantation and was approved for this indication in 2017. It is interesting to note that ATG also causes sustained and rapid expansion of regulatory T cells, which play an important part in maintaining immune homeostasis and limiting antigraft immunity. The approved dose of rabbit-derived thymoglobulin is 1.5 mg/kg daily for 4 to 7 days. Alemtuzumab (Campath-1H; Sanofi Genzyme) is a humanized anti-CD52 monoclonal antibody that targets lymphocytes, monocytes, macrophages, and NK cells and causes prolonged B and T cell depletion. Alemtuzumab is also used off-label as induction therapy in about 10% of kidney transplants, particularly as part of steroid-sparing protocols. It is usually given as a single dose of 30 mg intraoperatively when infusion-related events are often masked by general anesthesia. Campath-1H was withdrawn from markets in the US and Europe in 2012 to prevent off-label use in multiple sclerosis, but can be obtained directly from the manufacturer by institutions that have established inventory for solid organ transplant induction. ATGAM, an equine ATG, is rarely used in the United States because of its poorer efficacy. Muronomab-CD3 (Orthoclone OKT3; Janssen-Cilag), a murine monoclonal antibody to CD3, was associated with significant acute side effects, such as cytokine release syndrome, and was withdrawn from the market in 2010.

Depleting agents can elicit major side effects, including fever, chills, and hypotension. The polyclonal agents are xenogeneic proteins. Cell death and cytokine release peak with the first infusion and diminish substantially with subsequent doses. Reactions can be minimized by premedication with corticosteroids, acetaminophen, and an antihistamine along with slow infusion (over 4 to 6 hours) through a large-diameter vessel. Other side effects include leukopenia, thrombocytopenia, serum sickness, glomerulonephritis, and, rarely, anaphylaxis. In the long term, depleting agents have been associated with a higher incidence of infections and malignancy, particularly posttransplant lymphoproliferative disorders (PTLDs).

IL-2 receptor antagonists do not deplete T cells, with the possible exception of T regulatory cells; rather, they block IL-2–mediated T cell activation. Daclizumab (Zenapax) and basiliximab (Simulect) are chimeric and humanized monoclonal antibodies, respectively, that bind to the α chain of the IL-2 receptor, thus blocking IL-2–mediated responses. Daclizumab has a longer half-life ($T_{1/2}$) than basiliximab (20 days vs. 7 days), and the typical dosing schedule results in longer saturation of the IL-2Rα on circulating T cells (120 days vs. 30 to 45 days). However, saturation of the IL-2Rα may not prevent rejection and was noted to be similar in patients with or without an acute rejection episode. Rejection in patients despite IL-2R blockade may occur through a mechanism that bypasses the IL-2 pathway as a result of cytokine-cytokine receptor redundancy (i.e., IL-7, IL-15). Both drugs are fairly well tolerated, and no cytokine release syndrome has been observed, although anaphylaxis may occur rarely. Following the withdrawal of daclizumab from the market in October 2008, basiliximab is the only anti-IL2R antibody currently available for use as induction therapy.

More aggressive approaches to induction therapy have been used in patients with high levels of anti-HLA antibodies, donor-specific antibodies, or previous humoral rejection. These include plasmapheresis and intravenous immune globulin (IVIG), to reduce the levels of preformed antibodies, and rituximab, a chimeric anti-CD20 monoclonal antibody, to selectively deplete B cells.

Maintenance Immunosuppression

The basic immunosuppressive protocols use multiple drugs simultaneously. Therapy typically involves a CNI, glucocorticoids, and MMF, each directed at a discrete site in T cell activation. Protocols using rapid steroid withdrawal (within 1 week) are used in over one-third of kidney transplant recipients with good short-term results, although the effects on long-term graft function are not known. Azathioprine has mostly fallen out of favor, except for use during pregnancy and sometimes as part of lower-cost regimens. Sirolimus and everolimus have been used mostly in de novo or conversion regimens that spare/minimize CNI exposure. Maintenance biologic therapy with belatacept, in combination with a steroid and an antiproliferative agent, permits complete avoidance of calcineurin inhibition and has been associated with superior kidney function, improved metabolic parameters, and improved graft survival in recipients at low immunologic risk.

Glucocorticoids

Glucocorticoids are used in high doses as part of induction protocols, for the treatment of acute rejection episodes, and in low doses for maintenance immunosuppression. Steroids exert broad antiinflammatory effects on multiple components of cellular immunity but have little effect on humoral immunity. They lyse (in some species) and redistribute lymphocytes, causing a rapid transient lymphopenia. To effect long-term responses, steroids bind to intracellular receptors and downregulate the transcription of numerous genes such as IL-1, IL-2, IL-3, IL-6, TNF-α, and IFN-γ, thereby inhibiting T cell activation. Neutrophils and monocytes display poor chemotaxis and decreased lysosomal enzyme release. In addition, steroids curtail the activation of NF-κB, thus increasing the apoptosis of activated cells.

The long-term use of steroids is associated with several adverse effects, including growth retardation in children, avascular osteonecrosis, osteopenia, increased risk for infection, poor wound healing, cataracts, hyperglycemia, and hypertension. Steroid minimization (avoidance and withdrawal) protocols are associated with comparable short-term graft survival and improved metabolic parameters achieved at the cost of higher acute rejection rates and unknown long-term effects on the graft.

Calcineurin Inhibitors

Cyclosporine A ushered in the modern era of organ transplantation, increasing the rates of early engraftment, extending kidney graft survival, and making heart and liver transplantation possible. Cyclosporine and tacrolimus are structurally unrelated agents that bind to distinct molecular targets (cyclophilin and FK-binding protein [FKBP] 12, respectively), blocking calcineurin and selectively inhibiting signal transduction in activated T cells. Cyclosporine also increases the expression of transforming growth factor-β (TGF-β), which inhibits IL-2 and the generation of cytotoxic T cells.

Cyclosporine is a lipophilic and highly hydrophobic cyclic polypeptide of 11 amino acids produced by the fungus *Beauveria nivea*. Cyclosporine, as supplied in the original soft gelatin capsule (Sandimmune; Novartis Pharmaceuticals Corporation), is absorbed slowly, with 20% to 50% bioavailability. A modified microemulsion formulation (Neoral; Novartis Pharmaceuticals Corporation) with improved bioavailability was approved in 1995 and became the most widely used preparation. Generic preparations of both are available and are bioequivalent to the original formulation but not to each other. The initial dose is usually 6-12 mg/kg/day, divided into two doses. The administration of cyclosporine with food delays and decreases its absorption, and it can lower the peak concentration by 33% and the area under the drug concentration curve (AUC) by 13%. The elimination of cyclosporine from the blood is generally biphasic, with a terminal $T_{1/2}$ of 5 to 18 hours. It is metabolized extensively in the gut and the liver by CYP3A and P-glycoprotein. Cyclosporine and its metabolites are excreted principally through the bile into the feces, with 6% being excreted in urine. Dosage adjustments are required for liver dysfunction but not for reduced glomerular filtration rate. Despite being the most commonly used monitoring tool, 12-hour trough cyclosporine levels (C0 level) are poorly reflective of the AUC and, thus, are not an accurate indication of cyclosporine exposure in individual patients. Drug levels 2 hours after Neoral dose administration (C2 levels) have shown better correlation with the AUC but are difficult to obtain in routine clinical practice.

The principal adverse reactions to cyclosporine therapy are kidney dysfunction and hypertension. Tremor, hirsutism, hyperlipidemia, hyperuricemia, and gingival hyperplasia are also frequently encountered. Nephrotoxicity occurs in the majority of patients and is the major reason for the cessation or modification of therapy. Cyclosporine causes a dose-related, reversible renal vasoconstriction that particularly affects the afferent arteriole. In the long term, fibrosis occurs as a consequence of both chronic ischemia and cyclosporine-enhanced TGF-β expression. The increased production of TGF-β also promotes cancer progression through its effect on the proliferation of tumor cells. Thrombotic microangiopathy (TMA) is an uncommon but distinct form of CNI-induced endothelial toxicity. It can be systemic or limited to the kidney, and it usually responds to withdrawal of the CNI.

Tacrolimus (FK506; Prograf; Astellas Pharma Us, Inc.), a macrolide antibiotic produced by *Streptomyces tsukubaensis*, was approved for the prophylaxis of kidney transplant rejection in 1997. Because of slightly greater efficacy, particularly in African-American recipients and those with delayed graft function, and ease of blood level monitoring, tacrolimus has become the preferred CNI. Oral bioavailability is about 25%, and $T_{1/2}$ of tacrolimus is 8 to 12 hours. As with cyclosporine, tacrolimus is extensively metabolized in the gut and liver by CYP3A, and the majority is excreted in the feces. The recommended initial oral dose is 0.1 mg/kg/day in two divided doses, when used in combination with mycophenolate. Trough tacrolimus levels seem to correlate better with the drug AUC and with clinical events than they do for cyclosporine. The first generic tacrolimus product gained US Food and Drug Administration (FDA) approval in August 2009. Dose requirements and trough levels are similar between brand and generic tacrolimus, but postconversion monitoring is prudent because patients may require dose titration. Care should also be taken when switching from one generic version to another. Two extended release formulations of tacrolimus, which allow once-daily dosing, have been approved by the FDA for use in kidney transplant recipients: Astagraf XL (Astellas Pharma Us, Inc.) in 2013 and Envarsus XR (Veloxis Pharmaceuticals, Inc.) in 2015. Compared with both immediate release tacrolimus and Astagraf XL, Envarsus XL demonstrates greater bioavailability (higher AUC_{24}) and a flatter pharmacokinetic profile (lower C_{max} and more prolonged time to peak of 6 hours), which can help attenuate the higher peak concentrations in CYP3A5 expressers. Of note, when converting from immediate release tacrolimus to an extended release formulation, a conversion factor (approximately 1.25 for Astagraf XL and 0.8 for Envarsus XR) needs to be applied to the total daily dose due to the difference in pharmacokinetics. Similar to cyclosporine, nephrotoxicity is a limiting factor with tacrolimus. Neurotoxicity (e.g., tremor, headache, paresthesias, seizures), hyperglycemia, hypomagnesemia, and gastrointestinal (GI) complaints tend to occur more commonly in patients on tacrolimus as compared with cyclosporine, whereas elevations in uric acid and low-density lipoprotein (LDL) cholesterol are less common. Diarrhea and alopecia are common in patients on both tacrolimus and mycophenolate. Unlike cyclosporine, tacrolimus does not cause hirsutism or gingival hyperplasia.

Both cyclosporine and tacrolimus are extensively metabolized by hepatic microsomal enzymes, especially CYP3A, as well as through P-glycoprotein, and interact with a wide variety of commonly used drugs. These interactions are better characterized for cyclosporine but usually apply to both drugs. CYP3A inhibitors can decrease cyclosporine metabolism and increase blood cyclosporine concentrations (Table 61.2). These include nondihydropyridine calcium channel blockers (e.g., verapamil, diltiazem), antifungal agents (e.g., fluconazole, ketoconazole), antibiotics (e.g., erythromycin), human immunodeficiency virus protease inhibitors (e.g., ritonavir), and other drugs (e.g., amiodarone). Grapefruit juice inhibits CYP3A and the P-glycoprotein multidrug efflux pump and can increase the blood concentrations of both CNIs. In contrast, hepatic microsomal inducers, such as some antibiotics (e.g., nafcillin, rifampin), anticonvulsants (e.g., phenobarbital, phenytoin), and St. John's wort (*Hypericum perforatum*), can decrease cyclosporine and tacrolimus blood levels. Cyclosporine and tacrolimus also affect the concentration of other drugs by competing for the hepatic microsomal system and plasma protein binding, and they decrease the clearance of drugs, such as statins, digoxin, and methotrexate. Close monitoring of drug levels and attention to dosage are required when such combinations are used. CNI nephrotoxicity can also be exaggerated by the combination with amphotericin, aminoglycosides, and nonsteroidal antiinflammatory drugs.

Antiproliferative/Antimetabolite Agents

Azathioprine (Imuran; Prometheus Laboratories Inc.) is an imidazolyl derivative of 6-mercaptopurine, which inhibits de novo purine synthesis. Cell proliferation is thereby blocked, impairing a variety of lymphocyte functions. Azathioprine was the first chemical immunosuppressive agent used in organ transplantation. It has been superseded by mycophenolate in current clinical practice, except in women who are pregnant or desirous of pregnancy, in whom the use of mycophenolate is contraindicated. Oral bioavailability of azathioprine is about 50%, and it is metabolized by oxidation and methylation in the liver and/or erythrocytes. The

TABLE 61.2	Notable Drug Interactions with Cyclosporine	
Drug Class	**Agents**	**Effect on Cyclosporine Level**
Anticonvulsants	Barbiturates, phenytoin, carbamazepine, oxcarbazepine	↓
Antibiotics	Nafcillin, IV trimethoprim, imipenem, cephalosporins, terbinafine	↓
	Clarithromycin, erythromycin, telithromycin	↑
Antifungals	Ketoconazole, fluconazole, itraconazole, voriconazole	↑
Antimycobacterials	Rifampin, rifabutin (to a lesser extent)	↓
	Pyrazinamide	↑
Antiretrovirals	Efavirenz, etravirine, nevirapine	↓
	Atazanavir, boceprevir, darunavir, delavirdine, fosamprenavir, indinavir, ritonavir, saquinavir, telaprevir	↑
Antiarrhythmics	Amiodarone, dronedarone, quinidine	↑
Calcium channel blockers	Diltiazem, nicardipine, verapamil	↑
Food and herbs	St. John's wort	↓
	Grapefruit juice	↑
Glucocorticoids	Methylprednisolone, prednisone	May ↓ or ↑ via CYP3A4 induction or competitive inhibition

major side effect is myelosuppression, which can be severe if it is used in combination with allopurinol. Allopurinol inhibits the enzyme xanthine oxidase, which converts azathioprine to inactive 6-thiouric acid. Other adverse effects of azathioprine include hepatotoxicity, alopecia, GI toxicity, pancreatitis, and increased risk for neoplasia.

MMF (CellCept; Roche Laboratories Inc.) is a prodrug that is rapidly hydrolyzed to the active drug mycophenolic acid (MPA), a selective, noncompetitive, reversible inhibitor of inosine monophosphate dehydrogenase (IMPDH). B and T cells lack nucleotide salvage pathways, are highly dependent on de novo purine synthesis for cell proliferation, and are, therefore, selectively inhibited by this drug. MMF is indicated for the prophylaxis of transplant rejection and is typically used in combination with a CNI and glucocorticoids. In addition, it has benefits in the treatment of acute and chronic rejection, which arise from its ability to inhibit the recruitment and interaction of mononuclear cells and to prevent the development and progression of proliferative arteriolopathy, respectively. The typical starting dose is 1 g twice daily, although a higher dose (1.5 g twice daily) often is recommended for African-American recipients. The parent drug is cleared from the blood within a few minutes, and MPA in turn is conjugated to glucuronide (MPAG) before excretion in bile. Enterohepatic cycling of MPAG occurs, producing a second peak at 5 to 6 hours, after which MPAG is excreted in the urine. Although oral bioavailability is about 90% with a $T_{1/2}$ of 12 hours, plasma concentrations of MPA after a single dose in kidney transplant patients within the first month are about half of those found in healthy volunteers or long-term transplant recipients. A generic version of MMF was approved in 2009 and can be safely substituted for Cellcept. As with the use of tacrolimus and cyclosporine generics, it is important to ensure that patients consistently receive the same generic product, that patients and clinicians are aware when substitutions occur, and that enhanced vigilance is provided during the transition.

The principal toxicities of MMF are GI and hematologic. These include leukopenia, anemia, diarrhea, abdominal pain, and vomiting. An enteric-coated form of MPA (Myfortic; Novartis Pharmaceuticals Corporation) is also available, which anecdotally has superior GI tolerability, although this has not been demonstrated convincingly in controlled studies. There is also an increased incidence of certain infections with MMF, especially sepsis associated with cytomegalovirus (CMV) and an association with progressive multifocal leukoencephalopathy (PML) caused by John Cunningham (JC) virus. Because of the higher potency of cyclosporine in interrupting enterohepatic circulation, the combination of MMF with tacrolimus leads to higher AUC for MPA and is more immunosuppressive than the combination with cyclosporine. The use of MMF in pregnancy is associated with congenital malformations and increased risk for pregnancy loss. Women of childbearing potential must adhere to a Risk Evaluation and Mitigation Strategy (REMS) and use effective contraception while taking MMF.

Sirolimus or rapamycin (Rapamune; Wyeth Pharmaceuticals Inc.) is a macrocyclic lactone produced by *Streptomyces hygroscopicus*. It also forms a complex with FKBP-12, but unlike with tacrolimus, this complex binds to and inhibits the protein kinase mTOR, leading to a cell-cycle arrest in the G1 phase. It is absorbed rapidly after an oral dose, and bioavailability is about 15%. It is extensively metabolized in the liver by CYP3A4 and P-glycoprotein. The blood $T_{1/2}$ after multiple doses in stable kidney transplant patients is 62 hours. It is usually dosed once daily, with target trough blood levels of 5 to 15 ng/mL. Everolimus (Zortress;

Novartis Pharmaceuticals Corporation) is closely related chemically and clinically to sirolimus, but has a shorter $T_{1/2}$ (23 hours) and, therefore, a shorter time to achieve steady-state drug concentrations. Both sirolimus and everolimus are indicated for the prophylaxis of kidney transplant rejection in combination with a reduced dose of a CNI and glucocorticoids.

Although earlier protocols focused on using mTOR inhibitors (mTOR-i) in combination with early or late CNI withdrawal or minimization, enthusiasm has dampened because of higher rates of acute rejection and graft loss when compared with CNI and an antimetabolite, possibly due to the expansion of CD8 memory T cells. Use of an mTOR-i with a CNI potentially offers an alternative to an antimetabolite with CNI as rates of graft loss and acute rejection are similar and mTOR-i regimens are associated with a reduced risk of CMV infections. The anti-CMV effect of mTOR inhibitors noted in clinical trials may arise from stimulation of interferon-γ–producing T-cells and virus-specific CD8+ T-cells as well as the need for host mTOR activity to produce CMV proteins. Sirolimus has also been associated with the expansion of CD4 regulatory T cells and, therefore, may find utility as part of regimens that promote transplant tolerance. One unique advantage of mTOR-i is its antitumor effect, which arises from inhibition of angiogenesis and G1 to S cell cycle transition. mTOR inhibition has shown clinical benefit in both primary and metastatic Kaposi sarcoma and renal cell carcinoma, and it shows promise in the treatment of other solid and hematologic malignancies. A clinical trial (TUMORAPA study) of conversion from a CNI-based regimen to sirolimus-based regimen in kidney transplant recipients showed a reduction in the incidence of repeat skin cancers without any increase in the risk of acute rejection or graft dysfunction.

The major adverse effects of sirolimus in the early posttransplant period arise from its antiproliferative actions, including impaired wound healing and wound dehiscence, prolonged delayed kidney graft function, and a higher incidence of lymphoceles. Hypercholesterolemia and hypertriglyceridemia, hyperglycemia, bone marrow suppression, oral ulcers, and GI side effects are well known. Rarely, it can cause localized limb edema, angioedema, and interstitial pneumonitis. Due to these adverse effects, the use of an mTOR-i is associated with treatment discontinuation rates of 20%-30%. Sirolimus given alone does not produce acute or chronic decreases in kidney function; however, it can cause direct tubular and podocyte toxicity resulting in hypokalemia and *de novo* or worsened proteinuria, occasionally sufficiently severe to reach criteria for nephrotic syndrome. When mTOR-i are used in combination with standard doses of CNI, there is a potentiation of nephrotoxicity beyond that expected by their pharmacokinetic interaction. For this reason, it is recommended that the CNI dose be reduced when mTOR-i is added. Sirolimus and everolimus are embryotoxic, and their use is contraindicated in pregnancy. Women must use effective contraception while on sirolimus. Reversible oligospermia and reduced testosterone levels have also been described.

Biologics for Maintenance Immunosuppression

Abatacept or CTLA4-Ig (Orencia; Bristol-Myers Squibb Company) contains the binding region of CTLA4 and the constant region of human IgG_1, and it competitively inhibits CD28 (Fig. 61.5). However, CTLA4-Ig was less effective when used in nonhuman primate models of kidney transplantation. Belatacept, or LEA29Y (Nulojix; Bristol-Myers Squibb Company), is a second-generation CTLA4-Ig with two amino acid substitutions

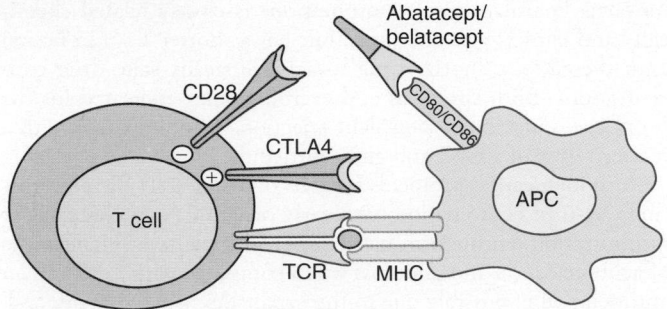

• **Fig. 61.5** Abatacept and belatacept bind to CD80 and CD86 and block costimulation. *APC,* Antigen-presenting cell; *MHC,* major histocompatibility complex; *TCR,* T cell receptor. (From Vincenti F. Costimulation blockade in autoimmunity and transplantation. *J Allergy Clin Immunol* 2008;121:299–306.)

that has higher affinity for CD80 (twofold) and CD86 (fourfold), yielding a 10-fold increase in potency.

Preclinical studies showed that belatacept did not induce tolerance but did prolong graft survival. BENEFIT and BENEFIT-EXT were two randomized, multicenter trials in which adult patients receiving a kidney transplant were randomized to one of three regimens for maintenance immunosuppression: a more intensive (MI) regimen of belatacept, a less intensive (LI) regimen of belatacept, or cyclosporine (Fig. 61.6). Patients in all treatment arms received basiliximab induction and were maintained on MMF and corticosteroids. The demonstration of comparable efficacy to cyclosporine associated with superior kidney function and metabolic parameters led to the LI belatacept regimen receiving FDA approval in 2011 for maintenance immunotherapy in kidney transplantation. The more intense regimen was associated with more infections and PTLD, and, therefore, belatacept is not approved for use in Epstein-Barr virus (EBV)-negative patients. Although belatacept was associated with more rejection episodes, which were also histologically more severe when compared with

those in cyclosporine-treated patients, these rejection episodes lacked other characteristics that are usually associated with poor outcomes, such as the development of donor-specific antibodies. A preexisting repertoire of memory T cells, which are resistant to costimulation blockade and may not be affected by anti-IL2-receptor antibodies, may be responsible for the difference in acute rejection rates. Interestingly, graft function in patients with acute rejection was nevertheless superior to cyclosporine-treated patients without rejection at 1 and 3 years. Further, an analysis of safety and efficacy data at 7 years of follow-up showed a 43% reduction in the risk of death or graft loss for both belatacept regimens as compared with the cyclosporine regimen, again underscoring the contribution of CNI nephrotoxicity to graft dysfunction, graft loss, and cardiovascular disease.

The risk of early acute rejection can be abrogated using belatacept in combination with a depleting induction agent and an mTOR inhibitor, and this strategy could further improve long-term graft outcomes. Belatacept has also been used as part of a CNI-free conversion strategy in stable kidney transplant recipients and has demonstrated superior improvement in GFR with conversion versus CNI continuation.

A second costimulatory pathway involves the interaction of CD40 on activated T cells with CD40 ligand (CD154) on APCs. Two humanized anti-CD154 monoclonal antibodies have been used in clinical trials in kidney transplantation and autoimmune diseases but were associated with thromboembolic events. An alternative approach with monoclonal antibodies to CD40 is more attractive. Although clinical trials of bleselumab (ASKP1240 or 4D11; Astellas Pharma US, Inc.), a fully human anti-CD40 monoclonal IgG4 antibody, provided evidence of efficacy with reduced-dose tacrolimus and steroids, there was an unacceptably high rate of acute rejection, and additional studies in transplantation were placed on hold. Iscalimab (CFZ533; Novartis Pharmaceutical Corporation), a fully human, Fc-silent, nondepleting monoclonal antibody to CD40, has been found to be safe and effective when compared to tacrolimus in early trials; these findings need to be confirmed in an ongoing phase 2 trial.

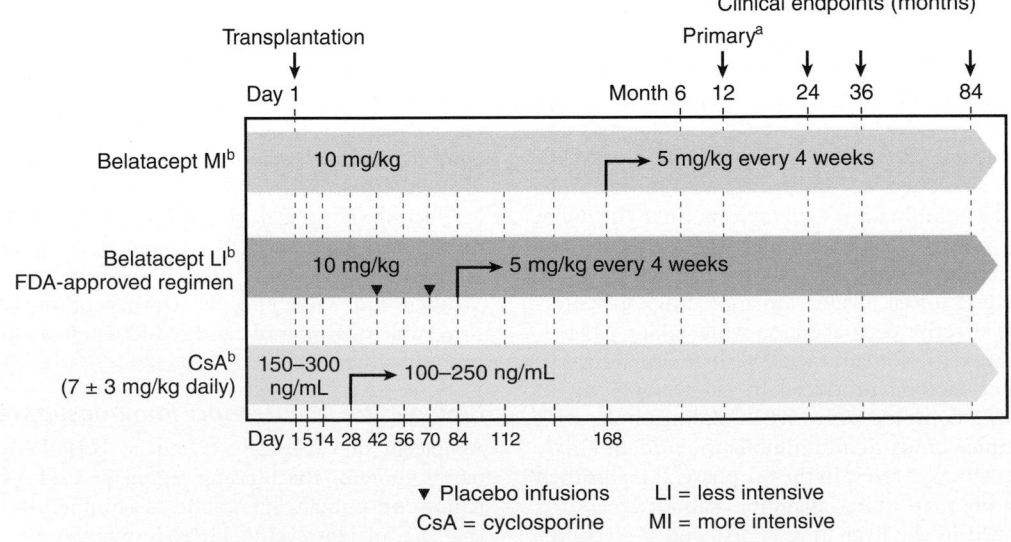

aBelatacept arms unblinded at 12 months.
bAll patients received basiliximab induction, mycophenolate mofetil, and corticosteroid taper.

• **Fig. 61.6** BENEFIT and BENEFIT-EXT study design and medication dosing.

Small Molecules

Cytokine receptors are enticing targets for modulation by new small molecules. Janus kinases (JAK) are important cytoplasmic tyrosine kinases involved in cell signaling. Tofacitinib, or CP-690550 (Xeljanz XR; Pfizer Inc.), inhibits JAK3, which is expressed on NK cells, activated T cells, B cells, and myeloid cells. In clinical trials, it was noninferior to tacrolimus in terms of rejection rates and graft survival. It also showed a lower rate of hyperglycemia but a trend toward more infections including CMV and polyomavirus, and has not currently received approval for use in kidney transplant recipients.

Targeting B Cells and Human Leukocyte Antigen Antibody

Most of the advances in transplantation can be attributed to drugs designed to inhibit T cell responses. As a result, T cell–mediated acute rejection has become much less of a problem. Disappointingly, long-term graft loss rates did not change substantially, even with the reduction in 1-year acute cellular rejection rates to <10% with newer protocols. The development of newer methods to identify donor-specific anti-HLA antibodies (DSA) using single-antigen beads, the recognition histologic features of antibody-mediated injury (C4d staining), and the characterization of gene expression profiles associated with rejection has led to the understanding that a chronic injury mediated by preexisting or de novo alloantibody is the major cause of late graft loss. Therefore, therapies that address B cell responses and the humoral response to the graft are critical not only for the treatment of acute AMR, which is rare, but also to address the larger problem of late graft attrition. Current strategies include B cell depletion, modulation of B cell activation and survival, plasma cell depletion, antibody removal, and inhibition of antibody effector function (Fig. 61.7).

Rituximab (Rituxan; Genentech, Inc.), a chimeric monoclonal antibody directed against CD20 on B cells, causes rapid sustained depletion of circulating and lymphoid B cells for more than 6 months. Because CD20 is not found on pro-B cells or plasma cells, rituximab does not prevent the regeneration of B cells from precursors and does not directly affect immunoglobulin levels, although some studies have reported a reduction in DSA. It has been used pretransplant to reduce high levels of preformed anti-HLA or ABO antibodies, as well as posttransplant to treat acute AMR. It has not yet been rigorously tested in clinical trials. Infusion reactions can occur and are usually prevented by premedication. Rare cases of PML have been associated with its use. Newer, fully human, and humanized monoclonal anti-CD20 antibodies are less immunogenic, more efficacious, and can overcome rituximab resistance. Obinutuzumab (Gazyva; Genentech), also known as *afutuzumab* until 2009, is a fully humanized monoclonal antibody to CD20 on mature B cells that is currently approved by the FDA for the treatment of chronic lymphocytic leukemia in combination with chlorambucil. In an open-label, phase Ib study of 25 highly sensitized patients with ESRD awaiting transplant, obinutuzumab plus IVIG resulted in profound peripheral B cell depletion and reduction of B cells in retroperitoneal lymph nodes. However, reductions in anti-HLA antibodies were limited and not clinically meaningful for most patients.

IVIG is a preparation of human polyclonal IgG (95%) derived from the pooled plasma of adults. The mechanism of action of high-dose IVIG in immune modulation is complex and involves multiple pathways. It provides anti-idiotypic antibodies, reduces

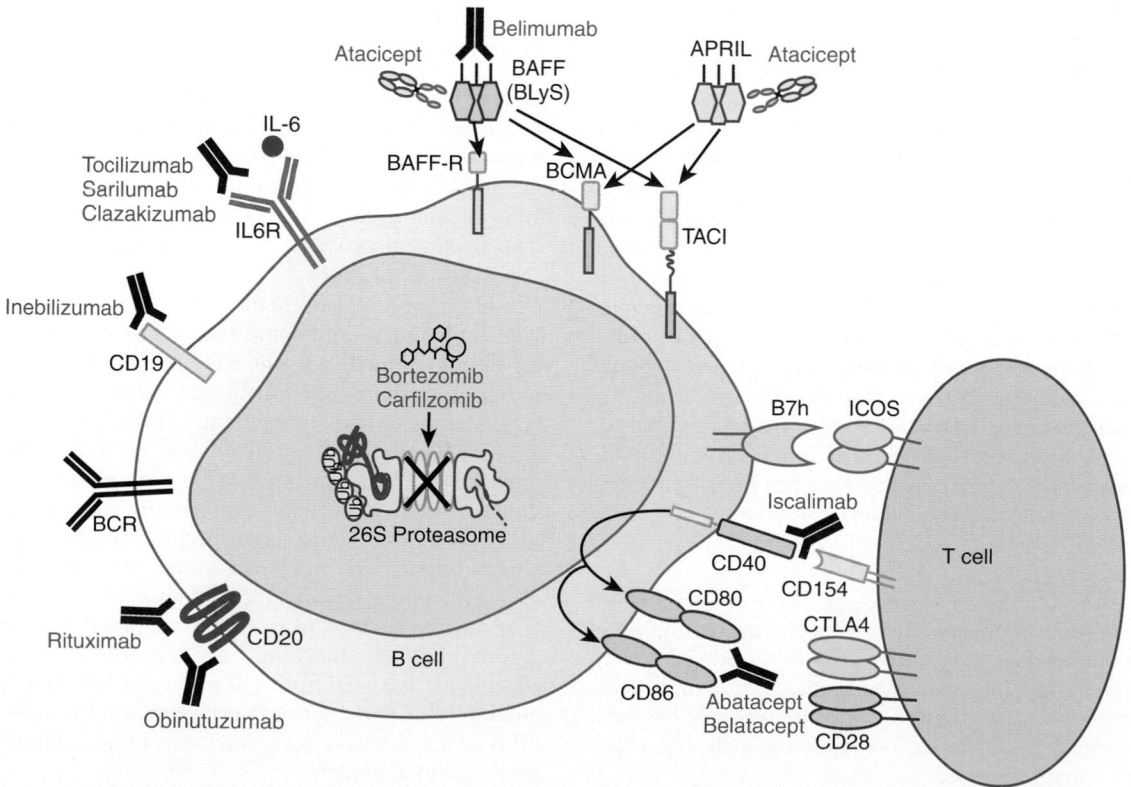

• **Fig. 61.7** Novel strategies targeting humoral alloimmunity. (From Webber A, Hirose R, Vincenti F. Novel strategies in immunosuppression: issues in perspective. *Transplantation.* 2011;91:1057–1064.)

the expression and function of Fc receptors on leukocytes and endothelial cells, increases IgG clearance, downregulates the activation and effector function of T and B cells, and inhibits complement activation and cytokine production. IVIG causes a rapid reduction in DSA and has shown efficacy in clinical trials as part of the desensitization strategies. The standard dose is 2 g/kg up to a maximum of 140 g in a single administration infused over 4 to 8 hours. Minor reactions, such as flushing, chills, headache, nausea, myalgia, and arthralgia, are common; these are reduced with premedication and by slowing the infusion rate. Hemolytic anemia, aseptic meningitis, and thrombotic complications are rare. Acute kidney injury, due to osmotic nephrosis from the sucrose or sorbitol vehicle, is usually self-limited.

Bortezomib (Velcade; Millennium Pharmaceuticals, Inc.) is a 26S proteasome inhibitor that is approved for the treatment of multiple myeloma. Proteasomal inhibition results in the accumulation of misfolded IgG and causes apoptosis of plasma cells. Bortezomib also reduces NF-κB activity by inhibiting the degradation of IκB, which then leads to the reduced transcription of IL-6, a potent plasma cell survival factor. Bortezomib has been used for desensitization, the treatment of acute AMR, and in the experimental protocols of transplant tolerance. The main toxicity of bortezomib is neurologic, with de novo or worsened peripheral neuropathy being common. Hematologic and GI toxicity can also occur. Carfilzomib (Kyprolis; Amgen Inc.) is a second-generation proteasome inhibitor that irreversibly binds to and inhibits the chymotrypsin-like activity of the 20S proteasome. An advantage of carfilzomib over bortezomib is the reduced risk of neuropathy, although cardiac toxicity persists. A prospective trial of desensitization using carfilzomib and plasmapheresis in 15 patients with ESRD showed a significant initial reduction in HLA antibody, but it was followed by a rapid rebound. Based on experimental data from nonhuman primates, the key to preventing rebound is to avoid activation of memory B cells and re-expansion of the germinal center. This is being attempted in early trials using a combination of plasma cell depletion (with proteasome inhibitors or anti-CD28 antibodies) and costimulation blockade.

Eculizumab (Soliris; Alexion Pharmaceuticals, Inc.) is a monoclonal antibody to the complement protein C5, which blocks C5 cleavage and halts the formation of the membrane attack complex. It is approved for the treatment of paroxysmal nocturnal hemoglobinuria and is emerging as a novel therapy for the treatment of acute AMR due to its ability to arrest complement-mediated injury. This creates a window of opportunity for other therapies to clear DSA. Because eculizumab diminishes the defense against encapsulated bacteria, especially meningococci, patients should ideally undergo meningococcal vaccination before receiving the first eculizumab treatment. Plasma-derived C1 esterase inhibitor (Cinryze; Shire Viropharma Inc.) showed initial promise in the treatment of acute AMR, but a phase 3 trial was prematurely terminated due to an interim analysis showing futility.

Treatment of Rejection

Maintenance immunosuppression is effective in preventing acute cellular rejection; however, it is less effective in blocking activated T cells and, thus, in treating established acute rejection or preventing chronic rejection. After the acute rejection episode has been treated, intensification of the maintenance regimen and closer monitoring are often indicated.

Treatment of acute cellular rejection requires the use of agents directed against activated T cells. These include glucocorticoids in high doses (pulse therapy), polyclonal antilymphocyte antibodies, or muromonab-CD3. Steroids reverse about 75% of first acute rejections and are typically tapered down over a few weeks to maintenance doses of 5 to 10 mg/day. Rabbit anti-thymocyte globulin (Thymoglobulin; Genzyme Corporation) has largely replaced OKT3, and it reverses about 90% of severe acute rejections. The treatment of acute AMR consists of strategies to remove DSA (plasmapheresis), decrease antibody production (IVIG, rituximab, and bortezomib), and inhibit complement activation (eculizumab). More recently, the combination of bortezomib with belatacept was found to reverse acute AMR in a case series of six kidney transplant recipients. Further studies are needed to confirm the efficacy and long-term results of this strategy.

The management of chronic allograft rejection is difficult because the histologic changes seen are often irreversible and lead to the progression of kidney disease, regardless of the original injury. Intensification of calcineurin inhibition is generally not effective. C4d positivity or microvascular inflammation in patients with chronic rejection is a marker for ongoing humoral injury, and these patients may benefit from intensification of immunosuppression and IVIG. Treatment with IL-6 blockade using tocilizumab (Actemra; Genentech, Inc.), a monoclonal antibody to the IL-6 receptor, showed significant reductions in DSA and stabilization of kidney function at 2 years in a cohort of 36 kidney transplant recipients with chronic AMR. A phase 3 trial of clazakizumab, a humanized rabbit monoclonal antibody to IL-6, to treat chronic active antibody-mediated rejection in kidney transplant recipients, is currently underway. The risks and benefits of immunosuppression must be weighed carefully at every stage. If graft function continues to deteriorate, immunosuppression should be withdrawn in a stepwise fashion to avoid precipitating acute rejection, and the patient should be prepared for dialysis, preemptive transplant, or comprehensive conservative care.

Tolerance

Operational transplant *tolerance* is defined as prolonged survival of a transplanted organ in the absence of immunosuppression, without evidence of a destructive response. In addition, the recipient should be able to respond normally to immune stimuli, such as infection and tumors. Transplant tolerance is, therefore, an active state of antigen-specific nonresponsiveness, rather than a failure to respond to the allograft.

Chimerism (coexistence of cells from two genetic lineages in a single individual) can be induced by first dampening or eliminating immune function in the recipient and then providing a new source of immune function by adoptive transfer (transfusion) of bone marrow or hematopoietic stem cells. Upon reconstitution of immune function, the recipient no longer recognizes new antigens provided during a critical period as non-self. Early animal studies showed that fetal/neonatal exposure to donor blood cells led to hematopoietic chimerism and specific transplant tolerance. In the precyclosporine era, improved kidney transplant outcomes were seen with donor-specific blood transfusions. These disappeared after the introduction of cyclosporine, presumably due to the efficacy of this drug in blocking T cell activation. It is possible that the effect may have been from cell surface or soluble HLA molecules. Soluble HLA and peptides corresponding to linear sequences of HLA molecules have been shown to induce immunologic tolerance in animal models.

The creation of bone marrow chimeras as a tool for transplant tolerance was first demonstrated when patients who had undergone bone marrow transplantation (BMT) for the treatment of hematologic malignances subsequently underwent successful kidney transplantation for kidney failure from their original BMT donor, without the requirement for maintenance immunosuppression. However, the toxicity of the myeloablative therapy and the risk of lethal graft-versus-host disease (GVHD) precludes this protocol for routine transplantation. Two approaches to reduce toxicity involve the creation of a mixed allogeneic chimera using (a) cytotoxic drugs and thymic irradiation in combination with a limited course of immunosuppression or (b) total lymphoid irradiation (TLI) that targets the thymus, spleen, and supradiaphragmatic lymph nodes. TLI, compared with total body irradiation, resulted in a markedly reduced incidence of GVHD by sparing recipient NK cells, but neither approach has been reliable in achieving durable operational tolerance in HLA-mismatched patients.

Several combinations of biologics can be envisioned as potentially inducing tolerance. Although preclinical trials of a monoclonal antibody to CD40 ligand (CD40L) with CTLA4Ig were promising, clinical trials were halted due to increased thromboembolic events. The combination of belatacept and anti-CD40 antibody may be useful.

Regulatory T cells (T_{regs}) were found to suppress the rejection response of naive T cells in adoptive transfer assays. T_{regs} express the transcription factor FOXP3 that is responsible for their suppressive functions, whereas activated effector T cells do not stably express FOXP3. Several studies involving the use of T_{regs} in kidney transplant recipients as either tolerogenic agents or immunotherapy for graft inflammation are currently under way.

Operational tolerance in transplantation has not yet been routinely achieved. The development of new agents and improved understanding of transplant immunology are now allowing us to create simplified immunosuppressive regimens with low toxicities that have the potential to improve long-term patient and graft survival.

Immune Monitoring

Current monitoring of kidney transplant recipients consists primarily of serial measurements of kidney function and of immunosuppressive drug levels. These methods have limited sensitivity and specificity for the diagnosis of rejection, which is usually made by kidney biopsy. However, a kidney biopsy is invasive, cannot be used for frequent monitoring, and only identifies an established rejection process.

Biomarkers may serve not only as diagnostic parameters but also as predictive tools that anticipate the subsequent development of subclinical and clinical acute rejection. The identification of biomarkers of immune alloreactivity in blood, urine, and tissue would allow the early identification of patients at risk for rejection, the optimization of drug regimens, and the monitoring of responses to changes in therapy. Biomarkers could also guide the development of novel therapies. Studies in human kidney recipients suggest unique protein and genetic signatures that may identify biomarkers of injury as well as potential targets of therapy.

Preformed and de novo anti-HLA antibodies are associated with both acute and chronic AMR and graft loss. Serial monitoring of DSA is used mostly in highly sensitized patients. Recent studies suggest that the development of *de novo* DSA, which occurs in approximately 20% of kidney transplant recipients by 1 year, predicts subsequent development of rejection and graft loss. *De novo* DSA development correlates strongly with HLA eplet mismatch

and immunosuppression non-adherence, and routine monitoring could identify patients at high risk of graft loss and allow for application for mitigation strategies. Further studies are needed to identify the populations that would benefit most from screening and to establish the cost effectiveness of this approach.

Cell-based assays aim to measure recipient T cell reactivity. The cell-mediated lympholysis (CML) assay primarily measures class I alloreactivity through the direct pathway, whereas the mixed lymphocyte culture (MLC) test recognizes class II differences between the recipient and the donor by both direct and indirect recognition pathways. Alloreactive T cells can be measured with flow cytometry-based assays, as well as with HLA class I and class II tetramers. An enzyme-linked immunosorbent spot assay (ELISPOT) can measure the secretion of cytokines, such as IFN-γ from T cells after alloantigen stimulation, and provides a useful means of assessing the indirect pathway. ELISPOT may identify recipients at risk for acute rejection posttransplant, and further testing is under way to establish its role. The ImmuKnow assay (Cylex, Inc.) quantifies the amount of intracellular ATP that is released from CD4 T cells in response to a nonspecific mitogenic stimulus. It is less specific, and changes in test values may be more predictive than single time point assessments. The kidney solid organ response test (kSORT; Immucor, Inc.) is a 17-gene set detected using quantitative polymerase chain reaction (PCR) on peripheral blood samples that is able to predict acute rejection on kidney biopsy up to 3 months in advance.

Donor-derived, cell-free DNA (dd-cfDNA) has emerged as a useful biomarker of allograft injury. In prospective studies, plasma levels of dd-cfDNA have been found to correlate with active rejection, more strongly with antibody-mediated than cellular rejection. This assay is available commercially as AlloSure (CareDx, Inc.) and Prospera (Natera, Inc.). Urine proteomics, as well as messenger RNA (mRNA) isolation, have been proposed as another means of identifying acute rejection, graft IF/TA, and drug toxicity. Urinary mRNA levels of several cytolytic proteins, such as granzyme B and perforin, have been demonstrated to significantly discriminate acute rejection from stable allograft function or tubular necrosis, and are currently undergoing development in commercial assays.

Microarray analysis and real-time PCR of candidate transcripts in allograft tissue obtained from kidney biopsy have demonstrated unique findings in clinical settings, such as ischemia-reperfusion injury, stable graft function, acute rejection, subclinical rejection, and polyomavirus infection. A common rejection module consisting of 11 genes that are significantly overexpressed in acute rejection was initially identified in four different types of transplanted organs. Expression of 10 of these 11 genes was found to be elevated in the urinary cell sediment of kidney transplant patients with acute rejection, and this urinary, 10-gene, expression-based score is being developed further as a urinary biomarker. Transcriptomic analysis of microarray data from >1000 kidney transplant biopsies was used to create classifier scores predicting the presence or absence of rejection. These scores were further analyzed to create "archetypes" which showed 32% disagreement with existing histologic Banff categories (Reeve et al., 2017). Interestingly, graft survival for biopsies with antibody-mediated rejection was better predicted by the molecular archetype than the Banff classification. This assay is now available commercially as the Molecular Microscope Diagnostic System for Kidney Transplant biopsies or MMDx-Kidney (Transcriptome, Inc.).

The development of reliable biomarkers is crucial for individualizing therapy aimed at extending allograft survival and improving patient health, particularly when incorporating novel immunosuppressive agents, implementing drug minimization protocols, and selecting patients for transplant tolerance trials.

Complete bibliography is available at Elsevier eBooks for Practicing Clinicians.

Key Bibliography

Alloway RR, Woodle ES, Abramowicz D, et al. Rabbit anti-thymocyte globulin for the prevention of acute rejection in kidney transplantation. *Am J Transplant.* 2019;19(8):2252–2261.

Bloom RD, Bromberg JS, Poggio ED, et al. Circulating Donor-Derived Cell-Free DNA in Blood for Diagnosing Active Rejection in Kidney Transplant Recipients (DART) Study Investigators. Cell-free DNA and active rejection in kidney allografts. *J Am Soc Nephrol.* 2017;28(7):2221–2232.

Halloran PF. Immunosuppressive drugs for kidney transplantation. *N Engl J Med.* 2004;351(26):2715–2729.

Redfield RR, Jordan SC, Busque S, et al. Safety, pharmacokinetics, and pharmacodynamic activity of obinutuzumab, a type 2 anti-CD20 monoclonal antibody for the desensitization of candidates for renal transplant. *Am J Transplant.* 2019;19(11):3035–3045.

Reeve J, Böhmig GA, Eskandary F, et al. Assessing rejection-related disease in kidney transplant biopsies based on archetypal analysis of molecular phenotypes. *JCI Insight.* 2017;2(12):e94197.

Scandling JD, Busque S, Shizuru JA, et al. Induced immune tolerance for kidney transplantation. *N Engl J Med.* 2011;365(14):1359–1360.

Tremblay S, Driscoll JJ, Rike-Shields A, et al. A prospective, iterative, adaptive trial of carfilzomib-based desensitization. *Am J Transplant.* 2020;20(2):411–421.

Vincenti F, Rostaing L, Grinyo J, et al. Belatacept and long-term outcomes in kidney transplantation. *N Engl J Med.* 2016;374(4):333–343.

Vincenti F, Silva HT, Busque S, et al. Evaluation of the effect of tofacitinib exposure on outcomes in kidney transplant patients. *Am J Transplant.* 2015;15.1644–1653.

Wiebe C, Gibson IW, Blydt-Hansen TD, et al. Rates and determinants of progression to graft failure in kidney allograft recipients with de novo donor-specific antibody. *Am J Transplant.* 2015;15(11):2921–2930.

62

Infectious Complications of Kidney Transplantation

MICHAEL G. ISON

Infections are among the more common complications following kidney transplantation. While advances in surgical techniques and modern induction and maintenance immunosuppression regimens have improved the outcomes of the allograft, they have also changed the risk of posttransplant infections over time. For example, lymphocyte depletion induction combined with tacrolimus-mycophenolate-based maintenance has resulted in an increase in the frequency of BK virus nephropathy. To counter the enhanced risk of infection, broader use of modern antimicrobial prophylaxis is deployed in an attempt to delay and reduce the incidence of posttransplant infections. This chapter will summarize the timing of infectious complications, discuss key issues related to donor-derived disease transmission and methods to mitigate the risk of these events, review key strategies to minimize the risk of infectious complications following kidney transplantation, and finish with focused reviews of common infections complicating kidney transplantation (BK virus nephropathy [BKVN], cytomegalovirus [CMV] diarrhea, and urinary tract infections [UTI]).

Timing of Infectious Complications in Kidney Transplantation

Infectious complications typically occur in one of three time periods posttransplant: early posttransplant, during peak immunosuppression, and late onset. A number of donor- and recipient-specific factors impact the timing of infections, including preexisting infection or immunity, the use of antimicrobial prophylaxis, and the net state of immunosuppression. Of these, the net state of immunosuppression requires the closest consideration as there are no direct measures to assess the impact of various factors on risk of rejection or infectious complications. Instead, the clinician must assess a variety of factors including current and past immunosuppression; underlying immunodeficiency; neutropenia; lymphopenia; complex metabolic conditions, such as presence of uremia, malnutrition, poorly controlled diabetes mellitus, and cirrhosis; and replication of immunomodulatory viruses, including HIV, CMV, Epstein-Barr virus (EBV), hepatitis B, and hepatitis C. Review of immunosuppression must keep in mind both medications that may not be readily apparent on the patient's medication list (i.e., alemtuzumab for induction or rituximab for the treatment of antibody-mediated rejection as such antibody-based immunosuppression may have longstanding impacts of components of

the immune system) as well as the impact of recent immunosuppression, such as recent rejection treatment, high plasma levels of tacrolimus, or recent conversion from one immunosuppression agent to another. For example, with many immunosuppression conversions, the patient is effectively exposed to multiple agents with effective immunosuppression as one agent is titrated off and another is titrated on. Taken together, these inform the net state of immunosuppression for an individual patient.

Early posttransplant infections are infections that occur in the first 30 days after transplantation. The majority of such infections (~98%) are those one would see in any surgical patient, but they may be more severe or more common. The most common postsurgical infections include deep and superficial surgical site infections, hospital-acquired pneumonias as a consequence of mechanical ventilation, urinary tract infections due to bladder catheterization, bacteremia secondary to use of intravenous catheters, and *Clostridium difficile* colitis as a complication of perioperative antimicrobial utilization. Management approaches for such infections are consistent with the local epidemiology and susceptibility of predicted pathogens and published guidelines. Rarely, donor-derived infections may present during the first 30 days posttransplant, as discussed in greater detail below. Finally, recipient-origin infections may manifest in the first 30 days. These include respiratory viral infections, such as influenza, or occult bacteremia that were incubating in the candidate at the time he or she presented for the transplant procedures.

Infections during peak immunosuppression are typically opportunistic infections or pathogens that reactivate from latent infection in the recipient; these generally occur between 30 days and 6 months posttransplant, or within 3 months of treatment of rejection. Use of prophylactic antimicrobials may delay the onset of such infections, resulting in later than typical onset. For example, high-risk CMV donor seropositive, recipient seronegative (D+/R–) patients frequently will be given 6 months of anti-CMV prophylaxis, and, as a result, CMV incidence peaks 1–3 months after such prophylaxis is discontinued. Examples of infections that typically occur during the period of peak immunosuppression include BK virus, CMV, HSV, VZV, HBV, HCV, tuberculosis, Listeria, Strongyloides, and Chagas.

Late-onset infections are infections that typically present greater than 6 months posttransplant, or greater than 3 months after treatment for a rejection episode. Most late-onset infections are community-acquired infections, such as community-acquired pneumonia, respiratory viral infections including influenza, and urinary tract infections. Such infections may lead to hospitalization or require aggressive antimicrobial therapy for treatment. Patients may acquire infections from exposure to the environment or travel, which increases over time as the patient returns to normal function. Examples of environmental exposures include endemic mycoses, including histoplasmosis, blastomycosis, and coccidiomycosis, West Nile Virus, and travel-associated malaria. Some opportunistic infections notoriously present late, including Nocardiosis, mucormycosis, and JC virus-mediated progressive multifocal leukoencephalopathy (PML). Lastly, some infections such as CMV, EBV-positive and EBV-negative posttransplant lymphoproliferative disorder (PTLD), hepatitis, and TB may present in this late period. *Pneumocystis jirovecii* (PCP) historically was an infection complicating the period of peak immunosuppression, although, with universal prophylaxis, most cases of PCP occur late posttransplant in the current era.

Donor-Derived Infections and Risk Mitigation Strategies

Donor-derived infections are defined as any infection present in the donor that is transmitted to the recipient with the transplanted organ or vessels. Donor-derived infections can be categorized as either expected disease transmissions, where the pathogen is known to be present in the donor at the time of procurement and steps are taken to mitigate the disease transmission, or unexpected disease transmissions, when the donor is not recognized to have an infection that is identified after resulting in clinical disease in one or more of the transplant recipients. Examples of expected disease transmissions include CMV or EBV, in which the donor is recognized to have an infection and the recipient is either monitored for evidence of disease or given prophylactic medications to prevent clinical diseases. Examples of unexpected disease transmissions include bacteria (*E. coli*, Mycobacteria tuberculosis, and *S. aureus*), fungi (Candida, Cryptococcus, and Histoplasmosis), parasites (Chagas, Strongyloides, and Acanthamoeba), and viruses (lymphocytic choriomeningitis virus (LCMV), rabies, HIV, and HCV). In the United States, any documented or suspected unexpected donor-derived disease transmissions need to be reported to the Organ Procurement and Transplantation Network (OPTN) as soon as possible, but not greater than 24 hours after initially suspecting transmission (OPTN Policy 15.4); the report is made through the Patient Safety Portal. Timely reporting of suspected transmissions is essential to facilitate communication and rapidly allow screening and treatment of recipients of other organs from the same donor. Data on such disease transmissions have been collected and categorized based on standardized methodologies.

There are several ways in which potential living and deceased donors can be screened to mitigate the risk of disease transmission. All prospective donors should undergo a careful review of their medical and social history, have a physical examination of the donor and the potential organs, and receive a thorough testing of blood. The donor medical and social history should be reviewed for history of documented infection or exclusion from blood donation. The donor's social history should be reviewed for residence or travel to regions of endemicity for potentially transmissible infections, including Chagas, Coccidiomycosis, *Mycobacteria tuberculosis*, Strongyloidosis, Toxoplasmosis, and West Nile Virus. Patients with evidence of prior exposures to such potentially transmissible diseases should be screened for latent infection, and such

TABLE 62.1	US Public Health Service Definitions of Donors at Increased Risk of HIV, HBV, and HCV Transmission

All Age Groups

- Sex (i.e., any method of sexual contact, including vaginal, anal, and oral) with a person known or suspected to have HIV, HBV, or HCV infection
- Man who has had sex with another man
- Sex in exchange for money or drugs
- Sex with a person who had sex in exchange for money or drugs
- Drug injection for nonmedical reasons
- Sex with a person who injected drugs for nonmedical reasons
- Incarceration (confinement in jail, prison, or juvenile correction facility) for ≥72 consecutive hours
- Unknown medical or social history

Pediatric Donors

- Child breastfed by a mother with HIV infection
- Child born to a mother with HIV, HBV, or HCV infection

HIV, Human immunodeficiency virus; *HBV,* hepatitis B virus; *HCV,* hepatitis C virus. For all risk factors, incident to have occurred within 30 days of organ donation.

screening is required for living donors (OPTN Policy 15.3). The social history should also be reviewed for risk factors that place the donor at increased risk of transmission of HIV, HBV, and HCV, as defined by the US Public Health Services, as summarized in Table 62.1. Recently, OPTN policy markedly changed the approach to categorizing donors at increased risk of infection transmission and how they are handled. Historically, these donors required special informed consent and focused posttransplant testing. With the most recent revisions, the period of risk in the donor was reduced to 30 days, education about risks was incorporated into standard education on all patients, and all patients are to have HIV, HBV, and HCV polymerase chain reaction (PCR)-based testing at 4-6 weeks posttransplant; liver transplant patients are also required to have HBV testing at 1 year. There is no longer a requirement for special informed consent.

Donors with recognized infections require additional attention (Table 62.2). While full discussion of relevant risk and prevention strategies are available elsewhere, three unique situations warrant review here: HBV infection in the donor, bacteremic donors, and donors with meningitis or encephalitis. Required screening of donors includes hepatitis B surface antigen (HBsAg) and hepatitis B core antibody (HBcAb); many donors may also have HBV nucleic acid testing (NAT) available. Donors with detectable virus by positive HBV NAT or HBsAg have active infection and can transmit infection to kidney recipients. As such, these are typically reserved for recipients with preexisting HBV infection, typically with the use of HBV-active antivirals to prevent replication. Transplant of HBV-infected donor kidneys in select hepatitis B surface antibody (HBsAb)-positive recipients has been described with typically excellent outcomes, but in the setting of careful monitoring, antiviral medication, and informed consent. Donors with HBcAb positivity alone have a history of infection with HBV, which remains latent. Since these individuals account for up to 15% of the donor population, there is a greater body of evidence on the outcomes of recipients of such donors. Typically, HBcAb+ donors are utilized in recipients with prior HBV vaccination and positive HBsAb titers of >10 IU/L (although optimal protection is with ≥100 IU/L). Outcomes of such transplants are generally excellent without the need for

TABLE 62.2	Screening Assays for Living and Deceased Organ Donors

Required Screening for All Living and Deceased Donors

- Anti-HIV I, II, or Combined HIV Antibody-Antigen Assay
- HIV NAT
- Hepatitis B: HBsAg, HBcAb, HBV NAT
- Hepatitis C: Anti-HCV, HCV NAT
- Syphilis screening
- Anti-CMV
- EBV serological testing
- Blood and urine cultures (deceased donors only)
- Toxoplasmosis

Screening for Endemic Infections (Required for Living Donors with Relevant Risks)

- Strongyloides
- Tuberculosis
- *T. cruzi* (Chagas disease)
- West Nile virus

Optional Screening Test

- HSV (herpes simplex) IgG antibody
- Varicella-zoster virus antibody
- Measles antibody
- Mumps antibody
- Rubella antibody
- HHV8 serology

HIV, Human immunodeficiency virus; *HBV,* hepatitis B virus; *HCV,* hepatitis C virus; *EBV,* Epstein Barr virus; *HHV,* human herpesvirus; *CMV,* cytomegalovirus; *NAT,* nucleic acid testing.

antivirals with a low rate of HBV transmission, typically 4% or lower. Such patients should be monitored for HBV replication posttransplant. If HBcAb+ donors are used in HBsAb-negative recipients, antivirals can be considered until vaccination is given to the recipient.

Donors with bacteremia are another group that requires careful consideration as they compromise up to 5% of organ donors. Donors with active bacteremia pose a clear risk of disease transmission, and use of these organs requires careful consideration, informed consent of the recipient, and posttransplant antibacterial therapy. Most cases of transmission have involved resistant bacteria or recipients who receive inadequate therapy. Generally, it is recommended that the bacteremic donor receives effective antimicrobial treatment (targeted at the causative bacteria with known susceptibility patterns) for at least 24–48 hours and that the donor has ideally some degree of clinical response (improved white blood cell count, improved hemodynamics, defervescence). The donor should be carefully assessed for the presence of metastatic infection, particularly in the organ to be transplanted, and for endocarditis when there is more than transient bacteremia or risk factors (i.e., intravenous drug use, recent dental work). Use of donors with gram-negative bacteria producing carbapenemases, which usually exhibit extended drug-resistant phenotypes and remain susceptible to only a few antibiotics, must be done with caution and with active engagement of Transplant Infectious Diseases experts as these pose the highest rates of disease transmission and active agents may be associated with nephrotoxicity. Recipients are typically treated for at least 14 days of active antibiotic posttransplant and then monitored closely for evidence of recrudescent bacteremia.

Organs from donors with documented bacterial meningitis, with or without bacteremia, can generally be safely utilized with little risk of disease transmission. Generally, donors are treated for 24–48 hours with antibiotics directed at the identified bacteria prior to procurement, optimally with evidence of clinical improvement. The recipient is typically treated for 7–14 days posttransplant with antibiotics directed at the cultured bacteria. Meningitis caused by highly virulent or intracellular organisms such as *Listeria* species or *Mycobacteria* are considered a contraindication. Donors with a clinical diagnosis of bacterial meningitis but without positive bacterial cultures have been known to transmit infections and malignancies, and should generally be avoided. Donors with encephalitis, particularly with fever, without a documented cause are frequently associated with disease transmission. Transmission of rabies, parasitic infections, lymphomas, and leukemias has occurred when donors with encephalitis without a proven cause were accepted as organ donors. As such, donors dying of encephalitis without a proven cause should likely be avoided. The one exception are donors with documented *Naegleria fowleri* meningitis/meningoencephalitis in which the risk of disease transmission is low and such donors can generally be safely used.

Infectious Disease Prevention Strategies

While available therapies have improved the outcome of infectious complications of kidney transplantation, prevention remains the key to optimize care of these patients. Prevention strategies include thorough recipient screening, optimization of vaccination of recipients and their contacts, and use of selected antimicrobial prophylaxis. All recipients should be screened pretransplant for HIV, HBV, HCV, CMV, EBV, VZV, measles, mumps, rubella, tuberculosis (with either a PPD or interferon-gamma release assay), and relevant latent endemic infections, including Chagas disease, Coccidiomycosis, and Strongyloides. Patients who plan to travel to underdeveloped regions of the world posttransplant should be seen by travel medicine experts for consideration of protective vaccines prior to transplant and at least 30 days prior to any such travel. Candidates should have a thorough screening to ensure their vaccine status is up to date prior to transplant. Special attention should be paid to candidates with negative VZV serology, who should receive pretransplant varicella vaccine, patients with negative measles, mumps, or rubella titers, who should receive the MMR vaccine, and patients with negative HBsAb who should receive the three-dose HBV vaccine series. Pre- and posttransplant, candidates and their family members should have up-to-date influenza (annually), tetanus-diphtheria-acellular pertussis (Tdap, once every 10 years), and pneumonia vaccine (Table 62.3).

Selected antimicrobial prophylaxis should be given to patients beginning at the time of transplantation. Published guidelines recommend cefazolin or vancomycin plus either aztreonam or a fluoroquinolone given no more than 60 minutes before the skin incision as a single dose. *Pneumocystis jirovecii* prophylaxis consists of trimethoprim-sulfamethoxazole (TMP-SMX) single or double strength daily to three times per week for the first 6–12 months posttransplant; for sulfa-allergic patients, atovaquone 1500 mg daily, dapsone 50–100 mg daily (must not be used with G6PD deficiency), or pentamidine 300 mg nebulized every 4 weeks are alternatives. Prophylaxis for CMV is discussed below, although CMV D-/R- recipients need prevention of VZV and HSV with acyclovir, valacyclovir, or famciclovir for 3-6 months posttransplant. Kidney recipients benefit from UTI prophylaxis while ureteral stents are in place; TMP-SMX daily or cephalexin 500 mg daily is adequate.

TABLE 62.3	Vaccines for Transplant Candidates, Recipients, and Contacts			
Vaccine	**Type**	**Recommended Pretransplant**	**Recommended Posttransplant**	**Safe for Contacts of Transplant Recipients**
Influenza – Injectable	I	YES	YES	YES
Influenza – Intranasal	LA	YES	NO*	NO*
Hepatitis A	I	YES	YES	YES
Hepatitis B	I	YES	YES	YES
Tdap	I	YES	YES	YES
H. influenzae	I	YES	YES	YES
Conjugated S. pneumoniae	I	YES	YES	YES
Polysaccharide S. pneumoniae	I	YES	YES	YES
N. meningitidis	I	YES	YES	YES
Human papillomavirus (HPV)	I	YES	YES	YES
Rabies	I	YES	YES	YES
Varicella	LA	YES	NO	YES
Rotavirus	LA	YES	NO	YES
MMR	LA	YES	NO	YES
BCG	LA	YES†	NO	YES
Anthrax	I	NO	NO	YES
Smallpox	LA	NO	NO	NO
SARS-CoV-2	I	YES	YES	YES

For all vaccines, follow recommended dose and frequency, consistent with national guidelines.
Tdap, Tetanus, diphtheria, acellular pertussis; *MMR,* measles, mumps, rubella; *I,* inactivated; *LA,* live attenuated.
*Can use if no other alternative vaccine available, but monitor for clinical disease.
†Use only if recommended by national guidelines.

Common Infectious Complications of Kidney Transplantation

BK Virus Nephropathy

BK virus is a polyoma virus that infects most children by 3-4 years of age and remains latent in the uroepithelium for the remainder of an individual's life. Immunosuppression results in increased frequency of replication and, in some patients, damage to the kidney and graft loss. Such BK virus nephropathy occurs in 4%–8% of kidney transplant recipients. Rarely, a related polyoma virus, JC virus, can cause similar disease that is clinically indistinguishable from BK virus nephropathy other than levels of JC virus are detected in the blood and urine instead of BK virus. Replication begins in the uroepithelium with initial detection of virus or shed infected cells (decoy cells). This typically precedes spillover of the virus into the blood compartment by 3–6 months. Viremia, without intervention, leads to subsequent development of BK virus nephropathy 1–3 months after initially being detected. As a result of these replication characteristics, routine screening of kidney transplant recipients can identify those at risk. Screening of blood monthly for 9 months then every 3 months until year 2 posttransplant is currently recommended. Screening should also be performed with any rise in creatinine and at the time of any for cause or protocol biopsy. While the gold standard to diagnose BK virus nephropathy (BKNV) is biopsy with immunohistochemical stains for

the large T antigen, plasma viral loads >10,000 are utilized by many to diagnose BK virus nephropathy. Detection of replication should typically prompt reduction of immunosuppression, which has been demonstrated to reduce progression to BKVN. Optimal strategies for reduction of immunosuppression have not be defined in prospective studies; the overall goal is to reduce the net state of immunosuppression. If viruria or viremia persists despite reduction of immunosuppression, further reduction of immunosuppression and use of systemic cidofovir, leflunomide, or intravenous immunoglobulin infusions can be considered; prospective studies have not documented superiority of any specific interventions. Fluoroquinolones have been tried in the past, but multiple prospective, randomized studies failed to demonstrate clinical success so these are not recommended currently for the prevention or management of BK viremia.

Cytomegalovirus

Cytomegalovirus (CMV) remains the most common viral infection complicating kidney transplants. The risk is highest among seronegative recipients of seropositive donor organs (CMV D+/R–). Intermediate risk of CMV is present in the seropositive recipient with slightly higher risk in donor seropositive than donor seronegative. The lowest risk is among D-/R–, which still have an incidence of ~2% due to false-negative serology or posttransplant acquisition of infection. Given the high prevalence of CMV in the donor and recipient populations and the efficacy of antiviral therapy, serologic matching is typically not utilized. Instead, prevention of CMV is achieved with one of three approaches: universal prophylaxis, preemptive monitoring, or a hybrid approach. With universal prophylaxis, all at-risk patients receive prophylaxis with either ganciclovir, valganciclovir, or valacyclovir for a fixed period of time. For preemptive monitoring, patients have regular (weekly or twice weekly) CMV viral load measurements and only receive antivirals when there is documented replication. The hybrid approach applies universal prophylaxis for a period of time and follows it with preemptive monitoring. Universal prophylaxis is frequently the easiest to implement in most settings and is associated with superior graft outcomes but is associated with the high cost of the drug and complications of prophylaxis, including neutropenia, late-onset CMV replication, and development of resistance. Preemptive monitoring requires logistic systems to optimize consistent monitoring but is associated with high rates of rejection and graft loss and can result in emergence of resistance. The hybrid approach intuitively would be the optimal approach, although prospective studies have failed to document consistent superiority to clinical monitoring.

While valacyclovir has been shown to be effective in preventing CMV, it requires high doses with high rates of neurologic side effects. Given the ease and efficacy, most centers use valganciclovir. While approved at 900 mg daily or the GFR-adjusted equivalent dose for prevention, some centers use a lower dose of 450 mg daily or the GFR-adjusted equivalent. This is associated with less neutropenia but may result in high rates of clinical failure. Among high-risk patients, 6 months of valganciclovir is associated with 16% of patients developing CMV. Current guidelines recommend CMV D+/R– and patients given lymphodepleting induction receive 6 months of prophylaxis while lower-risk patients receive 3–6 months of prophylaxis.

In patients who develop CMV viremia or tissue invasive disease, treatment is with full-dose valganciclovir or intravenous ganciclovir. A randomized, controlled trial demonstrated similar outcomes with either approach except in patients with severe CMV, defined as CMV pneumonitis, CMV colitis, or high level CMV replication (>50,000-100,000 copies/mL). As a result, oral valganciclovir 900 mg twice daily or the GFR-adjusted equivalent is preferred for most patients. Intravenous therapy is generally reserved for patients with severe disease or CMV colitis. Treatment is continued until patients have no evidence of CMV end-organ disease and undetectable CMV viral load(s). Historically, a period of secondary prophylaxis has been used after completing therapy. Several studies have raised questions about the utility of secondary prophylaxis and it is generally reserved for selected settings or if CMV-specific immunity remains deficient. Full details on diagnostics and treatment are available in published guidelines. Patients who fail to have clinical or virologic response should be tested for resistance. Management of resistance is complex and is best done by an experienced Transplant Infectious Diseases expert.

Diarrhea

Diarrhea is a frequent complication of kidney transplantation and can be the result of drug side effects, infection, or other causes, including graft-versus-host disease or malignancy, especially PTLD. The optimal approach to diarrhea begins with an initial evaluation of stool for *C. difficile*, Norovirus PCR, stool cultures, Giardia and Cryptosporidium enzyme immunoassay (EIA), and serum CMV viral load. If diarrhea persists with negative studies, reduction of mycophenolic acid can be attempted; if diarrhea persists,

colonoscopy with random biopsies for pathology that includes immunohistochemical stains for CMV should be performed. *C. difficile* is the most common infectious cause of diarrhea among transplant patients and can happen in the context of recent antibiotics or without obvious inciting events. Treatment is consistent with published guidelines, which typically includes either metronidazole, vancomycin, or fidaxomicin. Novovirus is the second most common infectious cause of diarrhea in transplant patients and can result in chronic, often prolonged, diarrhea that may be relapsing and remitting in nature. Reduction of immunosuppression typically does not have a significant impact on viral shedding or diarrhea. Although IVIG, oral immunoglobulin, breast milk, and nitazoxanide have been tried to treat chronic norovirus, superiority or efficacy has not been clearly demonstrated for any one intervention. The focus of therapy should be aggressive hydration and antimotility agents to control diarrhea. The third most common infectious cause of diarrhea is CMV colitis. Approximately 15% of cases of CMV colitis may be demonstrated in the absence of systemic viremia, highlighting the need for colonoscopy for diagnosis. Treatment is with IV ganciclovir, as previously outlined.

Urinary Tract Infections

Urinary tract infections (UTIs) are common among kidney transplant recipients, particularly in patients with frequent pretransplant UTIs, female patients, and patients with foreign material such as stents and drains in the urinary tract. Asymptomatic bacteriuria is a frequent occurrence in transplant patients that does not warrant treatment. Only patients with abnormal urinalysis, symptoms, and >100,000 CFUs of bacteria or Candida on urine culture should be treated with antibiotics. Given rising resistance to fluoroquinolones among enteric gram-negative bacteria, the preferred first-line therapy is cephalexin dosed to kidney function. Definitive therapy is dictated by the specific susceptibility patterns of the cultured organism. Patients with limited cystitis likely can be treated with 3–7 days of antibiotics while patients with bacteremia or signs or symptoms of pyelonephritis, which is more frequent among transplant patients, require a longer course of 14–21 days of therapy. Patients with recurrent UTIs should undergo urologic evaluation for correctable issues in the urinary tract, although surgically addressable problems are rarely identified. While antibiotic-based suppression can be considered, this frequently leads to prolonged worsening resistance and challenges in managing subsequent infections. Nonantibiotic preventative strategies including methenamine hippurate can be tried, and use is associated with a significant reduction in the frequency of UTIs and associated hospitalizations.

Complete bibliography is available at Elsevier eBooks for Practicing Clinicians.

Key Bibliography

Angarone M, Snydman DR. Diagnosis and management of diarrhea in solid-organ transplant recipients: Guidelines from the American Society of Transplantation Infectious Diseases Community of Practice. *Clin Transplant.* 2019;33:e13550.

Danziger-Isakov L, Kumar D. Vaccination of solid organ transplant candidates and recipients: Guidelines from the American Society of Transplantation Infectious Diseases Community of Practice. *Clin Transplant.* 2019;33:e13563.

Dorschner P, McElroy LM, Ison MG. Nosocomial infections within the first month of solid organ transplantation. *Transpl Infect Dis.* 2014;16:171–187.

Echenique IA, Penugonda S, Stosor V, Ison MG, Angarone MP. Diagnostic yields in solid organ transplant recipients admitted with diarrhea. *Clin Infect Dis.* 2015;60:729–737.

Fernandez-Ruiz M, Rodriguez-Goncer I, Parra P, et al. Monitoring of CMV-specific cell-mediated immunity with a commercial ELISA-based interferon-gamma release assay in kidney transplant recipients treated with antithymocyte globulin. *Am J Transplant.* 2020;20:2070–2080.

Fishman JA. Infection in solid-organ transplant recipients. *N Engl J Med.* 2007;357:2601–2614.

Garzoni C, Ison MG. Uniform definitions for donor-derived infectious disease transmissions in solid organ transplantation. *Transplantation.* 2011;92:1297–1300.

Goldman JD, Julian K. Urinary tract infections in solid organ transplant recipients: Guidelines from the American Society of Transplantation Infectious Diseases Community of Practice. *Clin Transplant.* 2019;33:e13507.

Huprikar S, Danziger-Isakov L, Ahn J, et al. Solid organ transplantation from hepatitis B virus-positive donors: consensus guidelines for recipient management. *Am J Transplant.* 2015;15:1162–1172.

Ison MG, Nalesnik MA. An update on donor-derived disease transmission in organ transplantation. *Am J Transplant.* 2011;11:1123–1130.

Jones JM, Kracalik I, Levi ME, et al. Assessing solid organ donors and monitoring transplant recipients for human immunodeficiency virus, hepatitis B virus, and hepatitis C virus infection—U.S. Public Health Service Guideline, 2020. *MMWR Recomm Rep.* 2020;69:1–16.

Kaul DR, Vece G, Blumberg E, et al. Ten years of donor-derived disease: A report of the disease transmission advisory committee. *Am J Transplant.* 2021;21(2):689–702.

Kotton CN, Kumar D, Caliendo AM, et al. The Third International Consensus Guidelines on the Management of Cytomegalovirus in Solid-Organ Transplantation. *Transplantation.* 2018;102:900–931.

Kumar D, Chin-Hong P, Kayler L, et al. A prospective multicenter observational study of cell-mediated immunity as a predictor for cytomegalovirus infection in kidney transplant recipients. *Am J Transplant.* 2019;19:2505–2516.

Malinis M, Boucher HW. Screening of donor and candidate prior to solid organ transplantation: Guidelines from the American Society of Transplantation Infectious Diseases Community of Practice. *Clin Transplant.* 2019;33:e13548.

Razonable RR, Humar A. Cytomegalovirus in solid organ transplant recipients: Guidelines of the American Society of Transplantation Infectious Diseases Community of Practice. *Clin Transplant.* 2019;33:e13512.

van Delden C, Stampf S, Hirsch HH, et al. Swiss Transplant Cohort Study. Burden and timeline of infectious diseases in the first year after solid organ transplantation in the Swiss transplant cohort study. *Clin Infect Dis.* 2020;71(7):e159–e169.

Wolfe CR, Ison MG. Donor-derived infections: Guidelines from the American Society of Transplantation Infectious Diseases Community of Practice. *Clin Transplant.* 2019;33:e13547.

PART 12

Hypertension

63

Pathogenesis of Hypertension

CHRISTOPHER S. WILCOX, WEN SHEN

Hypertension implies an increase in either cardiac output or, more typically, in systemic vascular resistance (SVR). Essential hypertension developing in young adults may be initiated by an increase in cardiac output, associated with signs of overactivity of the sympathetic nervous system; the blood pressure (BP) is labile, and the heart rate is increased. Later, the BP increases further because of a rise in SVR, with return to a normal cardiac output. Most patients in clinical practice with sustained hypertension have an elevated SVR. Over time, vascular remodeling and microvascular rarefaction (loss of vessels and capillaries) contribute a structural component.

The abrupt left ventricular systole creates a shock wave that is reflected back from the peripheral resistance vessels and reaches the ascending aorta during early diastole and is visible in tracings of aortic pressure as the dicrotic notch. With aging, there is loss of elasticity of the conduit vessels that transport the pressure wave more rapidly and an increase in the tone of the resistance vessels that provides the reflected shock wave. Eventually, this shock wave in the aorta coincides with the upstroke of the aortic systolic pressure wave, leading to an abrupt increase in the height of the systolic BP. This accounts largely for the frequent finding of isolated, or predominant, systolic hypertension in the elderly. In contrast, systolic hypertension in the young usually reflects an enhanced cardiac contractility and output.

Pathophysiology of Hypertension

Integration of Cardiorenal Function

The integration of cardiorenal function is illustrated by the response of a normal person to standing. Upon standing, there is an abrupt fall in venous return and, hence, in cardiac output; this elicits a baroreflex response, as resistance vessels constrict to buffer the immediate fall in BP, and capacitance vessels contract to restore venous return, resulting in only a small drop in the systolic BP with a modest rise in heart rate. During prolonged standing, increased renal sympathetic nerve activity enhances the reabsorption of sodium chloride (NaCl) by the kidney tubules, as well as the release of renin from the juxtaglomerular apparatus. Renin release and the subsequent generation of angiotensin II and aldosterone maintain systemic BP and circulating volume. In contrast, the BP of patients with autonomic insufficiency declines progressively upon standing, sometimes to the point of syncope. Patients with autonomic failure vividly illustrate the crucial importance of a stable BP for efficient function of the brain and kidneys. Therefore, it is no surprise that evolution has provided

multiple, coordinated BP-regulatory processes. The understanding of the cause of a sustained change in BP, such as hypertension, requires knowledge of a number of interrelated pathophysiologic processes. The most important and best understood of these are discussed in this chapter.

Kidney Mechanisms and Salt Balance

The kidney has a unique role in BP regulation. Kidney salt and water retention sufficient to increase the extracellular fluid (ECF) volume, blood volume, and mean circulatory filling pressure enhances venous return, cardiac output, and BP. The kidney is so effective in excreting excess fluid during periods of surfeit, or retaining fluid and electrolytes during periods of deficit, that the ECF volume and, specifically, the blood volume normally vary less than 10% with changes in salt intake. Consequently, the role of body fluids in hypertension is subtle. For example, a 10-fold increase in daily NaCl intake in normal subjects increases ECF volume by only about 1 L (about 6%) and normally produces no change, or only a small increase, in BP. Conversely, a diet with no salt content leads to the loss of approximately 1 L of body fluid over 3 to 5 days with only a trivial fall in BP. Different effects can be seen in patients with chronic kidney disease (CKD) whose BP often increases with the level of salt intake. This "salt-sensitive" component to BP increases progressively with the loss of kidney function. Among normotensive subjects, salt-sensitive BP is apparent in about 30% and appears to have a genetic component. Salt sensitivity is almost twice as frequent in patients with hypertension and is particularly common among Black persons, the elderly, and those with CKD. It is generally associated with a lower level of plasma renin activity (PRA).

What underlies salt sensitivity? Normal kidneys are exquisitely sensitive to BP. A rise in mean arterial pressure (MAP) of as little as 1 to 3 mm Hg elicits a subtle increase in kidney NaCl and fluid elimination. This "pressure natriuresis" also works in reverse and conserves NaCl and fluid during decreases in BP. It is rapid, quantitative, and fundamental for normal homeostasis. It is primarily a result of changes in tubular NaCl reabsorption rather than total renal blood flow (RBF) or glomerular filtration rate (GFR). Indeed, kidney autoregulation maintains RBF and GFR remarkably constant during changes in BP. It is the pressure natriuresis mechanism that accurately adjusts salt excretion and body fluids in persons with healthy kidneys across a range of BPs. Two primary mechanisms of pressure natriuresis have been identified.

First, a rise in kidney perfusion pressure increases blood flow selectively through the medulla since medullary blood flow is not as tightly autoregulated as cortical blood flow. These increases in pressure and flow enhance kidney interstitial hydrostatic pressure throughout the kidney, which is an encapsulated organ. This rise in interstitial pressure reduces proximal tubule reabsorption, increases salt excretion, and impairs fluid return to the bloodstream. Second, the degree of stretch of the afferent arteriole regulates the secretion of renin into the bloodstream and, hence, the generation of angiotensin II. Thus, an increase in BP that is transmitted to this site reduces renin secretion. Angiotensin II coordinates the body's salt and fluid retention mechanisms by stimulating thirst and enhancing NaCl and fluid reabsorption in the proximal and distal nephron segments. By stimulating secretion of aldosterone and arginine vasopressin, and inhibiting atrial natriuretic peptide (ANP), angiotensin II further enhances the reabsorption in the distal tubules and collecting ducts. Thus, during normal homeostasis, an increase in BP is matched by a decrease in PRA that reduces sodium reabsorption. It follows that a normal or elevated value for PRA in hypertension is effectively "inappropriate" for the level of BP, and is thereby contributing to the maintenance of hypertension.

The relationships among long-term changes in salt intake, the renin-angiotensin-aldosterone system (RAAS), and BP are shown in Fig. 63.1. Healthy people regulate the RAAS closely with changes in salt intake. An increase in salt intake brings about only a modest rise in MAP, because the RAAS is suppressed and the highly effective pressure natriuresis mechanism rapidly increases NaCl and fluid elimination in the urine sufficiently to restore a near-normal blood volume and BP. Expressed quantitatively in Fig. 63.1, the slope of the long-term increase in NaCl excretion with BP is normally almost vertical. One factor contributing to the steepness of this slope, or the gain of the pressure natriuresis relationship, is the reciprocal changes in the RAAS with BP that dictate appropriate alterations in salt handling by the kidney. Therefore, when the RAAS is artificially fixed, the slope of the pressure natriuresis relationship flattens, resulting in salt sensitivity,

displacement of the set point, and a change in ambient BP. For example, an infusion of angiotensin II into a normal subject raises the BP. Because angiotensin II is being infused, the kidney cannot suppress angiotensin II levels appropriately by reducing renin secretion. Therefore, one component of the pressure natriuresis mechanism is prevented and the BP elevation is sustained without an effective kidney compensation. In contrast, normal individuals treated with an angiotensin-converting enzyme (ACE) inhibitor to block angiotensin II generation or an angiotensin receptor blocker (ARB) to block AT$_1$ receptors have a fall in BP. Again, the kidney cannot stimulate an appropriate effect of angiotensin II and aldosterone that would be required to retain sufficient NaCl and fluid to buffer the fall in BP. Therefore, when the RAAS is fixed, the BP changes as a function of salt intake and becomes highly "salt sensitive" (see Fig. 63.1). These studies demonstrate the unique role of the RAAS in long-term BP regulation and its importance in isolating BP from NaCl intake.

Some recent findings add complexity to these simple relationships. Renin is also generated within the connecting tubule and collecting ducts. This kidney renin may contribute to the very high level of angiotensin within the kidney that does not share the same relationship with dietary salt. Animal models of diabetes mellitus and chronic kidney disease (CKD) demonstrate an increase in local angiotensin generation and action in the kidneys that may contribute to the beneficial effects of ACE inhibitor and ARB therapy, despite often low circulating renin levels. Other studies have shown that prorenin, although not itself active, becomes activated after binding to a renin receptor in the tissues, notably the kidneys. This is important because conventional RAAS antagonists may not block these actions of prorenin.

Four compelling lines of evidence implicate the kidney and RAAS in long-term BP regulation. First, kidney transplant studies in rats showed that a normotensive animal that received a kidney from a hypertensive animal becomes hypertensive, and vice versa. Similarly, human kidney transplant recipients frequently become

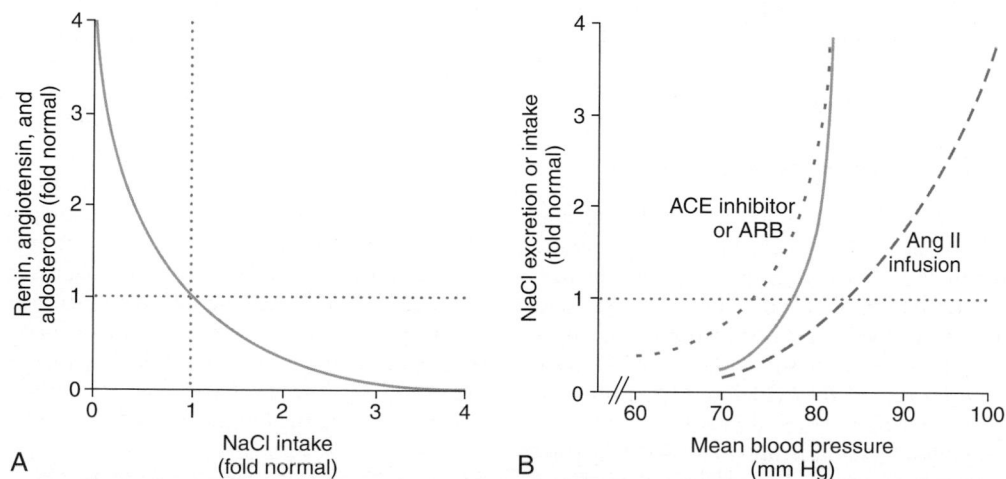

• **Fig. 63.1** (A) Normal steady-state relationship between plasma concentrations of renin, angiotensin II (Ang II), and aldosterone and dietary salt intake. (B) Relationships between sodium excretion relative to intake and mean arterial blood pressure in normal subjects *(solid line)*, in subjects given an angiotensin-converting enzyme (ACE) inhibitor or angiotensin receptor blocker (ARB; *short dashes*), and in subjects given an infusion of Ang II *(long dashes)* to prevent adaptive changes in Ang II levels. *NaCl,* Sodium chloride. (Modified from Guyton AC, Hall JE, Coleman TG, et al. The dominant role of the kidneys in the long-term regulation of arterial pressure in normal and hypertensive states. In: Laragh JH, Brenner BM, eds. *Hypertension, Pathophysiology, Diagnosis and Management.* New York: Raven; 1995:1311–1326.)

hypertensive if they receive a kidney from a hypertensive donor. Apparently, the kidney in hypertension is programmed to retain salt and water inappropriately for a normal level of BP, thereby resetting the pressure natriuresis to a higher level of BP and dictating the appearance of hypertension in the recipient, even if the neurohumoral environment is that of normotension. Nevertheless, recent studies in gene-deleted or transgenic mice subjected to kidney transplantation concluded that the increase in BP during prolonged infusion of angiotensin II was mediated by the combined effects of angiotensin on angiotensin receptors within the kidney and the systemic circulation, most likely involving the kidney afferent arterioles and the brain. A second observation was that the BP was normally reduced 5% to 20% by an ACE inhibitor, an ARB, an aldosterone receptor antagonist, or a renin inhibitor. The fall in BP was greatest in those with elevated PRA values, and it was enhanced by dietary salt restriction or concurrent use of diuretic drugs that stimulate the RAAS (see Fig. 63.1). Third, almost 90% of patients approaching end-stage kidney disease (ESKD) whose kidneys have lost most of their capacity to accurately adjust salt excretion have hypertension. Fourth, the major monogenetic causes of human hypertension involve genes that activate RAAS signaling (such as glucocorticoid-remediable hypertension) or kidney sodium transport (such as Liddle syndrome).

Recent studies have suggested that kidney also plays a role in the pathogenesis of hypertension through activation of ENaC in the collecting ducts by proteases including plasmins. Plasmin is a serine protease converted in the kidney from its precursor plasminogen. An ENaC activated by plasmin engages increased kidney sodium and fluid retention and a rise in BP.

Total-Body Autoregulation

An increase in cardiac output necessarily increases peripheral blood flow. However, each organ has intrinsic mechanisms that adapt its blood flow to its metabolic needs. Therefore, over time, this local tissue mechanism translates an increase in cardiac output into an increase in SVR. The outcome is that organ blood flow is maintained, but hypertension becomes sustained. This total-body autoregulation is demonstrated in human subjects who are given salt-retaining mineralocorticosteroid hormones. An initial rise in cardiac output is translated in most individuals into sustained hypertension from an elevated SVR over 5 to 15 days.

Structural Components to Hypertension

Hypertension causes not only remodeling in the distributing and resistance vessels and the heart, but also fibrotic and sclerotic changes in the glomeruli and interstitium of the kidney. Hypertrophy of resistance vessels limits the ratio of lumen to wall and dictates a fixed component to SVR. This is evidenced by a higher SVR in hypertensive versus normotensive individuals during maximal vasodilatation. Moreover, thickened and hypertrophied resistance vessels have greater reductions in vessel diameter during vasoconstrictor stimulation. This is apparent as an increase in vascular reactivity to pressor agents. Remodeling of resistance arterioles diminishes their response to changes in perfusion pressure. This manifests as a blunted myogenic response contributing to incomplete autoregulation of RBF, thereby adding a component of barotrauma to hypertensive kidney damage. Sclerotic and fibrotic changes in the glomeruli and kidney interstitium, combined with hypertrophy of the afferent arterioles, limit the sensing of BP in the juxtaglomerular apparatus and kidney parenchyma.

This blunts renin release and pressure natriuresis, thereby contributing to salt sensitivity and sustained hypertension. Rats receiving intermittent weak electrical stimulation of the hypothalamus initially had an abrupt increase in BP followed by a sudden fall after the cessation of the stimulus. However, eventually the baseline BP increased in parallel with the appearance of hypertrophy of the resistance vessels, suggesting that vascular remodeling can sustain hypertension. These structural components may explain why it often takes weeks to achieve maximal antihypertensive action from a drug, a reduction in salt intake, or correction of a renal artery stenosis or hyperaldosteronism. Vascular and left ventricular hypertrophy is largely, but usually not completely, reversible during treatment of hypertension, whereas fibrotic and sclerotic changes are not.

Sympathetic Nervous System, Brain, and Baroreflexes

A rise in BP diminishes the baroreflex, thereby reducing the tone of the sympathetic nervous system and increasing the tone of the parasympathetic nervous system. Paradoxically, human hypertension is often associated with an increase in heart rate, maintained or increased plasma catecholamine levels, and an increase in directly measured sympathetic nerve discharge despite the stimulus to the baroreceptors. What is the cause of this inappropriate activation of the sympathetic nervous system in hypertension? Studies in animals show that the baroreflex "resets" to the ambient level of BP after 2 to 5 days. Thereafter, the baroreflex no longer continues to "fight" the elevated BP but defends it at the new higher level. Much of this adaptation occurs within the baroreceptors themselves. With aging and atherosclerosis, the walls of the carotid sinus and other baroreflex-sensing sites become less distensible. Therefore, the BP is less effective in stretching the afferent nerve endings, and the sensitivity of the baroreflex is diminished. This may contribute to the enhanced sympathetic nerve activity and increased plasma catecholamines that are characteristic of elderly hypertensive subjects. Additionally, animal models have identified central mechanisms that alter the gain of the baroreflex process, and, therefore, the sympathetic tone, in hypertension. The importance of central mechanisms in human hypertension is apparent from the effectiveness of drugs, such as clonidine, that act within the brain to decrease the sympathetic tone. The kidneys themselves contain barosensitive and chemosensitive nerves that can regulate the sympathetic nervous system. In one study, hemodialysis patients experienced an increased sympathetic nervous system discharge and increased BP that were not apparent after bilateral nephrectomy. This suggests that the renal nerves were maintaining enhanced sympathetic tone. Based on this pathophysiology, radiofrequency ablation of the renal nerves has successfully improved BP control in some, but not all, studies of patients with drug-resistant hypertension, further illustrating the importance of the renal nerves in setting the long-term level of BP in human subjects.

Endothelium and Oxidative Stress

Calcium-mobilizing agonists, such as bradykinin or acetylcholine, as well as shear forces produced by the flow of blood result in the release of endothelium-dependent relaxing factors, predominantly nitric oxide (NO). NO has a half-life of only a few seconds because of inactivation by oxyhemoglobin or reactive oxygen species (ROS), such as superoxide anion (O_2^-). People with essential hypertension have defects in endothelium-dependent relaxation of peripheral vessels and also diminished NO generation. One underlying mechanism is oxidative stress, with excessive O_2^- formation inactivating NO and leading to functional NO deficiency. Another mechanism is the appearance of inhibitors of nitric oxide synthase (NOS), including asymmetric dimethyl arginine (ADMA). Finally, atherosclerosis, prolonged hypertension, or the development of malignant hypertension causes structural changes in the endothelium that limit endothelial function further. NO inhibits NaCl reabsorption in the loop of Henle and collecting ducts of the kidney. Therefore, NO deficiency not only induces endothelial dysfunction and vasoconstriction but also reduces pressure natriuresis. Functional NO deficiency in large blood vessels contributes to vascular inflammation and atherosclerosis.

Genetic Contributions

The heritability of human hypertension can be assessed from differences in the concordance of hypertension between identical twins (who share all genes and a similar environment) versus nonidentical twins (who share only a similar environment). These studies suggest that genetic factors contribute less than half of the risk for developing hypertension in modern humans. Studies in mice with targeted disruption of individual genes or insertions of extra copies of genes provided direct evidence of the critical regulatory roles for certain gene products in hypertension. Deletions of the gene in mice for endothelial NOS lead to salt-dependent hypertension, and the BP of mice decreases with the number of copies of the gene encoding ACE. While these are compelling examples of circumstances in which a single gene can sustain hypertension, there is increasing recognition of the complexity and importance of gene–gene interactions and the crucial effects of the genetic background on the changes in BP that accompany insertion or deletion of a gene.

Currently there is evidence that certain individual gene defects can contribute to human essential hypertension. However, the net effect on BP is small. Certain rare forms of hereditary hypertension are caused by single-gene defects. For example, glucocorticoid-remediable hyperaldosteronism (GRA) is caused by a chimeric rearrangement of the gene encoding aldosterone synthase that renders the enzyme responsive to adrenocorticotropic hormone (ACTH). Liddle syndrome is caused by a mutation in the gene encoding one component of the endothelial sodium channel that is expressed in the distal convoluted tubule. The mutated form has lost its normal regulation, leading to a permanent "open state" of the sodium channel that dictates inappropriate kidney NaCl retention and salt-sensitive, low-renin hypertension (see Chapters 9, 37, and 65).

Implicated Mediators of Hypertension

Alterations in the synthesis, secretion, degradation, or action of numerous substances are implicated in hypertension. Some of the most important mediators are described in the following paragraphs.

Renin, Angiotensin II, and Aldosterone

The PRA is not appropriately suppressed in most patients with essential hypertension and is above normal values in approximately 15%. Individuals with normal or high PRA have a greater antihypertensive response to single-agent therapy with an ACE inhibitor, an ARB, or a beta-blocker than patients with low-renin hypertension, who respond notably to salt restriction and diuretic therapy. The RAAS is particularly important in the maintenance of BP in patients with renovascular hypertension, although its importance wanes during the chronic phase when structural alterations in blood vessels or damage in the kidney dictate an RAAS-independent component to the hypertension.

Sympathetic Nervous System and Catecholamines

Pheochromocytoma is a catecholamine-secreting tumor, often occurring in the adrenal medulla, which increases plasma catecholamines 10- to 1000-fold. However, even such extraordinary increases in pressor amines are rarely fatal because there is downregulation of the catecholamine receptors. Moreover, an intact pressure natriuresis mechanism reduces the blood volume, thereby limiting the rise in BP. Indeed, such patients can have orthostatic hypotension between episodes of catecholamine secretion (see Chapter 65).

Increased sympathetic nerve tone of resistance vessels in human essential hypertension causes α_1-receptor-mediated vasoconstriction of the blood vessels and β_1-receptor-mediated increases in contractility and cardiac output; these are incompletely offset by β_2-receptor–mediated vasorelaxation of peripheral blood vessels. Increased sympathetic nerve discharge to the kidney leads to α_1-mediated enhancement of NaCl reabsorption and β_1-mediated renin release.

Dopamine

Dopamine is synthesized in the brain and kidney tubular epithelial cells independent of sympathetic nerves. Dopamine synthesis in the kidney is enhanced during volume expansion and contributes to decreased reabsorption of NaCl in the proximal tubule. Defects in tubular dopamine responsiveness are apparent in genetic models of hypertension. Recent evidence relates single-nucleotide polymorphisms of genes that regulate dopamine receptors to human salt-sensitive hypertension.

Arachidonate Metabolites

Arachidonate is esterified as a phospholipid in cell membranes. It is released by phospholipases that are activated by agents such as angiotensin II. Three enzymes principally metabolize arachidonate. Cyclooxygenase (COX) generates unstable intermediates whose subsequent metabolism by specific enzymes yields prostaglandins that are either generally vasodilative (e.g., prostaglandin I_2 [PGI_2]), vasoconstrictive (e.g., thromboxane), or of mixed effect (e.g., PGE_2). COX-1 is expressed in many tissues, including platelets, resistance vessels, glomeruli, and cortical collecting ducts. Inflammatory mediators induce COX-2. However, the normal kidney is unusual in expressing substantial COX-2, which is located in macula densa cells, tubules, medullary interstitial cells, and arterioles. The net effect of blocking COX-1 generally is to retain NaCl and fluid while raising BP and dropping PRA. Blockade of COX-2 has little effect on normal BP, but it can increase BP in those with essential hypertension. Nonsteroidal antiinflammatory agents exacerbate essential hypertension, blunt the antihypertensive actions of many commonly used agents, predispose to acute kidney injury during periods of volume depletion or hypotension, and blunt the natriuretic action of loop diuretics.

In contrast, aspirin reduces BP in patients with renovascular hypertension, testifying to the prohypertensive actions of thromboxane and other prostanoids that activate the thromboxane-prostanoid receptor in this condition. Metabolism of arachidonate by cytochrome P-450 monooxygenase yields 19,20-hydroxyeicosatetraenoic acid (HETE), which is a vasoconstrictor of blood vessels but inhibits tubular NaCl reabsorption. Metabolism of arachidonate by epoxygenase leads to epoxyeicosatrienoic acids (EETs), which are powerful vasodilators and natriuretic agents. Arachidonate metabolites act primarily as modulating agents. Their role in human essential hypertension remains elusive.

L-Arginine–Nitric Oxide Pathway

NO is generated by three isoforms of NOS that are widely expressed in the body. NO interacts with many heme-centered enzymes. Activation of guanylyl cyclase generates cyclic guanosine monophosphate, which is a powerful vasorelaxant and inhibits NaCl reabsorption in the kidney. Defects in NO generation in the endothelium of blood vessels in human essential hypertension may contribute to increased peripheral resistance, vascular remodeling, and atherosclerosis, whereas defects in NO generation in the kidney may contribute to inappropriate NaCl retention and salt sensitivity. NOS activity is reduced in hypertensive human subjects and in those with CKD.

Reactive Oxygen Species

The incomplete reduction of molecular oxygen, either by the respiratory chain during cellular respiration or by oxidases such as nicotinamide adenine dinucleotide phosphate (NADPH) oxidase, yields ROS including superoxide (O_2^-) and peroxynitrite ($ONOO^-$). $ONOO^-$ has long-lasting effects through oxidizing and nitrosylating reactions. Reaction of ROS with lipids yields oxidized low-density lipoprotein (LDL) that promotes atherosclerosis and isoprostanes that cause vasoconstriction, salt retention, and platelet aggregation. Hypertension, especially in the setting of CKD, is a state of oxidative stress. Drugs that effectively reduce O_2^- lower BP in animal models of hypertension, but they are largely unexamined in human hypertension.

Endothelins

Endothelins are produced primarily by cells of the vascular endothelium and collecting tubules. Discrete receptors mediate either increased vascular resistance (type A) or the release of NO and inhibition of NaCl reabsorption in the collecting ducts (type B). Endothelin type A receptors potentiate the vasoconstriction accompanying angiotensin II infusion or blockade of NOS. Endothelin is released by hypoxia, specific agonists such as angiotensin II, salt loading, and cytokines. Nonspecific blockade of endothelin receptors lowers BP in models of volume-expanded hypertension, whereas collecting duct-specific deletion of endothelin B (ETB) receptors increases BP. The role of endothelin in human essential hypertension is unclear.

Atrial Natriuretic Peptide

ANP is released from the heart during atrial stretch. It acts on receptors that increase GFR, decrease NaCl reabsorption in the distal nephron, and inhibit renin secretion. ANP is released during volume expansion and contributes to the natriuretic response. Its role in essential hypertension is unclear. Endopeptidase inhibitors that block ANP degradation are natriuretic and antihypertensive, but also inhibit the metabolism of kinins. Although an increase in kinins may contribute to the fall in BP with endopeptidase or ACE inhibitors, kinins can cause an irritant cough or a more serious anaphylactoid reaction.

Plasminogen and Plasmin

Urinary plasminogen derives from glomerular filtration in proteinuric states. It is converted into plasmin in the tubular lumen by urokinase-type plasminogen activator (uPA). Plasmin is the major protease that activates ENaC and results in sodium and fluid retention. Kidney excretion of plasmin(ogen) correlates with albuminuria, 24-hour ambulatory blood pressure, and, in individuals with CKD and proteinuria, is an independent predictor of hypervolemia. This indicates that activation of ENaC by filtered plasmin(ogen) may contribute to hypertension.

Pathogenesis of Hypertension in Chronic Kidney Disease

The prevalence of salt-sensitive hypertension increases proportionally as GFR declines. Hypertension is almost universal in patients with CKD caused by primary glomerular or vascular disease, whereas those with primary tubulointerstitial disease may be normotensive or, occasionally, salt losing.

With declining nephron number, CKD limits the ability to adjust NaCl excretion rapidly and quantitatively during changes in intake. The role of ECF volume expansion is apparent from the ability of hemodialysis to lower BP in patients with kidney failure.

Additional mechanisms besides primary fluid retention contribute to the increased SVR and hypertension in patients with CKD. In dialysis patients, the kidneys generate abnormal afferent nerve impulses, which entrain an increased sympathetic nerve discharge that is reversed by bilateral nephrectomy. Plasma levels of endothelin increase with kidney failure. CKD also induces oxidative stress, which contributes to vascular disease and impaired endothelium-dependent relaxation. A decreased generation of NO from L-arginine follows the accumulation of ADMA, which inhibits NOS. The thromboxane-prostanoid receptor is activated and contributes to vasoconstriction and structural damage.

Clearly, hypertension in CKD is multifactorial, but volume expansion and salt sensitivity are predominant. Pressor mechanisms mediated by angiotensin II, catecholamines, endothelin, or thromboxane-prostanoid receptors become more potent during volume expansion. This fact may underlie the importance of these systems in patients with kidney failure. Finally, many of the pathways that contribute to hypertension in kidney failure (such as impaired NO generation and excessive production of endothelin, ROS, and ADMA) also contribute to atherosclerosis, cardiac hypertrophy, and progressive kidney fibrosis and sclerosis. Indeed, kidney damage in poorly treated hypertension further enhances hypertension, which itself engenders further kidney damage, generating a vicious spiral culminating in accelerated hypertension, progressively diminishing kidney function, and the requirement for kidney replacement therapy. Therefore, rational management of hypertension in CKD first entails salt-depleting therapy with a salt-restricted diet and diuretic therapy. Patients frequently require additional therapy to combat the enhanced vasoconstriction and to attempt to slow the rate of CKD progression.

Bibliography

Araujo M, Wilcox CS. Oxidative stress in hypertension: role of the kidney. *Antioxid Redox Signal*. 2014;20(1):74–101.

Carlestrom M, Wilcox CS, Arendshorst W. Renal autoregulation in health and disease. *Physiol Rev*. 2015;95:405–511.

Navar LG. The role of the kidneys in hypertension. *J Clin Hypertens*. 2005;7:542–549.

Wilcox CS. ADMA and ROS Unwelcome twin visitors to the cardiovascular and kidney disease tables. *Hypertens*. 2012;59:375–381.

Wilcox CS. Oxidative stress and nitric oxide deficiency in the kidney: a critical link to hypertension? *Am J Physiol Regul Integr Comp Physiol*. 2005;289:R913–R935.

64

Evaluation and Management of Hypertension

DEBBIE L. COHEN, RAYMOND R. TOWNSEND

Hypertension remains the leading cause of cardiovascular (CV) mortality and morbidity including stroke, heart disease, kidney disease, and other vascular disease. The relationship between blood pressure (BP) and CV risk is linear, continuous, and additive to other well-known risk factors including diabetes, dyslipidemia, obesity, and cigarette smoking. For individuals aged 40 to 69 years, each increment of either 20 mm Hg in systolic BP or 10 mm Hg in diastolic BP doubles the mortality risk related to stroke, ischemic heart disease, and other vascular causes across the entire BP range from 115/75 to 185/115 mm Hg. Hypertension affects more than 100 million US adults and more than 80 million qualify for treatment with antihypertensive medications. The prevalence of hypertension continues to increase steadily because of aging and increasing obesity in the US population. The lifetime risk of developing hypertension is about 90%.

In 2017 the ACC/AHA Hypertension Guidelines for Clinical Practice classified BP into four strata: normal, elevated BP, hypertension stage 1, and hypertension stage 2, with hypertension defined at a lower threshold than in prior guidelines (Table 64.1). The elevated BP category, defined by a SBP of 120 to 129 mm Hg and a DBP < 80 mm Hg, replaced the prior "prehypertension" category that was created to reflect its association with higher CV risk compared with normal BP and affects, on average, about a quarter of the US adult population. This reclassification of BP increases the prevalence of hypertension in the general population from approximately 32% to 46% and increases prevalence in all genders and racial groups as shown in Table 64.2. Correctly assessing BP status and overall CV risk is key to optimizing therapy to reduce CV morbidity and mortality. At first diagnosis, a comprehensive evaluation is usually undertaken in those with a consistent systolic BP greater than 140 mm Hg and/or diastolic BP greater than 90 mm Hg, or in those with established CV disease or an estimated 10-year ASCVD risk of ≥10% and a consistent systolic BP greater than 130 mm Hg and/or diastolic BP greater than 80 mm Hg.

Evaluation of Hypertension

Three key questions are addressed when assessing each hypertensive patient. The first is whether the BP increase is essential (primary) or represents a secondary form of hypertension. Most hypertensive patients have primary or essential hypertension and are likely to remain hypertensive for life. However, some patients have identifiable, or secondary, causes for their elevated BP that may warrant specific therapy in addition to antihypertensive medications to address the underlying specific or dominant pathology and offer possible cure. The clinical clues suggesting the possible presence and cause of secondary hypertension are discussed in Chapter 65.

The second question assesses the presence of other CV risk factors, as summarized in Table 64.3. CV risk factors are defined as modifiable, such as smoking, obesity, and inactivity, and nonmodifiable, including increased age, male sex, and a positive family history of premature cardiovascular disease (CVD). Defining overall CV risk is important in the choice of antihypertensive medications, BP target, and management of other treatable factors such as dyslipidemia.

The third question evaluates the presence of end-organ damage, defined as clinically evident sequelae of hypertension, as summarized in Table 64.4. The presence of end-organ damage redirects the goal of treating BP from primary prevention of target-organ integrity to the more challenging realm of secondary prevention.

Measuring Blood Pressure

Proper methods should be used to accurately measure and document blood pressure for the diagnosis, classification, and management of hypertension. Fig. 64.1 lists steps recommended to obtain reliable BP readings, and Table 64.5 lists common mistakes leading to inaccurate BP measurements as well as information regarding correct BP cuff selection. Key elements for success in office settings include proper preparation of the patient, use of a validated upper-arm BP measurement device, correct technique, and averaging of readings. During the initial visit, BP should be measured in both arms (and in the leg if aortic coarctation is suspected). For proper BP assessment, it is important to take the BP in the correct way at least twice on any occasion and on at least two, and preferably three, separate days for the initial diagnosis of hypertension. The 2015 US Preventive Services Task Force (USPSTF) guidelines on hypertension recommend that all individuals 18 years or older be screened for elevated BP, and the ACC/AHA guidelines suggest the use of out-of-office blood pressure measurements to confirm the diagnosis of hypertension and to titrate medications.

Pseudohypertension is a problem occasionally encountered in examining patients with very stiff and difficult-to-compress blood vessels due to arterial wall calcification. The pressure required to

| TABLE 64.1 | Classification of Blood Pressure Status |

BP Classification	Systolic BP (mm Hg)		Diastolic BP (mm Hg)
Normal	<120	and	<80
Elevated	120–129	or	<80
Hypertension			
Stage 1	130–139	or	80–89
Stage 2	≥140	or	≥90

BP, Blood pressure.
Whelton PK, Carey RM, Aronow WS, et al. American College of Cardiology/American Heart Association Task Force on Clinical Practice Guidelines. *Hypertension.* 2018;71(6):e13–e115.

| TABLE 64.3 | Cardiovascular Risk Factors in Individuals with Hypertension |

Modifiable Risk Factors	Relatively Fixed Risk Factors
• Current cigarette smoking, second-hand smoking • Diabetes mellitus; fasting glucose >126 mg/dL • Dyslipidemia/hypercholesterolemia • Overweight/obesity; BMI >30 kg/m² • Physical inactivity/low fitness • Unhealthy diet	• Chronic kidney disease • Family history • Increased age • Low socioeconomic/educational status • Male sex • Obstructive sleep apnea • Psychosocial stress • Albuminuria ≥30 mg/g • Left ventricular hypertrophy

compress the stiff brachial artery and to stop the audible blood flow with a standard BP cuff can be much greater than the actual intraluminal BP obtained invasively. Osler's maneuver can be used to identify this condition by inflating the BP cuff at least 30 mm Hg above the palpable systolic pressure and then trying to "roll" the brachial or radial artery underneath the fingertips. Pseudohypertension may be present when something resembling a stiff tube is felt underneath the skin because a normal artery should not be palpable when empty. It is important to identify pseudohypertension as it tends to occur in the elderly and chronically ill, including those with chronic kidney disease (CKD), who are also more prone to orthostatic and postprandial hypotension, which can be aggravated by the unwarranted intensification of BP treatment.

Electronic oscillometric devices are increasingly used to measure BP at home and in the office setting, and have become the clinical standard for BP measurement. This is due to environmental

concerns about mercury toxicity, the need for frequent calibration with aneroid sphygmomanometers, errors due to auscultation and inappropriately rapid deflation of the cuff, and the greater convenience and cost savings associated with use of oscillometric devices. The cuff is inflated until the disappearance of the brachial pulses is detected. Upon deflation, sensors detect the increasing amplitude in the brachial pulsation and measure the mean arterial pressure. The systolic and diastolic BP readings are then derived from the mean arterial BP. Typically, systolic BP is slightly lower and diastolic BP is slightly higher when measured with electronic devices when compared to invasively measured arterial pressure.

Also available are specialized electronic devices to perform automated office blood pressure monitoring (AOBP) in the office setting. With AOBP, multiple BP readings are recorded using a fully automated sphygmomanometer with the patient resting quietly and sitting alone. Proper timing, patient positioning, cuff size,

| TABLE 64.2 | Prevalence of Hypertension After Reclassification Following Release of the 2017 ACC/AHA Guidelines |

	SBP/DBP ≥130/80 mm Hg OR ANTIHYPERTENSIVE MEDICATION		SBP/DBP ≥140/90 mm Hg OR ANTIHYPERTENSIVE MEDICATION	
Overall, crude	46%		32%	
	Men (n = 4717)	Women (n = 4906)	Men (n = 4717)	Women (n = 4906)
Overall, age-sex adjusted	48%	43%	31%	32%
Age group, yr				
20–44	30%	19%	11%	10%
45–54	50%	44%	33%	27%
55–64	70%	63%	53%	52%
65–74	77%	75%	64%	63%
75+	79%	85%	71%	78%
Race-Ethnicity				
Non-Hispanic White	47%	41%	31%	30%
Non-Hispanic Black	59%	56%	42%	46%
Non-Hispanic Asian	45%	36%	29%	27%
Hispanic	44%	42%	27%	32%

Whelton PK, Carey RM, Aronow WS, et al. American College of Cardiology/American Heart Association Task Force on Clinical Practice Guidelines. Hypertension. 2018;71(6):e13–e115.

TABLE 64.4 **Target-Organ Effect of Hypertension**

Organ	History/Symptom(s)	Physical Examination	Laboratory
Retina	Blurry vision, headache, disorientation	Retinopathy	—
Brain	Stroke, TIA, confusion/disorientation	Signs of stroke, carotid bruits	MRI, CT, or ultrasound
Heart	Angina, MI, heart failure, cardiac arrest, atrial fibrillation	Cardiomegaly, S4, rales, irregular heartbeats	ECG may show LVH and/or prior MI
Kidney	Chronic kidney disease, polyuria, nocturia, anorexia, nausea, weight loss, peripheral edema	Epigastric bruits	Elevated creatinine, proteinuria, hematuria; ultrasound may show small kidneys with increased echogenicity
Circulation	Peripheral arterial disease, claudication, ioohomio digito	Femoral bruits, diminished or absent pedal pulses	Ankle-brachial index <0.9

CT, Computed tomography; *ECG*, electrocardiogram; *LVH*, left ventricular hypertrophy; *MI*, myocardial infarction; *MRI*, magnetic resonance image; *TIA*, transient ischemic attack.

1. Have patient relax for at least 5 minutes before taking blood pressure. Feet should be on the floor, with the back supported.

2. The patient's arm should be supported (i.e., resting on a desk) for the measurement.

3. The stethoscope bell, not the diaphragm, should be used for auscultation.

4. Blood pressure should first be checked in both arms with the patient sitting. Note which arm gives the higher reading. This arm (with the higher reading) should then be used for all other (standing, lying down) and future readings.

5. All measurements should be separated by 2 minutes.

6. Measure the blood pressure in the sitting, standing, and lying positions.

7. Use the correct cuff size, and note if a larger or smaller than normal cuff size is used.

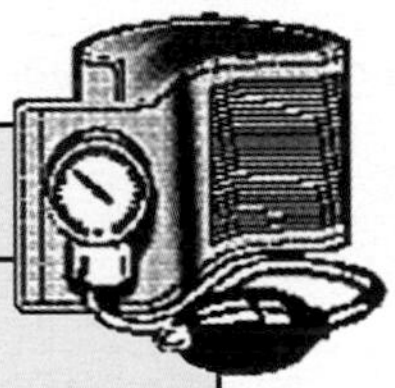

Blood Pressure Cuff Size Criteria

Arm Circumference	Weight Female	Weight Male	Cuff Size to Use
24–32 cm	<150	<200	REGULAR
33–42 cm*	>150	>200	LARGE
38–50 cm*	–	–	THIGH

Either cuff is acceptable in the overlap diameter zone

8. Record systolic (onset of first sound) and diastolic (disappearance of sound) pressures.

9. Do not round off results to zeros or fives. Record exact results to nearest even number.

10. Average the readings.

11. Provide BP readings to patient.

• **Fig. 64.1** Instructions for taking blood pressure. Steps in obtaining accurate blood pressure measurements by aneroid sphygmomanometry.

TABLE 64.5	Common Causes Contributing to Inaccurate Blood Pressure Readings
Failure to sit quietly for 5 min before a reading is taken	
Lack of arm and foot support	
Too small a cuff size relative to the arm (cuff bladder should encircle ≥80% of upper arm circumference)	
Too rapid cuff deflation (i.e., >2 mm Hg/sec)	
Ongoing conversation	
Recent caffeine intake or cigarette smoking	
Talking or using a cellular device	

and placement are still necessary to be certain that the readings are accurate. There are currently three validated devices available for performing AOBP, and each can be programmed to take multiple consecutive BP measurements in intervals of typically 1 to 2 minutes. The devices differ in the number of readings taken and the number of minutes before the first BP measurement is recorded. Ideally, oscillometric devices should be preprogrammed (when possible) to record repeated measurements at 1-minute intervals after the 5-minute rest period. AOBP has the same cutpoint as home BP and awake ambulatory BP (130/80 mm Hg) for defining hypertension because systolic pressure readings typically are 5 to 10 mm Hg lower with AOBP than with auscultatory measurement. In 2011 the Canadian Hypertension Education Program recommended AOBP for the diagnosis of hypertension, in 2013 the European Society of Hypertension recommended using AOBP if feasible, and in 2017 the ACC/AHA stated that there is a growing evidence base to support the use of AOBP measurements.

AOBP has some specific advantages, including that AOBP is not associated with the white-coat effect (the response in some patients in which BP readings taken by doctors and nurses tend to be higher because of increased patient anxiety), multiple readings are obtained, and readings better correlate with awake ambulatory BP readings when compared with manual office readings, as demonstrated in the Conventional Versus Automated Measurement of BP in the Office (CAMBO) study. Results from the Systolic Blood Pressure Intervention Trial (SPRINT) also indicate that unattended and attended automated office BP measurements result in similar BPs when the core recommendations for accurate BP measurement are followed.

Assessing Cardiovascular Risk and End-Organ Damage

The evaluation of each hypertensive patient should include a detailed personal and family history, thorough physical examination, and selected tests focused on addressing the above three key questions. Key components of the history and physical examination are listed in Table 64.6.

A detailed personal history of hypertension includes its onset, duration, severity and related symptoms, presence of other CV risk factors, and target-organ complications. The medication history should include the prior and current use of any prescription and over-the-counter agents. Special attention should be paid to antihypertensive medications with their related clinical responses and adverse effects, as well as common offending agents, such as nonsteroidal antiinflammatory drugs (NSAIDs), oral contraceptives, and cold/cough remedies. NSAIDs can increase BP directly and can decrease the efficacy of antihypertensive medications by inhibiting the vasodilatory and natriuretic effects of prostaglandins and

potentiating vasoconstrictive effects of angiotensin-II. Dietary salt intake, alcohol consumption, tobacco use, physical activity, and weight changes should be recorded. With the increasing prevalence of obesity, essential hypertension manifests at a younger age, often in the 30s. In addition, more elderly patients are expected to develop essential hypertension as systolic BP increases throughout life. Family history of hypertension, diabetes, and related CV complications should also be noted, as a positive family history further increases the individual's CV risk. Excluding monogenic causes of hypertension, available data suggest that the heritability of essential hypertension ranges from 20% to 40%.

Physical examination should start with measurement of height, weight, and waist circumference, and calculation of body mass index (BMI). BP is usually measured in sitting and standing positions on the initial evaluation, and at least once in both arms (and at least one leg if aortic coarctation is suspected). Subsequent BP measurements are obtained in the seated position from the arm with the higher initial BP reading.

The optic fundi are the only places where blood vessels can be directly examined. The fundoscopic examination looks for arteriolar narrowing (grade 1), arteriovenous compression (grade 2), hemorrhages and/or exudates (grade 3), and papilledema (grade 4), which not only provide information on the degree of target-organ damage related to BP but also provide important prognostic information on overall CV outcomes.

Bruits in the neck, abdomen, and groin should be noted. Bruits may simply result from vascular tortuosity, particularly with high-flow vessels. However, they may be a sign of vascular stenosis and irregularity and be a clue to vascular damage leading to future loss of target-organ function. The radial artery is similarly distant from the heart as the femoral artery, and the pulse should arrive at approximately the same moment when palpating both sites simultaneously. In aortic coarctation, a palpable delay in the arrival of the femoral pulse compared with the radial pulse supports this diagnosis, as does an interscapular murmur heard during auscultation over the back of the patient. A systolic BP in the leg behind the knee (popliteal) lower than the brachial value suggests the presence of aortic or iliac obstruction, but it may also reflect more peripheral arterial disease in certain patients, such as smokers and those with target-organ damage. Patients should be advised that measuring leg BP may be uncomfortable given the large cuff and the amount of pressure required to occlude the femoral artery.

Cardiac examination by palpation may reveal a displaced apical impulse, indicative of left ventricular enlargement. A sustained apical impulse may suggest left ventricular hypertrophy (LVH). Auscultation should focus on listening for an S4 that is heard with left ventricular stiffness. An S3 indicates impairment in left ventricular function and usually underlying heart disease when crackles are present on lung examination, although the presence of S3 and crackles is uncommon on initial office evaluation of new hypertensive patients. The lower extremities should also be examined for peripheral arterial pulses and edema. The loss of pedal pulses is a sign of peripheral vascular disease (target-organ damage) and is associated with higher CV risk.

Finally, a brief neurologic examination for evidence of remote stroke should assess gait, bilateral grip strength, speech, memory, and mental acuity. Given the link between hypertension and future loss of cognitive function, it is useful to establish the baseline cognitive function before starting antihypertensive medications, as some patients may complain of memory loss after starting pharmacotherapy.

TABLE 64.6 Key Elements of History and Physical in Evaluating Hypertensive Patients

Key Elements	Evaluation
History	
Age of onset, duration, and severity	Onset at younger age (<30 years) or older age (>55 years) suggests secondary causes; new onset of severe hypertension also suggests a secondary cause
Contributing factors	Dietary salt intake, physical inactivity, psychosocial stress, symptoms of sleep apnea
Concomitant medications	Common offenders include NSAIDs, oral contraceptives, corticosteroids, licorice, cough/cold/weight-loss sympathomimetic agents (pseudoephedrine, ma huang, ephedrine)
Risk factors for cardiovascular disease	Diabetes, smoking, family history of premature cardiovascular disease particularly in a first-degree relative (parent or sibling)
Symptoms suggestive of secondary causes	Palpitations or tachycardia, spontaneous sweating, migraine-like headaches in paroxysms (catecholamine excess); muscle weakness, polyuria (decreased potassium from aldosterone excess); personal or family history of kidney disease or findings (proteinuria, hematuria), or symptoms like ankle swelling (edema); thinning of skin and stigmata of cortical excess; snoring and daytime somnolence (sleep apnea); heat intolerance and weight loss (hyperthyroidism)
Target-organ damage	Chest pain or chest discomfort (possible coronary artery disease); neurologic symptoms consistent with stroke or transient ischemic attack; dyspnea and easy fatigue (possible heart failure); claudication (peripheral arterial disease)
Physical Examination	
General appearance, skin lesions, distribution of body fat	Patient may fit criteria for metabolic syndrome (increased cardiovascular risk); evidence of prior stroke from gain/station; rarely secondary forms as striae (Cushing syndrome) or mucosal fibromas (MEN II)
Fundoscopy	See text for lesion grades; retinal changes reflect severity of hypertension (target-organ damage to the eyes) and future cardiovascular risk
Neck	Diffuse multinodular goiter indicating Graves disease; presence of carotid bruits suggests potential stroke risk
Cardiopulmonary examination	Rales and cardiac gallops consistent with target-organ damage (heart enlargement or heart failure), interscapular murmur during auscultation of the back for aortic coarctation
Abdominal examination	Palpable kidneys suggest polycystic kidney disease; mid-epigastric bruits indicate renal artery disease
Neurologic examination	Signs of previous stroke (reduced grip, hyperreflexia, spasticity, Babinski sign, muscle atrophy, and gait disturbances) reflect target-organ damage
Pulse examination	Delayed or absent femoral pulses may reflect coarctation of the aorta or atherosclerosis

MEN, Multiple endocrine neoplasia; *NSAIDs,* nonsteroidal antiinflammatory drugs.

Several laboratory studies are recommended in the routine evaluation of the hypertensive patient. Testing should include hemoglobin or hematocrit, urinalysis with microscopic examination, serum potassium, bicarbonate, creatinine, fasting glucose, lipid profile, and 12-lead electrocardiogram (ECG). Assessing albuminuria is important as albuminuria has been associated with increased CV risk and may warrant more aggressive BP reduction. Assessing kidney function is also an important part of the evaluation as CKD is not only a sign of target-organ damage but also a common cause of hypertension. Depending on the degree of glomerular filtration rate (GFR) loss, up to 90% of patients with advanced CKD or end-stage kidney disease (ESKD) have hypertension. Uric acid may be checked in those with a history of gout as diuretics can increase uric acid level and lead to gouty flares. In some cases, checking calcium, thyroid-stimulating hormone (TSH), or other thyroid studies may be reasonable when clinically indicated.

Plasma renin activity and serum aldosterone levels are useful in screening for aldosterone excess and salt sensitivity. However, these measurements are usually reserved for patients with hypokalemia or metabolic alkalosis or those who fail to achieve BP control on a three-drug regimen (that includes a diuretic). A suppressed renin activity level with a normal aldosterone level and an increased aldosterone-to-renin ratio supports a contribution of dietary sodium excess to hypertension; this scenario should respond well to dietary salt restriction and diuretics. It is worth noting that primary aldosteronism is more common than previously thought. In patients referred to one hypertension center in Italy, 11% had primary hyperaldosteronism, with 5% having a potentially curable aldosterone-secreting adenoma and 6% having idiopathic hyperaldosteronism. In the same study, only 50% of patients with a confirmed aldosterone-producing adenoma had hypokalemia, underscoring the importance of considering this diagnosis in patients with normal levels of potassium. A recent study that included participants with normotension ($n = 289$), stage 1 hypertension ($n = 115$), stage 2 hypertension ($n = 203$), and resistant hypertension ($n = 408$) showed that for every BP category there was a continuum of renin-independent aldosterone production, where greater severity of production was associated with higher BP. Adjusted prevalence estimates of biochemically overt primary aldosteronism were present in 11.3% of normotensives, 15.7% of stage 1 hypertensives, 21.6% of stage 2 hypertensives, and 22.0% of resistant hypertensives. This indicates that prevalence of primary aldosteronism is high and largely unrecognized.

Additional testing may be indicated in some patients depending on the clinical situation. Limited echocardiography is more sensitive than an ECG for detection of LVH. The presence of LVH, a sign of target-organ damage, can help establish or reinforce the need of antihypertensive therapy, especially in those who have borderline BP and/or are reluctant to start antihypertensive medications.

Ambulatory and Home BP Monitoring

Since BP can be influenced by an environment such as an office or hospital, ambulatory BP monitoring (ABPM) or home BP monitoring (HBPM) is useful in establishing or excluding the diagnosis of hypertension in those with white-coat hypertension or masked hypertension (Fig. 64.2). ABPM and HBPM are also useful in assessing the adequacy of BP control in outpatients and helping identify those with morning surges in BP (i.e., >55 mm Hg increase in systolic BP during the early waking hours compared with sleeping). The morning surge has been associated with increased risk of cerebrovascular diseases, including brain white matter lesions and stroke. In addition, ABPM is helpful in screening for nocturnal hypertension or nondipper status (i.e., <10% reduction in nighttime BP compared with daytime). Data from large ABPM cohorts suggest that nighttime BP provides the greatest information regarding CV risk. CV risks associated with elevated nighttime BP levels outweigh the risks associated with elevated routine office BP measurements and those of the cumulative daytime hours. In addition, the BP variability data from ABPM suggest that a greater degree of BP variability during the 24 hours of monitoring is associated with a greater risk of CV target-organ damage. ABPM is typically programmed to take BP measurements every 15 to 30 minutes during awake hours and every 30 to 60 minutes during sleep hours. It is important for patients to complete the diary correctly so that the hours of sleep (including naps) can be incorporated into the ABPM report.

Current estimates suggest that more than half of hypertensive patients measure their BP at home. Home BP monitors are relatively inexpensive and reasonably accurate. An updated list of validated devices can be found at www.validatebp.org. Specific recommendations have been published on how to incorporate HBPM into overall BP assessment. For the diagnosis of hypertension, it is recommended to take two BP readings in the morning between 7 a.m. and 10 a.m. and two measurements in the evening between 7 p.m. and 10 p.m. for 7 consecutive days.

Values from the first day are discarded, and the subsequent 6 days' values are averaged. For the diagnosis of hypertension in untreated patients, hypertension is not present if the average is less than 120/80 mm Hg, but hypertension is likely present if the value is greater than 130/80 mm Hg. Suggested corresponding values for clinic, HBPM, daytime, nighttime, and 24-hour ambulatory blood pressure measurements are listed in Table 64.7. When patients are using HBPM for monitoring and titrating medications it is recommended that they measure BP in the morning before taking antihypertensive medications and in the evening before dinner, with two readings at each time of day 1 minute apart. Patients do not need to measure home BPs daily but should obtain readings for 3 to 7 days a few weeks after initiating or changing medication and before clinic visits. Clinicians should adjust hypertension therapy based on the average of all readings over the 3- to 7-day monitoring period (minimum of 12 readings).

ABPM and HBPM have important similarities, but they also have meaningful differences. They are viewed as complementary rather than alternative techniques because they provide different information regarding BP. Table 64.8 compares similarities and differences among the various techniques available for BP measurement.

The National Center for Health and Clinical Excellence (NICE) in the United Kingdom recommended using ABPM or HBPM to confirm all new diagnoses of hypertension. Similarly, the 2015 USPSTF guidelines recommended that the diagnosis of hypertension be confirmed with ABPM. However, the USPSTF and, more recently, the ACC/AHA guidelines recognize that ABPM is not widely available because of equipment cost and lack of widespread insurance coverage; these guidelines, therefore, state that out-of-office blood pressure measurements are required to confirm the diagnosis of hypertension and that either HBPM or ABPM is

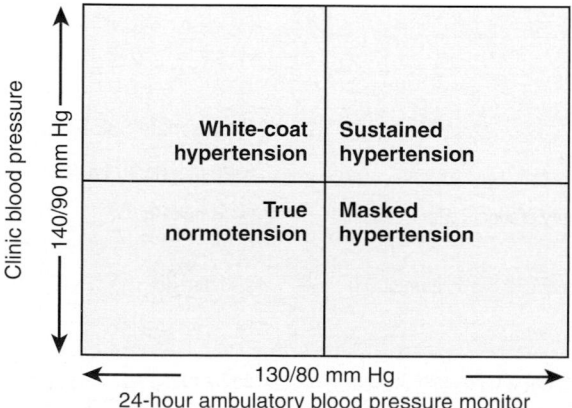

• **Fig. 64.2** Use of ambulatory blood pressure monitoring in diagnosing hypertension. This grid helps to integrate ambulatory blood pressure (BP) monitor data with office BP results. Sustained hypertension is diagnosed if office BP is ≥140/90 mm Hg and 24-hour average of ambulatory BP is ≥130/80 mm Hg. White-coat hypertension is diagnosed when office BP is ≥140/90 mm Hg but 24-hour average of ambulatory BP is <130/80 mm Hg. Masked hypertension is diagnosed when office BP is <140/90 mm Hg but 24-hour average of ambulatory BP is ≥130/80 mm Hg.

TABLE 64.7	Clinic, Ambulatory, and Home Blood Pressure Value Equivalents			
Clinic	HBPM	Daytime ABPM	Nighttime ABPM	24-Hour ABPM
120/80	120/80	120/80	100/65	115/75
130/80	130/80	130/80	110/65	125/75
140/90	135/85	135/85	120/70	130/80
160/100	145/90	145/90	140/85	145/90

HBPM, Home blood pressure monitoring; *ABPM,* ambulatory blood pressure monitoring.
Whelton PK, Carey RM, Aronow WS, et al. American College of Cardiology/American Heart Association Task Force on Clinical Practice Guidelines. Hypertension. 2018;71(6):e13–e115.

TABLE 64.8	**Comparison of Ambulatory, Home, and Office Blood Pressure Monitoring**		
	ABPM	Home	Office
Detects WCH and masked HTN	Yes	Yes	No
Multiple measurements	Yes	Yes	Yes
Evaluates circadian rhythm of BP	Yes	No	No
Predicts events	Yes	Yes	Yes
Evaluates BP variability	Yes	No	No
Improves compliance and BP control	?	Yes	Yes
Cost	High	Low	Low
Reimbursement	Partial	No	Yes

ABPM, Ambulatory blood pressure monitoring; *HTN*, hypertension; *WCH*, white-coat hypertension.

acceptable to make the diagnosis. Currently, Medicare and most insurance companies do not provide financial coverage for ABPM in patients with established hypertension but provide coverage for its use to diagnose white-coat hypertension and, more recently, coverage for masked hypertension has been added. The Centers for Medicare & Medicaid Services (CMS) recently proposed expansion of Medicare coverage for ABPM and may soon announce a decision regarding coverage for such monitoring for patients with established hypertension. Since January 2020, there is now a CPT code to bill for HBPM or self-monitored BP (SBPM). The 2020 CMS fee schedule includes reimbursement for HBPM, including billing for one-time patient education and training using a validated device provided by the patient. Monthly reimbursement requires documentation of a minimum of 12 readings reported to the physician and communication of a treatment plan by the physician to the patient.

Management of Hypertension

Lifestyle Modifications

Several nonpharmacologic approaches are used in lowering BP. In obese patients, the most effective measure to reduce BP is weight loss. For all patients, reducing dietary sodium intake to less than 100 mmol/day (2300 mg of sodium) and increasing physical activity to at least 30 minutes daily on most days of the week are high-yield lifestyle modifications. Finally, limiting alcohol intake to two drinks a day for men (one drink a day for women) helps reduce BP. Other approaches, including modification of intake of fish oil, garlic, and green tea and supplementation of potassium, magnesium, and calcium, have had variable success in managing BP. Although they do not appear harmful, these approaches lack robust data to support their widespread use in the management of patients with elevated BP or sustained hypertension. Table 64.9 summarizes the effects of various lifestyle modifications on BP.

There is evidence for the benefit of lifestyle measures in hypertension management. The Dietary Approaches to Stop Hypertension (DASH) Study showed that a diet low in sodium and high in fruits, vegetables, and calcium is effective in lowering BP. In addition, the Trials of Hypertension Prevention (TOHP2) and Trials of Non-Pharmacological Interventions in the Elderly (TONE) reported that in middle-aged (TOHP2) and elderly (TONE) subjects with mild to moderate hypertension, diet, exercise-induced weight loss, and sodium restriction can be sustained and are associated with significant BP reductions. A meta-analysis of 24 randomized, controlled trials showed that dietary modifications are associated with significant incremental reductions in BP. The authors found that the net reduction in systolic and diastolic BP was 3.1 mm Hg and 1.8 mm Hg, respectively. From this same analysis, it appears that some dietary patterns are more effective than others, as the DASH diet was associated with the greatest overall reduction in BP with a net reduction in systolic and diastolic BP of 7.6 mm Hg and 4.2 mm Hg, respectively.

The effect of aerobic exercise was evaluated in a meta-analysis of 54 randomized, controlled trials and demonstrated that aerobic

TABLE 64.9	**Lifestyle Modification to Manage Hypertension**		
Modification	**Recommendation**		**Approximate SBP Reduction**
Weight reduction	Maintain normal body weight (BMI 18.5–24.9)		5–20 mm Hg/10-kg weight loss
Adopt DASH eating plan	Consume a diet rich in fruits, vegetables, and low-fat dairy products with a reduced content of saturated and total fat		8–14 mm Hg
Dietary sodium reduction	Reduced dietary sodium intake to no more than 100 mmol/L (2.3 g sodium or 6 g sodium chloride)		2–8 mm Hg
Physical activity			
Aerobic	Engage in regular aerobic physical activity such as brisk walking (at least 30 min/day, most days of the week)		5–8 mm Hg
Dynamic	90–150 min/wk; 6 exercises, 3 sets/exercise, 10 repetitions/set		4 mm Hg
Isometric	4 × 2 min (hand grip), 1 min rest between exercises, 3 sessions/wk; 8–10 wk		5 mm Hg
Moderation of alcohol consumption	Limited consumption to no more than two drinks per day for most men and no more than one drink per day for most women and lighter-weight persons		2–4 mm Hg

For overall cardiovascular risk reduction, stop smoking. The effects of implementation of these modifications are dose- and time-dependent and could be higher for some individuals.
BMI, Body mass index, *DASH*, Dietary Approaches to Stop Hypertension.

exercise reduces systolic and diastolic BP by 3.8 mm Hg and 2.6 mm Hg, respectively. This BP reduction was noted in both overweight and normal-weight participants, as well as in normotensive individuals. Dynamic resistance exercises (such as weight lifting and circuit training) and isometric exercises (such as handgrips or weighted resistance machines) have also been shown to effectively reduce BP, and it is recommended they are performed 3 to 5 times per week.

Viewed in sum, these studies demonstrate the importance of individually evaluating the various lifestyle factors associated with hypertension in all patients as part of the initial management.

Medication Nonadherence

An important and underappreciated cause of poor BP control and apparent resistant hypertension is medication nonadherence. Medication nonadherence in hypertensive patients has been shown to be present in up to 50% of patients when using prescription claims data over the course of 2 years in Germany. Failure to recognize medication nonadherence early in the disease course may result in unnecessary testing, complications of polypharmacy, inappropriate treatment, and worse patient outcomes. Multiple studies have demonstrated that a significant fraction of patients referred for resistant hypertension are either partially or completely nonadherent. Similarly, when urinary drug metabolites were measured in patients with apparent resistant hypertension, 25% were at least partially nonadherent. Clinicians must be aware of potential barriers to adherence and routinely minimize these barriers for patients. Remediable barriers include socioeconomic factors, treatment complexity, adverse medication effects, and patient motivation. Motivation is commonly affected by depression, lack of belief in the benefit of treatment, and lack of insight into illness. Medications should preferentially include low-cost and generic antihypertensives. Adherence is inversely proportional to the frequency of dosing; so, once-daily medications and combination antihypertensive formulations should be used when available. Adverse medication effects should be addressed since patients may be reluctant to continue intolerable therapies for an otherwise asymptomatic disease. Patients require education and should be empowered in management decisions, which may improve adherence.

Principles of Pharmacologic Care

Many patients with hypertension find it difficult to make or sustain the necessary lifestyle modifications to effectively lower BP. Treatment with antihypertensive medications is recommended when BP remains above the goal despite lifestyle modifications.

Major classes of antihypertensive medications with their mechanism of actions, common side effects, and compelling indications are listed in Table 64.10. Heart failure and stroke are the types of end-organ damage most reduced with long-term antihypertensive therapy. A large meta-analysis suggests that all five major classes of antihypertensive agents (angiotensin-converting enzyme [ACE] inhibitor, angiotensin II receptor blocker [ARB], beta-blocker, calcium channel blocker [CCB], and diuretic) can reduce target-organ damage when used to control BP effectively. Choosing an agent involves a decision-making process that takes into account demographics (age and ethnicity), drug cost, and the anticipated side-effect profile. Use of long-acting agents that can

be dosed once or, at most, twice a day and use of combination therapies are preferred as this simplifies the regimen and increases adherence. The usual response to a single antihypertensive agent is a reduction in systolic BP of 12 to 15 mm Hg and diastolic BP of 8 to 10 mm Hg. Follow-up visits for BP assessment and dose titration are often scheduled in 2 to 4 weeks for single-agent therapy as most agents will exert their antihypertensive effects at that dose by then.

In patients with systolic BP greater than 20 mm Hg and/or diastolic BP greater than 10 mm Hg above the goal, beginning treatment with combination drug therapy can shorten the time to achieve BP goal, require less dose titration of antihypertensive agent, and increase the likelihood of achieving BP goal. Combination therapy is often more desirable than a stepwise approach of maximizing one agent before adding another agent because of the better efficacy in BP control and side-effect profile.

A useful approach in building an effective combination therapy is based on a convenient model, shown in Fig. 64.3. This approach is similar to the popular "Birmingham Square" used in the United Kingdom to develop combination regimens. The art in building or adjusting a combination antihypertensive regimen is to use medications with complementary, and not overlapping, mechanisms of action and to try to minimize side effects by leveraging known pharmacology. Examples include adding an ACE inhibitor to a diuretic to reduce occurrence of hypokalemia or adding an ACE inhibitor (or an ARB) to a CCB to reduce CCB-associated edema.

Major Classes of Antihypertensive Agents and Associated Cardiovascular Benefits

Diuretics

Diuretics are proven antihypertensive agents and play a key role in building a successful combination regimen. They work mostly by inhibiting kidney sodium reabsorption. There is abundant evidence to support the benefit of diuretics compared with placebo in reducing CV morbidity and mortality, including ischemic heart disease, heart failure, stroke, other vascular disease, and death. Data from the Antihypertensive and Lipid-Lowering Treatment to Prevent Heart Attack Trial (ALLHAT) suggest that thiazide diuretics are as effective as CCBs and ACE inhibitors in lowering BP and reducing coronary events. Despite the concern of higher incidence of new onset of diabetes with diuretics, secondary analyses from ALLHAT found a diuretic to be equally effective as an ACE inhibitor and a CCB in reducing CV risk, including ischemic heart disease, heart failure, stroke, kidney disease, and death in both diabetic and nondiabetic patients. The published data on long-term outcomes of the Systolic Hypertension in the Elderly Program (SHEP) further affirm the benefits of diuretic therapy in reducing CV endpoints.

Hydrochlorothiazide (HCTZ) is the most commonly prescribed diuretic for hypertension. Chlorthalidone is a nother common thiazide-like diuretic. HCTZ and chlorthalidone are pharmacologically different. Chlorthalidone has a duration of action of 48 to 72 hours versus 16 to 24 hours for HCTZ. The longer duration of action may explain the observation of improved mean 24-hour ambulatory BPs (including daytime and nighttime) with chlorthalidone versus HCTZ and the superiority of chlorthalidone in preventing CV events when compared with HCTZ in one meta-analysis.

TABLE 64.10 Major Classes of Available Antihypertensive Medications With Their Mechanisms and Side Effects

Class	Mechanisms	Side Effects	Compelling Indications
Diuretics	Reduce kidney sodium absorption	—	Heart failure, high CAD risk, diabetes, stroke
[a]Thiazide diuretics	Inhibit sodium and chloride cotransporter in the distal convoluted tubule; more effective in BP control than loop diuretics	Hypokalemia, hyponatremia, hypomagnesemia, hyperuricemia, photosensitivity, and metabolic effects including dyslipidemia and impaired glucose tolerance	
Loop diuretics	Inhibit sodium, potassium, and chloride cotransporter in the thick ascending limb of the loop of Henle	Hypokalemia but fewer other metabolic side effects	
Potassium-sparing diuretics	Inhibit the epithelial sodium channel in the distal tubule	Hyperkalemia	
Renin Angiotensin System Blockers	Dampen arterial wave reflections, increasing aortic distensibility and venodilation	—	Heart failure, post MI, high CAD risk, diabetes, CKD, stroke
[a]ACE inhibitors	Block the conversion of angiotensin I to angiotensin II	Cough, hyperkalemia, elevated creatinine, fetal toxicity, angioedema	
[a]ARB	Block binding of angiotensin-II to the type 1 angiotensin receptor	Similar to ACE inhibitors except no cough	
Direct renin inhibitor (aliskiren)	Block conversion of angiotensinogen to angiotensin I	Similar to ARB; diarrhea at high doses	
[a]Calcium Channel Blockers	Inhibit the L-type voltage-gated plasma membrane channel	—	High CAD risk, diabetes
Dihydropyridine	Vasodilatation	Dependent edema, gingival hyperplasia	
Diltiazem	Vasodilation and AV nodal blockade	Bradycardia	
Verapamil	Vasodilation and AV nodal blockade	Bradycardia, constipation	
Beta-Blockers	Inhibit adrenergic receptors	Reduced exercise tolerance, depression, bronchospasm	Heart failure, post MI, high CAD risk, diabetes, stroke
Nonselective beta-blockers	Inhibit both beta 1 and 2 receptors	More bronchospasm	
Selective beta-blockers	Block beta 1 receptors	Less bronchospasm	
Combined alpha- and beta-blockers	Block both beta and alpha receptors	—	
Aldosterone Blocker	Block aldosterone receptor	—	Heart failure, post MI
Spironolactone	—	Androgen-blocking effect including irregular menses, gynecomastia, impotence	
Eplerenone	—	Less potent but fewer side effects related to androgen blocking	
Direct Vasodilators	Smooth muscle relaxant	Peripheral edema	
Alpha-1 Blockers	Vasodilatation	Postural hypotension	
Central Adrenergic Agonists	Inhibit central adrenergic tone	Drowsiness, fatigue, and dry mouth	
SGLT2 Inhibitors	Decreases glucose reabsorption in the proximal tubule with resultant natriuresis	Genital fungal infections, urinary tract infections, increased thirst	CKD, heart failure

ACE, Angiotensin-converting enzyme; *ARB*, angiotensin II receptor type I blocker; *AV*, atrioventricular; *BP*, blood pressure; *CAD*, coronary artery disease; *CKD*, chronic kidney disease; *MI*, myocardial infarction; *SGLT2*, sodium glucose transport inhibitors
[a]First-line agents that should be used as the first three agents added, in no particular order, taking into account patient's underlying comorbidities.

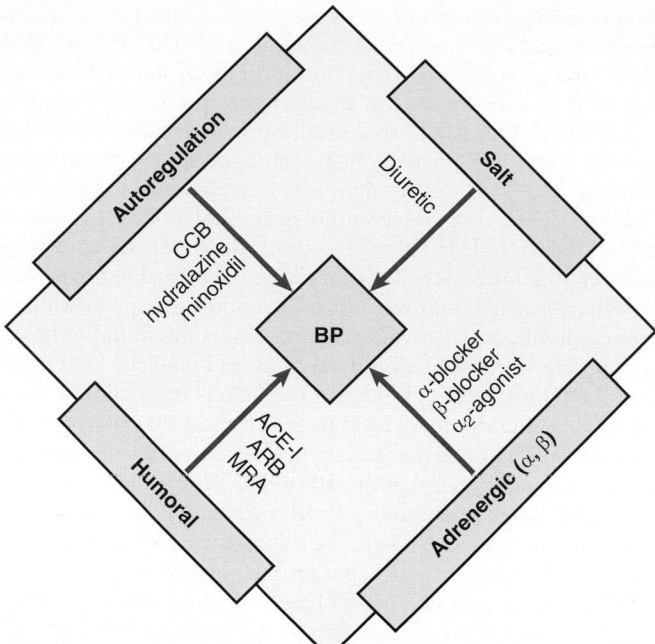

• **Fig. 64.3** Building successful combination antihypertensive therapy. The diagram emphasizes four basic physiologic processes that regulate blood pressure (BP) and places the major classes of antihypertensive medications along the side, corresponding to the process responsible for the primary antihypertensive effect of the class. Combining agents to control hypertension is usually more effective when drugs are chosen from different sides (e.g., diuretic plus ARB) as opposed to the same side (e.g., beta-blocker plus alpha$_2$-agonist) of the diagram. *ACE-I,* Angiotensin-converting enzyme inhibitor; *ARB,* angiotensin receptor blocker; *CCB,* calcium channel blocker; *MRA,* mineralocorticoid antagonist.

Renin-Angiotensin-Aldosterone System (RAAS) Blockade

ACE inhibitors, ARBs, direct renin inhibitors, and spironolactone/eplerenone block the conversion of angiotensin I to II, the binding of angiotensin II to its receptor, the conversion of angiotensinogen to angiotensin I, and the binding of aldosterone to the mineralocorticoid receptor, respectively. ACE inhibitors and ARBs have been shown in many studies to reduce CV events, prevent stroke, improve kidney outcomes, and lower the incidence of new-onset diabetes. Aliskiren, a direct renin inhibitor, is an effective antihypertensive agent with a side-effect profile that appears similar to ARBs, but it lacks evidence of benefit in hard endpoint outcome trials. Although spironolactone and eplerenone both have potential benefits in congestive heart failure, they are currently used as third- or fourth-line antihypertensive agents. The PATHWAY-2 Study found that spironolactone, when compared with bisoprolol and doxazosin, was more effective for BP lowering among patients with resistant hypertension already on a three-drug regimen, indicating that spironolactone is an effective fourth-line agent after the three first-line agents.

Calcium Channel Blockers

CCBs inhibit the L-type voltage-gated channels resulting in vasodilatation (and decreased cardiac output with nondihydropyridine CCBs). Data from ALLHAT suggest that dihydropyridine CCBs are as effective as thiazide diuretics and ACE inhibitors in lowering BP and reducing CV events, including myocardial infarction (MI), stroke, and overall mortality. In addition, data from the

Anglo-Scandinavian Cardiac Outcomes Trial (ASCOT) showed that a combination of CCB with ACE inhibitor was superior in reducing stroke than a combination of beta-blocker with ACE inhibitor. Data from the Avoiding Cardiovascular Events through Combination Therapy in Patients Living with Systolic Hypertension (ACCOMPLISH) trial demonstrated that, despite identical BP control, combination therapy with an ACE inhibitor and a CCB seemed superior to the combination of an ACE inhibitor and a diuretic in hypertensive patients at high CV risk.

Beta-Blockers

Beta-blockers generally decrease cardiac output, but several beta-blockers also show vasodilatory effects, either from a combined alpha blockade (labetalol and carvedilol) or through nitric oxide potentiation (nebivolol). Beta-blockade is useful in treating ischemic heart disease and congestive heart failure. However, in older patients, beta-blockers have been increasingly replaced by other classes of agent because of concerns that beta-blockade does not prevent stroke as effectively as other agents. Although ASCOT suggests the combination of dihydropyridine CCB plus ACE inhibitor is better than the selective beta-blocker atenolol plus diuretic, the newer generation of beta-blockers with combined alpha- and beta-blocking activities or nitric oxide-potentiating effect may provide benefit in lowering CV events, although this remains speculative at present.

Sodium-Glucose Co-Transporter 2 (SGLT2) Inhibitors

SGLT2 inhibitors are a relatively new class of drugs that primarily reduce blood sugar but also have a BP-lowering effect. The SGLT2 receptor is expressed in the proximal tubule of the kidney and mediates reabsorption of approximately 90% of the filtered glucose load. SGLT2 inhibitors promote the kidney excretion of glucose and thereby modestly lower elevated blood glucose levels. SGLT2 inhibitors modestly decrease BP by approximately 4/2 mm Hg. The mechanism of BP lowering is thought to be due to modest natriuresis and weight loss. Although the BP lowering is modest, these agents are increasingly being used due to impressive reductions in cardiovascular outcomes, heart failure, and progression of CKD.

Other Agents

Alpha$_1$-blockers and other direct vasodilators are used as add-on therapy in resistant hypertension. However, as previously mentioned, the PATHWAY-2 study found that spironolactone is more effective than doxazosin (an alpha$_1$-blocker) for BP lowering in patients with resistant hypertension. In addition, the doxazosin arm in ALLHAT was terminated early because of its inferior CV outcomes, particularly for the risk of new heart failure, compared with the diuretic, ACE inhibitor, and CCB arms. Because of these studies, alpha$_1$-blockers are not commonly prescribed for BP lowering as the initial or even the second agent.

Vasodilators such as minoxidil and hydralazine are used in resistant hypertension if the preferred drugs are not efficacious. Hydralazine needs to be dosed 3–4 times per day and compliance is often difficult; however, these agents may be useful in Blacks with heart failure. Minoxidil is a potent agent but causes significant fluid retention and needs to be used together with a loop diuretic; it causes facial hirsutism and can infrequently cause a pericardial effusion. Centrally acting sympatholytics are used less often and are also reserved for resistant hypertension. Clonidine is available in oral form or transdermal patch. The oral form particularly is associated with dry mouth and lethargy that can be quite debilitating. It is also short acting, needs to be dosed 2-3 times per day, and is associated with rebound hypertension if not dosed regularly. It is not recommended to use clonidine as a rescue agent for BP spikes as this causes a rapid decrease in BP with a dramatic rebound about 6 hours later, which often results in multiple emergency room visits for patients. The clonidine patch has a steady release of the drug and appears to be better tolerated than the oral form and is particularly useful in dialysis patients and patients with poor adherence as it is only applied once a week. Guanfacine is a centrally acting alpha$_{2A}$-adrenergic receptor agonist and is generally better tolerated than other agents in this class, is available in extended release forms, and can be dosed once a day.

Novel Antihypertensive Therapies

Baroreceptor Activation Therapy (BAT)

Several device-based interventions are under investigation to treat hypertension either alone or as a complement to standard antihypertensive medications. One approach uses the known effects of carotid baroreceptor activation therapy (BAT) to reduce sympathetic output and lower BP. This requires surgical implantation of a pacemaker-like device that has an electrode placed on the carotid body in the neck. When the signal generator is activated, it stimulates the carotid baroreceptors to reduce signals to the brain stem, resulting in lower BP and heart rate. Feasibility studies have shown reductions in BP after implantation of different devices designed to stimulate the carotid baroreflex system. Initial experience with the Rheos device showed significant and sustained mean reduction in BP of 21/12 mm Hg at 3 months and 33/22 mm Hg at 2 years; however, a recent pivotal study of 265 patients with drug-resistant hypertension failed to achieve two of its five primary endpoints. This study observed that 35% of patients had a serious procedure-related adverse event, including nerve injury. A second device using baroreflex amplification (MobiusHD) is inserted into the carotid sinus by endovascular deployment (rather than surgical implantation) and amplifies carotid stretch signals. An initial pilot study lowered 24-hour ambulatory BP at 6 months by 21/12 mm Hg in 30 patients with apparent resistant hypertension, with serious adverse events in four patients. An open-label study was recently closed due to low recruitment. These devices are not currently approved for the treatment of hypertension in the United States.

Renal Denervation (RDN)

Another approach uses either radiofrequency energy from an intravascular signal source or focused ultrasound for delivery of an ablative chemical such as alcohol into the perivascular renal nerve supply. The procedure usually takes less than an hour to complete and reduces sympathetic flow into (efferent) and out of (afferent) the kidneys. Initial studies suggested that RDN could substantially lower BP in patients with drug-resistant hypertension. This early progress came to a standstill with the surprising negative results of the sham-controlled SYMPLICITY HTN-3 Trial. These results were attributed to the confounding effects of antihypertensive medication changes, technical limitations in the catheter technology, and the experience of the proceduralists, which may have limited the ability to achieve satisfactory nerve ablation.

There has been renewed interest in RDN after recent sham-controlled trials used an updated radiofrequency ablation technology with a new Spyral catheter design that provides a more comprehensive ablation of the sympathetic nerve plexus around the main renal artery as well as branch arteries. The SPYRAL OFF MED trial demonstrated reduction in both 24-hour ABPM and office BP in patients not on medical therapy for hypertension. The SPYRAL ON MED trial examined the efficacy of RDN in patients already on pharmacologic antihypertensive therapy and demonstrated statistically significant reduction in office and 24-hour ABPM in the intervention arm. Similar results were seen in the RADIANCE-HTN SOLO trial, which utilized ultrasound ablation. The DENERHTN trial also standardized antihypertensive therapy in the control and intervention groups before and after randomization. The intervention group was found to have a 5.9-mm Hg larger reduction in daytime ambulatory SBP. Finally, the RADIOSOUND-HTN study evaluated both radiofrequency and ultrasound techniques head to head against sham controls and demonstrated improvement in hypertension across all intervention groups and superior mean BP reduction for the ultrasound-based approach. The durability of BP reduction remains unknown, although the Global SYMPLICITY registry has demonstrated persistent decreases in office and ambulatory BP in patients followed for up to 3 years post-RDN. Animal models have shown regrowth of both afferent and efferent sympathetic fibers, but this has not been demonstrated in humans having undergone RDN procedures. There is a need for further study in order to improve patient selection for these promising technologies, particularly with respect to patients with resistant hypertension in whom these techniques would be most beneficial. RDN is not currently approved for use in the United States.

Goal Blood Pressure Levels

In 2003, JNC 7 recommended a BP goal of less than 140/90 for patients less than 80 years of age in the absence of comorbidities or compelling indications. A revised recommendation, published in 2014 by members of the Joint National Committee (JNC 8), suggested a goal of less than 140/90 mm Hg for the general population under 60 years of age and a goal of less than 150/90 mm Hg for those aged 60 years and older. In addition, they recommended a goal of less than 140/90 mm Hg in those with diabetes and in those with CKD, representing a change from prior recommendations. The JNC 8 members based their recommendations for raising the BP goal among patients aged greater than 60 years on several studies including the Principal Results of the Japanese Trial to Assess Optimal Systolic Blood Pressure in Elderly Hypertensive Patients (JATOS) Study, the Target Blood Pressure for Treatment of Isolated Systolic Hypertension in the Elderly: Valsartan in Elderly Isolated Systolic Hypertension (VALISH) Study, the Treatment of Hypertension in Patients 80 Years of Age or Older (HYVET) Study, the Randomised Double-Blind Comparison of Placebo and Active Treatment for Older Patients with Isolated Systolic Hypertension (SYST-EUR) Study, and SHEP. The recommendation for raising the goal systolic BP in this group was not unanimous and remains controversial.

In 2015, the Systolic Blood Pressure Intervention Trial (SPRINT) was published. SPRINT was a large, multicenter, randomized, controlled trial that enrolled 9361 patients aged 50 years or older who had a systolic BP of 130 to 180 mm Hg plus one or more of the following additional risks factors for CVD: age 75 years or older; clinically evident CVD; an estimated GFR (eGFR) of 20 to 59 mL/min; or a 10-year Framingham Risk Score ≥15%. SPRINT excluded patients with diabetes, prior stroke, polycystic kidney disease (PKD), greater than 1 g of proteinuria, or an eGFR of less than 20 mL/min. Automated oscillometric BP was used to measure BP in the study.

SPRINT tested whether a systolic BP goal of less than 120 mm Hg compared with less than 140 mm Hg would reduce the occurrence of CVD and CKD events in a moderately high-CV-risk population. The SPRINT study was terminated early when it was observed that the patients in the lower SBP target group had significantly lower rates of heart failure and death. However, there were more acute kidney injury events and electrolyte disturbances in the lower SBP goal group, suggesting that patients who were targeted more aggressively require closer monitoring. Several meta-analyses since SPRINT have overall concluded that intensive BP control reduces CV risk and mortality in the general population of ambulatory adults 50 years and older, in diabetes, CKD, and the elderly (these populations are addressed separately below).

Based largely on the findings from SPRINT, the ACC/AHA recommended a BP goal of <130/80 mm Hg and advocated starting BP-lowering medications at an average BP ≥130/80 mm Hg for secondary prevention of CVD events in patients with CVD and for primary prevention of CVD in adults with an estimated 10-year ASCVD risk of ≥10%. In adults with no history of CVD and a 10-year ASCVD risk of <10%, they suggest starting BP-lowering medications at an average BP ≥140/90 mm Hg for primary prevention of CVD and suggest a BP target of <130/80 mm Hg may be reasonable in this population. These guidelines cannot be applied to every patient, and goal BP still needs to be individualized in patients who may not be able to achieve these goals or may be unable to tolerate these lower goals, including those susceptible to falls or AKI.

Special Populations

Women

Women show similar BP response to antihypertensive agents as men. Before menopause, women have lower BP than men of a similar age. This trend reverses after menopause, and Black women tend to have the highest BP. In women of childbearing age, ACE inhibitors and ARBs are usually avoided because of the risk of fetal malformation. Women tend to have a higher risk of hypokalemia when treated with diuretics and a greater risk of hyponatremia when treated with thiazide diuretics, more cough with ACE inhibitors, and more edema with CCBs, but show similar benefits from antihypertensive agents as men.

Blacks

Hypertension is more prevalent in Black populations, tends to be more salt sensitive, and responds better to diuretics and CCBs than ACE inhibitors, ARBs, or beta-blockers when used as monotherapy. In addition, Blacks tend to experience higher rates of target-organ damage than Whites at any level of BP. The reason is not entirely clear, but recent advances in genetic predisposition, particularly the presence of APOL1 risk alleles, explain part of this enhanced predisposition. Compared with Whites, Blacks have more frequent CV complications, such as heart failure, and about a fourfold higher risk of kidney failure. In 2017, the ACC/AHA guideline recommended a goal BP less than 130/80 mm Hg in Black patients. The BP control rate in Black hypertensive patients (~44%) is not as high as in, for example, White hypertensives (~54%). Judging by awareness and treatment data, which appear as high in Black as in White hypertensive populations, the reduced

BP control rates in Black populations seem to be due to more resistance to antihypertensive therapy and not a lack of awareness or treatment.

Elderly

The pattern of BP elevation in older patients is characterized predominantly by systolic hypertension. This relates in large part to the significant role of vascular stiffness, which also contributes to a decline in diastolic BP and, therefore, an increase in the pulse pressure. With low diastolic pressure, concern exists with further therapeutic lowering of DBP while targeting SBP, especially in those with existing coronary artery disease due to increasing CV events below a certain DBP threshold. Current recommendations are to avoid lowering diastolic BP less than 70 mm Hg in those with active coronary artery disease at any age.

Moderate discordance exists among guideline-recommended BP goals. The ACP/AAFP guidelines recommend a goal of <150 mm Hg systolic while the ACC/AHA 2017 guideline recommends a goal of <130 mm Hg systolic. Among patients 75 years of age and older who participated in SPRINT, targeting intensive BP control reduced mortality and CV events even among those who were frail or had decreased gait speed. In addition, there was no increase in serious adverse events, falls, or orthostatic hypotension with intensive BP control. The results suggest that older patients with similar characteristics as those included in SPRINT can benefit from intensive BP lowering. Challenges in managing hypertension in older patients include polypharmacy due to comorbidities, frailty and falls, cognitive impairment, and threats to life expectancy from nonhypertensive disorders like cancer.

Diabetes Mellitus

The presence of both diabetes mellitus (DM) and hypertension represents a substantial CV risk. Treating hypertension is an effective way of reducing this risk. An ACE inhibitor or ARB is preferred as initial therapy in a hypertensive diabetic patient with albuminuria to slow progression of kidney disease. Several studies have indicated that a combination of ACE inhibitor *and* ARB is *not* superior to monotherapy with one of these agents and is associated with more side effects.

Although most guidelines suggest a goal BP in patients with DM of less than 130/80 mm Hg, the 2019 statement from the American Diabetic Association (ADA) recommended a BP goal of <140/90 mm Hg in diabetic patients with <15% 10-year ASCVD risk, reserving the 130/80 mm Hg goal for those patients with >15% 10-year ASCVD risk. The Action to Control Cardiovascular Risk in Diabetes (ACCORD) trial greatly influenced current recommendations about target goals in diabetics. In ACCORD, the intensive group with SBP goal less than 120 mm Hg did not experience an improvement in the primary outcome of composite fatal and nonfatal CV events despite a SBP that was 14 mm Hg lower than the standard group. Stroke, a prespecified secondary outcome, however, was significantly reduced in the lower BP goal group. As in SPRINT, the increased medication requirement in the lower BP group resulted in more side effects, including reduced kidney function.

Follow-up data from the ACCORD BP trial were recently published in the Action to Control Cardiovascular Risk in Diabetes Follow-Up Study (ACCORDION). The ACCORDION trial looked at 3957 participants from the ACCORD BP trial who were followed for an additional 5 years. Results showed that during a median follow-up of 8.8 years, there remained a nonsignificant reduction in the primary outcome of CVD with intensive lowering of BP. In addition, the stroke benefit that was observed in ACCORD did not persist after BP differences waned.

There are theories as to why the SPRINT study demonstrated lower CV and mortality rates with an SBP target under 120 mm Hg, whereas the ACCORD trial failed with intensive treatment to the same target in diabetes. The factorial design of ACCORD with randomization to intensive versus standard glucose control and differences in patient population may have contributed to the discrepant results.

Chronic Kidney Disease

Hypertension is a frequent finding in both acute and chronic kidney diseases. Mortality and morbidity from CVD are high among those with CKD, and CKD is an independent risk factor for coronary heart disease. The risk of death, particularly due to CVD, is typically higher than the risk of eventually requiring kidney replacement therapy. Risk factor modification, including BP lowering, can reduce the CV complications associated with CKD. Abundant evidence supports the current recommendation of using ACE inhibitors and ARBs in patients with CKD, especially those with proteinuria. The current ACC/AHA 2017 guideline-recommended BP goal is <130/80 mm Hg.

Findings from SPRINT indicate that patients with an eGFR of 20 to 59 mL/min and less than 1 g of proteinuria had a lower rate of fatal and nonfatal CV events and death when targeted to a lower SBP goal of less than 120 mm Hg. However, as in the ACCORD trial, the increased medication requirement in the lower BP group resulted in an increased risk of reduced kidney function. Because the trial was stopped early, long-term outcomes for CKD events (doubling of serum creatinine or development of end-stage kidney disease) were not significant. This may be due to the low event rates of the CKD endpoint in both the standard and intense BP-lowering groups. More aggressive BP therapy in SPRINT was associated with a lower eGFR during the trial in that group. However, there was no loss of CVD benefit despite the presence of CKD at the time of randomization or in association with the lower eGFR during follow-up in the more intensive BP goal group.

As the SPRINT trial excluded patients with PKD, eGFR less than 20 mL/min, kidney transplants, and proteinuria greater than 1 g per 24 hours, findings cannot be applied to these patient groups. There are no randomized trials examining the optimal BP targets in kidney transplant recipients. Patients with PKD were studied in the Halt Progression of Polycystic Kidney Disease (HALT-PKD) Study, which showed that rigorous BP control was associated with a slower increase in total kidney volume, no overall change in the estimated GFR, a greater decline in left ventricular mass index, and greater reduction in albuminuria.

With respect to proteinuria, some guidelines have recommended a lower BP goal in this population. Much of the data that support this recommendation in patients with nondiabetic CKD come from the Modification of Diet in Renal Disease (MDRD) trial that assessed the effect of more aggressive BP lowering in patients with CKD. This study suggested that with increasing degrees of proteinuria at baseline more aggressive BP lowering was associated with a slower rate of GFR loss, compared with less aggressive BP lowering.

Heart Disease

Hypertension is a major risk factor for ischemic heart disease and heart failure. Beta-blockers and renin-angiotensin system blockers have been shown to reduce morbidity and mortality associated

with acute MI and high-risk ischemic heart disease. Although beta-blockers may worsen acute congestive heart failure, beta-blockade remains a key agent in managing chronic congestive heart failure. Diuretics also play an essential role in managing patients with congestive heart failure.

The 2017 guidelines from the ACC/AHA recommend a BP target of less than 130/80 mm Hg in patients with hypertension and coronary artery disease. In patients with stable ischemic heart disease, the use of beta-blockers or RAAS blockers like ACE-inhibitors or ARBs is recommended as initial antihypertensive therapy, followed by addition of CCB and diuretics if still uncontrolled.

In patients with heart failure, the BP goal is also <130/80 mm Hg. This area of treatment remains fluid. As of 2020, the only guidance for those with preserved ejection fraction is the use of diuretics to control volume, followed by ACE inhibitor or ARB and beta-blockade to achieve goal BP. For those with reduced ejection fraction, there is little guidance on specific agents, but there is a recommendation to avoid nondihydropyridine CCB like verapamil and diltiazem due to negative inotropy.

Stroke

Hypertension is the most common and most important risk factor for ischemic stroke, the incidence of which can be markedly reduced by effective antihypertensive therapy. Hypertension is also an important risk factor for hemorrhagic stroke. The approach to BP management of a stroke patient differs in the acute and chronic phases of stroke and depends on whether a patient has an acute ischemic versus acute hemorrhagic stroke. This is beyond the scope of this chapter.

Persons who survive a stroke or TIA are at increased risk of experiencing another stroke. Treatment of hypertension with diuretics, renin-angiotensin blockers, CCBs, and beta-blockers is beneficial for reducing risk of recurrent stroke. As mentioned previously, beta-blockade may not provide *as much* benefit in stroke reduction as other forms of antihypertensive drug therapy. Current guidelines recommend restarting antihypertensive therapy when a hospitalized stroke patient is stable, with a goal of <140/90 mm Hg

The optimal SBP targets to prevent recurrent stroke were tested in the Secondary Prevention of Small Subcortical Strokes (SPS3) trial, which studied 3020 patients with recent lacunar infarctions. Patients were randomized to an SBP target of 130 to 149 mm Hg versus a lower target of less than 130 mm Hg. There was a nonsignificant reduction in recurrent stroke in the group randomized to the lower SBP goal. The AHA/ASA recommends a target BP level <140/90 mm Hg for secondary prevention of stroke/TIA, but it suggests that a target systolic BP less than 130 mm Hg is not unreasonable given the SPS3 trial findings.

Resistant Hypertension

The definition of resistant hypertension was recently updated after the publication of the 2017 ACC/AHA guidelines. It is now defined as a BP that remains above "current guideline BP goal" in spite of concurrent use of three antihypertensive agents of different classes, with one of the three agents a diuretic (if tolerated), and all agents prescribed at optimal doses (50% or more of the maximum recommended antihypertensive dose) or maximally tolerated doses, with BP elevation confirmed outside the clinic (by HBPM or ABPM) with attention paid to ensuring adherence to medication. The true prevalence of resistant hypertension is not known, with estimates ranging from 2% to 20% of treated hypertensives. These patients are more likely to have target-organ damage and are at greater risk of stroke, MI, heart failure, and CKD compared with patients who have more easily controlled hypertension.

Pseudoresistance or *apparent resistant hypertension* refers to poorly controlled hypertension that appears resistant to treatment but is actually attributable to other factors, including inaccurate BP measurement, poor adherence, and white-coat effect. Out-of-office BP monitoring is a valuable tool to determine the presence of true drug resistance, including both ABPM and HBPM.

Medication adherence (taking medication as prescribed) and persistence (refilling prescriptions) data increasingly indicate that patients prescribed antihypertensive regimens with multiple drugs take either no drug or fewer than the prescribed number of drugs in about half of the cases of drug-resistant hypertension. These are important factors to consider before making a diagnosis of resistant hypertension.

Mineralocorticoid receptor antagonists like spironolactone and eplerenone are evidence-based treatment options for patients with resistant hypertension. The antihypertensive effect of spironolactone was evaluated in the ASCOT in which the addition of spironolactone (median dose of 25 mg daily) as a fourth drug was associated with a mean 22/10-mm Hg reduction in BP at 1-year follow-up. In addition, the previously mentioned PATHWAY-2 study was the first randomized, controlled trial comparing multiple different agents with placebo for resistant hypertension. The mineralocorticoid antagonist spironolactone was the most effective agent.

Obstructive Sleep Apnea

Obstructive sleep apnea (OSA) is common among patients with hypertension, especially in resistant hypertension. Both of these highly prevalent conditions contribute to an increased CV risk. Patients with more severe OSA are also more likely to have abnormal nocturnal BP patterns. Although OSA increases the risk of CV disease through a number of mechanisms, repetitive cycles of hypoxemia and re-oxygenation probably play a central role in increasing CV risk by augmenting sympathetic nervous system activity, systemic inflammation, and oxidative stress. The effects of continuous positive airway pressure (CPAP) on BP reduction are modest, and use of supplemental nocturnal oxygen as salvage therapy has been shown to be ineffective for BP reduction in patients with OSA for whom CPAP is problematic. Combining weight loss with CPAP has been shown to be more effective in reducing SBP than either intervention alone. CPAP has also been shown to restore nocturnal dipping in resistant hypertensive patients, and the number of hours of CPAP use is correlated with the degree of BP improvement. Patients with OSA and either resistant hypertension or frequent apneic episodes are also more likely to have a greater reduction in BP from use of CPAP.

Obesity

Obesity (body mass index >30 kg/m²) is a global pandemic. As the prevalence of obesity increases, so does its associated comorbidities, including hypertension. Resistant hypertension and OSA are common in obese patients. The mechanism by which obesity raises BP is not completely understood. Theories implicate insulin resistance and hyperinsulinemia, adipokines that are secreted by adipose tissue, and elevated plasma aldosterone levels that are often found in obese patients. All of these factors contribute to impaired sodium excretion, increased sympathetic nervous system activity, reduced vascular compliance, and activation of the renin-angiotensin-aldosterone system (RAAS).

The approach to lowering BP in obese patients includes treating sleep apnea if present, weight loss, lower-sodium diet, encouraging exercise, and pharmacologic therapy. Again, the goal BP is <130/80 mm Hg. In addition, bariatric surgery may be helpful. Bariatric surgery (e.g., Roux-en-Y gastric bypass [RYGB], sleeve gastrectomy [SG], and adjustable gastric band [AGB]) is increasingly being used as a therapeutic option for controlling obesity. In a meta-analysis of 136 studies, average weight loss and improvement in hypertension control with several bariatric procedures were significant, with 78.5% of patients categorized as having resolved or improved BPs. In a prospective study comparing the various bariatric surgery approaches, resolution or remission of hypertension at 1 year after the procedure occurred in 79% of patients managed with an RYGB, 68% undergoing a SG, and 44% undergoing an AGB.

Conclusion

Hypertension is common, and the prevalence continues to rise with an increasingly older and obese population. Adequate treatment of hypertension remains the key to lowering CV morbidity and mortality. Correctly assessing BP status, CV risk, and the presence of target-organ damage is important in optimizing therapy to reduce CV morbidity and mortality. Recent studies have suggested that intensive BP reduction reduces CV morbidity and mortality in most adults with hypertension, and a goal BP of <130/80 mm Hg is advocated by many society guidelines in adults 50 years or older, diabetics, in individuals with CKD, and in ambulatory elderly patients. The most effective approach to BP lowering is addressing lifestyle factors, secondary causes of hypertension, and medications that are complementary in action. Medication adherence is a major problem that should be addressed with all patients to improve BP control. Novel therapies with devices may provide additional options in managing the truly resistant hypertension with renal denervation being the most promising.

Bibliography

American Diabetes Association. 2. Classification and diagnosis of diabetes: *standards of medical care in diabetes-2019. Diabetes Care.* 2019;42(Suppl 1):S13–S28.

Böhm M, Kario K, Kandzari DE, et al. Efficacy of catheter-based renal denervation in the absence of antihypertensive medications (SPYRAL HTN-OFF MED Pivotal): a multicentre, randomised, sham-controlled trial. *Lancet.* 2020;395(10234):1444–1451.

Brown JM, Siddiqui M, Calhoun DA, et al. The unrecognized prevalence of primary aldosteronism: a cross-sectional study. *Ann Intern Med.* 2020;173(1):10–20.

Carey RM, Calhoun DA, Bakris GL, et al. Resistant hypertension: detection, evaluation, and management: a scientific statement from the American Heart Association. *Hypertension.* 2018;72(5):e53–e90.

DASH Collaborative Research Group. A clinical trial of the effects of dietary patterns on blood pressure. *N Engl J Med.* 1997;336:1117–1124.

Drawz PE, Beddhu S, Kramer HJ, Rakotz M, Rocco MV, Whelton PK. Blood pressure measurement: a KDOQI perspective. *Am J Kidney Dis.* 2020;75(3):426–434.

Gay H, et al. Effects of different dietary interventions on blood pressure: systemic review and meta-analysis of randomized controlled trials. *Hypertension.* 2016;67:733–739.

Hameed MA, Tebbit L, Jacques N, Thomas M, Dasgupta I. Non-adherence to antihypertensive medication is very common among resistant hypertensives: Results of a directly observed therapy clinic. *J Hum Hypertens.* 2016;30(2):83–89.

James PA, et al. Evidence-based guidelines for the management of high blood pressure in adults (JNC 8). *J Am Med Assoc.* 2014;311:507–520.

Kandzari DE, Böhm M, Mahfoud F, et al. Effect of renal denervation on blood pressure in the presence of antihypertensive drugs: 6-month efficacy and safety results from the SPYRAL HTN-ON MED proof-of-concept randomised trial. *Lancet.* 2018;391(10137):2346–2355.

Kernan WN, et al. Guidelines for the prevention of stroke in patients with stroke and transient ischemic attack: a guideline for healthcare professionals from the American Heart Association/American Stroke Association. *Stroke.* 2014;45:2160–2236.

McMurray JJV, Solomon SD, Inzucchi SE, et al. Dapagliflozin in patients with heart failure and reduced ejection fraction. *N Engl J Med.* 2019;381(21):1995–2008.

Myers MG, et al. Conventional versus automated measurement of blood pressure in the office (CAMBO) trial. *Fam Pract.* 2012;29:376–382.

Perkovic V, Jardine MJ, Neal B, et al. Canagliflozin and renal outcomes in type 2 diabetes and nephropathy. *N Engl J Med.* 2019;380(24):2295–2306.

Rossi GP, et al. A prospective study of the prevalence of primary aldosteronism in 1,125 hypertensive patients. *J Am Coll Cardiol.* 2006;48:2293–2300.

Siu A. Screening for high blood pressure in adults: U.S. preventive services task force recommendation statement. *Ann Intern Med.* 2015;163:1–9.

The Sprint Research Group. A randomized trial of intensive versus standard blood-pressure control. *N Engl J Med.* 2015;373:2103–2116.

Whelton PK, Carey RM, Aronow WS, et al. ACC/AHA/AAPA/ABC/ACPM/AGS/APhA/ASH/ASPC/NMA/PCNA guideline for the prevention, detection, evaluation, and management of high blood pressure in adults: a report of the American College of Cardiology/American Heart Association Task Force on clinical practice guidelines [published correction appears in *Hypertension.* 2018 Jun;71(6):e140–e144]. *Hypertension.* 2018;71(6):e13–e115.

Whelton SP, et al. Effect of aerobic exercise on blood pressure: a meta-analysis of randomized, controlled trials. *Ann Intern Med.* 2002;136:493–503.

Williams B, et al. Spironolactone versus placebo, bisoprolol, and doxazosin to determine the optimal treatment for drug-resistant hypertension (PATHWAY-2): a randomised, double-blind, crossover trial. *Lancet.* 2015;386:2059–2068.

Zinman B, Wanner C, Lachin JM, et al. Empagliflozin, cardiovascular outcomes, and mortality in type 2 diabetes. *N Engl J Med.* 2015;373(22):2117–2128.

65
Secondary Hypertension

ALDO J. PEIXOTO

Definition and Prevalence of Secondary Hypertension

Secondary hypertension is generally defined as hypertension associated with a specific cause and, therefore, potentially curable if that cause is removed. The use of this definition generates two separate lines of diseases. The first are considered "classic" causes of secondary hypertension, which, if diagnosed in a timely manner, can be effectively cured. Examples include acute glomerulonephritis, primary aldosteronism, renal artery stenosis, pheochromocytoma, Cushing syndrome, hypothyroidism and hyperthyroidism, and coarctation of the aorta. Other conditions may be associated with higher BP levels; however, given complex pathophysiologic mechanisms and the association with multiple other cardiovascular risk factors, their correction does not necessarily result in resolution of hypertension. Examples in this category include chronic kidney disease, sleep apnea, and obesity.

The prevalence of secondary hypertension is estimated at around 10% of all cases of hypertension in adults. Absent from most prevalence studies, all of which were conducted from the 1970s through the 1990s, is the recognition that primary aldosteronism was underdiagnosed, that the definitions of kidney disease were too conservative, and that sleep apnea was not considered as a diagnosis. Therefore, it is likely that an updated survey of the prevalence of secondary hypertension would result in higher prevalence estimates.

The relationship between age and prevalence of secondary causes must be acknowledged. Among hypertensive children, secondary causes are the rule rather than the exception with up to 90% of young children having an identifiable secondary cause, most commonly structural kidney disease. The prevalence of "classic" causes of secondary hypertension among hypertensive adolescents had been about 65% in older observations, although the obesity epidemic has somewhat masked this relationship. While obesity is associated with a higher prevalence of primary hypertension in children and adolescents, its presence does not exclude the presence of a typical secondary cause (~30%). The 2018 Clinical Practice Guidelines from the American Academy of Pediatrics does not recommend screening for secondary causes in obese children aged 6 years or older. I do not find these recommendations consistent with the available data, and my interpretation of the same literature in proposing recommendations to the care of young adults is that the coexistence of obesity should not prevent the clinician from investigating secondary hypertension.

The transition point of prevalence rates from childhood/adolescence numbers to more typical adult numbers is unknown.

In several small cohorts including adolescents, the prevalence of secondary causes is between 25% and 80%. I believe these are large numbers that deserve the attention of the treating clinician. In my personal opinion, until there are large cohort studies defining which adolescents/young adults should and which should not be investigated, we should err on the side of an approach that includes a basic evaluation of renoparenchymal, renovascular, and mineralocorticoid hypertension. The only study that investigated the effect of age on the prevalence of secondary hypertension in adults was unable to show a higher prevalence among patients aged 18–29 years (5.6%) compared with any other age bracket; in fact, because of the high rate of renovascular disease and primary aldosteronism in older patients, the prevalence of secondary hypertension was lowest among the youngest group. Mindful of these somewhat unexpected data, we must recognize that there is a transition period and that ignoring it would inevitably lead to frequently missing the diagnosis of a secondary cause. Accordingly, our search for secondary hypertension in younger adults, especially those under the age of 30 years, is always more "aggressive" than in older patients. In this chapter, we will restrict our discussion of secondary hypertension to adults.

Clinical Opportunites To Diagnose Secondary Hypertension

There are two critical opportunities to identify secondary hypertension during the evaluation and management of hypertensive patients. First, and most important, is during the initial evaluation of a patient diagnosed with hypertension. It is important to consider the breadth of possibilities at this time, especially as patients are not on pharmacologic antihypertensive treatment, so diagnostic tests often perform at their best. Table 65.1 lists clinical features suggestive of each of the major causes of secondary hypertension. The clinician should explore the presence of these different clinical signs and symptoms in every patient. The list of general diagnostic tests recommended as part of the initial evaluation of hypertensive individuals (see Table 65.1) addresses the identification of secondary causes. It should be reviewed carefully for every patient, and further investigations should be pursued if suggested by this initial review.

The second occasion to explore secondary causes is when patients are noted to be resistant to therapy. Resistant hypertension, identified in 10%-15% of treated patients with hypertension, is defined as BP that remains above target (in general, above 140/90 mm Hg) despite the use of three adequately dosed drugs of

TABLE 65.1	Clues That Suggest Secondary Hypertension Based on Simple Diagnostic Tests That Are Routinely Recommended for the Initial Evaluation of Hypertensive Patients

Test	Possible Causes of Secondary Hypertension
Basic Metabolic Panel	
eGFR (based on creatinine)	Low: chronic kidney disease (any etiology), renal artery stenosis
Potassium	Low: aldosterone excess (primary or secondary), hypercortisolism, apparent mineralocorticoid excess syndromes, primary reninism High: familial hyperkalemic hypertension (Gordon syndrome), CKD
Bicarbonate	High: aldosterone excess (primary or secondary), apparent mineralocorticoid excess syndromes, primary reninism Low: familial hyperkalemic hypertension (Gordon syndrome), chronic kidney disease (any etiology)
Calcium	High: hyperparathyroidism
Urinalysis	
Hematuria	Glomerulonephritis, interstitial nephritis
Proteinuria	Glomerulonephritis
Complete Blood Count	
Hematocrit/hemoglobin	High: sleep apnea, any polycythemic disorder (e.g., polycythemia vera)

synergistic drug classes, at maximal or maximally tolerated doses, preferably including a diuretic. Patients with resistant hypertension have higher rates of secondary hypertension, in particular, primary aldosteronism (~20%), renovascular disease (~25%), and obstructive sleep apnea (>50%). Therefore, every patient with resistant hypertension should be reconsidered for secondary causes, and, if not previously screened, objective testing for these conditions should be pursued.

Clinical Syndromes Suggestive of Secondary Hypertension

Hypertension and Hypokalemia

The coexistence of hypertension and spontaneous hypokalemia should always raise the possibility of secondary causes of hypertension. The approach should start with a clinical evaluation that confirms that the kidney is the source of potassium wasting. This can be achieved with measurement of the transtubular potassium gradient (TTKG) ([urine potassium/plasma potassium]:[urine osmolality/plasma osmolality]) or the urine potassium/creatinine ratio. In the presence of hypokalemia, a TTKG greater than 2 or a urine potassium/creatinine ratio greater than 13 mEq/g is diagnostic of renal potassium wasting. Once renal potassium wasting is confirmed, paired measurement of plasma renin activity (in ng/mL/h) and plasma aldosterone (in ng/dL) allows us to create a

thoughtful differential diagnosis according to three different diagnostic patterns:
1. *High aldosterone (>15 ng/mL) with high plasma renin activity (>1.5 ng/mL/h).* This combination results in a variable aldosterone-to-renin ratio, but it is usually <20. These patients have secondary hyperaldosteronism, commonly caused by diuretic therapy (thiazides, loop diuretics), renal artery stenosis (particularly unilateral), malignant hypertension (of any etiology), or the rare syndrome of primary reninism, which is usually caused by a benign renin-producing tumor of the juxtaglomerular cells, though several extrarenal tumors have been reported (teratomas, adenocarcinomas of the adrenal, lung, pancreas or ovary, or hepatocellular carcinoma).
2. *High aldosterone with suppressed renin activity* (<0.6 ng/mL/h), leading to an aldosterone-to-renin ratio >30. This is diagnostic of primary aldosteronism and should lead to further subtype differentiation (see specific section below).
3. *Low aldosterone* (often suppressed to undetectable levels) *and low renin activity.* These patients behave clinically as if they had hyperaldosteronism but have undetectable aldosterone levels. This implicates one of three possibilities: (1) an alternative source of mineralocorticoid activity (e.g., deoxycorticosterone or cortisol from a tumor, or congenital adrenal hyperplasia due to 11-beta hydroxylase or 21-hydroxylase deficiency); (2) a disorder of impaired degradation of cortisol, thus leaving it available to activate the mineralocorticoid receptor (e.g., licorice ingestion, posaconazole, or primary 11-beta-hydroxysteroid dehydrogenase type 2 deficiency); or (3) mutations in the epithelial sodium channel (Liddle syndrome) or the mineralocorticoid receptor (Geller syndrome). Some of these conditions are briefly presented in Table 65.2.

Hypertension with a Strong Family History of Hypertension Early in Life

Hypertension has a significant genetic component, with multiple genes associated with small effects on BP. However, patients who have a strong family history of hypertension early in life should be approached more carefully, as they may have a genetic disorder responsible for the hypertension. The most common of these conditions is autosomal dominant polycystic kidney disease (1:500 to 1:1000 live births), which can result in hypertension several years before producing symptoms or causing loss of kidney function. There are several rare monogenic causes of hypertension that the clinician should entertain in the right clinical setting; Table 65.2 summarizes their key clinical and genetic features.

Hypertension and Obesity

Obesity is strongly associated with hypertension, mediated by increased activity of the renin-angiotensin system and sympathetic nervous system, increased production of aldosterone by adipocytes, and impaired production of natriuretic peptides. Localized fat accumulation in the liver (as in nonalcoholic steatohepatitis) or kidney (renal sinus fat) is also associated with an increased prevalence of hypertension.

Weight gain often results in loss of BP control, and weight loss, when significant, can lead to resolution of hypertension. This can be achieved with lifestyle changes (dietary caloric restriction, exercise, behavioral modification to adjust caloric intake patterns), with or without the addition of drugs (orlistat, phentermine/topiramate,

TABLE 65.2	Clinical Clues to Guide the Investigation in Young Hypertensive Patients With a Potential Hereditary Cause	
Possible Causes of Familial Hypertension		**Clinical Clues**
Catecholamine-Producing Tumors		
Pheochromocytoma/paraganglioma	Familial cases are responsible for up to 40% of cases	Paroxysmal palpitations, headaches, diaphoresis, pale flushing. Syndromic features of any of the associated disorders (see Pheochromocytoma/Paraganglioma section for details)
Neuroblastomas (adrenal)	1%–2% of neuroblastomas are familial	Symptoms of the abdominal tumor (pain, mass) or catecholamine release (same as PPGL)
Parenchymal Kidney Disease		
Glomerulonephritis	Alport disease (X-linked, AR or AD), familial IgA nephropathy (AD with incomplete penetrance)	Proteinuria, hematuria, low eGFR
Polycystic kidney disease	ADPKD type 1 or 2, ARPKD	Multiple kidney cysts (as few as three in patients under the age of 30)
Adrenocortical Disease		
Glucocorticoid-remediable aldosteronism (familial hyperaldosteronism type 1)	AD chimeric fusion of the 11-beta hydroxylase and aldosterone synthase genes	Cerebral hemorrhages at young age, cerebral aneurysms. Mild hypokalemia. High plasma aldosterone, low renin
Familial hyperaldosteronism type 2	AD. Unknown defect	Severe hypertension in early adulthood. High plasma aldosterone, low renin. No response to glucocorticoid treatment
Familial hyperaldosteronism type 3	AD mutation in the KCJN5 potassium channel	Severe hypertension in childhood with extensive target organ damage. High plasma aldosterone, low renin. Marked bilateral adrenal enlargement.
Congenital adrenal hyperplasia	AR mutations in 11-beta hydroxylase or 21-hydroxylase	Hirsutism, virilization. Hypokalemia and metabolic alkalosis. Low plasma aldosterone and renin
Monogenic Primary Renal Tubular Defects		
Familial hyperkalemic hypertension (Gordon syndrome)	AD mutations of KLHL3, CUL3, WNK1, WNK4. AR mutations of KLHL3	Hyperkalemia and metabolic acidosis with normal renal function
Liddle syndrome	AD mutations of the epithelial sodium channel	Hypokalemia and metabolic alkalosis. Low plasma aldosterone and renin.
Apparent mineralocorticoid excess	AD mutation in 11-beta-hydroxysteroid dehydrogenase type 2	Hypokalemia and metabolic alkalosis. Low plasma aldosterone and renin
Geller syndrome	AD mutation in the mineralocorticoid receptor	Hypokalemia and metabolic alkalosis. Low plasma aldosterone and renin. Increased BP during pregnancy or exposure to spironolactone
Unknown Mechanisms		
Hypertension-brachydactyly syndrome	AD mutation in the phosphodiesterase 3 (PDE3) gene	Short fingers (small phalanges) and short stature. Brainstem compression from vascular tortuosity in the posterior fossa

AD, Autosomal dominant; *Aldo,* aldosterone; *AR,* autosomal recessive; *PKD,* polycystic kidney disease; *PPGL,* pheochromocytoma/paraganglioma.
Modified from Peixoto AJ. Attending Rounds: A Young Patient with a Family History of Hypertension. Clin J Am Soc Nephrol. 2014; 9:2164–2172.

liraglutide, semaglutide naltrexone/bupropion) or bariatric surgery. It is important to remember that some drugs used to treat obesity, such as lorcaserin (a serotonin 5-HT2 receptor agonist no longer FDA approved), bupropion (a serotonin and dopamine reuptake inhibitor), and phentermine (a sympathomimetic amine), can induce significant hypertension in some patients. However, the net BP result of these drugs is usually favorable and reflects the achieved weight loss. Naltrexone/bupropion is the exception and should be avoided in obese patients with hypertension.

The impact of bariatric surgery on hypertension control in obese patients is well established. A meta-analysis of 57 studies in over 50,000 patients showed that 64% of patients had improved BP levels, and up to 50% were able to fully come off medications. In general, the amount of weight loss is greater with a Roux-en-Y gastric bypass than with other techniques that are purely restrictive (gastric banding, gastric sleeve) and, in many studies, this is also associated with greater BP reduction. However, a substantial portion of BP lowering occurs in the two initial postoperative weeks, before the majority of weight loss occurs. This implicates other mechanisms for BP reduction, such as decreased plasma leptin, leading to lower sympathetic tone, increased glucagon-like peptide 1 (GLP-1), and decreased reactive oxygen species as a result of caloric restriction, leading to improved endothelial function.

Drug-Induced Hypertension

Patients presenting with hypertension or whose BP control suddenly worsens should always be evaluated for exposure to hypertensogenic substances (Table 65.3). These include substances of abuse as well as over-the counter and prescription drugs. Oral contraceptive pills (OCP), especially earlier-generation pills that had higher estrogen and progesterone content, can cause hypertension. Modern low-estrogen pills can also produce hypertension, though at rates much lower than with older preparations. Stopping the OCP cures the hypertension after several weeks to months in most but not all women. Nonsteroidal antiinflammatory drugs (NSAIDs) result in a modest average hypertensive effect (up to ~5 mm Hg), but some patients can have very large BP responses. In addition, NSAID induced hypertension often presents as loss of BP control in patients taking a diuretic or a blocker of the renin-angiotensin system, whereas the antihypertensive effect of calcium channel blockers tends to be less affected in NSAID users.

Sympathomimetic amines (legal or illegal) usually cause hypertension acutely, close to the time of ingestion. Alcohol has an acute hypotensive effect, but chronic use in large amounts (>4–5 drink-equivalents per day) is associated with increased BP. Glucocorticoids and mineralocorticoids can produce a dose-dependent rise in BP. Although generally seen only with systemic treatment, there are isolated reports of hypertension resulting from high-exposure topical therapy. Glucocorticoids with low mineralocorticoid activity (dexamethasone, budesonide) induce less pressor responses. Selective serotonin reuptake inhibitors (SSRIs) and serotonin-norepinephrine reuptake inhibitors (SNRIs) can produce a modest increase in BP. SNRIs are more commonly culprits, and the hypertensive response in some patients can be severe. Interestingly, when used for hypertensive

patients with depression, BP often improves as depressive symptoms improve.

Angiogenesis inhibitors, such as anti-VEGF antibodies (bevacizumab, ramucirumab) and tyrosine kinase inhibitors (sorafenib, sunitinib, axitinib), can produce hypertension that often persists despite discontinuation. Most cases are related to systemic therapy, though there are isolated reports following intravitreal administration of bevacizumab. Because hypertension during the use of these drugs correlates with better tumor responses (likely a reflection of successful antiangiogenesis), treatment is usually continued unless BP control to acceptable levels is not achievable or if severe kidney injury develops.

Labile Hypertension or Hypertension With Symptoms of Catecholamine Excess

Some patients present with paroxysmal hypertension (isolated episodes interspersed with normotension), labile hypertension (wide fluctuations in BP during any given time interval), or hypertension accompanied by stereotypical spells suggestive of catecholamine excess (headaches, palpitations, diaphoresis, pallor). In these situations, ruling out pheochromocytoma/paraganglioma (PPGL) is the initial step. However, because these symptoms are nonspecific and PPGL is rare, most patients turn out to have either an alternative diagnosis or, quite often, no specific etiology identified. Important considerations to be entertained in patients presenting as "pseudopheochromocytoma" include sympathomimetic drug use, alcohol withdrawal, hyperthyroidism, renal artery stenosis, carcinoid, intracranial hypertension, neurovascular brainstem compression, panic disorder, and baroreflex failure (as in patients with bilateral carotid sinus injury due to trauma, surgery, or irradiation). Further testing is based on specific symptoms and signs associated with each of these conditions.

Specific Causes of Secondary Hypertension

Parenchymal Kidney Disease

Chronic kidney disease (CKD) of any etiology can lead to hypertension. Approximately 75% of patients with glomerular filtration rate (GFR) <45 mL/min are hypertensive. Patients with polycystic kidney disease and glomerulopathies tend to be hypertensive earlier in the course of the disease (at higher GFR) than patients with interstitial diseases. However, with progressive decline in kidney function, the prevalence of hypertension is relatively similar across all causes of CKD. Proteinuria is linked to increased sodium retention and hypertension. This relationship starts at relatively low levels of proteinuria and progressively strengthens with higher degrees of protein excretion. Low GFR and proteinuria have a synergistic association with higher BP.

The pathogenesis, diagnosis, and management of CKD (including hypertension), glomerular and interstitial diseases, and polycystic kidney disease are discussed elsewhere in this book.

Renovascular Disease

Renovascular hypertension due to renal artery stenosis (RAS) is present in 1%-5% of hypertensive patients. There are two main types of RAS that can lead to hypertension: atherosclerotic renal artery stenosis (ARAS, >90% of cases) and fibromuscular dysplasia (FMD, <10%). ARAS is an atherosclerotic process indistinctive from atherosclerosis in any other vascular bed, with similar

TABLE 65.3	Drugs Commonly Associated With Hypertension

Oral Contraceptives

Nonsteroidal antiinflammatory drugs (NSAIDs; selective, and nonselective)

Sympathomimetics: pseudoephedrine, phenylpropanolamine, phentermine, cocaine, amphetamines (prescription or illegal), yohimbine (alpha-2 antagonist)

Selective serotonin reuptake inhibitors (SSRIs) and serotonin-norepinephrine reuptake inhibitors (SNRIs)

Monoamine oxidase inhibitors (MAOIs)

Cyclosporine and tacrolimus

Erythropoietin and darbepoetin

Corticosteroids, mineralocorticoids (fludrocortisone)

Anti-VEGF antibodies (bevacizumab, ramucirumab) and certain tyrosine kinase inhibitors with anti-VEGF activity (e.g., sorafenib, sunitinib, axitinib)

Proteasome inhibitors (carfilzomib)

11-beta hydroxysteroid dehydrogenase type 2 inhibitors: Licorice, posaconazole

Ethanol

pathobiologic mechanisms. Conversely, FMD is a nonatherosclerotic, noninflammatory disease of the arterial wall that results in stenosis of the arterial lumen.

Many hypertensive patients may have renovascular atherosclerotic lesions without a role in the pathogenesis of hypertension. Renovascular atherosclerosis is associated with increased cardiovascular risk, but should be differentiated from renovascular hypertension. In this chapter, we refer solely to RAS (atherosclerotic or fibromuscular) that leads to hypertension through ischemia-induced activation of the renin-angiotensin-aldosterone system (RAAS) as well as progressive endothelial dysfunction, capillary rarefaction, and kidney injury. In animal models of arterial flow restriction, unilateral RAS results in ipsilateral ischemia and renin production, which leads to increased angiotensin II levels that produce a systemic pressor response. Because the other kidney is normal, there is pressure-induced natriuresis and the animals do not become volume overloaded. In contrast, in bilateral disease natriuresis is impaired so hypertension is initially driven by angiotensin II-stimulated vasoconstriction but is maintained by sodium retention, which ultimately leads to decreased renin production. However, in humans, perhaps reflecting the chronicity of this process, there is wide variability in plasma renin levels in bilateral disease, although it is generally accepted that kidney tissue renin levels are high.

Recent animal models have provided new insights, especially on atherosclerotic disease, demonstrating that renal artery flow restriction induces a proinflammatory and profibrotic environment that results in endothelial dysfunction, microvascular rarefaction, and interstitial fibrosis. The degree of flow restriction to trigger these responses in humans is a matter of debate. Available evidence from a study testing ipsilateral renin generation during balloon inflation indicates that a 20% drop in perfusion pressure is required and that renin generation progressively increases with greater degrees of hypoperfusion (Fig. 65.1). The degree of luminal stenosis necessary to produce this pressure gradient typically exceeds 70%, although it may occur with lesions in the 50%–70% range.

Diagnosis of RAS

Renovascular hypertension should be suspected in patients with hypertension and an unexplained decrease in GFR, hypokalemia due to secondary hyperaldosteronism (seen in unilateral RAS), worsening of kidney function with use of ACE inhibitors or ARBs (this suggests bilateral disease, unilateral stenosis in a single kidney, or unilateral stenosis accompanied by underlying parenchymal disease), kidney asymmetry (difference in kidney length of 1.5 cm or more), abdominal and/or flank bruits, generalized atherosclerosis, or unexplained acute pulmonary edema (particularly if recurrent).

Once suspected, the diagnosis of RAS is based on imaging tests. Renal angiography is the gold standard for the diagnosis of RAS; however, most patients are evaluated noninvasively prior to angiography. The three accepted noninvasive diagnostic modalities are computed tomography angiography (CTA), magnetic resonance angiography (MRA), and duplex renal ultrasound (DRU). All other tests, including renal scintigraphy and several previously used biochemical tests, should no longer be used for screening due to poor sensitivity and specificity.

CTA and MRA are preferred because they are easy to perform, are operator independent, and provide good anatomic detail, including visualization of plaque burden in ARAS, morphology of the renal artery in FMD, detailed information on degree of stenosis, and assessment of the typical poststenotic dilatation. Despite

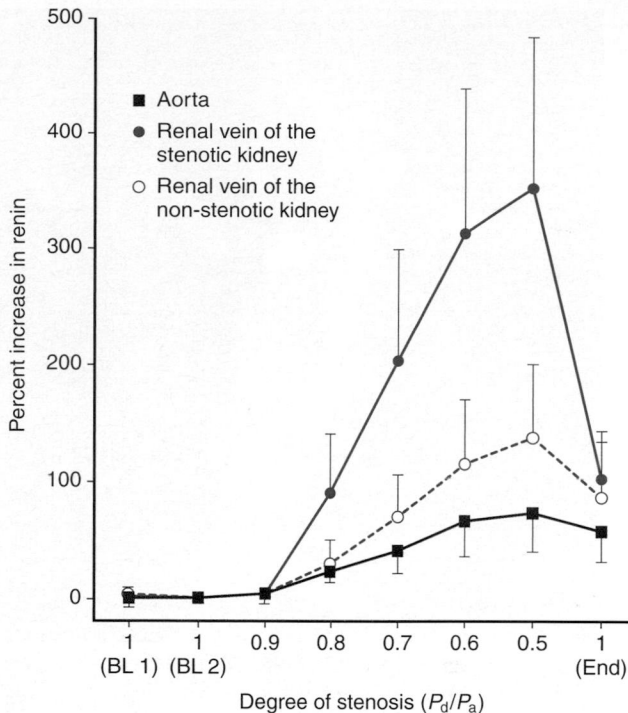

• **Fig. 65.1** Transstenotic pressure thresholds for renin secretion after graded renal artery occlusion in patients with unilateral renal artery stenosis. The experiment was performed after the lesion was treated with stenting. The pressure gradient was induced by progressive inflation of an angioplasty balloon. Pd/Pa indicates the systolic BP ratio between the renal artery (distal to the balloon) and the aorta. A ratio of 1.0 indicates no difference in BP (i.e., no stenosis). The graph shows significant increases in ipsilateral renin secretion with transstenotic systolic BP gradients >20% (i.e., ratio of 0.8 or lower). Renin data are presented for the aorta (*squares*), renal vein of the stenotic kidney (*closed circles*), and renal vein of the non-stenotic kidney (*open circles*). BL1 is the baseline before stenting; BL 2 is the baseline after stenting. (From De Bruyne et al. Assessment of Renal Artery Stenosis Severity by Pressure Gradient Measurements. J Am Coll Cardiol. 2006;48:1851.)

the fact that many in the past have used 50% stenosis as the cutoff for diagnosis, and that the presence of any atherosclerotic renal artery lesion (of any severity) is associated with increased cardiovascular mortality, current guidelines call for luminal occlusion >70% to be considered hemodynamically significant. The quality of the images using CTA (Fig. 65.2) is generally better than MRA, but its use may be precluded by the coexistence of impaired kidney function and the attendant risk of contrast-induced nephropathy. MRA has the caveat of requiring breath holding; accordingly, motion artefacts are common. Both CTA and MRA are limited by a tendency to overestimate lesions and the inability to provide any functional information.

Duplex ultrasound, in experienced hands, is ~90% accurate for the diagnosis of RAS. The diagnosis is not made through visualization of the stenosis, but by the detection of increased flow velocity at the site of stenosis compared to the adjacent aorta. A renal-to-aortic ratio >3.5 (peak systolic velocity within the renal artery divided by the peak systolic velocity in the aorta) accompanied by a peak systolic velocity >280 m/s is suggestive of >60% RAS on angiography (this was the cutoff utilized by the seminal validating studies). Additionally, functional information on the RAS can be derived from Doppler tracings obtained from the renal

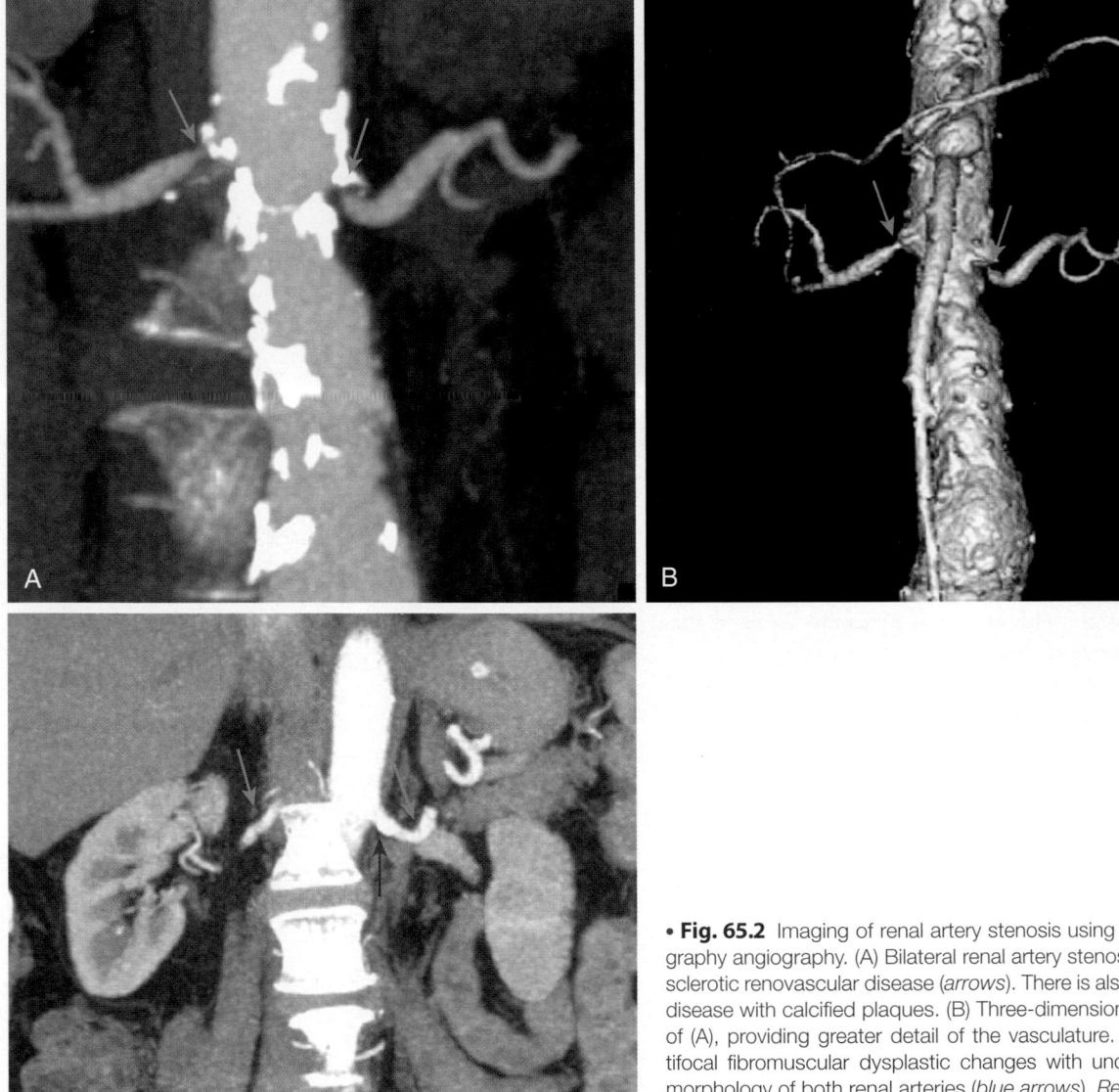

• **Fig. 65.2** Imaging of renal artery stenosis using computed tomography angiography. (A) Bilateral renal artery stenosis due to atherosclerotic renovascular disease (*arrows*). There is also extensive aortic disease with calcified plaques. (B) Three-dimensional reconstruction of (A), providing greater detail of the vasculature. (C) Bilateral multifocal fibromuscular dysplastic changes with undulating, saccular morphology of both renal arteries (*blue arrows*). *Red arrow*, left renal artery aneurysm, a relatively frequent complication of fibromuscular dysplasia.

parenchyma. Acceleration times reflect the time needed for the incident pulse wave to reach its peak. In conditions of restricted flow, the acceleration time is increased (>100 ms), which results in a pulse wave of decreased amplitude and late peak (i.e., a "pulsus parvus et tardus"). While this abnormality is insensitive for the diagnosis of severe RAS, it is quite specific for hemodynamically significant lesions, and the tracings should always be inspected to try to identify it. The resistive index ([peak systolic velocity – diastolic velocity]/peak systolic velocity) is a marker of increased parenchymal resistance to blood flow due to increased renovascular resistance but is also influenced by systemic factors such as heart rate, peripheral vascular resistance, and arterial stiffness. It can be increased (>0.8) in the setting of acute kidney injury or CKD of any cause. The resistive index is low in a kidney with a hemodynamically significant inflow restriction, and a low resistive index (<0.6) in a kidney with a visualized RAS suggests that the lesion is hemodynamically significant. If the contralateral kidney has a resistive index >0.8, the likelihood of clinical response

to revascularization is lower, as the high resistive index in the absence of a flow-limiting renal artery lesion in the contralateral kidney suggests systemic microvascular disease and parenchymal kidney damage. Because it does not involve contrast administration, DRU is often used in patients with advanced kidney disease. However, it is time consuming and dependent on both operator skill and patient body habitus, resulting in unreliable results in up to 25% of patients.

Novel techniques are under development to provide functional data in RAS. The most promising appears to be blood oxygen level-dependent MRI (BOLD-MRI), a technique that detects areas of ischemia (based on deoxyhemoglobin levels) in the kidney. This modality is being perfected to identify kidneys that remain viable despite underlying ischemia, allowing clinicians to identify good candidates for revascularization. Unfortunately, difficulties with protocol validation and lack of studies demonstrating its value are still restricted to small case series; thus, its use in clinical practice cannot yet be recommended.

Management of Atherosclerotic RAS

All patients with ARAS should receive maximal medical therapy including smoking cessation (if applicable), antiplatelet therapy, statins, and a blocker of the RAAS. Even though there are no data demonstrating a benefit from smoking cessation and antiplatelet therapy, there is general agreement based on the management of vascular disease in other arterial beds that smoking cessation, antiplatelet therapy (aspirin or clopidogrel), and statins should be offered to all patients. In one observational study, exposure to a beta-blocker was associated with lower risk of cardiovascular events and death. Therefore, it is reasonable to include a beta-blocker as part of the antihypertensive regimen in patients with ARAS.

Observational studies support the use of RAAS blockers (ACE inhibitors or ARBs) to improve cardiovascular and kidney outcomes in ARAS. This is important to recognize because clinicians are often fearful of using these agents in ARAS. In fact, ACE inhibitors are associated with lower risk of death and kidney failure in this population, even among patients with bilateral disease. Inability to tolerate a RAAS blocker (i.e., a drop in GFR >20%) in such patients is an indication of hemodynamic significance of the lesions and should lead the clinician to strongly consider revascularization.

There is little evidence from clinical trials to support an advantage of revascularization over medical therapy in patients with disease of mild severity (<70% stenosis), in those incidentally discovered without accompanying hypertension or kidney dysfunction, or in those with well-controlled hypertension and stable kidney function during follow-up. Although meta-analyses indicate that BP is ~7/3 mm Hg lower in patients randomized to revascularization compared with medical therapy, two randomized clinical trials, STAR (STent placement and blood pressure and lipid lowering for the prevention of progression of renal dysfunction caused by Atherosclerotic ostial stenosis of the Renal artery) and ASTRAL (Angioplasty and Stenting for Renal Artery Lesions), studied patients with relatively mild degrees of stenosis, stable clinical course, and reasonable BP control, and demonstrated no significant BP reduction, kidney function improvement, or effect on the occurrence cardiovascular events, end-stage kidney disease, or death associated with renal artery stenting. The Cardiovascular Outcomes in Renal Atherosclerotic Lesions (CORAL) trial was the most detailed trial comparing renal artery stenting with medical therapy in patients with hypertension and significant stenosis (>80% or 60%–80% with a transstenotic systolic BP gradient >20 mm Hg). In CORAL, renal artery stenting resulted in minimally lower systolic BP than medical therapy (2.3 mm Hg, P=0.03), but there was no difference in the occurrence of the composite primary endpoint of cardiovascular or kidney death, myocardial infarction, hospitalization for congestive heart failure, stroke, progressive kidney disease, and need for kidney replacement therapy (35.1% in the stent group, 35.8% in the medical group, P=0.58), any of the components of this composite outcome, or any secondary endpoints. Results did not differ between patients with unilateral or bilateral disease. Lastly, a meta-analysis of five randomized clinical trials revealed no role for intervention to reduce the occurrence of nonfatal myocardial infarction in ARAS (the risk ratio compared with medical therapy was 0.86 [0.51–1.43], P=.55), a finding that was independent of follow-up kidney function or duration of follow-up.

It is important to recognize that the available clinical trials excluded a large number of patients. For example, ASTRAL included only patients whose clinicians were "uncertain that patients would definitely benefit from revascularization." None of the studies included patients with rapid loss of kidney function or patients presenting with recurrent, unexplained pulmonary edema. Because of this, I believe that the triad of rapid loss of kidney function, resistant hypertension in the hands of a hypertension specialist, and unexplained recurrent pulmonary edema are acceptable indications for intervention in ARAS. I often recommend intervention in patients who have bilateral disease and develop kidney hypoperfusion and loss of kidney function upon achievement of adequate BP control and/or initiation of RAAS blockade. The 2018 Report on the Appropriate Use Criteria for Peripheral Artery Intervention sponsored by multiple cardiovascular societies supports these indications.

Revascularization is currently accomplished via percutaneous transluminal angioplasty and stenting (PTRAS) in 98% of patients who require an intervention. Angioplasty alone (without stenting) is not an adequate technique in ARAS due to the extensive amount of arterial recoiling following the procedure. This is due to the proximal nature of the lesions and shared plaque with the aorta. In addition, stent use results in significantly lower rates of restenosis compared to angioplasty alone. Surgical intervention is rarely needed and is left for patients with extensive aortic disease that would require simultaneous open correction.

Approximately one-third of patients undergoing intervention experience worsening kidney function. This may be the result of contrast nephropathy or atheroembolic kidney disease, which often goes unsuspected and undiagnosed.

Monitoring patients closely is extremely important. Patients with ARAS followed without intervention are at risk of occlusion and atrophy of the ipsilateral kidney (~10% and 22% over 3 years, respectively). However, studies of incidental ARAS suggest a stable kidney course over time, though patients with ARAS have high risk of cardiovascular events, likely a reflection of overall atherosclerotic disease burden. Current recommendations suggest yearly ultrasounds to monitor kidney size. My practice is to do so for 2–3 years, but if patients have stable BP and kidney function, I typically stop and reserve re-imaging to cases of loss of clinical stability. Following interventions, current guidelines call for imaging with renal duplex ultrasound within 30 days of the procedure, at 6 and 12 months, and yearly thereafter.

Fibromuscular Dysplasia

FMD predominantly affects younger women, most often diagnosed between 40 and 50 years old. The renal arteries are the vessels most commonly affected (80%–100% of patients, up to 60% bilateral), although many other sites can be involved, including the carotid and vertebral arteries (up to ~70% in some series, 20% to 30% in most). Most cases are sporadic, although ~10% are familial, and rare cases can be associated with specific genetic diseases such as neurofibromatosis, tuberous sclerosis, Ehlers-Danlos syndrome, Alagille syndrome, Williams syndrome, and Turner syndrome. Renal FMD is associated with smoking in about 30% of patients.

Renal FMD is subdivided according to its radiographic appearance as multifocal (~80% of cases, usually representing involvement of the media) or unifocal (~20%, usually due to intimal or perimedial disease). The radiographic appearance does not seem to affect the clinical presentation, which is one of hypertension, usually with preserved kidney function. However, data from the most comprehensive series indicate that, although the median BP response to angioplasty is similar for both FMD subtypes (~30 mm Hg), cure of hypertension is not the norm, occurring in 54% of patients with unifocal disease and 26% with multifocal disease.

The goal in FMD is early identification and treatment with percutaneous angioplasty, which is indicated in patients with hypertension as long as there is no significant atrophy of the affected kidney (e.g., kidney length less than 8 cm on ultrasound). Stenting is rarely necessary, and surgical correction is reserved for patients with complex anatomic lesions. Despite the absence of comparative trials, most believe that medical management is a less preferred option in FMD. In patients who opt against angioplasty, treatment is a drug regimen that includes an ACE inhibitor (or an ARB). Antiplatelet therapy with low-dose aspirin is recommended in the absence of contraindications. Statins are not necessary, but smoking cessation should be strongly encouraged.

The management of patients with renal FMD also includes screening for extrarenal disease. The International Consensus recommends at least a one-time screening CT or MR angiography from head to pelvis to screen for FMD in the brain (aneurysms), cervico-cranial, and splanchnic territories.

Primary Aldosteronism

Primary aldosteronism is a common cause of secondary hypertension, with an estimated prevalence of 5%–10% among hypertensive patients. In patients with resistant hypertension, that number approaches 20%. Most cases are due to adrenal hyperplasia (~60%), which is typically bilateral, or aldosterone-producing adrenal adenomas (~40%). Uncommon causes include adrenal carcinoma, unilateral adrenal hyperplasia, and glucocorticoid-remediable aldosteronism.

The pathobiology of adrenal proliferation and aldosterone excess in primary aldosteronism is linked to mutations affecting cation flux in the adrenal glomerulosa. Somatic mutations in the KCJN5 gene coding for an inward rectifying potassium channel in adrenal adenomas are present in about one-third of adenomas. These mutant channels expressed in the adrenal glomerulosa lose their specificity for potassium and allow inward flow (i.e., into the cell) of sodium, resulting in chronic cell depolarization and calcium inflow, which, in turn, stimulates cell proliferation and aldosterone production. The same mutation has been identified as a germline mutation in patients with a rare form of adrenal hyperplasia (familial aldosteronism type 3) and results in massive adrenal hyperplasia, aldosterone production, and severe hypertension with cardiovascular complications. Similar effects on cell depolarization and inward calcium inflow have been demonstrated with other somatic mutations in adenomas, such as in the CACNA1D gene coding a voltage-gated calcium channel, the ATP1A1 gene coding the alpha1 subunit of the Na/K ATPase, and the ATP2B3 gene encoding the plasma membrane Ca-ATPase 3. In addition, mutations in other pathways for adrenal adenoma formation have been recently described, such as those in the beta-catenin gene CTNNB1, leading to tumor growth and aldosterone secretion through mechanisms that are not yet fully understood but seem to involve overexpression of beta-catenin and, therefore, overactivity of the WNT signaling pathway. Approximately 80% of adenomas have one of these identifiable somatic mutation.

While hypokalemia is the most common clue to the diagnosis, its prevalence is quite variable and usually restricted to a minority of patients (only 9%–37% have serum potassium <3.5 mEq/L). It is more common in patients with adenomas (~50%) than bilateral hyperplasia, likely reflecting the generally higher plasma aldosterone levels in adenomas. Therefore, clinicians must be attuned to the possibility of primary aldosteronism in many other situations. Recognizing this, the Endocrine Society recommends screening for primary aldosteronism when hypertension is associated with one of seven specific circumstances: (1) BP consistently >150/100 mm Hg, (2) resistant hypertension (>140/90 mm Hg on >3 drugs), (3) spontaneous or diuretic-induced hypokalemia, (4) adrenal incidentaloma, (5) sleep apnea, (6) family history of early-onset hypertension or stroke at age younger than 40 years, or (7) family history of primary aldosteronism (of any type). Recent studies show higher risk of incident atrial fibrillation in patients with primary aldosteronism that can be mitigated by effective aldosterone suppression by adrenalectomy or mineralocorticoid receptor antagonism. These data have led to some experts recommending screening patients with hypertension and atrial fibrillation.

Biochemical Diagnosis

Screening is performed with simultaneous measurement of plasma aldosterone and plasma renin activity (PRA) and calculation of the aldosterone/renin ratio (ARR). It is important to analyze each of these components and not focus solely on the ARR. There are numerous factors that impact on this ratio, and it is particularly sensitive to the PRA, as small changes in value can result in significant changes in the ARR. In order to maximize the accuracy of the test, it is best to obtain it in the morning, after the patient has been out of bed for at least 2 hours, after 5–15 minutes in the seated position, and preferably under liberal salt intake and appropriate potassium repletion. While many drugs can impact the ARR (Table 65.4), most patients are screened while taking antihypertensive medications, with the exception of mineralocorticoid receptor antagonists (MRA) and other potassium-sparing

TABLE 65.4	Factors Impacting on the Interpretation of the Aldosterone/Renin Ratio	
	False Positives	**False Negatives**
Aldosterone relatively high	Potassium loading	
Renin relatively low	Beta-blockers Central antiadrenergics Direct renin inhibitors NSAIDS Chronic kidney disease Sodium loading	
Aldosterone relatively low		Hypokalemia
Renin relatively high		Diuretics (any type) ACE inhibitors Angiotensin receptor blockers Dihydropyridine calcium blockers Serotonin reuptake inhibitors Acute sodium depletion Estrogens, oral contraceptives Pregnancy

Direct renin inhibitors uniformly lower aldosterone levels. However, their effect on renin differs if measured as plasma renin activity (PRA falls) or plasma renin concentration (PRC increases).

diuretics, and renin inhibitors. Long-acting drugs such as spironolactone must be stopped for at least 4 weeks prior to testing.

If the ARR results (see later) obtained while the patient is receiving medications are counter to the clinical suspicion, patients should come off all drugs that can affect the ARR (see Table 65.4) for at least 2 weeks and undergo retesting. Medications with minimal or no effects on the ARR, such as nondihydropyridine calcium channel blockers (diltiazem, verapamil), alpha blockers (doxazosin, terazosin), and hydralazine, should be used as needed to control BP during this washout period.

An ARR >30 (using aldosterone measured in ng/dL and PRA measured in ng/mL/h) is suggestive of primary aldosteronism, especially if accompanied by plasma aldosterone levels >15 ng/dL. However, one must keep in mind that using higher aldosterone cutoff levels decreases the sensitivity of the approach, while improving specificity. Lowering the cutoff has the opposite effect, but may be worth considering, especially in high-risk patients. For example, 30%–40% with high ARR and plasma aldosterone between 10 and 15 ng/dL have positive confirmatory tests that assess aldosterone production; this number is ~4% if aldosterone <10 ng/dL. Therefore, it is plausible to consider a confirmatory test in patients with a high ARR and plasma aldosterone >10 ng/dL, especially in those with a high a priori probability of the diagnosis. Furthermore, a recent multicenter study showed that many patients with primary aldosteronism have low plasma aldosterone levels, raising concerns about using absolute plasma aldosterone levels to guide the need for confirmatory studies (see below). In patients with a high ARR, low PRA (<0.2 ng/mL/h), aldosterone >20 ng/dL, and hypokalemia, confirmatory testing is not necessary; these patients are virtually certain to have primary aldosteronism.

Confirmatory tests are designed to document persistent autonomous production of aldosterone despite the use of a physiologic factor that strongly suppresses aldosterone secretion (i.e., sodium loading). There are several accepted confirmatory tests, most importantly the oral sodium loading test (OSLT), the saline infusion test (SIT), and the fludrocortisone suppression test. I prefer either the OSLT or the SIT, both for ease of performance and overall safety. In the OSLT, sodium intake is liberalized in order to achieve >200 mEq/day sodium intake for 3 days. Potassium should be effectively replaced during the collection to avoid hypokalemia. A 24-hour urine collection is performed starting in the morning of the third day. I measure urine creatinine (to assess the completeness of the collection), sodium (to confirm >200 mEq/day intake), and aldosterone. Urine aldosterone excretion >12–14 mcg/day is confirmatory, while levels <10 mcg/day convincingly exclude the diagnosis. In cases of intermediate values, repeating the collection is necessary. In the SIT, the patient lies supine for 1 hour before administration of 2 L of normal saline over 4 hours with the patient remaining in the supine position. We measure pre- and postsaline plasma aldosterone. A postinfusion aldosterone >10 ng/dL confirms the diagnosis, while aldosterone <5 ng/dL rules it out. Levels between 5 and 10 ng/dL are considered indeterminate and require either repeat testing or an alternative confirmatory test. I also measure pre- and postpotassium and cortisol to exclude an effect of potassium or ACTH on the changes in aldosterone concentration. Because both tests involve the administration of substantial amounts of sodium, they are contraindicated in patients with congestive heart failure, severe hypertension, or severe hypokalemia. In such cases, a pragmatic decision is made regarding the likelihood of the diagnosis using simply the screening aldosterone and PRA.

Subtype Differentiation

Once the biochemical diagnosis of autonomous aldosterone excess is confirmed, the next step is subtype differentiation. The two most common subtypes are bilateral hyperplasia (~60% of cases) and adrenal adenomas (~40% of cases). Rare causes include adrenal carcinoma, unilateral adrenal hyperplasia, and glucocorticoid-remediable aldosteronism.

The differential diagnosis starts with a thin-cut adrenal CT. The major role of the CT is to rule out an adrenal carcinoma, which is typically a large mass (rarely <4 cm). Visualization of a small (<2 cm), hypodense (<10 Hounsfield units) adrenal nodule is virtually diagnostic of an adenoma. However, evidence based on adrenal venous sampling (AVS) studies suggests that nodules are nonfunctional in 20%–25% of cases. Moreover, a meta-analysis of older studies (using older imaging technology) showed that imaging (CT and MRI) and AVS data are discordant in almost 40% of cases. This includes not only the occurrence of nonfunctional adenomas but also cases when no adenoma was visualized but there was lateralization of aldosterone production on AVS (microadenomas or unilateral adrenal hyperplasia). Therefore, the most appropriate method to distinguish between the clinical subtypes is AVS, and, indeed, current recommendations call for AVS in almost all patients in whom surgical treatment of a possible functioning adenoma is being entertained. The only possible exception refers to patients who are younger than 35 years, have hypertension with hypokalemia and high aldosterone levels (>20 ng/dL), and have an adenoma on CT. This is justified by the very low rate of incidental adrenal masses in this age range. Patients who are not interested in or are at high risk for surgery do not require AVS and should be treated medically.

AVS should be performed by an experienced interventional radiologist who is familiar with the protocol and is skilled in the procedure, especially because of the angle of the right adrenal vein, which precludes successful catheterization in up to 25% of cases. The test starts with the administration of cosyntropin, which is used to produce maximal cortisol secretion from both adrenal glands in order to provide a good means for "adjustment" of the aldosterone results. I use a continuous infusion of 50 mcg/h intravenously, starting 30 minutes prior to the catheterization and continued until the end of the procedure. Blood is sampled from each of the adrenal glands and a peripheral site (can be the inferior vena cava or an upper extremity vein) and is sent for both aldosterone and cortisol.

Interpretation of AVS Results

First, each aldosterone and cortisol level should be analyzed as ratios of aldosterone to cortisol from each of the three sampling sites. Second, the aldosterone/cortisol ratio for the right adrenal vein is compared with the left adrenal vein, and both are compared with the peripheral ratio. If the aldosterone/cortisol ratio on one of the adrenal veins is greater than or equal to 4 times higher than the contralateral side, the diagnosis of lateralization is made, indicating the presence of an aldosterone-producing adenoma or, rarely, unilateral adrenal hyperplasia. Most adenomas have lateralizing ratios >10–20 times. In addition, patients with adenomas typically have suppressed secretion from the contralateral side (defined as aldosterone/cortisol ratio from the contralateral side lower than that from the periphery).

Other Testing

In the past, several biochemical tests and nuclear medicine imaging (iodocholesterol) were used to help in subtype differentiation. The accuracy of these tests is low, and they are no longer recommended. In patients suspected of having glucocorticoid-remediable aldosteronism (early hypertension, personal or family history of hemorrhagic strokes or brain aneurysms), the diagnosis should be made through formal genetic testing to identify the chimeric gene mutation (between the aldosterone synthase and 11-beta-hydroxylase genes). Indirect physiologic tests, such as the dexamethasone suppression test or the measurement of urinary hybrid steroids, are no longer recommended, though may still be used in resource-poor areas where genetic testing is not available.

Treatment of Primary Aldosteronism

Primary aldosteronism is associated with cardiovascular and kidney damage, likely related to aldosterone excess, and removal or blockade of this excess results in improved clinical outcomes. Patients with an aldosterone-producing adenoma or unilateral adrenal hyperplasia should be offered laparoscopic unilateral adrenalectomy. All adrenalectomized patients experience normalization of serum potassium levels. On the other hand, BP improvement occurs primarily in younger patients who are lean (body mass index <26 kg/m²), more often female, have a relatively recent history of hypertension (<5–6 years), require <2 drugs for treatment of their hypertension, and have normal kidney function. Patients who have few or none of these characteristics have poor BP response to adrenalectomy; accordingly, an initial attempt at medical therapy may be a more reasonable choice in the group.

Bilateral hyperplasia is managed medically, with an MRA as the backbone of therapy. A clinical trial showed that spironolactone was slightly better than eplerenone, though the doses may not have been precisely exchangeable. We typically start with spironolactone 25 mg once daily and escalate the dose as needed (typically 50–150 mg/day) to achieve BP and potassium control. For those patients who develop intolerable side effects to spironolactone, especially those related to its antiandrogenic effects, we substitute eplerenone using a 2:1 dosing ratio and twice-daily dosing. There are several new nonsteroidal MRAs under clinical testing, such as finerenone, and their role in treating primary aldosteronism awaits determination. The Endocrine Society guidelines recommend against the use of MRAs in patients with eGFR <30 mL/min. I disagree with this recommendation because MRAs are effective antihypertensive agents even in anephric patients. The risk of hyperkalemia obviously exists but can be mitigated with the use of smaller doses (e.g., starting at 12.5 mg daily) and closely monitoring serum potassium levels.

Aldosterone synthase inhibitors have been tested in patients with primary aldosteronism. The early experience indicates that, while successful in suppressing aldosterone levels, the efficacy of managing BP is significantly less than eplerenone. At the present time, they are not yet marketed and their role in treatment remains uncertain, although one could envision a situation in which they are used in combination with an MRA or other BP agents, especially as patients often need additional agents to reach BP control despite the use of an MRA. Amiloride is useful in patients who are intolerant to spironolactone and eplerenone, though less effective in BP control. Thiazide diuretics are often helpful, although potassium levels must be monitored closely as they may drop precipitously with the thiazide. Calcium channel blockers are also effective for BP control in primary aldosteronism.

Pheochromocytoma/Paraganglioma (PPGL)

Pheochromocytoma is a tumor arising from the adrenomedullary chromaffin cells. Paraganglioma is a tumor derived from extraadrenal chromaffin cells of the sympathetic paravertebral and neck ganglia. Pheochromocytomas are almost always biochemically active, producing epinephrine, norepinephrine, or dopamine, alone or in combination. Paragangliomas may be biochemically silent, especially when originating in the neck and base of the skull. Overall, pheochromocytomas represent ~80%–85% of these tumors, whereas paragangliomas account for ~15%–20%.

PPGL are rare tumors (incidence 2–8 cases per million per year). However, knowledge about their clinical presentation and the appropriate approach to diagnosis and management is important because of the cardiovascular risk they pose through severe hypertension. Most PPGL patients are hypertensive (~90%), particularly those with pheochromocytoma. Approximately one-third of patients have only paroxysmal BP elevations, and, of the two-thirds with sustained hypertension, about half also have episodic peaks. These paroxysms are associated with catecholamine release and are characterized clinically by the classic triad of headaches, palpitations, and diaphoresis. This diagnostic triad is present in the majority of patients but has limited specificity (positive predictive value 6%), so that most patients with the triad actually do not have PPGL. Other common symptoms are anxiety, tremulousness, pallor, flushing, and orthostatic hypotension. There is growing acknowledgement of the fact that PPGL may be asymptomatic more often that previously considered and needs to be entertained in the diagnostic approach to adrenal masses and other masses of the neck, abdomen, and pelvis with the right location and radiographic appearance.

Overall, 5%–10% of PPGL are extraabdominal, 10%–15% are multifocal (including bilateral adrenal lesions), and ~10% are malignant. Recent advances in genetic testing have significantly increased the percentage of patients with PPGL associated with a specific syndrome or germline mutations. In the past, genetic causes of PPGL had been restricted to syndromic forms of PPGL, such as multiple endocrine neoplasia type 2 (MEN2), hereditary retinoblastoma (RET), neurofibromatosis type 1 (NF1), and von Hippel-Lindau disease (VHL). However, current estimates are that up to 40% of PPGL patients have a germline mutation, even in patients with sporadic PPGL, a number that is likely to increase as novel mutations continue to be identified. Many germline and somatic mutations have already been described and have contributed to the understanding of the pathobiology of PPGL. For example, one cluster of germline mutations involves the VHL gene and the genes for the succinate dehydrogenase (SDX) units, and the somatic mutations of the hypoxia-induced factor 2A (HIF2A) gene are characterized by an impact on abnormal transcription in response to hypoxia. Another cluster of mutations that involve RET and NF1 among other genes is characterized by activation of kinase-mediated cell proliferation pathways such as the PI3/AKT/mTOR. These developments have not only diagnostic and important for genetic counseling, but also may have treatment implications in the future.

PPGL should be suspected in every hypertensive patient with symptoms suggestive of catecholamine excess. While there are several reports of hypertensive PPGL presenting without any symptoms, these are unusual (probably ~1%) and, as a general rule, I do not screen patients referred to us for the evaluation of nonparoxysmal hypertension who are fully asymptomatic. The exception are very young patients or those who have the sudden development of hypertension that is not explained by other, more common, secondary causes. It should also be suspected in patients with one of the syndromic forms of PPGL, such as multiple endocrine neoplasia type 2 (MEN2), hereditary retinoblastoma (RET), neurofibromatosis type 1 (NF1), and von Hippel-Lindau disease (VHL), and in adult patients with chronic congenital cyanotic heart disease, an association that has been based on the role of chronic hypoxia as a mediator of tumor development.

Biochemical Diagnosis and Imaging of PPGL

Biochemical documentation of catecholamine excess is essential during the evaluation of PPGL. No other tests (e.g., localizing imaging tests) should be performed until there is laboratory evidence of excessive catecholamine production and/or metabolism. The measurement of free metanephrines in serum or urine is the preferred diagnostic tests. Metanephrines are produced continuously within chromaffin cells (or chromaffin-derived PPGL); this is different and independent from the pattern of catecholamine release, which can be intermittent.

Plasma or urine free metanephrines are acceptable screening measurements, both having an accuracy in the 96%–99% range. Sensitivity is very high, although there are shortcomings in specificity due to substances that may cause falsely elevated levels. In the case of plasma metanephrines, false-positive normetanephrine can be observed with acetaminophen (only certain assays), tricyclic antidepressants, methyldopa, phenoxybenzamine, and sulfasalazine use, whereas buspirone may elevate plasma metanephrines. MAO-inhibitors, cocaine and other sympathomimetics, and levodopa can provoke false elevations of both plasma metanephrine and normetanephrine. Similar patterns are observed for urine metanephrine and normetanephrine levels. In addition, labetalol and sotalol can increase both urinary levels (but have no effect on plasma measurements).

Measurement of plasma free metanephrines requires cautious attention to position. When levels are obtained in the seated position, there is almost a three fold increase in false positives compared with supine measurements. The Endocrine Society recommends supine measurements. However, it recognizes the practical limitations of this recommendation as most laboratories are unable to accommodate this request; accordingly, it is acceptable to obtain samples in the seated position and, in case results are high, have them repeated in the supine position or corroborated by a 24-hour urine collection.

Most PPGLs result in metanephrine levels more than three times above the normal range. In such cases, anatomic localization is indicated. In patients with repeatedly borderline levels, the clonidine suppression test can be performed to distinguish between a normal variant (suppressible plasma metanephrines) and PPGL (nonsuppressible levels). In this test, clonidine 0.3 mg is given orally immediately after measurement of plasma metanephrines, which are measured again 3 hours later. Normally, clonidine lowers catecholamine and metanephrine levels by >40%; no such effect occurs in PPGL.

Once convincing biochemical evidence of PPGL is available, radiographic localization is indicated. The screening method of choice is a contrast-enhanced CT of the abdomen and pelvis, as 85% of PPGLs are intraabdominal. If negative, extension of imaging to the chest (CT) and neck (MRI) should be performed. In patients in whom a tumor cannot be identified despite the above approach, ^{123}I-metaiodobenzylguanidine (MIBG) scintigraphy is indicated as another method to locate the tumor. Other techniques, including ^{123}I-MIBG positron emission tomography (PET), 68-Gallium dotatate PET, and 5-fluorodopamine-PET, are not easily available outside of referral centers or research institutions.

Genetic Testing in PPGL

The Endocrine Society recommends the use of shared decision making with the patient regarding genetic testing. The guidelines suggest individual screening for mutations based on the familial distribution, presence of a defined syndrome, and guided choice of genes to be tested based on location and biochemical profile of the tumor. Because of the continued rise in identification of mutations in PPGL, many clinicians from several referral centers do not follow this approach and instead screen all patients (including those with sporadic PPGL) using a next-generation sequencing package that covers all known mutations (as of 2020, at least 22 susceptibility genes have been identified).

Treatment of PPGL

The treatment of choice for PPGL is surgical excision and should take place in referral centers with large experience with neuroendocrine tumors. Pheochromocytomas can be managed laparoscopically, whereas paragangliomas are usually resected with an open approach. All patients should be treated medically for at least 1–2 weeks in anticipation of surgery. The cornerstone of therapy is an alpha-blocker (either the nonselective phenoxybenzamine or a selective alpha-1 blocker such as doxazosin or terazosin). Calcium channel blockers (amlodipine or nifedipine) are the first option as add-on treatment if BP is not adequately controlled with an alpha-blocker, followed by the addition of a beta-blocker (propranolol or atenolol). Some clinicians also use metyrosine (a tyrosine hydroxylase inhibitor that blocks the first step in catecholamine synthesis) to improve BP control and intraoperative stability in these patients.

The evaluation and management of metastatic disease is nuanced and beyond the scope of this chapter. Follow-up is planned based on individual clinical and genetic characteristics. In most cases, biochemical screening is repeated 6 months following resection, then yearly. In high-risk patients, such as those with large pheochromocytomas, multifocal paragangliomas, and those with biochemically silent disease, yearly imaging is indicated.

Other Endocrine Causes of Hypertension

Cushing Syndrome

Approximately 80% of patients with glucocorticoid excess due to Cushing syndrome have hypertension. However, they typically come to medical attention due to other features of the syndrome (weight gain, fatigue, muscle weakness, skin changes, anxiety, glucose intolerance, hyperlipidemia, osteopenia) rather than hypertension. Patients with ectopic ACTH production tend to have more severe hypertension. In many cases, hypokalemia can be significant. It is important to always consider the possibility of glucocorticoid excess in patients with hypertension accompanied by low aldosterone and suppressed plasma renin activity.

Thyroid Disease

Hypertension may be observed both in hypothyroidism and hyperthyroidism, although the hemodynamic profile of each condition is quite distinct. Hypertension is seen in ~40% of patients with hypothyroidism and has a predominantly diastolic phenotype associated with increased systemic vascular resistance and decreased arterial compliance. Because of low cardiac output, patients may have a narrow pulse pressure despite stiff vessels. Subclinical hypothyroidism is also associated with hypertension, though the impact of its treatment on BP lowering is still uncertain. Hypertension in hyperthyroidism is primarily systolic and is related to increased cardiac output. Because vascular resistance is decreased, pulse pressure is often wide. Hyperthyroid patients may present with spells and paroxysmal features that, at times, resemble pheochromocytoma. Specific treatments for each thyroid disturbance are sufficient to normalize BP in most patients.

Primary Hyperparathyroidism

Up to 70% of patients with primary hyperparathyroidism due to a parathyroid adenoma are hypertensive. Despite the absence of a direct correlation between serum calcium or parathyroid hormone levels and BP in these patients, it is presumed that it is the increase in cytosolic calcium that results in hypertension due to increased vascular resistance and cardiac output. Hypercalcemia-induced renal vasoconstriction and kidney damage due to hypercalciuria are additional mechanisms that may mediate hypertension. Removal of the adenomatous gland cures or improves BP in most hyperparathyroid patients with a new diagnosis of hypertension.

Acromegaly

Hypertension is common in acromegaly, though much of its prevalence may be explained by age and sex. Despite this, BP decreases following successful treatment in many patients, thus raising the possibility that growth hormone and insulin-like growth factor 1 are indeed related to hypertension in this condition. BP elevations are seldom severe.

Obstructive Sleep Apnea

Obstructive sleep apnea (OSA) is a common disorder in the general population, and is associated with hypertension, in particular due to the shared common occurrence of obesity. OSA results not only in nocturnal but also diurnal elevations in BP, and there is a direct relationship between the severity of OSA and the frequency and severity of hypertension. In patients with resistant hypertension, the prevalence of OSA is 73%–82%.

OSA should be suspected in obese patients (men more so than women) who report severe snoring, daytime somnolence, witnessed nocturnal choking or gasping, and have a "crowded oropharynx" (limited or no visualization of the soft palate) on physical examination. The diagnosis of OSA is based on an ambulatory sleep study or in-center polysomnography (the gold-standard).

OSA can be considered a "non-classic" cause of secondary hypertension because its treatment with continuous positive airway pressure ventilation (CPAP) does not necessarily result in cure of hypertension. In fact, the overall BP-lowering effect of CPAP is low (~3/2 mm Hg). However, patients who have more severe hypertension (resistant hypertension with BP >145/85 mm Hg despite the use of three or more drugs), more severe OSA (apnea/hypopnea index >30), higher daytime sleepiness score (Epworth Sleepiness Score >10), and greater adherence to CPAP (average use >4 h per night) tend to have greater responses.

Despite the limited magnitude of the BP-lowering effect of CPAP, I still believe there is value in asking about and screening for OSA in hypertensive patients and referring those with high sleepiness scores for formal sleep testing. In nonsleepy OSA patients, the strength of the evidence for benefit on BP lowering is weak. Because the impact of CPAP treatment on cardiovascular outcomes and mortality in asymptomatic OSA patients is uncertain, I tend to pursue the diagnosis and treatment of OSA in nonsleepy patients only in the setting of resistant hypertension.

Aside from CPAP, patients with sleep apnea can benefit from medical therapy. Hypertension of OSA is associated with both sympathetic activation and aldosterone excess. While there is no definitive trial demonstrating the superiority of one drug class over another in OSA, there is some evidence that beta-blockers are particularly effective. In addition, spironolactone, either alone or in combination with a loop diuretic, can also be helpful, presumably mediated by improved volume status and decreased rostral airway edema, therefore improving not only BP but also OSA.

Coarctation of the Aorta and Other Aortopathies

Coarctation of the aorta (CoA) is a constriction of the descending thoracic aorta, most commonly distal to the left subclavian artery, but should be interpreted as a diffuse large vessel arteriopathy. It is an unusual cause of hypertension in adults and should be suspected in patients with hypertension in the arms but normal or low BP in the thigh/leg. A bicuspid aortic valve is a common accompaniment, present in 50% of CoA patients. Conversely, ~6% of patients with a bicuspid aortic valve have CoA. Therefore, in patients with a known bicuspid aortic valve who develop hypertension at a young age or have new, otherwise unexplained hypertension should have the possibility of CoA entertained, especially as bicuspid aortic valves are relatively common (1%–2% of the population). Hypertension is noted in the upper extremities due to mechanical obstruction to blood flow, which, in turn, results in renal ischemia and activation of the RAAS. The diagnosis is made using MR or CT angiography to locate and define the severity of the coarctation. Echocardiography is an alternative method, though not as accurate. Once diagnosed, patients should undergo angiography to define the translesional gradient and, if elevated (>20 mm Hg), should undergo repair either surgically or with balloon angioplasty with or without stenting. In recent years, percutaneous angioplasty has been increasingly used in lieu of open surgical techniques for the successful treatment of localized CoA in adults. Surgery is preferred for complex lesions not suitable for percutaneous management.

Stenotic lesions of the aorta due to other forms of aortic disease can be seen at any level and may result in hypertension through similar mechanisms as CoA. Though rare, the most common such aortopathy is Takayasu arteritis, which should be considered in patients with evidence of a systemic inflammatory disease with progressive involvement of the aorta and large branches. Populations at higher risk are women (~90%) of East Asian descent, though the disease has been identified with increasing frequency in the Indian subcontinent, the Middle East, and Central and South America.

Complete bibliography is available at Elsevier eBooks for Practicing Clinicians.

Key Bibliography

Brown JM, Siddiqui M, Calhoun DA, et al. The unrecognized prevalence of primary aldosteronism: a cross-sectional study. *Ann Intern Med.* 2020;173(1):10–20.

Buffet A, Burnichon N, Favier J, Gimenez-Roqueplo AP. An overview of 20 years of genetic studies in pheochromocytoma and paraganglioma. *Best Pract Res Clin Endocrinol Metab.* 2020;34(2):101416.

Caielli P, Frigo AC, Pengo MF, et al. Treatment of atherosclerotic renovascular hypertension: review of observational studies and a meta-analysis of randomized clinical trials. *Nephrol Dial Transplant.* 2015;30(4):541–553.

Cohen JB, Gadde KM. Weight loss medications in the treatment of obesity and hypertension. *Curr Hypertens Rep.* 2019;21(2):16.

Cohen JB, Geara AS, Hogan JJ, Townsend RR. Hypertension in cancer patients and survivors: epidemiology, diagnosis, and management. *JACC CardioOncol.* 2019;1(2):238–251.

Elliot WE, Peixoto AJ, Bakris GB. Primary and secondary hypertension. In: Yu ASL, Chertow GM, Luyckx V, Marsden PA, Skorecki K, Taal MW, eds. *Brenner and retor's the kidney.* 11th ed. Philadelphia: Elsevier; 2019.

Flynn JT, Kaelber DC, Baker-Smith CM, et al. Clinical practice guideline for screening and management of high blood pressure in children and adolescents. *Pediatrics.* 2017;140(3).

Funder JW, Carey RM, Mantero F, et al. The management of primary aldosteronism: case detection, diagnosis, and treatment: an endocrine society clinical practice guideline. *J Clin Endocrinol Metab.* 2016;101(5):1889–1916.

Gornik HL, Persu A, Adlam D, et al. First international consensus on the diagnosis and management of fibromuscular dysplasia. *J Hypertens.* 2019;37(2):229–252.

Gottlieb DJ, Punjabi NM. Diagnosis and management of obstructive sleep apnea: a review. *JAMA.* 2020;323(14):1389–1400.

Labarca G, Dreyse J, Drake L, Jorquera J, Barbe F. Efficacy of continuous positive airway pressure (CPAP) in the prevention of cardiovascular events in patients with obstructive sleep apnea: systematic review and meta-analysis. *Sleep Med Rev.* 2020;52:101312.

Liu L, Cao Q, Guo Z, Dai Q. Continuous positive airway pressure in patients with obstructive sleep apnea and resistant hypertension: a meta-analysis of randomized controlled trials. *J Clin Hypertens (Greenwich).* 2016;18(2):153–158.

Plouin PF, Amar L, Dekkers OM, et al. European Society of Endocrinology Clinical Practice Guideline for long-term follow-up of patients operated on for a phaeochromocytoma or a paraganglioma. *Eur J Endocrinol.* 2016;174(5):G1–G10.

Rimoldi SF, Scherrer U, Messerli FH. Secondary arterial hypertension: when, who, and how to screen? *Eur Heart J.* 2014;35(19):1245–1254.

Sander GE. Secondary hypertension: drugs and herbal preparations that increase pressure. *J Am Soc Hypertens.* 2014;8(12):946–948.

Wolley M, Thuzar M, Stowasser M. Controversies and advances in adrenal venous sampling in the diagnostic workup of primary aldosteronism. *Best Pract Res Clin Endocrinol Metab.* 2020;34(3):101400.

Index

Page numbers followed by *f* indicate figures; *t*, tables; *b*, boxes.